W0043083

MEDICAL RADIOLOGY
Diagnostic Imaging

Editors:
A.L. Baert, Leuven
F. H.W. Heuck, Stuttgart
J.E. Youker, Milwaukee

Springer-Verlag Berlin Heidelberg GmbH

E. Zeitler (Ed.)

Radiology of Peripheral Vascular Diseases

With Contributions by

E. Ammann · D. C. Baumgart · A. Beck · G. J. Becker · H. Berger · S. A. Beyer-Enke
U. Böttcher · D. Colombier · J. Cynamon · K. Detmar · D.-D. Do · H.-J. Fernholz
T. Fritsche · K. Gall · W. Gross-Fengels · P. Heilberger · R. Hildebrandt · B. Holik
K. Hüttl · F. Joffre · B. T. Katzen · J. Kirchner · W. Krause · J. Lammer · P. Leger
D. Liermann · W. Lösch · D. A. Loose · R. Loose · T.F. Lüscher · F. Mahler · M. L. Marin
M. Martin · K. Mathias · R. Möller · M. Mück-Weymann · T. Ohki · F. Olbert
M. Oldendorf · P. Otal · E. Paul · P. Perreault · P. Pickel · T. Pollack · D. Raithel
E.-I. Richter · W. Ritter · P. Romaniuk · H. Rousseau · T. Schmidt · C. Schunn · P. Soula
F. Stösslein · U. Szeimies · F. C. Tanner · F. J. Veith · U. Voss · K.-U. Wagenhofer
H.-J. Wagner · J. Weber · D. M. Williams · M. Wucherer · E. Zeitler · Ch. L. Zollikofer

Foreword by
A. L. Baert

With 495 Figures in 990 Separate Illustrations, 102 in Color and 198 Tables

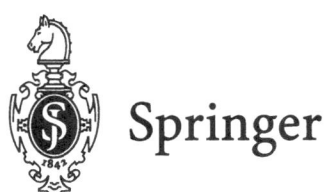

Springer

EBERHARD ZEITLER, MD
Professor
University Erlangen-Nürnberg
Wetterkreuz 21
D-91058 Erlangen-Tennenlohe
Germany

address for correspondence:
Virchowstrasse 13
D-90409 Nürnberg
Germany

MEDICAL RADIOLOGY · Diagnostic Imaging and Radiation Oncology

Continuation of
Handbuch der medizinischen Radiologie
Encyclopedia of Medical Radiology

ISBN 978-3-642-62936-5   ISBN 978-3-642-56956-2 (eBook)
DOI 10.1007/978-3-642-56956-2

Library of Congress Cataloging-in-Publication Data. Radiology of peripheral vascular diseases / (ed.) E. Zeitler ; with contributions by E. Ammann ... [et al.] ; foreword by A. L. Baert. p. cm. – (Medical radiology.) Includes bibliographical references and index. ISBN 978-3-642-62936-5 (alk. paper) 1. Peripheral vascular diseases–Imaging. 2. Peripheral vascular diseases–Treatment. I. Zeitler, E. (Eberhard), 1930– . II. Ammann, Ernst. III. Series. [DNLM: 1. Peripheral Vascular Diseases–diagnosis. 2. Peripheral Vascular Diseases–surgery. WG 500 R1295 1999] RC694.R33 1999 616.1'31–dc21 DNLM/DLC for Library of Congress 97-50385 CIP

© Springer-Verlag Berlin Heidelberg 2000
Originally published by Springer-Verlag Berlin Heidelberg New York in 2000
Softcover reprint of the hardcover 1st edition 2000

Typesetting: Best-set Typesetter Ltd., Hong Kong

SPIN: 104 707 36   21/3135 – 5 4 3 2 1 0

Foreword

Over the last decade, important advances have been made in the radiological management of peripheral vascular diseases. In the diagnostic field, the role of conventional angiography has diminished considerably in favor of new, non-invasive diagnostic modalities such as color Doppler imaging and magnetic resonance angiography.

Percutaneous radiological treatment of arterial diseases of the limbs has revolutionized therapeutic concepts in this area.

Professor E. Zeitler is a renowned international expert in the field of peripheral vascular diseases. He was one of the pioneers in investigating and developing percutaneous catheter treatment of arterial stenosis of peripheral arteries.

This volume is based upon his unique lifetime's experience of treating patients presenting with peripheral vascular diseases. Moreover, Professor Zeitler was very successful in engaging a group of excellent authors, all specialists in their field, to contribute individual chapters.

Together, they have suceeded in producing one of the most comprehensive books on the modern radiological approach to patients with peripheral vascular diseases.

It is my firm belief that this volume will be of great interest to radiologists, angiologists, and vascular surgeons alike by providing them with the latest knowledge and information in the field of radiology.

I wish this volume the same success as the many other volumes already published in the book series "Medical Radiology."

Any constructive criticism that the reader may wish to affer is welcomed.

Leuven

ALBERT L. BAERT
Series Editor

Preface

The increase in life expectancy not only in Europe and the US but also worldwide has also entailed an increasing number of persons suffering from arteriosclerosis at different locations. Besides coronary heart disease and cerebrovascular disease resulting in stroke. Progressive occlusive vascular disease is one of the threats mainly to young men, caused largely by cigarette smoking. In woman, this clinical picture manifests itself about 10 years later, after the menopause. While previously in addition to cigarette smoking the identified risk factors were mainly hypertension, hyperlipidemia and diabetes mellitus, nowadays additional risk factors, such as metabolic disorders, infections, and greater age are under discussion.

For angiologists and radiologists this means that they can no longer adhere to the principle of consultation upon demand.

The immense progress in diagnostic imaging modalities can only be used for the benefit of the individual and the community if all physicians are well informed about both the potential and the limitations of the new techniques. The trend towards diagnosis with ever-growing safety and less pain to the patient, however is so rapid that even the expert sometimes has difficulty choosing the individually appropriate method from the many available. Thus, the first aim of this volume is to offer up-to-date comparative information on the different imaging modalities, including controversial viewpoints.

Moreover, the prospects for the standard minimally invasive therapies performed under imaging guidance are described. In the next few years, the use of fluoroscopy with X-rays, enhanced by image-intensifier and television systems, will probably continue to dominate. On the horizon, however, future ultrasound-, magnetic resonance imaging- or angioscopy-guided interventions in ateries and veins, rendering X-rays superflous, are already taking shape. The recanalizing techniques, i.e., percutaneous transluminal angioplasty, clot lysis, and the implantation of stents or endoprostheses currently make up the lion's share of therapies for arterial and venous diseases. The benefits are that major operations can be avoided and on the other hand the minimal diseases can be treated at low risk in good time. The effect will be higher quality of life for the patients and, hopefully, their motivation to take secondary preventive measures.

Both aspects together – optimized early diagnosis of the disturbed peripheral perfusion and timely employment of all appropriate types of therapy, conservative, interventional or operative – have given the diagnostic radiologist spezialized in cardiovascular interventions a new role including a share in the clinical responsibility. To perform this task reliably, not only radiologic knowledge and skill are needed. This also applies to angiologists, cardiologists and vascular surgeons, who cannot ignore the process in diagnostic and interventional radiology.

When vascular surgeons write about the aim of developing reconstructive techniques according to the "3-s principle" – simpler, shorter, safer – it should not be forgotten that pioneers such as Dotter, Grüntzig and Palmaz had already initiated medical developments whose foremost aim was to help the ill. Exclusively this should be our motivation in striving for efficient interdisciplinary treatment, without "turf battles". Last but not least, this volume is designed to lead to mutual understanding among the medical specialties.

The rapid developments in some fields of radiology have delayed the publication of this book by 2 years. Nevertheless, it is highly topical, and one hopes that it will be a helpful guide not only to radiologists and angiologists but also to other physicians.

I wish to thank all authors who have contributed to this book. My thanks go also to Professor Loose at the Institute of Diagnostic and Interventional Radiology of the Nürnberg Clinic North, and Mr. Richard from the photographic department of that institute, for their continous support. I thank especially my secretaries, Mrs. Groschner and Mrs. Usinger, who have supported me in writing of my own chapters and in the compilation of the references and the index. I am particularly indepted to my colleague, Professor Baert, for having entrusted me with the editing of this volume. I wish him further success in his scientific endeavours. Springer-Verlag gave me necessary and valuable support. I wish to thank the many members of staff involved, represented by Ms. U. N. Davis and the publisher, Dr. Götze.

Many thanks to my wife

CHRISTINE

Nürnberg

EBERHARD ZEITLER

Contents

Abbreviations

AA	Aortic aneurysm	MIP	Maximum intensity projections
AAA	Abdominal aortic aneurysm	MPR	Multiplanar image reconstruction
AAS	Aortic arch syndrom	MR	Magnetic resonance
ABI	Ankle-brachial-index	MR-A	Magnetic resonance angiography
ABMS	American board of medical specialities	MRT/I	Magnetic resonance tomography / imaging
ABP	Ankle blood pressure	NIDDM	Non-insulin-dependent diabetes mellitus
ADA	American diabetic association	NIF	Neuroischemic foot
AGIR	Arbeitsgemeinschaft "Interventionelle Radiologie" in der Deutschen Röntgengesellschaft (DRG)	NIH	National Institute of Health
		NO	Nitric oxide
AMPPULSE	Âmplified protosystolic pulse	NPF	Neuropathic foot
AS	Arteriosclerosis	OGTT	Oral glucose tolerance test
ASA	Acetylsalicyclic acid	PA	Plasminogenactivator
AVF	Arteriovenous fistula	PAC	Pullback-atherectomy catheter
AVM	Arteriovenous malformation	PAES	Popliteal artery entrapment syndrom
BES	Brachial entrapment syndrom	PAT	Percutaneous aspiration thromboembolectomy
BMFT	Bundesministerium für Forschung und Technologie	PDAB	Patent ductus arteriosus Botalli
		PDGF	Platelet-derived-growth factor
BP	Blood pressure	PEP	Polyethylene perephtalat
BPP	Brightest pixel projection	PES	Post-embolization syndrom
BTS	Blue toe syndrom	POVD	Peripheral occlusive vascular disease
BVP	Brightest voxel projection	PSS	Progressive systemic sclerodermia
CAD	Cystic adventitia degeneration	PTA	Percutenous transluminal angioplasty
CAQ	Certificate of added qualifications	PTCA	Percutaneous transluminal coronary angioplasty
CCDS	Color-coded duplex-sonography	PTFE	Polytetrafluoroethylene
CEG	Corvita-endovascular-graft	PTR	Percutaneous transluminal recanalization
CHD	Coronary heart diseases	PTRA	Percutaneous transluminal rotational atherectomy
CLI	Critical leg ischemia		
CM	Contrast medium	PTRD	Percutaneous transluminal renal dilatation
COCERT	Comitee on certification, subcertification and recertification	PTT	Partial thrombin time
		PVC	Polyvinylchloride
CRAG	Cooperative rotablator atherectomy group	PVD	Peripheral vascular disease
CSQ	Certificate of special qualifications	PW Doppler	Pulsed-wave doppler
CT	Computertomography	RAS	Renal artery stenosis
CVD	Cerebrovascular disease	ROC	Receiver operator characteristic
CVTS	Chronic vibration trauma syndrom	ROI	Region of interest
CW Doppler	Continous-wave-doppler	RPM	Rotations per minute
DM	Diabetes mellitus	rt-PA	Recombinat tissue-plasminogenactivator
DNOAP	Diabetic-neuropathic osteo-arthropathies	RVH	Renal vascular hypertension
DSA	Digital subtraction angiography	SFA	Superficial femoral artery
EBT	Electron beam tomography	SLE	Systemic lupus erythematousus
EGS	Endovascular grafting system (before EVT)	SMA	Superior mesenteric artery
F	French (measurement of catheter diameter, 1 F = 0,33 mm)	SMC	Smooth muscle cells
		SSD	Surface shaded display
		SSS	Subclavian steal-syndrom
FMD	Fibromuscular dysplasia	TAR	Thoracic aortic rupture
GAMS	German-Angioplasty Multicenter-study	TAS	Tibialis anterior syndrom
GFR	Glomerular filtration rate	TEA	Thromboendarterectomy
HAES	Hydroxy aethyl starch	TEC	Transluminal extraction catheter
HDL	High-density lipoproteins	TEEC	Trans esophageal echocardiography
HHS	Hypothenar Hammer-syndrome	TFI	Thrombocyte function inhibitor
HIT	Heparin-induced thrombocytopenia	TOF	Time-of-flight-MRA
HITS	High intensity transient signals	TOS	Thoracic outlet syndrom
HU	Hounsfield units	TSBP	Transcutaneous oxygen pressure
IDDM	Insulin-dependent diabetes mellitus	UFH	Ultra-filtrated Heparin
IH	Intimal hyperplasia	UHSK	Ultrahigh streptokinase dosage regimen
IMA	Inferior mesenteric artery	VD	Venous diseases
INR	International normalized ratio	VRT	Volume rendering technique
IR	Interventional radiology	VS	Vasospastic syndromes
IVUS	Intravascular ultrasound	VSMC	Vascular smooth muscle cell
HDL	High-density lipoproteins	WHO	World Health Organization
LDL	Low-density lipoproteins		
LMWH	Low-molecular weighted Heparin		

Peripheral Vascular Diseases

1 Definition, Incidence, and Prevalence

E. Zeitler

CONTENTS

Since William Harvey's findings in 1628, it has been a recognized fact that the blood circulation between the heart, arteries, and veins in the pulmonary and general circulation, is the basis for blood flow insuring oxygen supply to all regions of the body, and that the backflow of the anoxemic blood, saturated with CO_2 through the veins, including the contact areas in the capillary region, is the so-called micro-circulation. Under these conditions, a periphery exists in the circulation, particularly in the extremities, the brain, and all parenchymal organs.

As a consequence, peripheral vascular diseases can occur both in the arterial and the venous vascular systems. While arteriosclerosis is the major cause of all arterial vascular diseases, orthostatic effects and physical stress in the low-pressure circulation are the most common causes of disorders in the venous vascular system.

Taking medical practice into account and the distribution of tasks in the diagnosis and treatment of patients by different specialists, such as cardiologists and angiologists, within internal medicine, and cardiac surgeons and vascular surgeons in operative medicine, the following differentation seems to be useful, irrespective of the joint efforts and shared common ground in the diagnosis and treatment of vascular diseases:
- Coronary heart diseases
- Cerebrovascular diseases
- Peripheral vascular diseases.

EBERHARD ZEITLER, MD, Professor, University Erlangen-Nürnberg, Germany
address for correspondence:
Virchowstraße 13, D-90409 Nürnberg, Germany

The peripheral vascular diseases dealt with in this book should be understood in that sense. They encompass disorders of the aorta and the branching arteries, of the arteries of the legs and arms, and common diseases of the venous system in the lower and upper extremities and the major veins of the body (venae cava cranialis and caudalis). Peripheral vascular diseases affecting organs, such as the liver or the brain, are not regarded as peripheral vascular diseases here.

As radiological imaging modalities for diagnosis and treatment in the microcirculation have only played a minor role to date, the issue is not addressed in this book.

Peripheral vascular diseases are therefore defined from the standpoint of diagnostic and interventional radiologists who have the responsibility of intervening at the order of, and in close cooperation with, internists, angiologists, vascular surgeons, and of course with all other physicians involved, including specialists in phlebology and cardiology. Thus, the most common diseases to be diagnosed using radiological procedures are complications resulting from arteriosclerosis in the aorta and leg and arm arteries, followed by congenital, posttraumatic, or inflammatory vascular diseases.

In the field of venous diseases primary varicosis and phlebothrombosis, including its complications, require the radiologist's contribution in the diagnosis, treatment, and assessment of the course of the vascular disease. Moreover, arteriovenous (AV)-malformations, mostly of congenital, but some also of an acquired nature are a challenge as regards precise pretherapeutic diagnosis and additional interventional treatment: for example, the occlusion of AV-shunts today plays a major role in interventional radiology.

Although diagnostics have been the major task of radiology, percutaneous interventional radiology in the vascular system as an ever growing field of activity has developed on the basis of the Seldinger technique (ABRAMS 1983; ATHANASOULIS 1982; COPE et al. 1990; DONDELINGER 1990; GÜNTHER and THELEN

1988; LAMMER and SCHREYER 1991; ZEITLER 1997). The various techniques carried out under the control of fluoroscopy or other monitoring imaging techniques have gained in importance in the field of minimally invasive medicine under the increasingly tightened economic conditions.

1.1
Definition

Peripheral occlusive vascular diseases (POVD) manifest themselves more frequently in legs than in arms. The causes differ as regards pathogenesis and etiology, but the symptoms are almost identical. The initiating cause may be located far from the diseased organ. For example, cardiac insufficiency can initiate disorders of the peripheral circulation, while clots carried from the heart or the aorta into the periphery (thrombus, plaque) can cause ischemia due to embolism. On the other hand, arteriosclerosis is the major cause of disturbed arterial circulation leading to hemodynamically significant narrowing of the vessel, i.e., stenosis or occlusion. Inflammations as first described as "thromboangiitis obliterans" by BUERGER (1924) are mainly located peripherally in the lower leg and the feet, affecting both arteries and veins.

The majority of chronic (POVD's) are, however, part of the generalized arteriosclerosis progressing with age. The time of their manifestation and their location – more peripheral or central – depend on the effects of the different risk factors. For example, the presence of multiple risk factors represents a much higher risk of developing the obliterating type of arteriosclerosis. The difference is that patients with the main risk factor of hypertension are likely to develop disturbed cerebrovascular circulation with carotid stenosis, patients with the main risk factor of elevated lipid values (such as cholesterol), possibly combined with cigarette-smoking, are often candidates for coronary heart disease (CHD), and patients with the main risk factor of cigarette-smoking are at risk of developing POVD, mostly located in the arteries of the thigh or the pelvis, while diabetes in addition to microangiopathy more frequently causes obliterations in tibial and foot arteries (KANNEL and SHURTLEFF 1973; WIDMER et al. 1981; WIDMER 1983).

1.2
Incidence and Prevalence

In patients with POVD the prevalence and incidence of coronary heart disease (CHD) and cerebrovascular disease (CVD) is high. While in POVD the main symptoms of ischemia in the sense of functio laesa are intermittent claudication, pain at rest, or gangrene, the effects of venous diseases (VD) are edemas, varicosis, swollen leg, and leg ulcers. The incidence of different diseases, compared to POVD and relevant venous diseases, is demonstrated in Fig. 1.1.

The *incidence* provides information about diseases occuring over a limited period of time in patients who were initially healthy (development over the time), while the *prevalence* provides information about the number of diseased persons at a certain time (momentary situation).

1.2.1
Arterial Diseases

The prevalence and incidence of POVD have been considerably underestimated in earlier years, since attention focused on the symptomatic forms associated with intermittent claudication. Only first systematic studies, as carried out for example by the National Institute of Health (NIH) in the United States on a randomized population of 5127 inhabitants of the town Framingham aged between 39 and 59 years, revealed a higher incidence (GORDON and KANNEL 1972). The analysis of the study included a

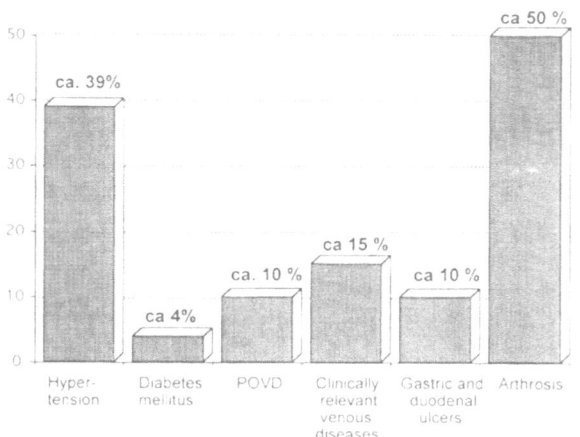

Fig. 1.1. Incidence of different diseases compared to peripheral occlusive vascular disease *(POVD)*

medical examination, in addition to a questionnaire for each individual. In Framingham, 43% of the patients with claudication were suffering simultaneously from CHD and/or CVD (KANNEL 1974; KANNEL et al. 1970, 1976).

Other important results, valuable mainly for European countries, were published in the "Basler Studie" (Basler Study), a study carried out on a large group of workers in the pharmaceutical industry in Switzerland (WIDMER et al. 1981). Prospective studies are more meaningful than retrospective analyses. A crucial aspect is the definition of the collective, i.e., (men, women, age, drop-out rate, etc). The Basler Study on arterial diseases included 2759 healthy men. Examination, including analysis of the anamnesis, the pulse status, oscillographies both at rest and under stress, and of the vascular auscultation were performed over a 5-year period. After these 5 years, 174 of the 2759 men had developed a POVD. The number of new diseases increased with age (Fig. 1.2).

The incidence of asymptomatic POVD was 81 out of 1000, and was four times higher in those men who were 60 years of age at the beginning of the study compared to those 40. Among all agegroups the asymptomatic form occurred three times as often as the symptomatic form with intermittent claudication.

In almost all age-groups, CHD developed as frequently as POVD. In patients with POVD, CHD was found 2.5 times more often than in persons with healthy arteries. In contrast, POVD occurred 2.3 times more frequently in patients with CHD than in persons without coronary symptoms (Fig. 1.3), but POVD was more often asymptomatic than CHD. Therefore, all patients with CHD require diagnosis of the peripheral circulation, and vice versa.

A global analysis of the prevalence of POVD on the basis of 50 international studies carried out between 1964 and 1992 on 108 000 patients has been published. The number of patients in the different studies varied between 184 and 18 403, and the methods for identification of the disease had been determined. The prevalence of POVD was 2.7% – without differentiation regarding age and sex.

In persons older than 60 years of age, one assumes a prevalence of 28%–30%. A steady increase has been observed from the age of 40. POVD of different etiology can also occur in young age (Fig. 1.4). This figure shows a slight difference in the prevalence for woman and men with increasing age. Between the ages of 70 and 79 the incidence of POVD is 9.8% in men and 7.7% in women.

The prognosis for POVD if untreated is bad. Ac-

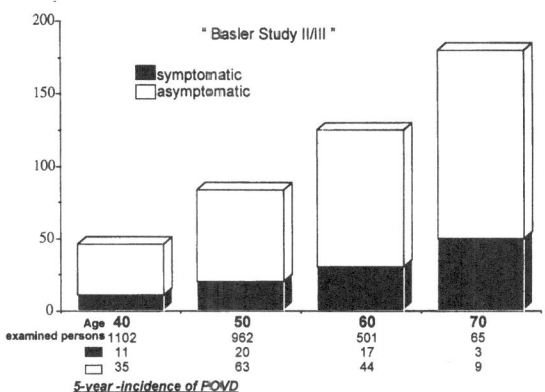

Fig. 1.2. 5-year incidence of peripheral occlusive vascular disease *(POVD)* according to Basler Study II/III

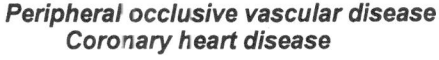

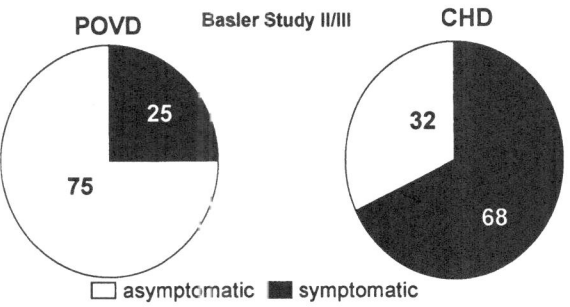

Fig. 1.3. Comparison of the course of peripheral occlusive vascular disease *(POVD)* and coronary heart disease *(CHD)* according to Basler Study II/III

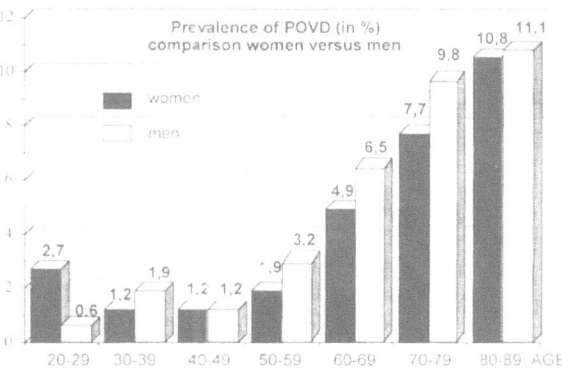

Fig. 1.4. Prevalence of peripheral occlusive vascular disease (in percent); comparison in women versus men

cording to various, mostly retrospective analyses, 25% of patients with POVD die within 5 years, and 17% suffer a leg amputation (HASSE 1959; JUERGENS et al. 1960; RATSCHOW 1959; WIDMER 1993).

Follow-up controls of patients in Fontaine stage II "intermittent claudication" have shown that 50% died within ten years, 20% did not change, and 20% experienced a deterioration. Only 10% improved spontaneously.

Of the patient group requiring leg amputation, rehabilitation, including the ability to walk, is only achieved in 25%, whereas 25% will remain in need of medical care for a long period of time.

In the prospective Basler Study a 5-year mortality rate of 17.5% was found. In comparisons with persons with healthy arteries, those with POVD had a two-fold higher mortality rate. In the age group of 35–44 years, the mortality rate was 4.5 times higher, the main cause of death being CHD. A total of 15% died from heart infarction and 5% from cerebral stroke (WIDMER et al. 1981; KANNEL 1976).

In cases of arterial stenoses in the superficial femoral artery one third of patients developed an arterial occlusion within 5 years. The number of stenoses at multiple locations increased from 52% to 87% within that period of time. In contrast to this, a regression could be angiographically identified in iliac arteries in only 5% (6 out of 116 arteries).

The 5-year amputation rate according to the Basler Study (2.1%) is significantly lower than that of basically symptomatic populations from several other clinics.

1.2.2
Venous Diseases

The Basler Study III, carried out on 3744 men and 785 women was the first study to provide profound, detailed knowledge on peripheral venous diseases, on the basis of anamnestic data and clinical angiological examinations. About 50% of these patients confirmed pain in the leg, 15% of whom were being treated for that reason. A mild varicosis was found in 45%, a severe one in 16%. Chronic venous isufficiency,. classified according to severity, was diagnosed in 8% as mild, in 6% as moderately severe, and in 1% as ulcus cruris. A total of 2% of the men and 3% of the women had suffered pulmonary embolism.

The 3% of patients with pathological varicosis had experienced complications 20 times as often. It is particularly difficult in venous diseases to dis-

tinguish between disease and disorder since both conservative and operative treatment are also performed simply for cosmetic reasons (Fig. 1.5).

Disorders comprise mild and severe forms of the reticular and asymptomatic varices. Diseases, in contrast, define the severe forms of combined varicose dilatations of the cutaneous veins, reticular varices, and varices of the vena saphena magna and parva. Peripheral venous diseases in the sense of "disease" were found in 12% of men and women, indicating that there is nearly no difference between sexes. In contrast, a clear correlation with age could be demonstrated. In the collective of 70-year-olds, a venous disease was found in 23% of men, and 34% of women, whereas in 40-year-old women it showed up in only 4%, compared to 7% in men of the same age.

Complications of the relevant pathological varicosis were found in a statistically more significant number of the population with pathological varicosis, compared to persons without varices of the same age (Fig. 1.6). Among the pathological subgroup, 14% had a leg ulcer, whereas in the patient population without varices no leg ulcer occurred in the follow-up.

The data regarding frequency of the various treatments performed during the Basler Study (Fig. 1.7) confirm the clinical and out-patient experience that compression treatment and sclerotherapy are performed in markedly higher numbers than operative stripping. The study also made an attempt to define the different stages of peripheral venous diseases. It was shown that in the majority of patients with uncomplicated venous disease an imaging diagnosis is required only for exclusion of complications, which

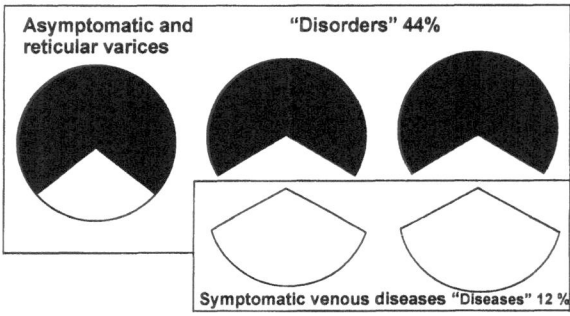

Fig. 1.5. Differentiation between varicose "disorder" and "disease" according to Basler Study III, significant and negligible varicosis of the saphenous veins ($n = 3744$)

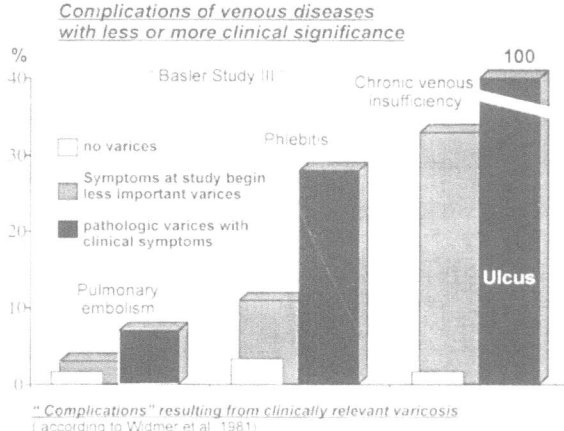

Fig. 1.6. Complications of venous disease resulting from clinically relevant varicosis (according to WIDMER et al. 1981; Basler Study III)

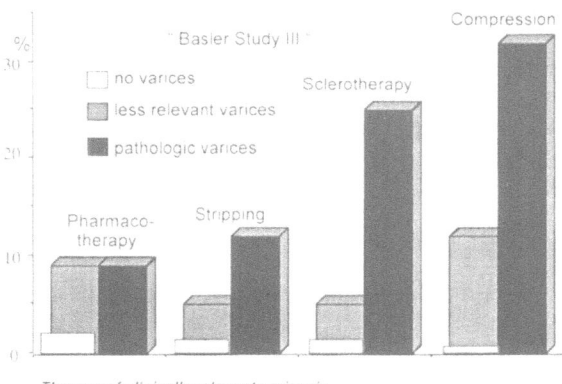

Fig. 1.7. Therapy for clinically relevant varicosis (Basler Study III)

eighth adult suffered from advanced chronic venous insufficiency, and every thirty-seventh presented an ulcus cruris. A total of 5% of the people questioned stated that their venous disease had led to interference with their profession. In the analysis based only on case history, 72% of the women and 54% of the men claimed to have suffered or to still be suffering from symptoms in the feet, the joints, or the legs. The underlying causes to which these symptoms were attributed are shown in Fig. 1.8.

One in six women, but only one in 25 men were said to have had a phlebitis. For thrombosis and ulcus cruris the difference in frequency between women and men is not that remarkable. The age-related effects of the mentioned venous diseases can be seen in Fig. 1.9.

From the age of 35, an age-related increase (40%–60% affected) becomes obvious. While varicosis, phlebitis, and swollen legs were observed between two and four times as often in women than in men, the data of men and women who had suffered pulmonary embolism were equal.

1.3
Summary

The epidemiologic data of both peripheral arterial and venous diseases show that a great proportion of the population is affected by these. This causes high costs, whereby those for peripheral venous diseases, which are mainly treated on an out patient basis, are higher than those for peripheral arterial diseases. As

is mainly done using ultrasound, whereas in patients with relevant and pathologic peripheral venous disease sophisticated diagnostic modalities such as color-coded duplex sonography, magnetic resonance imaging, or phlebography are recommended to decide on appropriate therapy.

In contrast to the Basler Study III, the Tübinger Study (FISCHER 1981) did not provide the same clear selection of subjects examined and controlled under long-term conditions. It was a population of 1522 men and 3008 women from urban and rural areas, not employees and workers in an industrial company as in the Basler Study.

The Tübinger Study showed that every second women and every fourth man had varices. Every

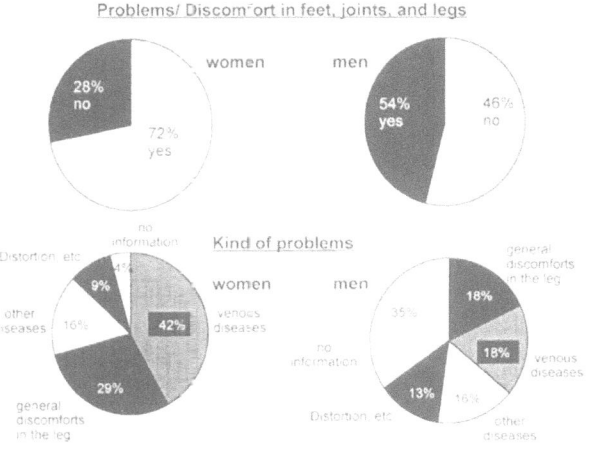

Fig. 1.8. Problems and discomfort in feet, joints, and legs (according to FISCHER 1981)

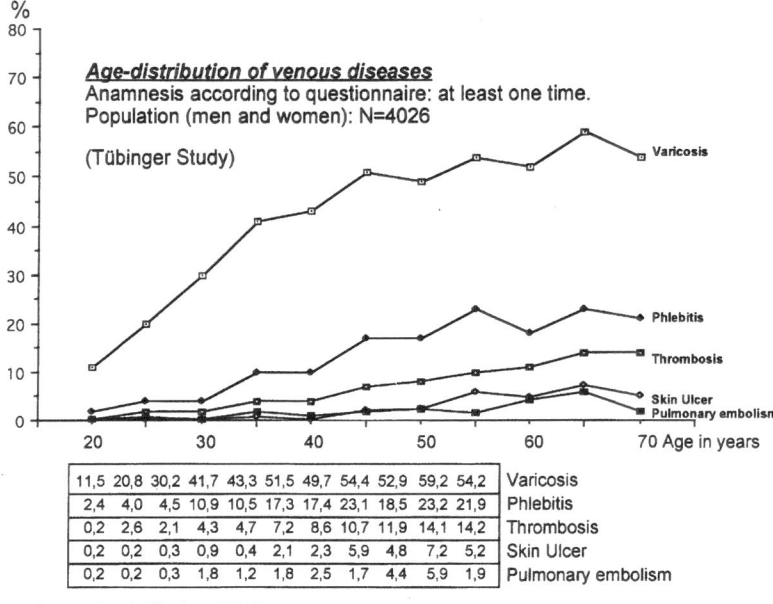

Fig. 1.9. Age-distribution of venous diseases. Anamnesis according to questionnaire which was answered at least once. Population (men and women): n = 4026. (According to FISCHER 1981; Tübinger Study)

11,5	20,8	30,2	41,7	43,3	51,5	49,7	54,4	52,9	59,2	54,2	Varicosis
2,4	4,0	4,5	10,9	10,5	17,3	17,4	23,1	18,5	23,2	21,9	Phlebitis
0,2	2,6	2,1	4,3	4,7	7,2	8,6	10,7	11,9	14,1	14,2	Thrombosis
0,2	0,2	0,3	0,9	0,4	2,1	2,3	5,9	4,8	7,2	5,2	Skin Ulcer
0,2	0,2	0,3	1,8	1,2	1,8	2,5	1,7	4,4	5,9	1,9	Pulmonary embolism

(according to Fischer, 1981)

regards the costs of arterial circulatory disturbances, it is difficult to give precise data as it is in the nature of generalized arteriosclerosis that in many cases an additional CHD or cerebrovascular disease is present, each of these adversely influencing one another when progressing.

An early diagnosis of arterial stenosis, followed by medical consultation and the appropriate treatment, can have a lasting impact on the patient's way of life by reducing or eliminating his/her risk factors. Physical activity is highly benificial. Through these measures, an improvement is achieved in general by the slowed-down progression of the disease, combined with simple local treatment measures.

To identify a clinically suspected arterial stenosis or obliteration, imaging modalities play an important role. Of the currently available technical equipment, (color-coded) duplex sonography is the most important to complete clinical angiologic examinations and to determine the ankle brachial index. For confirmation of a diagnosis and decision on active therapy, the use of an imaging modality with low risk for the patient is indicated.

In peripheral venous diseases medical care, inspection, and analysis including palpation dominate, whereby for detection of deep venous thrombosis duplex sonography has proven to be very reliable. In complex cases involving patients who are difficult to examine and where a method of treatment involving a certain risk is planned, the combined fluoroscopically-controlled ascending press phlebography still plays an important role. It will become all the more necessary the more the therapeutic aim will be one of restitutio ad integrum.

References

Abrams H (1983) Angiography, 3rd edn, vol III. Little Brown, Boston

Athanasoulis CH, Pfister RC, Greene RE, Roberson GH (1982) Interventional Radiology. WB Saunders, Philadelphia

Buerger L (1924) The circulatory disturbances of the extremities including gangrene, vasomotor and trophic disorders. WB, Saunders, Philadelphia

Cope C, Burke DR, Meranze S, Baum ST (1990) Atlas of interventional radiology. Lippincott, Philadelphia

Dondelinger RF, Rossi P, Kurdziel JC, Wallce S (1990) Interventional radiology. Thieme, Stuttgart

Fischer H (1981) Venenleiden. Eine repräsentative Untersuchung in der Bevölkerung der Bundesrepublik Deutschland (Tübinger Studie). Urban & Schwarzenberg, Munich

Gordon T, Kannel WB (1972) Predisposition to atherosclerosis in the head, heart and legs - the Framingham Study. JAMA 221:661-666

Günther RW, Thelen M (1988) Interventionelle Radiologie. Thieme, Stuttgart

Hasse HM (1959) Statistische Daten zur Prognose der arteriellen Verschlußkrankheiten In: Ratschow M (ed) Angiologie, Pathologie, Klinik und Therapie der peripheren Durchblutungsstörungen. Thieme, Stuttgart, pp 609-622

Juergens JL, Barker NW, Hines EA (1960) Arteriosclerosis obliterans: review of 520 cases with special reference to pathogenic and prognostic factors. Circulation 21:188

Kannel WB (1974) Role of blood pressure in cardiovascular morbidity and mortality. Prog Cardiovasc Dis 17:5-24

Kannel WB, Skinner JJ, Schwartz MJ, Shurtleff D (1970) Intermittent claudication. Incidence in the Framingham Study. Circulation 41:875-883

Kannel WB, Shurtleff D (1973) Cigarettes and development of intermittent claudication. The Framingham Study. Geriatrics 28:61-68

Kannel WB, McGee D, Gordon T (1976) A general cardiovascular risk profile: the Framingham Study. Am J Cardiol 38:46-51

Lammer J, Schreyer H (1991) Praxis der Interventionellen Radiologie. Hippokrates, Stuttgart

Ratschow M (1959) Angiclogie, Pathologie, Klinik und Therapie der peripheren Durchblutungsstörungen. Thieme, Stuttgart

Widmer LK, Stähelin HB, Nissen C, da Silva A (eds,) (1981) Basler Studie. Huber, Bern

Widmer LK (1993) Prävelenz der Gefäßkrankheiten: Alexander K (ed) Gefäßkrankheiten. Urban & Schwarzenberg, Berlin

Zeitler E (1997) Klinische Radiologie: Arterien und Venen. Springer, Berlin Heidelberg New York

2 Diagnostic Principles

E. Zeitler

CONTENTS

2.1
Introduction

The tasks of general health care, patient care, and medical personnel are manifold with regard to vascular disease (WIDMER et al. 1994). As a matter of priority, not only do patients' symptoms need to be alleviated and the progression of localized disease, and severe complications arising there from, need to be avoided, but also the existence of arteriosclerotic disease in other vascular territories, e.g., in the coronary arteries or the cerebrovascular system, must be checked with non-invasive methods (ALEXANDER 1994; BOLLINGER 1979; VERSTRAETE 1980). This is all the more important since coronary and cerebrovascular complications of generalized arteriosclerotic disease are also the main reason for which people suffering from peripheral arterial occlusive diseases (POVD) have life expectancy 10 years lower than a comparable group of individuals with healthy arteries (LEVY and SCHOOP 1982; WIDMER et al. 1994). A total of 20% of male and 30% of female patients die as a result of these complications within 8 years (PEABODY et al. 1974), while 50% of patients with intermittent claudication at the time of first symptoms are already suffering from coronary heart disease (CHD).

Improving health awareness should be a task undertaken both at home and at school, by family practitioners and social institutions, by informing young people about the main risk factors of arteriosclerosis, such as cigarette smoking, poor diet, and insufficient physical activity, and its complications, with the aim of preventing such diseases in later years.

It is important to establish an appropriate diagnostic procedure for each person suffering from vascular disease and risk patient, taking his/her complaints into full consideration. The appropriate plan of treatment will be determined mainly by the urgency of non-invasive medical investigation, followed by the appropriate imaging method.

In situations with no acute risk of death or loss of an organ (which would be the case, for example, in aortic ruptures, critical limb ischemia, pulmonary embolism, or similar critical situations), diagnosis should be oriented by the clinical symptoms. The diagnostic procedure is influenced by: (a) Local complaints, (b) spreading of vascular changes, (c) risk factors, and (d) dominant, non-vascular underlying causes.

Prior to selecting the imaging modality best suited to localizing and determining the severity of vascular changes, a physical examination for arterial and venous diseases is also essential for the cardiovascular radiologist (GÜNTHER and THELEN 1995; LANZER and RÖSCH 1994). The steps of such an examination include:

- Taking the patient's medical history, including main complaints
- Taking the history of the present illness and the cardiovascular risk profile, including current medications and allergies (Table 2.1)
- Physical examination of the cardiovascular system, including inspection, pulse palpation, and auscultation of the heart, arteries and veins. The standard sites for pulse palpation, auscultation, and segmental blood pressure measurement with and without the Doppler technique are indicated in Fig. 2.1

EBERHARD ZEITLER, MD, Professor, University Erlangen-Nürnberg, Germany
address for correspondence: Virchowstraße 13, D-90409 Nürnberg, Germany

Table 2.1. Twelve questions which should be routinely put to the patient

- What are your complaints?
- When did you first become aware of them?
- Do they occur at rest or after exercise?
- Do you suffer from any heart problems (angina pectoris)?
- Is your sight impaired (amaurosis fugax)?
- Do you suffer from dizziness?
- Do you have problems with your legs (intermittent claudication, edema at the ankle, or others)?
- Do the complaints occur in particular situations, for example, when turning your head, when going upstairs, etc.?
- Have you sustained any injury or been involved in an accident?
- Have you undergone surgery because of these problems?
- Are you taking medication? If so, what medication?
- Does (or has) any member of your family suffer(ed) from similar complaints?

- Determination of the individual cardiovascular risk profile:
  - History of cigarette smoking (number of cigarettes/day)
  - History of diabetes mellitus
  - Control of lipoproteins:
    - Cholesterol (normal values without risk in men over 40 years of age: 200–240 mg/100 ml)
    - Triglycerides (normal values without risk: below 200 mg/dl)
    - High-density lipoproteins (normal values: men above 65 mg/dl, women above 55 mg/dl)
    - Low-density lipoproteins (normal values without vascular risk: below 150 mg/dl)
- Other information of importance may include a genetic familial predisposition, negative stress factors, or laboratory findings such as disturbance of homocystein and uric acid (normal for men: 3.4–7.0 mg/dl, for women: 2.4–5.7 mg/dl). Hyper-homocysteinemia is classified as:
  Mild: plasma/serum concentration less than 30 μmol/l
  Moderate: concentration 30–100 μmol/l
  Severe: concentration over 100 μmol/l (KANG et al. 1992)
- Physical skin and venous examination. This includes the definition of peripheral edemas, ulceration, and gangrene, as well as checking for the presence and location of varicose veins or signs of deep venous thrombosis.

The results of all these examinations help to define the clinical stage of arterial (Table 2.2), venous (Table 2.3), and coronary heart disease (Table 2.4).

Only in view of therapeutic measures can the diagnostic plan for the use of invasive or non-inva-

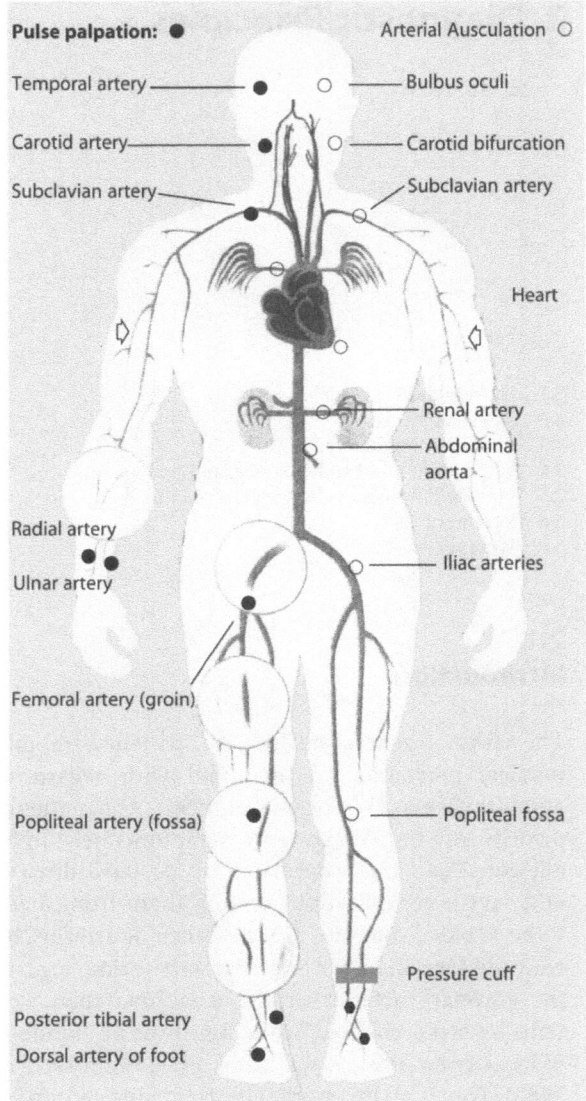

Fig. 2.1. Locations for pulse palpation (indicated by *filled dots*), auscultation of arteries (indicated by *open dots*), blood-pressure measurement with cuff (indicated by *filled arrow*) and Doppler technique (indicated by *filled pentagon*) (from KAPPERT 1985)

sive imaging modalities be established. The indications for the different imaging modalities are as follows: Doppler measurements and duplex sonography can be organized simultaneously with the initial physical examination (ALEXANDER 1994; BOLLINGER 1979; SIMON and SCHOOP 1986; KAPPERT 1985; VERSTRAETE 1980). However, angiography, computed tomography (CT) or spiral CT with contrast medium, or magnetic resonance angiography (MRA) (ARLART et al. 1996), require special indications in situations where an active treatment has to be decided upon – operation or

Table 2.2. Modified Fontaine classification of chronic POVD

Stage I	Asymptomatic
Stage II	Intermittent claudication
A:	Painless walking distance more than 2 blocks (over 200 m)
B:	Painless walking distance less than 2 blocks (under 200 m)
Stage III	Pain at rest
A:	ABP above 50 mm Hg
B:	ABP below 50 mm Hg or/and TSP below 30 mm Hg
Stage IV	Ulceration or gangrene of foot or toes
A:	ABP above 50 mm Hg or 30 mm Hg TSP
B:	ABP below 50 mm Hg or below 30 mm Hg TSP

ABP, ankle blood pressure; TSP, toe systolic pressure.

Table 2.3. Classification of venous diseases

A Deep venous thrombosis
  1. Calf veins
  2. Thigh veins
  3. Pelvic veins
  4. Of multicentric origin
B Postthrombotic syndrome
C Primary varicose veins
  1. Asymptomatic
  2. Symptomatic
  3. Symptomatic, with ulceration at the ankle
D Miscellaneous venous disorders
  1. Venous aneurysm
  2. Malformations
  3. Extrinsic compression

Table 2.4. New York Heart Association classification of CHD

I	No symptoms
II	Restricted endurance
III	Highly restricted Endurance
IV	Angina pectoris at rest

interventional radiology, medical treatment over a long period of time, or treatment in the case of bleeding complications, for example under the use of thrombolysis and anticoagulation – (KONECNY et al. 1986; HEIMIG and MARTIN 1997).

The information which can be obtained from the different imaging modalities varies. Some methods provide the same information with varying degrees of accuracy; others provide less or more important additional details [e.g., angioscopy, intravascular ultrasound (IVUS)]. Finally, cost, availability, and the experience of the respective physician also have an influence on the imaging method ultimately used.

2.2
Angioscopy

This modality demonstrates the free lumen and the condition of the intima, including possible changes in color caused by white or yellow plaque, and red (hyaline) or white (blood-platelet) thrombus (BECK 1993; SIGWART et al. 1996; REES et al. 1989). Thus, it is particularly useful when deciding on subsequent thrombolysis or atherectomy, and in detecting dissections. It has opened up the possibility of quality control of surgical and interventional therapies by immediately detecting suboptimal treatment, such as incomplete endarterectomy, dissection, intimal involution, or inaccurate sutures. Moreover, angioscopically controlled service interventions are a useful complement to the various treatments. After operation and angioplasty, angioscopy shows dissection or thrombus which now can be optimally treated for instance by secondary surgery or stenting.

Angioscopy is, however, not capable of visualizing the artery distal to an occlusion. Information can only be obtained on the basis of the vasa vasorum, but not on direct and indirect collateral circulation.

2.3
Roentgen Angiography

This technique (see also Chap. 8) provides information on severe complications of arteriosclerosis, such as vascular *occlusion* and vascular *stenosis*. It depicts multiple obliterations in succession (occlusion, stenosis, tandem stenoses, aneurysm, etc.) as clearly as isolated pathologic conditions and extravascular compression (ABRAMS 1983; ZEITLER 1997).

The presence and extent of collateral circulations can be demonstrated by various angiographic techniques. Multiple collateral circulations can be better visualized after a proximal administration of contrast medium than with selective angiographic methods. Early, uncomplicated arteriosclerosis can only be identified by localized or multiple irregularities in the vascular wall (see Fig. 2.2a,b).

For quantitative measurements, biplanar or multiplanar angiography is required for a precise demonstration of each individual stenosis and the degree of arteriosclerosis by its longitudinal extension. The angiographic techniques used for detecting and interpreting vascular changes in the different territories are dealt with in Chap. 8. It is important to document pelvic arteries, the femoral bifurcation,

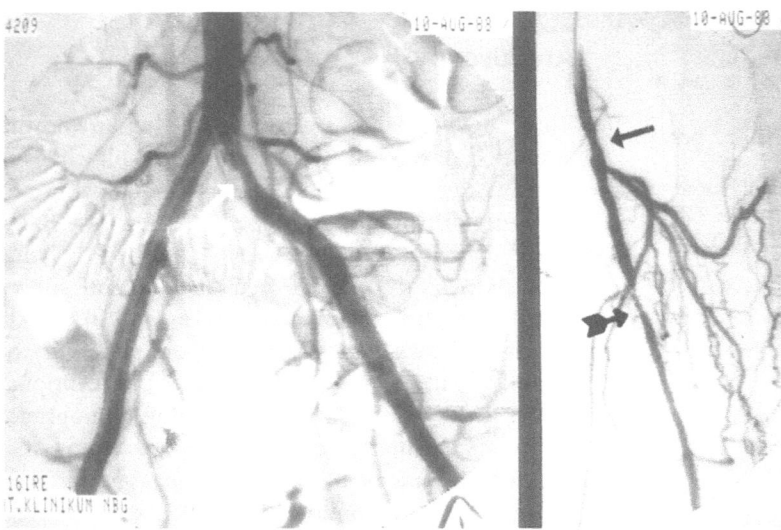

a   b

Fig. 2.2 a,b. Arteriosclerotic changes of iliac and femoral arteries. a Aorto-iliac bifurcation with common iliac artery stenosis on the left (*arrow*). b Superficial femoral artery left with 80% superficial femoral artery stenosis (*reverse arrow*) and arteriosclerotic irregularities without (*arrow*) hemodynamic effect and collateral arteries. Digital subtraction angiography of a 63-year-old man with risk factors of cigarette smoking and arterial hypertension

and the origin of renal arteries in oblique projections between 30° and 45°.

Prerequisites for angiography are the puncture and catheterization of the artery (transarterial angiography) or vein (phlebography or transvenous angiography), with subsequent contrast medium injection and the use of X-rays. In the majority of cases today, angiography (arteriography or phlebography) is performed as digital subtraction angiography (DSA); conventional angiography is only carried out in special cases. However, the clinical information obtained from conventional angiography and DSA does not differ to a great exent.

When assessing stenoses, the different types – circular or excentric – need to be considered. The correlation between the diameter and degree of stenosis can be seen in Fig. 2.3a,b.

Angiography is the appropriate technique for planning therapy in symptomatic patients and often indispensable. Patients with critical limb ischemia, suspected aneurysm, or arteriovenous malformations require in all cases, firstly, admission to hospital and, secondly, angiography prior to active treament. Angiography is also a prerequisite for emergency service operations in cases of post-therapeutic complications and is useful for the assessment of vascular disease in progression. It is the most common method and any physician treating vascular diseases should be familiar with the interpretation of the images. The points of information obtained are objective, but can be individually interpreted. Angiography is the best basis on which to make important therapeutic decisions and is still the gold standard for arterial disease, much like

Concentric regular stenoses

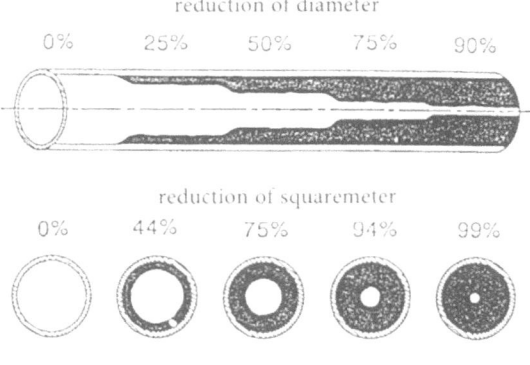

Excentric irregular stenoses

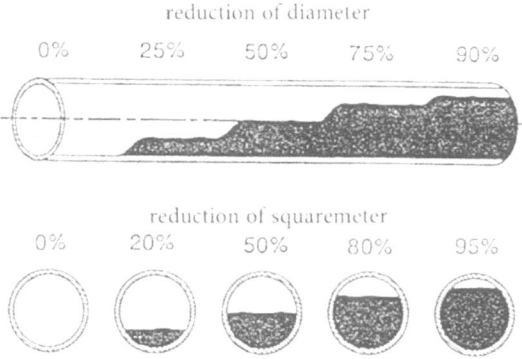

Fig. 2.3 a,b. Angiographic view of arterial narrowing and cross-sectional documentation. a Concentric regular stenoses of varying degrees. b Excentric irregular stenoses of varying degrees

phlebography (under optimal conditions) is for venous disease.

Regarding analysis over several or more years, angiography provides the best opportunity for defining qualitative and quantitative progression, outcome of treatment, and possible regression of vascular changes. With small 3- and 4-F catheters, transfemoral and transbrachial arteriography can be acquired in many cases at outpatient follow-up.

Roentgen angiography requires the use of X-rays and the application of iodinated contrast medium. Modern contrast media still carry the risk of adverse reactions, which can be reduced by using non-ionic contrast media and/or premedication with H_1- and H_2-antagonists. The stochastic and deterministic risk of angiography in the extremities due to the use of X-rays is very low (see Chap. 8.6).

The quantitative determination of arterial vascular changes in the lower extremities is possible using the Bollinger score (see Fig. 8.58) or analogous schemata which consider both local and multiple pathological changes (BOLLINGER et al. 1981, 1982).

Angiography offers clear information about changes to the vessel lumen on the basis of comparison with normal patency without any narrowing. In addition, angiography can demonstrate the collateral circulation in arteries and veins.

2.4
Ultrasound and Duplex Sonography

Sonography (see also Chap. 10) can be used simultaneously for the analysis of arteries and veins since it is an external, non-invasive technique. Its great advantages include its non-invasiveness and, depending on existing equipment (which can be the more expensive the more precise the information provided), its ability to carry out morphological analysis of the vascular wall, the vascular lumen, and flow characteristics. Highly accurate information can be obtained in localized regions (e.g., the carotid bifurcation, the arteries and veins of the groin, and the fossa poplitea).

For vascular analyses, duplex sonography (see Chap. 10.4) is excellent for the diagnosis of acute thrombotic occlusions of arteries and veins in the thigh, the popliteal area, and – with some limitations – in iliac vessels. Duplex scanning, either in grey scale or color-coded, provides the clearest infor-mation about acute deep venous thrombosis and insufficient perfo-

rating veins (SIMON and SCHOOP 1986; STRAUSS and NEUERBURG-HEUSLER 1997).

In the diagnosis of peripheral arterial diseases, it is possible to define stenoses in the leg and changes following recanalization procedures, and to determine the patency of arteries, or restenosis, on the basis of long-term posttherapeutic checks with duplex sonography and other non-invasive methods (HENNERICI and NEUERBURG-HEUSLER 1988; KAPPERT 1984; VERSTRAETE 1980).

The simplest technique with great practical importance to all patients is the quantification of peripheral blood pressure using the Doppler technique with a blood pressure cuff above the ankle. In all individuals without calcification of the arteries the blood pressure at the ankle is about 10–20 mmHg higher than at the brachial arteries (BOLLINGER 1979; SIMON and SCHOOP 1986). Mönckeberg's calcification, which is very common in patients with diabetic macroangiopathy, can be diagnosed by simple X-ray imaging or fluoroscopy.

Determining the ankle brachial index (ABI) using the Doppler technique is more precise for therapeutic indications or for comparisons between different therapies (e.g., vascular surgery versus angioplasty). With the blood pressure cuff above the ankle, blood pressure can be measured behind the medial malleolus at the posterior tibial artery and at the back of the foot, in the area of the dorsal pedal artery (BOLLINGER 1979). The gradient between ankle blood pressure and brachial blood pressure gives the relative values of the ankle brachial index.

$$\text{For example,} \frac{\text{ankle blood pressure}: 70}{\text{brachial blood pressure}: 140}$$
$$= \text{ABI}: 0.5$$

The ABI makes it possible to follow the course of the disease over a certain period without invasive methods. In addition, valuable information can be obtained by determining post-exercise ankle blood pressure. Also, segmental blood pressure indices provide particular information about the degree of vascular disease. The pressure cuff is placed above the knee at different levels and the Doppler controls are measured at the popliteal artery.

The Doppler method is an important tool in determining the stages of chronic limb ischemia according to the modified FONTAINE classification (FONTAINE et al. 1954) (see Table 2.2), or the RUTHERFORD gradings (RUTHERFORD and BECKER 1991) (see Table 5.10).

Spiral CT Angiography

Spiral CT (see also Chap. 9) as a new CT technique (KALENDER and POCLAIN 1991; ZEMAN et al. 1995) does not only provide cross-sectional images of arteries and veins, demonstrating the lumen and vascular wall, but also includes the possibility of obtaining three-dimensional documentation of the entire arterial and/or venous vascular system through a longitudinal section of the body of 40–80 cm. This requires only one contrast medium injection. It is the best method for detecting aneurysms and aortic dissections. Spiral CT provides rapid information when an intravenous contrast medium injection is used, allowing simultaneous artificial respiration and emergency reanimation.

2.5
Magnetic Resonance Angiography

Like duplex sonography, MRA (see also Chap. 12) is non-invasive. It requires neither the puncture and catheterization of the vessels, nor the application of iodinated contrast medium. The morphological information obtained, however, is better with the use of MR contrast agents, the side-effects of which are less than those of iodinated contrast agents (ARLART et al. 1991, 1996; DETMAR et al. 1997; WALLNER 1993).

By using MRA, arteries and veins can be visualized in different modes, whereby it is very important to choose the appropriate imaging technique to avoid artifacts or misinterpretation. Most common are the time-of-flight (TOF) and phase-imaging (PhI) techniques (EDELMANN et al. 1991). Its advantage over ultrasound techniques is the exclusion of subjective interpretation, while its disadvantage is the need for more costly technical equipment. The examination technique requires, in contrast to ultrasound, a clear measurement protocol, so that there is no need for specially qualified examiners. The individual imaging modalities of MRA enable larger areas to be examined than in ultrasound. The functional parameters, however, clearly differ between ultrasound and MRA; while ultrasound enables the precise determination of the parietal layer at limited areas (e.g., atheromatous ulcer, local dissection), information on the condition of the vascular walls of arteries and veins is different with MRA and can be obtained over larger sections. However, calcifications are not accurately visible on MRI, but can be well detected with ultrasound.

While ultrasound techniques are particularly suited to vascular analyses of the extremities and neck vessels, MRI and MRA provides overall better results in the head, pelvis, abdomen, and body trunk. It gives very precise information in the intracranial regions and is likely to play an important role in the future in the analysis of coronary vessels too. MRA also provides valuable information on calf and foot arteries.

2.6
Summary

The prerequisites of any useful and economical indication for the use of imaging modalities include a carefully established individual history and a physical examination. In addition, some laboratory data, the ABI, and ultrasound as a screening technique help in choosing the imaging technique on an individual basis.

When selecting the appropriate imaging modality for the diagnosis of disturbed arterial circulation, the prompt use of angiography is indicated in acute situations. If the situation permits, angiography can be preceded by one of the non-invasive imaging methods. In non-acute situations and for follow-up controls, color-coded or grey-scale duplex sonography is useful as a first imaging method and is sometimes fully sufficient. Simple therapeutic interventions can sometimes be performed on the basis of a correlation between a clinical examination, anamnesis, and the findings of duplex sonography. However, in the interests of quality assurance and to avoid complications and false indications, angiography is indispensable prior to invasive therapeutic measures – medicamentous, interventional, or surgical. If minimal changes to the wall need to be identified, duplex sonography can provide more detailed information than angiography. In special situations, IVUS or angioscopy are useful as complementary methods; they are mainly used within the framework of therapeutic interventions and basic science. For the analysis of complications, progression, regression, or recurrence, angiography should be preceded, however, by one of the non-invasive imaging methods, such as ultrasound sonography or MRA.

References

Abrams H (1983) Angiography, 3rd edn. volume III. Little Brown, Boston

Alexander K (1994) Gefäßkrankheiten. Urban und Schwarzenberg, München

Arlart JP, Guhl L, Fauser L, Edelmann RR, Kim D, Laub G (1991) MR-Angiographie (MRA) der Abdominalvenen. Radiologe 31:192–201

Arlart JP, Bongartz GM, Marchal G (1996) Magnetic resonance angiography. Springer, Berlin Heidelberg New York

Beck A (1993) Percutaneous transluminal angioscopy (1993) Springer, Heidelberg Berlin New York

Bollinger A (1979) Funktionelle Angiologie. Lehrbuch und Atlas. Thieme, Stuttgart

Bollinger A, Breddin K, et al (1981) Semiquantitative assessment of lower-limb atherosclerosis from routine angiographic images. Atherosclerosis 38:339–346

Bollinger A, Schneider E, Pouliadis G, Torres CH, Schlumpf M (1982) Erfolgsbeurteilung der peripheren transluminalen Angioplastie (PTA) mit einem computerfähigen, arteriographischen Score-System. VASA 11:309–312

Detmar K, Hildebrandt R, Loeffler W, Zeitler E (1997) Magnetische Resonanztomographie (MRA). In: Zeitler E (ed) Klinische Radiologie: Arterien und Venen. Springer, Berlin Heidelberg New York, pp 143–164

Edelmann RR, Chien D, Atkinson DJ, et al (1991) Fast time-of-flight magnetic resonance angiography with improved background suppression. Radiology 179:867–870

Fontaine R, Kim M, Kieny R (1954) Die chirurgische Behandlung der peripheren Durchblutungsstörungen. Helv Chir Acta 21:499–515

Günther RW, Thelen M (1995) Interventionelle Radiologie, 2nd edn. Thieme, Stuttgart

Heimig T, Martin M (1997) Thrombolyse. In: Zeitler E (ed) Klinische Radiologie: Arterien und Venen. Springer, Berlin Heidelberg New York, pp 193–198

Hennerici M, Neuerburg-Heusler D (1988) Gefäßdiagnostik mit Ultraschall. Thieme, Stuttgart

Kalender WA, Poclain A (1991) Physical performance characteristics of spiral CT-scanning. Med Phys 18:910–915

Kappert A (1985) Lehrbuch und Atlas der Angiologie, 12th edn. Huber, Bern

Konecny H, Ehringer H, Marosi L, Minor E, Ahmadi R (1986) Complications of thrombolysis with streptokinase (SK) or urokinase (UK) in peripheral arterial occlusive disease (POVD). In: Trübestein G (ed) Conservative therapy of arterial occlusive disease. Thieme, Stuttgart New York, pp 396–400

Kang SS, Wong PWK, Malinow MR (1992) Hyperhomocysteinemia as a risk factor for occlusive vascular disease. Ann Rev Nutr 12:279–298

Lanzer P, Rösch J (eds) (1994) Vascular diagnostics. Springer Berlin Heidelberg New York

Levy M, Schoop W (1982) Lebenserwartung bei Männern mit peripherer arterieller Verschlußkrankheit. Lebensversicherungsmedizin 5:98–102

Peabody CN, Kannel WB, McNamara PM (1974) Intermittent claudication – surgical significance. Arch Surg 109:693

Rees MR, Gehani AA, Ashley S, et al (1989) Percutaneous video angioscopy in peripheral vascular disease. Clin Radiol 40:347

Rutherford RB, Becker GJ (1991) Standards for evaluating and reporting results of surgical and percutaneous therapy for peripheral arterial disease. J Vasc Interv Radiol 2:169–174

Sigwart U, Bertrand M, Serruys PW (eds) (1996) Handbook of cardiovascular interventions. Churchill Livingstone, New York

Simon H, Schoop W (eds) (1986) Diagnostik in der Kardiologie und Angiologie. Thieme, Stuttgart

Strauss AL, Neuerburg-Heusler D (1997) Doppler- und Duplexsonographie. In: Zeitler E (ed) Klinische Radiologie: Arterien und Venen. Springer, Berlin Heidelberg New York, pp 593–606

Verstraete M (ed) (1980) Methods in angiology. Instrumentation and techniques in clinical medicine, vol 2. Martinus Nijhoff, The Hague

Wallner B (1993) MR-Angiographie. Thieme, Stuttgart

Widmer LK, da Silva A, Widmer MT (1994) Epidemiologie und sozialmedizinische Bedeutung der peripheren arteriellen Verschlußkrankheit. In: Alexander K (ed) Gefäßkrankheiten. Urban und Schwarzenberg, München, pp 16–24

Zeitler E (1997) Klinische Radiologie: Arterien und Venen. Springer, Berlin Heidelberg New York

Zeman RW, Bergman PM, Sulverman PM, et al (1995) Diagnosis of aortic dissection: value of helical CT with multiplanar reformation and three-dimensional rendering. AJR 164:1375–1380

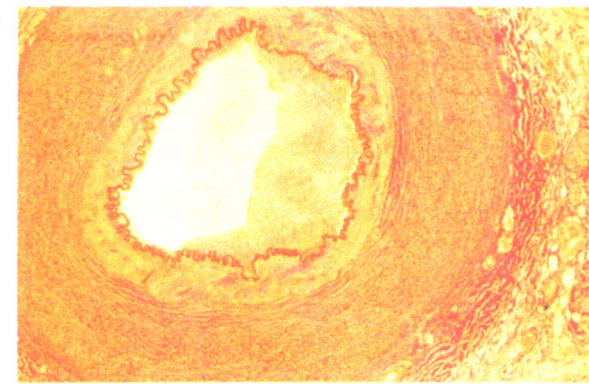

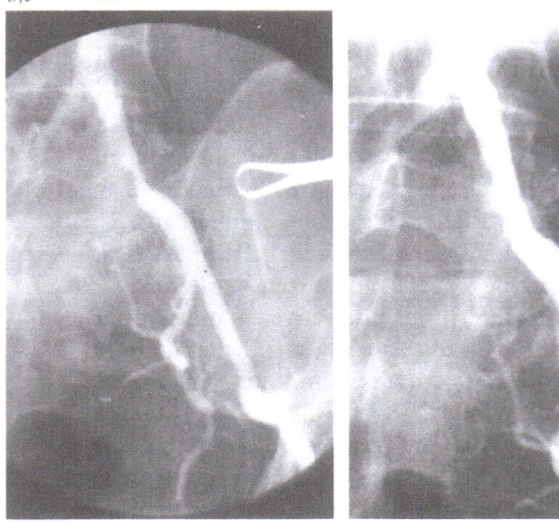

Fig. 3.1. Arterial Stenosis. **a** Histology. Cross-sectional image of a stenosed renal artery in a 30-year-old woman (Prof. WÜNSCH, Nürnberg) **b** Angiography of the left common iliac arteries with excentric stenosis **c** Angiography of the left common iliac arteries (zoom technique) after succesful balloon angioplasty

posed areas, whereby the natural aging process, metabolic disorders, physical hemodynamic effects, and influences of the coagulation system seem to be interacting (ALEXANDER 1993; FRY 1968; HINES and BARKER 1940; KEATINGE et al. 1986; RATSCHOW 1959; ROACH and SMITH 1983; ROBBINS and COTRAN 1979). *The arteries harden first, and then the fibrous plaques begin to be laid down. Without arteriosclerosis*, there will be *no atherosclerosis* in general. The pathoanatomical stages of arteriosclerosis are local edema, followed by arterial thickening which, with time, frequently changes into calcified plaques and occluded arteries. These steps are shown schematically in Fig. 3.3.

According to their varying pathomechanisms, three distinct but overlapping types of arteriosclerosis can be distinguished (EGNER et al. 1997), although precise definitions are not possible:

1. *The centrifugal-senile type* which has its origin in the abdominal aorta and spreads into the peripheral arteries. This type is most influenced by hypertension, blood-pressure changes, and cigarette smoking
2. *The multifocal-juvenile type* associated with disturbed lipid metabolism and progressing with cigarette smoking
3. *The centripetal-progressive type* with rapid, diffuse spreading in peripheral arteries in patients with diabetes mellitus.

The macromorphology of arteriosclerosis and occlusive vascular disease can be diagnosed with several imaging systems (ALEXANDER 1993; DEJDAR et al. 1967; RATSCHOW 1959; SCHETTLER 1961; ZEITLER 1997) with varying degrees of qualitative and quanti-

acetylsalicylic acid (ASA), this thrombocyte adhesion can be reduced to a large extent.

Following the rupture of atheroma with the formation of an atheromatous ulcer, the direct result is the development of a thrombus at its surface. This begins with platelet adhesion and aggregation and is followed by the formation of a white, hyaline thrombus (BENEKE 1975; BREDT 1963; KEATINGE et al. 1986; PACKMAN and MUSTARD 1986; ROKA 1967; ROSS and GLOMSET 1976; WIDMER et al. 1969). Gradually, this may be followed by cholesterol deposition (Fig. 3.2) and localized calcification (GOLDSTEIN and BROWN 1985; MEYER and LIND 1972; SCHETTLER 1961).

Arteriosclerosis is a multicausal process with the morphological picture of focal changes in predis-

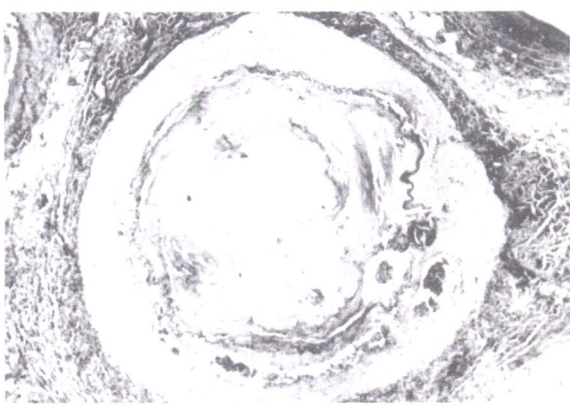

Fig. 3.2. Severe atherosclerosis in the popliteal artery (amputation of the lower leg).Multiple vasa vasorum in the media and cholesterol deposition

3 Arteriosclerosis and Its Risk Factors

E. ZEITLER

CONTENTS

3.1 Morphology

The aorta and its major branches are elastic-type arteries; their intima is thicker than that of the extremity arteries. The extremity arteries are of a muscular structure, characterized by a media full of muscle. Around several layers of muscle cells there is elastic and collagenous tissue (EGNER et al. 1997; WOLF and WERTHESSEN 1979).

The main cause of common arterial vascular disease is arteriosclerosis (ALLEN et al. 1946; BELL 1950; BREDT 1963; COWDRY 1967; DOERR 1963a, b; EGNER et al. 1997; HAUST 1971; RATSCHOW 1959; SCHETTLER 1961). The "response-to-injury" hypothesis of its atherogenesis as established by ROSS in 1973 has been widely accepted, but has since been updated (ROSS 1993) on the basis of various experimental studies partly stimulated by results using endoluminal techniques.

Manifold causes lead to the adhesion and aggregation of blood platelets on the intima, leading to the release of platelet-derived growth factor. In experiments, these causes included: local cold injuries, mechanical trauma caused by a balloon, dabbing with adrenalin solution (1:1000), elevated lipid intake, and inhalation of cigarette smoke (HESS 1970; HESS et al. 1975), as well as absorption of tobacco products by salivation. This causes an ingrowth of smooth muscle cells from the media into the intima, with a subsequent overreaction in the form of fibrous fatty and fibrous intimal pads. The localized intimal edema ("grey gelatinous deviations") can be considered as one early stage of arteriosclerosis. Through defective endothelial cells, proteins, lipids, and proteoglycans penetrate to the subendothelial space. After the transition of lipids into the subendothelial space, the intima thickens by forming fatty streaks, and later the atheromatous plaque. Monocytes then migrate between and below the endothelium cells, creating macrophages which absorb lipids and change into foam cells (BENEKE 1971; BETZ 1993). These, together with lymphocytes, form the fatty streaks. The increased ingrowth of smooth muscle cells from the media into the intima on the one hand, and the increased deposition of thrombocytes on the other result in a gradual narrowing of the arterial lumen, developing into hemodynamically effective stenoses (Fig. 3.1a,b) (ALLEN et al. 1946; BENEKE 1971; DOERR 1963a, b; HAUST 1971; LIEBEGOTT 1976; PACKMAN and MUSTARD 1986; ROBBINS and COTRAN 1979; ROKA 1967; ROSS 1993; SINZINGER et al. 1980; SCHETTLER 1961). Moreover, the formation of subendothelial sclerosis causes hardening of the artery. Under physiological conditions, the homeostatic mechanisms of the vascular wall prevent the adhesion of thrombocytes and other blood cells (ROKA 1967).

With raster screen electron microscopy (HESS 1970; HESS et al. 1975) it was possible to clearly demonstrate, on the example of mini-pigs, that inner and outer noxae disturb homeostasis, with adhesion of thrombocytes on the intima as a primary mechanism. In the example of carotid and femoral specimens it could be shown that, through the use of

EBERHARD ZEITLER, MD, Professor, University Erlangen-Nürnberg, Germany
address for correspondence: Virchowstraße 13, D-90409 Nürnberg, Germany

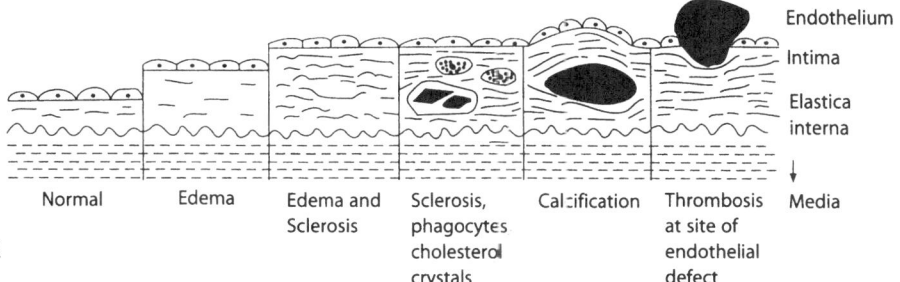

Fig. 3.3. Stages of arterio- and atherosclerosis

tative precision: (a) Angiography using X-rays, (b) duplex sonography using ultrasound, (c) magnetic resonance angiography (MRA), (d) spiral computed tomography (CT) angiography using X-rays, and (e) angioscopy using light.

In addition to macromorphology and histology, all of these imaging modalities are helpful in obtaining detailed information about changes in different parts of the vessel wall and lumen.

3.2
Progression and Regression

The progression of arteriosclerosis is, no doubt, a multifactorial process which has been studied in many experiments, as well as in epidemiologic studies (CAMPBELL and CAMPBELL 1980; CARO et al. 1971; CARTWRIGHT et al. 1985; GOLDSTEIN and BROWN 1985; KEATINGE et al. 1986; PACKMAN and MUSTARD 1986; ROSS 1986; SCHWARTZ et al. 1965; WEISS 1972; WIDMER et al. 1964). The *progression factors* can be summarized in five major parts:

- Arterial wall
- Blood pressure changes due to mechanical stress
- Blood factors: Platelets and clotting system
- Metabolism: Lipids, diabetes, homocysteine levels, infection
- Rheologic determinants: Viscosity, hematocrit

Morphological and clinical examinations have always confirmed a typical distribution and formation of arterial stenoses and occlusions (SPAIN 1966), which RATSCHOW (1959) called the "Lokalisatoreffekt" (localization-determining effect). The known primary obliterations in the different regions (Fig. 3.4) are attributable to adaptive "adjustments" to increased tensile stress, which is accompanied by intimal thickening with age (COTRAN et al. 1989). Arteries respond to chronic injury by strengthening adaptive mechanisms which cause them to thicken

and harden in order to maintain their structural functions. Injury to the arteries (CARO et al. 1971; FRY 1968; JONES et al. 1990; Ku et al. 1985; VITA et al. 1989; V.R. VEUSEY, Y.J. CHO 1993, personal communication) is caused by two types of stress: (1)*Tensile stress* on the arterial wall due to arterial pressure; (2) *shear stress* on the intima due to flow.

To avoid rupture, the artery wall adapts to excessive tensile stress by thickening and hardening, thus reducing vessel compliance and lumen size (CHO and KENSEY 1991). Shear stresses in site-specific areas increase in magnitude at high shear and oscillate in directions more rapidly in low-shear regions. Two types of shear stress cause injuries to the intima under amplified protosystolic pulse (AMPPULSE) circulation.

Compared with the normal pulsatile pressure-wave form, arteriosclerotic patients have abnormal pressure-wave forms (Fig. 3.5) with AMPPULSE, which occurs when the arterial wall loses compliance.

Both, artery hardening and plaque formation begin with mechanical injury rather than biochemical damage. Arteriosclerosis occurs in specific predictable regions. *Atherosclerosis* tends to occur at specific sites, such as bifurcations and bends.

Many arteriosclerotic lesions develop in high-shear areas (MEYER and LIND 1972; ROACH and SMITH 1983; SINZINGER et al. 1980), others in low-shear areas (CARO et al. 1971; DAVIS et al. 1986; MEYER and NAUJOKAT 1964; STEHBENS and MARTIN 1989; VITA et al. 1989; ZARINS et al. 1983). Low-shear areas are "turbulent" and characterized by flow separation and recirculation.

When the shear stress exceeded 390 dyne/cm^2, FRY (1968) found histological and biochemical changes in endothelial cells of the aorta. This critical shear stress strongly depended on exposure time, and may vary from patient to patient.

According to the hypotheses by CHO and KENSEY (1991) (see also Fig. 3.6) and K.R. KENSEY (1997, personal communication), the main causes of vascu-

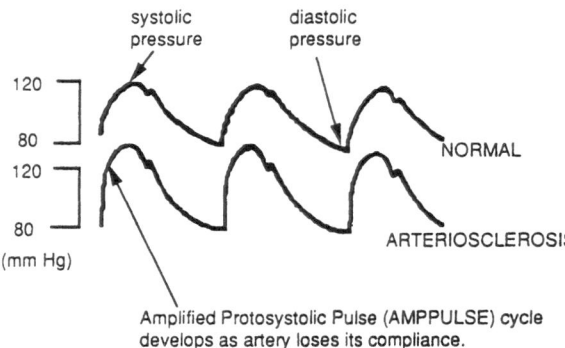

Fig. 3.5. Amplified protosystolic pulse (AMPPULSE) in arteriosclerotic arteries in contrast to non-arteriosclerotic arteries

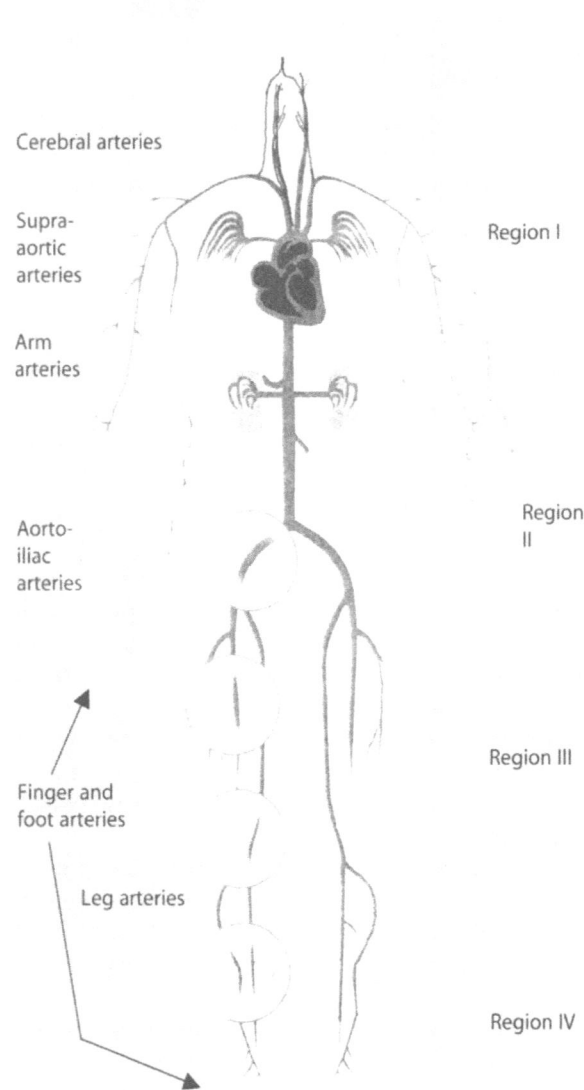

Fig. 3.4. Arteries divided into four regions depending on the energy source of injury and the preferred locations of arteriosclerotic diseases

lar injury have three key parameters: (1) Arterial pressure, (2) blood viscosity, (3) magnitude of protosystolic acceleration.

A regression in the long term can only be expected if all risk factors are completely eliminated. On angiogram, regression is rather the spontaneous lysis of thrombotic plaque, or plaque retraction (DEJDAR et al. 1967). An objectifiable regression in people following a strict diet remains to be proven by clinical studies. The cumulative effects of these factors, such as lipid and cholesterol levels, hematocrit, red blood cell deformability, and heart rate all contribute to the three parameters mentioned above.

Computer simulations with non-Newtonian blood viscosity, and the results of streamlines and wall shear stress demonstrate the location of high force exerted on localized areas and have shown the importance of rheological blood properties (Fig. 3.7).

Thickening of the artery creates turbulent flow, with its high and low shear forces.

Wall shear stresses calculated from an AMPPULSE cycle are significantly larger than those calculated from a non-AMPPULSE cycle. For example, distal branch wall AMPPULSE cycles yield shear stresses of $140\,dyne/cm^2$, whereas non-AMPPULSE cycles give $100\,dyne/cm^2$. Therefore, intima in high-shear regions absorbs greater quantities of energy during AMPPULSE circulation via increased wall shear stress. Similar results were demonstrated by DAVIS et al. (1986), who found turbulent flow to be a major determinant of hemodynamically-induced endothelial cell turnover.

PACKMAN and MUSTARD (1986) investigated the role of platelets in the development of atherosclerosis and concluded that thrombi can form at sites injured by disturbed blood flow.

Many experimental and in-patient studies have shown that the intima thickens when injured. Thus the "response-to-injury" hypothesis of Ross (1986, 1993) is widely accepted and new results can give detailed answers to open new questions. Injury to the intima is multifactorial and AMPPULSE circulation identifies one cause of specific localizations of atherosclerotic obliterative diseases.

One factor influencing blood viscosity is hematocrit (normal in men: 37%–49%, normal in women: 34%–46%). Blood viscosity is mostly determined by the concentration of blood cells and the deformability of red blood cells. The absolute viscosity of blood at 37°C is $2.30–2.72 \times 10^{-3}\,pa \times$ seconds. Relative viscosity can be measured in vitro at 18°C compared to water and is 4.75 pa.

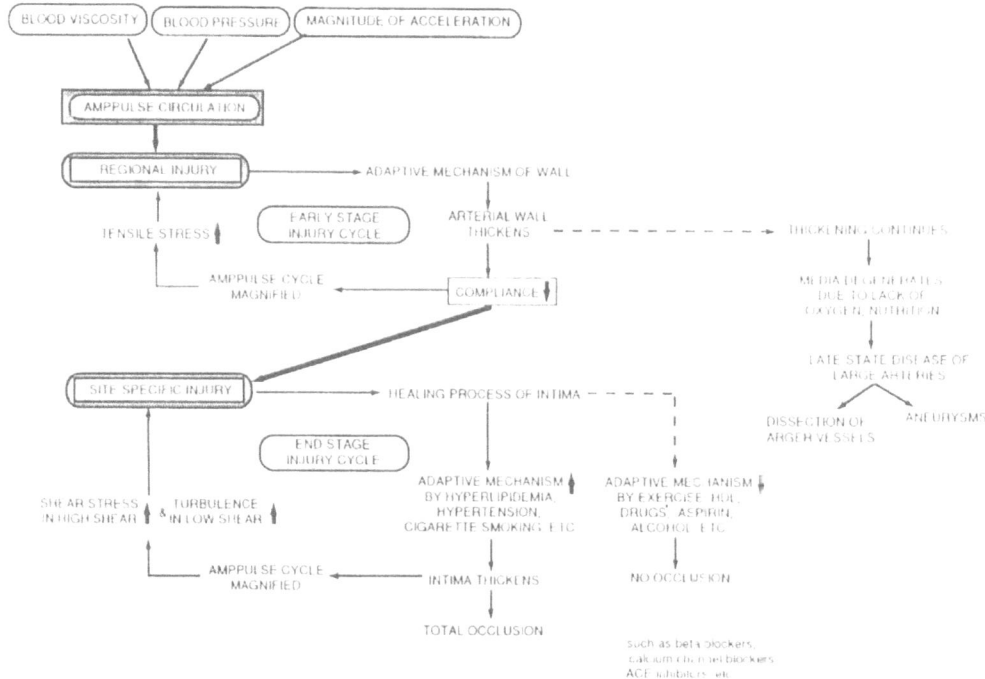

Fig. 3.6. Theory of progression of arteriosclerosis according to Cho and Kensey (1991). *HDL*, high-density lipoprotein

Cigarette smoking impairs all three factors which contribute to a properly functioning heart: (1) Viscosity, (2) blood pressure, and (3) Contraction force of the left ventricle. The topography of morphologic changes can be attributed to localized metabolic variations in the arterial wall and specific hemodynamic tensile and shear stresses to the arterial tube with damage to the respective site.

3.3
Risk Factors

Risk factors are determinants affecting a "population at risk". Prospective studies on incidence have revealed a statistical difference in the occurrence of new diseases after several years of examinations using the same examination techniques. The risk factor itself is not an etiologic factor (Alexander 1993; Ratschow 1959; Schettler 1961; Widmer et al. 1981).

Crucial findings on risk factors have been obtained from differently organized epidemiologic studies, among which the Framingham Study (Kannel et al. 1970) and the Basler Study (Widmer et al. 1981) have most clearly demonstrated current knowledge based on comparisons between subjects with healthy and diseased arteries.

3.3.1
Cigarette Smoking

The Framingham Study found that heavy smokers (more than 20 cigarettes per day) developed intermittent claudication four times more often than non-smokers (Kannel et al. 1970; Kannel and Shurtleff 1973). In multifactorial analysis, cigarette smoking with a regression coefficient of 0.451 was risk factor number one (Gordon and Kannel 1972).

In the Basler Study, cigarette smokers developed peripheral occlusive vascular disease (POVD) 2.9 times more frequently than non-smokers. Those subjects who smoked in excess of 35 cigarettes per

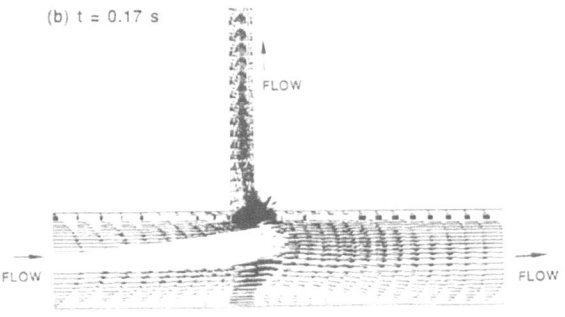

Fig. 3.7. Computer simulations demonstrate the location of high force against localized areas with the non-newtonian viscosity of blood (Cho and Kensey 1991)

day developed POVD 2.5 times more frequently than those who smoked five cigarettes per day, and three times more often than non-smokers (Fig. 3.8). The correlation is almost linear. Men who at the beginning of the study, smoked 35 or more cigarettes daily, developed POVD four times more than those who had initially been non-smokers. Deviations between the two 5-year periods are attributable to the fact that occasional smokers in the first Basler Study were classified as smokers, whereas in the second study they were regarded as non-smokers (WIDMER et al. 1981).

The study was based on the analysis of 2630 working men with healthy arteries who, at the outset, were between 35 and 64 years of age. In re-aortographed subjects and in subgroups – 248 males with confirmed stenoses or occlusions and 65 with re-angiographies after a 5-year interval – progression was observed in 63% of extremities; in 33% new additional stenoses, and in 30% fresh occlusions had developed. Progression was particularly marked at the femoral and lower-leg level and in the initially stenosed arteries.

By stopping smoking, the progression of POVD can be slowed down, leading to a lower risk of vascular surgery or amputation. JONASON and BERGSTRÖM (1987) found a reduction in cardiac fatalities to 46% in subjects who had given up smoking, compared to 82% in smokers. Cigarette smokers have a three-fold higher incidence of POVD than non-smokers and a higher death rate (HAMMOND and HORN 1954).

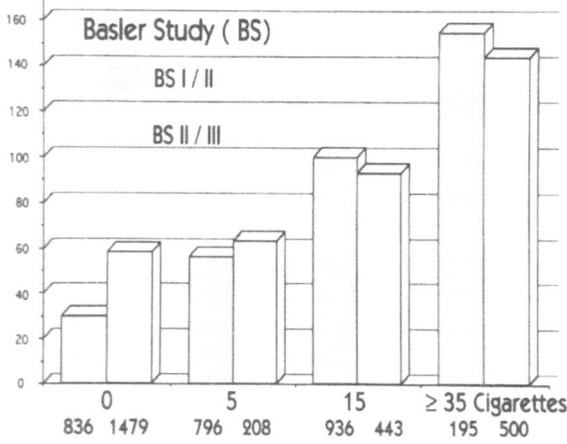

Fig. 3.8. Cigarette smoking and 5-year incidence of peripheral occlusive vascular disease

3.3.2
Hypertension

HINES and BARKER (1940) from the Mayo Clinic had already pointed out the correlation between POVD and arterial hypertension, stating: *It is a well established fact that arteriosclerosis develops prematurely among patients who have arterial hypertension.*

Prospective studies on prevalence (JÜRGENS et al. 1960; SCHWARTZ et al. 1965; WIDMER et al. 1981) have shown hypertension to be present in patients with POVD between two and three times more often than in people without arterial disease. In patients with POVD, hypertensive blood pressure values were found in 20%–30%, in contrast to 6%–14% in persons with healthy arteries.

However, in the multifactorial analysis carried out in the Framingham Study (GORDON and KANNEL 1972), the regression coefficient was only 0.178, i.e., lower than that of cigarette smokers.

In the Basler Studies II and III, patients with hypertension – elevated systolic blood pressure – developed POVD 1.7 times more often within 5 years than non-hypertensive patients (WIDMER et al. 1981).

3.3.3
Hyperlipidemia

As early as 1856, Rudolf VIRCHOW spoke of a "fat metamorphosis and imbibition from the blood into the arterial wall" (VIRCHOW 1856). In the Framingham Study, hypercholesterolemia was found to be the third leading risk factor. Its incidence is most apparent in cases of hypercholesterol combined with hypertriglyceridemia (HARTMANN et al. 1981).

In subjects who, at the beginning of the Basler Study, had both elevated cholesterol and triglyceride values, the incidence of POVD was three times higher than in comparative groups of the same age with normal cholesterol and triglyceride values.

3.3.4
Diabetes Mellitus

Diabetes mellitus is a common disease affecting 2%–5% of the general population (BELL 1950; COWDRY 1967; DOERR 1963b; KRAMER 1932). One serious complication of the disease is the development of POVD with ulcers and gangrene of the lower limb

(KRONE and MÜLLER-WIELAND 1990), in addition to diabetic nephropathy and retinopathy. As early as in 1932 it was recognized that the limbs of diabetics are threatened (KRAMER 1955). According to WIDMER (1993), prospective studies revealed a rapid increase in peripheral vascular diseases in diabetics (25%–58%). In 40% of these this led to critical leg ischemia, which was only found in 18% of non-diabetics.

In the Basler studies I and II ($n = 2759$ men) diabetics experienced an asymptomatic POVD 1.9 times more often than non-diabetics. In the Basler studies II and III ($n = 2630$ men) diabetics developed intermittent claudication 2.6 times more often, and asymptomatic POVD 2.3 times more often. The diagnostic and therapeutic management of diabetic patients with critical limb ischemia is an important health problem. The leg-amputation rate among diabetics is approximately 15 times higher than that among non-diabetics (KRONE and MÜLLER-WIELAND 1990; MOST and SINNOCK 1983).

Diabetes mellitus alone is a risk factor for POVD, but is frequently associated with other cardiovascular risk factors, such as hypertension, hyperlipidemia, and smoking. Up to 60% of diabetics have abnormal plasma lipoprotein levels. Patients with diabetes can have increased triglyceride levels and/or cholesterol levels, as well as low concentrations of high-density lipids (KRONE and MÜLLER-WIELAND 1990).

According to ALEXANDER (1993): "after 15 to 20 years of diabetes mellitus the likelihood of morphologically identifiable microangiopathy is present in nearly every case", particularly with diabetic nephropathy and retinopathy.

3.3.5
Infection

The currently practiced concept of prevention and treatment of arteriosclerosis and its complications is based on the knowledge gained from studies on large patient populations. It has been found that various risk factors greatly influence the manifestation and degree of arteriosclerosis associated with disturbed circulation in the coronary, cerebral, and peripheral vessels.

New findings on the basis of seroprevalence studies (MIETTINEN et al. 1996; SAIKKU et al. 1992) have led to the assumption that arteriosclerosis *might* be caused by *Chlamydia pneumoniae* bacteria.

The investigated serum of men with hypercholesterolemia (Helsinki Heart Study) showed that persons with continuously increasing sensitivity of specific IgG- and IgA-class antibodies to *C. pneumoniae*, or specific immunocomplexes, had a 2.6 times higher risk of experiencing heart infarction. In the case of additional smoking, the risk was elevated by a factor of 5.6. In men with hypercholesterolemia and serologic signs of a persisting *C. pneumoniae* infection, the risk of heart infarction increased as much as seven-fold. In patients with acute myocardial infarction, a seroconversion to lipopolysaccharide was identified.

Several working groups succeeded in directly identifying the bacteria in arteriosclerotic coronary vessels and aortas using electron microscopy, immunohistochemistry, polymerase chain reactions, and cell cultures of specimens from operations and autopsies. Under electron microscopy, *C. pneumoniae* elementary particles were found in macrophages that had changed into foam cells and in smooth muscle cells.

Moreover, using direct immunofluorescence, the *Chlamydia* species could be clearly identified in the arteriosclerotic tissue obtained by atherectomy in 71 out of 90 patients with coronary heart disease (CHD) (MUHLESTEIN et al. 1996). In non-sclerosed coronary tissue, by contrast, the chlamydia bacteria was only found in one case.

The various authors therefore assume that chlamydia infection could be one of the causes, or an additional risk factor, of arteriosclerosis. Several authors speculate that restenoses in bypasses and following stent implantation, as well as reocclusions, might be initiated by a chronic chlamydia infection. LÜDERITZ (1997), however, states that however much the hypothesis and its consequences may be plausible, or may even encourage the use of antibiotic therapy in the case of arteriosclerotic complications, they have not been proven as yet. Although there is great doubt as regards the involvement of inflammatory vascular disease (angiitis) in the formation of CHD, particularly instable angina pectoris, its causal genesis has not as yet been determined. Other studies have reported that the presence of C-reactive protein in cases of apoplexia and myocardial infarction suggests that a co-factor of inflammatory nature exists. Also, the clearly positive results of long-term treatment with aspirin with antiphlogistic effects might support this theory (RIDKER et al. 1997). In patients with POVD, no chlamydia infection was to date identified as an initiating cause.

The currently practiced, efective principles of primary and secondary prevention of CHD and POVD should, however, under no circumstances be given up. One aspect of paramount importance in the prevention of complications from arteriosclerosis is the prophylactic therapy of the relevant risk factors: hypertension, diabetes, and hyper-cholesterolemia. Smokers should stop smoking, and regular physical exercise is beneficial.

Only if the "chlamydia hypothesis" is clearly proven should adaptations to current therapies, i.e., the administration of antibiotics, be taken into consideration.

3.3.6
Combination of Risk Factors

The coincidence of several risk factors has a considerable influence on the likelihood of developing POVD (KANNEL et al. 1970; WIDMER et al. 1981; PUCHMAYER et al. 1974). There is a distinct correlation between a person's number of risk factors and the incidence of POVD (Fig. 3.9). For example, in the Basler Study men with three risk factors developed the disease between four and six times more frequently than those without risk factors (WIDMER et al. 1993).

Clinical angiographic examinations taking known risk factors into consideration, have emphasized that cigarette smoking, either as the only risk factor or combined with others, is linked in particular with arterial obliterations in the region of the superficial femoral artery in the peripheral vessels. The risk factor of hypertension, in contrast, tends to result mainly in stenotic arteriosclerotic changes in the cerebral arteries, as well as coronary, calf, and digital arteries (LIEBEGOTT 1976). When correlating the

angiographically identified pathologic findings to the risk factor of hypertension (DEMBSKI 1976), it was found that 25% of angiographically examined patients with hypertension as the sole risk factor had stenoses and occlusions of the feet and digital arteries. Only when additional risk factors are present does the likelihood of additional stenotic changes in the lower leg, thigh, and pelvic arteries increase. The influence of the severity of hypertension and its history could only be anticipated on the basis of these examinations since systematic angiographic studies on larger populations are not yet available.

Also, in post mortem angiographic studies (DEJDAR et al. 1967) attempts were made to explore the signs of a correlation between risk factors and to show the possibilities of documenting progression and regression in angiograms, in the interests of an objective assessment and for studies on the factors influencing the course of the disease. Color-coded duplex sonography, in contrast, enables the analysis of arteriosclerotic changes and localized stenoses, even with frequent examinations at different times. This provides the possibility of drawing further conclusions about the course of POVD in the future, not only in the area of the carotid bifurcation, but also in the extremities (ALEXANDER 1993; BOLLINGER 1979; JÄGER et al. 1985; NEUERBURG-HEUSLER and HENNERICI 1995; STRAUSS and NEUERBURG-HEUSLER 1997).

In addition to all risk factors, we know empirically that smokers without CHD or POVD exist. On the other hand, a small number of patients without any risk factors can develop POVD or CHD. In most cases these patients are of advanced years; therefore, being aged over 80 is also a risk factor. Furthermore, family histories have shown that there is also a genetic plus or minus as regards the development or non-development of arteriosclerosis as a clinical entity.

3.4
Recommendations

It is important for every physician to know the risk factors and pathophysiology in order to be able to give all patients, both healthy and diseased the following helpful recommendations:

1. Give up smoking!
2. Check blood pressure to prevent or treat hypertension.
3. Take regular exercise—at least one walk or jog daily, provided there is no contraindication.

Risk factors

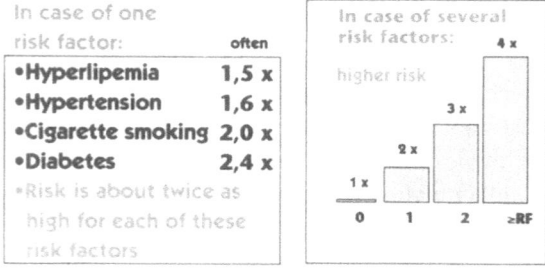

Basler Study ; Büchner, K. ;Widmer, L.1992

Fig. 3.9. Incidence of peripheral occlusive vascular disease with different single and several simultaneous risk factors

4. Check blood sugar; optimal treatment of diabetes mellitus (oral or subcutaneous) is necessary.

5. A low-fat diet with reduced calories can reduce composite blood viscosity.

6. Hydration lowers composite blood viscosity by making the red blood cells more deformable.

7. Regular checks by the doctor from the age of 50 at the latest.

References

Alexander K (ed) (1993) Gefäßkrankheiten. Urban and Schwarzenberg, Munich

Allen E, Barker W, Hines E (1946) Peripheral vascular diseases. Saunders, Philadelphia

Bell ET (1950) A post mortem study of 1214 diabetic subjects with special reference to the vascular lesions. Proc Diab Assoc 10:62

Beneke G (1971) Pathologische Anatomie der Arteriosklerose. Med Klin 66:729

Beneke G (1975) Pathophysiologische und pathomorphologische Betrachtungen zur Arteriosklerose. Ther Umsch (Bayer) 47:5–14

Betz E (1993) Experimentelle Grundlagen zur Atherogenese. In: Alexander K: Gefäßkrankheiten. Urban and Schwarzenberg, Munich pp 47–55

Bollinger A (1979) Funktionelle Angiologie. Lehrbuch und Atlas. Thieme, Stuttgart

Bredt H (1963) Morphologie und Pathogenese der Arteriosklerose. In: Schettler G (ed) Arteriosklerose Thieme, Stuttgart

Campbell GR, Campbell JH (1980) Spontaneous intimal loss in arteries of old hypertensive rats and the experimental production of similar lesions in young rabbits. Micron 11:1457–1458

Caro CG, Fitz-Gerald JM, Schroter RC (1971) Atheroma and arterial wall shear: observation, correlation and proposal of a shear dependent mass transfer mechnism for atherogenesis. Proc Roy Soc Lond B 177:109–159

Cartwright IJ, Pockley AG, Galloway JH, Greaves M, Preston FE (1985) The effects of dietary omega-3-polyunsaturated fatty acids on erythrocyte membrane phospholipids, erythrocyte deformability and blood viscosity in healthy volunteers. Atherosclerosis 55:267–281

Cho YJ, Kensey KR (1991) Effects of the non-Newtonian viscosity of blood on hemodynamics of diseased arterial flows: part 1, steady flows. Biorheology 28:241–262

Cotran RS, Kumar V, Robbins SL (1989) Robbins pathologic basis of disease, 4th edn, chap 12: blood vessels. Saunders, Philadelphia, pp 553–596

Cowdry S (1967) Atherosclerosis. Thomas, Springfield

Davis PF, Remuzzi A, Gordon EJ, Dewey CF (1986) Turbulent fluid shear stress induces vascular endothelial cell turnover in vitro. Proc Natl Acad Sci USA 83:2114–2117

Dejdar R, Roubkova A, Cachovan M, Kruml J, Linhart J (1967) Vergleich postmortaler Angiogramme mit makro- und mikroskopischen Befunden an A. femoralis und A. poplitea. Arch Kreislaufforschg 54:309–315

Dembski (1976) Angiographische Befunde an den Extremitäten bei Hypertonie. In: Zeitler E (ed) Hypertonie, Risikofaktor in der Angiologie. Wittstrock, Baden-Baden, pp 138–147

Doerr W (1963a) Perfusionstheorie der Arteriosklerose. Thieme, Stuttgart

Doerr W (1963b) Gangarten der Arteriosklerose. Klin Wochenschr 41:576–583

Egner E, Kraus-Huonder B, Markmann HU (1997) Grundlagen der Pathomorphologie der Blutgefäße. In: Zeitler E (ed) Arterien und Venen. Springer, Berlin Heidelberg New York, pp 3–56

Fry DL (1968) Acute vascular endothelial changes associated with increased blood velocity gradients. Circ Res 22:165–167

Goldstein JL, Brown MS (1985) Receptor-mediates endocytosis. Concepts emerging from the LDL receptor system. Annu Rev Cell Biol 1:1–39

Gordon T, Kannel WB (1972) Predisposition to atherosclerosis in the head, heart and legs – the Framingham Study. JAMA 221:661

Hammond EC, Horn D (1954) The relationship between human smoking habits and death rates. A follow-up study of 187766 men. JAMA 155:1316

Hartmann G, Stähelin HB et al. (1981) Die Hyperlipidämie als Risikofaktor. In: Widmer LK, Stähelin HB, Nissen C, da Silva A (eds) Venen-, Arterien-Krankheiten, koronare Herzkrankheit bei Berufstätigen. Prospektiv-epidemiologische Untersuchung Basler Studie I-III. Huber, Bern, pp 277–287

Haust MD (1971) Arteriosclerosis. In: Brunson JG, Gau A: (eds) Concepts of disease. MacMillan, New York

Hess H (1970) Neue Überlegungen zur Physiopathologie obliterierender Arteriopathien. Fortschr Med 88:833, 923

Hess H, Marshall M, Mallasch M (1975) Zur Verhütung von Thrombozytenabscheidungen durch ASS (Colfarit®) – tierexperimentelle Untersuchungen. Ther Umsch (Bayer) 47:15–21

Hines EA Jr, Barker NW (1940) Arteriosclerosis obliterans. A clinical and pathological study. Am J Med Sc 200:717

Jäger K, Phillip AD Martin RL et al. (1985) Noninvasive mapping of lower limb arterial lesions. Ultrasound Med Biol 11:515–521

Jonason T, Bergström R (1987) Cessation of smoking in patients with intermittent claudication. Acta Med Scand 221:253–260

Jones CJ, Singer DR, Watkins NV, MacGregor GA, Caro CG (1990) Abnormal arterial flow pattern in untreated essential hypertension: possible link with the development of atherosclerosis. Clin Sci 78(4):431–435

Jürgens JC, Barker NW, Hines EA Jr (1960) Arteriosclerosis obliterans: review of 520 cases with special reference to pathogenic and prognostic factors. Circulation 21:188

Kannel WB, Shurtleff D (1973) Cigarettes and development of intermittent claudication. The Framingham study. Geriatrics 28:61

Kannel WB, Skinner JJ, Schwartz MJ, Shurtleff D (1970) Intermittent claudication. Incidence in the Framingham study. Circulation 41:875

Keatinge WR, Coleshaw SR, Easton JC, Cotter F, Mattock MB, Chelliah R (1986) Increased platelet and red cell counts, blood viscosity, and plasma cholesterol levels during heat stress, and mortality from coronary and cerebral thrombosis. Am J Med 81:795–800

Kramer DW (1932) Diabetic gangrene: incidence and pathogenesis – an analysis of 58 cases among 1008 diabetics. Am J Med Sc 183:503

Kramer DW (1955) Peripheral vascular disorders in diabetes mellitus. A survey of 3000 cases. Angiology 6:408

Krone W, Müller-Wieland D (1990) Special problems of the diabetic patient. In: Dormandy JA, Stock G (eds) Critical leg ischemia. Springer, Berlin Heidelberg New York, pp 145–157

Ku DN, Giddens DP, Zarins CK, Glagov S (1985) Pulsatile flow and atherosclerosis in the human carotid bifurcation. Arteriosclerosis 5:293–302

Liebegott G (1976) Morphologie der hypertensiven Angiopathie. In: Zeitler E (ed) Hypertonie, Risikofaktor in der Angiologie. Witzstrock, pp 15–26

Lüderitz B (1997) Ist die Koronarsklerose eine Infektionskrankheit? Dtsch Arztebl 94:B-950–951

Meyer MW, Lind J (1972) Calcifications of iliac arteries in newborns and infants. Arch Dis Child 47:364–372

Meyer MW, Naujokat B (1964) Über die rhythmische Lokalisation der atherosklerotischen Herde im cervicalen Abschnitt der Vertebralarterie. Beitr Pathol Anat 130:24–39

Miettinen H, Lehto S, Saikku P, Haffner SM, Rönnemaa T, Pyörälä K, Laakso M (1996) Association of Chlamydia pneumoniae and acute coronary heart disease events in non-insulin-dependent and non-diabetic subjects in Finland. Eur Heart J 17:682–688

Most RS, Sinnock P (1983) The epidemiology of lower extremity amputation in diabetic individuals. Diabetic Care 6:87–91

Muhlestein JB, Hammond EH, Carlquist JF et al. (1996) Increased incidence of Chlamydia species within the coronary arteries of patients with symptomatic atherosclerotic versus other forms of cardiovascular disease. J Am Cardiol 27:1555–1561

Neuerburg-Heusler D, Hennerici M (1995) Gefäßdiagnostik mit Ultraschall. Thieme, Stuttgart

Packman MA, Mustard JF (1986) The role of platelets in the development and complications of atherosclerosis. Semin Hematol 23(1):8–25

Puchmayer V, Bazika V (1974) Analysis of risk factors in atherosclerosis obliterans. Cas Lék Ces 113:172–176

Ratschow M (1959) Angiologie. Pathologie, Klinik und Therapie der peripheren Durchblutungs-störungen. Thieme, Stuttgart

Ridker PM, Cushman M, Stampfer MJ, Tracy RP, Hennekens CH (1997) Inflammation, aspirin, and the risk of cardiovascular disease in apparently healthy men. N Engl J Med 336:973–979

Roach MR, Smith NB (1983) Does high shear stress induced by blood flow lead to atherosclerosis? Perspect Bio Med 26:287–303

Robbins SL, Cotran RS (1979) Pathologic basis of disease. Saunders, Philadelphia

Roka L (1967) Physiologische Wechselwirkung zwischen Gefäßinhalt und Gefäßwand. Dtsch Med J 18:349–355

Ross R (1986) The pathogenesis of atherosclerosis – an update. N Engl J Med 314(8):488–500

Ross R (1993) The pathogenesis of atherosclerosis: a perspective for the 1990s. Nature 362:801–809

Ross R, Glomset JA (1976) The pathogenesis of atherosclerosis. N Engl J Med 295(8):420–425

Saikku P, Leinonen M, Tenkanen L, Ekman MR, Linnanmärki E, Manninen V, Mänttäri M, Frick MM, Huttunen JK (1992) Chronic Chlamydia pneumoniae infection as a risk factor for coronary heart disease in the Helsinki Heart Study. Ann Intern Med 116:273–278

Schettler G (1961) Arteriosklerose – Ätiologie, Pathologie, Klinik und Therapie. Thieme, Stuttgart

Schwartz D, Lellough J, Angueira G, Richard JL (1965) Tabac et autres facteurs étiologiques dans l' arteriopathie oblitérante des membres inférieurs. Résultat d'une enquete retrospective. J Atheroscler Res 5:302

Sinzinger H, Silberbauer K, Auerwald W (1980) Quantitative investigation of sudanophilic lesions around aortic ostia of human fetuses, newborn, and children. Blood Vessels 17:44–52

Spain DM (1966) Atherosclerosis. Sci Am 215(2):49–56

Stehbens WE, Martin BJ (1989) Hemodynamically-induced atrophic lesions of atherosclerosis. Proceeding of the 2nd international symposium on biofluid mechanics and biorheology, blood flow in large vessels, 25–28 June 1989, Munich, pp 1–11 (also published by Springer, 1991)

Strauss AL, Neuerburg-Heusler D (1997) Doppler- und Duplexsonographie. In: Zeitler E (ed) Klinische Radiologie: Arterien und Venen. Springer, Berlin Heidelberg New York, pp 593–606

Virchow (1856) Gesammelte Abhandlungen zur Wissenschaftlichen Medizin. Meidinger, Frankfurt

Vita JA, Treasure CB, Ganz P, Cox DA, Fish RD, Selwyn AP (1989) Control of shear stress in the epicardial arteries of humans: impairment by atherosclerosis. J Am Coll Cardiol 14:1193–1199 (Also, Bing RB, Editorial Comments, vol 14, 1989, pp 1200–1201)

Weiss NS (1972) Cigarette smoking and arteriosclerosis obliterans – an epidemiologic approach. Am J Epidemiol 95:17

Widmer LK, Greensher A, Kannel WB (1964) Occlusion of peripheral arteries. A study of 6400 working subjects. Circulation 30:836

Widmer LK, Hartmann G, Duchosal F, Plechl Sch (1969) Risk factors in arterial occlusion of the limbs. German Med Monthly XIV:476

Widmer LK, Stähelin HB, Nissen C, da Silva A (1981) (eds) Venen-, Arterien-Krankheiten, koronare Herzkrankheit bei Berufstätigen. Prospektiv-epidemiologische Untersuchung Basler Studie I–III. Huber, Bern

Widmer LK, da Silva A, Widmer MT (1993) Epidemiologie und sozialmedizinische Bedeutung der peripheren arteriellen Verschlußkrankheit. In: Alexander K (ed) Gefäßkrankheiten. Urban and Schwarzenberg, Munich, pp 16–24

Wolf und Werthessen (1979) Dynamics of arterial flow, Chap 1: anatomical and physiological characteristics of arteries. Plenum, New York, pp 18–20

Zarins CK, Giddens DP, Bharadvaj BK (1983) Carotid bifurcation atherosclerosis: Quantitative correlation of plaque localization with flow velocity profiles and wall shear stresses. Circ Res 53:502–514

Zeitler E (ed) (1997) Klinische Radiologie: Arterien und Venen. Springer, Berlin Heidelberg New York

4 Pathophysiology of Intimal Hyperplasia

F.C. Tanner and T.F. Lüscher

CONTENTS

4.1 Atherosclerosis

Atherosclerosis accounts for about half of both morbidity and mortality in Western countries; its pathogenesis, however, is only incompletely understood. Cardiovascular risk factors such as hyperlipidemia, hypertension, diabetes mellitus and tobacco consumption are associated with atherogenesis. These risk factors induce progressive vascular injury and lead to vascular dysfunction resulting in atherosclerotic changes (Ross 1993). Features of dysfunctional arteries include platelet activation and aggregation, monocyte adhesion and invasion, vascular smooth muscle cell (VSMC) proliferation and migration, insudation of lipid substances and formation of extracellular matrix (Fig. 4.1). Accumulation of VSMC and monocytes, as well as deposition of matrix and lipids, indeed represent the main features of neointima formation during atherogenesis (Ross 1993).

4.1.1 Role of Endothelial Cells

The endothelium is the part of the vessel wall most exposed to mechanical forces of the blood and to the

effect of the substances therein. Morphological studies indeed demonstrate changes in endothelial morphology with cardiovascular disease. Associated with such changes are functional alterations which result in a decreased release of factors inducing relaxation and inhibiting proliferation such as nitric oxide (NO) or prostacyclin, while the release of factors inducing contraction and stimulating proliferation such as endothelin-1 or angiotensin II is enhanced (Lüscher and Vanhoutte 1990). Endothelial denudation does not occur except in late stages of atherosclerosis and during plaque rupture or percutaneous transluminal angioplasty. Both endothelial dysfunction and denudation lead to platelet deposition and monocyte invasion and thus initiate neointima formation (Ross 1993). Aggregating platelets cause contraction via the release of thromboxane and serotonin; furthermore, they stimulate proliferation and migration of VSMC via the release of thrombin and platelet-derived growth factor. Invading monocytes release many cytokines and growth factors as well; moreover, they accumulate lipid and cholesterol and are an important component of the atherosclerotic plaque (Ross 1993). Thus, it is conceivable that growth inhibitors prevail under normal conditions rendering the vessel wall quiescent, while various cytokines and growth factors are produced in the presence of cardiovascular risk factors or following endothelial denudation. Therefore, the endothelium is the major mediator of vascular homeostasis; due to its anatomic position it is exposed to cardiovascular risk factors so that it becomes dysfunctional and with that initiates atherogenesis (Lüscher and Vanhoutte 1990).

4.1.1.1 Endothelial Factors Inducing Relaxation and Inhibiting Proliferation

The endothelium can elicit vascular relaxation when stimulated by neurotransmitters, hormones, sub-

F.C. Tanner, MD, Cardiovascular Research, University Zürich-Irchel, CH-8057 Zürich, Switzerland
T.F. Lüscher, MD, Division of Cardiology, University Hospital Zürich, Rämistraße 100, CH-8091 Zürich, Switzerland

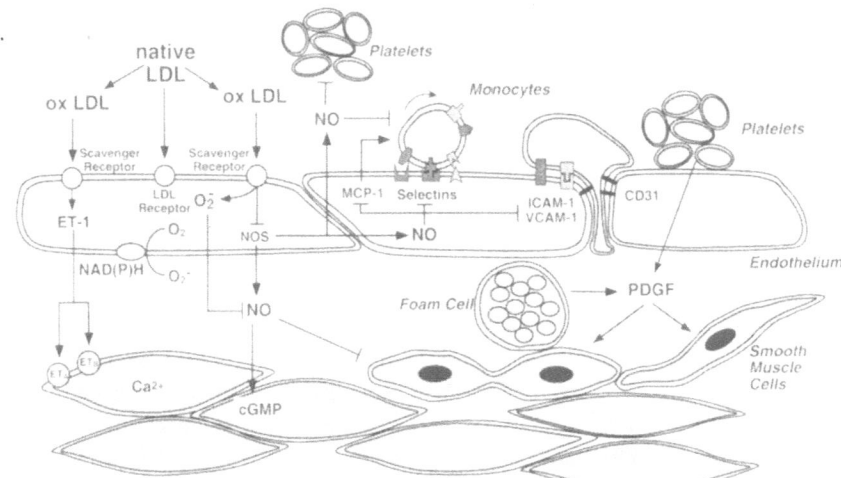

Fig. 4.1. Pathogenesis of neointima formation. Endothelial dysfunction due to cardiovascular risk factors such as low density lipoproteins (*LDL*) initiates the atherosclerotic lesion (LÜSCHER and VANHOUTTE 1990). LDL become oxidized and inhibit nitric oxide (*NO*) production by affecting NO synthase (*NOS*) expression (TANNER et al. 1991). NO is also inactivated by superoxide anions (O_2^-) generated by a nicotinamide adenine dinucleotide phosphate, reduced (*NAD(P)H*)-dependent enzyme. Furthermore, endothelin release is enhanced under such conditions (LERMAN et al. 1991). Moreover, endothelial expression of proteins such as MCP-1 and adhesion molecules such as intercellular adhesion molecule 1 (*ICAM-1*) or vascular cell adhesion molecule 1 (*VCAM-1*) is upregulated (Ross 1993). These changes favor vascular contraction, thrombus formation, monocyte invasion and smooth muscle cell proliferation as well as migration. Aggregating platelets release mitogens such as platelet-derived growth factor (*PDGF*) and with that enhance intimal smooth muscle cell accumulation (Ross 1993). Invading monocytes incorporate ox LDL and become foam cells which are an important source of mitogens or cytokines as well, and thus further stimulate intimal expansion (WITZTUM and STEINBERG 1991). *cGMP*, cyclic guanosine monophosphate

stances derived from platelets or the coagulation system and by shear stress (FURCHGOTT and ZAWADZKI 1980). The mediator of these responses is the free radical NO formed from L-arginine by oxidation of its guanidine – nitrogen terminal. Competitive inhibitors of NO synthase cause endothelium-dependent contraction in isolated arteries and long-lasting increases in blood pressure. This demonstrates that basal release of NO keeps the vasculature in a constant state of vasodilation (REES et al. 1989). NO also inhibits platelet adhesion and aggregation; as this occurs in response to platelet-derived substances such as serotonin or to coagulation products such as thrombin, the release of NO is a negative feedback mechanism preventing vasoconstriction and thrombus formation at sites of platelet activation (RADOMSKI et al. 1987). Furthermore, NO inhibits VSMC proliferation and migration by altering expression of cell-cycle regulatory proteins. This direct effect of NO is enhanced by the diminished release of mitogenic or chemotactic substances due to impaired thrombus formation (TANNER et al. 1998b). In addition to NO, endothelial cells release prostacyclin in response to many stimuli also producing NO. The platelet inhibitory effect of

prostacyclin is probably more important than its contribution to endothelium-dependent relaxation. NO and prostacyclin synergistically inhibit platelet aggregation, suggesting that the activity of both mediators is required to exert full antiplatelet activity (RADOMSKI et al. 1987).

Endothelium-dependent relaxation decreases with aging even in the absence of other risk factors, indicating that aging induces vascular dysfunction (ZEIHER et al. 1993). Furthermore, hypertension is associated with reduced endothelium-dependent relaxation; acetylcholine indeed causes paradoxical vasoconstriction and the acetylcholine-induced increase in blood flow is decreased in hypertension (LINDER et al. 1990). Moreover, endothelium-dependent relaxation is inhibited in hyperlipidemia and even more so in atherosclerosis; it is likely that the lysolecithin component of oxidized low-density lipoproteins mediates this phenomenon (TANNER et al. 1991). Studies in the hypercholesteremic or atherosclerotic rabbit aorta suggest that the overall NO production is not reduced, but rather that NO is inactivated by endothelial superoxide radicals leading to diminished concentration of biologically active NO (MINOR et al. 1990).

4.1.1.2
Endothelial Factors Inducing Contraction and Stimulating Proliferation

Endothelial cells can also mediate contraction under certain conditions (YANAGISAWA et al. 1988). Endothelium-derived contracting factors include the 21-amino-acid peptide endothelin, prostanoids such as thromboxane A_2 or prostaglandin H_2 and components of the renin angiotensin system (LÜSCHER and VANHOUTTE 1990). While endothelin exists in three isoforms, endothelial cells produce exclusively endothelin-1. Its release is stimulated by thrombin, transforming growth factor β, interleukin-1, epinephrine, angiotensin II, arginine vasopressin, calcium ionophore and phorbol ester (LÜSCHER and VANHOUTTE 1990). Endothelin-1 causes vasodilation at lower and marked contraction at higher concentrations. Two distinct endothelin receptors exist, namely ET_A and ET_B. Endothelial cells express ET_B which are linked to the formation of NO and prostacyclin mediating the transient vasodilation occurring when endothelin is infused into intact organisms. In contrast, VSMC express ET_A and in part ET_B which mediate contraction and proliferation (SEO et al. 1994). Particularly in the cerebral and ophthalmic circulation, agonists such as arachidonic acid, acetylcholine, histamine or serotonin evoke endothelium-dependent contraction mediated by thromboxane A_2 or prostaglandin H_2. Such prostaglandins activate the thromboxane receptor on VSMC or platelets counteracting the effect of NO and prostacyclin (LÜSCHER and VANHOUTTE 1990). The endothelium also regulates the activity of the renin angiotensin system. Angiotensin-converting enzyme is expressed on endothelial cells. Angiotensin II activates endothelial angiotensin receptors mediating endothelin release (LÜSCHER and VANHOUTTE 1990).

Endothelin release increases with age in most studies; the response to endothelin, however, decreases with age, presumably due to receptor downregulation. Endothelin plasma levels are normal in most patients with hypertension, except for those with renal failure or other end-organ damage. Endothelin release increases in hyperlipidemia and atherosclerosis, while expression of endothelin receptors is downregulated. Endothelin plasma levels indeed correlate with the extent of atherogenesis (LERMAN et al. 1991). A most likely stimulus for the increased endothelin production are oxidized low-density lipoproteins. VSMC, particularly those migrating into the intima during neointima forma-

tion, also produce endothelin. Endothelin is released by VSMC in response to platelet-derived growth factor, transforming growth factor β and arginine vasopressin (LÜSCHER and VANHOUTTE 1990). Thus, endothelin contributes to both vasoconstriction and VSMC proliferation during neointima formation.

4.1.2
Role of Vascular Smooth Muscle Cells

VSMC can form the major part of a lesion, especially in those without a necrotic core; proliferation indices in atherosclerotic lesions, however, tend to be less than 1%. This apparent paradox is solved by the observation that atherosclerotic lesions develop over decades, so that low proliferation rates at a given time point would be expected (GORDON et al. 1990). Intimal accumulation of VSMC is due to both proliferation and migration. The main mitogens and chemokines for VSMC are growth factors such as platelet-derived growth factor, insulin-like growth factor, basic fibroblast growth factor and heparin-binding epidermal growth factor, as well as cytokines such as interleukin-1 and tumor necrosis factor α (ROSS 1993). Interaction of VSMC with extracellular matrix is not only involved in regulating proliferation, it is also of major importance for migration; indeed, degradation of extracellular matrix by proteases is necessary for cell movement, and such movement is mediated by interaction of extracellular matrix with cell surface receptors linked to cytoskeleton components (LIBBY 1995). Most of the involved growth factors, cytokines and proteases are not expressed in the normal artery; during atherogenesis, however, they are released by aggregating platelets, invading monocytes, activated endothelial cells and by VSMC themselves. Overall, the development of the lesions is not only determined by growth factors, but also by growth inhibitors; indeed, cell cycle inhibitory proteins limit VSMC proliferation during neointima formation while having differential expression patterns, as well as differential regulatory roles (TANNER et al. 1998a).

Two different phenotypes of VSMC have been described based on the presence of cellular proteins and organelles. VSMC in the contractile phenotype express smooth muscle α actin and respond to substances affecting vascular tone such as NO, prostacyclin, endothelin-1 and angiotensin II. In contrast, VSMC in the synthetic phenotype harbor increased numbers of organelles for protein synthesis and secretion such as endoplasmic reticulum and Golgi apparatus; these cells release growth factors such as basic fibroblast growth factor, insulin-like growth factor and transforming growth factor β, as well as extracellular matrix components such as proteoglycan, collagen and elastin. In atherogenesis, VSMC change from the contractile into the synthetic phenotype, which determines both the reactivity and the development of the lesions (SJÖLUND et al. 1988). Thus, VSMC mediate the fibroproliferative aspect of atherosclerosis.

4.1.3
Role of Monocytes and Macrophages

Macrophages are present in all stages of atherogenesis. Circulating monocytes extravasate and, once in the artery wall, develop into macrophages residing in the tissue. Extravasation is increased in hyperlipidemia; NO is in part responsible as it regulates expression of endothelial adhesion molecules so that the diminished NO release in hyperlipidemic arteries leads to enhanced expression of these molecules favoring interaction of monocytes with the endothelium. Another factor involved are oxidized low density lipoproteins which induce expression of monocyte chemoattractant protein 1 and are chemotactic for monocytes by themselves (WITZTUM and STEINBERG 1991). Moreover, these lipoproteins are taken up by monocytes via the scavenger receptor leading to differentiation into macrophages.

Macrophages are not only important as scavenger cells, they also release a large number of growth factors and cytokines such as platelet-derived growth factor, transforming growth factor β, tumor necrosis factor α and interleukin-1 (Ross et al. 1990). Each of these molecules can lead to secondary release of platelet-derived growth factor, so that macrophages stimulate VSMC not only by releasing platelet-derived growth factor, but also by secreting these cytokines. Furthermore, macrophages are a major source of matrix degrading proteases and therefore important for the stability of atherosclerotic plaques. Whether a plaque ruptures is probably determined by the activity of VSMC secreting matrix forming substances versus that of macrophages releasing matrix degrading enzymes (LIBBY 1995). Moreover, macrophages act as antigen presenting cells to lymphocytes, which are found in low numbers in atherosclerotic plaques, indicating that there is not only an inflammatory, but also an immunologic reaction occurring. A specific antigen,

however, has not yet been found; in addition, the plaques formed in transplant atherosclerosis are concentric rather than eccentric and show very high numbers of lymphocytes (LIBBY and HANSSON 1991). Thus, macrophages act as scavengers, stimulate VSMC proliferation, regulate plaque stability and mediate the immunologic aspects of atherogenesis.

4.2
Restenosis

Invasive treatment of patients with atherosclerotic lesions consists of percutaneous transluminal angioplasty or bypass surgery. Neither procedure provides a definitive cure and both are associated with restenosis or bypass graft disease. Restenosis occurs within a few weeks to months following intervention and thus much faster than atherogenesis (MEIER 1991). As angioplasty induces arterial injury, restenosis can be seen as the response of the vessel wall to this injury; therefore, it is a repair process involving changes similar to those occurring in atherogenesis. Indeed, angioplasty induces de-endothelialization and platelet adhesion with thrombus formation. Endothelial cells regenerate within a few weeks; however, these cells exhibit functional alterations, particularly diminished release of NO and increased secretion of growth factors (SHIMOKAWA et al. 1989). Moreover, the presence of growth factors and cytokines released from aggregating platelets and invading monocytes, as well as the direct mechanical stimulation of the vessel wall, lead to VSMC proliferation, migration and the formation of extracellular matrix (LINDNER and REIDY 1991). Another major feature of restenosis is vascular remodeling; these changes consist of alterations in the diameter of the artery and can lead to increases or decreases in luminal diameter despite neointima formation (LAFONT et al. 1995). Thus, vascular remodeling and neointima formation occur in parallel; they are superimposed on each other and the luminal diameter of an artery is determined by both processes (Fig. 4.2). Animal studies indicate that proliferation rates of adventitial fibrocytes can be very high during the formation of restenotic lesions, suggesting that changes in adventitial cell numbers may affect vascular remodeling. This may be expected in so far as the extracellular matrix mediating the shrinkage phenomena is produced by adventitial cells. Thus, cellular proliferation leads to neointima formation in restenotic arteries and may also be important for vascular remodeling.

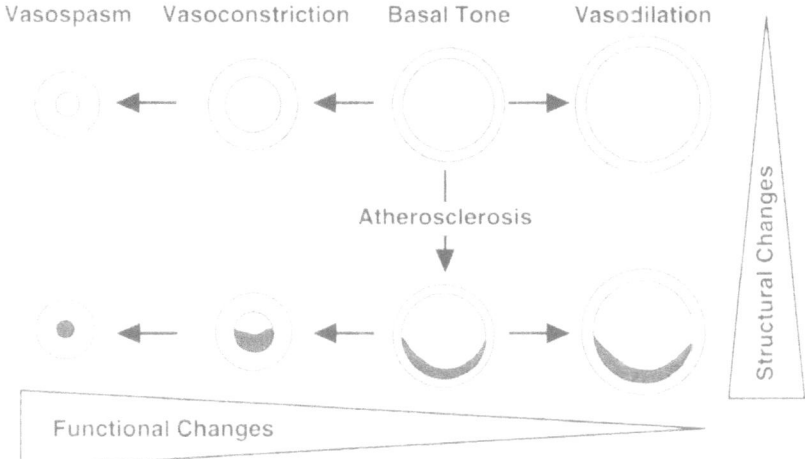

Fig. 4.2. Role of structural versus functional changes as a determinant of arterial obstruction. The luminal diameter can change due to vasodilation or vasoconstriction in both normal and atherosclerotic arteries. However, in atherosclerotic arteries, there is a higher tendency towards luminal narrowing (Lüscher and Vanhoute 1990). This effect is not only caused by functional changes with impaired release of relaxing factors and enhanced production of contracting factors, it is also related to structural changes with neointima formation and increased rigidity (Lafont et al. 1995)

4.3
Bypass Graft Disease

Bypass grafting with saphenous veins and internal mammary arteries is common practice for the treatment of patients with atherosclerotic coronary disease. The patency of mammary artery grafts, however, is better than that of saphenous veins (Loop et al. 1986). Neointima formation is indeed much less pronounced in mammary arteries than in saphenous veins. Consistent with this observation, endothelial and VSMC function is markedly different in these vessels. Mammary arteries exhibit pronounced endothelium-dependent relaxation to acetylcholine, bradykinin, thrombin and adenosine diphosphate. The latter is also responsible for endothelium-dependent relaxation to aggregating platelets. In contrast, endothelium-dependent relaxation of saphenous veins to acetylcholine is weak; furthermore, marked contraction occurs in response to thrombin and aggregating platelets (Yang et al. 1991). Consistent with these observations, flow-dependent vasodilation is stronger, while adhesion of platelets or monocytes is less pronounced in mammary arteries than in saphenous vein grafts. Moreover, thrombin and platelet-derived growth factor cause pronounced proliferation of VSMC obtained from saphenous veins, but not from mammary arteries. This difference is not related to differential activation of mitogen-activated protein kinase, but is caused by differential cell cycle regulation permitting higher proliferation rates in cells from saphenous veins as compared to those from mammary arteries (Yang et al. 1998). These differences are likely to be of great importance for graft patency and underscore the importance of endothelium and VSMC for neointima formation.

References

Furchgott RF, Zawadzki JV (1980) The obligatory role of endothelial cells in the relaxation of arterial smooth muscle by acetylcholine. Nature 299:373–378

Gordon D, Reidy MA, Benditt EP, Schwartz SM (1990) Cell proliferation in human coronary arteries. Proc Natl Acad Sci USA 87:4600–4504

Lafont A, Guzman LA, Whitlow PL, Goormastic M, Cornhill JF, Chisolm GM (1995) Restenosis after experimental angioplasty. Intimal, medial, and adventitial changes associated with constrictive remodeling. Circ Res 76:996–1002

Lerman A, Edwards ES, Hallett JW, Heublein DM, Sandberg SM, Burnett JJ (1991) Circulating and tissue endothelin immunoreactivity in advanced atherosclerosis. New Engl J Med 325:997–1001

Libby P, Hansson GK (1991) Involvement of the immune system in human atherogenesis: current knowledge and unanswered questions. Lab Invest 64:5–15

Libby P (1995) Molecular basis of the acute coronary syndromes. Circulation 91:2344–2850

Linder L, Kiowski W, Bühler FR, Lüscher TF (1990) Indirect evidence for release of endothelium-derived relaxing factor in human forearm circulation in vivo. Blunted response in essential hypertension. Circulation 81:1762–1767

Lindner V, Reidy MA (1991) Proliferation of smooth muscle cells after vascular injury is inhibited by an antibody against basic fibroblast growth factor. Proc Natl Acad Sci USA 88:3739–3743

Loop FD, Lytle BW, Cosgrove DM, Stewart RW, Goorastic M, Williams GW, Golding LAR, Gill CG, Taylor PD, Sheldon WC, Proudfit WL (1986) Influence of the internal mammary artery graft on 10-year survival and other cardiac events. New Engl J Med 314:1–6

Lüscher TF, Vanhoutte PM (1990) The endothelium: modulator of cardiovascular function. CRC Press, Boca Raton, pp. 1–228

Meier B (1991) Long-term results of coronary balloon angioplasty. Ann Rev Med 42:47–59

Minor R Jr, Myers PR, Guerra R Jr, Bates JN, Harrison DG (1990) Diet-induced atherosclerosis increases the release of nitrogen oxides from rabbit aorta. J Clin Invest 86:2109–2116

Radomski MW, Palmer RM, Moncada S (1987) Comparative pharmacology of endothelium-derived relaxing factor, nitric oxide and prostacyclin in platelets. Br J Pharmacol 92:181–187

Rees DD, Palmer RMJ, Moncada S (1989) Role of endothelium-derived nitric oxide in the regulation of blood pressure. Proc Natl Acad Sci USA 86:3375–3379

Ross R, Masuda J, Raines EW, Gown AM, Katsuda S, Sasahara M, Malden LT, Masuko H, Sato H (1990) Localization of PDGF-B protein in macrophages in all phases of atherogenesis. Science 248:1009–1012

Ross R (1993) The pathogenesis of atherosclerosis: a perspective for the 1990s. Nature 362:801–803

Seo B, Oemar BS, Siebenmann R, von Segesser L, Lüscher TF (1994) Both ET_A and ET_B receptors mediate contraction to endothelin-1 in human blood vessels. Circulation 89:1203–1208

Shimokawa H, Flavahan NA, Vanhoutte PM (1989) Natural course of the impairment of endothelium-dependent relaxations after balloon endothelium removal in porcine coronary arteries. Possible dysfunction of a pertussis toxin-sensitive G protein. Circ Res 65:740–748

Sjölund M, Hedin U, Sejersen T, Heldin CH, Thyberg J (1988) Arterial smooth muscle cells express platelet-derived growth factor (PDGF) A chain mRNA, secrete a PDGF-like mitogen, and bind exogenous PDGF in a phenotype- and growth state – dependent manner. J Cell Biol 106:403–413

Tanner FC, Noll G, Boulanger CM, Lüscher TF (1991) Oxidized low density lipoproteins inhibit relaxations of porcine coronary arteries. Role of scavenger receptor and endothelium-derived nitric oxide. Circulation 83:2012–2020

Tanner FC, Yang Z, Duckers E, Gordon D, Nabel GJ, Nabel EG (1998a) Expression of cyclin-dependent kinase inhibitors in vascular disease. Circ Res 82:396–403

Tanner FC, Greutert H, Nabel EG, Lüscher TF (1998b) Nitric oxide inhibits proliferation of human aortic vascular smooth muscle cells: role of cell cycle regulatory proteins (submitted)

Witztum JL, Steinberg D (1991) Role of oxidized low density lipoprotein in atherogenesis. J Clin Invest 88:1785–1792

Yanagisawa M, Kurihara H, Kimura S, Mitsui Y, Kobayashi M, Watanabe TX, Masaki T (1988) A novel potent vasoconstrictor peptide produced by vascular endothelial cells. Nature 332:411–415

Yang Z, Stulz P, von Segesser L, Bauer E, Turina M, Lüscher TF (1991) Different interactions of platelets with arterial and venous coronary bypass vessels. Lancet 337:939–943

Yang Z, Oemar BS, Carrel T, Kipfer B, Julmy F, Lüscher TF (1998) Different proliferative properties of smooth muscle cells of human arterial and venous bypass vessels: role of PDGF receptors, mitogen-activated protein kinase and cyclin-dependent kinase inhibitors. Circulation 97:181–187

Zeiher AM, Drexler H, Saurbier B, Just H (1993) Endothelium-mediated coronary blood flow modulation in humans. Effects of age, atherosclerosis, hypercholesterolemia, and hypertension. J Clin Invest 92:652–662

5 Interventional Radiology of Peripheral Vascular Diseases

E. Zeitler, R. Hildebrandt, P. Romaniuk, T. Fritzsche and D.C. Baumgart

CONTENTS

E. Zeitler, Prof., MD; Virchowstraße 13, D-90409 Nürnberg, Germany
R. Hildebrandt, MD; Institut für Diagnostische und Interventionelle Radiologie, Klinikum Nord, Flurstraße 17, D-90340 Nuremberg, Germany
P. Romanuik, MD; Charité-Humboldt Universität, Institut für Röentgendiagnostik, Schumannstraße 20/21, D-10098 Berlin, Germany
T. Fritzsche, MD; Universitätsklinikum der Humboldt-Universität zu Berlin, Campus Charité MiHe, Klinik für Anästhesiologie und operative intensivmedizin, Schumannstraße 20/21, D-10117 Berlin, Germany
D.C. Baumgart, MD; Georgetown University Hospital, Department of Medicine, 3800 Resevoir Rd NW, Washington DC 20007-2197, USA

Introduction

E. Zeitler

Interventional radiology (IR) of peripheral disesases comprises therapeutic measures with the use of imaging systems (Athanasoulis et al. 1982; Dondelinger et al. 1990; Dotter and Judkins 1965; Dotter et al. 1966; Günther and Thelen 1988; Lammer and Schreyer 1991; Zeitler 1997). IR includes:

- The recanalization of arteries and veins in symptomatic patients. Vascular obliterations can be the result of thrombus formation, arteriosclerosis or tumor infiltration. In these cases, IR uses different therapeutic principles: angioplasty, thrombolysis, percutaneous thrombus and embolus extraction, stent implantation, and others
- The occlusion of vessels in congenital and acquired arteriovenous shunts.
- The control of bleeding of varying nature, including traumata.
- The occlusion of tumor-feeding arteries.
- The extraction of foreign bodies, such as catheter material, broken guidewires, stents, and other material.

Such vascular interventions are mainly performed under roentgen-fluoroscopic control, whereby digital subtraction angiography (DSA) techniques are preferred. However, they can also be carried out under duplex sonography guidance, either in gray scale or color coded, and under magnetic resonance (MR) imaging control and MR angiography, depending on the respective case and the equipment available.

Thus, IR can be: (a) recanalization or occlusion of vessels, (b) application and extraction of materials in, or from vessels, and (c) pain control or tumor control combined with pharmacotherapy.

Special IR techniques also include percutaneous computed tomography (CT)-controlled interventions, among which the CT-guided sympathicolysis and the CT- or MR- guided puncture of vascular lesions in the diagnostic and therapeutic settings are most common.

The advantages of IR compared to open surgery include shorter hospitalization times and the lack of need for general anesthesia. Thus, even high-risk patients with cardiovascular or pulmonary insufficiency can be treated with IR procedures at reduced risk compared to surgery. Also, follow-up control in intensive care units is in general not necessary. Moreover, access to the diseased area in arteries and veins causes no skin or muscle damage, as the application of IR instruments requires only a small puncture hole in the artery or vein. Therefore, healing time is reduced and there is the possibility of spontaneous collateralization. There is no interference with the regeneration of the collateral vessels. Also, the risk of damaging nervous structures and lymphatic vessels is very low.

IR also offers the opportunity to repeat treatment in the same vascular territory, whereby open surgery is still possible after unsuccessful procedures, or in the case of complications.

The aim of interventional radiology is to achieve the optimum result with the lowest possible risk!

In general, the patients should be counseled 24h prior to the intervention, provided that it is not an emergency situation. Similarly, it is useful to provide the patient with an information leaflet on the symptoms of the disease, including explanations of the planned treatment and its risk. Part of the patient's personal history includes the question of any medication which he/she is possibly taking, e.g., anticoagulation, insulin therapy, or antihypertensives. During this information talk, alternative therapeutic methods of vascular surgery and internal medicine, including conventional physical therapy, as well as anticoagulation or thrombolysis, and the associated risks, need to be mentioned. The different steps of IR are shown in Table 5.1.

Table 5.1. The different steps of IR

IR includes:

1. Clinical examination
2. Interdisciplinary discussion of all aspects of the various possible therapeutic measures: conservative, surgical or interventional, and combined
3. Informed consent
4. Premedication
5. Intervention itself
6. Post-treatment care
7. Follow-up controls

THOMAS J. FOGARTY, of Stanford, USA, stated in 1997 (FOGARTY 1997):

The acute problem of arterial occlusion was remedied by a vascular surgeon using an embolectomy catheter, while the chronic problem of stenosis was addressed by an interventional radiologist.

Both concepts were developed one year apart and originated from the same institution, the University of Oregon, where both physicians conducted their research in separate departments.

As clinician and inventor I see a clear trend towards an escalation of endoluminal technology. It fits the model for technological success; it is simple, relatively easy to understand and learn, is minimally invasive and consequently less traumatic to the patient both physically and emotionally. It is clinically and economically effective.

5.1
Angioplasty

E. ZEITLER

5.1.1
Basic Information

Percutaneous transluminal angioplasty (PTA) is based on the diagnostic percutaneous catheter technique introduced by SELDINGER (1953) and was introduced by DOTTER and JUDKINS (1964) as a method to treat arteriosclerotic obliterations in arteries, primarily in the femoropopliteal area (DOTTER and JUDKINS 1965; DOTTER et al. 1966).

The original DOTTER method, developed from postmortem studies on coronary arteries, works on the principle that, after passage of the arterial obstruction under roentgen-fluoroscopic control with a guidewire, the coaxial Teflon catheter system is pressed corkscrew-like through the obstructed area upon the guidewire. First, the 8-F catheter passes the obstruction, followed by the 12-F outer catheter (3.6 mm) with higher power. This is also done with a screw-like advancing technique through the artery in a distal direction. In critically obliterated arteries, this was only achieved through an additional stabilization in longitudinal direction using a metal cannula in the space between the guidewire and the 8-F Teflon catheter, thus improving the pushability and better avoiding perforations.

The disadvantage with this 12-F coaxial catheter system was the big puncture hole at the entrance defect in the groin, which led to several post-treatment hematomas and bleeding complications. The inadequate friction of the outer Teflon catheter against the inner Teflon catheter led to several embolizations caused by the so-called snow-plug phenomenon (STAPLE 1968).

For this reason, the single Teflon catheters were introduced (STAPLE 1968; ZEITLER and MÜLLER 1969; VAN ANDEL 1976). Angioplasty and predilating catheters are listed in Table 5.2.

After experiences in some European departments, but non-acceptance in the US, two clinics started practicing the Dotter technique, including the evaluation of long-term results. These were the Charité Hospital in Berlin (WIERNY et al. 1974), and the Aggertal Clinic in Engelskirchen (ZEITLER and MÜLLER 1969; ZEITLER and MARESTA 1970; ZEITLER et al. 1971b; 1971; SCHMIDTKE et al. 1975).

Some small modifications to the Dotter technique at that time were the application of proximal side holes on the angioplasty Teflon catheter, a longer tapered catheter which, in the distal femoral popliteal artery, had a smaller, but proximal a larger diameter, the proximal use of a Y-connector for contrast medium injection at the time of guiding and catheter passage, enabling a more sophisticated fluoroscopic control than without contrast medium, and the additional use of Fogarty balloon catheters via the Teflon catheter (ZEITLER 1971; ZEITLER et al. 1971a). The modifications were first highlighted with the corset balloon catheter introduced by PORSTMANN in 1973 for dilatation of iliac artery stenoses, in arteries of diameters larger than 4 mm. This "caged balloon catheter" (DOTTER et al. 1974b) enabled the rupture of strongly calcified iliac artery stenoses, but at the same time led to several dissections in the iliac artery with reocclusions, necessitating surgical repair.

The year 1974 marked the beginning of a new era of percutaneous transluminal treatment with the introduction of the balloon catheter (GRÜNTZIG and HOPFF 1974) and selective intraarterial clot lysis with low-dose streptokinase (DOTTER et al. 1974b). With the smaller outer diameter of the balloon catheter, local complications at the puncture site could be reduced, and the dilatation force on stenotic lesions in arteries larger than 4 mm in diameter, like for example the common iliac artery, became more successful and low-risk than with the caged balloon catheter. From this time on, used in ever more departments and clinics, also in the US, the combined techniques with passage, bougieinage, and balloon dilatation, or in combination with intraarte-

rial application of streptokinase, helped improve the method with a reduction in complications, and higher success rates (SOBBE et al. 1973; HESS et al. 1978; DEMBSKI and ZEITLER 1978; HEIMIG and MARTIN 1997).

In 1977, at the first angioplasty symposium, the results of the cooperative study of PTA in 12 different clinics was put together, and it could be shown that the complication rate under use of the balloon catheter was low, primary success was high, but long-term results varied considerably.

The first histomorphologic studies (LEU and GRÜNTZIG 1978; JESTER and SINAPIUS 1978; HÖHN et al. 1975) showed that not only compression of the thrombus, plaque, and arterial wall is part of the mechanism of this treatment, but also intimal rupture and dissections – defects of the arterial wall with rupture of the intima and media – and also ectasia, such as the formation of small aneurysmal lesions (SANBORN et al. 1983; JESTER and SINAPIUS 1978).

Following the introduction of the catheter system for the treatment of coronary artery stenosis as well (GRÜNTZIG 1976b; GRÜNTZIG et al. 1976), followed by the first successful treatment of coronary heart disease using balloon dilatation (Grüntzig et al. 1979), PTA gained wider acceptance, also in the US (ALPERT et al. 1979; DIAMOND et al. 1979; KATZEN et al. 1979; ATHANASOULIS et al. 1982, WALTMANN et al. 1982; BECKER et al. 1989; CASTANEDA-ZUNIGA 1982, 1983; COPE et al. 1990; CAPEK et al. 1991; KUMPE 1981; KUMPE et al. 1988). Several types of balloon catheters offered by different companies are listed in Table 5.3.

After the introduction of percutaneous transluminal coronary angioplasty (PTCA), the balloon catheter technique was studied in more animal experiments (BLOCK et al. 1980; CASTANEDA-ZUNIGA et al. 1981; ZOLLIKOFER 1985, 1986). Independent of angioplasty with Teflon catheters and balloon catheters, the idea of applying intravascular tube grafts was first tried by DOTTER in 1969 in experiments. During the following years, several types of metallic stents for percutaneous application of endoprostheses were developed, demonstrated in animal experiments, and finally used in man in iliac, femoral, and coronary arteries (CRAGG et al. 1983; PALMAZ et al. 1985; ROUSSEAU et al. 1987; SIGWART et al. 1987; STRECKER et al. 1989; TRILLER et al. 1989; PALMAZ et al. 1988a; ZOLLIKOFER et al. 1988). The latest technique is the use of stents covered with a special fabric to treat aneurysms, arteriovenous fistulas, and vascular rupture (PARODI 1996; MARIN et al. 1994b; MAY et al. 1994; VOLODOS et al. 1991; RAITHEL et al. 1997; THOMAS and BELLI 1998). The most common vascular stents used in peripheral arteries are summarized in Table 5.4. Stents have their major indication in the treatment of complications of PTA, and critical obliterations in iliac and femoral arteries. Their primary indication is following recanalization of iliac artery occlusions longer than 5 cm. Indications also exist in patients with critical limb ischemia with femoropopliteal occlusion longer than 5 cm. Secondary indications include restenosis, reocclusion, and collapsing arteries in the iliac, femoral, and popliteal region.

With its impressive history that began in 1964, PTA, with several modifications, has meanwhile found worldwide acceptance in several arteriosclerotic and some non-arteriosclerotic arterial obliterations (DONDELINGER et al. 1990; GUNTHER and THELEN 1988; KADIR 1991; MAHLER and TRILLER 1990; LAMMER and SCHREYER 1991). In addition, balloon angioplasty, as well as the non-operative application of endoprostheses, have gained acceptance in veins, but also in non-vascular areas, such as the biliary tract, the esophagus, and the trachea.

The pathomorphologic mechanism can now be described as a controlled traumatic injury "which leads to dilatation with a free arterial lumen corresponding to that seen in histologic (ZOLLIKOFER et al. 1987) and angiographic examinations" (ROTH et al. 1983). The controlled traumatic injury can vary according to the location, extension, and age of the arteriosclerotic lesion and the balloon diameter used. The angioplastic result is not as good in long-distance lesions (MURRAY et al. 1987, 1995), in contrast to short stenotic lesions, with far more problems in calcified obliterations and in the recanalization of fresh thrombotic clots.

In atherosclerotic diseases with circular plaque formation, a luminal widening can be accomplished only by cracking or rupturing the plaque, with additional tears in the intima and media, as well as dilating the normal parts of the arterial wall (BLOCK et al. 1980, 1981; CASTANEDA-ZUNIGA et al. 1980; FAXON et al. 1984; ZOLLIKOFER et al. 1984, 1985).

In two thirds of dilated non-calcified arteries, short spasm-like luminal narrowings adjacent to the site of balloon dilatation were observed. In animal experiments, overdilation persisted on non-arteriosclerotic vessels for no longer than 18 h (ZOLLIKOFER 1985). In their animal experiments, FAXON et al. (1984) were able to show that aggregation inhibitors [acetysalicylic acid (ASA), sulfinpyrazone] significantly reduce intimal thickening,

restenosis rates, as well as the rate of thrombotic occlusions in the post-dilation period. Longitudinal clefts could be seen in the post-angioplasty angiography as "radiolucent linear defects" (ROTH et al. 1995). In excentric stenotic plaques, elastic stretching of the disease-free arch of the artery is an important part of lumen-widening (JESTER et al. 1976; BRUNNER and GRÜNTZIG 1975; BRUNNER et al. 1982; LEU 1982).

Experimental work in several laboratories on animals and in necropsies, was able to demonstrate the intended traumatic injury with the following *histologic changes after balloon PTA:*

- *Intimal rupture*
- *Fragmentation of the plaque and arterial wall*
- *Partial dehescence from the media*
- *Rupture of the media*
- *Stretching of the plaque-free arterial wall layers*
- *Increase in outer diameter.*

The theory is, and empirical controls with angiography and hemodynamic measurements (oscillography and ankle-pressure control at rest and after exercise) have shown that when lumen geometry and flow are optimal, shear stress is high and fluctuation in shear stress is low. In such circumstances, there is little or no restenosis. When lumen geometry and/or flow are suboptimal, shear stress is low and fluctuation in shear stress is great. Under these circumstances, there is a likelihood of restenosis (KU et al. 1985). This provides evidence for the strategy of optimizing both lumen geometry and the hemodynamic result of angioplasty (BECKER 1991). After several animal experiments with arteries of varying diameter, ZOLLIKOFER (1985) estimated that "possibly the stimulated intimal hyperplasia after PTCA in arteries of small diameter is of greater importance and may explain the higher restenosis rate in the coronary arteries, compared to iliac arteries".

5.1.2
The History of Interventional Radiology

1964 DOTTER and JUDKINS: New technique for treating arteriosclerotic obliterations with the coaxial Dotter set

1967 PORSTMANN and WIERNY: Recanalization of inoperable arterial obliterations

1968 DOTTER et al.: Non-operative, transluminal treatment of arteriosclerotic obliterations

1969 ZEITLER and MÜLLER: First results with the Dotter technique

1971 ZEITLER et al. (1971a): Catheter treatment of iliac artery stenosis

ZEITLER et al. (1971b): Treatment of occlusive arterial disease by transluminal catheter angioplasty

1973 WIERNY et al.: Long-term results of transluminal catheter recanalization

PORSTMANN: Corset balloon catheter for the treatment of iliac artery stenosis

ZEITLER et al.: ASA – first perioperative use in the Dotter technique

1974 GRÜNTZIG and HOPF: A new balloon dilatation catheter

DOTTER et al. (1974a): Transluminal iliac artery dilatation

DOTTER et al. (1974b): Intraarterial clot lysis

1975 OLBERT et al.: Austrian results with the angioplasty technique by Dotter

HORVARTH and ILLES: Hungarian results of transluminal angioplasty

VAN ANDEL: The Netherlands' results with transluminal angioplasty by Dotter

SCHMIDTKE et al.: Long-term results of percutaneous catheter therapy (Dotter technique) for stage II femoropopliteal arterial occlusions

1976 GRÜNTZIG: Clinical results with the new balloon dilatation catheter (GRÜNTZIG 1976a)

1977 GRÜNTZIG: Comparison between Dotter technique and balloon angioplasty

OLBERT and HANNEKA: Transluminal vascular dilatation with the modified dilatation catheter (Olbert catheter)

1978 SCHMIDTKE et al.: Long-term results of the Dotter technique in femoro-popliteal occlusions

HESS et al.: Combined treatment with percutaneous transluminal recanalization (PTR) and local thrombolysis

DEMBSKI and ZEITLER: Selective arterial clot lysis

GRÜNTZIG and ZEITLER: Cooperative study of PTR results in 12 clinics

LEU and GRÜNTZIG: Histopathologic aspects of transluminal recanalization

MAHLER et al.: Transluminal dilatation of stenoses in the deep femoral artery

MARTIN and ZEITLER: PTR and fibrinolysis

1979 MATHIAS et al. (1979a): Percutaneous recanalization of a posttraumatic popliteal occlusion

MATTHIAS et al. (1979b): Percutaneous transluminal revascularization of calf arteries

BACHMANN et al.: Iliofemoral angioplasty via the contralateral femoral artery

ROTH and CAPPIUS: Contralateral angioplasty of common femoral artery obliterations

GRÜNTZIG and KUMPE: Angioplasty with the GRÜNTZIG balloon catheter

MAHLER et al.: Treatment of renovascular hypertension by transluminal renal artery dilatation

FREIMANN et al.: Transluminal angioplasty of iliac, femoral, and popliteal arteries

TEGTMEYER et al.: Percutaneous transluminal dilatation of complete block in the iliac artery

KATZEN et al.: PTA with the GRÜNTZIG balloon catheter (70 cases)

SCHLOSSER et al.: Complications after PTR and surgical treatment

1980 MATHIAS et al.: Percutaneous catheter angioplasty of the subclavian artery

VELASQUEZ et al.: Non-surgical aortoplasty in Leriche's syndrome

BLOCK et al.: Histological and ultrastructural studies in animals after coronary angioplasty

MATHIAS and SCHLOSSER: Catheter recanalization of subclavian artery occlusion

MARTIN et al.: PTA in non-arteriosclerotic disease

INGRISCH et al.: Microdensitometric controls for quantification of the results in PTR of the femoral artery

CASTANEDA-ZUNIGA et al.: The mechanism of balloon angioplasty

COLAPINTO et al.: Percutaneous transluminal dilatation and recanalization in the treatment of peripheral vascular disease

MOTARJEME et al.: PTA of the deep femoral artery

ABELE: Balloon catheters and transluminal dilatation – technical considerations

BACHMANN and KIM: Transluminal dilatation for subclavian steal syndrome

MOTARJEME et al.: PTA of iliac arteries

STAIGER et al.: Peripheral occlusive disease – influence of platelet-aggregation inhibitors

WALTMANN: PTA – iliac and deep femoral arteries

TEGTMEYER et al.: Balloon dilatation of the abdominal aorta

ZEITLER: PTA – cooperation among specialities

ROTH and CAPPIUS: Simultaneous angioplasty in different territories (leg, renal, and supra-aortic) in one setting. Angioplasty of common femoral arterial obliterations

1981 TEGTMEYER: Removing the stuck, ruptured angioplasty balloon catheter

ZORN-BOPP et al.: Transluminal dilatation of distal abdominal aorta, common and external iliac artery

KATZEN and VAN BREDA: Low-dose streptokinase in the treatment of arterial occlusions

ROSEN et al.: A new exchange guidewire for transluminal angioplasty

JOFFRE: PTA

SOS and SNIDERMAN: GRÜNTZIG catheter with a 10-cm long balloon

COLAPINTO et al.: Percutaneous transluminal recanalization of complete iliac artery occlusions

RING and MCLEAN: Interventional radiology – principles and techniques

ZEITLER et al.: Techniques of PTA and additional treatment of leg arteries

ZÜHLKE et al.: Intraoperative transluminal angioplasty

1982 MOTARJEME et al.: PTA of brachiocephalic arteries

1985 PALMAZ et al.: Expandable intraluminal graft – a preliminary study

KREPEL et al.: PTA of the femoropopliteal artery – initial and long-term results

MCNAMARA and FISHER: Local thrombolysis of thrombosed grafts

1986 SCHNEIDER: Percutaneous extraction of thrombi and emboli

COLAPINTO et al.: Transluminal angioplasty of complete iliac obstructions

1987 JOHNSTON et al.: 5-year results of a prospective study of PTA

KALTENBACH and VALLBRACHT: Rotational angioplasty – a new catheter technique

KENSEY et al.: Recanalization of obstructed arteries with a flexible, rotating tip catheter

1988 PALMAZ et al. (1988b): Early endothelialization of balloon-expandable stents – experimental observations

TOENNESEN et al.: Transpopliteal angioplasty and chamber thrombolysis (see also TOENNESEN 1991)

SCHWARTEN and CUTCLIFF: Arterial occlusive disease below the knee – treatment with PTA performed with low-profile catheters and steerable guidewires

SCHWARTEN et al.: Simpson catheter for percutaneous trans-luminal removal of atheroma

1989 SCHROEDER: Transpopliteal catheter lysis

ROUSSEAU et al.: Treatment of femoropopliteal stenoses by "Wallstent" endoprostheses

TRILLER et al.: Vascular endoprostheses for treatment of femoropopliteal occlusive disease – results after 9 months of clinical application

1990 PALMAZ et al.: Placement of balloon-expandable intraluminal stents in iliac arteries – first 171 procedures

STRECKER et al.: Expandable tubular stents for treatment of arterial occlusive disease – experimental and clinical results

1994 LIERMANN et al.: Prophylactic endovascular radiotherapy to prevent intimal hyperplasia after stent implantation in femoropopliteal arteries

1995 HUSFELDT and ROTH: Competitive techniques in vascular surgery

ZEITLER et al. (1995a): PTA for crural obliterations

1996 SIGWART et al.: Handbook of cardiovascular interventions

HENRY et al.: Multidisciplinary angioplasty

DORROS: Coronary and carotid arteries

ROUBIN: Stent-supported PTA of carotid arteries

5.1.3
Angioplasty Procedure

Angioplasty is not only balloon dilatation; it is a combined procedure with the following steps, each of which are very important:

1. Premedication with aggregation inhibitors (ASA/clopidogrel).
2. Pre-treatment angiography and application of a sheath in the groin.
3. Guiding of the lesion (STRIBLEY and WILKINS 1987) and recanalization, i.e., the passage of the lesion using a guidewire, guiding catheter (sometimes a Cobra, otherwise a single Teflon catheter) after injection of 5000 IU of heparin. All this is done under roentgen-fluoroscopic control, after precise localization of the stenotic or occluded area.
4. Balloon dilatation: After precise localization of the obliterations with metallic markers, the guiding catheter is exchanged over the guidewire for the balloon catheter, and the appropriate balloon catheter is used for local dilatation of the lesion. Short lesions need one or two inflations of 20–30 in. at 5–7 atm. The appropriate balloon diameter leaves no residual kink. Long and calcified obliterations need between two and three over-

lapping inflations, sometimes up to 12 atm for 30 s at minimum, sometimes up to 2 min.

5. Control angiography: The control angiography provides information about the outcome of the intervention or the existence of intimal flaps, important dissections, collapsing arteries, and peripheral embolization. Depending on this result, the indication for additional techniques is made. This can be atherectomy, percutaneous aspiration thromboembolectomy (PAT), additional local intraarterial thrombolysis, or stent implantation.

6. Before the completion of the procedure, control angiographies demonstrate the result. Catheters, guidewires, and the sheath are removed from the groin and, by manual compression or application of a puncture-hole occluding system (Vasoseal Datascope, Bensheim, Germany, Angioseal Kensey Nash, Prostar, Perclose, Menlo Park, USA), the arterial wall defect needs to be controlled. Finally, the patient receives a hip-joint bandage.

7. Direct bedside follow-up controls under the advice of the IR team for 2–3 h. No intensive-care unit is necessary in most patients.

8. Hemodynamic control (ankle pressure) during the follow-up controls at several time intervals (first and third day, after 1, 3, and 6 months, and after the first, second, third, and fifth year).

Cooperation with internists and vascular surgeons is necessary. Independent of this, personal follow-up controls by the interventional radiologist between the first and third month, and after 1, 3, and 5 years is recommended in the interests of detecting any changes that might require a second intervention.

The objectives of vascular dilatation (angioplasty) include:

1. Technically:
   - To enlarge the vessel lumen and increase blood-flow
   - To keep the vessel open
   - To provide a smooth inner surface
   - Prevent distal embolization
2. Clinically:
   - To reduce clinical symptoms
   - To improve pain-free walking distance
   - To improve arterial blood flow
   - To heal ulcers
   - Prevent amputation.

5.1.4
Technical Equipment

In most situations, IR must be performed in an angiographic laboratory with high-resolution image-intensifier fluoroscopy, including digital angiography with last-image hold. The optimal equipment is described in Chap. 8, Sect. 8.5, including the problems of digital dynamic extremity angiography, spatial, and contrast resolution. Protecting the patient, doctor, and personnel from radiation is becoming increasingly important, especially in young patients (Chap. 8, Sect. 8.6). There is no doubt that safe percutaneous interventional radiology is only possible under X-ray control using the image-intensifier television technique. Only this can guarantee an aseptic and safe procedure. It is important for the interventionalist and his assistants to work in a clean and aseptic environment, similar to that of the aseptic operating room.

An aseptic working environment is imperative in procedures involving the implantation of foreign materials: stents, endoprostheses, coils, filters, and others, in order to prevent infection and aseptic reactions.

5.1.4.1
Standard Interventional Materials

In addition to the typical angiographic instrumentation (see Chap. 8, Sect. 8.3) individually adapted guidewires, guiding catheters, balloon dilatation catheters, catheters for atherectomy, and stents of different design are necessary. The technical instrumentation and equipment are given in Tables 5.2–5.4.

One highly important aspect is to have the optimal equipment and instrumentation for angioplasty available:

- *Angiographic unit with high-resolution image-intensifier fluoroscopy, last-image hold, and laser-printer film documentation*
- *Disposable syringes and needles for local anesthesia, contrast injection, and saline infusion*
- *Scalpels, clamps, seldinger needle, and catheter-adapters (Fig. 5.1)*
- *Dilator with tapered tip, sheaths of varying lengths for ipsi- and contralateral catheterization, sheaths with removable proximal membrane top (see Fig. 5.2)*
- *Different types of guidewires of varying tip configuration, diameter, and length*

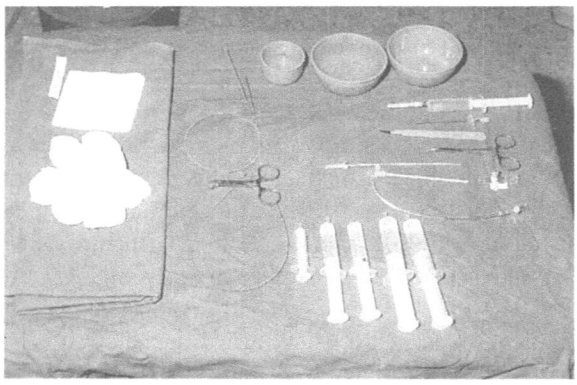

Fig. 5.1. Angio-table with scalpel, local anesthetic, syringes, needles, sponges, compresse, bottles for heparinized saline, and contrast medium

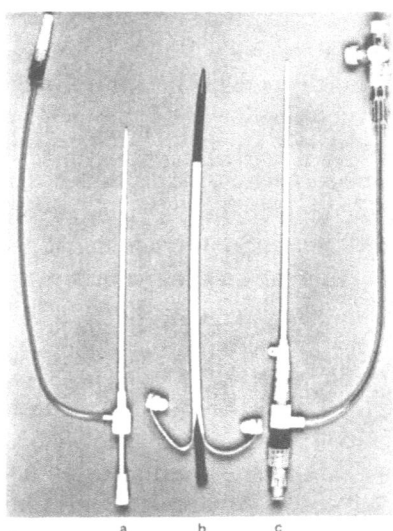

a   b   c

Fig. 5.2 a–c. Vascular sheaths. (**a**) Simple sheath with side-arm. (**b**) Simple sheath with tapered dilator. (**c**) Vascular sheath with removable valve and side-arm for infusion, as well as three-way stopcock

Table 5.2. Angioplasty and predilating catheters

Author/type	Characteristics
Dotter	Transluminal dilatation set CD-100
	Movable core guidewire, 0.047 in.
	Stiffening cannula GRM-16-921
	Coaxial catheter pair, 8 and 12 F
	Removable flushing hub
Zeitler	Dilatation catheter used before balloon dilatation
	Femoral
	Tapered Teflon catheter with 3-step dilatation
	(T 5.0–T 12.0) and four proximal side ports 2.5 cm distal of the final steps
	Iliac
	Teflon straight catheter with 2-cm tapered tip and four side holes
	proximal of the tip
	Stiffening cannula GRM-16-92
	Y-Connector
Van Andel	Dilatation catheters
	Teflon catheters for progressive dilatation by exchange
	Tapered tip (T 5.0–T 9.0), no side ports
Sos	Dilatation catheter
	Teflon catheter for pre-dilatation
	Two side ports, 1.5 cm behind the tip
Cope-Saddekni	Superficial femoral artery access dilator
	Angulated catheter with one proximal side port used for exchange of the guidewire
	from deep to superficial femoral artery
	ICD 5-35-25
Aspiration Catheter	Schneider: SCH-30141 and SCH-30435 (to order Boston Scientific)
Cook	Three-way-adapter, transparent
	TUOHY-BORST Adapter (order no.: PTBYC-RA)
Puncture occluder	DUETT, 5–9 F, 10 cm (Vascular Solutions, Cardiology)

- *Guiding catheters for first passage and selective catheterization with varying tip configurations, with and without proximal side holes and necessary adapters (see Table 5.2)*
- *Dilatation balloon catheters of different design*

(GRÜNTZIG 1977; OLBERT et al. 1984), with balloon diameters of 2.5–12 mm, and different lengths of between 2 and 12 cm (see Table 5.3)
- *Balloon-on-the-wire systems with balloon diameters of 3.4 and 6 mm*

Table 5.3. Balloon catheters for vascular dilatation

Trade name	Characteristics and coating	Manufacturer	Recommended for:
Diamond Back	5-F Shaft, 5-F introducer sheath for 3–6-mm ballons, 7-F introducer sheath for 9–12-mm balloons Rapid inflation and deflation, guidewire 0.035 in. Burst pressures up to 15 atm	Boston Scientific Meditech	Iliac, superficial femoral, popliteal, and subclavian arteries
Ultra-thin Diamond	5-F Shaft, 5-F introducer sheath, burst pressure of 15 atm, non-compliant UDT/6/4/5/75 and UDT 8/4/5/75, balloon material: Poly-Armor Balloon: diameters 3–12 mm, lengths 1.5–4 cm Guidewire 0.035 in.	Boston Scientific Meditech	Iliac, superficial femoral, and popliteal arteries
Blue Max 20	Material: two different polymers COEX Balloon: lengths 2, 4, 8, and 10 cm, diameters 4–10 mm Catheter: lengths 60–140 cm, shaft 5 and 8 F, High-pressure balloon (20 bar), non-compliant, quadro-fold technology, guidewire 0.035 in.	Boston Scientific Meditech	Calcified stenoses, highly resistant lesions, dialysis grafts, and venous dilatation
XXL	Balloon: lengths 2, 4, and 6 cm, diameters 12–18 mm Catheter: shaft 5 and 8 F, guidewire 0.035 in., sheath 7 and 8 F, balloon pressure 5 and 8 atm, quadro-fold technology	Boston Scientific Meditech	Large vessels, aorta, and vena cava
Symmetry	Glidex-coated shaft and balloon segment Non-compliant high-pressure balloon Excellent trackability and flexibility Balloon: diameters 1.5–6.0 mm, lengths: 2, 4, and 10 cm Introducer sheaths: 4 and 5 F Balloon pressure: 15 atm, guidewire 0.018 in.	Boston Scientific Meditech	Tibio-fibular and radio-ulnar arteries, tortuous anatomy
Olbert NoProfile	Rapid deflation design catheter: 4.8 F, guidewires: 0.025 in. Balloon: diameters 3–8 mm, lengths: 2 and 4 cm Balloon Pressure: 12 atm, introducer sheath 5 F	Boston Scientific Meditech	Localized stenoses in the superficial femoral and popliteal arteries
Tegwire ST	Balloon-on-the-wire for tibiofibular arteries, transpopliteal: 11–255 Balloon-on-the-wire for transfemoral use: 100 cm length 11-TW/4.0 – 2/100 11-STW/6.0 – 4/100	Boston Scientific Meditech	
Marshal	Material: Rawhide, non-compliant balloon, burst pressure 12 atm Gradual tapering to 5 F, lengths: 75, 90, and 135 cm Balloon: diameters 14–10 mm, lengths 2–10 cm, guidewire 0.035 in. Glidex hydrophilic shaft coating, balloon: quadro-fold technology Introducer sheath: 5–7 F, deflation time: 12 s	Boston Scientific Meditech	Stent delivery
		Schneider	Iliac and superficial femoral arteries
Smash	Controlled compliance Short shaft: Sch-50300–50373 (= 80 cm) Long shaft: Sch-50350–50367 (= 120 cm) e.g., SCH-50357 (balloon): diameter 5 mm, length 40 mm SCH-50360 (balloon): diameter 6 mm, length 40 mm	Schneider	Subclavian artery
Wanda	High-pressure balloon: 16 atm; nylon Low-profile balloon H965 SCH 505304	Schneider	Calcified lesions Assist stent dilatation

Table 5.3. *Continued*

Trade name	Characteristics and coating	Manufacturer	Recommended for:
Bijou	For small arteries: 12 atm; nylon PM 300, guidewire 0.018 in. Balloon diameter 1.5–5.0 mm; length 20–80 mm SCH-50224 (balloon): diameter 4 mm, length 40 (135 cm) SCH-50217 (balloon): diameter 3 mm, length 40 (135 cm)	Schneider	Tibio-fibular arteries Bifurcational Kissing balloons
Microporous-Match-35	For simultaneous drug application: SCH-40184 (through the balloon)	Schneider	Local application of drugs to prevent intimal hyperplasia Stent dilatation
Centurion	CT 5082, shaft 50 cm, balloon length 20 mm, diameter 8 mm, guidewire 0.035 in. CT 5084, shaft 50 cm, balloon length 40 m, diameter 8 mm Burst pressure 20 bar		
Tru-Trac	Non-compliant, three-ford, three-lumen, 6-F sheath, guidewire 0.035 in. High-pressure 15-bar crossover BARD: 0054062, 5-F catheter, 40-cm length; balloon diameter 6 mm, length 20 mm BARD: 0575810, 5-F catheter, 75-cm length; balloon diameter 8 mm, length 100 mm		High-pressure, 15-bar, crossover iliac artery occlusion
Opti-Plast	5 F "Smiling face": XT 75510, shaft length 75 cm, balloon diameter 5 mm, balloon length 10 mm XT, non-compliant, three-fold, two-lumen, gliding surface, 5-F sheath guidewire XT 7564, shaft length 75 cm, balloon diameter 6 mm, balloon length 40 mm		SFA long and short lesions
Ultraverse	PTA balloon catheter, 3.5-F shaft, 4- or 5-F sheath: PEB 4 F UV 10032, compliant, shaft 100 cm, balloon 3 mm, length 20 mm, guidewire 0.016 in. UV 10026, compliant, shaft 100 cm, balloon 2 mm, length 60 mm, guidewire 0.016 in. PAT – 21660050, application catheter, single lumen, 8-F catheter, length 80 cm 21660010, application catheter, single lumen, 5-F catheter, length 100 cm RAT – 21730050, rotation spiral, hand-controlled, placed through PAT catheter Dormio – 21922050 } flexible fragmentation basket 21922010 } Jet-Lyse catheters also available		Tibiofibular and pedal arteries
Opta 5	Quadro-fold design, diameters 6–10 mm, lengths 4, 6, and 8 cm	CORDIS Johnson & Johnson	Iliac and superficial femoral arteries
Power Flex	Diameters 6–10 mm, lengths 4, 6, and 8 cm	CORDIS Johnson & Johnson	Calcified lesions

– *Manometer-controlled pressure injector (see Fig. 5.3)*
– *Manometer to control blood pressure proximal and distal of obliterations before and after angioplasty – particularly recommended in iliac, subclavian, and renal PTA (see Fig. 5.4)*
– *Compresses, sponges, and electric pad or hot-water bottle to keep the feet warm before, during, and after PTA.*

5.1.4.2
Angioplasty Catheters – "POBA" (Plain Old Balloon Angioplasty)

The catheter types for vascular interventions include: catheters for sounding, Bougier catheters, balloon catheters for dilatation, catheters for occlusion, thrombolysis catheters, and catheters equipped

Table 5.4. Vascular stents

Stent	Characteristics	Manufacturer
Palmaz Stent	Balloon-expandable, length 10–33 mm Expansion: medium 4–9 mm, long Medium 6–10 mm, large 8–12 mm Stainless steel, different diameters and lengths Balloon: OPTA5 or Powerflex	Cordis Johnson & Johnson
Perflex	Premounted on OPTA5	Cordis Johnson & Johnson
Smart Stent	Nitinol, self-expanding	Cordis Johnson & Johnson
Wallstent	With rolling membrane: Different diameters and lengths	Boston Scientific
Easy Wallstent	Short instrument: H. 965 SCH 643250: Diameter 8 mm length: 30 mm; sheath 6 F Catheter shaft: 75 cm H. 965 SCH 643340: Diameter 12 mm length 70 cm; sheath 8 F SCH-64335: diameter 8 mm, length 30 mm *Iliac and leg indication:* Long instrument: H. 965 SCH 643400: Diameter 6 mm, length 20 mm; sheath 6 F H. 965 SCH 643420: Diameter 6 mm; length 50 mm; sheath 6 F H. 965 SCH 643490: Diameter 10 mm length 30 mm; sheath 7 F *Subclavian and arm indication:* Self-expandable stent, guldewire 0.035 in. SCH-64349: diameter 10 mm, length 30 mm	Boston Scientific
Strecker Stent II	Balloon-expandable, tantalum; ultrathin Balloon catheter Iliac: 16–327 (8–4/5/95) Femoral: 16–317 (6–4/5/95)	Boston Scientific Meditech
Symphony – Nitinol Stent	M00160–2120 Diameter 6 mm, length 40 mm (self-expandable with thermo-memory) M00160–2240 Diameter 7 mm, length 60 mm metal-markers M00160–2320 Diameter 8 mm, length 44 mm on both ends M00160–2400 Diameter 10 mm, length 40 mm M00160–4500 Diameter 12 mm, length 20 mm	Boston Scientific Meditech
Passager (Vanguard)	Covered stent, sheath 18–12 F, flexible Diameters 6–12 mm, lengths 2 and 40, 60, 80, 100 mm Radial force three times higher than that of the Palmaz stent	Boston Scientific Meditech
Memotherm	Nitinol stent Iliac artery ipsilateral and crossover, self-expandable Femoral artery ipsilateral and crossover, thermo-memory	BARD
Instent		Vascucoil
Sinus Stent	Nitinol stent, self-expandable	Optimed
Bridge Stents	Stainless steel, balloon-expandable for iliac stenting	AVE
Peripheral AVE	Sheath size 7 F for 6–8 mm, 8 F for 9–10 mm Nominal balloon pressure: 8–10 atm Electro-polished stent surface	

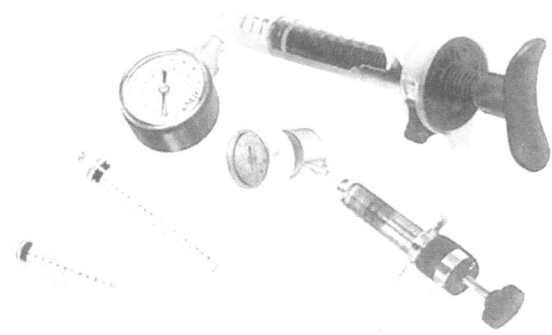

Fig. 5.3. Syringes with Luer-Lok connection, and syringes with manometer in direct or lateral arrangement

with specific instrumentation, as required for, e.g., atherectomies, thrombus aspiration, or declotting.

5.1.4.2.1
BOUGIER CATHETER SYSTEMS (see Table 5.2)

Dotter Coaxial Dilating Set. The first system was the Dotter coaxial dilating set (DOTTER 1964, 1966) consisting of an inner 8-F and an outer 12-F catheter (see Fig. 5.9), which are inserted via an "38"-type guidewire. For better stability, an inner metal cannula is used, through which a "35"-size Teflon-coated guidewire is advanced. We have started to use a Y-connector at the proximal Luer-lok end of the metal cannula (ZEITLER and MÜLLER 1996). The straight end houses the guidewire and the side port

enables the injection of saline solution or contrast agent for monitoring the whole procedure. The distal tip of the catheter is tapered resembling a frog's mouth. Recanalization is not effected through pushing-forward movements [due to the (risk of "snow-plug phenomenon" (STAPLE 1968)], but through rotational advancing. This screw-like technique helps achieve a more effective prevention of embolization which may be caused by larger ablated particles.

Zeitler Dilatation Catheters. The catheter has a tapered tip of 3 cm in length and widens from 5 F distally to 7 up to 12 F proximally (ZEITLER and MARESTA 1970). It has four side ports 2.5 cm distal of the final part, or 5 cm proximal of the tip. This provides the possibility of simultaneous opacification proximal and distal of the obstruction. The proximal connection with a Y-shaped connector and the use of a guidewire of 0.028 in. or 0.035 in. enables the dye injection at the time of recanalization. The diameter of the catheter changes in three steps, from the tip to the basic catheter.

Van-Andel Dilatation Catheters. These catheters have a tapered tip of 1.5–3.0 cm and are available in various diameters of 5–9 F (VAN ANDEL 1976).

Sos Dilatation Catheters. Straight Teflon catheters with two side ports behind the 1.5-cm tapered tip. These predilating catheters can be used for the first

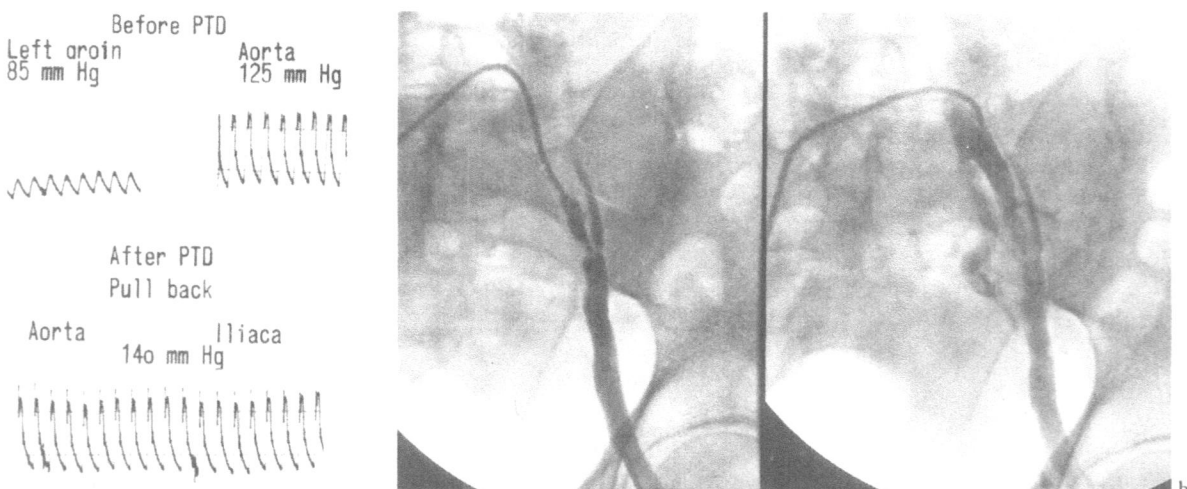

Fig. 5.4 a,b. Pressure curves before and after balloon dilatation of a stenosis in the left external iliac artery from the contralateral side. (**a**) Pressure-curves. *Upper curves,* pressure in the left groin before passage of the stenosis, and pressure in the aorta after catheterization from the contralateral side; *lower curve,* pressure in the aorta and iliac artery after balloon dilatation. (**b**) Angiography before and after balloon dilatation from the contralateral side. The images also show a subintimal channel resulting from a failed guiding attempt to the stenosis from the ipsilateral side

passage of stenotic lesions, or first recanalization in superficial femoral, popliteal, and proximal tibiofibular arteries, best in combinaton with catheters of 5- or 6-F diameter, through a 6-F sheath system.

After predilatation and safe passage over the guidewire distal to the obliteration, it is possible to use an appropriate balloon catheter in the selected diameter and length. The technique enables the precise measurement of the length and diameter of the obliteration.

Balloon Catheters (see Table 5.3). After the introduction of angioplasty by DOTTER and JUDKINS in 1964, some modifications perfected practice, such as the ZEITLER dilating catheters, and the VAN ANDEL Bougier catheters, both intended to reduce peripheral emboli and complications at the puncture site, whereby, whenever possible, catheters of less than 12 F were used. In addition, with the proximal side holes and the Y-connector, angioplasty became better controllable by fluoroscopy, since a dye injection was possible at the moment when the tip of the catheter was passing the obstruction in arteries.

Prior to the introduction of the GRÜNTZIG and OLBERT balloon catheters, I had been using FOGARTY balloon catheters through the 8-F Dotter catheter for iliac artery stenosis dilatation. PORSTMANN had published the corset balloon catheter which was modified by DOTTER and named the "caged balloon catheter". The caged balloon catheter, however, was associated with the risk of intimal dissection in the case of guidewire and balloon passage due to the slits in the outer Teflon catheter, but it was powerful in rupturing hard arteriosclerotic calcified iliac artery stenoses.

Therefore, a great breakthrough in this relatively new medical field was the GRÜNTZIG double-lumen balloon catheter. Nowadays, there is a remarkable variety of balloon catheters. Of course, the GRÜNTZIG balloon catheter and the OLBERT balloon catheter were the first to be used in practice. Both types of catheter underwent modifications during the time thereafter, not only by the companies Schneider in Zürich, Meadox in Copenhagen, and Meditech in Boston. Several types of therapeutic catheters for interventions in arterial and venous disease are presented in Table 5.2.

5.1.4.2.2
INDUSTRIAL INFORMATION

The typical *shaft materials* are thermoplastic elastomers. They provide a good combination of stiffness and flexibility. Polyvinylchloride (PVC) was one of the original-choice materials. As newer materials were developed, they were used in catheter-shaft applications. These include: plastics, nylon-chemistry-based TPE, urethane, hydrogel, polyester-chemistry-based, various derivatives and co-polymers of polyethylene, ethylene-vinyl-acetate, and graton-based materials, such as C-Flex and others.

Balloon materials are typically orientable materials, such as polyethylene and co-polymers of polyethylene, nylons, polypropylene, Poly-Armor or others. Also, all thermoplastic materials can be oriented to improve their film properties; amorphous materials lend themselves better to this process. Each material has its own processing problems which need to be understood and overcome. Polyethylene tetrachloride (PET) should be the ideal choice; it cannot be processed without its flaws, however. Newer materials are still on the way and in study programs. Most important is their diameter and biocompatibility, asepsis, and procedure-adjusted preparation.

The typical catheter characteristics important in proper selection prior to treatment of the different arterial lesions are:

- Pushability
- Trackability
- Flexibility
- Kink resistance
- Burst strength
- Column collapse
- Abrasion resistance
- Single- or multiluminal
- Outer diameter
- Diameter of the inner lumen
- Aseptic preparation

The different shaft materials, balloon materials, sterility, and ability to meet standard requirements demonstrate the high influence of excellent engineering cooperation between different institutions and clinics in basic science and technical knowledge, to produce safe products for medical use in diagnostics and treatment. The manifold, fruitful cooperation between physicians and industry over the years has been the guarantee for the rapid and successful advances in IR.

Inflation and Deflation of the Balloon. Dilating balloons can be inflated with a pump (see Fig. 5.3), or by manual pressure. Most users, for reasons of availability, simplicity, and tactile feed-back, seem to prefer a simple syringe and manual injection. For stent application, or in high-risk lesions, however, the pressure syringe with manometer control is recommended.

It is important to know that *the smaller the syringe diameter, the greater the pressure applied*. Therefore, a 2-ml syringe is very practical and 10–15 atm can be generated manually, whereas with a 20-ml syringe, no more than 5 atm can be generated by hand (ABELE 1980).

In applying suction, *a large syringe* displaces more volume, and more suction is produced. Therefore, with a 10-ml syringe, a suction of about 1.0 atm can be generated, whereas with the 2-ml syringe, only 0.5 atm suction can be generated (ABELE 1980). With modern-type balloon catheters, it is possible to work for inflation with a 2-cc syringe, and deflation with a 10-cc syringe. Therefore, the use of a two-way stopcock and pressure gauge are safe and very practical for quick deflation and prevention of over-inflation.

There is a significant difference regarding balloon dilatation in the different areas of the arterial systems – arteries in the peripheral circulation of the extremities, or coronary and cerebral arteries – because ischemia over a long period of time has different results. Therefore, the most important recommendations for balloon dilatation are:

- Select a balloon catheter of a diameter corresponding to the normal artery lumen measured angiographically directly before the stenosis (see Table 5.3).
- Balloon inflation must be controlled under roentgen fluoroscopy (Fig. 5.5).
- Start with low pressure and work up to the smooth outer diameter of the balloon, and thus the inner lumen of the artery.
- Dilatation time for short stenoses: 20 and 30 s
  Dilatation time for long stenoses or occlusions: 30 s at minimum, and up to 2 min.
- In the treatment of several overlapping stenotic areas, it is necessary to dilate the border of the obstruction at the beginning and at the end in addition. It is unclear, however, whether, in such situations, restenosis may develop in the area undergoing mechanical pressure injury to the normal arterial wall.

Therefore, if no short stenotic lesions exist, we perform at minimum three balloon dilatations in iliac and leg arteries. In short lesions of the supraaortic arteries, we perform one dilatation of 20–30 s only. The dilatation of stenoses in dialysis shunts requires one or two dilatation(s) of more than 1 min (each). Different technical systems of angioplasty in addi-

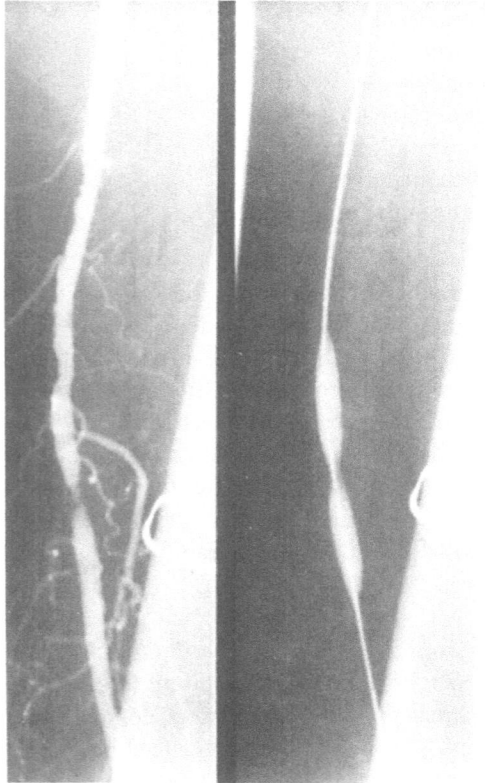
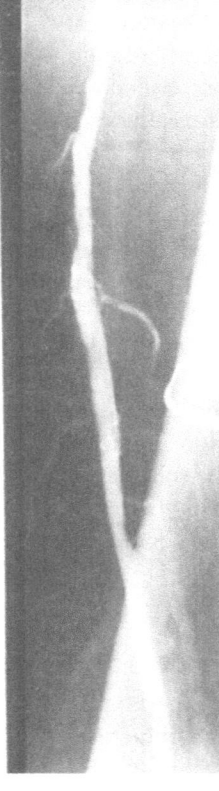

Fig. 5.5. Balloon dilatation of a concentric stenosis in the superficial femoral artery (SFA), before and at dilatation, and after successful plain old balloon angioplasty. Patient with claudication <200 m, arterial blood pressure index 0.6 before, and 0.9 after dilatation

tion to balloon dilatation can be used and are on the market.

I recommend in all patients the use of sheath systems and basic catheterization with a Cobra or Bougier catheter system. The original Dotter co-axial system is nowadays no longer indicated. Bougier catheters (see Table 5.2) and balloon catheters are available in different designs (see Table 5.3).

The GRÜNTZIG balloon catheter was originally a two-channel system, and it is possible to choose between balloon catheters with a short or long shoulder. In localized stenoses of short extension, a short shoulder should be preferred. Precise straight balloons are "sausage-like", while others bend on inflation, with a "banana-like" appearance.

In multiple stenoses, or long-distance stenoses, a long shoulder can sometimes also help in the basic dilatation without the risk of embolization (Fig. 5.6). Different balloon catheter systems have folded balloon material which may cause some problems after dilatation. Without good extraction of the fluid, the balloon can rupture at retraction through the sheath. Therefore, the sheath has to be chosen 1 F larger than the balloon catheter.

In tibiofibular arteries, in addition to classic small balloon catheter systems of 3–4 F, the Tegwire balloon-on-the guidewire, the Viper and Courier catheters with soft tips and gliding surfaces are less traumatic in the recanalization and dilatation of these obliterations. These special techniques and results are described in Chap. 33.

Under normal conditions, primarily a combination of recanalization and balloon dilatation is necessary to treat arteriosclerotic stenoses and occlusions in the iliofemoral and poplitotibial arterial system. If the control angiography of the primary result documents an improvement of the vessel diameter with less than a 20% residual stenosis without important dissection or collapsing arteries at the first time of treatment of the stenosis, balloon angioplasty alone is successful. But if, after control angiography, important dissections or collapsing arteries are found, or if there has been a recanalization of a total occlusion of more than 5 cm in length, the primary indication for implantation of a stent very often leads to better long-term results in iliac arteries (Fig. 5.7).

In femoropopliteal arteries, primary stent application is indicated after dissection, unsuccessful dilatation, or recanalization of occlusions longer than 5 cm, if poor angiographic results are found in patients with critical limb ischemia (PALMAZ

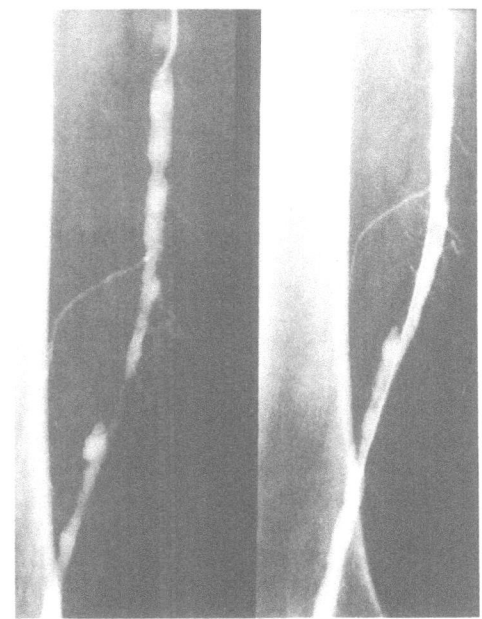

Fig. 5.6. Multiple stenoses in the superficial femoral artery with one long-distance stenosis at Hunter's channel before and after plain old balloon angioplasty. The patient is a 79-year-old man, with cigarette smoking and hypertension as risk factors

et al. 1988a; RICHTER et al. 1987, 1991, 1995; STRECKER et al. 1993; VORWERK and GÜNTHER 1990, 1995).

In contrast to this, the application of stents in the treatment of restenosis yields better early and long-term results. Various adjunctive treatments to prevent restenosis are undergoing prospective trials [radiotherapy (LIERMANN et al. 1994), drug application, and others (SCHNEIDER et al. 1987)].

Important are appropriate stent selection, the best-suited primary indication, and control of the final outcome. This is discussed in detail in the chapters dealing with iliac (Chap. 30), femoral (Chap. 31), tibioperoneal (Chap. 33), and supraaortic angioplasty (Chap. 35, Sect. 35.4).

5.1.4.2.3
ADJUNCTIVE DRUG THERAPY

Adjunctive treatment before, during, and after PTA has the following goals:

- To avoid platelet aggregation leading to early rethrombosis
- To avoid acute thrombosis during the procedure, when flow is reduced by the dilating catheter
- To avoid mechanically induced spasm

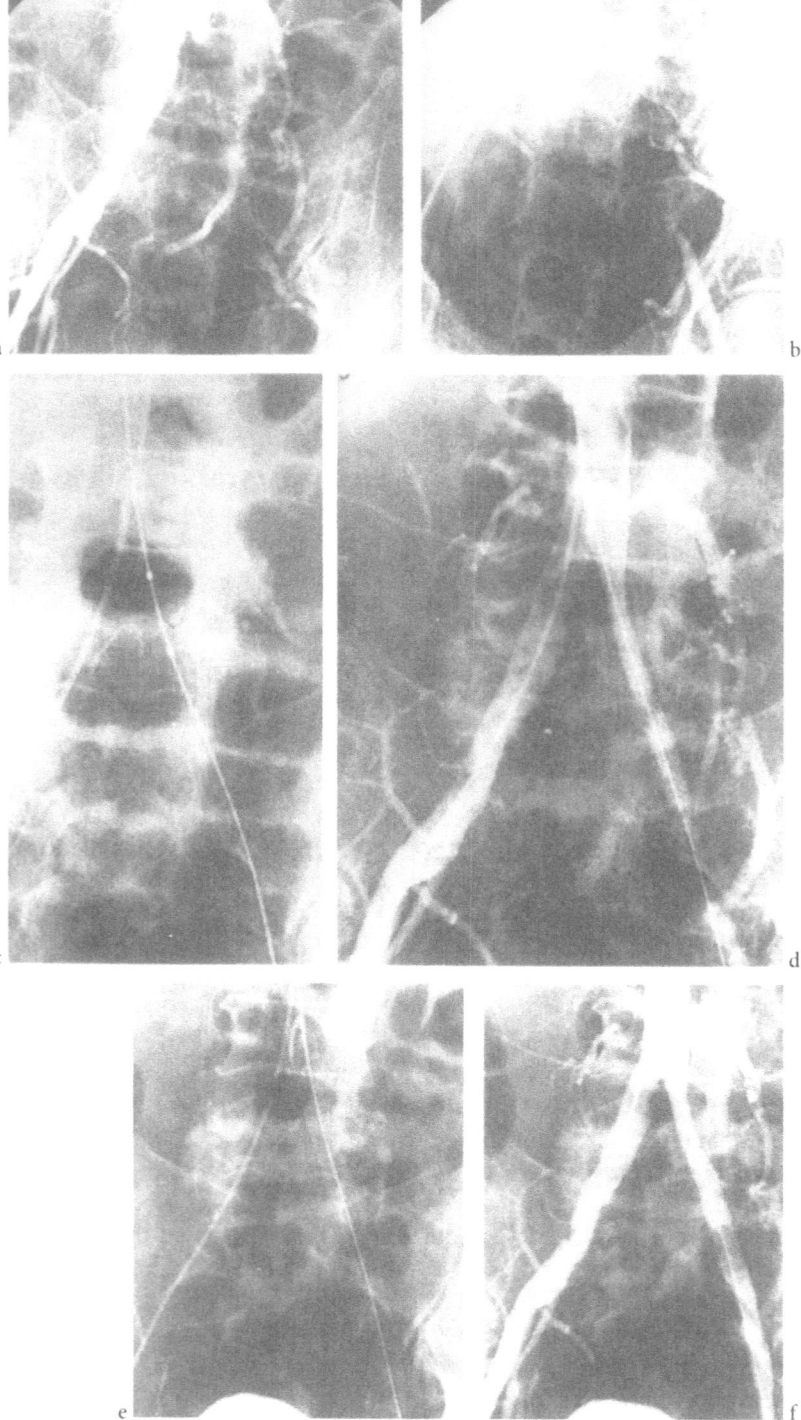

Fig. 5.7 a–f. Occlusion of the left common and external iliac arteries. **a,b** Angiography before angioplasty. **c,d** Documentation of bilateral catheterization just with guidewire and Cobra catheter, plus balloon dilatation (balloon catheter 8 mm in diameter and 4 cm in length). Overlapping dilatation. **e,f** In the interests of good long-term success, a Wallstent is placed. **e** Image without contrast medium. **f** Final angiographic control

– To maintain peripheral perfusion during catheter dilatation and subsequent manual compression of the arterial puncture site after catheter removal

Various forms of adjunctive drug therapy have been used to date. Any recommendations that can be given today reflect the best early and long-term results (Table 5.5). More information is given in Chap. 6.

5.1.4.3
Atherectomy Catheter Systems

The techniques of percutaneous atherectomy aim at the removal of material leading to the occlusion of vessels via access through a sheath. Without damaging the non-obliterated endovascular segments, these procedures imitate the surgical technique of thromboendarterectomy.

The employment of atherectomy techniques has to be considered whenever a proper recanalization with guidewire and a Bougier or balloon catheter has failed, or if the prospects of its success are poor. However, atherectomy was not found to be an alternative treatment with better long-term results (MAYNAR et al. 1989; KÜFFER et al. 1990). The major indications are calcified local, or extensively occluded, vascular segments which cannot be crossed by a guidewire. A particular indication is extraction of tissue from the artery for histologic analysis.

We differentiate as follows:
1. Techniques of local atherectomy
   - Peripheral Simpson atherectomy (P-SAC)
   - Pull-back atherectomy (FITCHELL and STADIUS 1991)
   - *Redha* atherectomy (REDHA et al. 1996)
2. Recanalization devices for total artery occlusions
   - Kensey high-speed rotational dynamic catheter
   - Transluminal endarterectomy catheter (TEC system, Interventional Technologies, San Diego, CA)
   - High-speed rotational atherectomy (AUTH Rotablator, Heart Technologies, Redmond, VA)
   - Vallbracht low-speed rotational system (Rotax).

5.1.4.3.1
SIMPSON ATHERECTOMY

The Simpson atherectomy catheter (SIMPSON et al. 1985; SCHWARTEN et al. 1988) is advanced via a 0.081-in. guidewire with the help of an introducer sheath. Close to the distal end of the catheter, there is a cylindrical metal chamber with openings on one side. In this chamber, a movable tube cutter, motor-driven from the proximal catheter end, is operated. After opening the chamber by withdrawing the tube cutter, a latex balloon at the opposite side is filled with contrast agent, at a pressure of 2 atm. Thus, the obliterating material can be pressed under fluoroscopic control into the open metal chamber. The catheter and the chamber are flushed via a side port with saline solution. The side port also enables the injecton of contrast agent to monitor the procedure. After safe placement (Fig. 5.8) of the metal chamber and entrance of the occluding material into the same, the tube cutter, rotating at 2000 rotations per minute (RPM), is manually advanced to shut the chamber. Atheromatous particles are thus cut off and get into the collecting chamber distal to the atherectomy chamber. After 2–3 cuts, the catheter has to be retracted, and the occluding material is removed from the collecting chamber. The catheter can then be inserted again if necessary via the guidewire.

If the control angiography reveals a residual stenosis, or vascular irregularity, an additional balloon angioplasty can follow. Figure 5.9 shows the outcome of a Simpson atherectomy with the atherectomized particles.

Results. Local excentric stenoses are safely removed in over 90% of cases (HÖFLING et al. 1988), complex stenoses or short occlusions are managed in 85% (MAYNAR et al. 1989; KÜFFER et al. 1990), but need additional balloon dilatation in more than 20% of cases. Complications such as embolism, dissection, and hematoma at the puncture site were observed in 5%–12% of patients (SCHWARTEN et al. 1988; HANSEN 1993).

Control angiographies showed that stenoses can be reduced to residual stenoses of less than 30% arterial narrowing in 90%–95% of cases. Clinical improvement of the Doppler index, and also of the painless walking distance according to the Rutherford criteria, was reported in all publications at a rate of up to 95% after primary treatment. Also in Nuremberg, our team was successful in 36 of 38

Table 5.5. Adjunctive drug therapy

Premedication
Aggregation inhibitors (orally): acetylsalicylic acid, 100–500 mg daily

At PTA
After arterial catheterization, to prevent early rethrombosis: 5000 IU of heparin injected intraarterially

To Prevent Arterial Spasm
Orally: calcium channel blockers, nifedipine or nitroglycerine spray,
1% lidocaine (3 ml) or nitroglycerine intraarterially

After successful PTA
Anticoagulation, heparin or low-dose heparin, 1–6 days depending on the severity of the obliteration: aggregation inhibitors,
    ASA 330 mg plus dipyridamole 75 mg once daily, acetylsalicylic acid 100–500 mg daily, or clopidogrel 75 mg daily

---

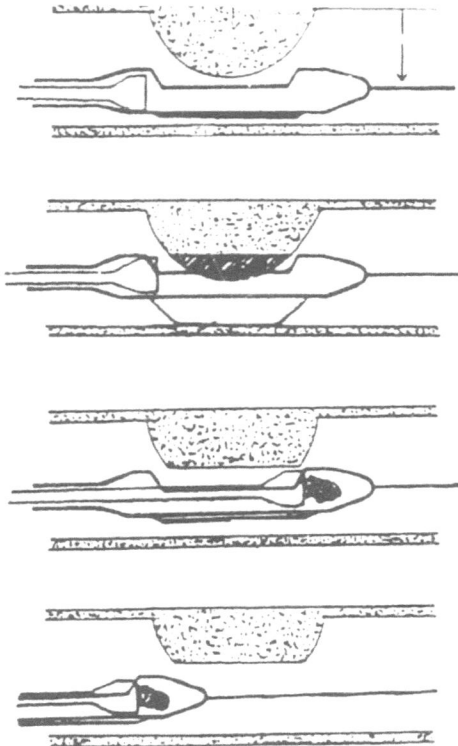

Fig. 5.8. The steps of Simpson atherectomy (according to HÖFLING et al. 1988)

treatments using Simpson atherectomy in the superficial femoral or popliteal arteries, with only one complication: dissection followed by thrombotic occlusion, which could be successfully lysed by intraarterial urokinase and was followed by stent application.

The restenosis rate after 3 years was 25% (9 of 36 cases). Irrespective of proper selection considering the type of obliteration, the main indications for Simpson atherectomy nowadays are restenoses after stent implantation at the border of stents, and within the stented lumen. Any traumatization of the stent filaments must then be avoided. The evaluation of histologic specimens is of importance for the assessment of new therapeutic strategies to reduce the restenosis rate and slow down, and where possible prevent, the progression of arteriosclerosis.

5.1.4.3.2
PULL-BACK ATHERECTOMY (PAC)

The Fitchell pull-back atherectomy catheter (PAC catheter) is an over-the-wire catheter designed to "circumferentially debulk" concentric arteriosclerotic obliterations (FITCHELL and STADIUS 1991). The device consists of the outer closing catheter and an inner movable cutting catheter which rotates

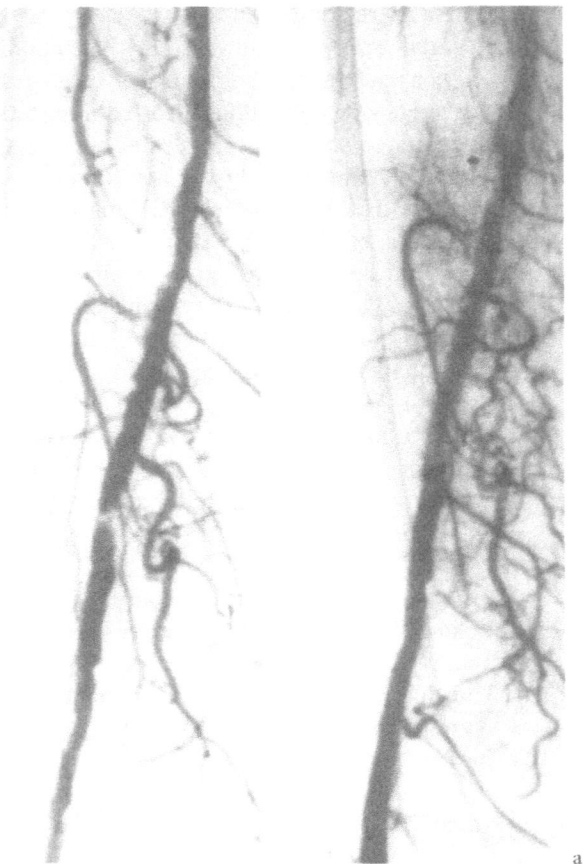

a,b

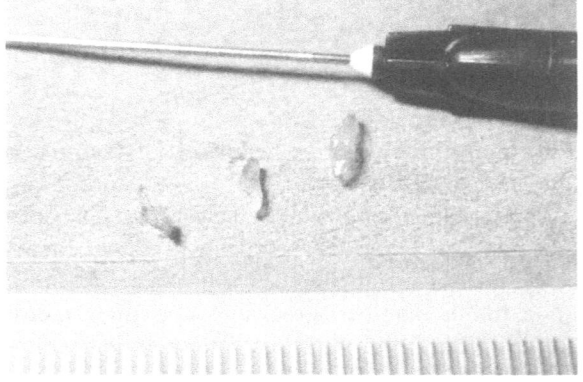

Fig. 5.9. Excentric superficial femoral artery stenosis. In the right leg of a 54-year-old woman, pain-free walking distance <100 m, with additional patency of only one tibioperoneal artery. Risk factors included diabetes, cigarette smoking, and overweight. **a** Antegrade femoral angiography before atherectomy, demonstrating an excentric stenosis of more than 80%. **b** Angiography after Simpson atherectomy, demonstrating irregularities only. The arterial blood pressure index was 0.42 before and 0.8 after atherectomy. **c** Atherectomized particles demonstrating organized plaque without fresh thrombus

at 2000 RPM. The cutting portion of the catheter is rotated by a battery-powered motor-drive.

Across the 0.018-in guidewire, through a 7–9-F vascular sheath, the PAC catheter is advanced to the lesion in "closed position". The catheter is then opened by advancing its distal portion. Before the motor-drive starts rotating the cutting blade and retracting the distal part of the instrument, external compression with a blood-pressure cuff stabilizes a large part of the atherosclerotic material of the superficial femoral artery into the capsule. Thus, pull-back atherectomy is completed. The same procedure can be repeated several times, with exchange over the guidewire. If necessary, atherectomy can be followed by balloon PTA.

Results. We employed this technique in eight patients with circumferential local stenoses of the superficial femoral artery (Fig. 5.10). We were successful in seven of the eight patients, once the guidewire had passed the obstructed area. The ankle-brachial index (ABI) improved from 0.62 to 0.89. After 2 years, two of the seven patients had a restenosis that was dilated with balloon PTA. We had no severe complications, neither during the primary procedure, nor during the follow-up period.

In the multicenter PAC trial (WHITE 1997) on 166 lesions, 165 could be passed by the guidewire followed by the atherectomy device. A total of 35% of these were treated without complementary balloon angioplasty. The mean lesion length was 2.2 cm (0.4–7.0 cm). Successful pull-back atherectomy was accomplished in 90% of the lesions (149

of 165). The ABI before treatment was 0.56 and improved to 0.87 after treatment. Follow-up studies showed restenoses in 58%. There were no major complications.

5.1.4.3.3
REDHA-CUT ATHERECTOMY
The Redha-cut is a percutaneous transluminal atherectomy device (REDHA et al. 1992). It consists of 4 or 6 cutting blades which, by moving the covering cylinder mechanically back and forth, can be opened and closed like an umbrella. The edge-to-edge distance varies for the four different sizes between 4 and 8 mm.

The device (Fig. 5.11) is available in diameters of 1.95 mm (6-F sheath) and 2.65 mm (8-F sheath). The 8-F device can be used in the femoropopliteal and iliac arteries, the smaller one in below-the-knee atherectomies.

The Redha catheter is maneuvered through the arterial stenosis over a thin guidewire (0.012 in.). After passage of the stenosis, the cutting blades are opened to their proper size. By gentle withdrawal of the cutter through the stenosis with open blades, pieces of the atherosclerotic material are cut and gathered within the device. The closed system is then

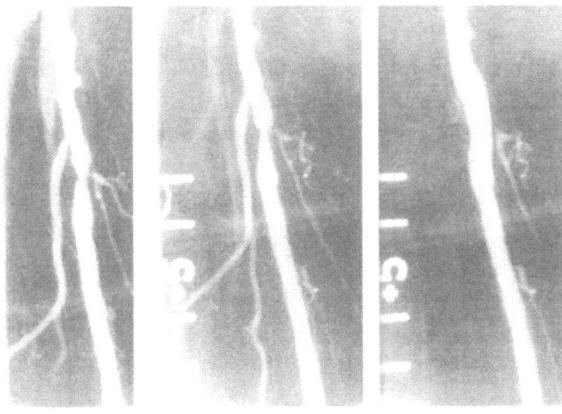

Fig. 5.10. Concentric superficial femoral artery stenosis before, after one, and after two additional atherectomies plus balloon dilatation. The successful final atherectomy was the result of additional pressure-cuff compression applied beforehand

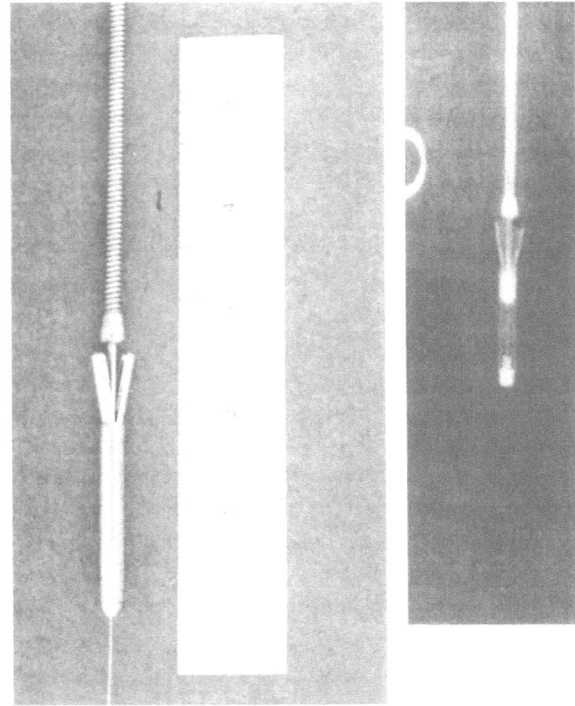

Fig. 5.11 a,b. Redha atherectomy catheter. **a** With open knife (four cutting blades). **b** Control during atherectomy under X-ray fluoroscopy

withdrawn from the vessel. Outside the artery it is opened, the plaque material is removed, and the instrument is flushed with sterile physiologic saline. If necessary, the procedure can be repeated.

In short, the steps of the procedure include:
- Advancing the device
- Opening it
- Retracting the device and cutting material
- Closing the device and extracting the ablated material.

Results. In the Nuremberg team (BEYER-ENKE et al. 1996), atherectomy performed on 20 patients using the Redha-cut was successful in 18 according to the Rutherford criteria, in 24 out of 25 lesions. The 6-month patency rate was 80% (16 of 20), the 1-year patency rate 76% (13 of 17).

REDHA et al. (1996) and DO, DO-DAI et al. (1996) treated 93 arteriosclerotic lesions in the femoropopliteal arteries in 70 patients with the Redha-cut device. The stenoses were reduced from 74% to 26%, and to 17% by additional balloon dilatation. No serious complications occurred. The cumulative patency rates were: 83% at 6 months and 66% at 1 year. BAUMGARTNER et al. (1996) have shown good results with color-coded duplex sonography controls and early demonstration of restenosis.

In contrast to the pull-back atherectomy device and Simpson atherectomy, the handling of the Redha-cut is simple and requires no auxiliary equipment such as a motor-drive system (DODER et al. 1996). Once the guidewire passes the lesion, it works very quickly, within minutes. The disadvantage is the risk of losing atherectomized particles on withdrawal of the device, which might cause embolism and have to be aspirated afterwards. In case of large ablated particles, the device may not close perfectly, so that at retraction problems may occur.

All three devices for local atherectomy are primarily important in isolated cases and for histologic studies in scientific problems. This has been confirmed by long-term follow-up which could not demonstrate better primary patency rates than balloon PTA alone (SCHWARTEN et al. 1988; HANSEN 1993; ROTH et al. 1988, 1995), or secondary patency after stent-assisted angioplasty (RICHTER et al. 1991; Palmaz et al. 1990).

5.1.4.3.4
HIGH-SPEED ROTATIONAL ANGIOPLASTY

The Kensey atherectomy catheter (KENSEY et al. 1987; ZEITLER 1988, 1989) consists of a flexible catheter with a high-speed rotational hummer. The high-speed rotations with 40 000 to 100 000 RPM are controlled by an electric motor. The metal tip has openings through which fluids are ejected from the catheter in a sharp jet, in the manner of a garden hose. This infusion quickly carries the ablated particles into the periphery, with the effect of further fragmentation. To flush the device, we used a mixture of HAES (hydroxyethyl starch) and 60% non-ionic contrast medium at a ratio of 1:1, with an additive of 100 000 IU urokinase. This solution is injected via a contrast medium injector at a speed of 0.5 ml/s.

Experiments on animals and clinical experience have shown that the catheter passes the arterial lumen without perforation. Histologic studies demonstrated a fragmentation of the intima in 30% of cases, and ablation of the endothelium in 38% (KENSEY et al. 1987). In vitro experiments (SCHMITZ-ROHDE and GÜNTHER 1991) have shown that the modified Kensey catheter, the Track-Wright catheter, and the Günther and Amplatz propellers produce the smallest particles, smaller than 400 μm. A cooperative study on 210 patients showed successful recanalization of chronic femoral artery occlusions in 157 cases (74%). The cumulative 1-year patency rate was 62%. Complications, mainly peripheral embolism, were observed in 11%. This type of dynamic angioplasty needs further improvements regarding the reduction of particle size to prevent peripheral embolism before deserving general acceptance. Without question, the handling of the Kensey or other recanalizational devices can also vary, and the embolization rate can be reduced with sufficient experience.

5.1.4.3.5
TRANSLUMINAL ENDARTERECTOMY CATHETER (TEC)

This type of atherectomy device was also developed on the hypothesis, that the removal of plaque, instead of its remodeling, would result in lower acute occlusion and restenosis rates than with PTA (BATES et al. 1988). After recanalization, the TEC device removes debris by a vacuum effect, with a low rate of embolization. The TEC system includes a cutter mounted on the distal end of the torque tube, which passes freely over a 0.014-in. steerable wire. The cutter consists of three blades which form the sides of a triangle. The tube cutter is connected to a motorized drive assembly and power source which rotates the torque tube at 750 RPM. The excised tissue is removed through the torque tube by an attached 125-ml vacuum bottle, under 1 atm negative pressure. The system exists in 5-, 7-, and 9-F sizes.

Results. Single department results (WHOLEY et al. 1989) with 52 obliterations in 45 patients reported successful treatment in 41 of these. In 69%, the patients had claudication, six complained of pain at rest, and eight had gangrene. Complications occurred in 9.6%.

A multicenter trial (WHOLEY 1997) with 132 patients and 204 lesions demonstrated technical success in 88%. Additional balloon PTA was necessary in 50% of the occlusions and 25% of short segmental stenoses.

In the multicenter trial, complications were observed at a rate of 23%. Most frequent were hematomas at the puncture site (8%), thrombosis, dissection, intimal flaps, and bleeding complications necessitating blood transfusion. The cumulative patency after 6 months was 84%, after 1 year 73%, and after 2 years 60%. WHOLEY (1997) recommends TEC atherectomy for total occlusions above and below the knee, with additional balloon PTA and stent application. Our team has no personal experience with this device.

5.1.4.3.6
AUT ROTABLATOR
The AUT Rotablator (AHN et al. 1988) is a high-speed rotational atherectomy device with a flexible non-radiopaque catheter fitted with a diamond-encrusted metal burr that selectively cuts away inelastic tissue during high-speed rotation. The catheter which tracks coaxially over a 0.009-in. (0.23-mm) guidewire to prevent deflection, is encased in a 4.3-F sheath that protects the vessel wall. During drive-shaft rotation, saline is infused through this sheath to lubricate and cool the catheter, burr, and guidewire. The drive shaft is connected to a compressed-air turbine that rotates the burr at speeds varying from 50 000 to 200 000 RPM. The diameters of available burrs range from 1.5 to 4.5 mm.

Results. The "Nine US Medical Centers' Trial" (THORPE 1988; THE COLLABORATIVE ROTABLATOR ATHERECTOMY GROUP 1994) represents 157 patients with 258 peripheral lesions. Claudication was present in 66% and critical limb ischemia in 34%. In 59%, there were single lesions, in 41% multiple tandem obliterations. In 99 patients there were tibiofibular and in 16% popliteal obliterations. Primary technical success was achieved in 77% without balloon PTA. The technical success rate using a combined treatment – Rotablator plus additional balloon PTA – was 93%.

The 6-month-cumulative patency rate was 80% in patients with claudication and 50% in patients with critical limb ischemia. In a European center (HENRY et al. 1995), 150 patients with 212 lesions were treated with the Rotablator. There were 193 stenoses (91%) and 19 chronic occlusions with significant calcification. More than 50% were localized below the knee. The immediate technical success rate was 95%. Residual stenoses after Rotablator treatment were more often observed in femoropopliteal than in tibioperoneal arteries. Primary success using a combination of Rotablator and balloon PTA for obliterations in 86 femoral, 19 popliteal, and 106 tibioperoneal arteries was 97% (HENRY et al. 1997).

The most important complications were spasms in 11% and acute thrombosis in 5.6%. The 6-month-follow-up patency rate was 66%. All papers up to now have described a higher complication rate during the learning phase. This risk of complications, together with cost, are the reasons for its lack of general acceptance, even though the use of the Rotablator in tibiofibular artery obliterations in patients with critical limb ischemia seems recommendable.

5.1.4.3.7
VALLBRACHT LOW-SPEED ROTATIONAL SYSTEM – "ROTACS"
The Rotacs system (VALLBRACHT et al. 1989) replaces the guidewire for the first passage of the obstruction as used in conventional PTA by a motor-driven shaft with a maximum rotation of 300 RPM. The catheter has a flexible tip with a metal, olive-shaped cap. The tip of the Rotacs fights its way through the obstruction where there is lowest resistance. Calcified lesions cannot be crossed.

Results. The multicenter trial (VALLBRACHT 1992) with 1252 angioplasties showed a primary success of 78%, at a complication rate of 1.5%–8% and a lethality of 0.1%. The best results (ROTH et al. 1995) were observed in the proximal third of the superficial femoral artery, with 64% for occlusions of 6 cm, and 67% for occlusions of on average 18 cm in length. In the medial third of the superficial femoral artery, the recanalization rate in short and long occlusions was 42% and 49%, respectively.

5.1.4.3.8
DISCUSSION
The development of the hydrophilic guidewires of the "Radifocus" type by companies such as Terumo and others, has restrained the use of the Rotacs device and a number of other general atherectomy

devices. Neither in the region of the pelvic arteries, nor of the superficial femoral artery, is there any need for an atherectomy device for short or normally long stenoses or occlusions, except if a histologic specimen is to be obtained. Only if there is a contraindication excluding surgical treatment with femoropopliteal or femorocrural bypass for extremely long femoropopliteal occlusions, the use of mechanical recanalization techniques, or additional laser-assisted angioplasty, may be indicated. This is all the more important since the long-term results of atherectomy and laser angioplasty have not been more favorable so far than those of balloon angioplasty.

Experience has shown that, even after use of the different atherectomy techniques (MCLEAN 1993, KÜFFER et al. 1990; REEKERS 1990) balloon angioplasty and, under certain circumstances also local thrombolysis, very often have to follow. Therefore, these special techniques belong – quite naturally – to the more expensive types of "combined angioplasty" compared to "plain old balloon angioplasty", which is capable of managing category I and II lesions with the appropriate guidewire, first-passage catheter, sheath, and balloon catheter. Only more extensive obliterations – categories III and IV – may justify the utilization of a combined treatment after interdisciplinary discussion, as an alternative to vascular surgery for the treatment of patients with critical limb ischemia.

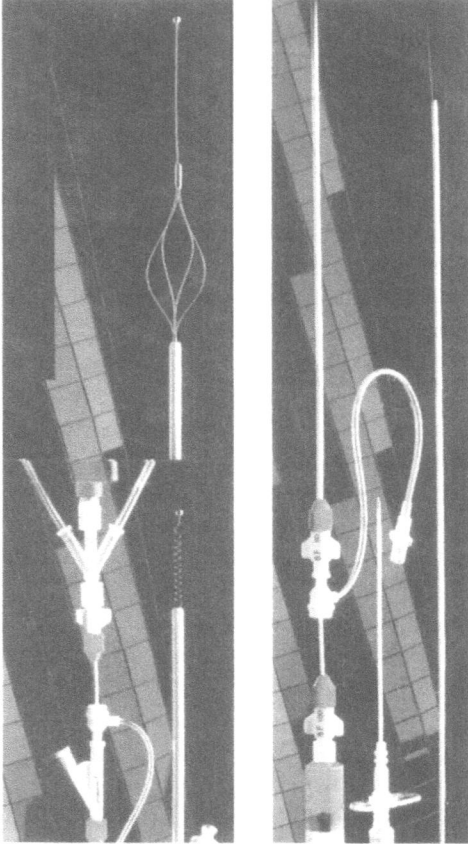

Fig. 5.12. Combined percutaneous aspiration thromboembolectomy-rotational aspiration thromboembolectomy instrument developed by Starck (1986)

5.1.4.4
Percutaneous Aspiration Catheter System

PAT was systematically introduced in 1985 by STARCK et al. into the therapy of pelvic and leg arteries, for acute and subacute thromboembolic occlusions. Irrespective of this, SCHNEIDER reported in 1986 on his experience with aspiration thrombectomy for subacute and chronic femoropopliteal occlusions SCHNEIDER and LARGIADÉR 1987; SCHNEIDER et al. 1987. The technique requires a vascular sheath, if necessary with a long catheter of 8–9 F with a proximal removable top cap, as well as the original aspiration catheter instrumentation. The aspiration catheter (Fig. 5.12) is open-ended, without side holes and untapered. For aspiration at the femoropopliteal level, an 8-F catheter should be preferred, whereas the distal popliteal artery and the tibiofibular arteries require a 5-F catheter. The rather rarely used aspiration in the region of the iliac arteries and in thrombosed bypasses necessitates 10-F aspiration catheters.

Definition: Acute leg ischemia and subacute thromboembolic occlusion have a history of up to 3 months.

The coaxial vascular sheath with the aspiration catheter is positioned closely above the lodged embolus or thrombus. The aspiration catheter is then pushed slowly into the occluded artery and, while suction is maintained with a 50-cc syringe, the catheter is gradually withdrawn. As soon as blood aspiration is no longer possible, the clot material is in the aspiration catheter. At this time, the catheter is removed and its contents expelled into a gauze-draped basin. While the vascular sheath catheter is clamped, the top cap including the valve is removed from the sheath and remaining clots within the sheath are aspirated to prevent them from getting into the artery and possibly causing embolization. When the vascular sheath has again been equipped with the top cap including the valve, a control angiography via the side-arm is performed. If necessary, aspiration can be repeated several times (STARCK et al. 1985, 1986). Clots that are fixed to the wall can be removed with mechanical auxiliary devices such as spherical tipped spirals or spherical baskets (rotational aspiration thromboembolectomy, RAT). In the course of further aspiration procedures, the femoropopliteal artery, and also the tibiofibular trunk, can be cleared of emboli, thrombi, or iatrogenic thrombi with the 8- and 5-F aspiration catheters.

Results. In 1989, STARCK and WAGNER (1990) published results on 114 procedures on 111 extremities in 109 patients. The mean length of the thromboembolic occlusions was 13.8 cm. Technical success was at that time achieved in 80%. In 10% of cases, additional local thrombolysis and in 29%, balloon PTA became necessary. Until 1992, he used his experience with PAT in more than 700 patients. In addition to aspiration, he very often used the spherical basket. Full clinical success, including local thrombolysis and balloon angioplasty – combined angioplasty type I – up to the patient's discharge from hospital was then achieved in 95%. In 50%, the use of thrombolytic agents could be avoided, while in the others the dose of lytic agents could be reduced.

In Nuremberg, we have successfully treated 18 of 24 femoropopliteal embolic occlusions (Fig. 5.13), without additional urokinase or other thrombolytic agents. In several other cases, we used the "combination type I angioplasty" for subacute thromboembolic occlusions and also chronic occlusions. In several cases, in addition to balloon angioplasty after PAT, the application of stents also became necessary. Therefore, in patients with acute and subacute total artery occlusions, we are always prepared for combined PTA type I, which means PAT, the administration of thrombolytic agents, and the application of balloons and stents can become necessary. In contrast, we see no indication for PAT in long chronic occlusions. The Auth Rotablator has its best indication in such cases, combined with balloon and stent application, unless vascular surgery with one of the bypass techniques is indicated and possible.

5.1.5
Angioplasty with Stents[1]

Intravascular stents are used as a mechanical device to solve problems arising at or after balloon angioplasty in case of intimal dissection, elastic recoil, or to improve long-term patency, as a primary type of angioplasty.

The original idea of placing stents in vessels with a percutaneous catheter under X-ray fluoroscopy

control must be accredited to Charles T. DOTTER (1969). His experiments in a canine popliteal artery demonstrated long-term patency after the application of a coil-spring tube graft. In 1983, he introduced the concept of a thermoplastic stent consisting of a small-diameter coil made of the alloy nitinol (nickel plus titanium), which has the ability to change shape when exposed to increased temperatures (around 37–38°C; 98.4°–100°F) (DOTTER 1983). In the same year, and independent of this, CRAGG et al. (1983) published their experimental results with the non-surgical placement of an arterial endoprosthesis, also made of the thermoplastic material nitinol. MAASS et al. from Zürich reported in 1984

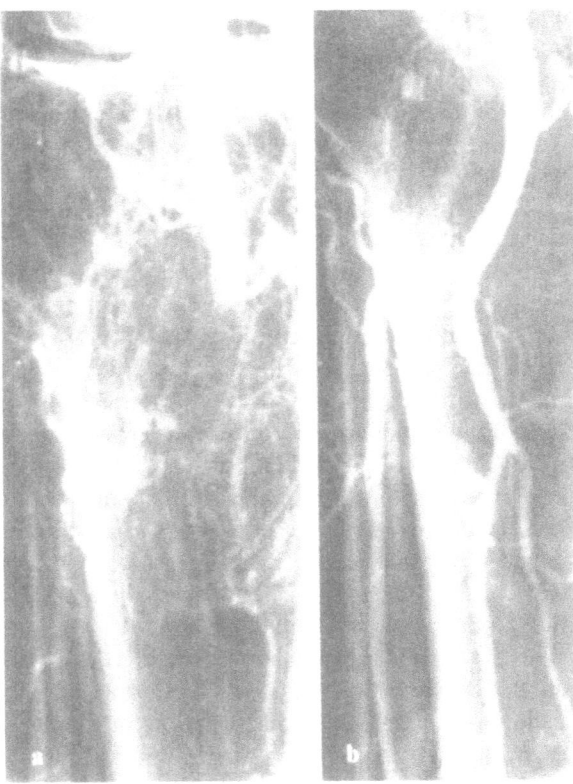

Fig. 5.13 a,b. Acute popliteal embolism in a 77-year-old woman with atrial fibrillation. **a** Angiography before percutaneous aspiration thromboembolectomy. **b** Angiography after successful percutaneous thromboembolectomy, plus local thrombolysis with 100 000 IU of urokinase

---

[1] Stents are named after the British dentist, C. R. Stent, who lived at the end of the 19th century. Stent's contribution was the invention of a dental impression material that was later used to promote the healing of skin grafts. The word "stent" was applied later on to all devices used for the support of living tissues during the healing phase, including internal structures (PALMAZ 1992).

on their experimental results with spring-loaded stainless steel coils that increase their diameter by unwinding after release.

WRIGHT et al. (1985) published their first experiments with an elastic stent consisting of a tempered, stainless-steel wire bent into a zig-zag tubular configuration. In the same year, PALMAZ et al. (1985) introduced the balloon-expandable stent which consists of a tubular meshwork of annealed stainless steel that is deployed by inflation of a coaxial balloon. In 1988, STRECKER et al. published their first experimental results with the balloon-expandable tantalum-woven stent. In the same years, RABKIN et al. (1984, 1989) presented their clinical experience with the nitinol stent in Russia, and SIGWART et al. (1987) published their results with a spring-loaded meshwork as an intravascular stent to prevent re-occlusion and restenosis after PTA, with a first application even in the coronary artery. The deployment of this device is accomplished by withdrawing a rolling membrane, allowing the stent to expand its diameter.

Meanwhile, between 1987 and 1999, numerous papers (RICHTER et al. 1987, 1991; JOFFRE and ROUSSEAU 1989; TRILLER et al. 1989) were published on the subject and the safe and successful application of stents in peripheral and coronary arteries was reported on at several symposia, as was more experimental work. Several companies have tried to bring new, more sophisticated stents onto the market, but up to now the final problem: which stent in which arteries, veins, or other channels (biliary, urogenital, bronchial, or gastrointestinal system) offers the best chance for good endothelialization (incorporation) without side-effects, but with long-term patency, has not yet been solved.

In the peripheral vascular system, there is experience with a few types of stents (see Table 5.4): the balloon-expandable Palmaz stent, the balloon-expandable Strecker stent made of tantalum, the self-expanding Easy Wallstent with a rolling membrane, and several self-expanding stents made of nitinol (Cragg stent, Symphony stent, Bard stent, InStent, and others).

Most experimental work dealing with the problems of intravascular stent material, early stent failure, and factors which influence the complete endothelialization of the stent, came from a small number of experimental working groups (PALMAZ et al. 1985, 1988a,b, 1990; ROUSSEAU et al. 1987, 1989; STRECKER 1988; LIERMANN 1990).

PALMAZ (1997) recommends the final expansion of the stent to be 10%–15% larger than the matched diameter of the vessel adjacent to the target point, to achieve embedment of the stent struts. If the stent is deployed without this slight overexpansion, the struts will not become embedded and thrombus formation occurs between and behind the struts, and re-endothelialization is much slower. Slower re-endothelialization results in increased thrombus deposition, proliferation of muscle cells, and decreased luminal diameter.

In small arteries, there is a correlation between slow flow and intimal hyperplasia, because slow flow induces subocclusive thrombus formation (PALMAZ et al. 1988b). Also, in arteries with larger diameters, low flow induces the same amount of thrombus, but the result is a lower reduction of the vessel diameter, and therefore the patency rate is higher than after thrombus formation in small arteries. With this theory in mind, prolonged anticoagulation with coumarin was recommended in situations with slow flow in arteries.

The following uncovered stents have been fitted to date in hundreds of patients, without high-risk complications.

The Strecker Stent (Boston Scientific) (Fig. 5.14). The Strecker stent is balloon-expandable and consists of a single tantalum wire woven in loosely connected loops. It is mounted on an ultra-thin balloon-angioplasty catheter with silicon sleeves at both ends. At dilatation, the stent does not shorten since the meshes of the stent are pushed together in a longitudinal direction and interlock when dilated. The Strecker stent has a good radiation absorption

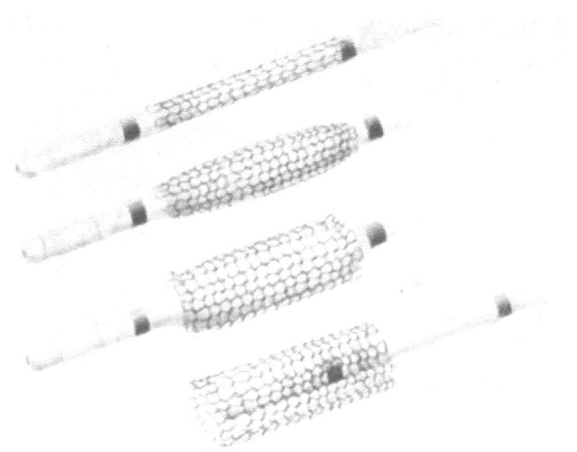

Fig. 5.14. Balloon-expandable Strecker stent made of tantalum. *Top to bottom*, stent fixed on the balloon catheter with metal marker, gradual deployment of the stent, and fully deployed stent, allowing the catheter to be withdrawn

during fluoroscopy and can be easily detected, even in the abdomen and pelvis. In imaging studies with magnetic resonance tomography (MRT), no artifacts are produced (Matsumoto et al. 1989; Liermann 1995). There is no contraindication for MRT examinations, as this stent is not ferromagnetic.

The Wallstent (Boston Scientific) (Fig. 5.15). The Wallstent is a self-expanding device, made of a tubular-woven wire net of medical-grade stainless-steel filament (non-soldered wires). It is attached to the catheter by a double membrane, thus rendering its surface smooth and atraumatic. On withdrawal of the protective membrane, the stent can increase its diameter. The stent then shortens from distal to proximal, in relation to the catheter tip, and exerts force on the inner wall of the vessel. The woven wire net does not absorb very much radiation, and the stent is not easily identifiable in the abdomen and pelvis.

The Easy Wallstent, with optimized radiopacity, is high flexible in positioning around the bifurcation. It is easy to use, with the option to reposition the stent following partial deployment. Thorough preparation is required prior to application in order to avoid dislocation of the stent while the membrane is pulled back.

The newer "Easy Wallstent", in contrast, has higher radio-absorption and can be better controlled under fluoroscopy, and preparation before application causes no problems. Additionally, application is much easier.

The Palmaz Stent (Johnson & Johnson/Cordis) (Fig. 5.16). The Palmaz stent is a balloon-expandable stent that consists of a thin-walled tube of stainless steel with longitudinal slits. When dilated by the balloon, it reveals a net-like structure. Stents of 40 mm in length shorten only by a few millimeters when dilated.

The long medium-spiral "Palmaz-Schatz" stent is also balloon-expandable, and the wall thickness could be reduced to 0.1397 mm. Three lengths are available: 42, 56, and 78 mm. The diameter corresponds to the diameter of the artery to be treated. The Palmaz stent was very stiff, whereas the long medium-spiral stent is a little more flexible. Its application in and over strongly angulated bifurcations is impossible.

The Bard Stent (Memotherm); (Angiomed, Karlsruhe) (Fig. 5.17). The Memotherm is a self-expanding stent made of nitinol shape-memory

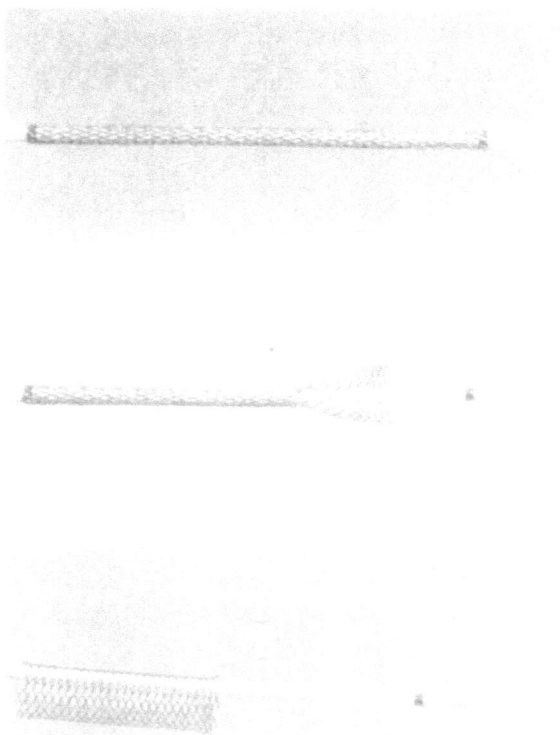

Fig. 5.15. Self-expanding Wallstent. *Top*, a protective membrane fixes the stent on the catheter. By withdrawal of the protective membrane, the stent is enabled to fully deploy, whereby it slightly shortens. *Bottom*, fully deployed and shortened stent

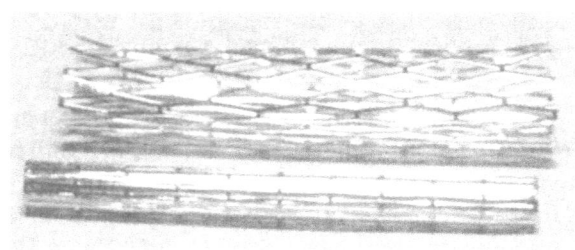

Fig. 5.16. Balloon-expandable Palmaz stent in closed and deployed state. Perflex stent, flexible stainless-steel stent with spined sinusoidal wave pattern, recommended for contralateral iliac stenting

metal. The special diamond-shape reconstruction shows no shortening during placement. The stent is flexible, has a smooth surface and a low profile. The stents are delivered with the aid of a delivery device. They have low radiopacity, which renders the correction of the stent position during placement impossible. One must therefore position the stent with the aid of the radiopaque markers. The markers reflect the true length of the deployed stent. When the most

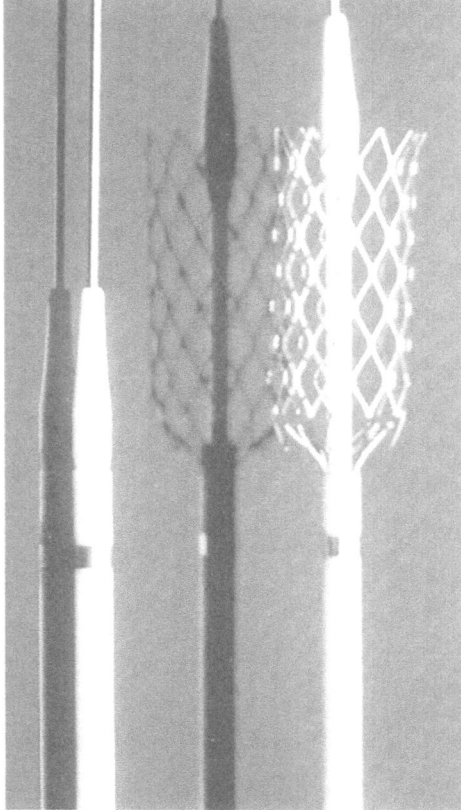

Fig. 5.17. Bard-Stent "Memotherm"

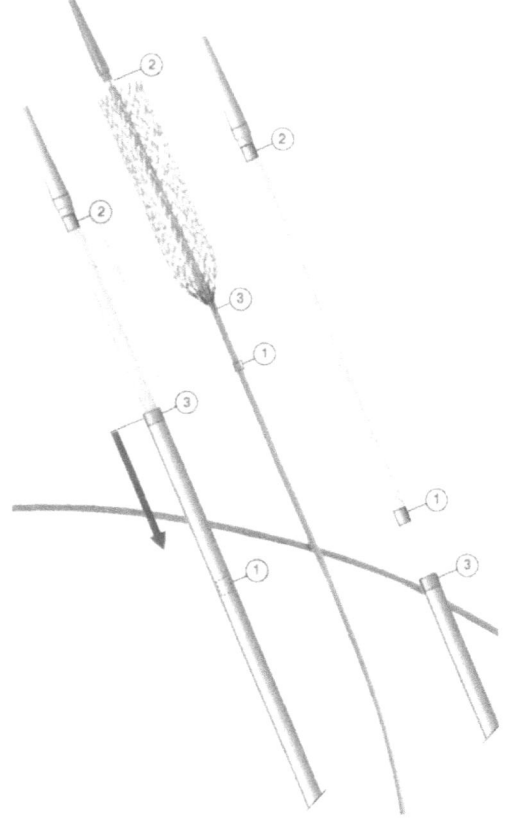

Fig. 5.18. SMART (shape-memory alloy recoverable technology) nitinol stent (Cordis and Johnson & Johnson

distal mark has passed the proximal marker, the stent is fully released.

The InStent (Vascu-Coil) (Fig. 5.20) The InStent, a self-expanding nitinol stent, is a simple coil with two terminal end balls that are used for mounting it on the catheter. There are loose windings in the middle of the stent which correspond to the released stent length, which are embraced by dense windings proximal and distal of the stent. A fixed marker assures precise positioning of the distal end of the stent.

Provided it is true that the least metal used in the application of an endovascular stent as possible, the lower the risk of intimal hyperplasia formation, the InStent would be of particular advantage.

The Sinus Nitinol Stent (Opti-Med, Ettlingen) (Fig. 5.19). The Sinus stent is a nitinol self-expanding, shape-memory stent. The diameter ranges between 4 and 12 mm, and it is 0.21 mm thick. The stent has good radiopacity once it is deployed. A total of 91% of the arterial surface remains free from metal con-

tact. The diameter should be 10%–20% larger than that of the artery. Before and after stent placement, balloon dilatation is recommended. The Sinus stent also has a small amount of metal. Extensive prospective studies have not been conducted as yet.

The "Symphony" Nitinol Stent (Boston Scientific) (Fig. 5.21). This stent has a constant self-expansion with excellent radial force, in balance with natural vessel compliance, it overcomes recoil, and maintains luminal patency. The open stent geometry minimizes neointimal accumulation, promoting maximal luminal size and side-branch patency. Its reduced metallic content minimizes turbulent flow through the stented segment. Rounded ends promote an atraumatic transition from stent to vessel wall and minimize abrasion of dilatation balloon surfaces at post-dilatation. In contrast to early nitinol stents, the Symphony offers precise positioning, accurate placement with a low-profile delivery system, and excellent trackability. Stent diameters are between 6 and 14 mm and lengths between 22 and 60 mm. The delivery-catheter shaft length is 75 or

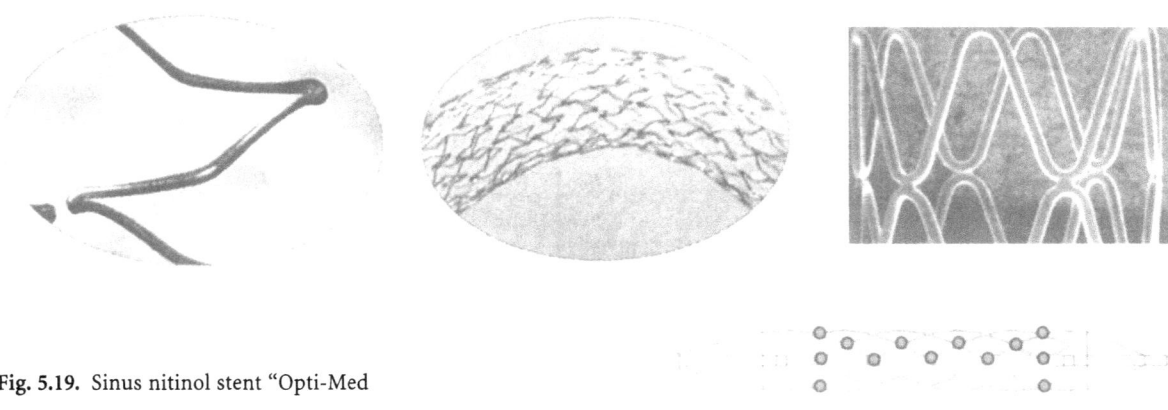

Fig. 5.19. Sinus nitinol stent "Opti-Med

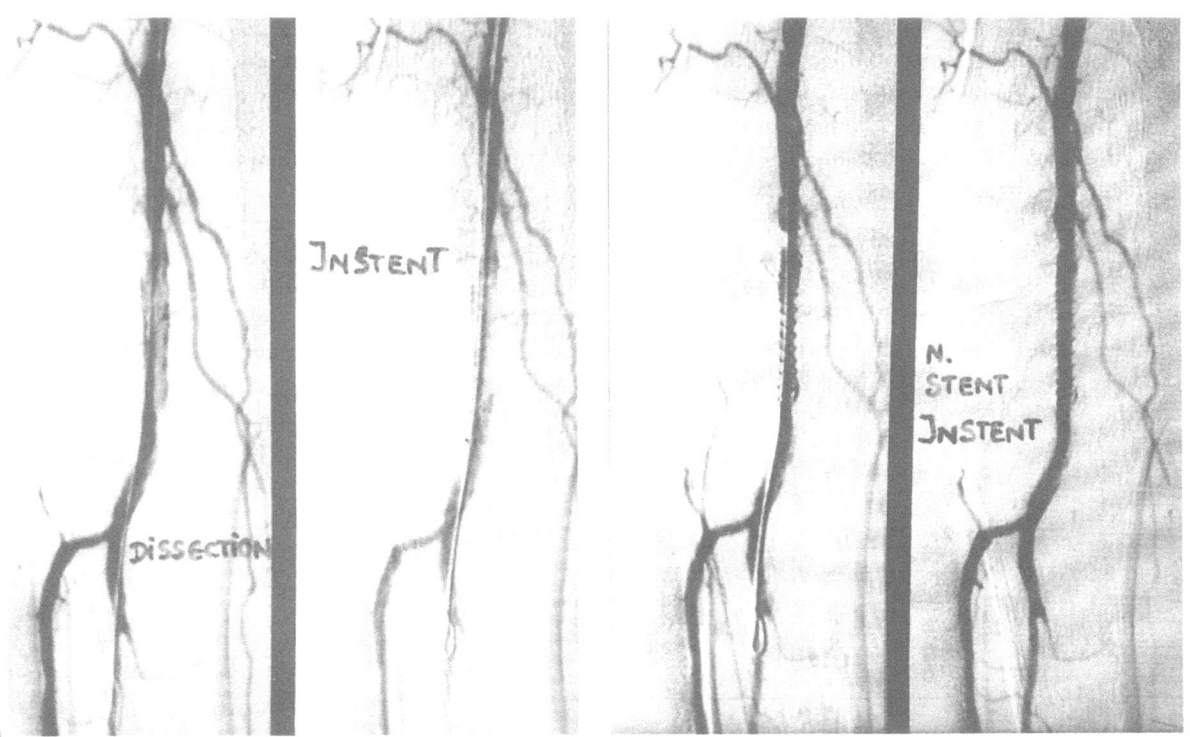

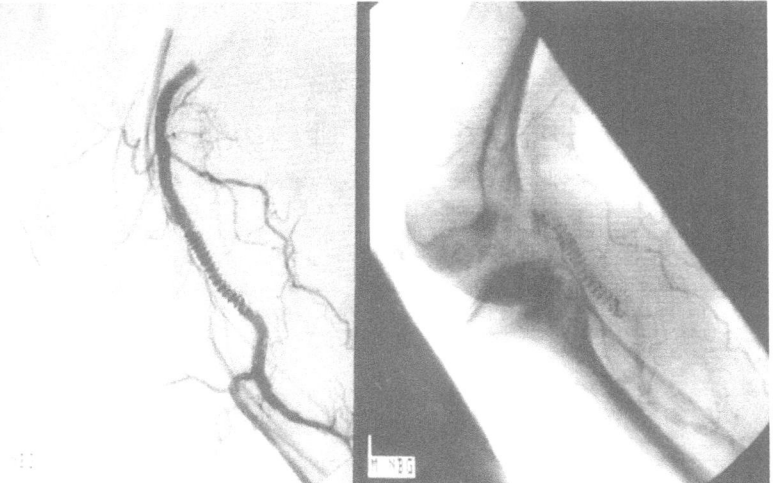

Fig. 5.20 a–c. Application of an InStent (Vascu-Coil) in the popliteal artery of a 65-year-old woman with popliteal stenosis and only one patent tibioperoneal artery. **a** High-grade dissection at the site of stenosis after balloon dilatation, and placing of the low-metal spiral InStent. **b** First angiography with the stent in place, followed by additional balloon dilatation inside the stent, showing no residual stenosis and good flow. **c** No kink in the popliteal artery before and in the area of the placed stent, at bended knee, both with and without subtraction

110 cm and the recommended sheath is 7 F, with a 0.035-in. guidewire.

5.1.5.1
Clinical Results

Some prospective and more retrospective controlled trials in balloon and stent PTA (CAPEK et al. 1991; GALLINO et al. 1984; ROCKE et al. 1987; SOULEN and GROFFISKY 1995; SCHNEIDEK et al. 1982; JOHNSTON et al. 1987; RICHTER et al. 1991; HENRY 1998; VORWERK and GÜNTHER 1997; STRECKER et al. 1993; VOGELZANG 1996), in addition to more practical experience from European and US hospitals, demonstrated excellent results in iliac arteries and less favorable results in femoral and popliteal arteries.

Between 1987 and 1992, during which time we placed 201 stents in 117 patients (2.8% of all PTA patients) at our department in Nuremberg, many papers were published about stent placement in different population groups. The results of a literature search, together with the data published in the paper by KOLLATH and LIERMANN in 1995, give us information about the mean complication and restenosis rates (Table 5.6), independent of the indication, length, and number of stents in one artery.

In the years 1990–1994, the central documentation of the German Working Group on Interven-tional Radiology (AGIR) was able to collect data on 886 patients with stent placement in iliac arteries, showing primary success in 89.5%, 6.9% complications, and a total fluoroscopy time per procedure of 17 (±11.4) min.

In 366 patients who received stents in the femoropopliteal arteries, clinical success was documented in 80.8%, with a complication rate of 7.9%, and a fluoroscopy time for the complete angioplasty, including stent application, of 20.2 (±13.6) min.

Whereas primary technical success in iliac and femoropopliteal arteries varies between 92% and 99%, clinical success has a wide range in different lesions and patient population groups of between 80% and 100% (VORWERK 1997). According to the Rutherford criteria, it is important to clearly differentiate between primary and secondary, or assisted cumulative patency rates. To compare the results in different lesions and anatomical areas, Table 5.7 gives an overview. But it is without question that also the learning period and the control method used during follow-up (clinical, hemodynamic, or angiographic studies), the use of anticoagulation with coumarin/warfarin, the administration of ASA alone, or additional ticlopidine hydrochloride, clopidogrel, or others, have a considerable influence on the results. Prospective trials alone can clearly document which stent yields the best final results in which anatomical location.

Table 5.6. Complications and restenosis rates after stent treatment

Patients (n)	Complications (%)	Restenosis rate (%)	Artery
>1800	7	8	Iliac artery
>500	15	27	Femoro popliteal artery
≈200	12	24	Renal artery

Table 5.7. Results of stent-assisted PTA in different peripheral arteries. (According to Knowledge Finder, 1994, and HENRY et al. 1998)

Location in different arteries	Primary technical success (%)	Primary patency rate		Secondary patency rate
		1 year (%)	2 years (%)	1 year (%)
Common iliac	95	94	85	98
External iliac	90	88	75	95
SFA proximal	90	80	66	82
SFA distal	85	65	49	80
Popliteal	70	50	40	76
Subclavian	95	90	86	92

SFA, superficial femoral artery.

The comparison of our initial results with stents in iliofemoral arteries (ZEITLER et al. 1995b) between the first 40 and the second 40 patients have provided some information on technical aspects. The population consisted of 70 men and 10 women, with a mean age of 59 (37–82) years. We applied 136 stents in the following locations:

- Common iliac arteries: 46
- External iliac arteries: 36
- Superficial femoral arteries: 49
- Popliteal arteries: 3
- Common femoral artery: 1
- Deep femoral artery: 1.

The 136 stents implanted in the course of this study consisted of 98 Strecker stents and 38 Wallstents. The mean follow-up control was 22.3 months in group 1, and 6 months in group 2.

In group I, stent occlusions occurred in six patients in the iliac (19%), and in five patients (31%) in the femoropopliteal arteries. In group II, stent occlusions occurred in five (15%) in the iliac, and in two (15%) in the femoropopliteal arteries. Re-occlusions in iliac arteries occurred only in patients after treatment of occlusions. Restenoses and re-occlusions without acute thrombosis in the first days showed up mainly between months 6 and 12. The re-occlusion rate in group I in total was 30% and could be reduced to 16% in group II, which represents a learning curve in the application of stents, especially close to the aortic bifurcation and with problems in the overlapping of two stents in one artery.

As regards long-term results, additional medicamentous treatment with or without anticoagulation (Marcumar) has shown better long-term primary cumulative patency rates in iliac and femoropopliteal stenting in patients with Marcumar. Also, the 1- and 2-year secondary patency rates were significantly better in patients who received Marcumar during follow-up. After 1 year, however, Marcumar administration was interrupted for various reasons such as bleeding or operations for other diseases.

Comparing the two stent types in iliac arteries, the 1- and 2-year secondary patency rates after Wallstent application was 100%, whereas after Strecker stent application it was 80%.

MATHIAS (Chap. 35, Sect. 35.4) has shown that in the subclavian and brachiocephalic arteries, stents help to reduce the occurrence of residual stenoses. Also, in the US, KUMAR et al. (1995) demonstrated good results after primary stenting with the Palmaz stent for the treatment of subclavian artery obstructions.

In more peripherally located arteries (arm, brachial, and forearm arteries), as well as in the tibiofibular region, no important study has been published as yet. However, to prevent acute thrombotic occlusion after dissection, or in the event of collapsing arteries after balloon dilatation or recanalization with the Rotablator or other atherectomy devices, the new nitinol stents with their small diameter and minimally thin metal seem to be useful.

5.1.5.2
Covered Stents

The idea of transluminally placed endovascular stent grafts was initially conceived by CHARLES DOTTER (1969). Some investigators followed his proposal with feasibility research, using experimental animal models of abdominal aortic aneurysms (PARODI et al. 1991; CHUTER et al. 1993; BALDO et al. 1986). Recently, the clinical use of endovascular stent grafts was described for the treatment of abdominal aortic aneurysm, subclavian artery aneurysm, arteriovenous fistula (Table 5.8), and is discussed in Chap. 17 in the section by HEILBERGER et al.

The endovascular application of covered stents is now of great interest also in the treatment of peripheral vascular disease and not only in the treatment of aortic dissections and aneurysms, with cut-down of the femoral artery in the groin or subclavian artery near the axilla. There are several important indications for the use of covered stents in iliac, femoral, popliteal, subclavian, carotid, and brachial arteries, with the possibility of reducing operative risks, hospitalization times, and possibly costs. These include:

- Arterial injury or iatrogenic rupture of arteries
- Arteriovenous fistulas, as these can be the result of trauma, surgery, interventional radiology, or tumor
- Aneurysms of the iliac, subclavian, femoropopliteal, and other arteries

In addition, there is great interest in the management of long occlusions of the superficial femoral artery with covered stents as an alternative to bypass surgery. Balloon PTA and uncovered stents had shown high and early restenosis and re-occlusion rates in these extensive obliterations.

The covered stents first used for the treatment of arterial and aortic rupture, or the treatment of abdominal or thoracic aortic aneurysms (dissections) were the PALMAZ, CRAGG, or GIANTURCO-RÖSCH-Z stents (GRZ-stents). These stents have been rendered non-porous, their outer surface having attached classical polyesters, well-known in surgery and as vascular prosthetic material (Dacron, PTFE, or autogenous veins) (VOLODOS et al. 1991; PARODI et al. 1991; SAYERS et al. 1993; MAY et al. 1994; MARIN et al. 1994b; HAGEN et al. 1993; RICHTER et al. 1994; DAKE et al. 1994).

The use of stent grafts for occlusive arterial disease is still controversial, since the healing modes and efficacy of these devices have not yet been defined. The use of stent grafts for aneurysmal and occlusive arterial disease has caused systemic reactions, e.g., fever, blood sedimentation rate (BSR) elevation, and pain lasting over days and weeks, which still remain unexplained.

The materials used for the manufacture of covered stents are widely known, but their use in combination with other materials needs futher experimental and clinical studies. The classic materials used to cover metal stents include Dacron, PET and expanded Teflon, or PTFE. In direct comparison with PTFE, PET absorbs more protein and blood cells in particular macrophages. The lower thrombogenicity of PTFE has favored this material for small-caliber bypass surgery. Dacron, however, is preferred for large conduit bypasses, because of its superior handling characteristics (PALMAZ 1997).

The various covered stents or endovascular grafts for percutaneous application can still not be considered as final products, but demonstrate the beginning of a new era of endovascular treatment of obliterations, aneurysms, and arteriovenous fistulas.

The most experience has been gained to date with the following devices:

Passager (formerly Endopro I- and II-Stent). The nitinol Cragg stent is covered with polyester on the outside. The stent is loaded on a special cartouche and, with the help of a pushing device, the stent is deployed under fluoroscopy (Fig. 5.21). Percutaneous application through a long vascular sheath and precise placement in iliac, femoral, and popliteal arteries is possible with up to 10 F. For the application of endovascular grafts to treat aortic aneurysms, open surgery of the femoral artery in the groin is necessary since the application device has a diameter of 20–24 F.

Smaller stent grafts can be introduced through a 7-F sheath with a long 7-F application catheter, as well as through the femoral artery in retro- and antegrade directions, or in a retrograde direction from the popliteal artery (CRAGG et al. 1983; HENRY et al. 1994, 1996). The stent graft is presented in compressed form in a loading cartridge, and for use in the superficial femoral artery it is available in 3–20 cm lengths. The application system is a 50-cm long introducer sheath, varying between 7 and 10 F, depending on the size of the stent graft to be implanted. For occlusive disease, balloon angioplasty

Table 5.8. Covered stents – endografts (see also Chap. 17, Sect. 17.4) -CEG-

Stent type	Material	Manufacturer	In use
Cragg-EndoPro	Nitinol, self-expanding with polyester	Mintec, Boston Scientific	-
Vanguard	Nitinol, self-expanding Sutured to the skeleton	Boston Scientific	+
EGS (*formerly EVT*) (Endovascular Grafting System)	Self-expanding, zig-zag attachments with polyester	Endovascular Technologies	++
Hemobahn	Self-expanding nitinol with ultra-thin PTFE	W.L. GoreProgaft	++
Talent	Nitinol (balloon-expandable) with Dacron	World Medical	++
Zenith	Self-expanding external stent with Dacron	Cook	++
AneuRx	Self-expanding external stent with Dacron	Stentgraft	++
Wallgraft	Covered Wallstent	Boston Scientific	

Characteristics of optimal endografts:
  Flexible, over-the-wire use
  dequate self-expansion power
  olid metal cylinder, break-resistant
  Good radiopacity in important parts
  Biocompatibility
  Low thrombogenicity
  Easy handling
  Small application system

PTFE, polytetrafluoroethylene.

Fig. 5.21. Different types of modifications of the Vanguard-endovascular graft (Meadox Boston Scientific, formerly Stentor-Mintec Company). *1* Bifurcated aortoiliac graft; *2* long and short covered grafts (iliac artery and superficial femoral artery); *3* straight covered aorta graft; *4* uncovered nitinol stent. The covered stents are covered with 0.1-mm thin uncrimped Dacron on the outside

has to be performed first in order to enlarge the arterial lumen. HENRY recommends debulking techniques using the Rotablator before application of the stent graft in the superficial femoral artery (HENRY et al. 1993a). Platinum markers at both ends of the stent assist in the precise positioning of the device. Once the stent graft is in position, the sheath is withdrawn and an internal positioning catheter is used to fix the stent graft in place. The stent graft expands by means of the thermal memory characteristics of its nitinol frame. This is usually followed by dilatation with an angioplasty balloon catheter at pressures of between 10 and 16 atm, which fixes the graft against the arterial wall and helps unwrinkle the fabric. When several grafts are needed to cover a lesion, it is important that the prostheses overlap one another by at least 5 mm, so that the fabric portion of the graft covers the entire arterial lumen.

The Corvita-Endovascular Graft (CEG). This graft consists of two components:

1. A self-expanding cylindrical wire structure made of a braided wire mesh
2. A highly porous and elastic coating on the inner surface of the structure, made of layers of polyurethane fibres in which blood can coagulate and which can seal the CEG to form a new blood-tight vessel wall.

This flexible CEG can be compressed into between 8- and 10-F introducer sheaths, allowing a percutaneous entry. It can be produced in various lengths (3–30 cm) and diameters (4–40 mm), cut to length by the user, and is released from the introducer sheath at the intended site by coaxial introduction of a "holding" catheter and slow pull-back of the introducer sheath.

Up to now, experience with percutaneous application has been gained in only a small number of departments and some of the most significant results have been published by HENRY et al. (1998). They presented their results with the Cragg EndoPro system/Passager system in 142 locations, including 20 aneurysms, with excellent patency rates up to 2 years in the iliac artery after treatment of stenotic and occlusive lesions (primary patency 94%, secondary patency 100%), whereas in the superficial femoral artery, the primary and secondary patency rates for occlusive and stenotic lesions after 2 years were 64% and 76%, respectively.

HENRY et al. have also published the results of their treatment of 64 lesions with the CORVITA graft, with a patency rate at the iliac level of 88.2% primary, and a 93.2% secondary cumulative patency rate, and at the femoropopliteal level, a 1-year patency rate of 76.8% primary and a 84.3% secondary cumulative patency rate.

Hemobahn Endovascular Graft. The pro-graft "Hemobahn" is a self-expanding endovascular stent graft, composed of 30-μm intranodal, ultra-thin-wall PTFE graft material on the inner surface, and a self-expanding nitinol stent on the exterior. This device has excellent flexibility both in the deployed and non-deployed state, excellent kink resistance, and good radial stiffness (DAKE 1998) (Fig. 5.22). Initial results in three departments in the US and 30 European centers included 106 patients. In the iliac artery, the average device diameter was 8.4 mm (range, 6–13 mm) and the average device length was 7.0 cm (range, 5–15 cm). The average number of devices used per limb treated was 1.24 (range, 1–3). The averae device diameter in the femoral group was 6.3 mm (range, 6–7 mm), and the average device length was 12.3 cm (range, 5–15 cm). The primary technical success was 99%, the primary and secondary iliac cumulative patency rate at 6 months was 98%, and the primary patency for treated femoral arteries at 6 months was 83%. Procedure-related complications included distal embolization in 4.4%, groin hematoma in 2.7%, and iliac artery rupture in 0.9% of cases.

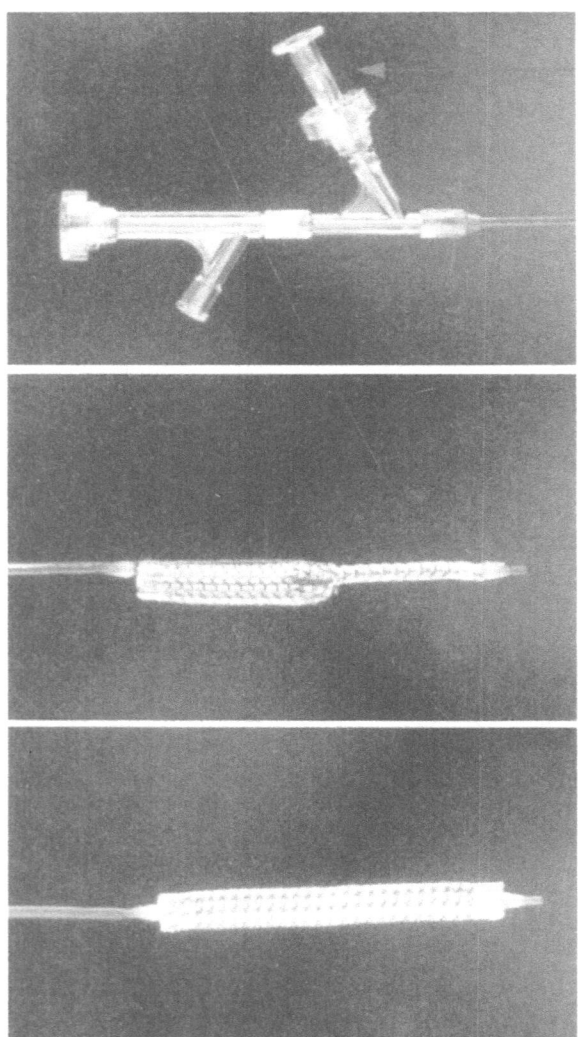

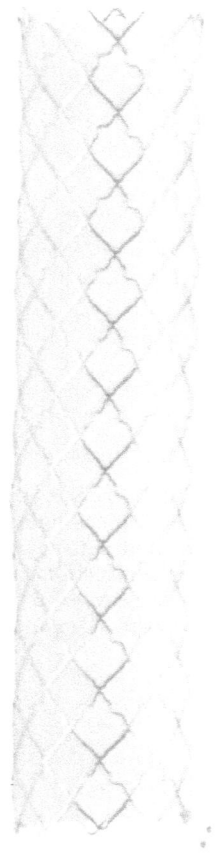

Fig. 5.22. Hemobahn endovascular graft with an inner fabric (ultra-thin PTFE) and outer self-expanding nitinol stent

Covered endoprostheses enable a true internal bypass using the percutaneous access to be performed. The indications might become an alternative to surgery. The most important indications are: iliac, femoral, and popliteal aneurysms, as well as subclavian aneurysms, or aneurysms in the carotid arteries in the neck. They are also under discussion for the treatment of superficial femoral artery obliterations longer than 10 cm, to improve long-term patency rates. Several experimental and clinical investigations are still necessary before the general application of covered stents in femoropopliteal arteries can be recommended.

The new product "Wallgraft" is recomended to treat aneurysms av-shunts and critical obliteriontions (e. g. carotid and SFA-obliterations).

5.1.6
Classification of Arterial Obliterations

There are several classifications of arterial obliterations in the different areas of the arterial system which serve as a basis to distinguish between acute and chronic obliterations suited for thromboembolectomy, primary bypass-surgery, primary interventional techniques, combined procedures, or conservative methods alone.

In Tables 5.9–5.11, clinical categories of acute and chronic limb ischemia according to Rutherford and Becker summarize all clinical possibilities. The Society of Cardiovascular and Interventional Radiology (SCVIR Syllabus 1994) and the German Working Group on IR (AGIR) have published recommendations for percutaneous angioplasty techniques in classes I–IV in an attempt to avoid surgery. These form the basis of our recommendations as summarized in Figs. 5.23–5.27. In general, in each region, class I is an excellent indication for PTA, whereas class IV is a primary indication for vascular surgery, provided there is no contraindication. In classes II and III, no general recommendations are possible since the individual situation, for example additional coronary heart disease, diabetes, or renal insufficiency, has great bearing on the procedure to be preferred.

In patients with intermittent claudication, in the case of single-level lesions, especially in the superficial femoral artery, a 3-week course of physical therapy with exercise in several cases, in addition to the treatment of the risk factors, brings the patient into an acceptable condition with no operation or intervention.

On the other hand, in patients with isolated stenoses in the iliac or popliteal arteries, early dilatation in the hands of an experienced radiologist very quickly re-establishes a good condition, and exercise treatment, as well as the treatment of risk factors, can follow. In this situation, the patient has less pain and the duration of the disease is shortened. However, it is important to prevent complications, which is of utmost importance in patients with a bad run-off

condition. In this case, direct intraarterial administration of urokinase (up to 1 000 000 IU) can follow a PTA procedure to explore for local emboli.

In patients with critical limb ischemia (Fontaine classification III and IV or Rutherford classes 4 to 6) or in young patients with two or three run-off arteries, however, the indication for bypass-surgery, if feasible, is the better solution because of excellent long-term patency rates. But in all other cases with critical limb ischemia, or claudication in patients aged over 60 years, angioplasty has a primary indication in class I–III obliterations.

Without question, in each patient and clinic the best type of treatment is judged on an individual basis and is the result of interdisciplinary cooperation. Figures 5.23–5.27 can be used as widely accepted indications with some personal modifications. It is also important to consider that class I and II lesions can be treated as outpatient procedures, whereas classes III and IV require stationary control and additional therapy (ZEITLER 1988).

Note: References for Sects 5.1–5.3 can be found at the end of Sect. 5.3.

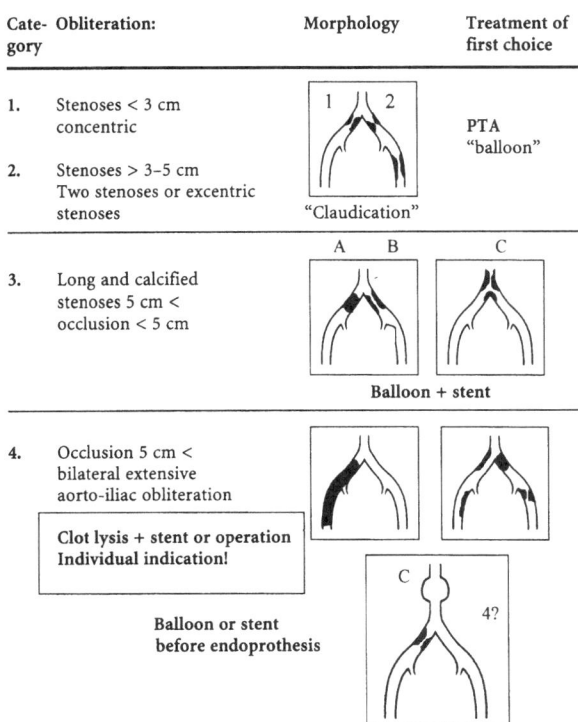

Fig. 5.23. Categories of obliteration (SCVIR/AGIR Guidelines 1998) in iliac arteries

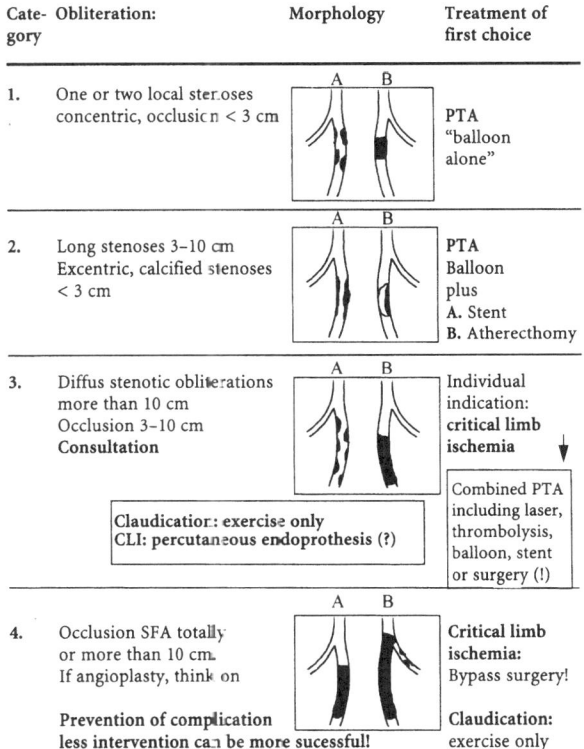

Fig. 5.24. Categories of obliteration (SCVIR/AGIR Guidelines 1998) in femoral arteries. *CLI,* critical limb ischemia, *SFA,* supeficial femoral artery

Cate-gory	Obliteration:	Morphology	Treatment of first choice
1.	Isolated stenoses Short occlusion < 3 cm **After imaging in B:** Atherectomy or balloon		A. Angioplasty B. Imaging; US, MRI or CT! individual
2.	Long stenoses 3 cm < Occlusion 3 cm < Also obliterations below knee **Critical limb ischemia: femoro-crural bypass**		A. PTA B. Combined PTA including clot lysis and balloon and aspiration (RAT-PAT)
3.	Diffus stenotic obliterations One stenosis + short occlusion **Critical limb ischemia: femoro-crural bypass**		A. Conservative or laser-assisted PTA B. PTA + urokinase 100 000 IU(?)
4.	Total occlusion Aneurysmatic stenoses Individual indication **Age! Symptoms! Endoprothesis Femoro-crural bypass**		A. **Surgery** or conservative B. Surgery or conservative or endo-prothesis

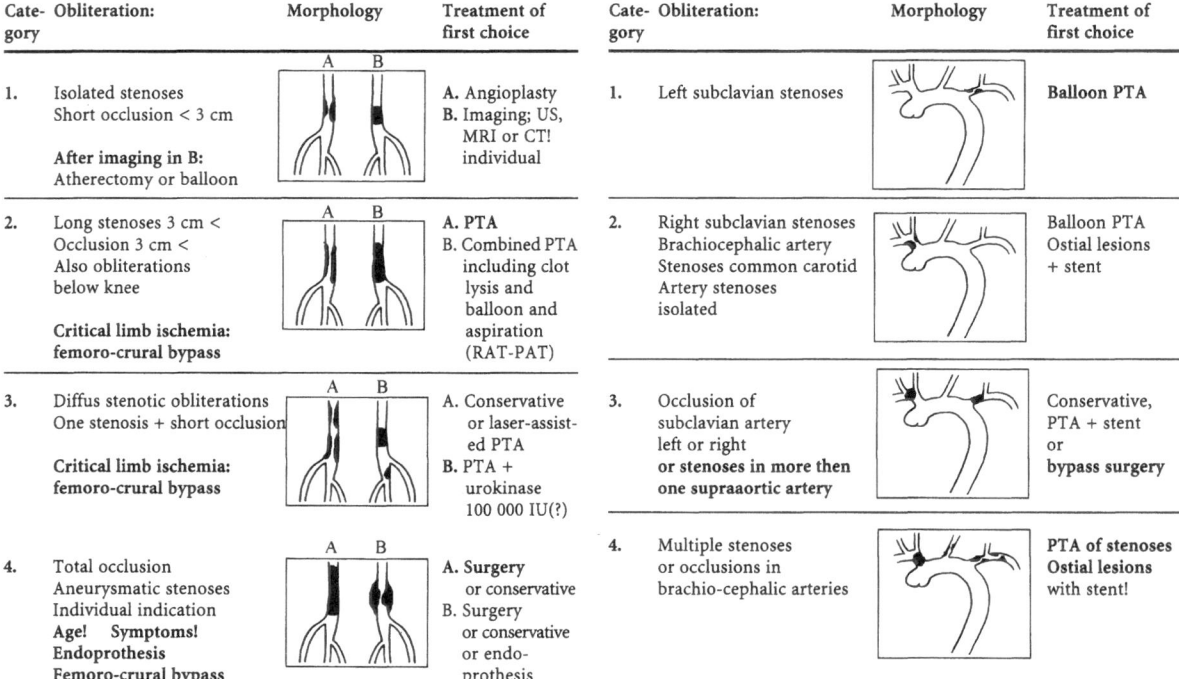

Fig. 5.25. Categories of obliteration (SCVIR/AGIR Guidelines 1998) in the popliteal artery. *US*, ultrasonography; *MRI*, magnetic resonance imaging; *CT*, computed tomography; *RAT-PAT*, rotational aspiration thromboembolectomy-percutaneous AT

Cate-gory	Obliteration:	Morphology	Treatment of first choice
1.	Isolated stenoses **Exercise!**		Only in addition to femoro-pop-liteal PTA and rest pain or CLI: balloon PTA small balloons
2.	Two or more stenoses **Treatment of risk-factors!**		A. As in Category 1 B. Conservative or femoro-crural bypass
3.	Occlusion < 3 cm Two or three stenoses in two tibio-fibular arteries Individual indication **Critical limb ischemia: femoro-crural bypass**		A. As in Category 1 B. small-balloon PTA small balloons or laser-assisted PTA
4.	Multiple occlusions Diffuse arteriosclerosis of two or three arteries If last alternative in patients interest after consultation: **Rotablator!**		A + B CLI: femoro-pedal bypass and/or sympathicolysis or laser-assisted PTA

Fig. 5.26. Categories of obliteration (SCVIR/AGIR Guidelines 1998) in infrapopliteal arteries. CLI, critical limb ischemia

Cate-gory	Obliteration:	Morphology	Treatment of first choice
1.	Left subclavian stenoses	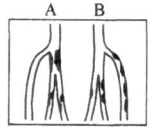	**Balloon PTA**
2.	Right subclavian stenoses Brachiocephalic artery Stenoses common carotid Artery stenoses isolated		Balloon PTA Ostial lesions + stent
3.	Occlusion of subclavian artery left or right **or stenoses in more then one supraaortic artery**		Conservative, PTA + stent or **bypass surgery**
4.	Multiple stenoses or occlusions in brachio-cephalic arteries		**PTA of stenoses Ostial lesions** with stent!

Fig. 5.27. Categories of obliteration (SCVIR/AGIR Guidelines 1998) in brachio-cephalic arteries

5.2
Pharmacological Thrombolysis

E. ZEITLER

Different techniques may be used:

1. Systemic thrombolysis: With intravenous long-term infusion of fibrinolytic agents (strep-tokinase, urokinase, plasminogen) (HEIMIG and MARTIN 1997).
2. Intraarterial thrombolysis: The thrombolytic agent is infused via a catheter placed in the artery (MCNAMARA and FISCHER 1985; LAMMER et al. 1986) in the area supplying the thrombotic occlusion or embolus for a few hours, if necessary some days, under simultaneous heparinization.
3. *Intrathrombotic "clot lysis"*: A catheter with side ports (Fig. 5.28) in varying formation is advanced directly into the occluding thrombus. The fibrinolytic agent can then be released in continuous or pulsed mode, whereby the pulsed application can be effected manually or mechanically (HESS et al. 1978; HESS and MIETASCHK 1982; BOOKSTEIN and VALJI 1992; TOENNESEN and HOLSTEIN 1992; LAMMER et al. 1985).

Table 5.9. Categories of acute ischemia according to the International Society of Cardiovascular Surgery. [from SCVIR SYLLABUS (1994)]

Category	Sensory loss	Muscle weakness	Doppler signal	
			Arterial	Venous
Viable	None	None	+	+
Threatened				
– Acutely	None or minimal (toes)	None	-	+
– Immediately	More than toes with pain at rest	Mild, moderate	-	-
Irreversible	Profound, anesthetic	Profound, paralysis	-	-

Table 5.10. Rutherford categories of chronic limb ischemia. [from DURHAM and RUTHERFORD (1994)]

Categories	Clinical criteria	Treadmill + AP
0	Asymptomatic	Normal treadmill test[a] Normal walking test[b]
1	Mild claudication	Test completed AP after exercise $\geq$ 50 mmHg
2	Moderate claudication	
3	Severe claudication	Treadmill cannot be completed AP after exercise < 50 mmHg Resting ABI < 0.8
4	Rest pain	Resting AP $\leq$ 40 mmHg
5	Minor tissue loss	Resting AP $\leq$ 60 mmHg Resting ABI < 0.5
6	Major tissue loss	Same as for Category 5

[a] Treadmill exercise test: 5 min at 3 km/h on a 12° incline.
[b] Walking test: 110 steps/min for 5 min, metronome-controlled.
ABI, ankle brachial index; AP, ankle pressure.

Table 5.11. Scale for gauging the degree of improvement

Score	Degree of Improvement	Symptomatic changes
+3	Markedly improved	Symptoms gone/markedly improved ABI increased to >90
+2	Moderately improved	Symptomatic, but at least single category improvement ABI increased by >0.10
+1	Minimally improved	ABI increased by >0.1, but no categoric improvement or deterioration

ABI, ankle brachial index.

While systemic fibrinolysis always requires the control of the coagulation parameters, this is only the case for intraarterial thrombolysis if performed as long-term treatment with high doses of a thrombolytic agent. Intrathrombotic clot lysis, which should be completed within 2, at maximum 4 h, does not require such strong controls in most circumstances. Special indications, for example the thrombolysis of thrombosed bypasses, require longer clot thrombolysis times. The control of the coagulation parameters, however, is imperative in these cases, as systemic thrombolysis may occur.

While short-term low-dose thrombolyses are performed in the interventional angio-suite only, long-term thrombolyses need to be observed later on in the intensive care unit (DEMBSKI and FEITLER 1978; MCNAMARA and FISHER 1985; HESS et al. 1987). The different principles of thrombolysis also result from the varying amounts of thrombolytic agents applied (Table 5.12).

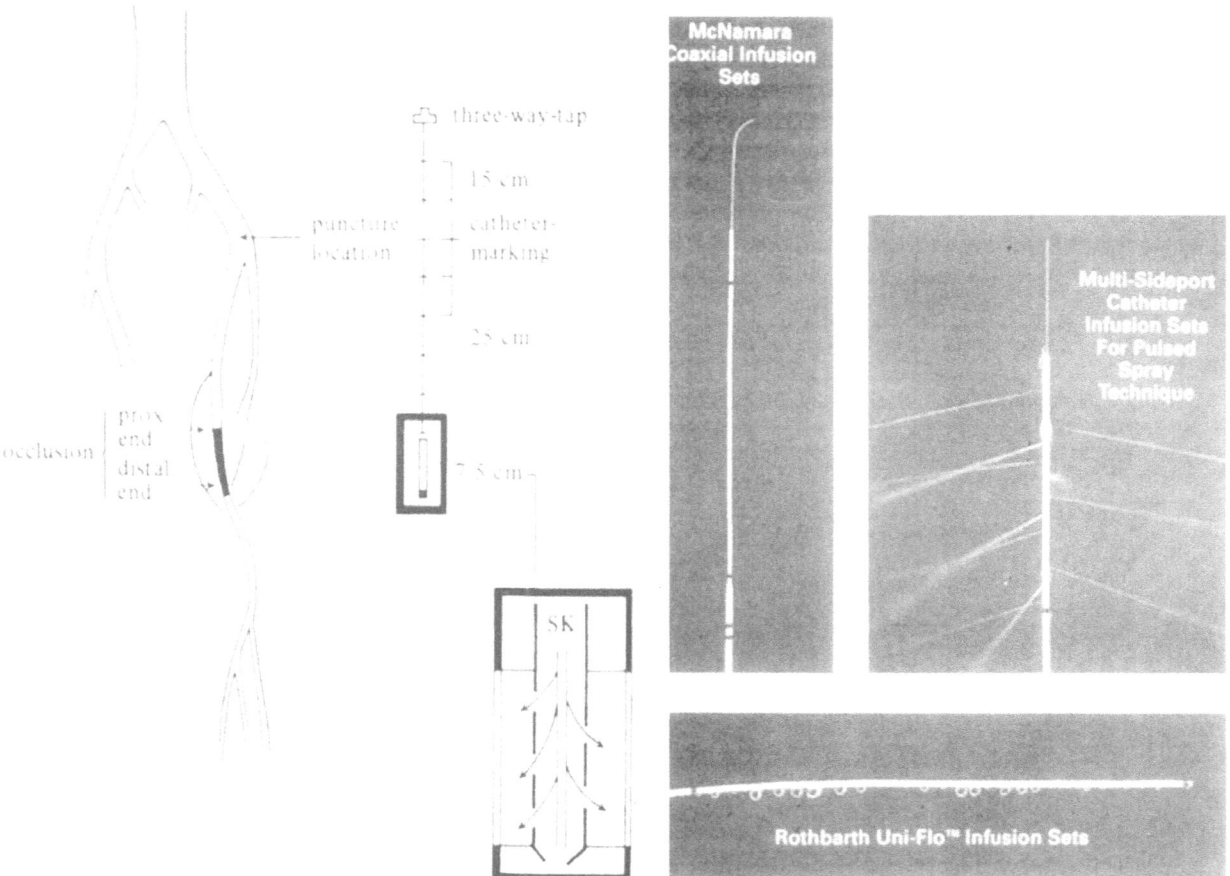

Fig. 5.28 a,b. Ideas of and different catheters for intrathrombotic administration of drugs, especially thrombolytic agents. **a** Idea of clot lysis with multiple side ports in the catheter by DEMBSKI and ZEITLER (1978). **b** Multiple side-port catheters, closed and during infusion (McNamara and Rothbart infusion sets)

Table 5.12. Local thrombolytic therapy in peripheral arteries

Thrombolytic agent	Administration	Technique	Dose
Urokinase	Intraarterial	Continuous infusion	ID: 5–10 000 IU TD: 1 million IU (50–100 000 IU/h)
Tissue-plasminogen activator (rt-plasminogen)	Intraarterial	Continuous infusion	ID: 0.15 mg–2 mg/h TD: 10 mg
Streptokinase	Intraarterial	Continuous infusion	ID: 10 000 IU TD: 250 000 IU
Urokinase	Intrathrombotic "clot lysis" with multiple side-hole catheters	Pulse-spray infusion	ID: 10 000 IU (50–100 000 IU/h) TD: 1 million IU
Tissue-plasminogen activator (rt-plasminogen)	Clot lysis	End-hole catheter (Hess technique)	ID: 1.0 mg TD: 3.0 mg
Urokinase	Clot lysis	End-hole catheter (Hess technique)	ID: 10 000 IU TD: 75–100 000 IU

ID, initial dose; TD, total dose.

Pharmacothrombolysis is capable of dissolving non-organized thrombi only. As a rule, thrombotic occlusions of arteries in the pelvis and thigh with a history of up to 6 weeks can be dissolved in large segments. Chronic thrombotic occlusions, or thromboembolic occlusions with a history of over 3 months can only be partially lysed. These cases often require complementary measures, such as PAT, balloon angioplasty, or stent application.

The contraindications to systemic thrombolysis are described in Chaps. 22 and 23. The primary results of intraarterial thrombolysis and clot lysis are mainly dependent on the location of the thrombus, history, and observance of a reliable therapeutic procedure as regards the duration of infusion and the additional administration of heparin. Primary success rates of 46%–96% are feasible. Critical complications include bleeding, embolism, and death as a result of bleeding, especially intracerebral bleeding. The incidence of such complications is higher in systemic thrombolysis than in intraarterial thrombolysis under control of the coagulation parameters, and with clot lysis at low doses of thrombolytic agents. The mechanical methods of thrombolysis have fewer bleeding complications.

5.3
Occlusion and Embolization

E. Zeitler

Transvascular percutaneous embolization can be used for controlling bleeding and for closing arteriovenous malformations or fistulas in the pelvis, shoulder, and upper and lower extremities. Whereas for neuro-embolization and embolization of parenchymal organs there is a great variety of embolic materials for temperorary and permanent vessel occlusion, in the embolotherapy of peripheral vessels, restriction to a small number of embolic materials (Table 5.13) is necessary.

Knowledge of the vascular anatomy, including variations, and the collateral circulation is essential for the prevention of complications and early recidivism. The post-embolization syndrome of fever, pain, and leucocytosis may last for several days.

There is a difference in embolization of pelvic vessels compared to arteries of the leg and arm. Indications for pelvic embolization include: Hemorrhage in pelvic fractures, tumor treatment, and congenital arteriovenous malformations.

Arterial intrapelvic hemorrhage with severe arterial, parenchymal, or venous bleeding is the most common cause of severe shock. Therefore, localization of the hemorrhage and its treatment take high priority, and the pelvic arterial hemorrhage should be replaced by transarterial hemostasis in conjunction with the reduction and internal fixation of the pelvic ring fracture (BENMENACHEM 1990).

As an embolization material, Gelfoam, either as a gel or in the form of superselective small particles, is recommended.

5.3.1
Pelvic Embolization as a Treatment of Hemorrhage in Cancer Patients (Urinary Bladder, Prostate, and Gynecological Tumors)

NOVAK (1990b) collected data from 693 patients who had pelvic embolizations. Complications occurred in 35 (5.1%), including three deaths (0.4%). Death was only seen in patients with urinary bladder tumors and hemorrhage [$n = 396$, complications 20 (5.1%), three deaths (0.8%)]. It is important to note that hemiplegia and/or paresis were encountered in 15 of 35 patients, leg ischemia in seven, skin necrosis in six, and urinary bladder gangrene in four. Complications occurred in four of 51 patients following bilateral occlusion of the hypogastric arteries in the form of uncontrollable hematuria and gynecological bleeding.

5.3.2
Selective and Superselective Embolization of Arteriovenous Malformations

Pelvic arteriovenous malformations are mainly inoperable and different symptoms can occur. Embolization can be palliative by reducing the clinical symptoms, but also pre-operative. As embolization materials, the proximal application of coils or detachable balloons cannot be recommended. Peripheral application with n-butyl-2-cyanoacrylate

Table 5.13. Embolization materials

Permanent	Temporary
Ethibloc and glucose	Ivalon
Histoacryl	Gelfoam
	Fibrospum
Detachable balloons	Coils, microcoils

(Histoacryl), Ethibloc occlusion gel, peripheral application of mini-coils or small detachable balloons close to the nidus are recommended. In addition, sclerosing therapy of draining veins can reduce the arteriovenous malformation before final surgical extirpation.

In the arm and leg, the main indications are congenital arteriovenous malformations (see Chap. 16). The aim of embolization of arteriovenous malformations in the extremities is to occlude the shunt at the level of the nidus, and to considerably diminish the blood volume shunting into the venous circulation. The primary approach should therefore be carried out using mircoparticles (150–250 µm), followed via the tracker catheter by particles of increasingly larger size. Should it become necessary, the embolization procedure can be completed by the use of mini-coils or a detachable balloon in a proximal direction; however, not at the ramification of major feeding arteries.

References

Abele JE (1980) Balloon catheters and transluminal dilatation. AJR 135:901–906

Abele JE (1983) Basic technology of balloon catheters. In: Dotter CT, Grüntzig A, Schoop W, Zeitler E (eds) Percutaneous transluminal angioplasty. Springer, Berlin Heidelberg New York, pp 31–36

AGIR Arbeitsgemeinschaft für Interventionelle Radiologie (1997) Leitlinien: 1. Gefäßrekanalisation, Röfo L4–L13

Ahn SS, Auth D, Marcus DR, Moore WS (1988) Removal of focal atheromatous lesions by angioscopically guided high-speed rotary atherectomy: Preliminary experimental observations. J Vasc Surg 7:292–300

Alpert JR, Ring EJ, Berkowitz HP, et al. (1979) Treatment of vein graft stenoses by balloon catheter dilatation. JAMA 242:2769–2771

Athanasoulis CH, et al. (eds) (1982) Interventional radiology. Saunders, Philadelphia

Bachmann DM, Casarella WJ, Sos TA (1979) Percutaneous iliofemoral angioplasty via the contralateral femoral artery. Radiology 130:617–621

Baldo A, Piasecki GZ, Shah DM, et al. (1986) Transfemoral placement of intraluminal polyurethane prosthesis for abdominal aortic aneurysm. J Surg Res 4:305–309

Bachman DM, Kim RM (1980) Transluminal dilatation for subclavian steal syndrom. SJR 135:995–996

Bates ER, O'Neill WW, Topol EJ (1988) Percutaneous atherectomy catheters. Cardiol Clin 6:373–382

Baumgartner I, Zwahlen I, Do DD, Redha F, Mahler F (1996) Color-coded duplex sonography for evaluation of femoropopliteal restenosis after percutaneous catheter atherectomy and subsequent transluminal balloon angioplasty. J Vasc Invest 2:125–130

Becker GJ (1991) Advances in angioplasty: theoretical and practical "interventional radiology". In: Mueller P (ed) Diagnostic radiology (syllabus). RSNA Publ 127–140

Becker GJ, Katzen BT, Dake MD (1989) Non-coronary angioplasty. Radiology 170:921

Ben-Menachem (1990) Bleeding from trauma. In: Dondelinger RF, Rossi P, Kurdziel JC, Wallace S (eds) Interventional Radiology. Thieme, Stuttgart, pp 378–395

Beyer-Enke SA, Loose R, Zeitler E (1996) Nurembery experience with the Redha-cut. Abstract, IMAGO 96, Nurnbery

Beyer-Enke SA, Adamus R, Loose R, Zeitler E (1997) Indikation und Erfolg der retrograden transpoplitealen Angioplastie. Aktuel Radiol 7:297–300

Block PC, Fallon JT, Elmer D (1980) Experimental angioplasty: lessons from the laboratory. AJR 135:907–912

Block PC, et al. (1981) Morphology after transluminal angioplasty in human beings. N Engl J Med 305:382–385

Bookstein JJ, Valji K (1992) Pulse-spray pharmacomechanical thrombolysis. Cardiovoasc Intervent Radiol 15:228–232

Brunner U, Grüntzig A (1975) Das Dilatationsverfahren nach Dotter in gefäßchirurgischer Sicht. Vasa 4:334–337

Brunner U, Schneider E, Gygax P (1982) Kombination der PTA mit chirurgischen Eingriffen im femoropoplitealen Bereich. Vasa 11:278–281

Capek P, McLean GK, Berkowitz HD (1991) Femoropopliteal angioplasty. Circulation 83[Suppl 1]:170–180

Castaneda-Zuniga WR (1983) Transluminal agioplasty. Thieme, Stuttgart

Castaneda-Zuniga WR, et al. (1980) The mechanism of balloon angioplasty. Radiology 135:565–571

Castaneda-Zuniga WR, et al. (1981) Mechanics of angioplasty: an experimental approach. Radiographics 1(3):1–14

Castaneda-Zuniga WR, Lock JE, Vlodaver, et al. (1982) Transluminal dilatation of coarctation of the abdominal aorta. An experimental study in dogs. Radiology 143:693–697

Chuter TA, Green RM, Ouriel K, et al. (1993) Transfemoral endovascular aortic graft placement. J Vasc Surg 18:185–195

Colapinto RF (1980) Inadvertent percutaneous transluminal dilatation of renal artery with a four year follow-up Radiology 135:605–606

Colapinto RF, Harries-Jones EP, Johnston KW (1980) Percutaneous transluminal dilatation and recanalization in the treatment of peripheral vascular disease. Radiology 135: 583–587

Colapinto RF, Haries-Jones EP, Johnston KW (1981) Percutaneous transluminal recanalization of complete ilioic artery occlusions. Arch Surg 116:277–281

Colapinto RF, Stronell RD, Johnston WK (1986) Transluminal angioplasty of complete iliac obstructions. AJR 146:854–862

Cope C, Dana R, Burke R, Meranze S (1990) Interventional radiology. Lippincott, Philadelphia

Cragg AH, Lung G, Rysavy JA, Salomonowitz E, Castaneda-Zuniga WR (1983) Percutaneous arterial grafting. Radiology 147:261–263

Dake M, Miller C, Semba CP, et al. (1994) Transluminal placement of endovascular stent-grafts for the treatment of descending thoracic aortic aneurysms. N Engl J Med 331:1729–1734

Dake MD, Semba CP, Kee ST, et al. (1998) Early results of hemobahn for the treatment of peripheral arterial disease. In: Henry M, Amor M (eds) Ninth int. course book of peripheral vascular intervention. Poris pp 259–260

Dembski JC, Zeitler E (1978) Selective arterial clot lysis with angiography catheters. In: Zeitler E, Grüntzig A, Schoop W (eds) Percutaneous vascular recanalization. Springer, Berlin Heidelberg New York, pp 157–159

Diamond NG, Casarella WJ, et al. (1979) Dilatation of critical transplant renal artery stenosis by percutaneous transluminal angioplasty. AJR 133:1167–1169

Do Dai-Do, Triller Y, Banmgartner J, Freiburghaus AU, Mahler F (1996) Percutaneous atherectomy of femoropopliteal arteries with a new atherectomy device (Redhacut): initial results. Abstract IMAGO 96, Nurnberg

Do Dai-Do, Triller J, Mahler F (1996) Erste Erfahrungen mit einem modifizierten Redha-cut zur perkutanen, transluminalen Atherektomie von femoropoplitealen Stenosen. Schweizer Gesellschaft für Angiologie, 29th annual meeting, Warth

Doder A, Zauner B, Lorenz M, Schulze-Bauer C, Pilger E (1996) Redha-cut versus balloon angioplasty in patients with femoropopliteal artery stenosis: a prospective randomized trial. Abstract IMAGO 96, Nurnberg

Dondelinger RF, Rossi P, Kurdziel JC, Wallace S (1990) Interventional Radiology. Thieme, Stuttgart

Dorros G, Jyver S, Zaitoun R, et al. (1991) Acute angiographic and clinical outcome of high-speed percutaneous rotational atherectomy (Rotablator). Cathet Cardiovasc Diagn 22:157-166

Dorros G (1996) Percutaneous Transluminal carotid PTA. Symposium on Transcatheter cardiovascular Therapies, Washington

Dotter CT (1969) Transluminally placed coil springs and arterial tube grafts. Long-term patecny in the canine popliteal artery. Invest Radiol 4:329-332

Dotter CT (1983) Transluminal angioplasty: results and future outlook. In: Dotter CT, Grüntzig A, Schoop W, Zeitler E (eds) Percutaneous transluminal angioplasty. Springer, Berlin Heidelberg New York, pp 337-338

Dotter CT, Judkins MP (1964) Transluminal treatment of arteriosclerotic obstruction: description of a new technique and a preliminary report of its application. Circulation 30:654-670

Dotter CT, Judkins MP (1965) Percutaneous transluminal treatment of arteriosclerotic obstruction. Radiology 84:631-643

Dotter CT, Judkins MP, Frische LH, Mueller R (1966) The "nonsurgical" treatment of ilio-femoral arteriosclerotic obstruction. Radiology 86:871-875

Dotter CT, Judkins MP, Rösch J (1968) Nichtoperative transluminale Behandlung bei arteriosklerotischen Verschlußaffektionen. RoFo 109:125-133

Dotter CT, et al. (1974a) Transluminal iliac artery dilatation – nonsurgical catheter treatment of atheromatous narrowing. JAMA 230:117-124

Dotter CT, Rösch J, Seaman AJ (1974b) Selective clot lysis with low-dose streptokinase. Radiology 111:31-37

Durham JD, Rutherford RB (1994) Standards for reporting lower extremity ischemia. In: Laberge JM, Darcy MD (eds) Peripheral vascular interventions. SCVIR-Syllabus, Fairfax, pp 206-215

Faxon DP, Sanborn DP, Haudenschild TA, et al. (1984) Effect of antiplatelet therapy on restenosis after experimental angioplasty. Am J Cardiol 53:72c-76c

Faxon DP, Sanborn TA, Haudenschild CC (1987) Mechanisms of angioplasty and its relation to restenosis. Am J Cardiol 60:5B-9B

Ferris EJ, Ledor K, Ben Avi DD, et al. (1985) Percutaneous Angioscopy. Radiology 157:319-322

Fogarty TJ (1997) Editorial. Endovasc Multimed Rev 1:5-8

Fontaine R, Kim M, Kieny R (1954) Die chirurgische Behandlung der peripheren Durchblutungsstörungen. Helv Chir Acta 5/6:499-533

Fitchell TA, Stadius ML (1991) New technologies for the treatment of obstructive arterial disease. Cath Cardiovasc Diagn 22:205-233

Freimann DB, Ring EZ, Oleaga JA, Berkowitz H, Roberts B (1979) Transluminal angioplasty at the iliac, femoral and popliteal arteries, Radiology 132:285-288

Freiman DB, Spence R, Gatenby R, et al. (1981) Transluminal angioplasty of the iliac and femoral arteries: follow-up results without anticoagulation. Radiology 141:347-350

Gailer H, Grüntzig A, Zeitler E (1983) Late results after percutaneous transluminal angioplasty of iliac and femoropopliteal obstructive lesions – a cooperative study. In: Dotter CT, Grüntzig A, Schoop W, Zeitler E (eds) Percutaneous transluminal angioplasty. Springer, Berlin Heidelberg New York, pp 215-218

Gallino A, Mahler F, Probst P (1983) Progression to total occlusion of lower limb artery stenoses selected for perctuaneous transluminal angioplasty. Lancet 1983 I:59-60

Gallino A, Mahler F, Probst P, Nachbar B (1984) Percutaneous transluminal angioplasty of the arteries of the lower limbs: a 5-year follow-up. Circulation 70:619-623

Grüntzig A (1976a) Die perkutane Rekanalisation chronischer arterieller Verschlüsse (Dotter-Prinzip) mit einem neuen doppellumigen Dilatationskatheter. RoFo 124:80-86

Grüntzig A (1976b) Perkutane Dilatation von Koronarstenosen. Beschreibung eines neuen Kathetersystems. Klin Wochenschr 54:543-545

Grüntzig A (1977) Die perkutane transluminale Rekanalisation chronischer Arterienverschlüsse mit einer neuen Dilatationstechnik. Witzstrock, Baden-Baden

Grüntzig A, Kumpe DA (1979) Technique of percutaneous transluminal angioplasty with the Grüntzig balloon catheter. AJR 132:547-552

Grüntzig A, et al. (1973) Perkutane Rekanalisation chronischer arterieller Verschlüsse nach Dotter – eine nichtoperative Kathetertechnik. Schweiz Med Wochenschr 103:825-831

Grüntzig A, Hopff H (1974) Perkutane Rekanalisation chronischer arterieller Verschlüsse mit einem neuen Dilatationskatheter. Dtsch Med Wochenschr 99:2502-2505

Grüntzig A, Reidthammer HH, Turina M, Rutishauser W (1976) Eine neue Methode zur perkutanen Dilatation von Koronarstenosen – tierexperimentelle Prüfung. Verh Dtsch Ges Kreislaufforsch 42:282-285

Grüntzig A, Zeitler E (1978) Cooperative study of results of PTR in twelve different clinics. In: Zeitler E, Grüntzig A, Schoop W (eds) Percutaneous vascular recanalization. Technique, application, clinical results. Springer, Berlin Heidelberg New York, pp 118-119

Grüntzig A, Senning A, Siegenthaler WE (1979) Non-operative dilatation of coronary artery stenoses – percutaneous transluminal coronary angioplasty. N Engl J Med 301:61

Günther RW, Thelen M (1988) Interventionelle Radiologie. Thieme, Stuttgart

Guidelines for percutaneous transluminal angioplasty (1990) Standards of Practice Commitee of the SCVIR. Radiology 177:619-626

Hagen B, Harnoss BM, Trabhardt S, et al. (1993) Self-expandable macroporous nitinol stents for transfemoral exclusion of aortic aneurysms in dogs: preliminary results. Cardiovasc Interv Radiol 16:339-342

Hansen RB (1993) Die direktionale Atherektomie bei peripherer aVk. Inaugural dissertation, Munich

Hausegger KA, Lammer J, Klein GE, et al. (1991) Percutaneous recanalization of pelvic artery occlusions – fibrinolysis, PTA, stents Fortschr. Röntgenstr 155:550-554

Heimig T, Martin M (1997) Thrombolyse. In: Zeitler E (ed) Klinische Radiologie - Arterien und Venen. Springer, Berlin Heidelberg New York, pp 193-198

Henry M, Amor M, Ethevenot G, et al. (1993a) Percutaneous peripheral rotational ablation using the rotablator: immediate and mid-term results. Single center experience concerning 146 lesions treated. Int Angiol 12:231-244

Henry M, Amicabile C, Amor M, et al. (1993b) Angioplastie artérielle périphérique. Intérêt de la voie poplitée. A propos de 30 cas. Arch Anat Coeur 88:463–469 (abstract)

Henry M, Amor M, Hentry I, et al. (1994) Percutaneous transluminal angioplasty of peripheral arteries with retrograde catheterization through the popliteal artery: series of 53 cases. Radiology 193:192

Henry M, Amor M, Ethevenot G, et al. (1995) Palmaz stent placement in iliac and femoropopliteal arteries: primary and secondary patency in 310 patients with 2–4-year follow-up. Radiology 197:167–174

Henry M, Amor M, Cragg A, et al. (1996) Clinical experience with a new stent-graft for treatment of occlusive and aneurysmal peripheral arterial disease. Radiology 201:712–724

Henry M, Amor B, Mentre B, Henry I, Gerber L, Tzvetanov K (1997) The contralateral approach. In: Henry M, Amor M, Diethrich EB, Katzen BT (eds) (1997) Endovascular therapy course. Europa Organisation, Paris, pp 87–99

Henry M, Amor M, et al. (1997) Percutaneous peripheral atherectomy using the Rotablator. In: Henry M, Amor M, Diethrich EB, Uatzen BT (eds) Eighth complex peripheral angioplasty course. Paris, pp 135–147

Henry M, Amor M, Diethrich EB, Katzen BT (1998) Endovascular therapy course. Coronary and Peripheral Congress, Paris, May 1997. Europa Organisation, Paris

Hess H, Mietaschk A (1982) Rezidivprophylaxe nach PTA: Antikoagulation oder Aggregationshemmer. Vasa 11:344–346

Hess H, Müller-Fassbender H, Ingrisch H, Mietaschk A (1978) Verhütung von Wiederverschlüssen nach Rekanalisation obliterierter Arterien mit der Katheter-Methode. Dtsch Med Wochenschr 103:1994–1997

Hess H, Mietaschk A, Brückl R (1987) Peripheral arterial occlusions: a 6-year-experience with local lowdose thrombolytic therapy. Radiology 163:753–758

Höfling B, Backa D, Lauterjung L, Pölnitz AV, von Arnim TH, Jauch KW (1988) Percutaneous removal of atheromatous plaques in peripheral arteries. Lancet 1988 I:354–386

Höhn P, Wagner R, Zeitler E (1975) Histologische Befunde nach der Katheterbehandlung arterieller Obliterationen nach Dotter und ihre Bedeutung. Herz Kreislaufforsch 7(11):13–23

Horsch S, Claeys L (1995) Critical Limb Ischemia. Steinkopff, Darmstadt/Springer, Berlin Heidelberg New York

Horvath L, Jlles, J (1975) A combveroer-elzarodas kezelese kateteres modozerrel, transluminalis angioplasty et kozverlen erdmenyei, Magy Radiol 27:203–211

Husfeldt KJ, Roth FJ (1995) Konkurrierende Verfahren in der Gefäßchirurgie. Steinkopff, Darmstadt

Ingrisch H, Häzlin M (1980) Percutane transluminale angioplasty einer stenose in einem aortorenalen Veneninterpositionstransplant Fortschr. Röntgenstr 133:493–495

Ingrisch H, Schatzl M, Hess H, Mietaschk A, Frey KW (1980) Microdensitometric controls for quantification of the results in percutaneous transluminal recanalization of the femoral artery. Ann Radiol 23:283–285

Jester HG, Sinapius D (1978) Morphologic alterations after percutaneous transluminal recanalisation of chronic femoral atherosclerosis. In: Zeitler E, Grüntzig A, Schoop W (eds) Percutaneous vascular recanalisation. Springer, Berlin Heidelberg New York, pp 51–56

Jester HG, et al. (1976) Morphologische Veränderungen nach transluminaler Rekanalisation chronischer arterieller Verschlüsse. In: Zeitler E (ed) Hypertonie – Risikofaktor in der Angiologie. Witzstrock, Baden-Baden

Joffre F (1981) Percutaneous transluminal angioplasty – Personal experience. Applications clinique de rayans et des àutres et physiques de exploration et de traitment. J Radiol 62:514–519

Joffre F, Rousseau H (1989) Autoexpandable vascular endoprosnesis. In: Zeitler E, Seyferth W (eds) Pros and cons in PTA. Springer, Berlin Heidelberg New York

Johnston KW, Rae M, Hogg-Johnston SA, et al. (1987) 5-year results of a prospective study of percutaneous transluminal angioplasty. Ann Surg 206:403–413

Kadir S (1991) Current practice of interventional radiology. Decker, Philadelphia

Kaltenbach M, Vallbracht C (1987) Rotationsangioplastik – ein neues Katheterverfahren. Fortschr Med 105:36–38

Katzen BT, van Breda A (1981) Low-dose streptokinase in the treatment of arterial occlusions. AJR 136:1171–1178

Katzen BT, Chang J, Know WG (1979) Percutaneous transluminal angioplasty with the Grüntzig balloon catheter. A review of 70 cases. Arch Surg 114:1389–1397

Kensey KR, Nash JE, Abrahams C, Zarins CK (1987) Recanalization of obstructed arteries with a flexible, rotating tip catheter. Radiology 165:387–389

Kollath J, Liermann D (1995) Stents III. Entwicklung, Indikationen und Zukunft. Schnetztor, Konstanz

Krepel VM, van Andel GJ, von Erp WFM, Breslau PJ (1985) Percutaneous transluminal angioplasty of the femoropopliteal artery: initial and long-term results. Radiology 156:325–328

Krings W, Roth FJ (1986) Die Angioplastie bei Rezidiven nach gefäßchirurgischen Eingriffen. In: Trübestein G (ed) Konservative Therapie Arterieller Durchblutungsstörungen. Thieme, Stuttgart, pp 486–491

Ku DN, Giddens DP, Zarins CK, Glagov S (1985) Pulsatile flow and atherosclerosis in the human carotid bifurcation. Arteriosclerosis 5:293–302

Küffer G, Spengel FA, Hansen R, et al. (1990) Simpson Atherektomie peripherer Arterien: Frühergebnisse und Nachkontrollen. RoFo 153:61–67

Kumar M, Dorros G, et al. (1995) PTA of carotid arteries with Palmaz stent presented at the catheter Therapy Symposium, Washington

Kumar S (1989) Percutaneous transluminal angioplasty in nonspecific aortoarteritis (Takayasu's disease): experience in 16 cases. CVIR 12:321–325

Kumpe DA (1981) Percutaneous dilatation of an aortic abdominal stenosis: three-balloon-catheter technique. Radiology 141:536–538

Kumpe DA, Zwerdlinger S, Griffin DJ (1988) Blue digit syndrome: treatment with percutaneous transluminal angioplasty. Radiology 166:37–44

Laborde JC, Parodi JC, Clem MF, et al. (1992) Intraluminal bypass of abdominal aortic aneurysm: feasibility study. Radiology 184:185–190

Lammer J, Schreyer H (1991) Praxis der Interventionellen Radiologie. Hippokrates, Stuttgart

Lammer J, Pilger E, Justich E, et al. (1985) Fibrinolysis in chronic arteriosclerotic occlusions: intrathrombotic injection of streptokiase. Radiology 157:45–50

Lammer J, Pilger E, Neumayer K, et al. (1986) Intraarterial thrombolysis: long-term results. Radiology 161:159

Leu HJ (1982) Morphologie der Arterienwand nach perkutaner transluminaler Dilatation. Vasa 11:265–269

Leu HJ, Grüntzig A (1978) Histopathologic aspects of transluminal recanalisation. In: Zeitler E, Grüntzig A, Schoop W (eds) Percutaneous vascular recanalization. Springer, Berlin Heidelberg New York, pp 39–50

Liermann D, Strecker EP, Vallbracht C, Kollath J (1990) Indikation umol klinischer Einsatz des strecker-stents. In: Kollath J, Liermann D (eds) Stents-ein aktrieller Überblick, Schnetzter, Konstanz, pp 24–37

Liermann D, Strecker EP, Peters J (1992) The strecker stent: indications and results in iliac and femoropopliteal arteries. Cardiovasc Intervent Radiol 15:298–305

Liermann D (1995) Stents – state of the art and future developments. Polyscience. Morin Heights, Canada

Liermann D, Böttcher MD, Kollath J, et al. (1994) Prophylactic endovascular radiotherapy to prevent intimal hyperplasia after stent implantation in femoropopliteal arteries. Cardiovasc Intervent Radiol 17:12–16

Maas D, Zollikofer CL, Largiadèr F, Senning A (1984) Radiological follow-up of transluminally inserted vascular endoprothesis: an experimental study using expanding spirals. Radiology 152:659–663

Mahler F, Krneta A, Haertel M (1979) Treatment of renovascular hypertension by transluminal renal artery dilatation. Ann Intern Med 90:56–57

Mahler F, Triller J (1990) Katheterinterventionen in der Angiologie. Thieme, Stuttgart

Mahler F, Grüntzig A, Schlumpf M (1978) Transluminal dilatation of a stenosis in the deep femoral arter. In: Zeitler E, Grüntzig A, Schoop W (eds) Percutaneous vascular recanalization. Springer, Berlin Heidelberg New York, p 141

Marin ML, Veith FJ, et al. (1994a) Transfemoral endoluminal stented graft repair of a popliteal artery aneurysm. JVIR 5:794

Marin ML, Veith FJ, Cynamon J, et al. (1994b) Transfemoral endoluminal repair of a penetrating vascular injury. JVIR 5:592

Martin EC, Diamon NG, Casarella WJ (1980) Percutaneous transluminal angioplasty in atherosclerotic disease. Radiology 135:27–33

Martin M, Zeitler E, (1978) Percutaneous transluminal recanalization (PTR) and fibrinolysis: fibrinolytic treatment of femoral reocclusions subsequent to PTR procedures. In: Zeitler E, Grüntzig A, Schoop W (eds) Percutaneous vascular recanalization techniques, application, clinical results. Springer, Berlin Heidelberg New York, pp 152–156

Mathias K, Nöldge G, Konrad-Graf S, Kiefer S (1979a) Percutane transluminale Katheter-rekanalisation eines post-transmatischen Popliteaverschlusses. Dtsch Med Wschr 104:60–61

Mathias K, Staiger J, Thron A, Spillner G, et al. (1980) Percutane Katheterangioplastik der Arteria subclavia, Dtsch Med Wschr 105:16–18

Mathias K, Schlosser V, Reinke M (1980) Katheterrekanalisation eines Subklavia-Verschlusses. Fortschr Röntgenstr 132:346–347

Mathias K (1997) Phänomenologie von Gefäßerkrankungen. In: Zeitler E (ed) Arterien und Venen. Springer-Verlag, Berlin Heidelberg New York, pp. 129–142

Matsumoto A, Barth K, Lutz RJ, Miller DL (1989) Hepatic artery model for evaluating the distribution of intraarterial chemotherapy infusion: non-pulsed versus pulsed infusion. Radiology 170:1077–1080

May J, White G, Waugh R, Yu W, Harris J (1994) Treatment of complex abdominal aortic aneurysms by a combination of endoluminal and extraluminal aortofemoral grafts. J Vasc Surg 19:924–933

Maynar M, Reyes R, Cabbera, et al. (1989) Percutaneous atherectomy as an alternative treatment for postangioplasty obstructive intimal flaps. Radiology 170:1029–1031

McLean PK (1993) Percutaneous peripheral atherectomy. J Vasc Intervent Radiol 4:465–480

McNamara TO, Fisher JR (1985) Thrombolysis of peripheral arterial and graft occlusions: improved results using high-dose urokinase. AJR 144:769

Mewissen MW, Minor PL, Beyer GA, Lipchik EO (1990) Symptomatic native arterial occlusions: early experience with over-the-wire thrombolysis. J Vasc Intervent Radiol 1:43

Minar E, Ahmadi RA, Ehringer H, Marosi L, Czembirek H, Konecny U (1986) Perkutane transluminale Angioplastie (PTA) bei peripherer arterieller Verschlußkrankheit der unteren Extremitäten. Wien Klin Wochenschr 98:33–39

Motarjeme A, Keifer JW, Zuska AJ (1980) Percutaneous transluminal angioplasty of the deep femoral artery. Radiology 135:613–617

Motarjeme A, Keifer JW, Zuska AJ (1982) Percutaneous transluminal angioplasty of the brachiocephalic arteries. AJR 138:457–462

Murray JG, Apthorp LA, Wilkins RA (1995) Long segment femoropopliteal angioplasty: improved technical success and long-term patency. Radiology 195:158–162

Murray RR, et al. (1987) Long-segment femoropopliteal stenoses: is angioplasty a boon or a bust? Radiology 162:473–476

Novak D (1990a) Embolization materials. In: Dondelinger RF, Rossi P, Kurdziel JC, Wallace S (eds) Interventional radiology. Thieme, Stuttgart, pp 295–313

Novak D (1990b) Complications of arterial embolization. In: Dondelinger RF, Rossi P, Kurdziel JC, Wallace S (eds) Interventional radiology. Thieme, Stuttgart, pp 314–324

Olbert F, Hanecka L (1977) Transluminale Gefäßdilatation mit einem modifizierten Dilatations-katheter. Wien Klin Wochenschr 89:281–284

Olbert F, Orgis E, Denck H, et al. (1975) Die percutane, transluminale Dilatation nach Dotter – eine radiologische Methode zur Wiederherstellung der arteriellen Strombahn. Österr Arztetg 30/19:1226

Olbert F, Kasparzak Muzika N, Schlegl A (1984) Percutaneous transluminal dilatation and recanalization. Long-term results and report on experience with a new catheter system. Ann Radiol (Paris) 27:349–356

Palmaz JC, Sibbitt RR, Reuter SR, Tio FO, Rice WJ (1985) Expandable intraluminal graft: a preliminary study. Radiology 156:73–77

Palmaz JC, Richter GM, Noeldge G, et al. (1988a) Intraluminal stents in atherosclerotic iliac artery stenosis: preliminary report of a multi-center study. Radiology 168(3):727–731

Palmaz JC, Tio FO, Schatz RA, Alvarado R, Rees C, Gareis FS (1988b) Early endothelialisation of balloon-expandable stents: Experimental observations. J Intervent Radiol 3:119–124

Palmaz JC, Garcia OJ, Schatz RA, et al. (1990) Placement of balloon-expandable intraluminal stents in iliac arteries: first 171 procedures. Radiology 174:969–975

Palmaz JC, Reuter SR (1997) Intravascular stents: basic physical and biological properties. In: Henry M, Amor M, Diethrich EB, Katzen BT (eds) Eight international course of peripheral vascular intervention. Paris pp 149–158

Parodi JC (1996) Use of transluminally placed endovascular grafts in abdominal aortic aneurysms and vascular trauma. Lecture held at IMAGO, 4th international congress of angiography and vascular intervention, July 1996, Nuremberg

Parodi JC, Palmaz JC, Barone HD (1991) Transfemoral intraluminal graft implantation for abdominal aortic aneurysms. Ann Vasc Surg 5:491–499

Patel RI, Gardiner GA, Bonr J, Donovan ME (1995) Causes and consequences of balloon angioplasty failure in peripheral arteries. Radiology 197:142

Porstmann W (1973) Ein neuer Korsett-Ballonkatheter zur transluminalen Rekanalisation nach Dotter unter besonderer Berücksichtigung von Obliterationen an den Beckenarterien. Radiol Diagn (Berl) 2:239–244

Porstmann W, Wierny L (1967) Intravasale Rekanalisation inoperabler arterieller Obliterationen. Zentralbl Chir 92:1586–1591

Rabkin JH (1987) Extremities revascularization by means of roentgen endovascular prosthetics of vessels. XXIV Congress of Radiology, GDR. Akademie-Verlag, Leipzig, p 36

Rabkin JK, Zaimovsky VA, Khmelevskaya JY, et al. (1984) Experimental ground and first clinical experience of roentgen endovascular prosthetics (in Russia) Herald Roentgenol Radiol (Moscow) 4:59–64

Rabkin JK (1989) Endovascular prosthesis: experimental study and clinical use. In: Zeitler E, Seyferth W (eds) Pros and cons in PTA and auxiliary methods. Springer, Berlin Heidelberg New York, pp 139–147

Raithel D, Ritter W, Zeitler E (1997) Endovaskuläre Chirurgie. In: Zeitler Z (ed) Klinische Radiologie: Arterien und Venen. Springer, Berlin Heidelberg New York, pp 247–255

Redha F, Uhlschmid GK, Antonucci F, Zollikofer CL (1992) New device for peripheral atherectomy: experimental results. 78th RSNA. Radiology 185(P)[Suppl]:229

Redha F, Do DD, Mahler F, Triller J, Freiburghaus AU, Uhlschmid GK (1996) First clinical results of the treatment of peripheral arterial stenosis with a novel percutaneous atherectomy device (REDHA-CUT). Swiss Surg 2:102–104

Reekers J (1990) Percutaneous interventional extraluminal recanalization ("PIER"). Cardiovasc Intervent Radiol 13:

Richter GM, Roeren TH, Noeldge G, Kauffmann GW, Wenz W (1987) Erster klinischer Fallbericht über eine ballon-expandierte Gefäßprothese. Radiologe 27:560–563

Richter GM, Roeren TH, Noeldge G, et al. (1991) Superior clinical results of iliac stent placement versus percutaneous transluminal angioplasty: four-year success rates of a randomized study (abstract). Radiology 181(P):161

Richter GM, Palmaz JC, Allenberg JR (1994) Die transluminale Stent-Prothese beim Bauchaortenaneurysma. Radiologe 34:511–518

Richter GM, Noeldge G, Palmaz JC, et al. (1995) Weitere Analysen einer randomisierten Studie: Primäre Stentimplantation in der Beckenarterie versus PTA. In: Kollath J, Liermann D (eds) Stents III, Entwicklung, Indikation, Zukunft. Schnetztor, Konstanz, pp 24–29

Ring EJ, McLean PK (1981) Interventional radiology: principles and techniques. Little Brown, Boston

Ring EJ, Freiman DB, McLean GK, Schwarz W (1982) Percutaneous recanalization of common iliac artery occlusions: an inacceptable complication rate? AJR 139:587–589

Rocke TW, Stanson A, Johnson CM, Sheedy U, Miller WE, Osmundson PJ (1987) Percutaneous transluminal angioplasty in the lower extremities: a 5-year experience. Mayo Clin Proc 62:85–90

Rollins, et al. (1987) ••

Rosen RJ, Mclean GK, Oleaga JA, Freiman DB, Ring EJ (198) A new exchange guide wire for transluminal angioplasty. Radiology 140:242–243

Roth FJ, Cappius (1980) Die Angioplastie der in der Leiste gelegenen Arterienabschnitte. In: Müller-Wiefel H, Barras JP, Ehringer H, Krüger M (eds) Mikrozirkulation und Blutrheologie. Therapie der peripheren arteriellen Verschlußkrankheit. Witzstrock, Baden-Baden, pp 429–432

Roubin G (1996) Carotid stent supported angioplasty: the exciting field of neurovascular intervention, Symposium on Transcatheter Cardiovascular Therapies, Washington

Roth FJ, Cappius G, Fingerhut E (1983) Radiologic pattern at and after angioplasty. In: Dotter CT, Grüntzig A, Schoop W, Zeitler E (eds) Percutaneous transluminal angioplasty. Springer, Berlin Heidelberg New York, pp 78–83

Roth FJ, Heining T, Berliner P, et al. (1988) Perkutane Rekanalisation peripherer Gefäße. In: Günther RW, Thelen M (eds) Interventionelle Radiologie. Thieme, Stuttgart, pp 20–44

Roth FJ, Sommer B, Grün B, Barthen I (1995) Die Angioplastie der Oberschenkelarterien. In: Husfeldt KJ, Roth FJ (eds) Konkurrierende Verfahren in der Gefäßchirurgie. Steinkopff, Darmstadt, pp 187–200

Rousseau H, Puel J, Joffre F, Sigwart U, DuBoucher C, Wallsten H, et al. (1987) A new type of selfexpanding endovascular stent prosthesis: experimental study. Radiology 164:709–714

Rousseau HP, Raillat CR, Joffre F, et al. (1989) Treatment of femoropopliteal stenoses by means of self-expandable endoprostheses: midterm-results. Radiology 172:961–964

Rutherford RB, Becker GJ (1991) Standards for evaluating and reporting the results of surgical and percutaneous therapy for peripheral arterial disease. JVIR 2:169–174 and Radiology 181:271–281

Sanborn TA, et al. (1983) The mechanism of intraluminal angioplasty: evidence for formation of aneurysms in experimental atherosclerosis. Circulation 68:1136–1140

Sayers RD, Thompson MM, Bell PRF (1993) Endovascular stenting of abdominal aortic aneurysms. Eur J Vasc Surg 7:225–227

Schlosser V, Spillner G, Mathias K (1979) Komplikationen nach perkutaner transluminaler Gefäßrekanalisation (PTR) und ihre clirurgische Behandlung. VASA 5:324–325

Schmidtke I, Zeitler E, Schoop W (1975) Langzeitergebnisse der perkutanen Katheterbehandlung (Dotter-Technik) bei femoropoplitealen Arterienverschlüssen im Stadium II. Vasa 4:210–226

Schmidtke I, Zeitler E, Schoop W (1978) Spätergebnisse (5–8 Jahre) der perkutanen Katheterbehandlung (Dotter-Technik) bei femoropoplitealen Arterienverschlüssen im Stadium II. Vasa 7, 4–15

Schmitz-Rohde T, Günther RW (1991) Percutaneous mechanical thrombolysis: a comparative study of various rotational catheter systems. Invest Radiol 26:557–563

Schneider E (1986) Percutaneous extraction of thrombi and emboli. In: Maurer PC, Becker MM, Heidrich H, Hoffmann G, Kriessmann A, Müller-Wiefel M, Prätorius C (eds) What is new in angiology? Zuckschwerdt, Munich, p 180

Schneider E, Largiadèr J (1987) Therapiekonzept beim akuten Verschluß von Extremitätenarterien. Ther Umsch 44:653–660

Schneider E, Grüntzig A, Bollinger A (1982) Langzeitergebnisse nach perkutaner transluminaler Angioplastie (PTA) bei 882 konsekutiven Patienten mit iliakalen und femoro-poplitealen Obstruktionen. Vasa 11:322–326

Schneider E, Pfyffer M, Jäger K, Küpferle L, Bollinger A (1987) Lokale Thrombolyse (LTL), perkutane transluminale Angioplastie und perkutane Thrombenextraktion (TE) bei akuten und subakuten Beinarterienverschlüssen. Früh- und Spätergebnisse. Schweiz Med Wochenschr 117:7–11

Schröder J (1989) Catheter lysis and percutaneous transluminal angioplasty below the knee via the popliteal artery in a patient with femoral artery obstruction: technical note. Cardiovasc Intervent Radiol 12:344–345

Schwarten DE, Cutcliff WB (1988) Arterial occlusive disease below the knee: treatment with PTA performed with low-profile catheters and steerable guide wires. Radiology 169:71–74

Schwarten DE, Katzen BT, Simpson BJ, Cutcliff WB (1988) Simpson catheter for percutaneous transluminal removal of atheroma. Am J Roentgenol 150:799–801

SCVIR Syllabus (1994) Peripheral vascular interventions. In: La Berge JM, Darcy MD (eds). Library of Congress Catalog card number 94–069675

Seldinger SI (1953) Catheter replacement of the needle in percutaneous arteriography. A new technique. Acta Radiol 39:368–376

Seyferth W, Ernsting M, Grosse-Vorholt R, Zeitler E (1983) Complications during and after percutaneous transluminal angioplasty. In: Dotter CT, Grüntzig A, Schoop W, Zeitler E (eds) Percutaneous transluminal angioplasty. Springer, Berlin Heidelberg New York, pp 161–169

Sigwart U, Puel J, Mirkovitch V, Joffre F, Kappenberger L (1987) Intravascular stents to prevent occlusion and restenosis after transluminal angioplasty. N Engl J Med 316:12

Sigwart U, Bertrand M, Serruys PW (1996) Handbook of cardiovascular interventions. Churchill Livingstone, New York

Simonetti G, et al. (1983) Iliac artery rupture: a complication of transluminal angioplasty. AJR 140:989–990

Simpson LJ, Johnson DE, Thapliyal HV, et al. (1985) Transluminal atherectomy: a new approach to the treatment of atherosclerotic vascular disease. Circulation 72[Suppl]2:3–146

Sobbe H, Martin M, Trübestein G (1973) Besondere Aspekte der transluminalen Katheterbehandlung nach Dotter. RöFo 118:682–690

Sos TA, Sniderman KW (1981) Percutaneous transluminal angioplasty. Semin Roentgenol 16:26–41

Soulen MC, Groffisky CJL (1995) Superficial femoral and popliteal artery angioplasty: results from a transluminal angioplasty and revascularisation registry. Radiology 197:142

Staiger J, Mathias K, Friedrich M, Heiss HW, Konrad S, Spillner G (1980) Perkutane Katheterrekanalisation (Dotter-Technik) bei peripherer arterieller Verschlußkrankheit. Herz/Kreislauf 12:383–386

Standards of Practice Committee of the Society of Cardiovascular and Interventional Radiology (1990) Guidelines for percutaneous transluminal angioplasty. Radiology 177:619–626

Staple TW (1968) Modified catheter for percutaneous transluminal treatment of arteriosclerotic obstructions. Radiology 91:1041–1043

Starck EE, Wagner HJ (1990) Rotations-Aspirations-Thromboembolektomie. Dtsch Med Wschr 116:1–6

Starck EE, McDermott JC, Crummy AB, Turnispeed WD, Acher CW, Burgess JH (1985) Percutaneous aspiration thromboembolectomy. Radiology 156:61–66

Starck EE, McDermott JC, Crummy A, Holzman P, Herzer M, Kollath J (1986) Die perkutane Aspirations-Thromboembolektomie: eine weitere transluminale Angioplastiemethode. Dtsch Med Wschr 111:167–172

Strecker EP, Berg G, Schneider B, Freudenberg N, Weber H, Wolf HRD (1988) A new vascular balloon expandable prosthesis: experimental studies and first clinical results. J Intervent Radiol 3:59–62

Strecker EP, Schneider B, Wolf HRD, Zeitler E, et al. (1989) Flexible, Percutaneously Insertable, Balloon-Expandable Arterial Prosthesis. In: Zeitler E, Seyferth W (eds) Pros and cons in PTA and auxiliary methods. Springer, Berlin Heidelberg New York, pp 17–187

Strecker EP, Liermann D, Barth KM, et al. (1990) Expandable tubular stents for treatment of arterial occlusive disease: experimental and clinical results. Radiology 175:97–102

Strecker EP, Hagen B, Liermann D, Schneider B, Wolf HR, Wambsganss J (1993) Iliac and femoropopliteal vascular occlusive disease treated with flexible tantalum stents. Cardiovasc Intervent Radiol 16:158–164

Stribley K, Wilkins RA (1987) Techniques of superficial femoral artery catheterization prior to percutaneous transluminal angioplasty. J Intervent Radiol 2:99–104

Sultzmann J, Probst P (1987) A new puncture needle (Seldinger technique) for antegrade catheterization of the superficial femoral artery. Eur J Radiol 7:53–55

Tegtmeyer CJ, Moore TS, Chandler JG, Wellons HA, Rudolf LE (1979) Percutaneous transluminal dilatation of a complete block in the right iliac artery. AJR 133:532–535

Tegtmeyer G, Bezirdjian DR (1981) Removing the strick, ruptured angioplasty balloon catheter. Radiology 139:231–232

Tegtmeyer CJ, Wellons HA, Thompson RN (1980) Balloon dilatation of the abdominal aorta. J Am Med Assoc 244:2636–2637

The Collaborative Rotablator Atherectomy Group (CRAG) (1994) Peripheral atherectomy with the Rotablator. A multicenter report. J Vasc Surg 19:509–515

Thomas S, Belli AM (1998) Endovascular methods of retrieving a failing graft. Critical Ischaemia (8) 1:19–29

Thorpe PE, Ginsburg R, Wright AM, Kusnick CA, Baxter R, Wittich GR, Jenkins N, Wexler L (1988) Evolution of lower extremity angioplasty: Stanford experience comparing the use of laser, Kensey catheter, Rotablator and atherectomy catheter as adjuncts to Balloon angioplasty for vascular occlusions. Radiology 169[Suppl]:306

Thorpe PE (1992) Percutaneous transluminal rotational atherectomy (PTRA). International Andreas Grüntzig Society Meeting, Nurnberg

Toennesen KH, Holstein P (1992) Femoropopliteal artery occlusions treated by percutaneous transluminal angioplasty and enclosed thrombolysis. J Cardiovasc Intervent Radiol 3:441–447

Toennesen KH, Sager P, Karle A, et al. (1988) Percutaneous transluminal angioplasty of the superficial femoral artery by retrograde catheterization via the popliteal artery. Cardiovasc Intervent Radiol 11:127–131

Toennesen KH, Holstein F, Andersen E (1991) Femoropopliteal artery occlusions treated by percutaneous transluminal angioplasty and enclosed thrombolysis. J Vasc Intervent Radiol 3:441–447

Triller J, Mahler F, Do DD, Thalmann A (1989) Die vaskuläre Endoprothese bei femoro-poplitealer Verschlußkrankheit. Ergebnisse nach 9 Monaten klinischen Einsatzes. RoFo 180:328–334

Triller J, Mahler F, Do DD, Thalmann R, Wallstén H (1989) Vascular Endoprothesis (stents) in the treatment of femoropopliteal occlusions. In: Zeitler E, Seyferth W (eds) Pros and cons in PTA: Springer, Berlin Heidelberg New York

Vallbracht C, Kampf AH, Liermann D, Beinborn W, Roth FJ, Kollath J (1992) Low-speed rotational angioplasty in chronic peripheral occlusions. Experience in 1252 patients. Radiology 185:229

Vallbracht C, Liermann D, Prignitz J, et al. (1989) Low-speed rotational angioplasty in chronic peripheral arterial occlusions: experience in 83 patients. Radiology 172:327–330

Van Andel GZ (1975) Transluminale angioplastiek volgens Dotter. Ned Tijdschr Geneeskd 119:343–344

Van Andel GJ (1976) Percutaneous transluminal angioplasty. The Dotter procedure. Excerpta Medica, Amsterdam

Velasquez G, Castaneda-Zuniga WR, Formanek A (1980) Non-surgical aortoplasty in Leriche syndrome. Radiology 134:359–360

Vogelzangich (1996) Long-term results of angioplasty. JVIR 7:179–180

Volodos NL, Karpovich IP, Troyan VI, et al. (1991) Clinical experience of the use of self-fixing synthetic prostheses for remote endoprosthetics of the thoracic and abdominal aorta and iliac arteries through the femoral artery and as intraoperative endoprosthesis for aorta reconstruction. VASA 33[Suppl]:93–95

Vorwerk D, Guenther RW (1997) Arterial stent placement pp 3–20 In: Adam A, Dondelinger RF, Mueller PR (Editors) Textbook of Metallic Stents. Isis Medical Media, Oxford

Vorwerk D, Günther RW (1990) Mechanical revascularization of occluded iliac arteries with use of self-expandable endoprostheses. Radiology 175:411–415

Vorwerk D, Günther RW (1995) Der Stent beim Beckenarterienverschluß – eine Alternative zur operativen Therapie? In: Husfeldt KJ, Roth FJ (eds) Konkurrierende Verfahren in der Gefäßchirurgie. Steinkopff, Darmstadt

Waltman AC (1980) Percutaneous transluminal angioplasty: iliac and deep femoral arteries. AJR 135:921–925

Waltman AC, Greenfield AJ, Athanasoulis CA (1982) Transluminal angioplasty: general rules and basic considerations. In: Athanasoulis CA, Pfister RC, Greene RE, Roberson GH (eds) Interventional radiology. Saunders, Philadelphia, pp 253–272

White CJ (1997) Pullback atherectomy: the technique indications and results. In: Henry M, Amor M, et al. (eds) Eighth complex peripheral angioplasty course, Poris, pp 129–134

Wholey MH, Jarmolowski CR (1989) New reperfusion devices: the Kensey catheter, the atherolytic reperfusion wire device, and the transluminal extraction catheter. Radiology 172:947–952

Wholey MH (1997) The TEC: technique, indications, results. In: Henry M, Amor M, Diethrich EB, Katzen BT (eds) Eighth complex peripheral angioplasty course. Europa Organisation, Poris. pp 117–128

Wierny L, Plass R, Porstmann W (1973) Langzeitbeobachtungen nach transluminaler katheterrekanalisation arterieller obliterationen nach Dotter und Judkins Zentralbl Chir 98:1761–1772

Wierny L, Plass R, Porstmann W (1974) Long-term results in 100 consecutive patients treated by transluminal angioplasty. Radiology 112:543–548

Wright KC, Wallace S, Charnsangavej CH, Carasco CH, Gianturco C (1985) Percutaneous endovascular stents: an experimental evaluation. Radiology 156:69–72

Yakes WF, Kumpe DA, Brown SB (1989) Percutaenous transluminal aortic angioplasty: techniques and results. Radiology 172:965–970

Zeitler E (1971) Perkutane transluminale Verschlußrekanalisation und Stenosedilatation bei Angiopathia obliterans. Actuel Chir 6:143–154

Zeitler E (1980) PTA cooperation among specialties. Cardiovasc Intervent Radiol 3:207–212

Zeitler E (1981) Percutaneous dilatation and recanalization of iliac and femoral arteries. In: Athanasoulis CA, Abrams HL, Zeitler E (eds) Therapeutic angiography. Springer, Berlin Heidelberg New York, pp 11–16

Zeitler E (1988) Dymanische Angioplastie und Atherektonie. In: Günther RW, Thelen M (eds) Interventionelle Radiologie. Thieme, Stunttgort, pp 117–124

Zeitler E (ed) (1997) Klinische Radiologie: Arterien und Venen. Springer, Berlin Heidelberg New York

Zeitler E (1998) PTA is an outpatient procedure. J Invasive Cardiol 10:410–414

Zeitler E, Maresta A (1970) Ricanalizzazione transluminale percutanae delle occlusioni e delle stenosi arteriose nella arteriopatia aterosclerotica obliterativa. Gior Clin Med 51:381–399

Zeitler E, Müller R (1969) Erste Ergebnisse mit der Katheter-Rekanalisation nach Dotter bei arterieller Verschlußkrankheit. RoFo 111:345–352

Zeitler E, Roth FJ (1982) Technik und Instrumentarium für periphere perkutane transluminale Angioplastie (PTA). Vasa 11:250–257

Zeitler E, Grosse-Vorholt R, Richter EJ, Saida Y (1981) Technique of Percutaneous transluminal angioplasty (PTA) and additional treatment of leg arteries. Ann Radiol 24:361–364

Zeitler E, Seyferth W (1989) Pros and cons in PTA and auxiliary methods. Springer, Berlin Heidelberg New York

Zeitler E, Hüring HG, Schoop W, Schmidtke I (1971a) Mechanische Behandlung von Beckenarterienstenosen mit der perkutanen Kathetertechnik. Verh Dtsch Ges Kreislaufforsch 37:402–407

Zeitler E, Schoop W, Zahnow W (1971b) The treatment of occlusive arterial disease by transluminal catheter angioplasty. Radiology 99:19–26

Zeitler E, Reichold J, Schoop W, Loew D (1973) Einfluß von Acetylsalicylsäure auf das Frühergebnis nach perkutaner Rekanalisation arterieller Obliterationen nach Dotter. Dtsch Med Wochenschr 98:1285–1288

Zeitler E, Grüntzig A, Schoop W (1978) Percutaneous vascular recanalization. Springer, Berlin Heidelberg New York

Zeitler E, Ernsting M, Richter EI, Seyferth W (1982) Komplikationen nach PTA femoraler und iliakaler Obstruktionen. Vasa 11:270–273

Zeitler E, Richter E, Roth F, Schoop W (1983) Results of percutaneous transluminal angioplasty. Radiology 146:57–60

Zeitler E, Beyer-Enke SA, Ritter W (1995a) Percutaneous transluminal angioplasty for crural obliterations. In: Horsch S, Claeys L (eds) Critical limb ischemia. Steinkopff, Darmstadt/Springer, Berlin Heidelberg New York, pp 71–80

Zeitler E, Beyer-Enke SA, Ritter W, Rompel O (1995b) Stents: future developments. In: Liermann D (ed) Stents – state of the art and future developments. Polyscience, Morin Heights, pp 401–403

Zollikofer CL (1985) Experimentelle Grundlagen der perkutanen transluminalen Angioplastie. Habilatationsschrift, University of Zürich

Zollikofer CL, et al. (1984) Transluminal angioplasty evaluated by electron microscopy. Radiology 153:369–374

Zollikofer CL, Salomonowitz EK, Brühlmann WF, Frick MP, Castaneda-Zuniga WR, Amplatz K (1985) Significance of balloon pressure recording during angioplasty. Fortschr Roentgenstr 142:527–530

Zollikofer CL, et al. (1986) Dehnungs-, Verformungs-, und Berstungs-Charakteristika häufig verwendeter Ballon-Dilatationskatheter. In vivo Untersuchungen an Hundegefäßen, part 2. RoFo 144:189–195

Zollikofer CL, et al. (1987) Acute and long-term effects of massive balloon dilation on the aortic wall and vasa vasorum. Radiology 164:145–149

Zollikofer CL, Largiadèr J, Brühlmann WF, Uhlschmid GK, Marty AH (1988) Endovascular stenting of veins and grafts: preliminary clinical experience. Radiology 167:707–712

Zollikofer CL, Tentonucci F, Stuckmann G (1990) Die Entwicklung endovaskularer Stents. In: Kollath J, Liermann D (eds) Stents – ein Aktueller Überblick. Schnetztor Verlag, Konstanz, pp 10–17

Zorn-Bopp E, Ingrisch H, Mietaschk A, Frey KW (1981) Transluminale Gefäßdilatation der distalen Bauchaorta, der Arteria iliaca communis und externa. Fortschr Roentgenstr 134:471–478

Zühlke HV, Sürensen R, Hering R, Konradt J (1981) Die intraoperative offene transluminale Angioplastie (IOTA). Chimny 52:265–270

5.4
Sympathicolysis

R. Hildebrandt

At the late stages of arteriosclerotic disease or endangiitis obliterans, when severe stenosis or occlusion of arteries has developed, sufficient reconstruction is not always possible by means of surgical or angiographic-angioplastic procedures. As far as extremities are concerned – usually the lower limb – rest pain, gangrene, or ulcerations arise and amputation becomes imminent. It has long been common practice in such cases to carry out operative sympathectomy in order to reduce rest pain, heal gangrene, and prevent, or at least delay, imminent amputation.

In comparison to this method, CT-guided chemo-induced sympathicolysis is a real alternative. It has also been available for a long time, but first received greater attention due to its CT-guided puncture facilities. Both operative sympathectomy and chemo (phenol or ethanol)-induced sympathicolysis achieve the same objective following the same therapeutic principle with identical indications.

5.4.1
Indications and Principles

Sympathicolysis is indicated if there is no, or insufficient, peripheral blood supply attainable by surgical or angiographic-angioplastic intervention. At late stages III and IV of arteriosclerotic disease or endangiitis obliterans, the perfusion rate in the periphery finally decreases to below the critical level, to the extent that finally, even in rest, a sufficient blood supply is no longer available. Even in this situation, there remains a certain basic vasoconstrictive stimulation caused by sympathic nerve structures. Under normal conditions, this is a very useful preparative mechanism, but in the end-stages of arteriosclerotic disease it influences the situation adversely. Operative sympathectomy, as well as CT-guided

sympathicolysis, aim to eliminate the corresponding sympathic nerve structures (for the leg the lumbar sympathic chain at the level of L2–L4) and thereby improve peripheral blood supply by eliminating remaining basal vasoconstriction (Figs. 5.29, 5.30). The global effect of sympathicolysis includes different components as follows:

1. The main effect is a maximal dilatation of arteries in the dependent area. Peripheral flow resistance in the poststenotic area is influenced more intensively than flow-resistance in collateral vessels at the level of stenosis (early effect immediately after sympathicolysis).

2. Although global blood supply will increase in the poststenotic periphery, the effective blood pressure will nevertheless decrease. This effect will be the stronger the more stenoses present one after another. Therefore, a monostenotic situation is considered more advantageous than a multi-stenotic one. Thus, it is to be considered that by sympathicolysis blood pressure can indeed be reduced to below a critical minimum level. This is to be expected if, prior to sympathicolysis, blood

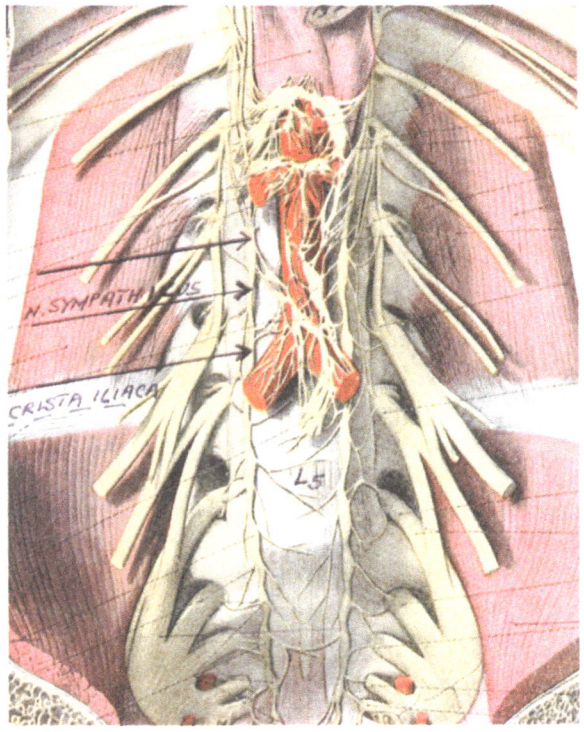

Fig. 5.29. The lumbar sympathic chain (*arrows*) and connecting nerve structures at the level of ganglion lumbale II–IV. Note the close position to the femoral plexus and great vessels (aorta at the right vena cava inferior is not shown)

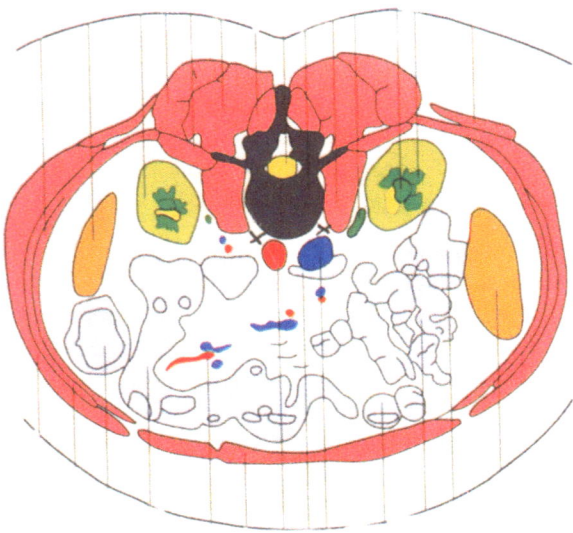

Fig. 5.30. Important landmarks of the target area for sympathicolysis (*crosses*). Patient in prone position

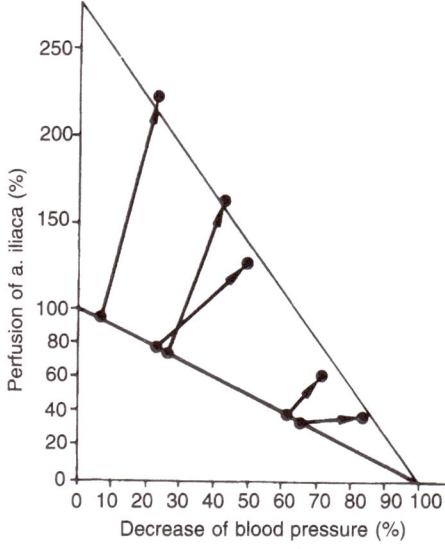

Fig. 5.31. Effect of sympathicolysis on the relation of perfusion rate vs poststenotic fall of pressure at increasing grades of stenosis. The lower the poststenotic pressure, the less the increasing effect on perfusion after sympathicolysis

pressure in the poststenotic area is at the critical level of 40–60 mmHg. In these cases, an acute deterioration is possible. Primarily this fact received too little attention for a long time, leading to unfortunate results (Figs. 5.31, 5.32).

3. Local sympathicolysis also simultaneously eliminates local pain-afferent fibers running together with the efferent vasomotoric-vasoconstrictive fibers of the sympathic chain. Rest pain is blocked, thus creating the most impressive effect for the patient, and usually occurring promptly after application.

4. In some cases, a late effect of sympathicolysis may be an increase in blood pressure to even higher levels than before. This can take place if growth of collaterals at the stenotic level is induced by a long-standing increase in peripheral blood supply (such as in muscular training late effect of sympathicolysis).

5. Also, sudomotoric efferent fibers will be involved. Sympathicolysis, therefore, also leads to a decrease, or even stop, in sudation and skin becomes dry. This effect represents a particular indication in hyperhydrotic disease.

It must be considered that in long-term diabetes distinctly lower success rates are to be expected. This disadvantageous situation is due to diabetic polyneuropathy in which the sympathicolytic reserve can already have been consumed, almost as diabetic autosympathicolysis (Table 5.14).

5.4.1.1
Technique

1. The patient is placed in a prone position; alternatively, puncture can also be carried out in a lateral or prone-oblique position.

2. The target level (for the lower limb at lumbar vertebra 3, alternatively 2 and/or 4) is determined by corresponding CT slices.

3. At this level, a deep local anesthesia is given along the final route of the puncture needle.

4. The puncture needle (diameter 0.6–0.7 mm, length 150–180 mm) is pushed forward to the target area just immediately anterior to the psoas muscle, just latero-anterior to the corresponding vertebra, and posterior to the aorta or vena cava inferior, keeping a reliably safe distance from the

Table 5.14. Indication for sympathicolysis. Arteriosclerotic disease stages III–IV if sufficient reconstruction of vessel is not possible

Advantageous:
Peripheral obstruction
in rest pain: BP above 40 mmHg
in gangrene: BP above 60 mmHg

Disadvantageous:
Proximal or multiple obstructions, diabetes
in rest pain: BP below 40 mmHg
in gangrene: BP below 60 mmHg

BP, blood pressure.

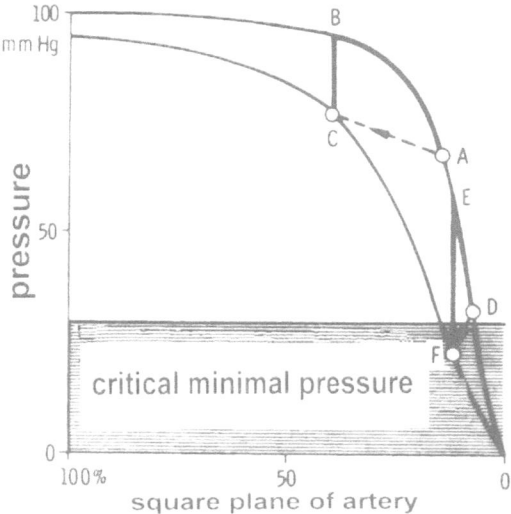

Fig. 5.32. Effect of sympathicolysis on poststenotic arterial pressure in different previous grades of arterial stenosis. *Outer curve*, poststenotic pressure before sympathicolysis, i.e., at normal peripheral flow resistance. *Inner curve*, poststenotic pressure after sympathicolysis, i.e., at (maximal) peripheral vasodilatation. *A–C*, sympathicolysis reduces flow-resistance of collaterals – poststenotic pressure could rise to *B*. Simultaneously, the peripheral resistance decreases and, peripheral pressure finally falls to *C*. In this situation a real, effective increase of peripheral pressure would result and limb ischemia (rest pain etc.) would be released. *D–F*, If poststenotic pressure is already at a low level, sympathicolysis reduces flow resistance of collaterals (*E*) but also of peripheral arteries (*F*). In this disadvantageous initial situation, the global result of sympathicolysis would be a fall in peripheral pressure to below the critical occlusive level. Acute aggravation of symptoms will arise. Between these two extremes, any transition is possible

kidney and ureter. Marking these structures by the application of contrast medium i.v. is recommended. The correct site should be established by a control CT slice by means of a small deposit of contrast medium at the needle tip to avoid hazardous misinjection (Fig. 5.33a,b).

5. If distribution of the contrast probe confirms a correct position, 6–8 ml of a 6.7% solution of phenol in glycerin or, as favored more in recent publications, 6–8 ml of 98% (pure) ethanol is injected, together with an adequate volume of local anesthetic. To avoid dislocation of the needle tip, the syringe should be attached to the needle by a small connection tube.

6. Still kept in the same position, the puncture needle is washed out with a small volume of saline before final retraction.

5.4.2
Results

Results are presented in Tables 5.15–5.19. They compare well to surgical sympathectomy and even to recent modalities of surgical implantation of a spinal cord stimulator. The advantage of these CT-guided chemo-induced sympathicolysis scores is markedly less complications, and in particular no cases of death. In addition, lower costs, time, and staff are required.

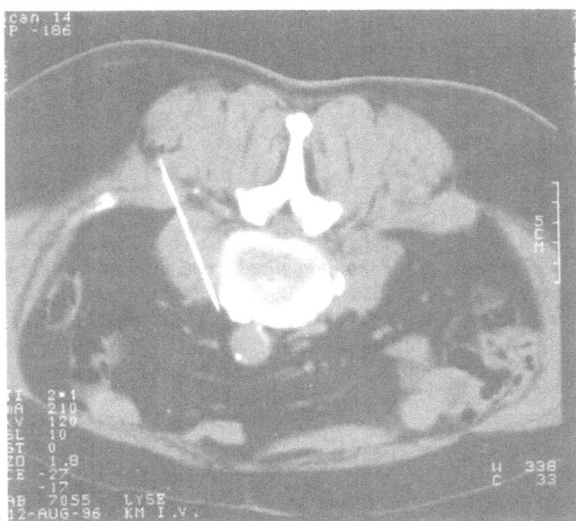
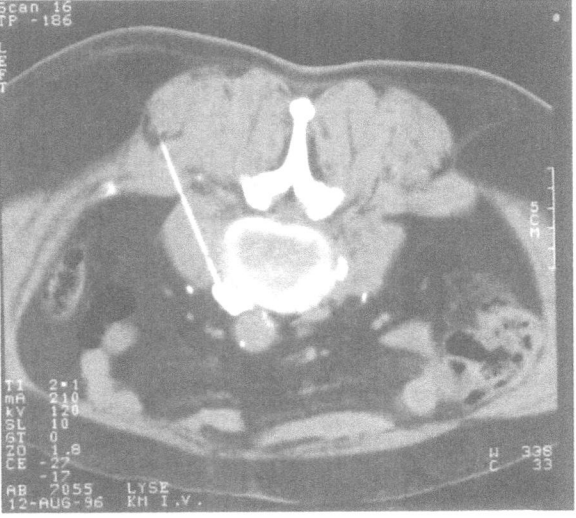

Fig. 5.33 a. Patient in prone position. The needle tip is exactly in the target area, closely anterior to the psoas muscle and posterior to the aorta (for comparison see Fig. 5.30). The sympathetic structures are not usually directly visible. **b** small volume of contrast medium confirms correct position. None of the surrounding vascular structures (including the ureter) shows misinjection. Application of ethanol or phenol can be carried out

Table 5.15. Complications in sympathectomy/sympathicolysis

	Operative sympathectomy BAUMGARTL et al. (1975)	Phenol – induced sympathicolysis			
		REID et al. (1970)	WALKER et al. (1978)	DONDELINGER and KURCTRID (1983)	NÜRNBERG (1987)
Mortality	0–4.4%	0.1%	0	0	0
Neuritis	2–55%	15%	35%	14%	3.6%
Organ lesion	Mentioned, no numbers	0.5%	0	0	0
Pleural effusion	0	0.6%	0	0	0
Peritonitis	Mentioned, no numbers	0	0	2%	0
n =	No numbers	1028	50/127	69	54

Table 5.16. Prospective study of sympthicolysis in 50 patients (WALKER et al. 1978)

Rest pain	$n = 32$	Success	No success
BP above 35 mmHg	25	23	2
BP below 35 mmHg	7	0	7
Gangrene of the toes	$n = 11$		
BP above 60 mmHg	6	6	0
BP below 60 mmHg	1	0	1
Diabetes/infection	$n = 4$	0	4
Gangrene of the heel	$n = 7$	1	6
Total	$n = 50$	30 (60%)	20 (40%)

BP, blood pressure.

Table 5.17. Results of CT-guided sympathicolysis ($n = 69$). (From DONDELINGER and KURDZIEL 1984)

Before treatment	Stage IV	31/69	45.0%
After lysis	II	12	38.7%
	III	5	16.1%
	Improved	4	12.9%
	No success	10	32.3%
Before treatment	Stage III	19/69	27.5%
After lysis	II	15	78.9%
	Improved	1	5.3%
	No success	3	15.8%
Before treatment	Stage II	19/69	27.5%
After lysis	I	2	10.6%
	Improved	14	73.7%
	No success	3	15.7%

Table 5.18. Results of CT-guided sympathicolysis ($n = 72$). (Results obtained at KLINIKUM NÜRNBERG, 1985–1988)

Prestage	IV	31/72	43.0%
After lysis	II	17	55.0%
	II–III	3	9.6%
	Improved	8	26.8%
	No success	3	9.6%
Prestage	III	39/72	55.0%
After lysis	I/II	20	51.5%
	II–III	1	2.5%
	Improved	13	33.0%
	No success	5	13.0%
Prestage	II	2	3.0%
	Improved	2	

Table 5.19. Results of spinal cord stimulation ($n = 94$). (KASPRZAK and RAITHEL 1994)

Surgical correction	13.8%
Septic complications	5.3%
No function	4.3%
Success III/IV → II	64.9%
No success	12.8%
Following extensive amputation	22.3%

Late results, 3 months–5 years.

Finally, of course, it must be kept in mind that arteriosclerotic disease is of a progressive nature. This means that CT-guided sympathicolysis, as well as the other relevant methods, usually yield more temporary and palliative rather than curative effects. Nevertheless, long-term healing of rest pain and even of long-standing ulcerations/gangrene was observed in numerous cases when other treatment methods were not available.

References

Baumgartl •• (1975) ••

Dondelinger R, Kurdziel JC (1984) Percutaneous phenol neurolysis of the lumbar sympathic chain with computed tomography control. Ann Radiol (Paris) 27:376–379

Kasprzak P, Raithel D (1994) Can SCS (spinal cord stimulator) reduce the amputation rate in patients with CLI (critical limb ischaemia)? In: •• (ed) Spinal cord stimulation. Steinkopff, Darmstadt

Rau G (••) Sympathektomie. In: Schoop, Heberer (eds) Angiologie. ••

Reid W, Watt JK, Gray TG (1970) Phenol injection of the sympathic chain. Br J Surg 57:45–50

Schild H (1988) Perkutane Neurolyse des lumbalen Sympathikus. In: Günther RW, Thelen M (eds) Interventionelle Radiologie. Thieme, Stuttgart, pp 409–415

Walker PM, MacKay IM, Johnston KW (1978) Phenol sympathectomy for vascular occlusive disease. Surg Gynecol Obstet 146:741–744

5.5
Laser-Assisted Angioplasty and New Developments

P. ROMANIUK, TH. FRITZSCHE, and
D.C. BAUMGART

5.5.1
Introduction

Soon after the development of laser energy sources, and at about the time of the first reports on percutaneous catheter-assisted repair of atheromatous lesions (LINDBLOM and FERNSTRÖM 1962; DÖRSCHEL 1989; DOTTER and JUDKINS 1964; GRUNKEMEIER and GREGORY 1992; GRUNTZIG and HOPFF 1974; ZEITLER and MÜLLER 1969), McGUFF et al. (1963) showed that atheromatous lesions in vessels can be vaporized by laser energy. The first clinical use of laser angioplasty in human coronary arteries and femoral vessels was described by CHOY (CHOY) 1988; CHOY et al. 1982, 1984; CHIESA et al. 1990) and GINSBURG et al. (1984, 1985; GIZSBERG et al. 1991). These momentous results with intravascular laser application went almost unnoticed at that time since mechanical recanalization of vessels by balloon catheterization was widely accepted as the established procedure (DÖRSCHEL 1989; PORSTMANN 1973; PORSTMANN and WIERNY 1967; GRÜNTZIG and HOPFF 1974; ZEITLER 1980, 1985; ZEITLER and MÜLLER 1969; VAN ANDEL 1975). Investigators started to question and reassess the efficiency of mechanical angioplasty only when extensive follow-up studies revealed that mechanical recanalization or dilatation of vascular lesions was associated with a range of severe complications (ZOLLIKOFFER 1985), such as large areas of dissection involving all vessel layers; failure to pass vascular occlusions depending on the age, length, and site of the lesion (ROMANIUK et al. 1986, 1987); limited dilatation of fibrotic or calcified vessel segments; occurrence of complex wall lesions in tortuous, angular, or kinked vessel segments; relatively high rates of reocclusion or reconstruction. Experimental studies have established that the dilatation of stenotic or recanalized vessel segments is based on various mechanisms. These include compression of atheromatous material by squeezing of lymphatic fluid; development of local fissures in the vessel wall; superficial, deep, or spiral dissections; flattening of fatty atheromatous pads by cold flowing; fracture of calcified plates; and irreversible overextension of

circular fiber bundles (DOTTER and JUDKINS 1964; GÜNTZIG and HOPFF 1974; ZOLLIKOFFER 1985). Dilatation of vessels by mechanical angioplasty creates an endovascular and intramural wound surface and is achieved without extraction or removal of atheromatous and thrombotic material (DOTTER and JUDKINS 1964). Furthermore, histological studies elucidated how complications develop in mechanical angioplasty, and thus paved the way for the introduction of ablation techniques such as laser interventions (AHMED et al. 1996; ALT et al. 1992; BERLIEN et al. 1993; BERLIEN and MÜLLER 1989; CUMBERLAND et al. 1986a,b; DIETHRICH 1990b, 1991; DIETRICH et al. 1991; GESCHWIND et al. 1987; GINSBURG et al. 1984, 1985; ILEGBUSI and NOSOVITSKY 1997; LEE et al. 1993; LUFT et al. 1993; NISHIOKA and DAMANKEVITZ 1990; PEACOCK 1981; PREISACK et al. 1997; ZWAAN et al. 1996a; WERNER et al. 1986).

The general assumption used to be that the local application of ablative laser energy was comparable to surgical ablation, such as endarterectomy, and that removal of part of the atheromatous and thrombotic material by laser ablation would create a stable vessel lumen (ABELE et al. 1985b; AHMED et al. 1996; POYEN et al. 1991). It was furthermore expected that the long-term results would be better following laser angioplasty (BAURIEDEL 1998; BAURIEDEL et al. 1992; BIAMINO 1990; CARAVELLO et al. 1990; CARLSSON 1998; COX and JACOBS 1987; ESCOJIDO et al. 1996; FRÖHLICH 1998; HAASE and KARSCH 1996; HAASE et al. 1997; HABERBOSCH 1998; ILEGBUSI and NOSOVITSKY 1997; ISNER et al. 1985; JEANS et al. 1990; KAMINOW et al. 1984; KATUS 1998; LEE 1986; LEEUWEN et al. 1996; LINSKER et al. 1984; PETIT et al. 1993; PILGER et al. 1991; STILLE 1998), as it was hoped that vaporization, photodisruption, or photoablation occurring at the site of laser exposure would destroy local atherogenic agents (such as growth hormones released by cells of the vessel wall or thrombocytes, proinflammatory adhesion molecules from monocytes, or atherogenic pathogens such as herpes virus, cytomegalovirus, *Heliobacter pylori, Chlamydiae pneumoniae* (MEHRAN et al. 1997; MINICK et al. 1979; MORGUET et al. 1997b; NILSSON et al. 1993; PEACOCK 1981; PREVOSTI et al. 1937; RIAMBAU-ALONSO et al. 1991; ROMANIUK 1996).

5.5.2
General Aspects of Laser Techniques

The competent application of laser-assisted angioplasty without complications is based on a range of physical and technical prerequisites (BERLIEN and MÜLLER 1989).

5.5.2.1
Physical Aspects of the Laser Generator

The induced emission of photons or quantum particles in a high-frequency feedback transmitter is referred to as:

- *Laser* (light amplification of stimulated emission of radiation)
- *Maser* (microwave amplification of stimulated emission of radiation)
- *Graser* (gamma-ray amplification of stimulated emission of radiation)

depending on the wavelength of the radiation generated (DÖRSCHEL 1989; GARRAND et al. 1991; GERTHSEN 1966). In a laser generator, the first step is to raise molecules from a lower to a higher energy plateau by means of inversion in a so-called three- or four-level system. This step is accomplished by means of a weak amplifier operating in an appropriate surrounding laser medium (free atoms, free ions, molecules, molecule ions in gases, molecule ions in vapors, dye molecules in fluids, ions in solid bodies, etc.).

The laser medium is excited either by optical pumping, i.e., by intermittent application of high-intensity light energy, or by particle acceleration in a gas discharge tube (Fig. 5.34). In either case, the kinetic energy of the electrons is transferred to the collision particles. A laser resonator (plane parallel or confocal arrangement of mirrors) redirects the photons back into the laser medium. At a very high overall amplification, the system thus assumes a self-excited state. The laser radiation is emitted in an avalanche-like fashion when the higher energy plateau is left (MÜLLER-STOLZENBURG et al. 1989; ODINK et al. 1995; OEZISIK 1985). The laser radiation at the resonator is characterized by two different intensity distributions: (1) One depending on the wavelength (so-called longitudinal mode), and (2) one depending on geometric or spatial properties (so-called transverse electromagnetic mode). It must be borne in mind that the emitted laser radiation reflects the energy development inside the resonator. The latter determines the focus of the beam with respect to its size, shape, and boundaries by intensity differences in terms of the longitudinal and transverse mode. Irregular boundaries of the focus will result in an uneven transmission of the laser energy via the light guides of multiple-fiber catheters (see Fig. 5.37c). Additional components inserted along the feedback pathway of the laser generator can alter the quality of feedback and thus release the stored energy as induced emission at different time intervals (BERLIEN and MÜLLER 1989). The radiation emitted by the resonator has three major properties that exist simultaneously (DÖRSCHEL 1989): (1) coherence, (2) extreme collimation (maximal deviation of the beam direction: 1 cm at a length of 10 km), and (3) monochromasy. These special properties account for the high local effects of laser energy (ABELE et al. 1985b; ALT et al. 1992; ASADA et al. 1993; ASHLEY et al. 1990; BAO et al. 1993; BATCHELOR et al. 1996; BERLIEN et al. 1993; BHATA et al. 1989; BITTL 1996; CLARKE et al. 1987; CRAZZOLARA et al. 1991; DAIKUZONO and JOFFE 1985; DUDA et al. 1993; FANKHAUSER et al. 1994; GROSS 1996; HAASE and KARSCH 1996; HELFMANN 1989; ISNER et al. 1985; KAR and RINGELHAN 1992; LEE 1986; LINSKER et al. 1984; McKENZI 1984; MÜLLER-STOLZENBURG et al. 1989; PETIT et al. 1993; SATHYAM et al. 1996; SRINIVASAN and LEIGH 1986; YANG et al. 1991; YEH 1986).

5.5.2.2
Laser Parameters

The mean power densities of laser beams are listed in Table 5.20. The tissue effect depends on the power density (watt/cm^2) and exposure time (to be derived from the absorption coefficient) as the two major biological parameters (Table 5.21). Additional beam parameters are used for a more detailed description and quantitative characterization of the tissue effect of laser energy:

Table 5.20. Power densities of different lasers

Light source	Light output	Power density
He-Ne laser	1 mW	4×10^4 W/cm^2
Argon laser	10 W	4×10^8 W/cm^2
Nd:YAG laser	100 W	4×10^5 W/cm^2
CO$_2$ Laser metal finishing	10 kW	10^8 W/cm^2
Pulsed lasers	1000 MW	10^{14} W/cm^2

Table 5.21. Absorption coefficients of laser radiation

Wavelength		Absorption coefficient		Mean wavelength	
		Water	Blood	Water	Blood
10 600 nm	(CO$_2$ laser)	103 cm^{-1}	103 cm^{-1}	0.001 cm	0.001 cm
1 060 nm	(Nd:YAG laser)	0.1 cm^{-1}	4 cm^{-1}	10 cm	<0.2 cm
500 nm	(Argon laser)	0.001 cm^{-1}	330 cm^{-1}	10 000 cm	0.003 cm

- T (laser pulse duration), (temporal extension of an individual impulse)
- W (laser pulse energy)
- P (t) (momentary laser pulse power)
- P (pulse power averaged over time)
- f (pulse sequence frequency)
- Ps (mean power of a pulse sequence)
- I (t) (momentary laser pulse intensity)
- I (intensity averaged over time in watt/cm^2)
- E (field strength averaged over time)
- N (photon density averaged over time).

5.5.2.3
Technical Aspects of the Transmission and application of Laser Energy

The mode of laser generation (in gases, dye solutions, or solid bodies) results in a range of laser systems that differ considerably in terms of mobility, size, and technical complexity (e.g., maintenance-intensive inert gas circuits, water cooling) (Figs. 5.35). The systems preferred for medical applications are mobile solid-body lasers without cooling (BERLIEN and MÜLLER 1989). The tissue effect or application of a laser beam depends on the type of procedure used (ABELA et al. 1985a; ASADA et al. 1993; ASHLEY et al. 1990; BAO et al. 1993; BAUER et al. 1996; BECKER et al. 1989; COX and JACOBS 1987; CREA et al. 1986; CUMBERLAND et al. 1986a; DECKER-DUNN et al. 1990; DIETHRICH et al. 1991; FANKHAUSER et al. 1994; FIELD et al. 1995; FOURRIER et al. 1987; GANDY et al. 1990; GMITO et al. 1988; ODINK et al. 1995; ILEGBUSI and NOSOVITSKY 1997; KLOCEK and SIGEL 1989; LEE et al. 1990; LITVACK et al. 1987; MCMATH et al. 1990; MÜLLER-STOLZENBURG et al. 1989; NORDSTROM et al. 1988; SATHYAM et al. 1996; SIEVERT et al. 1995, 1996; SINGLETON et al. 1987; VINCENT et al. 1990; WILMS et al. 1990; YANG et al. 1990; YEH 1986; ZEITLER 1985; ZWAAN et al. 1996a):
- Energy application without direct tissue contact
- Energy application with direct tissue contact
- Energy application via single fibers (WHITE et al. 1991, 1993; WOLLENEK et al. 1988; CHOY et al. 1982, 1984; CHOY 1988)
- Energy application via single fibers with metal caps (CUMBERLAND et al. 1986a; SPIES 1990; OBIS 1989; WHITE 1990)
- Energy application via single fibers with sapphire lenses (WHITE et al. 1991, 1993; SANBORN et al. 1985, 1988, 1989a,b; VERDAASCONK 1987)
- Energy application via single fibers with fenestrated metal caps and sapphire lenses (BELLI et al. 1991; POYEN et al. 1991)
- Energy application via multiple-fiber catheters (LITVACK et al. 1987, 1989; DECKELBAUM et al. 1985; GESCHWIND et al. 1984, 1987, 1989, 1991, 1992)
- Energy application via gas as the medium
- Energy application via sodium chloride as the medium
- Energy application via radiographic contrast agents as the medium
- Energy application via blood as the medium (static or flowing)
- Continuous energy application (LAMMER et al. 1991; LAMMER and JOHANNES 1995; PILGER et al. 1991)
- Pulsed-energy application (DECKELBAUM 1989, 1994a,b; DECKELBAUM et al. 1985, 1987, 1995a,b)
- Ultrashort pulsed energy application (Q-switch technique) (KOPCHOK et al. 1990).

Only light guide systems are used nowadays in angiology and cardiology. The light guides consist of highly purified, water-free quartz fibers (ABELA et al. 1985a; ANDERSON et al. 1983; ASHLEY et al. 1990; BAO et al. 1993; BERLIEN and MÜLLER 1989; BIAMINO 1990; KLOCEK and SIGEL 1989; MÜLLER-STOLZENBURG et al. 1989; SCHÖNBORN 1989; SOWADA et al. 1988; SRINIVASAN et al. 1990), which allow transmission of the laser energy over a wide frequency range (Figs. 5.36–5.38; see Fig. 5.40). Lightwave guides always consist of a two-component glass body (core and cladding) with different refraction indices (for transportation of the laser beam by total reflection) and a synthetic coating (see Fig. 5.39). The quality of laser energy transmission is determined by (MÜLLER-STOLZENBURG et al. 1989):

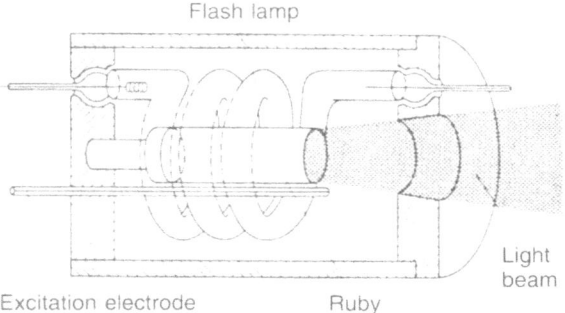

Fig. 5.34. Ruby laser according to Maibach (GHAZZAL et al. 1995)

- The type of coupling optics inserted between the generator and the glass fiber
- The efficiency of fiber coupling
- The linearity of the fiber course (bending losses).

Damping losses occur even with optimal light guidance in a totally reflecting light guide. They are caused by:

- The innate damping of the quartz glass material
- The additional damping resulting from unavoidable flaws in the material (pores, cracks, glass bubbles)
- The additional damping resulting from the geometric arrangement (bending or torsion of the fibers).

Further sources of energy loss include:

- Disturbed coherence during passage of the light guide
- Restricted focusing of light guide transmission
- Reflection due to long fibers
- Reflection due to insufficiently de-reflected fiber ends
- Reflection due to insufficient preparation of the fiber ends
- Reflection due to high refraction indices.

Of practical relevance are scratches on the light guide surfaces or organic impurities, such as blood or tissue fragments, on the light guide surfaces of bare fibers, or when multiple-fiber catheters are used (Fig. 5.38). Such impurities may result in excessive local energy absorption with subsequent breaking of the light guide (Figs. 5.37, 5.38).

Inaccurate fiber coupling (location of the focus in the proximal fiber segment and not at the coupling interface), or inadequate preparation of the fiber surface at the coupling interface may likewise lead to the breakage, fusion, or complete destruction of fibers resulting from increased local heat absorption

(Figs. 5.36, 5.38). The threshold of destruction is especially low for laser energy in the lower short-wave range (excimer technique). Bare-fiber systems require continuous rinsing with a saline solution to prevent local overheating (CROSS et al. 1988; GRUNKEMEIER and GREGORY 1992; HAASE et al. 1997; PIZZULLI et al. 1996; PREISACK et al. 1992; SCHOMAKER et al. 1997; ZWAAN et al. 1996a).

The initial euphoria over bare-fiber ablation was soon superseded by a very critical attitude, but the recent introduction of a special laser wire (diameter 0.01 in., 11 microfibers) has led to a revival of the bare-fiber technique in the area of the coronary vessels (ESCOJIDO et al. 1996; ISCHINGER 1990; SIEVERT et al. 1995, 1996).

Another technique for the planar application of laser energy to biological tissue is to use multiple-fiber catheters (COTHREN 1986; DECKELBAUM 1989, 1994a,b; DECKELBAUM et al. 1985, 1987, 1995a), in which varying numbers of fibers and fiber diameters are radially incorporated into between 6 and 10-F angiography catheters (Figs. 5.36, 5.37, 5.40). The flexibility of multiple-fiber catheters (Fig. 5.39) has facilitated medical laser application, especially in angiology, allowing access to arteries and veins in various regions of the body (upper and lower leg, pelvic vessels, renal vessels, vena cava) (ROMANIUK 1996).

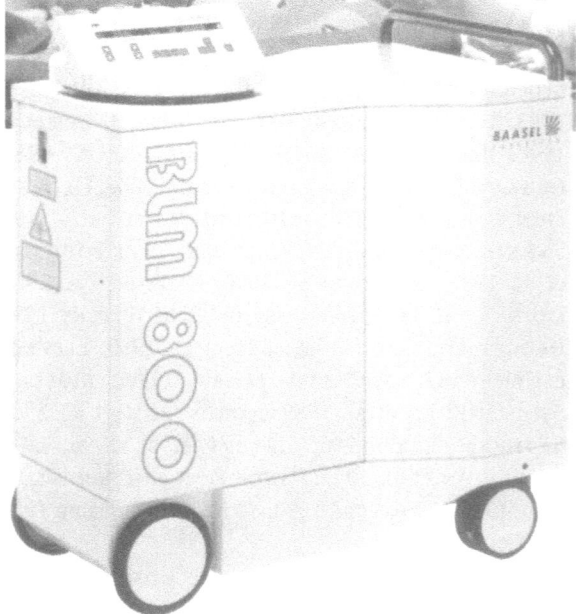

Fig. 5.35. BLM 800 holmium laser (Baasel, Starnberg). Maximal pulse rate, 50 Hz; pulse duration of up to 1000 µs or 0.02 µs in Q-switch technique; peak pulse power, 3 kW

When multiple-fiber catheters are used, the laser energy is applied simultaneously via all radially arranged fibers or in a sector-wise rotating fashion, depending on the control of the laser generator (XIE et al. 1993; SCULPER et al. 1996). This technique is aimed at reducing the shock waves. The individual fibers are glued into the catheter tip (see Fig. 5.36). Higher ablation energies can be applied only with the use of a thermostable glue, metal tubes for the central guiding wire, and continuous rinsing with a saline solution (ROMANIUK 1996). The diameters of multiple-fiber catheters range from 1.5–3.3 mm; they are inserted by means of the so-called over-the-wire technique, and are advanced for ablation at a mean velocity of 0.5–1.0 mm/s.

To minimize the risks of multiple-fiber catheter application in vessel repair, it is necessary to pass the laser system through the site of the lesion. This is achieved by prior mechanical recanalization by

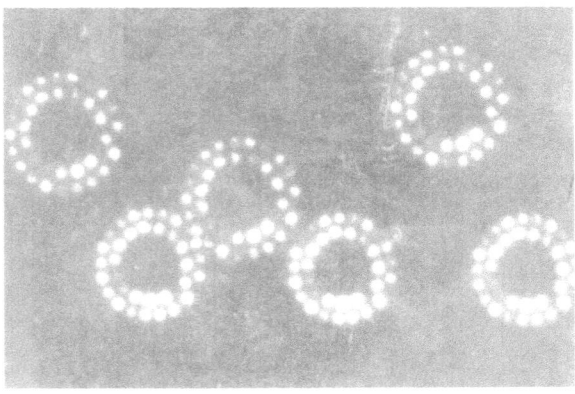

Fig. 5.37. a Exposure experiments with a 7-F multiple-fiber catheter (on blackened photographic paper) showing irregular transmission of laser energy (holmium laser) caused by either broken fibers or inhomogeneities at the laser focus

means of guiding wires, for instance wires with a sliding coat (Terumo system). Stand-alone techniques (ROSENTHAL et al. 1991; STONE et at. 1997), i.e., management of vessel lesions exclusively by laser ablation, only rarely create an adequately wide vessel lumen even when large 10-F multiple-fiber catheters are used; secondary dilatation with conventional balloon catheters is required in most cases (COOK et al. 1991; DECKER-DUNN et al. 1990; KENT et al. 1991; LEE et al. 1990; ROSENTHAL et al. 1991; SAFIAN et al. 1993; SCHMID et al. 1995; SCHOFER et al. 1996; SIEVERT et al. 1995, 1996; TOPAZ 1995; TORRE et al. 1990a; VINCENT et al. 1990; WHITE et al. 1991; MARGOLIS 1996; MARGOLIS et al. 1990; BITTL et al. 1992, 1993, 1994, 1995). Another technique is the so-called step-by-step technique, in which the multiple-fiber catheter is advanced into the occluded area 1 cm at a time without using guiding wires. However, this latter technique is associated with a higher incidence of complications (see Table 5.24) (Table 5; ABELA et al. 1985a; ABELA 1992; APPELMAN et al. 1996a,b; BARBIERI et al. 1990; CHIESA et al. 1990; EIBERG et al. 1995; GESCHWIND et al. 1984; GUINTINI et al. 1994; HAASE et al. 1991b; HENRY et al. 1990; JEANS et al. 1990; LEE et al. 1990; POYEN et al. 1991; ROSENTHAL et al. 1991; SANBORN et al. 1989a; SIEVERT et al. 1995, 1996; STRAUSS et al. 1995).

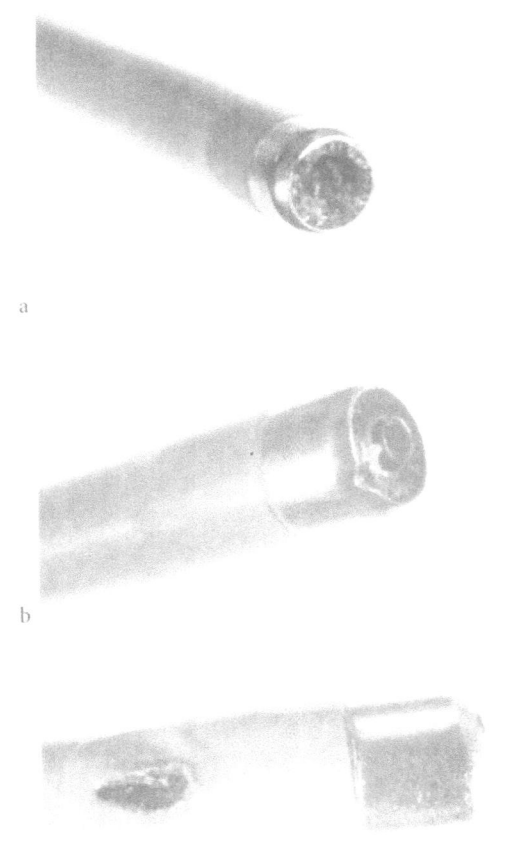

Fig. 5.36 a–c. Lesions of multiple-fiber catheters (holmium laser application) at the shaft (a), around a single fiber (b), and through consumption of several fibers (c) at high energy application with simultaneous leakage of thermo-unstable glue

5.5.3
Biological Action of Laser Radiation

Two basic properties determine the effects of laser energy on tissue (DÖRSCHEL 1989; WALTER 1989;

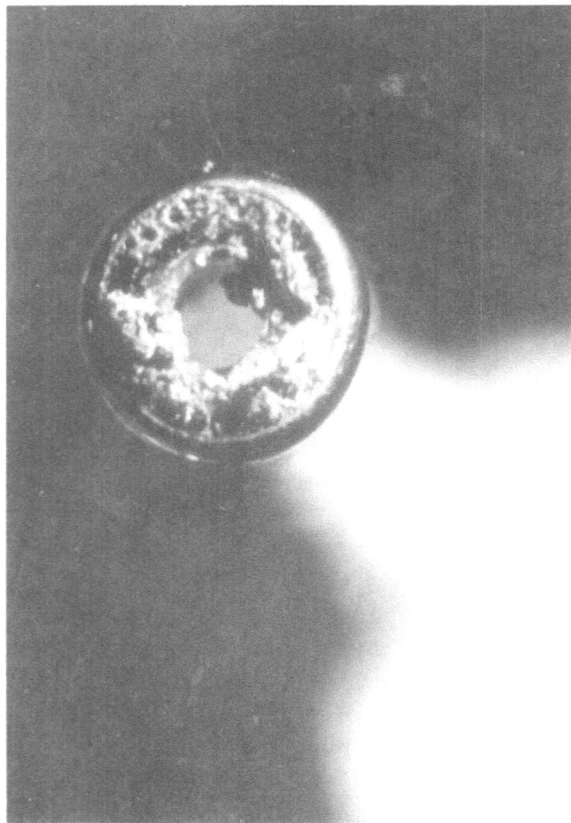

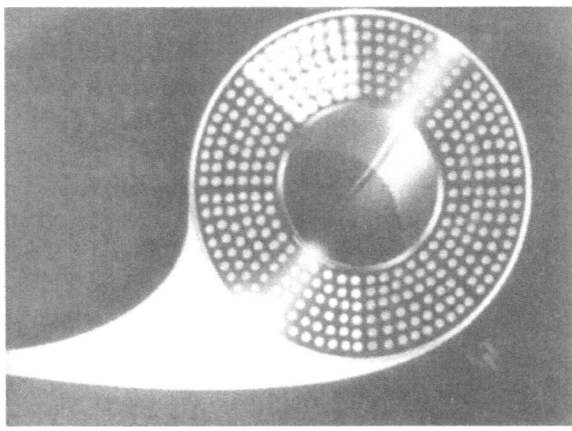

Fig. 5.40. Sector-wise sequentially controlled multiple-fiber catheter (Spectranetics, Nieuwegein,

Fig. 5.38. Organic deposits of fresh, soft atheromatous material on the frontal surface of a multiple-fiber catheter (following femoral holmium ablation)

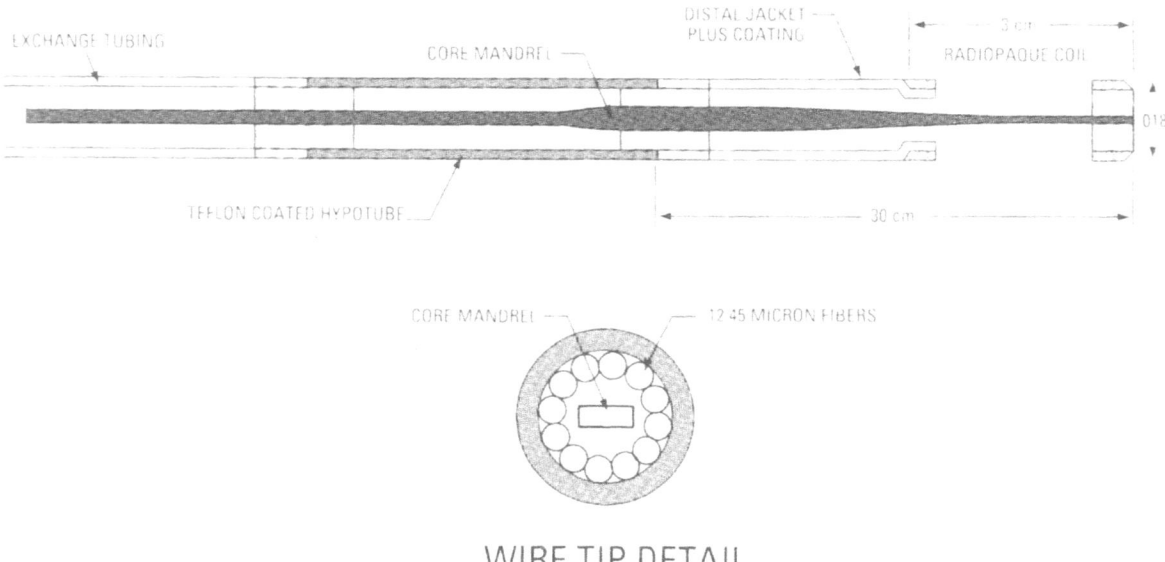

WIRE DETAIL

WIRE TIP DETAIL

Fig. 5.39. Laser wire (Spectranetics, Nieuwegein, NL). Diameter, 0.018 in, 12 light guides of 12.45 µ each

Asada et al. 1993; Gross 1996; Grundfest et al. 1985a; Hassenstein et al. 1992; Helfmann 1989; Huppert et al. 1992b; Ilegbusi and Nosovitsky 1997; Odink et al. 1995; Oezisik 1985; Poyen et al. 1991; Preisack et al. 1997): (1) The property of the laser radiation, (2) the property of the biological material.

The properties of the laser energy are determined by the following factors:

- The wavelength of the laser energy
- The energy density of the laser beam
- The duration of exposure
- The repetition frequency of the individual laser impulses.

In addition, the effects of the laser energy are also determined by the following basic properties of the exposed tissue (Prince and Athanasoulis 1992; Quan and Hodgson 1996; Reichel et al. 1987; Scheinert et al. 1998; Walsh et al. 1989; Walter 1989; Yang et al. 1991; Yeh 1986): (a) Tissue absorption, (b) tissue scattering, and (c) tissue density.

From a physicochemical perspective, the tissue effect is further influenced by: (a) the optical properties and (b) the thermal properties of the biological material.

netic spectrum, the physical absorption of the tissue determines the mean penetration depth, which is:

- Approximately 3 µm for the excimer laser (spectral range from 193 to 351 mm)
- Approximately 0.5–2.5 mm for the argon laser (spectral range from 450–590 nm)
- Approximately 10.6 µm for the holmium laser (spectral range around 2060 nm).

The degree of absorption and scattering is determined by the water content of a biological tissue in the infrared range and by its protein content in the ultraviolet range. These properties are crucial for laser applications in medicine and biology. The maximal absorption of important organic molecules is as follows: Protein (mean value), 100–300 nm; hemoglobin, 400–700 nm. These values explain the high energy uptake and energy binding of proteins including hemoglobin when argon lasers, dye lasers, and neodymium: ytlrium aluminum garnet (YAG) lasers are used. The latter are thus especially useful for tissue coagulation (Van Leeuwen et al. 1993). In contrast, erbium:YAG lasers and holmium lasers are preferentially used for tissue separation due to their high water absorption capacity (Fankhauser et al. 1994; McKenzi 1989; Torres et al. 1990).

5.5.3.1
Optical Properties of Tissue

Three effects can be observed when a biological tissue is exposed to laser energy (Dörschel 1989; Kar and Ringelhan 1992; Walsh et al. 1989; Walter 1989): (1) Tissue reflection, (2) tissue absorption, and (3) tissue transmission. Tissue reflection is high and amounts to about 60% of the applied laser energy. Cardiovascular laser application typically uses three ranges from the electromagnetic spectrum: (1) The infrared range (Geschwind et al. 1991; Heuser and Mehta 1991; Holmes et al. 1997; Ragosta et al. 1995; Romaniuk 1996; Teitelbalim 1992; Topaz et al. 1996; Quan and Hodgson 1996; White et al. 1991, 1993); (2) the ultraviolet range (Litvack et al. 1987, 1989; Huppert et al. 1990, 1991, 1992a,b, 1994; Duda et al. 1990a,b, 1993; Reeders 1996; Rosenfeldt et al. 1992; Sanborn et al. 1990; Vogl et al. 1996); (3) and the visible range (Geschwind et al. 1984, 1987, 1989, 1992; Duda et al. 1990a,b; Prince and Athanasoulis 1992; Yang et al. 1990, 1991; De Marchena et al. 1996; Anderson et al. 1983). In all of these three ranges of the electromag-

5.5.3.2
Thermal Properties of Tissue

The high absorption and scattering of laser energy in biological tissue induces a considerable increase in temperature. The following thermal properties of tissue need to be distinguished (Walter 1989; Yang et al. 1991): (a) The heat conduction capacity of the tissue, (b) the heat storage capacity, and (c) the heat dispersion capacity of the tissue. The heat conduction capacities of important biological tissues and media are compiled in Table 5.22.

In physical terms, the heat storage capacity of a tissue is a constant of the material. The value gives the amount of heat stored per unit of temperature increase and mass, for instance (Walsh et al. 1989): 3.22 KJ/Kg × K for blood and 3.0 KJ/Kg × K for fatty tissue.

Table 5.23 shows how heat conduction depends on blood flow. The mean perfusion rates of important biological tissues serve as a general orientation for laser application. The values show that tissues with low perfusion have a higher thermal penetration depth than tissues with high perfusion. Tissues with low perfusion are thus more susceptible to thermal damage. Noteworthy are the following effects that depend on the type of energy radiation: (a) Low power densities of a laser will induce photochemical effects at long exposure times (RÜCK 1989); (b) high power densities of a laser will produce thermal effects at short exposure; and (c) very high power densities (above 10^7 W/cm^2) will produce nonlinear effects in tissue at ultrashort exposure times (e.g., in the Q-switch mode) (TAYLOR et al. 1990; TOMARU et al. 1991, 1992; REICHEL et al. 1987).

Photochemical reactions are associated with biostimulation of cellular metabolism and photodynamic destruction of cells, thermal reactions induce tissue coagulation or evaporization, and nonlinear processes lead to photoablation of the tissue as a result of microexplosions in the tissue or disruption of the tissue texture with optical eruptions (BERLIEN and MÜLLER 1989). In detail, the following optical and structural changes can be observed in tissue relative to the temperature reached (DÖRSCHEL 1989):

- 37–60°C: Rise in tissue temperature (no apparent optical and mechanical changes in tissue texture)
- 60–65°C: Denaturation of tissue proteins (optically, greyish-white discoloration; mechanically, loosening of the tissue texture)
- 90–100°C: Tissue desiccation (optically, pronounced scattering; mechanically, tissue shrinkage detectable)
- Around 150°C: Tissue carbonization (optically, blackening of the tissue with increased absorption; mechanically, pronounced damage of the texture)
- Around 300°C: Optically, generation of gas; mechanically, tissue detachment
- Around 300°C–1000°C: Plasma formation in the tissue – optical eruption (optically, explosive tissue ablation; mechanically, disruption of molecular bonds in the tissue).

Regarding the undesired effects of laser radiation on the tissue immediately adjacent to the target area

Table 5.22. Heat conduction capacities of different substances

Substance	Watt/m·K
Air	0.02
Ethyl alcohol	0.16
Water	0.58
Blood	0.62
Steel	46.02
Copper	418.00
Fatty tissue	0.30
Tissue, water-containing	0.50

Table 5.23. Perfusion rates of important biological tissue

Biological tissue	ml × min × g Tissue
Kidney (dog)	3.3
Kidney (human)	3.4
Thyroid (mouse)	3.24
Thyroid (human)	4.0
Heart (dog)	0.6
Brain (human)	0.46
Skin (human)	0.15
Muscle (dog)	0.11
Arm muscle (human)	0.02
Fatty tissue (human)	0.012

Fig. 5.41 a,b. Human aortic wall (reflected-light microscopy). **a** Ostium of an intercostal artery (for comparison). **b** Status post athermal holmium laser ablation (single fiber; energy, 2008 mJ; power, 10 W; energy density, 245 J/cm^2; 12 individual impulses; pulse width, 500 µs; pulse frequency, 3 Hz)

Fig. 5.42. Human aortic wall (reflected-light microscopy). Athermal holmium laser ablation (single fiber, laser beam parameters as in Fig. 5.41b). Fissures in the marginal zone of the ablation canal induced by shock waves

Fig. 5.44 a,b. Human aorta (scanning electron microscopy). a Athermal holmium laser ablation (F-7 multiple-fiber cather; 19 fibers; beam parameters as in Fig. 5.43a; fiber direction as in Fig. 5.43b – central segment removed for preparation). b Slight thermal changes of the marginal zone (lesion as in (a), with magnification)

Fig. 5.43 a,b. Human aorta (reflected-light microscopy). a Athermal holmium laser ablation (F-7 multiple-fiber catheter; 19 fibers; energy, 1280 mJ; pulse duration, 240 µs; 20 individual impulses; pulse width, 240 µs; pulse frequency, 3 Hz; prograde catheter pressure without rotation). b As in (a), prograde catheter direction with rotation. Deep ring-shaped athermal ablation

(e.g., the edges of ablation areas), a distinction is made between thermal and athermal ablation (Figs. 5.41–5.45).

It is to be noted, however, that all laser spectra (both in the infrared and in the ultraviolet ranges) involve thermal effects on tissue (Huppert et al. 1991, 1992a,b, 1994; Duda et al. 1990a,b, 1993; Chiesa et al. 1990; Welsch et al. 1987).

Heat absorption at the cutting edge of a tissue lamella, which roughly corresponds to the optical penetration depth of the laser energy (e.g., approximately 286 µm at an energy of 2060 nm), will result in marginal coagulation. Deposition of thermal energy likewise involves the adjacent lamella (Linsker et al. 1984; Grundfest et al. 1985a,b; Isner et al. 1985). This observation explains that thermal effects such as coagulation and carbonization are not primarily dependent on the wavelength of the applied energy, but rather on the repetition frequency of the laser pulse and the heat conduction capacity of the tissue (Grundfest et al. 1985a; McKenzi et al. 1989).

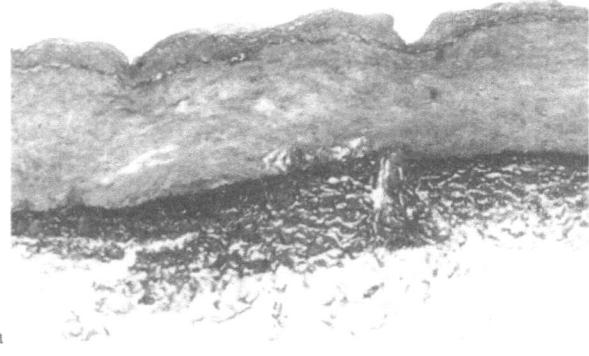

a

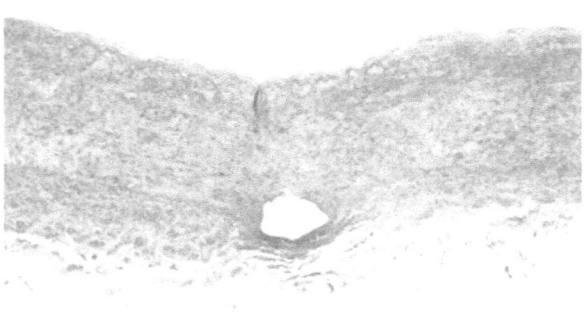

b

Fig. 5.45. **a** Athermal laser ablation (human aorta, Elastica staining, multiple-fiber catheter applied with slight pressure – early phase). **b** As in (**a**). Human aorta, hematoxylin and eosin staining, oblique section, bare fiber application, beam parameters as in Fig. 5.39b

The term "athermal ablation" is applied when the coagulation necrosis is less than 20 nm in size (Figs. 5.41, 5.44, 5.45).

The positive effect of athermal ablation occurs both in the infrared and in the ultraviolet ranges when very short individual impulses are applied. The required depth of ablation is achieved by increasing the number of impulses (KNOPF et al. 1992). The thermal effects can be reduced for all laser energies by using ultrashort individual impulses. However, this requires special switches (so-called Q-switch technique) (STRIKWERDA et al. 1995a; ROMAIUK 1996; CLARKE et al. 1987; DECKELBAUM et al. 1985; SATHYAM et al. 1996; SRINIVASAN et al. 1990; SRINIVASAN and LEIGH 1982, 1986; TAYLOR et al. 1990; GRUNDFEST et al. 1985a,b; ISNER et al. 1985). But there is as yet no system on the market that allows an easy transition from the regular pulse mode to the Q-switch mode without rearrangement of components.

5.5.3.3
Nonlinear Processes and Special Effects on Vessel Walls

Nonlinear processes occur when laser energy is applied with very short pulse durations and very high power densities (ASADA et al. 1993; BLOEMBERGEN 1974; CLARKE et al. 1987; CROSS et al. 1988; DÖRSCHEL 1989; GIJSBERS et al. 1991; GRUNDFEST et al. 1985a; HAASE et al. 1993a,b; HELFMANN 1989; JUDY et al. 1992; LEE 1986; MCKENZIE 1984; MURPHY-CHUTORIAN et al. 1986; OOMEN et al. 1990a; ORAEVSKY et al. 1992; PREISACK et al. 1992; REICHEL et al. 1987; REICHEL and SCHMIDT-KLOIBER 1989; SAPIENZA et al. 1994; SATHYAM et al. 1996; SRINIVASAN and LEIGH 1986). These effects were first described by SRINIVASAN and colleagues (SRINIVASAN et al. 1986; SRINIVASAN and LEIGH 1982, 1986) and are referred to as "photoablation". With the proper selection of laser parameters, these processes can be used for very precise tissue ablation with only little thermal damage to the tissue surrounding the target site. Photoablation occurs at an energy density of about $10 \, J/cm^2$ with laser pulse durations in the nanosecond range. Further increases in energy (e.g., above $10^{11} \, J/cm^2$) lead to plasma formation from ionization of matter (HASSENSTEIN et al. 1992). Plasma formation results in tissue ablation via explosive detachment of tissue particles. This process is associated with a specific opto-acoustic phenomenon, the formation of shock waves (Fig. 5.42).

Closer analysis (EISENMENGER 1962) of laser-induced optical eruptions in tissue (by high-frequency photography of the tissue surface or registration of acoustic signals by hydrophone) has shown that the shock or detonation waves lead to the formation of gas bubbles in fluid as the contact medium (ASADA et al. 1993; BARBEAU et al. 1990; BLOEMBERGEN 1974; CLARKE et al. 1987; CROSS et al. 1988; DIETHRICH 1991; EISENMENGER 1962; FROEHLICH et al. 1995; GIJSBERS et al. 1991; GRUNKEMEIER and GREGORY 1992; HAASE et al. 1993a,b; JUDY et al. 1992; KAR and RINGELHAN 1992; REICHEL et al. 1987; SATHYAM et al. 1996; TOMARU et al. 1991; VAN LEEUWEN et al. 1991, 1992, 1993, 1996; ZWAAN et al. 1991). In particular, when holmium and excimer lasers are used (TOMARU et al. 1991, 1992, 1995; QUAN and HODGSON 1996; YOSHIKAWA et al. 1992) ablation of atheromatous foci is associated with photoacoustic effects. Excimer-induced pyrolytic gas bubbles (VAN LEEUWEN et al. 1992, 1993, 1996), for instance, contain methane, acetylene, ethane, and tissue water. Bubble formation is associated with the generation of shock waves, which produce ablation of atheromas, as well as lamellar dissection and tissue swelling (VAN ERVEN et al. 1992; VAN LEEUWEN et al. 1991, 1992, 1993, 1996; HAASE et al. 1990, 1991a,b, 1993a,b, 1994, 1997; HAASE and KARSCH 1996). Excimer lasers (wavelength 308 µm) generate peak pressures of 1.3 MPA at the normal vessel wall and of 2.0 MPA at the calcified aortic wall (TCHENG et al. 1995). Such high pressures cause focal fragmentation of calcified plates (DUDA et al. 1990a,b, 1993; ESCOJIDO et al. 1996; LUFT et al. 1993; VAN LEEUWEN et al. 1992, 1993).

Studies with the pulsed PD-2 dye laser (wavelength 630 µm) using a single fiber with a diameter of 275 µm have shown that gas bubbles of up to 3 mm in diameter are generated at the calcified aortic wall and that these bubbles move at a velocity of 10 m/s (VAN LEEUWEN et al. 1991, 1992, 1996; BAUER et al. 1996; BAUMBACH et al. 1991; ZWAAN et al. 1991, 1996a,b; DE MARCHENA et al. 1996; DUDA et al. 1990a,b, 1993; HUPPERT et al. 1994).

Comparison of different laser systems (continuous-wave argon laser, continuous-wave neodymium:YAG laser, pulsed excimer laser, pulsed erbium:YAG laser) has shown that only the pulsed mode allows ablation of calcifications (TOMARU et al. 1992; HAASE et al. 1990, 1991, 1993a,b, 1994, 1997; HAASE and KARSCH 1996; STERENBORG et al. 1990). This observation is confirmed by our experimental investigations with holmium laser ablation using bare fibers with diameters of 200 nm–800 µm (ROMANIUK 1996). The higher percentage of wall irregularities demonstrated by coronary angiography after bare-fiber laser application is attributable to the shock waves (Fig. 5.43). The photoacoustic effects associated with bare-fiber laser treatment also induce vascular spasms and wall distentions with changes in vasomotor tone (TOMARU et al. 1991, 1992, 1995; VAN LEEUWEN et al. 1992, 1993).

Wound healing after holmium laser angioplasty occurs in two stages: Following formation of necrosis (around the third day), the wall lesions will be completely filled with proliferating smooth muscle cells within 2–4 weeks (HANKE et al. 1991a; HASSENSTEIN et al. 1992; KARSCH et al. 1991; PEACOCK 1981). Histologic studies after laser ablation of experimentally created vascular stenoses have shown that intimal hyperplasia and smooth muscle cell proliferation are similar to the effects observed after conventional balloon angioplasty (VAN ERVEN et al. 1992;

PREVOSTI et al. 1987; OOMEN et al. 1990b). The question as to whether laser angioplasty is associated with a lower incidence of elastic recoiling of the vessel wall is not answered uniformly (DE MARCHENA et al. 1996; PIZZULLI et al. 1996; STRIKWERDA et al. 1995a). Regarding the optical medium to be used for laser-assisted angioplasty, numerous experimental studies (TOMARN et al. 1991, 1992, 1995) have shown that the best results are obtained when a saline solution (BAUMBACH et al. 1991) is used for rinsing, since the latter reduces the incidence of adverse thermal effects and slows down excessive nonlinear processes compared to blood and contrast agents (GREGORY et al. 1990, 1994; GRUNKEMEIER and GREGORY 1992; SCHOMAKER et al. 1997; TCHENG et al. 1995). Mention should also be made of the positive adjuvant effects of heparin in laser-induced angioplasty (SCRIVEN et al. 1991). Recent studies show that heparin blocks the vascular receptors of thrombus formation, reduces lysyl oxidase-mediated collagen cross-linking, suppresses collagen fibrillogenesis, inhibits fibroblast proliferation and migration, decreases cellular inflammatory reactions, and reduces monocyte adhesion, thereby promoting endothelial wound healing (GLAZIER et al. 1997).

5.5.4
Clinical Significance

5.5.4.1
Indications for Laser Angioplasty

The general and specific guidelines pertaining to the indications for laser angioplasty on the basis of clinical, functional, clinicochemical, and imaging findings differ only little from the generally accepted guidelines for balloon angioplasty (ZEITLER 1997; HENRY et al. 1990; ROMANIUK et al. 1985, 1987; ROMANIUK 1996). The following describes the clinical staging of peripheral arterial occlusive disease:

- Stage I   No symptoms
- Stage IIa   Intermittent claudication
                 Walking range above 200 m
- Stage IIb   Intermittent claudication
                 Walking range below 200 m
- Stage IIIa   Rest pain
                 Blood pressure at the ankle joint above
                 50 mmHg

- Stage IIIb Rest pain
          Blood pressure at the ankle joint below
          50 mmHg
- Stage IV   Necrosis, gangrene.

Planning of percutaneous angioplasty (conventional or laser-assisted) should comprise a determination and classification of the degree of the vessel lesion, including its localization in accordance with generally accepted criteria in order to select the optimal access (EUROPEAN WORKING GROUP ON CRITICAL LEG ISCHEMIA 1991; STANDARDS OF PRACTICE COMMITTEE 1990).

In the iliac region, the following stages are distinguished:

- Stage I Noncalcified concentric stenosis, less than 3 cm in length
- Stage II Concentric noncalcified stenosis ranging in length from 3–5 cm or calcified eccentric stenosis with a length of up to 3 cm
- Stage III Stenoses ranging in length from 5–10 cm, or occlusions with a length of less than 5 cm
- Stage IV Stenoses or occlusions with a length of more than 5 cm after attempted lysis or extensive bilateral stenoses or stenoses complicated by aneurysm.

Laser angioplasty may be considered for stages II and III. Staging in the femoropopliteal area is as follows:

- Stage I Unilateral stenosis or occlusion less than 3 cm in length without impairment of the origin of the superficial femoral artery or of the distal segment of the popliteal artery
- Stage II Unilateral stenoses or occlusions ranging in length from 3–10 cm and freely patent popliteal artery, calcified stenoses of less than 3 cm, or multiple stenoses or occlusions of less than 3 cm in length
- Stage III Unilateral lesion ranging in length from 3–5 cm with involvement of the distal popliteal artery, multiple focal and partly calcified lesions ranging in length from 3 to 5 cm, or unilateral stenoses or occlusions up to 10 cm in length
- Stage IV Total occlusions of the common, superficial, or popliteal femoral artery with involvement of the proximal segment of the trifurcation of the lower leg.

In this area, laser angioplasty may be considered, in particular, for stages II and III.

The following stages are distinguished in the area of the lower leg and foot:

- Stage I Unilateral total stenosis of the anterior/posterior tibial artery or of the fibular artery with a length of less than 1 cm
- Stage II Multiple focal stenoses of one lower leg artery of up to 1 cm in length, one or two focal stenoses less than 1 cm in length in the lower leg trifurcation, or multiple stenoses in the middle third of the tibial or fibular artery
- Stage III Moderate stenosis (1–4 cm) or moderate occlusion (1–2 cm) in the area of the lower leg arteries or severe stenoses in the area of the lower leg trifurcation
- Stage IV Tibial or fibular occlusions with a length of more than 2 cm or diffuse stenoses of all lower leg arteries.

Laser angiography in this area is indicated in exceptional cases only. The classification of peripheral bypass lesions is as follows:

- Stage I Focal stenoses of the distal anastomosis, femoropopliteal, or femorocrural bypass
- Stage II Focal stenoses of proximal anastomoses, femoropopliteal, or femorocrural bypass, short stenoses of up to 5 cm in length at shunts, stenoses at the aortofemoral or aortoiliac bypass, or stenoses at the extra-anatomical bypass
- Stage III Medium-length stenoses (up to 5 cm) at the venous bypass
- Stage IV Long stenoses (over 10 cm) at the venous bypass.

Bypass stenoses, just as stent-in stenoses, are less frequently and more critically submitted to laser ablation (NATARAJAN et al. 1996; DIETHRICH 1990b, 1991; DIETHRICH et al. 1991; KÖSTER et al. 1997; Oz et al. 1990). The following, anatomically unfavorable vascular sites with lesions such as secondary stenoses require special attention and care in the planning of interventional procedures:

- Common femoral artery
- Deep femoral artery
- Bifurcation lesions:
  Aortoiliac bifurcations
  Iliac bifurcations
  Femoral bifurcations
  Lower leg trifurcations
- Peripheral ostium lesions:
  Ostium of common iliac artery
  Ostium of superficial femoral artery
  Ostium of deep femoral artery
  Ostium of lower leg arteries
- Residual stenoses persisting after balloon angioplasty.

The grades of vessel dissections or flow disturbances can be assessed and classified by applying the angiographic criteria used in cardiology to peripheral vessels. The angiographic classification of dissections is as follows:

- Type A Small bright area within the lumen; disappears after passage of the contrast agent
- Type B Filling defect parallel to the vessel lumen; disappears after passage of the contrast agent
- Type C Dissection outside the vessel lumen; persists after passage of the contrast agent
- Type D1 Spiral-shaped filling defect with normal drainage of the contrast agent
- Type D2 Spiral-shaped filling defect with delayed drainage of the contrast agent
- Type E Persisting filling defect with delayed drainage of the contrast agent
- Type F Filling defect with complete vascular occlusion.

The angiographic classification of flow grades corresponds to the following:

- TIMI 0 No perfusion, no antegrade flow behind the occlusion
- TIMI 1 Moderate passage of the contrast agent, adherence of contrast agent, no opacification of the distal vessel
- TIMI 2 Partial perfusion, opacification of the entire vessel, influx of the contrast agent slower than in a comparable, normal vessel
- TIMI 3 Normal and complete influx and passage of the contrast agent.

Part of the above-listed vascular lesions can only be managed by vascular surgery, another group by combined surgical and angioplastic techniques, and yet another by interventional means such as recanalization and angioplasty including stent implantation. Details of determining the most suitable approach will not be discussed here.

The proper site for the insertion of the laser instruments in the different regions listed above is determined by the site of the lesion, the extent of the lesion, the presence of single or multiple lesions, the assumed size of the opening in the vessel wall, and the stasis of blood circulation resulting from the need for long-term compression bandages or from hemostasis achieved by means of modern percutaneous vessel suture techniques.

5.5.5
Comparison of Results, Complications

The primary success rates of laser angioplasty in peripheral vessels (iliac and SFA) with additional balloon angioplasty (HARRINGTON et al. 1990; STRICKWERDA et al. 1995a,b) in most cases range from 70% to 95% (Table 5.24; Fig. 5.46). When the indication is based on strict guidelines, laser angioplasty of vessel wall lesions, such as shorter and longer occlusions, yields reliable short-term and long-term results that are comparable to those of balloon catheter angioplasty (FISHER et al. 1996; DECKELBAUM et al. 1987; DECKELBAUM 1989;

Fig. 5.46. a Long occlusion (approximately 11 cm) of the left superficial femoral artery. b Status post mechanical recanalization (Terumo wire) and laser ablation (7-F multiple-fiber catheter). c Status post additional balloon dilatation

Table 5.24. Efficiency of laser angioplasty (survey)

Author	Laser type	Region	Patients (n)	Primary success, recanalization (%)	Reduction of stenosis (%)	Follow-up (%)/(months)	Total complications (%)	Early occlusions (%)	Vessel proliferation (%)	Dissection	Embolism, peripheral	Remarks
SANBORN (1988)	Argon (BF; hot-tip)	Femoral	107	71		71/12						
NORDSTROM (1988)	Argon (BF; lens)	Femoro-popliteal	23	87		50/3						
DECKELBAUM (1989)	Argon (BF; CW)	Coronary			100							
COTE (1989)	Argon (CW)	Coronary			100							
LITVAK (1989)	Excimer (BF)	Femoro-popliteal	22	85		59/9						
MURRAY (1989)	Dye (40 nm) (BF; cap)	Femoro-popliteal	24	88		67/6						
GESCHWINDT (1989)	Dye (480 nm) (BF)	Femoral	12	95								
LEON (1990)	Dye (480 nm) (BF)	Femoro-popliteal	70	83								
DOUER (1990)	Dye (480 nm)	Femoro-popliteal	129	72			19					
CHIESA (1990)	Nd:YAG (BF; hot-tip)	Iliac and femoro-popliteal	20	95								5% No passage (calcifications)
GOMES (1990)	Dye (480 nm) (BF)	Iliac and femoro-popliteal	12	92								
MAST (1990)	Argon (BF; CW)	Coronary	30	60 (RCA, 55; LAD, 71)				3.3 (Infarction)				
PEENE (1991)	Excimer	Femoral	12	75				8.3	8.3			
HUPPERT (1991)	Excimer	Femoral	65	89							16.7	
PILGER (1991)	Nd:YAG	Femoro-popliteal	167	79					9			
LAMMER (1991)	Nd:YAG	Femoro-popliteal	338	85		70/12						
POYEN (1991)	Nd:YAG (hybrid system)	Femoro-popliteal	31	72 (occlusions)	91 (stenoses)							
ARLART (1991)	Nd:YAG (BF; sapphire)	Femoral	40	77.5					12.5		7.5	
RIAMBAU-ALONSO et al. (1991)	Nd:YAG	Femoral	39	89								5% No passage (calcifications)
KVASNICKA (1991)	Nd:YAG (BF; sapphire)	Femoral	22	92								

Reference	Laser type	Vessel	n	Success (%)	Patency (%)	Patency ratio	Complications				
DUDA (1993)	Dye or excimer (MF)	Femoro-popliteal	25	96							3.3
HUNDT (1993)	Argon (BF; hot tip) or excimer (MF)	Iliac, Femoro-popliteal	56	83.9							
LUFT (1993)	Nd:YAG (BF; sapphire)	Femoro-popliteal	108	Femoral, 87; popliteal, 93				7.3	4.5	0.8	
SAPIENZA (1994)	Nd:YAG	Femoro-popliteal	124	66		23/40					
HUPPERT (1994)	Excimer or dye	Iliac, Femoro-popliteal, Crural	134	81: iliac, 95; femoro-popliteal, 90; crural, 77		Iliac, 89/24; femoro-popliteal, 63/24; crural, 50/24				Iliac, 9.5; femoro-popliteal, 20.9; crural, 4.5	
HAASE (1994)	Excimer (MF; rotating sector)	Coronary	32		100			16	3	Minor, 28; major, 3	
ODINK (1995)	Nd:YAG	Femoral	47	0 < 5 cm, 90; 5–10 cm, 66.7; 0 > 10 cm, 42.9	100	53/36 < 5 cm, 66.4/12; 5–10 cm, 0/12; >10 cm, 0/12					
FIELD (1995)	Excimer	Femoral	33 (diabetics)								
ESCOJIDO (1996)	Excimer	Coronary	89		95.5		Acute bypass, 1.1; infarction, 2.2				
FISCHER (1996)	Excimer	Femoro-popliteal	90		100	43/24		Acute occlusions, 18			
BARBEAU (1996)	Excimer	Femoral	104	75							
RUMANIUK (1996)	Holmium: YAG (MF)	Iliac, Femoro-popliteal	30	86							
SCHEINERT et al. (1998)	Excimer (MF; step-by-step)	Iliac	152	92		80/24		1	1	2	

CW, continuous wave laser radiation; BF, bare fiber; MF, multiple-fiber catheter; RCA, right coronary artery; LAD, left anterior descending artery.

DIETRICH 1990a,b; POKORNY et al. 1990; ROMANIUK 1996; HUPPERT et al. 1990, 1991, 1992a,b, 1994; LUFT et al. 1993; ESCOJIDO et al. 1996; CHIESA et al. 1990; BARBEAU et al. 1990, 1996; BELLI et al. 1991; HARTNELL 1991; RIAMBAU-ALONSO et al. 1991; PEENE et al. 1991; WERNER et al. 1989; BITTL et al. 1992, 1993, 1994, 1995; BITTL 1996; FIELD et al. 1995; PILGER et al. 1991; MATSUMOTO et al. 1989, 1990; MOTZ 1997; ODINK et al. 1995; ARLART et al. 1991; SCHNEIDER and OSTHEIM-DZEROWYCZ 1990; DE MARCHENA et al. 1996; APPLEMAN et al. 1996a,b; HAUDE et al. 1997) (Table 5.25). What continues to be a problem is the reopening of very long vascular occlusions by means of the laser technique

Table 5.25. Efficiency of laser angioplasty (survey)

Author (year)	Laser type	Region	Patients (n)	Primary Success, recanalization	Reduction of stenosis	Follow-up/% Months	Complications total	Early Occlusion
LAMMER (1988)	Nd: Yag cw (bf)	Femoro-popliteal		82%				
SANBORN et al. (1988)	Argon (BF) (Hot Tip)	Femoral	107	71%		71% (12 months)		
NORDSTROM et al. (1988)	Argon (Bf) (Lens)	Femoro-popliteal	23	87%		50% (3 months)		
DECKELBAUM (1989)	Argon (Bf) CW	Coronary			100%			
COTE (1989)	Argon CW	Coronary			100%			
LITVAK et al. (1989)	Excimer (BF)	Femoro-popliteal	22	85%		59% (9 months)		
MURRAY (1989)	Dye (40 nm) (BF) (Cap)	Femoro-popliteal	24	88%		67% (6 months)		
GESCHWINDT et al. (1989)	Dye (480 nm) (BF)	Femoral	12	95%				
LEON et al. (1990)	Dye (480 nm) (BF)	Femoro-popliteal	70	83%				
DOUER (1990)	Dye (480 nm)	Femoro-popliteal	129	72%			19%	
CHIESA et al. (1990)	Nd:YAG (BF) (Hot-Tip)	Iliac and femoro-popliteal	20	95%				
GOMES (1990)	Dye (480 nm) BF	Iliac and femoro-popliteal	12	92%				
MAST et al. (1990)	Argon (BF) CW	Coronary	30	60% RCA= 55% RIVA= 71%				3.3% infarction
PEENE (1990)	Excimer	Femoral	12	75%				8.3%
HUPPERT et al. (1991)	Excimer	Femoral	65	89%				
PILGER (1991)	Nd:YAG	Femoro-popliteal	167	79%				
LAMMER et al. (1991)	Nd:YAG	Femoro-popliteal	338	85%		70% (12 months)		
POYEN et al. (1991)	Nd:YAG (hybrid system)	Femoro-popliteal	31	72% (occlusions)	91% (stenoses)			
AHLART (1991)	Nd:YAG (BF) (sapphire)	Femoral	40	77.5%				

Table 5.25. *Continued*

Author (year)	Laser type	Region	Patients (n)	Primary Success, recanalization	Reduction of stenosis	Follow-up/% Months	Complications total	Early Occlusion
RIMBO-ALONSO (1991)	Nd:YAG	femoral	39	89%				
KVASNICKA et al. (1991)	Nd:YAG (BF) (sapphire)	femoral	22	92%				
DUDA et al. (1993)	Dye or Excimer (MF)	femoro-popliteal	25	96%				
HUNDT (1993)	Argon (BF) (Hot Tip) or Excimer (MF)	iliac femoro-popliteal	56	83.9%				
LUFT et al. (1993)	Nd:YAG (BF) (sapphire)	femoro-popliteal	108	femoral =87% popliteal =93%				
SAPIENCA et al. (1994)	Nd:YAG	femoro-popliteal	124	66%		23% (40 months)		
HUPPERT et al. (1994)	Excimer or Dye	iliac femoro-popliteal crural	134	Ø iliac 81%	95% fem.-popl. 90% crural 77%	iliac	89% (24 months) fem.- popl. 63% (24 months) crural 50% (24 months)	
HAASE et al. (1994)	Excimer (MF) rotating sector	coronary	32			100%		
ODINK et al. (1995)	Nd:YAG	femoral	47			100%	53% (36 months)	
FIELD et al. (1995)	Excimer	femoral	33 (diabetics)	O < 5 cm = 90% 5–10 cm = 66.7% O > 10 cm = 42.9%			<5 cm = 66.4 (12 months) 5–10 cm = 0% (12 months) > 10 cm = 0% (12 months)	
ESCOJIDO et al. (1996)	Excimer	coronary	89			95.5%		1.1% acute bypass 2.2% infarction
FISCHER et al. (1996)	Excimer	femoro-popliteal	90		100%	43% (24 months)		18% acute occlusions
BARBÉAU et al. (1996)	Excimer	femoral	10 4	75%				
ROMANIUK (1997)	Holmium: YAG (MF)	iliac femoro-popliteal	30	86%			Ø	Ø
SCHEINERT et al. (1998)	Excimer (MF)	iliac Step-by-step	15 2	92%		80% (24 months)	1%	1%

Abbreviations:
CW   = continuous wave laser radiation
BF   = bare fiber
MF   = multiple-fiber catheter

(BIAMINO 1990; SCHEINERT et al. 1998). It seems that, under special circumstances (SCHEINERT et al. 1998), better primary patency can be achieved with the excimer laser and the step-by-step technique, than with classic angioplasty. This, however, needs to be controlled by a prospective randomized trial. But even with a primary success rate of 72.9%, a total complications rate of 16.3% was observed, including 6.4% perforations. With a 2-year patency rate of 55.7%, the authors reported a secondary patency rate of 87.5%. This group has also published a 92% primary and 80% secondary patency rate in iliac artery occlusions. This result, however, can also be achieved with hydrophilic guidewires, guiding and balloon catheters, and stent application.

Furthermore, there are as yet no conclusive results clearly demonstrating a lower rate of reocclusion after laser angioplasty (BUCHWALD et al. 1990). The clear decline in the use of laser angioplasty is primarily due to the high costs of disposable laser catheters and not to the lower primary or long-term efficiency of the procedure (SCULPHER et al. 1996).

The laser technique has an enormous therapeutic potential, such as spectroscopically-guided ablation or vital labeling and selective ablation of labeled plaques (KITRELL et al. 1985), as well as ablation of thromboses, that urgently requires further study and development (BLOEMBERGEN 1974; BOSSHART et al. 1992; BRINKER 1992; CLARKE et al. 1987; DECKELBAUM et al. 1987, 1995b; ESTELLA et al. 1993; GARRAND et al. 1991; GESCHWIND et al. 1989; GMITRO et al. 1988; GREGORY et al. 1994; HAASE et al. 1997; LEE et al. 1993; LEON et al. 1990; MCMATH et al. 1990; MORGUET et al. 1997a; NILSSON et al. 1993; PREVOSTI et al. 1987; PRINCE and ATHANASOULIS 1992; RENAULT et al. 1984; SCOTT et al. 1993; TOMARU et al. 1995; ZWAAN et al. 1991) (Fig. 5.47). To date, however, laser-assisted PTA has only been used in controlled prospective trials. There is a need for carefully controlled clinical studies in clearly defined lesion models.

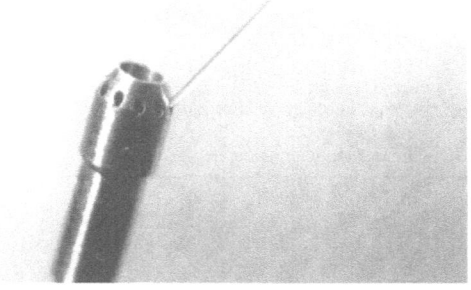

Fig. 5.47 a,b. Head (a) for a new multiple-fiber catheter (b) with the ablation axes of the light guides directed progradely in the center and laterally at the periphery

References

Abela GS, Fenech A, Crea F, Conti CR (1985a) Hot tip: another method of laser recanalization. Laser Surg Med 5:327–335

Abela GS, Crea F, Seeger JM, Franzini D (1985b) The healing process in normal canine arteries an in atherosclerotic monkey arteries after transluminal laser irradiation. Am J Cardiol 56:983–988

Abela G (1992) Abrupt closure after pulsed laser angioplasty: Spasm or "mille feuilles" effect? J Intervent Cardiol 5:259–262

Ahmed WH, Al Anazi MM, Bittl JA (1996) Excimer laser-facilitated angioplasty for undilatable coronary narrowings. Am J Cardiol 78(9):1045–1046

Alt E, Mentrup H, Matula M, Funk A, et al. (1992) Erste Untersuchungen zur Möglichkeit einer selektiven Ablation arteriosklerotischer Gefäßveränderungen mit Hilfe laserinduzierter Stosswellen. Z Kardiol 81(6):331–338

Anderson RR, Jaenke KF, Parrish JA (1983) Mechanism of selective vascular changes caused by dye lasers. Laser Surg Med 3:211–215

Appelman YEA, Piek JJ, Strikwerda S, Tijssen JGP, et al. (1996a) Randomised trial of excimer laser angioplasty versus balloon angioplasty for treatment of obstructive coronary artery disease. Lancet 347(8994):79–84

Appelman YE, Koolen JH, Piek JJ, et al. (1996b) Excimer laser angioplasty versus balloon angioplasty in functional and total coronary occlusions. Am J Cardiol 78:757–762

Arlart IP, Gerlach A, Grass HG (1991) Laser-assisted balloon angioplasty in complete femoropopliteal occlusions: preliminary results. Cardiovasc Intervent Radiol 14(4):233–237

Asada M, Kvasnicka J, Geschwind HJ (1993) Effects of pulsed lasers on agar model simulation of the arterial wall. Lasers Surg Med 13(4):405–411

Ashley S, Brooks SG, Gehani AA, Kester RC, et al. (1990) Experimental analysis of saphire contact probes for Nd-YAG laser angioplasty. Angiology 41(6):453–462

Bao SH, Zhang DS, Yu GR, Lu HH, Gai BK (1993) Assessment of Nd: YAG laser via cap and saphire tip delivery system. An experiment and clinical investigation. Chin Med J Engl 106(1):61–64

Barbeau GR, Abela GS, Seeger JM, Friedl SE, et al. (1990) Temperature monitoring during peripheral thermo-optical laser recanalizaion in humans. Clin Cardiol 13(10):690–697

Barbeau GR, Seeger JM, Jablonski S, Kaelin LD, et al. (1996) Peripheral artery recanalization in humans using balloon and laser angioplasty. Clin Cardiol 19:232–238

Barbieri E, Perbellini A, Taddei G, Scuro A, et al. (1990) Evaluation of complications during laser angioplasty with a hot tip system in the treatment of peripheral arteriopathy. Cardiologia 35(6):503–509

Batchelor WB, Chisholm RJ, Strauss BH (1996) Dissections following excimer laser assisted angioplasty of saphenous vein bypass grafts: analysis of incidence and effect of adjunctive balloon angioplasty. J Intervent Cardiol 9(3):265–269

Bauer J, Jiang XY, Wen Y, Yan W, Dal E, Liu LY, Tulip J, Lucas AR (1996) Comparative study of Nd: YAG laser angioplasty at 1.06 microns, 1.32 microns, and 1.44 microns wavelengths: decreased vascular spasm and early mortality with 1.44 microns laser ablation. Lasers Surg Med 19(3):299–310

Baumbach A, Wachter C, Haase KK, Hanke H, et al. (1991) Acute and long-term results of coronary Excimer laser angioplasty. Z-Kardiol. 1991 Ded; 81(12):656–663

Baumbach A, Haase KK, RC MSC, et al. (1994) Formation of pressure waves during in vitro excimer laser irradiation in whole blood and the effect of dilution with contrast media and saline. Lasers Surg Med 14:3–6

Bauriedel G, Windstetter U, Demaio SJ Jr, et al. (1992) Migratory activity of human smooth muscle cells cultivated from coronary and peripheral primary and restenotic lesions removed by percutaneous atherectomy. Circulation 85:554–564

Bauriedel G, Hutter G, Schmidt T (1998) Cheamydia pneumoniae in koronarem Plaquesgewebe: vermehrter Nachweis bei instabiler Angina. Herzmedizin 15:114

Becker GJ, Katzen BT, Dake MD (1989) Noncoronary angioplasty. Radiology 170:921–940

Belli AM, Cumberland DC, Procter AE, Welsh CL (1991) Total peripheral artery occlusions: conventional versus laser thermal recanalization with a hybrid probe in percutaneous angioplasty – results of a randomized trial. Radiology 181(1):57–60

Berlien H-P, Philipp C, Engel-Murke F, Fuchs B (1993) Laseranwendungen in der Gefäßchirurgie. Zentralbl Chir 118:383–389

Berlien HP, Müller G (1989) Angewandte Lasermedizin. Ecomed, Landsberg

Bhata KM, Rosen DI, Dretler SP (1989) Acoustic and plasma-guided laser angioplasty. Lasers Surg Med 9:117–123

Biamino G (1990) Coronary and peripheral laser angioplasty. Interventional cardiology. Hogrefe and Huber, Göttingen, pp 243–260

Bittl JA (1996) Excimer laser angioplasty: focus on total occlusions. Am J Cardiol 78:823–824

Bittl JA, Sanborn RA, Tcheng JE, Siegel RM, Ellis SG (1992) Clinical success complications and restenosis rates with excimer laser coronary angioplasty. Am J Cardiol 70:1533–1539

Bittl JA, Ryan TJ, Keaney JF, Tcheng JE, Ellis SG, Isner JI, Sanborn TA (1993) Coronary artery perforation during excimer laser angioplasty. JACC 21:1158–1165

Bittl JA, Kuntz RE, Estella F, Sanborn TA, Baim DS (1994) Analysis of late lumen narrowing after excimer laser-facilltated coronary angioplasty. J Am Coll Cardiol 23:1305–1313

Bittl JA, Brinker JA, Sanborn TA, Isner JM, Tcheng JE (1995) The changing profile of patient selection, procedural techniques, and outcomes in excimer laser coronary angioplasty. J Intervent Cardiol 8:653–660

Bloembergen N (1974) Laser-induced electric breakdown in solids. IEEE J Quant Electron QE-10(3):375

Bosshart F, Utzinger U, Hess OM, Wyser J, et al. (1992) Fluorescence spectroscopy for identification of atherosclerotic tissue. Cardiovasc Res 26(6):620–625

Brinker JA (1992) Laser angioplasty: the great "light" hope. Am J Cardiol 70(20):1605–1606

Buchwald A, Werner G, Unterberg C, Voth A (1990) Malignant restenosis after primary successful excimer laser coronary angioplasty. Clin Cardiol 13(6):397–400

Caravello J, Abela G, Barbeau F, Friedl S (1990) The effect of mechanical force with laser-thermal probes on the vaporization of atherosclerotic plaque. SPIE Proc 1201:114–128

Carlsson I, Miketic SV, Essen R (1998) Infektion mit Cytomegalievirus oder Helicobacter pylori und Risiko einer Restenose nach PTCA. Herzmedizin 15:116–118

Chiesa R, Castrucci M, Spiegel P, Melissano G, et al. (1990) Treatment of obliterating arteriopathies of the lower limbs using angioplasty. Comparision of 2 techniques of recanalization: Nd-YAG laser and radiofrequency thermal probe Minerva Chir 45(20):1303–1307

Choy DS, Stertzer SH, Rotterdam HZ, Bruno MS (1982) Laser coronary angioplasty: experience with 9 cadaver hearts. Am J Cardiol 50(6):1206–1208 (I); 1209–1211 (II)

Choy DSJ (1988) History of lasers in medicine. Thorac Cardiovasc Surg 36:114–117

Choy DSJ, Stertzer SH, Myler RK, Marco J, et al. (1984) Human coronary laser recanalization. Clin Cardiol 7:377–381

Clarke RH, Isner JM, Donaldson RF, et al. (1987) Gas chromatographic-light microscopic correlative analysis of excimer laser photoablation of cardiovascular tissues: evidence of a thermal mechanism. Circ Res 60:429–437

Cook SL, Elgler N, Shefer A, Goldenberg T, et al. (1991) Percutaneous excimer laser coronary angioplasty of lesions not ideal for balloon angioplasty. Circulation 84:632–643

Cote G, Smith A, Andrus S (1989) Immediate results of percutaneous argon laser coronary angioplasty. Circulation 80[Suppl II]:477

Cothren RM, Hayes GB, Cramer JR, Sacks B, et al. (1986) A multifiber catheter with an optical shield for angiosurgery. Laser Life Sci 1:1–12

Cox JL, Jacobs CP (1987) Laser-assisted angioplasty. Treating peripheral vascular disease AORN J 46(5):835–846

Crazzolara H, Muench W, Rose C, Thiemann U, Haase KK, et al. (1991) Analysis of the acoustic response of vascular tissue irradiated by an ultraviolet laser pulse. J Appl Phys 70:1847

Crea F, Davies G, Mckenna W, Pashazade M, et al. (1986) Percutaneous laser recanalization of coronary arteries. Lancet 2:214–215

Cross FW, Al-Dahir RK, Dyer PE (1988) Ablative and acoustic response of pulsed UV laser-irradiated vascular tissue in a liquid environment. Appl Phys 64:2194–2201

Cumberland DC, Tayler DI, Procter AE (1986a) Laser-assisted percutaneous angioplasty: initial clinical experience in peripheral arteries. Clin Radiol 37(5):423–428

Cumberland DC, Tayler DI, Welsh CL, et al. (1986b) Percutaneous laser thermal angioplasty: initial clinical results with a laser probe in total peripheral arterial occlusions Lancet 1:1457–1459

Daikuzono N, Joffe SN (1985) An artificial saphire probe for contact photocoagulation and tissue vaporization. Med Instrum 19:173–178

De Marchena E, Larrain G, Posada JD, Tang S, et al. (1996) Holmium laser-assisted coronary angioplasty in acute ischemic syndromes. Clin Cardiol 19:315–319

Deckelbaum LI, Isner JM, Donaldson RF, Clarke RH, et al. (1985) Reduction of laser-induced pathologic tissue injury using pulsed energy delivery. Am J Cardiol 56:662–667

Deckelbaum LI, Lam JK, Cabin HS, et al. (1987) Discrimination of normal and atherosclerotic aorta by laser-induced fluorescence. Laser Med Surg 7:330–335

Deckelbaum LI (1989) Laser-assisted angioplasty of inferior vena caval obstructions: what's good for the artery is good for the vein. Hepatology 9(2):338–339

Deckelbaum LI (1994a) Cardiovascular applications of laser technology. Lasers Surg Med 15(4):315–341

Deckelbaum LI (1994b) Coronary laser angioplasty. Lasers Surg Med 14:101–110

Deckelbaum LI, Natarajan MK, Bittl JA, et al. (1995a) Effect of intracoronary saline infusion on dissection during excimer laser coronary angioplasty: a randomized trial. The Percutaneous Excimer Laser Coronary Angioplasty Investigators. J Am Coll Cardiol 26:1264–1269

Deckelbaum LI, Desai SP, Kim C, Scott JJ (1995b) Evalution of a fluorescence feedback system for guidance of laser angioplasty Lasers Surg Med 16(3):226–234

Decker-Dunn D, Christensen DA, Vincent GM (1990) Multifiber gradient-index lens laser angioplasty probe. Lasers Surg Med 10(1):85–93

Diethrich EB (1990a) Laser angioplasty: a critical review based on 1849 clinical procedures. Angiology 41(9 Pt 2):757–767

Diethrich EB (1990b) Expanded indications for laser-assisted balloon angioplasty in peripheral arterial disease. J Vasc Surg 12(6):762–763

Diethrich EB, Santiago O, Bahadir I (1991) Laser-assisted angioplasty in the treatment of prosthetic graft stenosis. Angiology 42(7):576–580

Diethrich EB (1991) Temperature monitoring during peripheral thermo-optical laser recanalization in humans. Clin Cardiol 14(2):95, 184

Dörschel K (1989) Laserstrahlung; thermische Wirkungen; Verstärker. II-2.3; p. 1–4; II. 3.3.1; pp. 1–8; II. 2.1, pp. 1–2; III. 2.2, pp. 1–8. In: Berlien H, Müller P (eds) Angewandte Lasermedizin. Ecomed, Landsberg

Dotter CT, Judkins MP (1964) Transluminal treatment of arteriosclerotic obstruction. Circulation 30:654–670

Douek P, Leon MB, Geschwind H, Cook P, Neville RF, Keren G, Bonner RF (1990) Multicenter trial of fluorescence-guided, pulsed-dye laser-assisted ballon angioplasty in 129 patients with peripheral vascular occlusive disease. Radiology 177:102

Duda SH, Karsch KR, Haase KK, Huppert PE (1990a) Laser ring catheters in excimer laser angioplasty. Radiology 175(1):269–270

Duda SH, Wehrmann M, Haase KK, Huppert P, et al. (1990b) Excimer laser angioplasty I: The tissue effects of a ring catheter system on peripheral arterterial vessels. Rofo Fortschr Geb Rontgenstr 152(2):163–167

Duda SH, Huppert PE, Arndt V, Wehrmann M, et al. (1993) Experimental and clinical results with a pulsed dye laser for angioplasty. Eur Radiol 3:12–18

Edholm P, Fernström I, Lindblom K, Seldinger SI (1962) Roentgentelevision in practice with special regard to puncture examinations. ACTA Radiol (Stockholm) [Suppl]:216

Eiberg JP, Rasmussen JB, Schroeder TV (1995) Laser-assisted balloon angioplasty of occlusions in the femoropopliteal segment. Ugeskr Laeger 157:2840–2843

Eisenmenger W (1962) Eine Kontrollschallquelle für breitbandige Mikrofone zur Messung von Druckimpulsen in Flüssigkeiten. Acustica 12:165–172

Escojido H, Boyer C, Nebunu JC, Bouharaoua A, et al. (1996) Excimer laser assisted angioplasty. Immediate results in the treatment of complex coronary lesions. Arch Mal Coeur Vaiss 89:407–415

Estella P, Ryan RJ, Landzberg JS, Bittl JA (1993) Excimer laser-assisted coronary angioplasty for lesions containing thrombus. JACC 21:1550–1556

European working group on critical leg ischemia (1991) Second European consensus document on chronic critical leg ischemia. Circulation 84[Suppl 4, IV]:1–26

Fankhauser F, Schmoker R, van der Zypen E, England CS, et al. (1994) Lasermethoden in der chirurgischen Zungenplastik: grundsätzliche Betrachtungen bei der Anwendung eines neuen Laserskalpells. Lasermedizin 10:35–43

Field CK, Matsumoto T, Kerstein MD (1995) Nd: Yag laser-assisted balloon angioplasty of superficial femoral artery occlusions in a diabetic population. J Diabetes Compl 9(3):186–189

Fisher CM, Fletcher JP, May J, et al. (1996) No additional benefit from laser in balloon angioplasty of the superficial femoral artery. Eur J Vasc Endovasc Surg 11:349–352

Fourrier JL, Brunetaud JM, Prat A, Marache P, et al. (1987) Percutaneous angioplasty with sapphire tip. Lancet 1:105

Froehlich JJ, Möckel JW, Azumi N, Barth KH (1995) Analysis of particle size generated during plaque ablation with a flashlamp pumped pulsed dye laser. Cardiovasc Intervent Radiol 18(1):35–38

Fröhlich M, Sund M, Döring A (1998) C-reaktives Protein als Risikofaktor koronarer Ereignisse. Herzmedizin 15:118–119

Gandy KL, Hartz RS, Shih SR, Roth SI (1990) CO2-laser radiation damage of the arterial wall. Virchows Arch B Cell Pathol Incl Mol Pathol 58(6):411–416

Garrand TJ, Stetz ML, O'Brien KM, Gindi GR, et al. (1991) Design and evaluation of a fiberoptic flourescence guided laser recanalization system. Lasers Surg Med 11(2):106–116

Gerthsen C (1966) Physik – ein Lehrbuch zum Gebrauch neben Vorlesungen, 9th edn. Springer, Berlin Heidelberg New York

Geschwind HJ, Boussignac G, Teisseire B, Benhaiem N, et al. (1984) Conditions for effective Nd: YAG laser angioplasty. Br Heart J 52:484–489

Geschwind HJ, Blair JD, Mongolsmai D, Kern MJ, Stern J, et al. (1987) Development and experimental application of contact probe catheter for laser angioplasty. J Am Coll Cardiol 9:101–107

Geschwind HJ, Dubois-Rande JL, Shafton E, Boussignac G, Wexman M (1989) Percutaneous pulsed laser-assisted balloon angioplasty guided by spectroscopy. Am Heart J 117(5):1147–1152

Geschwind HJ, Dubois-Rande JL, Zelinsky R, Morelle JF, Boussignac G (1991) Percutaneous coronary mid-infra-red laser angioplasty. Am Heart J 122(2):552–558

Geschwind HJ, Nakamura F, Kvasnicka J, Dubois-Randé JL (1992) Excimer and holmium: YAG laser coronary angioplasty. SPIE 1642:82–86

Ghazzal ZM, Burton E, Weintraub WS, et al. (1995) Predictors of restenosis after excimer laser coronary angioplasty. Am Cardiol 75:1012–1014

Gijsbers GHM, van den Broecke DG, van Wieringen, et al. (1991) 308 nm excimer laser ablation with a contact beam delivery system: effects of applied force and gaseous debris. Lasers Surg Med [Suppl] 3:15

Ginsburg R, Kim DS, Guthaner D, Tots J, Mitchell RES (1984) Salvage of an ischemic limb by laser angioplasty: description of a new technique. Clin Cardiol 7:54–58

Ginsburg R, Wexler L, Mitchell RS, Profitt D (1985) Percutaneous transluminal laser angioplasty for treatment of peripheral vascular disease. Radiology 156:619–624

Gmitro AF, Cutruzzola FW, Stetz ML, Deckelbaum LI (1988) Measurement depth of laser-induced tissue flourescence with application to laser angioplasty. Appl Opt 27(9):1844–1849

Gomes AS, Palos MM, Moore WS, Lois JF, Ahn SS (1990) Laser-assisted balloon angioplasty with a computerized plaque-detection laser system. Radiology 177:102

Gregory KW, Prince MR, Lamuraglia GM, Flotte TJ, et al. (1990) Effect of blood upon the selective ablation of atherosclerotic plaque with a pulsed dye laser. Lasers Surg Med 10:533–543

Gregory KW, Buckley LA, Haw TE, Grunkemeier JM, Chasteney EA, Qu Z, Tuke-Bahlman D, Fahrenbach H, Block PC (1994) Photochemotherapy of intimal hyperplasia using soralen activated by ultra-violet light in a porcine model. Lasers Surg Med [Suppl] 6:12

Gross CM (1996) Die photoablativen Effekte des Excimer-Lasers in der Angioplastie. Ecomed, Landsberg (Fortschritte in der Lasermedizin, vol 10)

Grundfest WS, Litvack IF, Forrester JS, Goldenberg T, et al. (1985a) Laser ablation of human atherosclerotic plaque without adjacent tissue injury. J Am Coll Cardiol 5:929–933

Grundfest WS, Litvack IF, Goldenberg T (1985b) Pulsed ultra-violet lasers and the potential for safe laser angioplasty. Am J Surg 150:220–226

Grunkemeier JM, Gregory KW (1992) Acoustic measurements of cavitation bubbles in blood, contrast and saline using an excimer laser. Circulation 86[Suppl 4]:16

Grüntzig A, Hopff H (1974) Perkutane Rekanalisation chronischer arterieller Verschlüsse mit einem neuen Dilatationskatheter. Dtsch Med Wochenschr 99:2502

Guintini G, Midiri M, Bentivegna E, Romano P, Lo-Bosco S, Talarico F, La-Gattuta F (1994) Laser-assisted angioplasty in chronic obliterative arteriopathies of the lower limbs. Radiol Med Torino 88(3) 277–284

Glazier JJ, Jiang AJ, Crilly RJ, et al. (1997) Laser balloon angioplasty combined with local intracoronary heparin therapy. Am Heart J 134:266–273

Haase KK, Wehrmann M, Duda S, Karsch KR (1990) Experimental intracoronary excimer laser angioplasty. Z Kardiol 70(3):183–188

Haase KK, Baumbach A, Wehrmann M, Duda S, et al. (1991a) Potential use of holmium lasers for angioplasty: evaluation of a new solid state laser for ablation of atherosclerotic plaque. Lasers Surg Med 11:212–237

Haase KK, Hassenstein S, Duda SH, Wehrmann, et al. (1991b) In vitro alexandrite laser angioplasty: a study on fibre conduction and tissue effects. Lasers Med Sci 6:183

Haase KK, Hanke H, Baumbach A, Wehrmann M, Rose C, Karsch KR (1993a) In-vitro-Untersuchungen zu Stoßwelleneffekten während der Ablation von normaler und atherosklerotischer Gefäßwand durch Excimer-Laser. Z Kardiol 82:87–93

Haase KK, Hanke H, Baumbach A, Hassenstein, S, et al. (1993b) Occurence, extent, and implications of pressure waves during excimer laser ablation of normal arterial wall and atherosclerotic plaque. Lasers Surg Med 13:263–270

Haase KK, Baumbach A, Spyridopoulos I, Oberhoff M, et al. (1994) Initial clinical experience with a modified excimer laser for coronary angioplasty. Laser Med Sci ••:7–15

Haase KK, Karsch KR (1996) Coronary laser angioplasty: clinical value and experimental progress. Z Kardiol 85[Suppl]:81–86

Haase KK, Rose C, Duda S, et al. (1997) Perspectives of coronary excimer laser angioplasty: multiplexing, saline flushing, and acoustic ablation control. Lasers Surg Med 21:72–78

Haberbosch W (1998) Nachwels von Chlamydia pneumoniae in Atherektomieproben von Patienten mit koronarer Herzkrankheit. Herzmedizin 15:108–110

Hanke H, Haase KK, Hanke S, Oberhoff M, Hassenstein, et al. (1991a) Morphological changes and smooth muscle cell proliferation after experimental eximer laser treatment. Circulation 83:1380–1389

Hanke S, Hanke H, Oberhoff M, Haase KK, et al. (1991b) Transluminale Excimer-Laserangioplastie von experimentell erzeugten atheromatosen Plaques: Morphologische Veränderungen und Bedeutung der Proliferation glatter Muskelzellen. Z Kardiol 80(6):404–411

Harrington ME, Schwartz ME, Sanborn TA, Mitty HA, et al. (1990) Expandes indications for laser-assisted balloon angioplasty in peripheral arterial disease. J Vasc Surg 11(1):146–154; discussion 154–155

Hartnell GG (1991) Conventional angioplasty versus percutaneous transluminal laser angioplasty. Circulation 84(5):

2204-2205

Hassenstein S, Hanke H, Kamenz J, Oberhoff M, et al. (1992) Vascular injury an time course of smooth muscle cell proliferation after experimental holmium laser angioplasty. Circulation 86(5):1575-1583

Haude M, Welge D, Koch L, Roth T, Ge J, Baumgart D, Erbel R (1997) Laserangioplastie und -rekanalisation, vol 22(6) Herz, Urban and Vogel, pp 299-307

Helfmann J (1989) Nichtlineare Prozesse. In: Berlien HP, Müller G (eds) Angewandte Lasermedizin. Ecomed, Landsberg, II-3.4, pp 1-5; II-3.3, pp 1-8

Henry M, Beron R, Chastel A, Voiriot P (1990) Role of laser angioplasty in the management of peripheral arteriopathies. Report of 79 cases. J Mal Vasc 15(4):326-330

Heuser RR, Mehta SS (1991) Holmium laser angioplasty after failed coronary balloon dilation: use of a new solid-state, infrared laser system. Cathet Cardiovasc Diagn 23(3):187-189

Holmes DRJ, Mehta S, George CJ, et al. (1997) Excimer laser coronary angioplasty: the new approaches to coronary intervention experience. Am J Cardiol 80:99-105

Hundt C, Berger H, Schmand I, Lauterjung L (1993) Therapy of peripheral arterial disease: laser assisted angioplasty. Vasc Surg 27:81-88

Huppert PE, Duda SH, Haase KK, Karsch KR, Claussen CD (1990) Excimer laser angioplasty II: Initial clinical experience with peripheral arterial occlusive diseases. Rofo Fortschr Geb Rontgenstr 152(3):259-263

Huppert PE, Duda SH, Seboldt H, Karsch KR, Claussen CD (1991) Periphere Excimer-Laserangioplastie. Indikationen, Methode und klinische Ergebnisse. Dtsch Med Wochenschr 116(5):116-167

Huppert PE, Seboldt H, Duda SH, Helber U, et al. (1992a) Stellenwert der Laserangioplastie beim Oberschenkelverschlußtyp. Vasa [Suppl] 35:194-195

Huppert PE, Duda SH, Helber U, Karsch KR, et al. (1992b) Comparison of pulsed laser-assisted angioplasty and balloon angioplasty in femoropopliteal artery occlusions. Radiology 184:363-367

Huppert PE, Duda SH, Kalighi K, Baumbach A, et al. (1994) Periphere gepulste Laserangioplastie-Erfahrungen nach 4 jährigem klinischen Einsatz. Rofo Fortschr Geb Rontgenstr 160(2):125-131

Ilegbusi OJ, Nosovitsky VA (1997) A model of blood interaction with optical-fluid guide for laser angioplasty. Ann Biomed Eng 25:653-664

Ischinger T, Coppenrath K, Weber H, Enders S, Ruprecht L, Unsöld E, Hessel S (1990) Laser balloon angioplasty: technical realization and vascular tissue effects of a modified concept. Lasers Surg Med 10:112-123

Isner JM, Donaldson RF, Decklebaum LI, Clarke RH, et al. (1985) The excimer laser: gross, light microscopic and ultrastructural analysis of potential for use in laser therapy of cardiovascular disease. J Am Coll Cardiol 6:1102-1109

Jeans WD, Murphy P, Hughes AO, Baird RN (1990) Randomized trial of laserassisted passage through occluded femoro-popliteal arteries. Br J Radiol 63:19-21

Judy MM, Matthews JL, Goodson JR, Hults DF, Vieherkoski E, Aronoff BL (1992) Thermal effects in tissues from combined simultaneous coaxial CO2 and Nd: YAG laser beams. Lasers Surg Med 12:222-230

Kaminow IP, Wiesenfeld JM, Choy SJ (1984) Argon laser disintegration of thrombus and atherosclerotic plaque. Appl Opt 23(9):1301-1302

Kar H, Ringelhan H (1992) Grundlagen und Technik der Photoablation. Ecomed, Landsberg

Karsch KR, Haase KK, Wehrmann M, Hassenstein S (1991) Smooth muscle cell proliferation and restenosis after stand alone coronary excimer laser angioplasty. J Am Coll Cardiol 17(4):991-994

Katus AT, Dalhoff K, Kothe H (1998) Infektionstheorie zur Pathogenese der Atherosklerose - aus Sicht der Kardiologen. Herzmedizin 15:107-108

Kent KM, Satler LF, Kehoe MK, Pichard AD (1991) Stand alone excimer laser angioplasty. Circulation 84(II):363

Kittrell C, Willett RL, de los Santos-Pancheo C, et al. (1985) Diagnosis of fibrous arterial atherosclerosis using fluorescence. Appl Opt 25:2280-2281

Klocek P, Sigel GH (1989) Infrared fiber optics. Bellingham, Watertown

Knopf W, Parr K, Moses J, et al. (1992) Holmium laser angioplasty in coronary arteries. JACC 19:352A

Kopchok GE, White RA, Tabbara M, Saadatmanesh V, et al. (1990) Holmium: YAG laser ablation of vascular tissue. Lasers Surg Med 10(5):405-413

Köster R, Hamm CW, Terres W, Koschyk DH, et al. (1997) Treatment of in-stent coronary restenosis by excimer laser angioplasty. Am J Cardiol 80:1424-1428

Krepel VM, van Andel GJ, van Erp WF, Breslau PJ (1985) Percutaneous transluminal angioplasty of the femoropopliteal artery: initial and long-term results. Radiology 156:325-328

Kvasnicka J, Boudik F, Stanek F, Kubecek V, et al. (1991) Percutaneous laser angioplasty with a pulsed Nd: YAG laser. Initial clinical experience and early follow-up. Int Angiol 10(1):29-33

Lammer J, Pilger E, Karnel F, Schurawitzki W, Horvath, Oertl, Riedl M, Umer H, Klein GE (1990) Femoro-popliteal laser recanalisation - a multicenter study. Radiologe 30:45-49

Lammer J (1995) Laser angioplasty of peripheral arteries: an epilogue? Cardio vasc Intervent Radiol 18:1-8

Lammer J, Pilger E, Karnel F, Schurawitzke H, et al. (1991) Laser angioplasty: results of a prospective multicenter study at 3-year follow-up. Radiology 178:335-337

Lamuraglia GM, Murray S, Anderson R, Prince MR (1988) Effect of pulse duration on selective ablation of atherosclerotic plaque by 480-nanometer laser radiation. Lasers Surg Med 8:18

Larrazet FS, Dupouy PJ, Dubois RJ, Ducot B, Kvasnicka J, Geschwind HJ (1997) Anigioscopy variables predictive of early angiographic outcome after excimer laser-assisted coronary angioplasty. Am J Cardiol 79:1343-1349

Lee G (1986) Thermal effects of laser and electrical discharge on cardiovascular tissues. J Am Coll Cardiol 8:193-200

Lee G, Pond G, Sacks E, Butman S, et al. (1990) Single-passage laser recanalization plus subsequent balloon angioplasty by (1) a novel detachable fiberoptic guide wire device or (2) a balloon catheter over-the-fiberoptic wire system. Am Heart J 120(6):1477-1481

Lee G, Ikeda R, Stobbe D, Ogata C, et al. (1993) Vaporization of human thrombus by laser treatment. Am Heart J 106(2):403-404

Leeuwen TG, Jansen ED, Welch AJ, Borst C (1996) Excimer laser induced bubble: dimensions, theory, and implications for laser angioplasty. Lasers Surg Med 18:381-390

Leon MB, Almagor Y, Bartorelli AL, et al. (1990) Flourescence-guided laser-assisted balloon angioplasty in patients with femoropopliteal occlusions. Circulation 81:143-155

Linsker R, Srinivasan R, Wynne JJ, Alonso DR (1984) Far ultraviolet laser ablation of atherosclerotic lesions. Lasers Surg Med 4:201-206

Litvack F, Grundfest W, Goldenberg T, Doyle C, et al. (1987) Comparison of acute and chronic effects of argon and excimer laser energy on canine aorta. JACC 9:178A

Litvack F, Grundfest WS, Adler L, Hickey AE, et al. (1989) Percutaneous excimer-laser and excimer-laser-assisted angioplasty of the lower extremities: results of initial clinical trial. Radiology 172(2):331–335

Luft C, Horvath W, Oertl M, Haidinger D (1993) Laser-versus Rotationsangioplastie bei der Rekanalisation chronischer femoropoplitealer Arterienvershlüsse. Rofo Fortschr Geb Rontgenstr 158(1):53–58

Margolis JR (1996) Excimer laser vs balloon angioplasty: (AMRO study) – what ist the relevance? Eur Heart J 17:807–808

Margolis JR, Litvack F, Krauthamer D, Trautwein R, Goldenberg T (1990) Excimer laser coronary angioplasty: American multicenter experience. Herz 15(4):223–232

Mast EG, Plokker HW, Ernst JM, Bal ET, et al. (1990) Percutaneous recanalization of chronic total coronary occlusion: experience with the direct argon laser assisted angioplasty system (LASTAC). Herz 15(4):241–244

Matsumoto T, Okamura T, Rajyaguru V (1989) Laser arterial disobstructive procedures in 148 lower extremities. J Vasc Surg 10(2):169–177

Matsumoto AH, Barth KH, Teitelbaum GP (1990) Percutaneous management of emboli associated with hot tip laser-assisted angioplasty. Cardiovasc Intervent Radiol 13(2):71–74

McGuff PE, Bushnell D, Soroff HS, et al. (1963) Studies of the surgical applications of laser. Surg Forum 14:143–145

McKenzie AL (1984) How to control beam profile during laser photoradiation therapy. Phys Med Biol 29:53–56

McKenzie AL (1989) An extension of the three-zone model to predict depth of tissue damage beneath Er: YAG and Ho: YAG laser exisions. Phys Med Biol 34:107–114

McMath LP, Kundu SK, Spears RJ (1990) Experimental application of bioprotective materials to injured arterial surfaces with laser balloon angioplasty. Circulation 82 [4, Suppl III]:72

Mehran R, Mintz GS, Satler LF, et al. (1997) Treatment of instent restenosis with excimer laser coronary angioplasty: mechanisms and results compared with PTCA alone. Circulation 96:2183–2189

Minick CR, Fabricant CG, Fabricant J, Litrenta MM (1979) Atherosclerosis induced by infection with a Herpes virus. Am J Pathol 96:673–706

Mintz GS, Kovach JA, Pichard AD, Kent KM, et al. (1996) Intravascular ultrasound findings after excimer laser coronary angioplasty. Cather Cardiovasc Diagn 37(2):113–118

Morguet AJ, Gabriel RE, Buchwald AB, Werner GS, et al. (1997a) Single laser approach for flourescence guidance of excimer laser angioplasty at 308 nm: evaluation in vitro and during coronary angioplasty. Lasers Surg Med 20(4):382–393

Morguet AJ, Andreas S, Gabriel RE, Nyga R, Kreuzer H (1997b) Development and evaluation of a spectroscopy system for classification of laser-induced arterial flourescence spectra. Biomed Tech 42:176–182

Motz W (1997) The role of laser angioplasty in the spectrum of interventional treatments of coronary heart disease. Internist 38(1):27–30

Müller-Stolzenburg N, Stein E, Belien H-P (1989) Medizinische Anwendungsprinzipien des Lasers. In: Berlien HP, Müller G (eds) Angewandte Lasermedizin, vol III/1. Ecomed, Landsberg, pp 1–5

Murphy-Chutorian D, Selzer PM, Quay SC, Profitt D, Ginsburg R (1986) The interaction between excimer laser energy and vascular tissue. Am Heart J 112:739–745

Murray A, Wood RFM, Mitchell DC, Edwards DH, Grassy M,

Batu R (1989) Peripheral laser angioplasty with pulsed dye laser and ball-tipped optical fibres. Lancet ii 1471–1474

Natarajan MK, Bowman KA, Chisholm RJ, et al. (1996) Excimer laser angioplasty vs. balloon angioplasty in saphenous vein bypass grafts. Cathet Cardiovasc Diagn 38:153–158

Nilsson J, Herzfeld I, Grip L, Aberg B, Ryden L (1993) Immunohistochemical analysis of a human coronary artery exposed to excimer laser angioplasty in vivo: evidence for release of fibroblast growth factor at the site of injury. Am Heart J 125(3):908–912

Nishioka NS, Damankevitz Y (1990) Comparison of tissue ablation with pulsed holmium and thulium lasers. IEEE J Q E 26:2271–2275

Nordstrom LA, Castaneda-Zuniga WR, Lindeke CC, Rasmussen TM (1988) Laser angioplasty: controlled delivery of argon laser energy. Radiology 167:463–465

Odink HF, de Valois HC, Eikelboom BC (1995) Femoropopliteal artery recanalization: factors affecting clinical outcome of conventional and laser-assisted balloon angioplasty. Cardiovasc Intervent Radiol 18:162–167

Oezisik MN (1985) Heat Transfer. A basic approach. Mc Graw-Hill, New York

Oomen A, van Erven L, Vandenbroucke WV, Verdaasdonk RM, et al. (1990a) Early and late arterial healing response to catheter-induced laser, thermal, and mechanical wall damage in the rabbit. Lasers Surg Med 10(4):363–374

Oomen A, van Erven L, Vandenbroucke WV, Verdaasdonk RM, Slager CJ, et al. (1990b) Early and late arterial healingg response to catheter induced, thermal, and mechanical wall damage in the rabit. Lasers Surg Med 10:363–374

Oraevsky AA, Jacques SL, Pettit GH, Saidi IS, et al. (1992) Laser ablation of atherosclerotic aorta: optical properties and energy pathways. Lasers Surg Med 12:585–597

Oz MC, Lemole GM, Treat MR, Trokel SL, et al. (1990) Effects of a 2.15-micron laser on human atherosclerotic xenografts in vivo. Angiology 41(9, 2):772–776

Peacock EE, Jr (1981) Control of wound healing an scar formation in surgical patients. Arch Surg 116:1325–1329

Peene P, Wilms G, Piessens J, Baert AL (1991) Percutaneous transluminal laserangioplasty with balloon centered direct argon laser light. Experience with 12 patients and a minimal follow-up of 6 months. Rofo Fortschr Geb Rontgenstr 154(2):176–179

Petit GH, Saidi IS, Tittel FK, Sauerbrey R, et al. (1993) Thrombolysis by excimer laser photoablation. Lasers Life Sci 5:1–13

Pilger E, Lammer J, Bertuch H, Stark G, Decrinis M, Pfeiffer KP, Kreijs GJ (1991) Nd: YAG laser with saphire tip combined with balloon angioplasty in peripheral arterial occlusions Longterm results. Circulation 83(1):141–147

Pizzulli L, Jung W, Pfeiffer D, Fehske W, Luderitz B (1996) Angiographic results and elastic recoil following coronary excimer laser angioplasty with Saline perfusion. J Intervent Cardiol 9(1):9–18

Pokorny E, Bauer R, Vonasek H, Muckenhuber P (1990) Initial experiences with transpopliteal, laser-assisted balloon angioplasty of femoral artery occlusions. Rofo Fortschr Geb Rontgenstr 153(4):438–441

Porstmann W, Wierny L (1967) Intravasale Rekanalisation inoperabler arterieller Obliterationen. Zentralbl Chir 92(26):1586–1591

Porstmann WF (1973) Ein neuerer Korsett-Ballon-Katheter zur transluminalen Rekanalisation nach Dotter unter besonderer Berücksichtigung von Obiterationen an den Beckenarterien. Radiol Diagn (Berl) 14:239–244

Poyen V, Alessandri C, Duport G, Bergeron P (1991) Primary

results of laser recanalization in the endovascular treatment of arterial stenosis and occlusion of the lower limbs. Apropos of 45 treated cases. Arch Mal Coeur Vaiss 84(11):1537–1541

Preisack MB, Neu W, Nyga R, Wehrmann M, et al. (1992) Ultrafast imaging of tissue ablation by an excimer laser in saline. Lasers Surg Med 12:520–527

Preisack MB, Liewald C, Athanasiadis A, Baumbach A, et al. (1997) Success and procedural outcome of excimer laser coronary angioplasty compared to conventional balloon angioplasty. J Invasive Cardiol 9(1):10–16

Prevosti JLG, Lawrence F, Leon MB, Kramer WS, Du DY, Smith PD, Bonner RF (1987) Reduced surface thrombogenicity after thermal ablation. Circulation 76:IV–408

Prince MR, Athanasoulis CA (1992) Fluorescence-guided pulsed dye laser-assisted angioplasty. Radiology 182(3): 896–897

Quan KJ, Hodgson JMcB (1996) Comparison of tissue disruption caused by excimer and midinfrared lasers in clinical simulation. Cather Cardiovasc Diagn 38:50–55

Ragosta M, Gertz SD, Sarembock IJ, et al. (1995) Effect of midinfrared holmium: YAG laser angioplasty with and without balloon angioplasty on acute outcome and restenosis in atherosclerotic femoral arteries in rabbits. Lasers Surg Med 16:235–245

Reeders GS (1996) Coronary intervention with the excimer laser: a current perspective J Intervent Cardiol 9(2):175–178

Reichel E, Schmidt-Kloiber H, Schöffmann H, Dohr G, Eherer A (1987) Interaction of short laser pulses with biological structures. Opt Laser Technol 19(1):40

Reichel E, Schmidt-Kloiber H (1989) Photodisruption. In: Berlien HP, Müller G (eds) Angewandte Lasermedizin. Ecomed, Landsberg, II-3.4.2, pp 1–13

Renault G, Raynal E, Sinet M, Muffat-Joly M, et al. (1984) In situ double-beam NADH laser fluorimetry: choice of a reference wavelength. Am J Physiol 15:H491–H499

Riambau-Alonso V, Masotti-Centol M, Latorre-Vilallonga J, Viver-Manresa E, et al. (1991) Recanalization of the peripheral arteries by laser thermal balloon angioplasty. 2 years of clinical experience. Angiologia 43(3):103–110

Romaniuk P, Wierny L, Münster W (1985) Langzeiteffektivität der angioplastischen Therapie iliakaler und femoropoplitealer Obstruktionen im Vergleich zur Operation. In: Oeser H (ed) Angiologischsr Symposium. Schering, Berlin, pp 39–48

Romaniuk R, Wierny L, Münster W, Bürger K (1987) Langzeiteffektivität der angioplastischen Therapie peripherer Gefäßobstruktionen im Vergleich zur Gefäßoperation. Radiol. Diagn. 28(4):477–488

Romaniuk P (1996) Weiterentwicklung der interventionellen Therapie peripher und zentraler Gefäßobstruktionen durch Kombination der Holmiumlaserablation mit der Ballonangiographie einschließlich Implantation oberflächenaktiver Endoprothesen. BMFT-Forschungsbericht (Projekt: 01 ZZ 9101; Thema 10). Berlin/Bonn

Rosenfeldt FL, Chi L, Black AJR, Waugh JR, Pedersen JS, et al. (1992) Excimer laser angioplasty in the artherosclerotic rabbit: comparison with balloon angioplasty Am Heart J 124:349–355

Rosenthal D, Wheeler WG, III, Seagraves A, Erdoes L, et al. (1991) Nd: YAG iliac and femoropopliteal laser angioplasty: results with large probes as "sole therapy". J Cardiovasc Surg-Torino 32(2):186–191

Rück A (1989) Photochemische Wirkungen. In: Berlien HP, Müller G (eds) Angewandte Lasermedizin. Ecomed, Landsberg, VI-1.3.2, pp 1–6

Safian RD, Freed M, Lichtenberg A, May MA, et al. (1993) Are residual stenoses after excimer laser angioplasty and coronary atherectomy due to inefficient or small devices? Comparison with balloon angioplasty. JACC 22(6):1628–1634

Sanborn TA, Alexopoulos D, Marmur JD, Kahn H, Badimon JJ, Fuster V (1990) Coronary excimer laser angioplasty: reduced complications and indium-111 platelet accumulation compared with thermal angioplasty. J Am Coll Cardiol 16(2):502–506

Sanborn TA, Faxon DP, Haudenschild CC, Ryan TJ (1985) Experimental angioplasty circumferential distribution of laser thermal injury with a laser probe. J Am Coll Cardiol 5:934–938

Sanborn TA, Cumberland DC, Greenfield AJ, Welsh CL, et al. (1988) Percutaneous laser thermal angioplasty: initial results and 1-year follow-up in 129 femoropopliteal lesions. Radiology 168:121–125

Sanborn TA, Cumberland DC, Greenfield AJ, Motarjeme A, Schwarten DE, et al. (1989a) Peripheral laser-assisted balloon angioplasty. Initial multicenter experience in 219 peripheral arteries. Arch Surg 124(9):1099–1103

Sanborn TA, Mitty HA, Train JS, Dan SJ (1989b) Infrapopliteal and below-knee popliteal lesions: treatment with sole laser thermal angioplasty. Work in progress. Radiology 172(1):89–93

Sapienza P, Mingoli A, McGill JE, Perdikis G, et al. (1994) Comparative long-term results of laser-assisted balloon angioplasty and atherectomy in the treatment of peripheral vascular disease. Am J Surg 168(6):640–644

Sathyam US, Shearin A, Chasteney EA, Prahl SA (1996) Threshold and ablation Efficiency Studies of Microsound ablation of Gelatin under water Lasers Surg Med 19(4): 397–406

Scheinert D, Ragg JC, Vogt A, Biamino G (1998) Excimer Laser assisted recanalization of chronic arterial occlusions. In: 9th international course book of peripheral vascular intervention. Europa Edition, Paris, pp 139–152

Schmid KM, Xie D, Voelker W, et al. (1985) Intracoronary ultrasound following excimer-laser angioplasty. An invitro study in human coronary arteries. Eur Heart J 16:188–193

Schneider B, Ostheim-Dzerowycz W (1990) Laser-Angioplastie der Femoralarterie nach Stent-Implantation. Rofo Fortschr Geb Rontgenstr 153(5):615–616

Schofer J, Kresser J, Rau T, Kunze KP, et al. (1996) Recanalization of chronic artery occlusions using laser followed by balloon angioplasty. Am J Cardiol 78(7):836–838

Schomaker KT, Walsh A, Gregory KW, Kochevar IE (1997) Cell damage induced by angiovist 970 and 308 nm excimer laser radiation. Lasers Surg Med 20(2):111–118

Schönborn K-H (1989) Lichtwellenleiter. In: Berlien HP, Müller G (eds) Angewandte Lasermedizin. Ecomed, Landsberg, II-4.2.2, pp 1–9

Scott J, Desai SP, Deckelbaum LI (1993) Optimization of laser angioplasty catheter position using arterial flourescence feedback Lasers Surg Med [Suppl]5:12

Scriven AJI, Lidbury PS, Nathan AW (1991) Effects of laser-generated tissue debris on aggregation of human platelets. Am Heart J 122:802–808

Sculpher M, Michaels J, McKenna M, Minor J (1996) A cost-utility analysis of laser-assisted angioplasty for peripheral arterial occlusions. Int J Technol Assess Health Care 12:104–125

Sievert H, Scherer D, Merle H (1995) Crossing chronic coronary artery occlusions with a "laser wir" after failed attempted recanalization with other techniques. Z Kardiol 84:373–376

Sievert H, Rohde S, Ensslen R, Merle H, et al. (1996) Recanalization of chronic coronary occlusions using a laser wire. Cathet Cardiovasc Diagn 37(2):220–222

Singleton DL, Paraskevopoulos G, Taylor RS, Higginson LAJ (1987) Excimer laser angioplasty: tissue ablation, arterial response, and fiber optic delivery. IEEE J Quant Electr QE-23:1772–1781

Sowada U, Kahlert HJ, Basting D (1988) Excimerlaser-Strahlung durch Quarzglasfasern – Grenzen und Möglichkeiten. Laser Optoelektr 20:32

Spies JB, Lequire MH, Brantley SD, Williams JE, et al. (1990) Comparison of balloon angioplasty and laser thermal angioplasty in the treatment of femoropopliteal atherosclerotic disease: initial results of a prospective randomized trial. J Vasc Intev Radiol 1(1):39–42

Srinivasan R, Leigh W (1982) Ablative photo decompensation: action of far ultraviolet (193 nm) laser radiation on poly films. J Am Chem Soc 104:6784–6785

Srinivasan R, Leigh WT (1986) Ablation of polymers and biological tissue by ultraviolett lasers. Science 234:559–565

Srinivasan R, Braren B, Dreyfus RW, Hadel L, et al. (1986) Mechanism of the ultraviolet laser ablation of polymethyl methacrylate at 193 and 248 nm: laser-induced fluorescence analysis, chemical analysis, and doping studies. J Opt Soc Am 3:785–791

Srinivasan R, Casey KG, Haller JD (1990) Subnasosecond probing of the ablation of soft plaque from arterial wall by 308 nm pulses trough a fiber. IEEE J Q E 26:2279–2283

Standards of Practice Committee of the Society of Cardiovascular and Interventional Radiology (1990) Guidelines for Percutaneous transluminal angioplasty. Radiology 177:619–626

Sterenborg DJCM, Erkens CR, Dereijke TM (1990) Laser lithotripsy with a 504 nm pulsed dye laser: in vitro fragmentation related to stone weight and pulse energy. Lasers Med Sci 5:65

Stille W (1998) Infektionstheorie zur Pathogenese der Atherosklerose – aus Sicht des Infektiologen Herzmedizin 15:106–107

Stone GW, de Marchena E, Dageforde D, et al. (1997) Prospective randomized, multicenter comparison of laser-facilitated balloon angioplasty versus stand-alone balloon angioplasty in patients with obstructive coronary artery disease. Cardiol 30:1714–1721

Strauss BH, Natarajan MK, Batchelor WB, et al. (1995) Early and late quantative angiographic results of vein graft lesions treated by excimer laser with adjunctive balloon angioplasty. Circulation 92:348–356

Strikwerda S, van Swijndregt EM, Melkert R, Serruys PW (1995a) Quantitative angiographic comparison of elastic recoil after coronary excimer laser-assisted balloon angioplasty and balloon angioplasty alone. Am Coll Cardiol 25:378–386

Strikwerda S, Montauban VS, Foley DP, et al. (1995b) Immediate and late outcome of excimer laser and balloon coronary angioplasty: a quantative angiographic comparison based on matched lesions. J Am Coll Cardiol 26:939–946

Taylor RS, Higginson LA, Leopold KE (1990) Dependence of the Excimer Laser cut rate of plaque on the degree of calcification, laser fluence, and optical pulse duration. Lasers Surg Med 10(5):414–419

Tcheng JE, Wells LD, Phillips HR, Deckelbaum LI, et al. (1995) Development of a new technique for reducing pressure pulse generation during 308-nm excimer laser coronary angioplasty. Cathet Cardiovasc Diagn 34:15–22

Teitelbaum GP (1992) Holmium: YAG laser recanalization. Lasers Surg Med 12(1):112–113

Tobis J, Smolin M, Mallery J, MacLeay L, et al. (1989) Laser-assisted thermal angioplasty in human peripheral artery occlusions: mechanism of recanalization. J Am Coll Cardiol 13(7):1547–1554

Tomaru T, Geschwind HJ, Lange F, Boussignac G (1991) Enhancement of pulsed-dye laser ablation of arterial tissues with blood medium: effects of laser-induced shock waves. Am Heart J 122(3 1):809–817

Tomaru T, Geschwind HJ, Boussignac G, Lange F, Tahk SJ (1992) Comparison of ablation efficacy of excimer, pulsed-dye, and holmium–YAG lasers relevant to shock waves. Am Heart J 123(Pt1):886–895

Tomaru T, Nakaura F, Yanagisawamiwa A, Fujimori Y, Omata M, Kawai S, Okada R, Uchida Y (1995) Reduced vasoreactivity and thombogenicity with pulsed laser angioplasty: comparison with balloon angioplasty. J Intervent Cardiol 8(6):643–651

Topaz O (1995) Whose fault is it? Notes on "true" versus "pseudo" laser failure Cathet Cardiovasc Diagn 36:1–4

Topaz O, Rozenbaum EA, Schumacher A, Luxenberg MG (1996) Solid-state mid-infrared laser facilitated coronary angioplasty: clinical and quantative coronary angiographic results in 112 patients. Lasers Surg Med 19:260–272

Torre SR, Sanborn TA, Sharma SK, et al. (1990) Percutaneous coronary excimer laser angioplasty quantative angiographic analysis demonstrates improved angioplasty results with larger laser catheters Circulation 82[Suppl 3]:III 671

Torres JH, Motamedi M, Welch AJ (1990) Disparate absorption of argon laser radiation by fibrous versus fatty plaque: implications for laser angioplasty. Lasers Surg Med 10(2):149–157

Van Andel GJ (1975) Transluminale angioplastik volgens Dotter Ned Tijdschr Geneeskd 119:343–344

Van Erven L, Van Leeuwen TG, Post MJ, Van Der Veen MJ, Velema E, Borst C (1992) Mid-infrared pulsed laser ablation of the arterial wall. Mechanical origin of "acoustic" wall damage and ist effect on wall healing. J Thorac Cardiovasc Surg 104(4):1053–1059

Van Leeuwen TG, Van Der Veen MJ, Verdaasdonk RM, Borst C (1991) Noncontact tissue ablation by holmium: YSSG laser pulses in blood. Lasers Surg Med 11:26–34

Van Leeuwen TG, Van Erven L, Meertens JH, Motamedi M, et al. (1992) Origin of arterial wall dissection induced by pulsed excimer and midinfrared laser ablation in the pig. J Am Coll Cardiol 19:1610–1618

Van Leeuwen TG, Meertens JH, Velema E, Post MJ, Porst C (1993) Intraluminal vapor bubble induced by excimer laser pulse causes microsecond arterial dilation and invagination leading to extensive wall damage in the rabbit. Circulation 87:1258–1263

Van Leeuwen TG, Jansen ED, Welch AJ, Borst C (1996) Eximer laser induced bubble: dimensions, theory, and implications for laser angioplasty. Lasers Surg Med 18(4):381–390

Verdaasdonk RM, Cross FW, Borst D (1987) Physical properties of sapphire fibre tips for laser angioplasty. Lasers Med Sci 2:183–188

Verdaasconk RM, Rienks R, Van Erven L, Borst C (1989) Saphire and metal tip recanalization: Implications for safety. Lasers Med Sci 4[Suppl]:119–127

Vincent GM, Fox J, Johnson MD, Strickland R, Garry SL, Hammond E (1990) Thermal laser probe angioplasty: influence of constant tip temperature, plaque composition, and probe vessel diameter ratio. Lasers Surg Med 10(5):420–426

Vogl TJ, König TJ, Böttcher H, Felix R (1996) Experimentelle Ergebnisse der Excimer-Laser-PTA an einem Ex-vivo-Gefäßmodell. RoFo Fortschr 165(6):568–573

Walsh JT, Flotte TJ, Deutsch TF (1989) Er: YAG laser ablation of tissue: effect of pulse duration and tissue type on thermal damage. Lasers Surg Med 9:314–326

Walter JH (1989) Eigenschaften von biologischen Geweben. In: Berlien HP, Müller G (eds) Angewandte Lasermedizin. Ecomed, Landsberg, II-31, pp 1–7

Welch AJ, Bradley AB, Torres JH, et al. (1987) Laser probe ablation of normal and atherosclerotic human aorta in vitro: a first thermographic and histologic analysis. Circulation 76:1353–1363

Werner GS, Buchwald A, von Romatowski J, et al. (1989) Excimer-Laserangioplastie bei arterieller Verschluß-krankheit. Dtsch Med Wochenschr 114:1271–1275

White CJ, Ramee SR, Collins TJ, Mesa JE, Paulsen DB, Murgo JP (1991) Recanalization of arterial occlusion with a lensed fiber and a holmium: YAG laser. Lasers Surg Med 11(3):250–256

White CJ, Ramee SR, Collins TJ, Mesa JE, Murgo JP (1993) Holmium: YAG laser-assisted coronary angioplasty with multifiber delivery catheters. Cathet Cardiovasc Diagn 30(3):205–210

White RA, White GH, Mehringer MC, Chaing FL, et al. (1990) A clinical trial of laser thermal angioplasty in patients with advanced peripheral vascular disease. Ann Surg 212(3):257–265

Wilms G, Peene P, Baert AL, Verhaeghe R, et al. (1990) Angioplasty using a Nd: YAG laser with a saphire probe. J Radiol 71(2):103–107

Wollenek G, Laufer G, Grabenwoger F (1988) Percutaneous transluminal excimer laser angioplasty in total peripheral artery occlusion in man. Lasers Surg Med 8(5):464–468

Xie DY, Hassenstein S, Oberhoff M, et al. (1993) In vitro evaluation of ablation parameters of normal and fibrous aorta using smooth excimer laser coronary angioplasty. Lasers Surg Med 13:618–624

Yang XM, Manninen H, Soimakallio S (1990) Percutaneous transluminal laser angioplasty. Progress over the past two years. Acta Radiol 31(1):3–12

Yang XM, Manninen H, Soimakallio S (1991) Laser ablation ability of different fiber tips on human arteries. The role of photothermal effect. Chin Med J (Engl) 104(9):721–727

Yeh JTC (1986) Laser ablation of polymers. J Vac Sci Techno A 4:653

Yoshikawa M, Nakajima A, Arai T, Kikuchi M, et al. (1992) Measurement of cavity collapse time by probe technique on water, agar, and vascular tissue during Ho: YAG laser contact ablation. In: Jacques SL, Katzir A (eds) Laser tissue interactions vol IV. Bellingham

Zeitler E, Müller R (1969) Erste Ergebnisse mit der Katheterrekanalisation nach Dotter bei arterieller Verschlußkrankheit. Fortschr Rontgenstr 11(3):345–352

Zeitler E (1980) Percutaneous dilatation and recanalization of iliac and femoral arteries. Cardiovasc Intervent Radiol 3:207–212

Zeitler E (1985) Die perkutane transluminale Rekanalisation chronischer Stenosen und Verschlüsse peripherer Arterien. Med Wochenschr 135:384–392

Zeitler E (1997) Angiologische Diagnostik. In: Zeitler E (ed) Arterien und Venen. Springer, Berlin Heidelberg New York, pp 167–177

Zollikoffer CL (1985) Experimentelle Grundlagen der perkutanen der perkutanen transluminalen Angioplastie. Habilitationsschrift, Zürich

Zwaan M, Scheu M, Weiss HD, Lebeau A, Gothlin JH (1991) Schockwellenangioplastie mittels eines gewebedifferenzierenden Farbstofflasers. Vasa [Suppl] 32:151–153

Zwaan M, Behnle U, Engelhardt R, Vogel A, et al. (1996a) In-vitro-Untersuchungen zur gepulsten laserangioplastie in flüssigem und gasförmigem Medium. Fortschr Rontgenstr 164(1):68–71

Zwaan M, Behnle U, Engelhardt R, Vogel A, Kloess W, Birngruber R, Weiss HD (1996b) In vitro studies in pulsed laser angioplasty in liquid and gaseous medium. Fortschr Rontgenstr 164(1):68–71

6 Peri-interventional Medication

W. Gross-Fengels and K.U. Wagenhofer

Contents

6.1
Premedication in Peripheral Interventions

In radiological interventions, complex pathophysiological changes may occur. Appropriate premedication can prevent or weaken these mechanisms. Moreover, the examination can be carried out more rapidly, presents less risks and is less unpleasant for the patient (Cunningham et al. 1984). Patients with peripheral vascular disease often present with further manifestations of arterial occlusive disease, usually have more than one type of disease, and are frequently also receiving several different drugs simultaneously, which need to be taken into consideration when administering premedication.

6.1.1
General Remarks

In both outpatients and inpatients, we recommend that no solid foods be consumed for 12 h prior to the intervention. Clear, noncarbonated beverages are permitted up to 2 h before the intervention and are actually advisable, as tolerance to contrast media (CM) is increased with adequate hydration. Any adjuvant medication being administered orally up until the intervention, particularly cardioactive and antihypertensive drugs, should be continued on the morning of the intervention itself. However, diuretics and laxatives should not be administered. Preinterventional treatment with platelet aggregation inhibitors should always be continued, as this also lowers the rate of acute reocclusion.

Depending on the indication in each case, the anticoagulative effect of coumarins can be counteracted by simply discontinuing treatment and waiting or by also administering vitamin K orally until a prothrombin time of less than 50% has been achieved. In patients with certain artificial cardiac valves, especially those with mitral valves or chronic atrial fibrillation, however, this is often not tolerated; in such cases, it is advisable to initiate systemic heparinization (with overlap) before the intervention and to follow a similar procedure afterwards. Should a patient already be receiving anticoagulative treatment with heparin for other reasons, the partial prothromboplastin time (PTT) should be reduced to approximately 45 s before inserting F6 or larger catheters, especially before puncturing the brachial or axillary artery. In order to avoid an additional risk of hemorrhage, the platelet count should not drop below 100 000 per μl. Furthermore, before beginning with the intervention, an isotonic NaCl solution (ap-

W. Gross-Fengels, MD, Prof., K. U. Wagenhofer, MD, Abteilung für Diagnostische und Interventionelle Radiologie, Gefäß-Centrum Hamburg-Harburg (GCH), Allgemeines Krankenhaus Harburg, Eißendorfer Pferdeweg 52, 21075 Hamburg, Germany

proximately 200 ml/h) should be infused via a peripheral vein (at least 20 G). If the intervention is to be a lengthy one, the patient should, if necessary, be fitted with a bladder catheter beforehand.

6.1.2
Chronic Renal Dysfunctioning

Even in cases of fairly mild renal dysfunctioning, care should be taken to ensure that the patient receives sufficient liquid (EISENBERG et al. 1981; GOLDMANN and ALMEN 1985). In such cases, diuresis can be increased by administering 10–25 g mannitol immediately after the intervention. However, in patients with cardiac insufficiency, particular caution is warranted to avoid acute volume loading and hence a dramatic deterioration in cardiac performance. If the glomerular filtration rate (GFR) sinks to as low as 25 ml/min, which approximately corresponds to a serum creatinine level of >3 mg/dl, the intervention should be performed only after consulting a nephrologist; with a CM volume greater than 50 ml, short-term hemodialysis should be carried out after the intervention via a Shaldon's catheter in the central vein, as even these volumes of CM are sufficient to cause irreversible tubule damage in patients with a reduced GFR, e.g., associated with diabetic or vascular arteriolonephrosclerosis.

6.1.3
Diabetes Mellitus

In both non-insulin-dependent (NIDDM/type II) and insulin-dependent (IDDM/type I) diabetes mellitus patients, interventions should be scheduled for as early as possible in the morning as the first of the day in order to avoid prolonged catabolism. Care should be taken to ensure adequate primary metabolic stabilization (serum glucose, 110-200 mg/dl; HbA_1, <10%). The preinterventional medication for diabetic patients is shown in Table 6.1 (RATZMANN 1991). On the morning of the intervention, NIDDM patients with a well-regulated metabolism should be fasting and should not take oral antidiabetic agents. In IDDM patients with a stable metabolism, a 5% glucose infusion (40 drops/min) and 50% of his or her usual morning dose of regular insulin before the intervention are sufficient.

6.1.4
Hyperthyroidism

In cases of nodular or diffuse toxic goiter, antithyroid drug treatment (e.g., thioimidazole) and metabolic compensation should be accompanied by medication with perchlorate (600–1200 mg per day) from 3 days before to 7 days after the intervention. This usually prevents iodine accumulation by the thyroid and thyrotoxicosis. However, newer CM only

Table 1. Diabetes treatment program prior to radiological interventions

Diabetes type	Treatment	Preinterventional measures
NIDDM	Diet	Monitoring of blood sugar, fasting
	Diet + sulfonyl urea	Blood sugar <200 mg%: last sulfonyl urea on the evening before interventional radiology
		Blood sugar >200 mg%: change to 3-4× regular insulin subcutaneously (e.g., 5/4/4/3 E per day)
	Diet + sulfonyl urea + biguanides or acarbose	Discontinue biguanides (beware of lactacidosis in interventional radiology) Discontinue sulfonyl urea + acarbose, 2-4× regular insulin subcutaneously (see above)
IDDM	Diet + delayed-onset regular insulin	Change to 4× regular insulin subcutaneously on the day of the intervention

NIDDM, non-insulin-dependent diabetes mellitus; IDDM, insulin-dependent diabetes mellitus.

contain very small amounts of free iodine and their molecules are highly biostable; thus CM-induced thyrotoxic crises are now only very occasionally observed.

6.1.5
Contrast Media Intolerance

In patients with CM intolerance, the following premedication should be initiated at an early stage: a_1-receptor antagonists (e.g., 2 mg clemastine), H_2 receptor antagonists (e.g., 40 mg ranitidine), and corticosteroids (e.g., 40 mg triamcinolone phosphate).

This standard premedication suppresses both histamine-mediating, anaphylactic and dose-independent, anaphylactoid side effects. It has proved useful in increasing tolerance to CM even in atopic and allergic patients without a strong history of CM intolerance.

6.1.6
Prophylactic Antibiotic Treatment

Antibiotic prophylaxis is not necessary in classical percutaneous transluminal angioplasty (PTA) (SPIES et al. 1988). This includes the application of endovascular stents, regardless of whether these are coated or uncoated. However, in a combined surgical and radiological approach, e.g., elimination of abdominal aneurysm using stent prostheses, we routinely carry out antibiotic prophylaxis in analogy to the classical surgical approach, although controlled studies are not available.

Suitable preparations include the second-generation cephalosporins, e.g., the cefoxitin or cefuroxime group, which show strong resistance to degradation by β-lactamase. Alternatively, certain penicillins (e.g., floxacillin) may be used. Antibiotic prophylaxis is also recommended if the approach used involves an artificial bypass. Antibiotic treatment is usually initiated during or up to 1 h after the intervention and is continued for 1–2 days. Patients with artificial cardiac valves undergoing complex interventions, e.g., local fibrinolysis or stent implantation should receive prophylactic antibiotic therapy in order to avoid a potentially lethal endocarditis

6.2
Peri-interventional Use of Special Drugs

6.2.1
Sedatives

Sedatives are intended to prevent patients from being frightened or agitated, to calm them, to facilitate the control of pain and blood pressure, to decrease vasovagal reflexes, and to improve cooperation during the intervention by decreasing resistance. In the context of radiological interventions, the endpoint of sedation is somnolence, e.g., as manifested by woolly speech; however, the patient should be able to be brought around at any time (ESSINGER and RAVISSIN 1993). The depth of sedation should thus be monitored, and deep sedation that is difficult to control should be avoided. In radiological interventions, diazepam and midazolam, in particular, can be used as sedatives (Table 6.2). Diphenhydramine has both an antihistaminic and a mildly sedative effect. Attention should be paid to the additive effects of sedatives and analgesics, and doses should be adjusted accordingly.

Table 2. Sedatives and narcotics

Substance	Trade name	Dose	Route
Diazepam	Valium	5-10 mg	i.v.
Midazolam	Dormicum	0.5-2.5 mg	i.v.
Ketamine	Ketanest	0.2-0.8 mg/kg	i.v.
Propofol	Disoprivan 1%	0.25-1 mg/kg	i.v.
Diphenhydramine	Dolestan	25-50 mg	p.o.
Alfentanil	Rapifen	0.25 mg	i.v.
Chloral hydrate	Chloraldurat	80 mg/kg	p.o., rectally
Chlorprothixene	Truxal	25 mg	i.v.

6.2.2
Analgesics

If technically perfect local anesthesia is induced, vascular interventions are not usually painful. Should pain suddenly occur during an intervention, it should be regarded as a warning signal, possibly indicating an open or concealed vascular rupture, spasm, or ischemia. However, interventions are sometimes performed in patients already experiencing pain at the outset, e.g., in disease stages III or IV. In such cases, analgesics (Table 6.3) are indicated to improve patient compliance; these should preferably be administered intravenously to allow easier regulation.

Table 3. Analgesics

Substance	Trade name	Dose	Route
Pentazocine	Fortral	30 mg	i.v.
Pethidine	Dolantin	25–100 mg	i.v.
Morphine	Morphin-Merck 10	1-5 mg	i.v.
Tramadol	Tramal	50–100 mg	i.v.
Piritramide	Dipidolor	7.5–15 mg	i.v.

6.2.3
Antihypertensive Drugs

Many of the patients who have to undergo vascular interventions have arterial hypertonia. In such cases, we recommend that the corresponding long-term medication be continued on the day of the intervention. Moreover, in the course of the intervention, blood pressure may increase considerably. The effect of intravenous sedation should be awaited before undertaking any specific therapeutic steps. Should it become necessary to lower the blood pressure, calcium channel blockers, dihydralazine, or alpha-mimetic drugs (Table 6.4) may be administered. A sudden drop in blood pressure should be avoided at all costs; instead, careful "titration" of the antihypertensive drug is recommended until the blood pressure required is obtained.

Table 6.4. Antihypertensives

Substance	Trade name	Dose	Route
Nifedipine	Adalat	10-20 mg	s.l.
Dihydralazine	Nepresol	12.5-25 mg	i.v.
Clonidine	Catapresan	0.15 mg	i.v.
Nitroprusside	Nipruss	5 mg/min	Infusion (titrate)[a]

[a]A nontransparent infusion system should be used.

6.2.4
Antihypotensive Drugs

A fall in blood pressure can occur during vascular interventions, e.g., as a result of vasovagal reactions or blood loss. In addition, cardiac causes, overshooting of antihypertensive drugs, sedatives, or side effects caused by CM should be considered. Vasovagal reactions are often accompanied by yawning, vomiting, and bradycardia. As a first step, crystalloid solutions (NaCl 0.9%) and atropine can be administered intravenously; oxygen should be supplied, e.g., by nasal probe, and the patient put in Trendelenburg's

position. If these measures have no effect, dopamine may be cautiously administered intravenously (Table 6.5). If the fall in blood pressure is due to arterial bleeding, the puncture site should, if possible, be manually compressed. In addition, crystalloid solutions and starch should be infused, blood should be taken for crossmatching, and a vascular surgeon should be informed as a precaution. The effect of heparin may be counteracted using protamine sulfate (approximately 1 mg per 100 IU heparin), but this is not recommended as a general measure due to its possible allergic and hypotensive side effects.

6.2.5
Spasmolytics and Vasodilators

Vascular spasms can occur as a result of selective probing, particularly in small-caliber arteries and veins. Spasms reduce flow and are conducive to secondary thrombosis. Thus vascular spasms may jeopardize the success of a radiological intervention or considerably lengthen the duration of the examination (LAURENT et al. 1993). Vascular spasms are observed in renal and popliteal PTA in up to 25% of cases and also frequently occur in association with intracranial embolization, for example. Animal experiments carried out by LEVEEN et al. (1985) showed that premedication with heparin reduced the incidence of spasms; calcium channel blockers, such as verapamil, were able to ease them. However, verapamil is only effective as prophylactic treatment in the presence of heparin. Tolazoline (Table 6. 6) increases flow in the dilated area by reducing the

Table 6.5. Antihypotensive drugs, infusion solutions, and oxygen

Substance	Trade name	Dose	Route
Hydroxyethyl starch	Expafusin sine	500–1000 ml/day	Infusion
Plasma proteins	Humanalbumin 5%	250–500 ml	Infusion
Ringer's lactate solution	Ringer's lactate solution Pharmacia	500–2000 ml/day	Infusion
0.9% NaCl	–	500-2000 ml/day	Infusion
Atropine sulfate	Atropine sulfate Braun 0.5 mg	0.5–1 mg	i.v.
Oxygen	–	3–5 l/min	Nasal probe
Dopamine	Dopamine Fresenius	0.3-1 mg/min	Infusion (titrate)

Table 6.6. Spasmolytic drugs and vasodilators

Substance	Trade name	Dose	Route
Tolazoline	Priscol	25 mg	i.a.
Nimodipine	Nimotop	1-2 mg/h	i.v.
		0.2-0.4 mg	i.a.
Nifedipine	Adalat	10-30 mg	s.l.
		0.1-0.2 mg	i.a.
Diltiazem	Dilzem	60 mg	p.o.
Verapamil	Isoptin	2.5-5 mg	i.a.
Lidocaine	Lidocaine Braun 1%	50 mg	i.a.
Glycerol trinitrate	Nitro Mack Nitrolingual	0.1-0.2 mg 2 cartridges	i.a. Inhalation

Table 6.7. Vasoactive substances (HEIDER et al. 1997)

Stage of disease[a]	Substances	Treatment criteria
II	Pentoxifylline, naftidrofuryl, buflomedil, prostaglandin E_1	Walking exercises not possible; PTA not appropriate; obliteration of femoral arteries and arteries of the lower leg; malleolar pressure >60 mmHg; no iliac obliteration; no cardiac insufficiency; patient cannot walk 300 m without pain
III/IV	Prostaglandin E_1, prostacyclin	Surgery or angioplasty not possible or not sufficiently successful; no cardiac insufficiency or arrhythmia

[a]According to the Fontaine classification of peripheral arterial occlusive disease.

peripheral resistance without directly affecting spasms. Furthermore, we use vasodilators when measuring intra-arterial pressure, e.g., before an iliac PTA; this reduces the peripheral resistance, thus simulating load, which makes it easier to assess the hemodynamic relevance of stenosis.

Vasoactive substances recommended for use in peripheral arterial occlusive disease (HEIDRICH et al. 1997) are shown in Table 6.7.

6.3
Restenosis After Percutaneous Transluminal Angioplasty

6.3.1
Pathophysiology

The pathophysiological mechanisms of restenosis are the inevitable result of the injury to the vascular wall that is necessary for successful angioplasty and can best be described as "response to injury." The course that this physiological repair cascade takes is nonspecifically uniform and does not depend on whether the vascular wall trauma is spontaneous, e.g., plaque eruption, or iatrogenic, e.g., balloon angioplasty. A distinction is made between early and delayed repair processes. The initial reaction at the site of angioplasty is the reactive vasoconstriction by the smooth muscle of the vascular wall, which lasts for a few seconds to minutes after PTA, with simultaneous thrombin activation and subsequent platelet adhesion and aggregation ("white clot"). This is followed by the formation of a dimerous fibrinogen network by the platelets. This red thrombus joins up

with the white thrombus to form a "mixed" thrombus with various periods of formation. Thromboxane A_2 (which is synthesized by platelets) is an extremely potent vasoconstrictor (MRUK et al. 1990), causing regional stasis and further platelet aggregation. The deeper the angioplastic lesion is, the larger the initial thrombus (BADIMON et al. 1986). The subsequent processes of reorganization in the vascular wall last for a period of weeks; they have been well documented in animal experiments and proceed via a cascade of migration and proliferation factors of the smooth muscle cells, spindle cells, and the collagen that has become exposed. In this context, platelet-derived growth factor (PDGF) appears to be particularly important for the mitogenic nature of the smooth muscle cells (WILEMSKY et al. 1995).

6.3.2
Predictive Factors

Factors predictive of restenosis are divided into pre- and postinterventional factors. Of the pre-interventional factors, high-grade stenoses, extended lesions, and chronic, calcified vascular occlusion are regarded as indicative of a particular risk for restenosis (JOST et al. 1991). The only concomitant disease recognized as a predictor of restenosis is a poorly regulated diabetes mellitus (ALDERMANN 1996). Results concerning the predictive value of the patient's age, sex, hyperlipidemia, nicotine abuse, or arterial hypertoension vary and therefore cannot be regarded as firmly established (MRUK et al. 1990). Following PTA, the probability of restenosis occurring correlates with an angiomorphologically documented restenosis and a persisting pressure gradient. Postinterventional occurrence of thrombi is considered to be an important predictor of an increased risk of restenosis. However, this does not apply to simple dissections after angioplasty (BOURUSSA et al. 1991.)

6.3.3
Pharmacologic Prevention of Recurrence

6.3.3.1
Unfractionated Heparin

Unfractionated heparin consists of a mixture of acidic mucopolysaccharides possessing an immediate anticoagulative effect as a result of their increased antithrombin III effect. The main targets of heparin are direct thrombin degradation and prevention of thrombin synthesis by neutralizing factor Xa (ROSENBERG and DAMUS 1975). By analogy to diagnostic angiography (WALLACE et al. 1972), it is now considered standard practice to ensure peri-interventional heparin protection (usually 5000–10 000 IU) in angioplasties, etc. In contrast, subsequent heparin treatment following simple PTA without complications is not necessarily indicated and appears to have a number of disadvantages. However, if the result obtained by PTA is not satisfactory and/or the velocity of peripheral flow-off is dramatically decreased, intravenous heparinization for 1-2 days (approximately 1000 IU/h) is recommended. After arterial femoral, popliteal, and renal stent implantation, as after venous stent implantation, systemic heparinization for more than 2 days is propagated to avoid early thrombosis and to reduce the risk of restenosis.

6.3.3.2
Acetylsalicylic Acid

Acetylsalicylic acid (ASA) is a standard substance that, by inhibiting cyclooxygenase, blocks the prostaglandin peroxides that are regarded as a preliminary stage of thromboxane A_2 (BECKER et al. 1989). As early as 1973, ZEITLER et al. were able to show that ASA treatment plays a decisive role in lowering the rate of early reocclusion. Provided that the patient is not receiving any long-term medication, preinterventional intravenous administration of 500-1000 mg ASA is sufficient to avoid acute reocclusion. This dose is also sufficient for the first few days after PTA, as ASA irreversibly blocks the enzyme and the platelet function does not return until after 4-5 days with cell desquamation. In patients with blue toe syndrome, premedication with ASA should be initiated 6-12 weeks prior to any intervention and, if necessary, should be combined with anticoagulative treatment before proceeding with PTA (BREWER et al. 1988).

Postinterventional dosages of 100(-325) mg ASA per day have proved to be effective and adequate, especially since such dosages are not antiphlogistic and have not been shown to inhibit the desired prostacyclin synthesis (MINAR et al. 1995). MINAR et al. (1995) treated 216 patients after femoropopliteal PTA with 100 or 1000 mg ASS. Complete follow-up was performed over a period of 24 months in 207 of these patients. Cumulative patency in the two groups was identical (62.5%), while the incidence of gastrointestinal side effects was five times higher in the high-dose group. The authors came to the conclusion that restenosis after femoropopliteal PTA occurs no less frequently in patients receiving high ASA doses than in those receiving low doses and that low doses result in fewer side effects.

6.3.3.3
Ticlopidine + Clopidogrel

Another approved platelet aggregation inhibitor is ticlopidine, a substance that appears to function as an antagonist of membrane-adapted ADP receptors and thus in a completely different way from ASA; this has led to combination therapy with the two substances. In several studies (HERRMAN et al. 1993) on percutaneous transluminal coronary angioplasty (PTCA) and stent implantation, combination treatment with ASA (100–325 mg per day) and ticlopidine (2×250 mg per day) appears to have resulted in significantly lower reocclusion rates than long-term anticoagulative treatment. SCHOMIG et al. (1996; Table 6.8) observed coronary stent occlusion within 30 days in 0.8% of patients receiving combination treatment and in 5.4% of patients receiving anticoagulative therapy. This procedure has also been adopted in peripheral arteries, particularly after renal and femoropopliteal and complicated iliac stent placement. It has been observed that the effect of ticlopidine is delayed and does not become apparent until after 4-5 days (MCTAVISH et al. 1990). Although it does not have the mucosa-damaging side effects of the salicylates, its side effects are at least as serious and include other gastrointestinal effects such as

Table 6.8. Platelet function inhibitors and anticoagulation

Reference	Area	Substances	Results
ZEITLER et al. (1973)	Extremities	ASA, heparin (i.a.)	Early reocclusion rate: 4.6%
		ASA, heparin (i.a., i.v.)	Early reocclusion rate: 7.0%
		Heparin (i.a., i.v.)	Early reocclusion rate: 21.0%
THRONTON et al. (1984)	Heart	ASA	Restenosis rate at 6 months: 21%
		Coumarins	Restenosis rate at 6 months: 44%
Do and MAHLER (1994)	Extremities	ASA and dipyridamole	Patency at 12 months: 69%
		Anti-coagulation	Patency at 12 months: 53%
SCHOMIG et al. (1996)	Heart	ASA + ticlopidine	Early occlusion rate: 0.8%
		Heparin + coumarins	Early occlusion rate: 5.4%

ASA, Acetylsalicylic acid.

nausea, emesis, and diarrhea. Reversible neutropenia is occasionally observed, albeit rarely, and weekly monitoring of the blood count is therefore indicated in patients on ticlopidine medication at the beginning of treatment. Moreover, a decision should be taken every 3 months on whether or not treatment should be continued. Significant less side-effects occur with Clopidogrel (Plavix) 75 mg per day.

6.3.3.4
Low-Molecular Heparin and Heparinoids

If a heparin-induced thrombocytopenia has already been known to occur, renewed administration of normal heparin is absolutely contraindicated to avoid the possibility of a very severe white clot syndrome, involving the loss of extremities and a fatal outcome. As an alternative, danaparoid sodium (Orgaran) can be used; however, it has not yet been approved in all countries. Due to the high degree of cross-sensitization observed, the use of low-molecular heparin is currently not advised (WARKENTIN and KELTON 1991; GREINACHER 1996). In the future, recombinant hirudin can be used in the treatment of some patients with heparin-induced thrombocytopenia.

6.3.3.5
Coumarin Derivatives

The use of coumarins in secondary prophylaxis of arterial occlusive disease should be viewed very critically. Do and MAHLER (1994) carried out a controlled study in 160 patients after femoropoliteal PTA, comparing the effect of oral anticoagulants with a low-dose combination treatment using ASA (25 mg) and dipyridamole (200 mg). Patency after 1 year was 53% in the coumarin group and 69% in the ASA/dipyridamole group (differences not significant). In the anticoagulant group, four cases of hemorrhage were observed, one of which had a fatal outcome, while only five minor complications occurred in the ASA/dipyridamole group. Thus coumarin treatment can only be recommended in a few exceptional cases, e.g., reocclusion with ASA treatment and distal recanalization. After laser-assisted femoropopliteal PTA, TETTEROO et al. (1995) also found that anticoagulative treatment with coumarins was not superior to treatment with platelet aggregation inhibitors.

6.3.3.5
Medication After Local Fibrinolysis Treatment

Medication administered after local fibrinolysis treatment should be judged somewhat less sweepingly. After a successful intervention, all patients are initially heparinized systemically for 2–3 days, whereby the PTT should exceed 45 s. If the vascular occlusion was caused by embolism, oral treatment with coumarin derivatives should be initiated and continued for a period of 6 months unless long-term anticoagulation is contraindicated. Patients with contraindications and those with thrombotic vascular occlusion should be given the medication described above after fibrinolysis treatment in conjunction with platelet function inhibitors for at least 12 months.

6.3.4
Future Outlook for Adjuvant Medication

Further substances for secondary prophylaxis have already entered clinical trials (RUTSCH et al. 1995; HERRMAN et al. 1993). In addition to hirudin, these include chimeric platelet antibodies, such as the glycoprotein IIb/IIIA platelet receptor antagonist abciximab (Reopro), which has already proved effective in PTCA studies involving fairly small numbers of patients. The effect of this antibody is based on the irreversible inhibition of the thrombocytic glycoprotein surface receptor with interruption of thrombus formation at a central point. In contrast to heparin and platelet function inhibitors, complete short-term absence of thrombogenesis can be assumed. Further developments can be expected from direct, local application of drugs, e.g., using treated balloon catheters or stents. Genetic engineering approaches using direct vascular gene transfer to prevent recurrence are also currently being discussed (VILLA et al. 1995; VON DER LEYEN and GIBBONS 1995).

References

Aldermann EL (1996) Comparison of coronary bypass surgery with angioplasty in patients with multivessel disease. N Engl J Med 335:217-225

Badimon L, Chesebro JH, Badimon JJ (1986) Thrombosis formation on ruptured atherosclerotic plaques and rethrombosis on evolving thrombi. Circulation Suppl 86:74-85

Becker GJ, Katzen BT, Dake MD (1989) Noncoronary angioplasty. Radiology 170:921-940

Bourussa MG, Cesperance J, Eastwood C, Schwartz L (1991) Clinical, physiological and procedural factors predictive of restenosis after PTCA. J Am Coll Cardiol 18:368-376

Brewer ML, Kinnison ML, Perler BA, White RI (1988) Blue toe syndrome: treatment with anticoagulants and delayed percutaneous transluminal angioplasty. Radiology 166:31-36

Cunningham D, Kumar B, Siegel B, Girla L (1984) Aspirin inhibition of platelet disposition at angioplasty sites. Radiology 151:487-490

Do DD, Mahler F (1994) Low-dose aspirin combined with dipyridamole versus anticoagulants after percutaneous transluminal angioplasty. Radiology 193:567-571

Eisenberg RL, Bank WO, Heydock M (1981) Renal failure after angiography can be avoided with hydratation. Am J Roentgenol 136:859-861

Essinger A, Ravussin P (1993) Analgesia and sedation in the hands of the interventional radiologist. In: Steinbrich W, Gross-Fengels W (eds) Interventional radiology: adjunctive medication and monitoring. Springer, Berlin Heidelberg New York, pp 15-19

Goldmann K, Almen T (1985) Contrast media-induced nephrotoxicity. Survey and present state. Invest Radiol 20:92-97

Greinacher A (1996) Heparin-induzierte Thrombozytopenien. Internist 37:1172-1178

Heidrich H (1997) Vasoaktive Substanzen bei paVk. Empfehlungen der Arzneimittelkommission der BRD. Dtsch Aerztebl 94:C-1718

Herrman JPR, Hermanns WR, Voa J, Serruys PW (1993) Prevention of restenosis following angioplasty - the search for the holy grail. Drugs 46:18-52

Jost S, Nolte CW, Simon R, Amenda I, Gulba DC, Wiese B, Lichtlen RR (1991) Angioplasty of subacute and chronic total coronary occlusions. Success, recurrence rate and clinical follow-up. Am Heart J 122:1509-1514

Laurent A, Gobin YP, Launay F, Aymard A, Casasco A, Bailly AL, Houdart E, Merland JJ (1993) Drug therapy, monitoring, and function testing in neuroradiologic interventions. In: Steinbrich W, Gross-Fengels W (eds) Interventional radiology: adjunctive medication and monitoring. Springer, Berlin Heidelberg New York,, pp 147-161

LeVeen RF, Wolf GL, Biery D (1985) Angioplasty induced vasospasm in rabbit model. Invest Radiol 20:938-944

McTavish D, Faulds D, Goa KL (1990) Ticlopidine. An updated review of its pharmacology and therapeutic use in platelet dependent disorders. Drugs 40:238-259

Minar E, Almadi A, Kappersteiner R, Maca R, Stumflen A et al (1995) Comparison of effects of high dose and low dose aspirin on restenosis after femoropopliteal percutaneous transluminal angioplasty. Circulation 91:2167-2173

Mruk JS, Chesebro JH, Webster MWJ (1990) Platelet aggregation and interaction with the coagulation system: implications for antithrombotic therapy in arterial thrombosis. Cor Art Dis 1:149-158

Ratzmann KP (1991) Perioperative Stoffwechselführung bei Diabetes mellitus. Med Aktuel 17:250-251

Rosenberg RD, Damus PS (1975) The purification and mechanisms of action of human antithrombin-heparin. N Engl J Med 292:146

Rutsch W, Brunckhorst C, Serruys PW et al (1995) Rekombinantes Hirudin zur Restenoseprophylaxe nach PTCA. Z Kardiol 84:82

Schomig A, Neumann FJ, Kastrati A, Schuhlen H,, Blasini R et al (1996) A randomized comparison of antiplatelet and anticoagulant therapy after the placement of coronary-artery stents. N Engl J Med 334:1126-1128

Spies JB, Rosen RF, Lebowitz AS (1988) Antibiotic prophylaxis in vascular and interventional radiology: a rational approach. Radiology 166:381-387

Tetteroo E, Mali WP, Rienks R, van Kester JA, Banga JD (1995) The significance of coumarin anticoagulation in laser assisted percutaneous transluminal angioplasty of femeropopliteal arterial obstructions. Eur J Radiol 19:86-90

Thornton MA, Gruentzig AR, Hollman J, King SB et al (1984) Coumadin and aspirin in prevention of recurrence after transluminal coronary angioplasty: a randomized study. Circulation 69:721-727

Villa AE, Guzman LA, Poptic EJ et al (1995) Effects of antisense-c-myb-oligonucleotides on vascular smooth-cell proliferation and response to vessel wall injury. Circ Res 76:505-513

Von der Leyen HE, Gibbons GH (1995) Gene therapy inhibiting neointimal vascular lesions: in vivo transfer of endothelial cell nitric oxide synthase gene. Proc Natl Sci Acad USA 92:1137-1141

Wallace S, Medellin H, DeJongh D, Gianturco C (1972) Systemic heparinisation for angiography. Am J Roentgenol 115:204-209

Warkentin TE, Kelton JG (1991) Heparin induced thrombocytopenia. Progr Hemost Thromb 10:1-34

Wilemsky RL, March KL, Tradus-Pizio J, Sandinsky G, Fineberg N, Hathaway PR (1995) Vascular injury repair and restenosis after percutaneous transluminal angioplasty in the atherosclerotic rabbit. Circulation 92:2995-3005

Zeitler E, Reichold J, Schoop W, Loew D (1973) Einfluß von Acetylsalicylsäure auf das Frühergebnis nach perkutaner Rekanalisationen arterieller Obliterationen nach Dotter. Dtsch Med Wochenschr 98:1285-1288

7 Informed Consent and Patient Background

E. Zeitler

Although angiography of the peripheral arteries and percutaneous vascular interventions are minor invasive procedures in most cases, the principle of the patient's "right of self-determination", as well as medical ethics are based on objective communication between the physician and the patient, or his/her legal representative's (REUTER 1987).

Angiography is performed following needle puncture or catheterization of the vessel and administration of contrast medium (CM), the diffusion of which is then documented by means of an imaging system. Consequently, in view of the patient's uninjured condition, he/she needs to be informed not only of the risk of actual physical injury which may be caused by puncture and catheterization, but also of the risks associated with the administration of CM and the use of X-rays. Interventional radiologic procedures also include the same risks in most situations, although different devices are used. The incidence of complications varies according to the type of procedure. Also, local complications are the same, albeit with perhaps a higher incidence, but the procedure is nevertheless intended to treat disease and reduce symptoms.

From a legal point of view, the term "informed consent" implies:

Full information regarding the indicated treatment, i.e., the benefit of the examination or treatment to the patient.

Full information regarding the intervention itself, which requires that the physician carrying out the examination or treatment advises the patient in general about the type and significance of the intervention, possible adverse effects and potential risks,

as well as alternative suitable therapies, in terms comprehensible to the layman, thus enabling him to reach a self-determined decision (WEISSAUER 1991).

"Spontaneous information" provided by the physician which also requires a discussion between the interventional radiologist and the patient, in the course of which the latter gives information regarding his/her disease and diseases among his/her family, experiences during the time of the disease, occupational diseases, and previous experience of aftereffects, such as allergy, bleeding, or others. The talk should also comprise future plans, such as change of occupation, holiday trips, or similar events. The physician's aim is not to provide the patient with full technical details which may then worry him/her or even cause fear of the intervention. Fear, according to LALLI (1980), may responsible for the occurrence of moderate or severe complications caused, for example, by the heat sensation that may be experienced during the administration of CM prewarmed to 37°C.

A history of allergic reactions following CM administration, or special risks in the form of existing nephropathies, are always important. In such cases, the talk should include a discussion about special premedication and the treatment of side effects and complications (FINK et al. 1991; PETERS and ZEITLER 1991; PETERS et al. 1992).

The greater the need for and urgency of the intervention, the more persuasive the physician needs to be to encourage the patient to agree. Should alternative diagnostic or therapeutic methods of equal benefit exist, the physician is obliged to inform the patient accordingly and to assist him in his decision-making, without the use of persuasion. The patient determines the extent of the information he requires to come to a mutually satisfying "informed consent". As far as cooperation between the referring physican and the radiologist performing the examination or intervention is concerned, it should go without saying that known, important details on the disease and the findings of previous examinations are available

E. ZEITLER, Professor, MD, Virchowstraße 13, 90409 Nuremberg, Germany

at the time of the information talk. The referring physician should also have informed the patient beforehand of the reasons for the planned examinations, including the tentative diagnosis or planned therapy. Patients who have been pre-informed in this way have a better understanding of the situation than patients who come to the interventional radiologist as a primary-care physician. As the responsible care of the patient within the framework of interventional radiologic measures includes both the intervention itself and the follow-up period, not only does a "medical treatment contract" need to be entered into, but also a relationship between physician and patient based on trust needs to be established, forming the most reliable basis for cooperation during and after the intervention.

Information regarding risks: This includes the fatal risks that cannot be controlled even under thorough medical care. Adverse reactions caused by CM, hematomas at the puncture site, peripheral embolism in the framework of angioplasties, or similar risks cannot be completely eliminated even when the safest precautionary measures are employed.

The patient should always be informed of the potential of these risks, even when they are very critical, whereby general risks, and risks directly associated with the specific intervention need to be valued differently (VOGEL 1986). Patients are generally not familiar with the "typical risks" of the intervention, whereas there is considerable knowledge of the general risks, such as pain during puncture, raised temperature following an intervention, or the effects of general anesthesia in our well-informed society. Rare and critical complications need special mention as these could influence the patient's decision, as well as his/her quality of life after the intervention. These include, for example, plexus paresis following axillary puncture, paraplegia following translumbar aortography, and renal insufficiency in patients with diabetic nephropathy.

The more urgent, however, the diagnostic or therapeutic intervention, the less strict are the requirements regarding patient information, even from a legal standpoint. If, for example, only an immediate intervention has the chance of being successful, information about possible risks need not be as detailed. Diagnostic procedures which are imperative to decide on a promising therapy cannot be subject to more stringent regulations regarding patient information about possible risks than the therapeutic intervention itself. Legal requirements regarding patient information about diagnostic methods, however, are particularly stringent.

Naturally, information about alternatives is very important and requires considerable experience and knowledge on the physician's part. Particularly regarding angiography, ultrasound and magnetic resonance angiography are capable of providing a diagnosis without the use of X-rays. Should the information obtained using these non-invasive modalities be unsatisfactory, the need for conventional angiography should be justified. The more complex the decision on subsequent therapeutic or diagnostic measures, the more important it is to consider possible alternative therapies, as well the available equipment.

In the case of suspected abdominal aortic aneurysm, for example, ultrasound in combination with spiral computed tomography may provide all the necessary information for proceeding with a therapy, without vascular catheterization. Only if the information obtained is not sufficient to plan an important intervention or surgery, the cautious, anxious, or well-informed patient will give his consent to the slightly higher risk, possibly associated with pain. On the other hand, in the framework of interventional radiologic measures, it should be assessed whether surgery, or no intervention at all – involving certain impairments to quality of life or other controllable risks – would be a better solution in the patient's interests.

Of course, the information talk is *not necessary* (NARR 1983; REUTER 1987) if:

- The patient is already well informed as a result of a similar measure performed at an earlier time
- The patient is a colleague familiar with the problems
- The patient expresses his confidence in such a way that makes detailed information superfluous. In any, as well as such, cases, written documentation about the information talk is necessary. It may then be recommended that the document be signed by both the patient and the physician.

The talk can be prepared using information pamphlets, which make the subject more accessible and easier to understand. However, no printed information can replace the information talk between physician and patient, which is imperative to obtain the legally relevant "patient's informed consent". Independent of this, talks with the patient prior to, during, and after diagnostic or therapeutic interventions should take place in such a way as to enable the patient to be convinced of what he has agreed to. They form part of what is considered socially relevant good clinical practice, which is also in line with the contract with the referring colleague or physician performing the aftercare. The responsibilities of the diagnostic and interventional radiologist include, besides the proper performance of a specialist's tasks, taking on the role of a primary-care physician for a limited period of time. On the other hand, it is essential that the patient be aware of the consequences of a possible refusal of the planned or suggested intervention (COPE et al. 1992).

References

Cope C, Burke DR, Meranze S (1992) Atlas der interventionellen Radiologie. VCH, Weinheim

Fink U, Jung D, Fink BK (1991) Prämedikation bei Risikopatienten: Ergebnisse einer prospektiven Studie mit nichtionischen Kontrastmitteln. In: Peters PE, Zeitler E (eds) Röntgenkontrastmittel, Nebenwirkungen, Prophylaxe, Therapie. Springer, Berlin Heidelberg New York, pp 205–209

Lalli AF (1980) Contrast media reactions: data analysis and hypothesis. Radiology 134:1–12

Narr H (1983) Die Aufklärungspflicht des Radiologen in der Praxis. Radiologe 23:241–247

Peters PE, Zeitler E (eds) (1991) Röntgenkontrastmittel, Nebenwirkungen, Prophylaxe, Therapie. Springer, Berlin Heidelberg New York

Peters PE, Zeitler E, Clauß W (eds) (1992) Qualitätssicherung bei der Anwendung von Röntgenkontrastmitteln. Springer, Berlin Heidelberg New York

Reuter SR (1987) An overview of informed consent for radiologists. AJR Am J Roentgenol 148:219–227

Vogel H (1986) Risiken der Röntgendiagnostik. Urban & Schwarzenberg, Munich

Weissauer W (1991) Arzthaftung und Eingriffsaufklärung. In: Peters PE, Zeitler E (eds) Röntgenkontrastmittel: Nebenwirkungen, Prophylaxe, Therapie. Springer, Berlin Heidelberg New York, pp 181–197

Zeitler E (1991) Prophylaxe gegen Kontrastmittel-Nebenwirkungen. In: Röntgenkontrastmittel: Nebenwirkungen, Prophylaxe, Therapie. Springer, Berlin Heidelberg New York, pp 198–204

Imaging Modalities

8 Roentgen Angiography

E. Zeitler, F. Olbert, K. Detmar, W. Krause, E. Ammann, F. Stösslein,
T. Pollack, T. Schmidt and M. Wucherer

CONTENTS

E. Zeitler, Professor, MD, Virchowstraße 13, D-90409 Nuremberg, Germany

F. Olbert, Professor of Radiology, MD, Department of Radiodiagnostics, Clinical Department of Angiography and Interventional Radiology, General Hospital, Währinger Gürtel 18-20, A-1090 Vienna, Austria

K. Detmar, MD, Institut für Diagnostische und Interventionelle Radiologie, Klinikum Nord, Flurstraße 17, D-90340, Nuremberg, Germany

W. Krause, Professor, MD, Schering AG, Contrast Media Research, Müllerstraße 170-178, D-13342 Berlin, Germany

E. Ammann, Dr.-Ing., Abteilungsdirektor, c/o Siemens AG, Medizinische Technik, Henkestraße 127, D-91052 Erlangen, Germany

F. Stösslein, MD, Radiologic Clinic, Städtisches Klinikum, Dresden-Friedrichstadt, Friedrichstraße 41, D-01067 Dresden, Germany

T. Pollack, MD, Radiologic Clinic, Städtisches Klinikum, Dresden-Friedrichstadt, Friedrichstraße 41, D-01067 Dresden, Germany

T. Schmidt, PhD, Klinikum Nürnberg, Institut für Medizinische Physik, Flurstraße 17, D-90340 Nuremberg, Germany

M. Wucherer, PhD, Klinikum Nürnberg, Institut für Medizinische Physik, Flurstraße 17, D-90340 Nuremberg, Germany

8.1
History

As early as in the first year following Roentgen's discovery of the "X-ray" (1895), an article designed to demonstrate the practical value of this new photographic technique was published (Haschek and Lindenthal 1896). It clearly depicted the vessels of the hand of a corpse after injection of a chalk and cinnabar suspension through the brachial artery. This suspension – Teichmann's mass – was used at that time in anatomy departments to better demonstrate vessels.

For the further development of angiography, particularly of the aorta and extremity arteries, three aspects were of key importance:

1. The creation of non-toxic contrast media suitable for intraarterial, and/or intravenous administration in living patients in sufficient doses
2. The appropriate technique of contrast medium administration by needles or catheters
3. The optimal "Roentgen" technique for a precise documentation of the vascular system using the appropriate flow-dependent imaging system, first without, and later with, digital technologies.

8.1.1
Contrast Media

In Frankfurt am Main in 1923, Berberich and Hirsch presented the results of their examinations using liquid solutions of various halogenous salts, and determining the degree of blackening under varying voltages. They found that particularly strontium bromide ($SrBr_2$) in a 10% solution and sodium iodide had the highest contrast density. For their first arteriograms and phlebograms of the hand, they used strontium bromide. As early as in 1924, Hirsch published his monograph *Die peripheren Blutgefäße im Röntgenbild* (The peripheral blood vessels in the X-ray picture). In the same year, Brooks published his results on arterio-graphies of the leg following intraarterial injection of sodium iodide (Brooks 1924).

Early successes in the development of better tolerated contrast agents were achieved by using Uroselektan, produced synthetically from 1926, and by the further development of similar, di-iodinated contrast agents such as Uroselektan B, Perabrodil, Diotrast, and Jod-uron. These contrast agents were employed by Ratschow (1930, 1937) for phlebographies, and by Sgalitzer (1931) for arteriographies.

Thorotrast, a 20% colloidal thorium dioxide solution, was introduced into diagnostics in 1932 by Bluhbaum et al. (1928). This substance, with its low radioactivity, gave very good contrasting quality and, at that time, hardly any local or general side effects were known. It was preferred for cerebral and peripheral angiographies.

Only when the potential of late injuries in the form of Thorotrast-induced tumors, such as thorotrastomas, and angiosarcomas had been reported (Bauer 1943; Mac Mahon et al. 1947), were there warnings against the in vivo use of Thorotrast.

As a further development, tri-iodinated contrast agents appeared on the market. The meglumine and sodium salt of amidotrizoate (Urografin) was the best-tolerated contrast agent for coronary, cerebral, abdominal, and peripheral angiography for many years, and became the elemental prerequisite for the introduction of selective coronary angiography. An aspect that deserved special attention, thus, was the appropriate composition of cations (sodium or methylglucamine) to avoid rhythmic disorders during selective coronary angiography.

In the interests of further improvements, compounds of better vascular and general tolerance were created by various substitutions in the side chains. The result was contrast agents such as iothalamate (Angiografin, Conray), ioxithalamate (Telebrix), or ioglycinate (Rayvist). With the use of these contrast agents, general anesthesia, as practiced before for translumbar and femoral or brachial arteriography, became increasingly superfluous. However, the observed pain reactions still required adequate premedication for angiography of the extremities. Pain was caused mainly by the hyperosmolarity of the triiodinated, water-soluble contrast agents.

A significant step forward was the introduction of an ionic dimer of considerably lower osmolarity (Hexabrix), which enabled almost pain-free angiographies of the extremities, even without additional premedication, and without the necessity for general anesthesia. This substance, Ioxaglat, has six iodine atoms, but only one group of acids per molecule. Due to its lower osmolarity, higher contrast amounts could be administered if necessary, thereby allowing the examination of practically all vascular regions in question; for example, the aorta and leg arteries, the renal arteries and brain-supplying arteries in one setting, with up to 250 ml of contrast agent. Tolerance could even be enhanced by the introduction of non-ionic, water-soluble contrast agents, due to the successful synthesis of the contrast agent metrizamide (Amipaque) by ALMÉN in 1969.

However, only the introduction of the water-soluble, non-ionic contrast agents Iopamidol (Solutrast) in 1977, iohexol (Omnipaque) in 1980, and iopromide (Ultravist) in balanced solutions, led to increased use of these low-osmolar, non-ionic compounds which, in addition to the low osmolarity of the dimer ioxaglate, have the advantage of substantially better general tolerance.

Research in the field of contrast agents, however, has continued, resulting in low-osmolar, non-ionic dimeric contrast agents such as iotrolan (Isovist) and Idoixanol (Visipaque). Nevertheless, the use of the latter for angiographies, in contrast to the non-ionic monomeric contrast agents, has not been recommended in general, due to the possibility of various mild and moderate late reactions in 1%–3% of cases. Personal studies of interventional arteriographies in more than 100 patients have shown the same incidence of late reactions (2.0%) as with other contrast media, but with no pain or early allergic reactions, so the rise in high-risk patients in arterial contrast medium administration has started.

8.1.2
Administration of Contrast Media

Until the introduction of the percutaneous catheterization technique by SELDINGER (1953), contrast media were administered exclusively in the framework of needle angiographies, i.e., puncture needles of varying length and diameter were used to puncture the femoral artery in the groin, the cubital artery in the arm, the axillary and carotid arteries, and the aorta. For translumbar aortographies, hollow needles with, or without, mandrin were available. Nearly all needles could be combined first with the "Record" nozzle, and later with the "Luer-Lok" extension. To ensure a stable connection between cannula and injection syringe, connecting tubes and adapters with a stopcock were developed to keep blood loss following vascular puncture as low as possible.

The administration of contrast media was greatly eased by percutaneous catheterization techniques, since the technique of contrast medium administration for intravenous aortography, according to ROBB and STEINBERG (1939), used at that time – contrast medium injection into both elevated arms – had been somewhat complicated. Experience gained from ureteral catheterization encouraged FORSSMANN in 1929, after experimental studies, to advance a catheter from the cubital vein, under fluoroscopic monitoring, into the right side of the heart in a self-experiment which was successful. An earlier report on the catheterization of blood vessels via the femoral vein or artery, with the aim of selectively delivering drugs as close as possible to the appropriate site of action by BLEICHRÖDER (1912) was then forgotten. Independent of that, ICHIKAWA (1938) reported on the visualization of the abdominal aorta and the renal arteries after contrast administration via the opened circumflexal femoral lateral artery, in a German-language journal. In 1941, FARINAS published his results on the catheterization of the abdominal aorta and its side branches for visualization in the arteriogram via a surgically opened access in the femoral artery (FARINAS 1941).

During this period, access for catheterization via opened veins in the angle of the elbow and the groin became more and more common, both among cardiologists in the framework of lesion diagnosis of congenital and acquired heart failure, and among surgeons, either immediately before an operation or for the diagnosis of acute and chronic obliterations. When PVC catheters became available, the technique of puncture with large-caliber needles through which catheters for angiography were insertable, was developed (PEIRCE 1951; LINDGREN 1953).

The date that marked the breakthrough in the percutaneous catheterization of arteries and veins was, without doubt, 1953, with SELDINGER's publication of his work on catheter insertion with the help of a previously-placed guidewire.

Manifold practical and technical developments of the catheter material, configuration of the catheter tip, and the employment of SELDINGER's technique for general, as well as selective angiographies, were made, particularly in Sweden at institutes in Lund and Stockholm. Both the introduction of the radiopaque catheters and the design of several tip configurations for visceral and supraaortic selective catheterization were published by OEDMAN (1956). The first roll- and cut-film changers came from Sweden (Elema). Various high-pressure injectors (GIDLUND 1956) marked the beginning of automatic contrast medium injections in larger amounts. Essential improvements in contrast medium administration were possible on the basis of controlled, even ECG-controlled, contrast medium administration, not only in continuous, but also pulsed injection (SCHAD 1967; FRANKEN and ZEITLER 1978). Moreover, new injectors provided the possibility of a programmed contrast injection at varying speeds during one application (AMPLATZ 1960; VIAMONTE and HOBBS 1967).

The availability of needle angiographies, translumbar angiographies, and the catheter angiography according to SELDINGER led to a wide application of arteriographic and phlebographic examinations in several acute and chronic diseases. Many publications focused on their safe application and lack of complications (PÄSSLER 1957; HETTLER 1969; WENZ et al. 1970; BAUM et al. 1966; HINCK et al. 1967). The risk of thrombus formation at the surface of the catheter or side ports during long examinations raised questions about the problem of catheter thromboses (ZEITLER 1970a,b; DERAY and JACOBS 1996; DAWSON 1988). As a consequence, catheters were developed with a very smooth surface which constituted only a small target for platelet adhesion. Further attempts to reduce the risk of catheter thromboses culminated in the idea of systematic heparinization during angiographic examination (AMPLATZ 1971; WALLACE et al. 1972), and of preparing the catheter surface with heparin.

8.1.3
Equipment and Imaging Systems

The manifold refinements of the X-ray technique led from the single-cassette X-ray image to cassette changers (JANKER–PÄSSLER, GÄRTNER–REISER, and WENZLIK changers), and film changers (AOT, Puck), reaching their technical peak with the intro-

duction of the digital subtraction angiography (DSA) (MISTRETTA et al. 1981; MEANY 1980; BRENNECKE et al. 1978; CRUMMY et al. 1980; SEYFERTH et al. 1982).

Today, the standard of angiographies of the extremities using DSA is the documentation of the arteries of the pelvis and leg within the framework of one contrast medium injection under electronic control (FINK 1991; HILBERTZ et al. 1992). Digital angiography or DSA can be performed both after intravenous and intraarterial contrast injection (RÜCKFORTH et al. 1998). However, it should not be used as a screening method. Nowadays, non-invasive and simple clinical methods are available for screening purposes. The optimum technical angiography is the digital angiography or DSA following an intraarterial contrast medium injection either into the aorta or, in selective techniques, into the required artery. Despite this, there are situations suggesting an intravenous contrast medium administration, to avoid complications at the puncture site, or through arterial catheterization. Previous punctures, hematomas, scars, infections, and the patient's immobility render access via the best-suited femoral arteries in the groin much more difficult. The transbrachial catheter angiography using 3- or 4-F catheters is preferable for outpatient studies, after the venous or arterial approach. In arterial transbrachial techniques, however, heparin is to be administered intraarterially in prolonged studies, since there is the risk of thrombosis of the brachial artery.

The following sections describe the different access sites with the aim of providing a guide. None of the techniques is suited for every case. The most suitable site for puncture and catheterization must be determined on an individual basis. Therefore, indications are given by obvious symptoms and the results of non-invasive investigation. The radiologist himself must investigate the patient's situation, his/her complaints, make sure the symptoms indicate an angiography, and, if so, which angiography is optimally suited.

8.2
Access to Arteries and Veins

8.2.1
Femoral Vessels in the Groin

The *femoral artery* is the most common access to the arterial system for diagnostic and therapeutic procedures. It is also the site of classic surgical anastomosis in vascular surgery for arterial and venous diseases. Therefore, the prevention of infections in the groin prior to vascular surgery and diagnostic intervention must be observed in all cases of diagnostic and therapeutic procedures (WAGNER et al. 1998).

Whether one or both walls are entered as the needle passes into the artery is of no significant consequence in diagnostic angiographies with small needles, followed by catheterization with catheters of between 3 and 7 F (WHITE 1976). In patients under anticoagulation with heparin or warfarin, however, the two-wall puncture with large needles may be followed by a higher incidence of hematomas.

Important aspects of the angiographer's tasks include:

- Familiarity with the anatomy of the groin and the pathophysiology of the peripheral circulation
- Adequate manual skills in puncture and guiding techniques
- Ability to prevent complications, including infection, and, if necessary, their management
- Optimal radiodiagnostic work-up with precise imaging and radioprotection.

The best access to puncture the inguinal artery is the common femoral artery, in the upper third of the distance between the inguinal ligament and the inguinal crease.

The common femoral artery just below the inguinal ligament is lateral to the femoral vein (Fig. 8.1) and runs straight from the groin downwards, in the direction of the medial part of the knee. In the case of chronic occlusion of the superficial femoral artery, however, the profunda, as an important collateral vessel, takes a straighter direction, simulating the superficial femoral artery. The bifurcation of the common femoral artery is below the inguinal crease in 20% of cases, above the same in 75%, and at the same level in 5%. LECHNER's distance between the inguinal crease and the inguinal ligament varies between 0 and 11 cm (average 6.7 ± 1.9 SD). Only in a minority of patients (about 5%) is the inguinal crease in the intimal vicinity of the inguinal ligament (<2 cm). In the remaining 95%, a distance of 3–5 cm is available for safe puncture (LECHNER et al. 1988).

The puncture of inguinal arteries in the groin is a prerequisite of direct needle arteriography, or arterial catheterization as the basis of selective or overview catheter angiographies, as well as of all arterial interventions.

To prepare a successful puncture of the common femoral artery, there are several helpful measures:

- Pulse palpation
- A cushion placed beneath the patient's pelvis
- Doppler localization of the artery
- Localization with X-ray fluoroscopy of calcifications and the femoral head
- Measurement of Lechner's distance
- Intravenous DSA.

The puncture of the femoral vein in the groin requires orientation by the artery. The vein is located medial to the artery, and in part behind. Venous puncture is necessary for all types of pelvic and abdominal phlebography, including caudal cavography and phlebography of the veins of the thigh using Valsalva's test, and it forms the basis of catheterization of the right heart and the pulmonary arteries for pressure measurements, angiography, as well as of procedures for documenting the cranial vena cava and cranial inflow veins. Transfemoral venous interventions can be indicated in patients with pulmonary embolism, for the extraction of foreign bodies out of the heart chambers or pulmonary arteries, or for clot removal, followed by stent application in the case of cranial vena cava syndrome. Also for selective catheterization of the renal or suprarenal veins, before blood-sampling, or for the application of vena

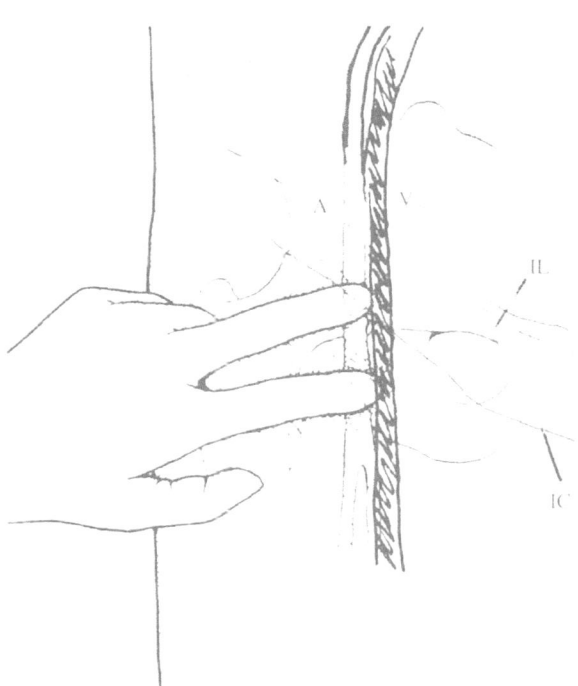

Fig. 8.1. Relationship between the femoral artery (*A*), vein (*V*), and the inguinal ligament (*IL*) and inguinal crease (*IC*). Positioning of the artery before retrograde common femoral puncture

cava filters, access via the femoral vein can be of importance as an alternative to the jugular or brachial veins. There are several indications where the jugular veins, as access to the cranial and caudal vena cava, should be chosen (GÜNTHER and THELEN 1996).

There are two puncture techniques in the groin from which to choose, both of which are mainly carried out under local anesthesia and which are painfree.

8.2.1.1
Retrograde Femoral Puncture Technique

Palpation and fixation of the femoral artery two fingers just below the inguinal ligament in the groin determines the place and direction of the puncture (Fig. 8.1). The cannula is advanced towards the artery at an angle of 45–60°, until a tiny pulsation is felt (Fig. 8.2). A dart-like puncture is then performed, seeking to perforate only a small segment of the anterior arterial wall and to avoid, wherever possible, perforation of the posterior wall through the oblique puncture direction. As soon as blood extravasates from the puncture needle without a mandrin, either a guidewire can be inserted, or the precise placement of the needle in the vessel can be checked by means of a contrast medium injection. Retroperitoneal bleeding can be avoided by safe

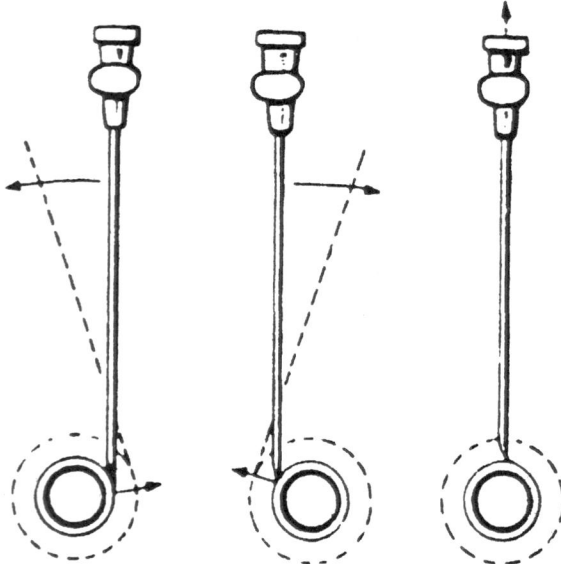

Fig. 8.2. Pulsation of the puncture needle according to its position in front, medial, or lateral of the artery. The cannula is approached synchronously with the pulse to the side where the artery is located. (According to Ratschow 1953)

infrainguinal puncture. The best site is 2–3 cm distal of the femoral head, which can be localized by X-ray fluoroscopy. The location of the artery, if no clear pulse can be localized, can be determined using the Doppler ultrasound technique.

8.2.1.2
Antegrade Femoral Puncture

This is the most common access to the femoropopliteal and tibioperoneal arteries (DOTTER and JUDKINS 1964; ZEITLER 1975; SADEKNI et al. 1985) (Fig. 8.3), as is the retrograde femoral puncture to the iliac and all arteries of the head and trunk for diagnostic and interventional procedures.

In all cases, it is important to place a cushion beneath the pelvis to stretch the inguinal vessels. The femoral artery is palpable directly below the inguinal ligament, or directly above (Fig. 8.4). With the second and third fingers, the artery is pressed against the pubic bone. The artery is punctured just above the two fingers, which controls the location of the artery in a caudal direction. The skin perforation is 1–3 cm above the point where the needle perforates the anterior wall of the artery. The antegrade puncture is more difficult, and in 5%–10% of cases – mostly obese patients – the tip of the needle may deviate into the deep femoral artery (ZEITLER 1975). Under fluoroscopy and dye injection, the needle tip can be directed back into the common femoral artery. As soon as it is in the common femoral artery or superficial femoral artery, the guidewire can be introduced or the angiography started. In case the needle tip lies in the deep femoral artery, attempts to retract it under fluoroscopy during the contrast dye injection and to correct the needle position can be made. Other possibilities include inserting a dilator or a catheter with a sharply angulated tip (right coronary artery catheter), or with a proximal side hole 3 cm behind the tip (COPE technique; COPE 1986), to continue, with the help of a guidewire, to proper placement and catheterization, without having to repeat the puncture.

8.2.1.2.1
COPE TECHNIQUE

Modified access technique. A 45° angulated dilator with a large side-port several centimeters distally of its tip is inserted into the deep femoral artery. Under fluoroscopic control, the dilator is retracted until the side-port releases contrast dye into the superficial femoral artery. Then, with the help of a preshaped

Access to the ilio-femoral Arteries
Incidence in Diagnostic and Interventionell Procedures

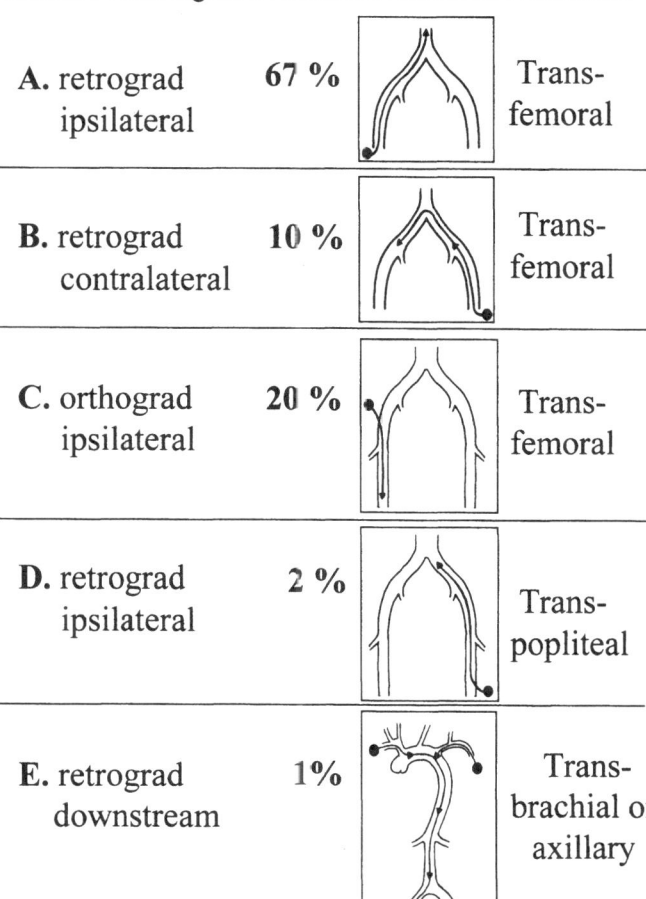

A. retrograd ipsilateral	67 %		Transfemoral
B. retrograd contralateral	10 %		Transfemoral
C. orthograd ipsilateral	20 %		Transfemoral
D. retrograd ipsilateral	2 %		Transpopliteal
E. retrograd downstream	1%		Transbrachial or axillary

Fig. 8.3 a–e. Acces to the iliofemoral arteries: incidence in diagnostic and interventional procedures. Different puncture techniques of the common femoral artery (a–e). The figure also shows the incidence in percent among patients hospitalized in the Nuremberg clinic in 1994

guidewire – most suitable is a bent-tip Terumo guidewire – the glide wire can be advanced directly into the superficial femoral artery. The dilator is then removed and a straight dilator inserted, through which the Terumo guidewire can be exchanged for a Teflon-coated safety J-guidewire. As soon as a sheath has been placed, an exchange of catheters, as required, is possible.

8.2.1.3
Contralateral Access from the Groin to Iliac and Femoral Arteries

In exceptionally complex situations, for example, after fresh operations in the groin, presence of large hematomas, or marked obesity, the antegrade catheterization of the femoral artery can be performed via access from the contralateral femoral artery (Fig. 8.3b), over the bifurcation. In such cases, it is necessary to ensure that, after precise sounding of the contralateral iliac artery with the help of a preshaped hook, sidewinder, or pigtail catheter, a long sheath is inserted, the tip of which is located in the side to be treated. Under these conditions, sounding in the contralateral femoral artery is also possible with a long guidewire (140 cm) and catheter.

The antegrade sounding of the femoral artery can also be carried out, if necessary, through the arm (brachial or axillary artery) (Fig. 8.3e), if an ipsilateral antegrade catheterization or contralateral puncture and catheterization are not feasible (Fig. 8.5). This is the case, for example, in unilateral occlusions of the pelvic arteries and after recent operations on the side to be treated, with fresh scars in the groin. Under such conditions, the use of extra-long guidewires (170–210 cm) and catheters enables catheterization of the femoral or popliteal artery even

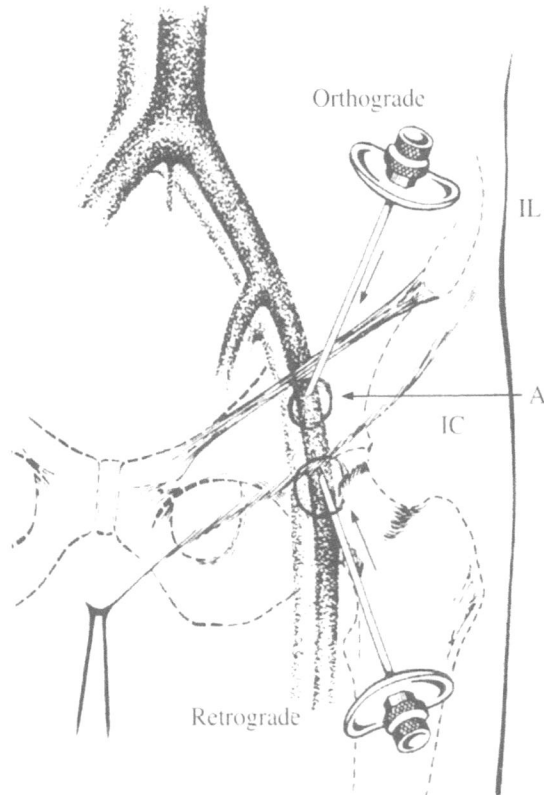

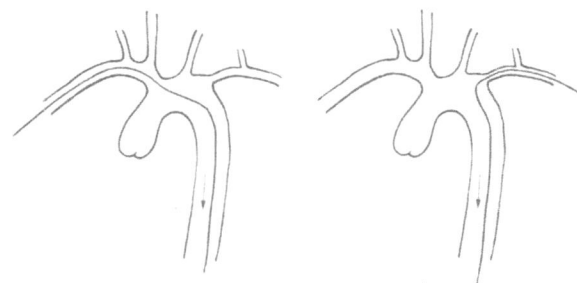

Fig. 8.5 a,b. Transthoracic catheterization of the descending thoracic and abdominal aorta from the left subclavian and right brachiocephalic artery. **a** Transinnominate (brachial or axillary access). **b** Transsubclavian

Fig. 8.4. Anatomical situation of the common femoral artery (*A*) between the inguinal ligament (*IL*) and inguinal crease (*IC*), demonstrating the different locations of retrograde and orthograde puncture

from the arm. It is, however, of vital importance in such cases to bear in mind that, in particular, sounding via the aortic arch and the brachiocephalic arteries involves the risk of cerebral complications (embolism). Due to the length of the catheter, thrombus formation is more likely, either on the outer surface or at the side-ports. For this reason, for angiographies of leg arteries started in the arm, the administration of 10 000 IU of heparin instead of 5000 is recommended, if the procedure exceeds 30 min.

8.2.1.3.1
PREVENTION OF COMPLICATIONS

The precautions to be taken to avoid complications during punctures – particularly in the region of the groin – include the following:

- Extensive shaving and cleaning of the groin
- Precise localization of the vessel, if necessary with Doppler technique
- Successful puncture, if possible at first attempt
- Avoidance of perforation of the posterior wall, if possible

- Utilization of a sheath to reduce trauma to the vessel
- To complete the procedure: compression as long as required, followed by a safe compression bandage or, alternatively, utilization of a percutaneous puncture-hole closure device (e.g., Angioseal, Vasoseal, Perclose).

The most common complications at the puncture site, altogether less than 3%, include:

- Post-procedure bleeding
- Hematoma
- Pulsating hematoma – false aneurysm
- Arteriovenous (av)-fistula
- Thrombus formation and occlusion
- Local infection or inflammatory hematoma
- Mechanically-induced neuralgia of the superficial femoral nerve.

These are minimal or moderate complications. Surgical repair is more common after prolonged interventions, to stop post-operative bleeding or treat thrombosed arteries. Pulsating hematomas can be managed by compression under ultrasound control.

As the groin is also the access site for heart catheterization, coronary angiography, and cardiac interventions, as well as for angiographies and interventions in the cerebrovascular system, the prevention of complications in this region deserves special attention. Instead of repeated attempts to puncture the vessel, the Doppler technique should be primarily applied for reliable localization of the vessel.

Compression following puncture using the needle technique alone can be performed manually, for about 10 min. After catheterization using catheter systems of 5 F and more, manual compression needs to be performed for at least 15–20 min to prevent the formation of periarterial hematomas. Compression is preferably performed by the physician who carried out the puncture as he is most familiar with the site of the puncture hole in the artery, which is not identical to the incision spot on the skin. Compression with two or three fingers first is preferable to wider compression, which might favor a seeping hemorrhage. To complete the compression, a hip-groin bandage (Fig. 8.6) is useful and should remain in place for 4–24 h, depending on the size of the puncture hole and the duration of the intervention. In obese patients, interventions of long duration, and when puncture systems of 8 F and over are used, a hemostatic puncture-hole closure device (Angioseal, Vasoseal, or Perclose) has considerable advantages over extended manual compression, due to its ability to ensure reliable compression. The application of such a device is demonstrated in Fig. 8.7.

Both in the patient's interests and in the interests of smooth organization of the proceedings in the "angio-interventional suite", the patient is placed – with the sheath inside the artery – either on a transport stretcher or into bed, where compression, including a compression bandage, is performed. This is more comfortable for the patient and the angio-table can be prepared in the meantime for the next procedure.

Optimum fluoroscopy, as ensured by appropriate X-ray units, is essential for the effective use of guidewires, catheters, and interventional instrumentation, not only in the patient's interests, but also in the interests of assistants and the physician himself. The requirements include: powerful X-ray tubes, suitable image-intensifier TV chains, appropriate filters and grids, the provision of pulsed fluoroscopy, and the necessary means of radiation protection for both patients and personnel, without which any fluoroscopy-controlled intervention involving the use of X-rays would be unacceptable.

In the near future, puncture, catheterization, diagnosis, as well as interventions will be performed increasingly under duplex sonography control. This requires highly sophisticated imaging units and, where possible, the intervention itself should be performed by one physician, while another physician operates the transducer.

8.2.2
Brachial

The retrograde puncture or catheterization of the brachial artery is started in the antecubital fossa, preferably with a very sharp needle of 18 or, even better, 21 gauge. Any damage to the posterior wall should be avoided. If there is free flow, a correction of the needle position is then possible. A preselected guidewire must then be inserted and, in the case of a cannula with a blunt surface being used, this has to be exchanged for a narrow-lumen dilator. Angiographies of the arteries of the arm, hand, and shoulder, as well as vertebral arteries, can then be safely performed through this narrow route. Unless the region to be examined has already been damaged due to several previous punctures, the problem that may be faced is a slight drifting away, and possibly a spasm of the artery. This is particulary the case when the first attempt to puncture has not been fully successful. Anatomic variations in the region of the bend of the elbow is a high-positioned bifurcation of the brachial artery into the radial and ulnar arteries. In patients who have received arteriovenous fistulas (Chimino shunt) for dialysis therapy, the individual anatomy is known due to previous operations. In such cases, however, the artery located in front is clearly palpable due to a mostly hard struc-

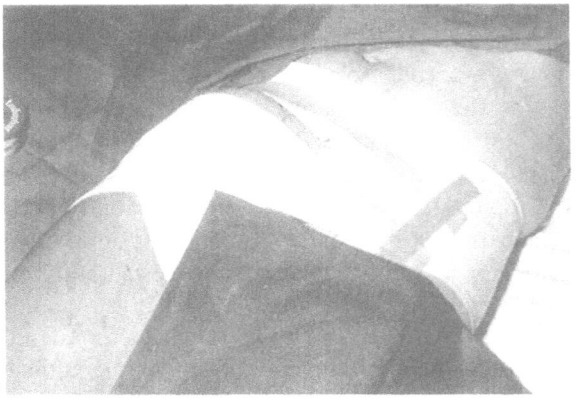

Fig. 8.6 a,b. Hip-joint bandage and styropor compressorium

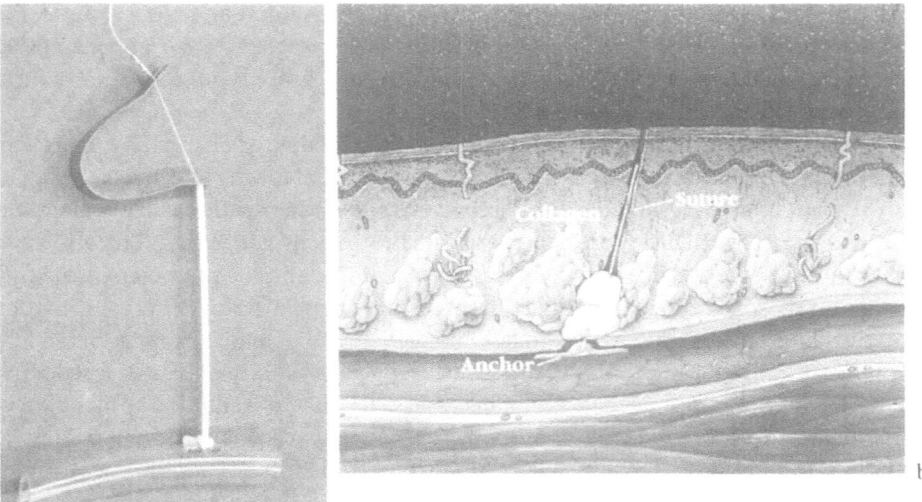

Fig. 8.7 a,b. Puncture-hole closure device (Angio-Seal)

ture caused by many previous punctures. Particularly in these cases, a very sharp-tipped cannula is essential.

For sounding of the supraaortic arteries from a brachial puncture site to the abdominal aorta and its branches, a guidewire with a preshaped tip and a preshaped catheter are required (see Fig. 8.5). Particularly in cases of severe aortic ectasia and elongation, the pigtail catheter, a sharply angled type, or a catheter for the left coronary artery can be very useful to successfully place the catheter in the thoracic descending aorta. As soon as the catheter has been safely advanced into the descending thoracic aorta, the extremely flexible Terumo guidewire has to be replaced by a more rigid, Teflon-coated safely J-guide, or a stiff Amplatz guidewire, if the branching point of the subclavian or anonyma artery forms an acute angle to the aorta. In diagnostic or interventional procedures of longer duration, it is essential to insert a guiding sheath via the guidewire for optimum prevention of any damage to the arterial wall. In addition, the placement of the sheath should be immediately followed by a heparin injection to prevent a thrombosis in the region of the brachial artery. After completion of transbrachial catheterizations, a control angiography of the arm is recommended to confirm free peripheral run-off in the region of the brachial artery.

8.2.3
Lumbar

Translumbar aortography was first described by the Portuguese surgeon Reynaldo Dos Santos in 1929

(Dos Santos et al. 1929a,b). It was the most common technique of aorto- and arteriography of the lower arteries for many years following the Second World War. It is a relatively fast, safe, and easy procedure for contrast visualization of the aorta and its lower branches. In most patients, percutaneous catheterization is nowadays applicable and translumbar access is unnecessary. However, there still remains a small group of patients with diffuse arterial occlusive disease and tortuosity which, in special situations, make catheterization impossible (Lipchik and Rogoff 1983).

Contraindications include hemorrhagic diathesis, anticoagulation therapy leading to prothrombin levels below 30%, or Quick's test below 40%. Seriously ill and dehydrated patients, or patients with renal insufficiency are also poor candidates for this technique, and the indication exists only prior to surgery.

The patient is in prone position and a pad is placed under the dorsum of the feet, another under the abdomen and pelvis. Puncture with a stiff needle (Dos Santos 1929a,b; Wellauer 1957; Loose and van Dongen 1976; Zeitler 1975), as suprarenal or infrarenal puncture (Fig. 8.8), is not necessary since the Teflon needle catheter set (Amplatz 1963; Gmelin 1986) provides more variability. Under fluoroscopy, the puncture is directed at an angulation of 45° directly before the vertebral column, at the height between the second to third lumbar spines. The instrument is 18 gauge in diameter and 18–24 cm in length. The tip of the catheter's Teflon sleeve should be positioned upstream or downstream. The flexible transparent tubing is connected to the needle. Luer-Lok fittings are used on all syringes, tubing, and needles to prevent the joints from opening during injection. Before the injection of 50 cl of dye through a pressure syringe, a control injection by hand is necessary under fluoroscopic control to prevent intramural or para-aortic contrast injection.

Before 1975, I used translumbar aortography in hundreds of patients, whereas in the 20 years between 1976 and 1996, in 12 patients only. During this period, femoral arteriography or abdominal aortography in combination with leg angiography were only performed after percutaneous catheterizations using the Seldinger or Hettler techniques, or with retrograde or antegrade needle angiography from the groin or arm. Needle angiography of the superficial femoral artery can be performed using Seldinger needles, or thin needles for lumbar myelography. Modern digital angiography DSA, contrast material of very low toxicity, and the percutaneous catheter technique with small needles and catheters have made arteriography of the peripheral vascular system very safe. Under these circumstances, it is unacceptable to speak of, or publish, works about "a diagnostic method with important complications". It has also been possible to reduce radiation exposure in recent years, and this constitutes neither a somatic, nor a stochastic risk for patients with arteriosclerotic diseases (see Sect. 8.6).

Note: References for Sects. 8.1–8.2.3 can be found at the end of Sect. 8.4.1.3.

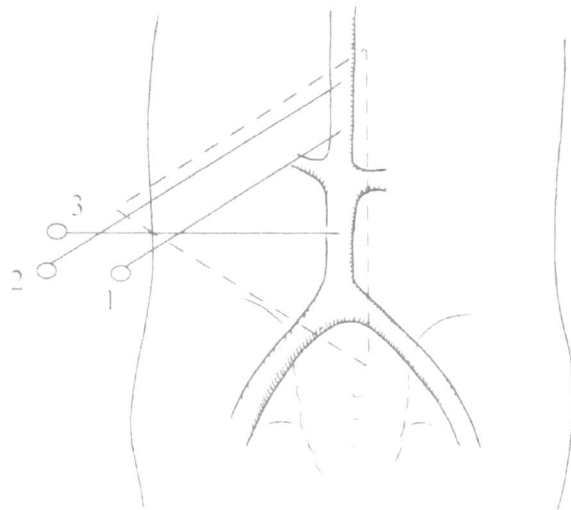

Fig. 8.8. Techniques of translumbar puncture of the abdominal aorta: (1) suprarenal, (2) subdiaphragmatic (high), (3) infrarenal (deep) aortic punctures. *Dotted lines*, lateral lumbar triangle

8.2.4
Axillary Access

F. Olbert

8.2.4.1
General Considerations

The vessels of the aortic arch, the arteries of the upper and lower extremities, the thoracic and abdominal aorta, and the visceral arteries are best and most safely visualized by using suitable catheters and by puncture of the femoral artery in the inguinal region. Hessel et al. (1981) found this approach to be associated with the lowest complication rate.

Alternatives to this approach are catheterization via the axillary (Hanafee 1963; Roy 1965) or brachial artery (Fergusson and Kamada 1981), and translumbar aortography (Dos Santos 1929; cited by Gammill and Craighead 1975).

Translumbar aortography requires general anesthesia and is therefore contraindicated in patients with coagulation defects, hypertension, aortic grafts, and aneurysmal dilatation of the abdominal aorta.

Digital intravenous subtraction angiography (Steinberg et al. 1959) should not be used in obese patients and in patients with poor cardiac performance because these states will reduce the quality of the images, especially those of the visceral and limb arteries (own experience).

8.2.4.2
Indication

A transaxillary angiography is indicated in the following situations:

1. When the aortic arch and its branches have to be visualized and the patient has no inguinal pulse
2. In cases of tumors or inflammatory changes in one groin with a non-palpable inguinal pulse on the contralateral side
3. Postoperative changes which make it impossible to puncture the femoral artery
4. In cases of infected aortic grafts
5. A non-infected aortic graft is a relative indication, since it can be safely punctured with a 4-F catheter
6. In cases of severe kinking of the pelvic arteries
7. When anatomic conditions hinder catheterization of visceral and/or renal arteries by the transfemoral approach (Roy 1965; Fig. 8.9).

In the course of a diagnostic intervention the radiologist may decide to perform a transaxillary angioplasty in cases of:

1. A stenosis or an occlusion of the subclavian artery
2. A stenosis in the visceral and/or renal arteries with anatomic conditions that prohibit employment of the transfemoral approach
3. A stenosis in the abdominal aorta (OLBERT et al. 1983; Fig. 8.10) and/or pelvic arteries (OLBERT et al. 1985; Fig. 8.11).

8.2.4.3
Anatomy

In the axillary fossa, the course of the axillary artery may be divided into three parts. The proximal part of the vessel lies medial to the pectoralis minor muscle; the middle part is located in the fascia of the brachial plexus (in most cases the median nerve arises in this region) and the distal portion of the artery (which is the most important part from the radiologist's point of view) lies lateral to the pectoralis minor muscle, immediately below the axillary fascia, pushing itself beneath the coracobrachial muscle. The ulnar nerve lies medial to the artery, the median nerve lateral, and the radial nerve dorsal to it.

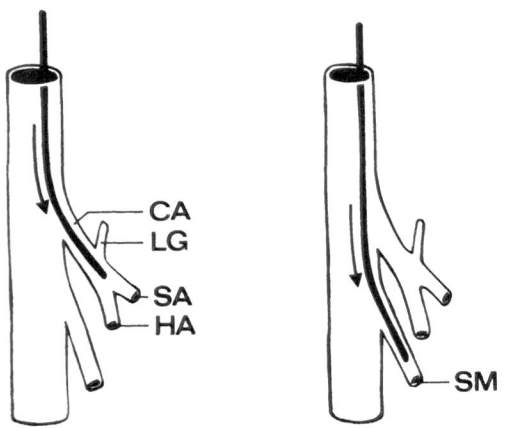

Fig. 8.9. Transaxillary catheterization becomes necessary for anatomic and/or technical reasons when the visceral or renal arteries arise at a sharp angle from the abdominal aorta. *CA*, celiac artery; *LG*, left gastric artery; *SA*, splenic artery; *HA*, hepatic artery; *SM*, superior mesenteric artery

8.2.4.4
Technique

The patient lies in supine position, the shoulder is raised with a pillow (the axillary artery is more easily palpable in this position) and the arm is extended cranially, nearly at right angles. The forearm is angulated with the head resting in the palm (OLBERT et al. 1985; Fig. 8.12).

After application of a local anesthetic, a 5-mm skin incision is made, the puncture site is tunnelled bluntly and the axillary artery is punctured using the Seldinger technique (SELDINGER 1953). A guide wire is introduced under fluoroscopic control. A catheter with a curved distal tip helps to manipulate the guide wire more easily into the ascending or descending aorta, depending on the indication (Fig. 8.13). An angiography is performed with a pigtail catheter, while a suitable dilatation catheter is employed for an angioplastic intervention. For exchanging the catheter we recommend a valve system. Five thousand units of heparin are administered intraarterially during the intervention. After withdrawal of the catheter and before placement of a compression bandage, the operator or his assistant exerts firm manual pressure (with appropriate caution) for 20–30 min on the puncture site. This is essential to prevent formation of a hematoma.

8.2.4.5
Own Experience

We performed a joint study with KASPRZAK et al. in 1982. Of 3662 angiographic studies performed in 1 year, the transaxillary approach was used in 150 examinations on 150 patients. The majority of patients had circulatory disorders in the upper and lower extremities. On retrospective review, the angiography could have been performed by the transfemoral approach in 27 patients (18%). In our own patients the indications for transaxillary angiography were as follows: Aneurysms in the abdominal aorta in eight cases, the absence of an inguinal pulse in 44 cases, after surgery in both groins in 36 cases, after surgery in one groin and an absent inguinal pulse on the contralateral side in 38 cases, in the presence of aortic grafts in 14 cases, and severe kinking of the pelvic arteries in ten cases. The patients comprised 127 men and 23 women (mean age 59 years). The right axillary artery was punctured in 50 patients and the left axillary artery in 100 patients. In some cases the distal celiac artery or pelvic arteries were dilated.

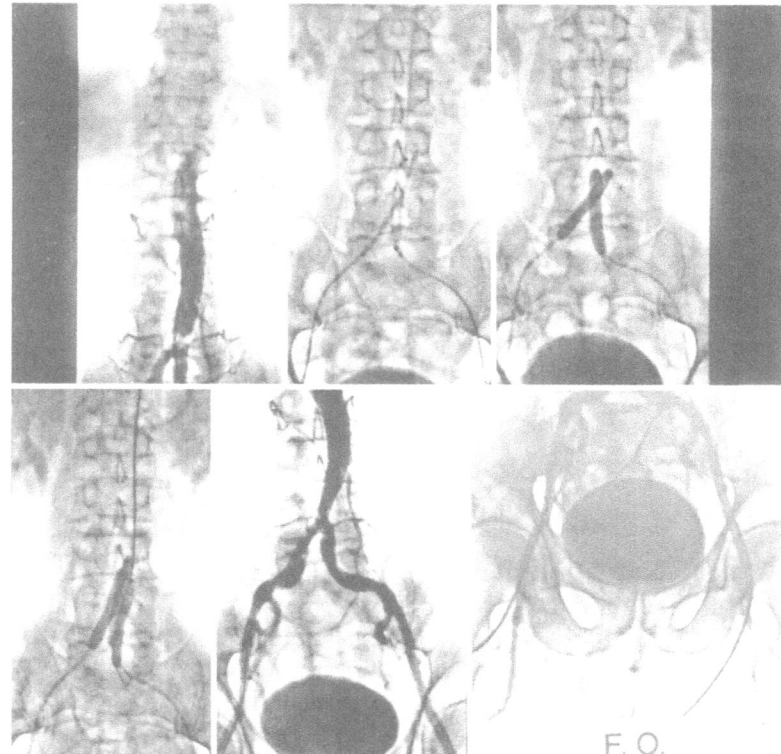

Fig. 8.10. Transaxillary angiography and the three-catheter technique in a distal stenosis of the abdominal aorta. Primary dilatation of the distal stenosis by means of transaxillary insertion of an 8-mm balloon results in moderate dilatation of the stenosis, such that the femoral artery becomes palpable in the inguinal region. An additional catheter introduced into the left and right groin removes the residual stenosis in the distal abdominal aorta

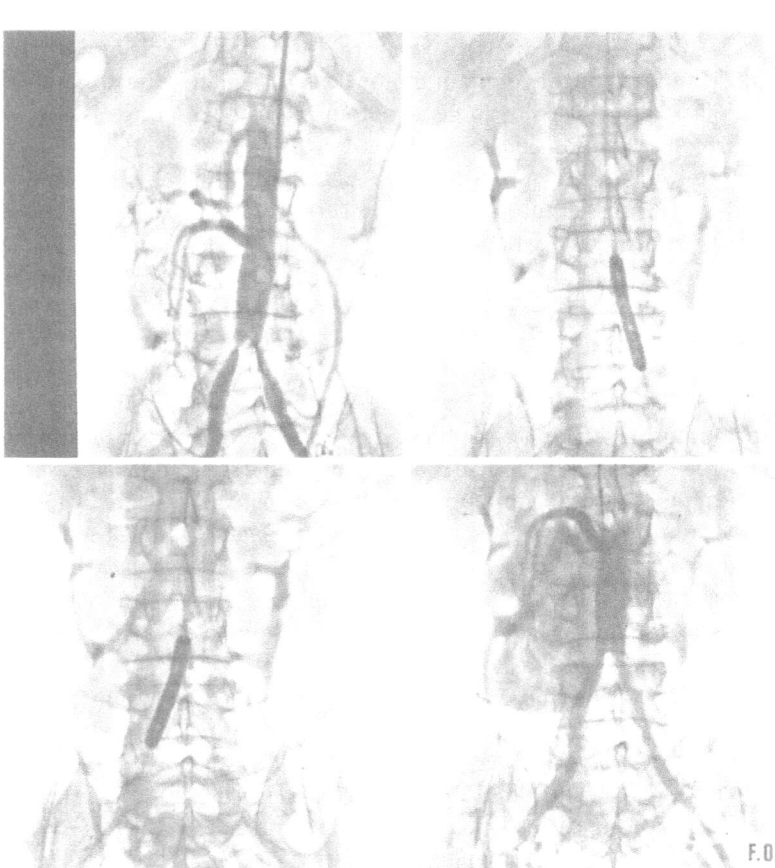

Fig. 8.11. Transaxillary catheterization for angiography and dilatation of a bilateral central stenosis of the common iliac artery

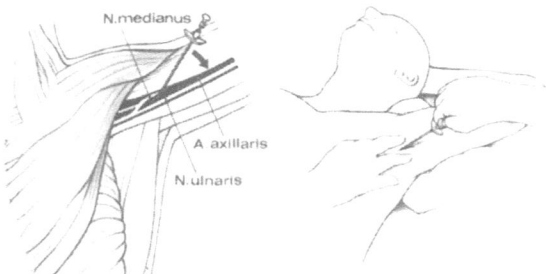

Fig. 8.12. Patient positioning and documentation of the puncture site in the distal part of the axillary artery in the immediate anterior axillary line

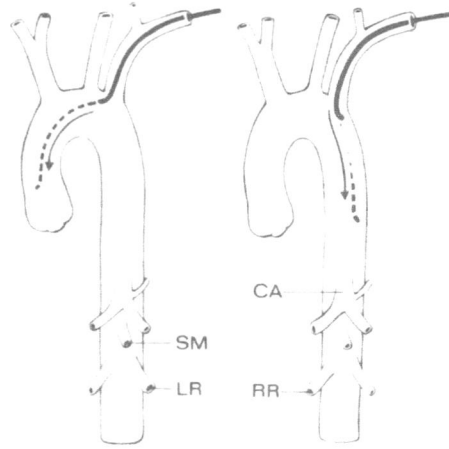

Fig. 8.13. A catheter curved at its distal tip is used to manipulate the guide wire into the ascending aorta (aortic arch angiography or selective visualization of the arteries to the brain) or the descending aorta for visualization of the abdominal aorta (selective visualization of the visceral and renal arteries) or the pelvic and limb arteries. *CA*, celiac artery; *SM*, superior mesenteric artery; *RR*, right renal artery; *LR*, renal artery

8.2.4.6
Complications (Own Patients)

Injury to the brachial plexus, large hematomas in the axillary region, acute vascular occlusions, and the formation of pseudoaneurysms were the most frequent serious complications. KASPRZAK et al. (1982) performed surgery after transaxillary angiography in 12 cases in order to remove large hematomas (two in cases of pseudoaneurysms), or sensory disturbances (three times with concomitant motor deficits) which had also been caused by large hematomas. Residual neurologic symptoms persisted for longer than 1 year in two patients. A transient weakness in the arm and a transient numbness in the fingers were observed in nearly all patients.

8.2.4.7
Literature Review

In 21 transaxillary angiographies, STAAL et al. (1966) observed injury to the brachial plexus in seven cases. Five patients were symptom-free after 1 year and only complained of weakness in the arm and sensory disturbances in the fingers; in two patients a severe injury to the plexus caused considerable residual symptoms. The subsequent operation revealed that the plexus damage had been caused by inflammatory changes and adhesions in the plexus region with the artery in one case, and by a pseudoaneurysm in the axillary artery in the other. A transient weakness in the arm and fingers and transient paresthesias were also observed and were attributed to the abnormal position of the arm during the examination.

In 200 angiographies, HANAFEE (1963) observed a temporary hemiparesis, the formation of a large hematoma in the axillary region, and an occlusion

of the subclavian artery in one case each. A transient plexus lesion with pain radiating into the third, fourth, and fifth fingers was also observed only in one case.

ROY (1965) performed 475 axillary angiographies. Apart from several small hematomas, the author encountered seven large local hematomas requiring surgery, and an occlusion of the axillary artery in eight cases, necessitating thrombectomy in three. Nearly all patients complained of weakness in the arm and numbness in the fingers. The symptoms persisted for up to 1 year in four patients (0.8%).

In a literature review O'KEEFE (1980) observed that plexus injury had involved the median nerve in 93% of cases, the ulnar nerve in 53%, and the radial nerve in 40%. According to surgery the plexus injury had been caused by a hematoma in the neurovascular sheath in 73%, and a pseudoaneurysm in 27% (SMITH et al. 1989). According to the report of O'KEEFE (1980) prompt surgery prevents a persistent nerve lesion, especially in the presence of motor dysfunction.

MCIVOR and RHYMER (1992) assess the risk of plexus injury as being less than 1%. In 245 transaxillary arteriograms, a thrombosis of the axillary artery requiring surgery was observed in two cases, while two patients suffered a cardiac arrest, which was successfully managed in both cases. A transient ischemic attack and plexus injury were encountered in one case each.

8.2.4.8
Discussion

Based on own experience and a review of the literature, it may be concluded that the lumen of the
catheter is closely related to the development of hematomas, pseudoaneurysms, and arterial occlusions
and is therefore indirectly related to severe plexus
injury. This explains the relatively high complication
rate reported by KASPRZAK et al. (1982). We used
7-F catheters for diagnostic angiography and 7.5-F
catheters for angioplasty (Olbert catheter system,
cited by OLBERT et al. 1985). Caution is advised in
patients with hypertension and deficient clotting, as
well as in patients who are undergoing anticoagulant
therapy.

8.2.4.9
Conclusion

Current levels of experience and research indicate
that the transaxillary approach using a catheter with
a narrow lumen may be recommended as an alternative to the transfemoral access. However, the transbrachial approach (Figs. 8.14–8.16) is preferred in
the majority of centers, including the Department
of Angiography and Interventional Radiology at
the Department of Radiodiagnostics, University of
Vienna. Nevertheless, the axillary artery with its
large lumen may well be given preference over the
brachial artery in the future for both diagnostic as
well as angioplastic interventions.

Acknowledgements. I thank Ms. Sujata Wagner for transla-
tion and preparation of the manuscript.

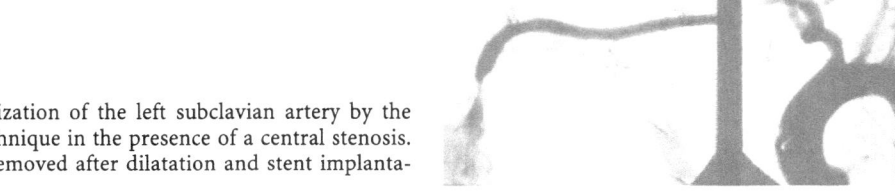

Fig. 8.14. Visualization of the left subclavian artery by the
transbrachial technique in the presence of a central stenosis.
The stenosis is removed after dilatation and stent implantation

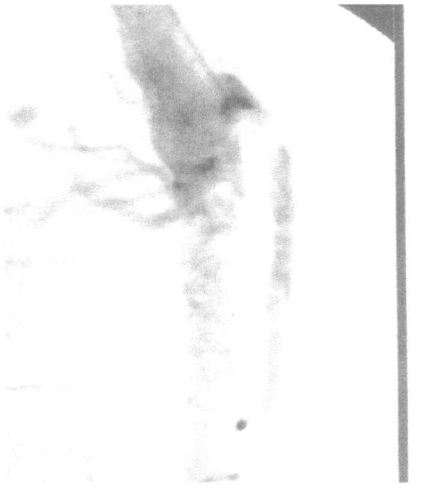

Fig. 8.15. Transbrachial angiography
and dilatation of a central stenosis in
the superior mesenteric artery

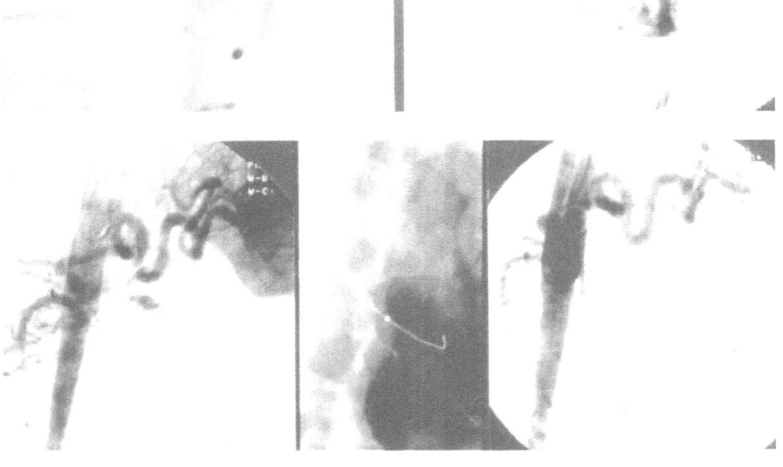

Fig. 8.16. Transbrachial angiography
and dilatation of a severe stenosis in the
left renal artery

References

Fergusson DJ, Kamada RD (1981) Percutaneous entry of the brachial artery for left heart catheterisation using a sheath. Catheterization Cardiovasc Diagn 7:111–114

Gammill S, Craighead C (1975) Translumbar aortography updated. Surg Gynaecol Obstet 140:59–64

Hanafee W (1963) Axillary artery approach to carotid, vertebral, abdominal aorta and coronary angiography. Radiology 81:559–567

Hessel SJ, Adams DF, Abrams HL (1981) Complications of angiography. Radiology 138:273–281

Kasprzak P, Olbert F, Muzika N (1982) Vergleichsstudie: Transaxilläre versus translumbale Aortographie. In: Denck H, Hagmüller GW, Brunner U (eds) Arterielle Durchblutungsstörungen der unteren Extremitäten "Grenzzonen der Therapieentscheidung". TM, Bad Oeynhausen, pp 1–34

McIvor J, Rhymer JC (1992) 245 transaxillary arteriograms in arteriopathic patients: success rate and complications. Clin Radiol 45:390–394

O'Keefe DM (1980) Brachial plexus injury following axillary arteriography: case report and review of the literature. J Neurosurg 53:853–857

Olbert F, Kasprzak P, Mendel H, Schlegl A, Denck H (1983) Perkutaner transluminaler angioplastischer Eingriff. Med Welt 34:180–183

Olbert F, Muzika N, Schlegl A (1985) Transluminale Dilatation und Rekanalisation im Gefäßbereich. In: Olbert F, Muzika N, Schlegl A (eds) Transluminale Dilatation und Rekanalisation der distalen Abdominalaorta (Transaxilläre Technik). Wacholz, Nürnberg, pp 51–53

Roy P (1965) Percutaneous catheterization via the axillary artery. A new approach to some technical roadblocks in selective arteriography. AJR Am J Roentgenol 94:1–18

Seldinger SI (1953) Catheter replacement of needle in percutaneous arteriography. Acta Radiol (Stockh) 39:368–376

Smith DC, Mitchell DA, Peterson GW, Will AD, Mera SS, Smith LL (1989) Medial brachial fascial compartment syndrome. Anatomic basis of neuropathy after transaxillary arteriography. Radiology 173:149–154

Staal A, van Voorthuisen AE, van Dijk LM (1966) Neurological complications following arterial catheterisation by the axillary approach. Br J Radiol 39:115–116

Steinberg I, Finby N, Evans JA (1959) Safe and practical intravenous method for abdominal aortography, peripheral arteriography and cerebral angiography. Am J Roentgenol 82:758–772

8.3
Angiography Materials

Diagnostic and therapeutic interventions require highly sophisticated instrumentation. This applies to both the techniques of needle angiography for the delivery of contrast medium, and the application of diagnostic and therapeutic adjunct devices, such as guidewires and diagnostic or therapeutic catheters, tubes, connectors, and adapters.

There is a wide range of industrial products of varying design to meet special needs within the framework of diagnostic or therapeutic interventions.

The differing designs are adapted to the specific field of application of the devices. For diagnostic examinations using selective or superselective catheterization, in particular, soft-tip catheters with a rigid shaft are required, with optimum rotational stability and maximum pushability. With its excellent technical memory, the catheter is best with a small outer diameter but large lumen. Due to a proximal Y-connector, the injection of contrast medium is possible with the guidewire in place.

Catheters for therapeutic interventions need to fulfil different objectives: for example, percutaneous thromboembolectomy, balloon dilatation, atherectomy, or the application of stents from covered or uncovered fabric. Aspects of crucial importance include high biocompatibility – for disposable instruments – and a guarantee of reestablishing total asepsis for those products which can be re-used, as well as catheter surfaces that do not favor thrombus formation. To achieve a perfectly smooth gliding of guidewires and catheters, a hydrophilic coating has proven advantageous. Both diagnostic and therapeutic catheter systems require good radiopacity, guaranteed by enhanced radiopaque tips or metal markers at the decisive sites.

8.3.1
Needles

Among the diverse types of puncture needles (Fig. 8.17) used as a basis for needle angiographies or catheter insertion, three techniques can be chosen from:

- The *Buchtala* or *Cournand needle* (puncture with open lumen). The Cournand extension is preferred in children for arteries and veins
- The *Seldinger needle* has a blunt outer cannula and a diamond-point obturator (double and triple cannula)
- The *Hettler triple cannula*, to start the insertion of closed-end catheters without guidewire
- The *Amplatz needle* has a bevelled cannula, obturator, and an outer Teflon sheath. The flange of the needle is either open-ended or with a Cournand extension.

Figure 8.17a,b shows four types of puncture needle and the modifications of the needle tips, respectively. The tip has either a sharp diamond point or is diagonally sharpened. One can use such diagonally sharpened puncture needles which persist after withdrawal of the stylet, but which need to be turned by 180° before advancing them in to the vessel after

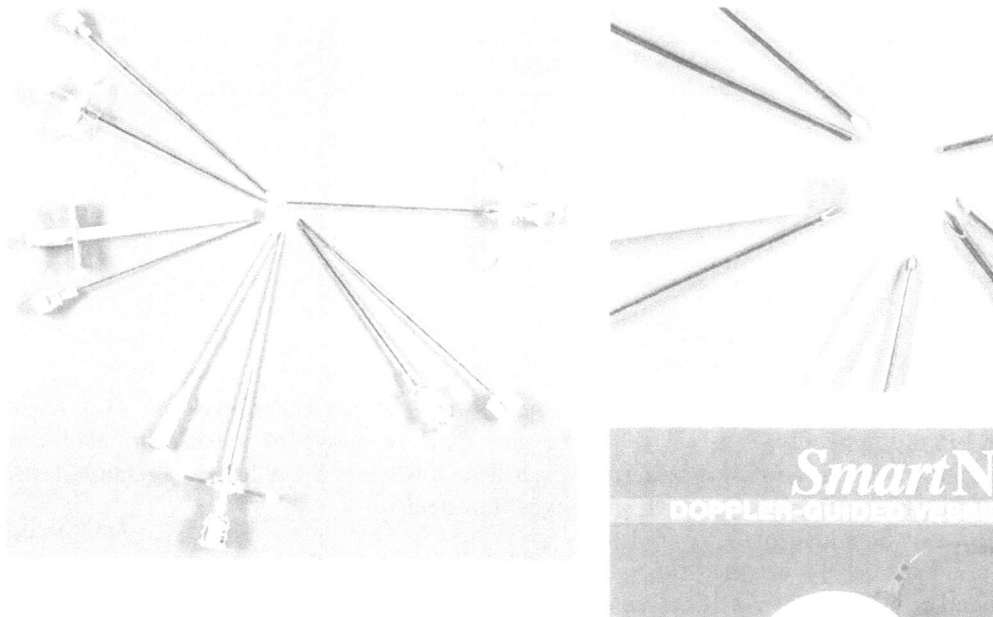

Fig. 8.17 a–c. Puncture needles. (a) general view, (b) needle tips, (c) Doppler-guided "Smart needle"

puncture. Others have a blunt cannula end after removal of the puncture stylet and thus an injury to the vascular wall when advancing it forward can be avoided.

Irrespective of the above, the guiding characteristics of the puncture needles vary according to their design and depending on whether they are used with or without a proximal wing. For arterial punctures, I myself prefer winged cannulas of the Seldinger type, whereas for venous punctures I prefer the Buchtala or Cournand needle without wing. This also helps avoid any confusion during special interventions. Moreover, the manufacturers offer a variety of modifications (Tables 8.1, 8.2).

The use of a puncture needle for translumbar aortography or catheterization is a rare exception today; nevertheless, its employment can become necessary.

Puncture needles are available in re-useable form, in a combination of metal and plastic, or as a disposable product with plastic as the outer material. The markings "standard" or "thin-walled" are important with regard to the inner lumen, allowing guidewires of different diameters to enter. Needles of 18 gauge ("standard") accept guidewires with a diameter of 0.035 in. (= 0.89 mm), this is the "35≤ guidewire". Puncture needles of 21 gauge ("thin-walled") take up guidewires of 0.018 in. diameter; this is type 18≤ For

Table 8.1. Puncture needles for vessel access

Needles
Seldinger
Cournand
Potts
Wilkov-Potts
Amplatz
Cope-Micropuncture Set
Translumbar Teflon-needle set

Table 8.2. Catheter introducer sheaths see Appendix

Sheaths
Hettler-triple-cannula
Desilets-Hofmann
Chek-flo-sets
Peel-away-sets
Balkin-up and over-set

converting French into gauge and inches into millimeters, see Table 1 in the Appendix.

Most commonly used for guiding purposes are puncture needles with a proximal wing which, in disposable systems, can be added or left out. The most important puncture needles are the Seldinger needle, the Cournand needle, and the Pott-Cournand needle with a hollow stylet design and open side-port for single-wall puncture. Initial flash-back through the side-port is visualized while maintaining the thumb position on the stylet. Modified Seldinger needles exist in two- or three-part versions with a blunt cannula, the inner pointed needle, and a needle stylet to occlude the hole of the inner pointed needle. The inner pointed needle, together with the needle stylet, can be exchanged for an operator to prevent bleeding.

The micropuncture introducer set (Cope) uses 21-gauge needles for introducing 0.035-in.-diameter guidewires. In this case, a 0.018-in. guidewire is first used to introduce a 4.0- or 5.0-F short catheter. Through this catheter, exchange for a stiffer guidewire (0.035 in. or 0.038 in.) is possible for all types of diagnostic selective procedures or interventions.

Localizing the artery or vein prior to puncture using the Doppler technique, and marking the most suitable point prior to actual puncture is a valuable aid. In particularly complex cases, e.g., obesity of the patient or puncture in an area with scaring, the Doppler-guided "Smart needle" (Fig. 8.17c) is recommended. Doppler guidance can be of some advantage as it helps reduce the number of attempts at access, and the incidence of bleeding in patients with multiple previous accesses or with scar formation. In most patients, however, this more expensive device is not required if the experienced interventionalist uses micro-puncture needles from the outset.

For differentiated atraumatic punctures, narrow-diameter cannulas are required. In order to enable a larger guidewire to follow a small puncture, there are combination sets, such as, for example, the Cope

system, which allows the conversion of a needle smaller than 16 gauge to a 0.035-in. guidewire, regardless of whether the guidewire is stainless steel or nitinol steel.

8.3.2
Guidewires

On the basis of relatively rigid guidewires that were originally used by the company KIFA, Sweden, for the Seldinger and Oedman catheters, or the Ulrich guidewires in combination with the HETTLER triple cannula, there are manifold high-quality guidewires on the market today (ABRAMS 1983; ZEITLER 1975).

The guidewire design enables the exchange of the puncture needle for catheters for percutaneous access. While in earlier years, guidewires were made only from stainless steel alloy, I myself have been preferring the safety Teflon-coated J-guidewire from Cook Company (Safe-T-J) since 1967. Meanwhile, several other companies are producing similar guidewires, and Cook have also brought newer modifications onto the market, such as the double-flexible tipped guidewire, and the movable-core guidewire in different variations (Tables 8.3 and 8.4). Guidewires are fragile instruments and the Teflon coating not only reduces the friction occurring in the catheter, but also the thrombogenicity of the guidewire itself. Nonetheless, all procedures exceeding 20 min require a heparin injection to prevent thrombus formation in and outside the catheter and on the surface of the guidewire. Under normal conditions, guidewires are safe instruments intended for single use. Re-use is not recommended due to the difficulties in re-establishing total asepsis (BECK 1993). Controls under microscope, electron microscope, and using X-rays have shown the damaged surface of used guidewires, with notches and uneven surfaces. Teflon-coated guidewires showed less

Table 8.3. Guidewires

Guidewire	Characteristics
Straight, heavy-duty fixed-core guidewire THSF-35-145	Teflon-coated, with 3 cm flexible tip
	Long flexible tip
Straight, fixed-core guidewires TSLF	Large diameter core with 20 cm flexible tip
	Diameter 18–38 in., length 80–145 in.
	20-cm Flexible tip
SAFE-T-J curved, fixed-core guidewires SCF, stainless steel uncoated	Tip-curve radius 3 mm
TSCF, Teflon-coated	Diameter 18–38 in., length 50, 180, 260 in.
Amplatz movable-core guidewires curved TCMTNA	Diameter 25–38 in., length 145 in.
	Tip-curve radius 3, 1.5 mm
Amplatz extra stiff THSCF	Diameter 25–38 in., length 145–300 in.
	(Boston Scientific 46–525, "J": 46–501)
Movable-core, curved Safe-T-J-guidewires TSCM	Diameter 25–28 in., length 80–145 in.
	Tip-curve radius 3, 1.5 mm
Steerable guidewires (modifications are Rosen, Moses, Allison)	
Magic Torque (0.035 in.)	Steerable guidewire with Hydromer coating and four platinum markers at 1-cm distance each
	(Boston Scientific: 46–591)
Platinum Plus (0.018 in.)	For small vessels and 3-F catheters
	(Boston Scientific: 46–604)
Roadrunner PC guidewire RLPC-35-180-7	Hydrophilic coating, distal platinum tip
Roadrunner extra-support guidewires RSTF	Diameter 14–18, length 180–300
	6-cm Flexible platinum spring coil
Terumo guidewire GT with gold coil RG-GA 1618 FM	The nickel-titanium alloy core provides excellent kink resistance and superior maneuverability
	– Radifocus guide wire –
Terumo guidewire M, stiff type RF-PA 35 183 M (several sizes available)	Hydrophilic polymer-coated surface makes the guidewire extremely smooth in contact with saline solution

deformities, when used exclusively through dilating catheters or sheaths.

The peeling-off of surface material was more obvious in guidewires than in catheter material. Damage to the surface in the form of peeling-off of coating material and breaking-up were also found in Terumo wires. Despite repeated sterilization using ethylene oxide, mechanical damage and contamination of the surface were still present. Therefore, the re-use of guidewires is not recommended in the interests of preventing mechanical damage to the vessel, thrombus formation, and transmission of infections. The more complex the instrumentation – as, for example, atherectomy devices or angioscopy catheters – the more care required when these are being re-used.

Guidewires that have either a fixed core or a tapered movable core (Fig. 8.18a–c) at the tip are suited for various purposes in the diagnostic catheterization of vessels in the framework of angiographies of the arteries, veins, and heart chambers. The safety-J guidewire in diameters of 3 or 6 mm excels with its atraumatic properties, protecting the intima, especially in the passage of thrombotic plaque in obliterated arteries or aneurysms, but also in the passage of the heart valves. Moreover, the use of Teflon-coated safety-J guidewires has proven advantageous in situations of a broken metal cannula, by stabilizing the same and preventing the broken particle from causing embolization. Another achievement is the reduction of thrombus formation at the surface of guidewires through the introduction of heparin-coated guidewires. The variety of guidewires on the market can be characterized in short as follows:

Exchangeable Guidewires. These have a straight or J-shaped tip, with a curvature radius of 3 mm. I myself prefer a diameter of 0.028 in. or 0.035 in., and a flexible tip of over 10 cm in length (these wires are available with flexible tips of 1–10 cm in length).

Table 8.4. Hand injectors

Boston-Scientific: S 15-102
SCIMED-Encore Inflation Device: 03205-01 with manometer
Le Veen Inflator: 15-101
Schneider International:
Breeze Inflation Device 98710001
Aria Inflation Device off-line 91600005

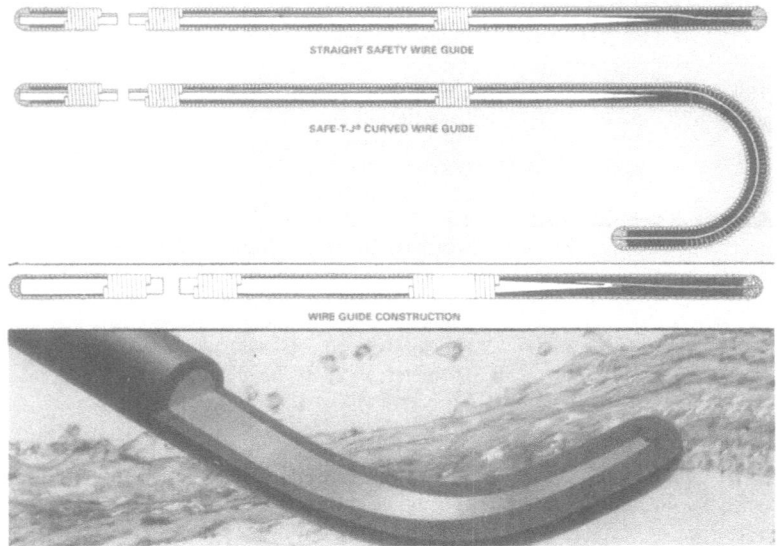

STRAIGHT SAFETY WIRE GUIDE

SAFE-T-J® CURVED WIRE GUIDE

WIRE GUIDE CONSTRUCTION

Fig. 8.18. Different guidewires with movable core. From *top* to *bottom*: Straight Safe-T guidewire, (TSM, 0.032" (0.81 mm), length, 100 cm); Safe-T-J-curved guidewire, "Rosen-wire", THSCF, 0.032 in. (0.81 mm), length 145 cm, tip curve, 1.5 mm; extra-stiff guidewire "Amplatz extra stiff", THSCF, 0.032 in, length, 180 cm (260 cm), tip curve, 3 mm; Terumo-Radifocus guidewire, "glidewire", RF × PS 35 15 3M. Diameter, 0.035 in, (0.89 mm), length, 150 mm, 3-cm flexible tip, RF × RB 16 18 8 M. Diameter, 0.016 in, (0.26 mm), length, 180 cm, 8-cm flexible tip, 70° angulated

The most common length of the wire is 180 cm, for the region of the pelvis and the legs. In the case of transfemoral catheterization of the upper extremities, or transbrachial approaches to the lower extremities, guidewires of 260 cm in length are necessary. For superselective catheterization in the region of the distal extremities, guidewires of 0.018 in. are preferred. The extension of guidewires using suture material and a knot is, in my opinion, only necessary when an inappropriate or excessively short guidewire has been chosen.

Steerable Guidewires. Guidewires of varying diameter and length, with a variety of tip configurations, can be chosen. A highly stable type is the Amplatz "extra-stiff" guidewire, which provides reliable stiffness to the catheter systems, guiding catheters, and therapeutic catheters, particularly for maneuvers crossing bifurcations and strongly bended curves. In the case of markedly elongated arteries, especially in the region of the iliac arteries, the use of movable-core guidewires is highly recommended, as these enable a safe "caterpillaring" through elongated, kinked arteries with additional atheromatous plaque. The introduction of the so-called glide wire, made from hydrophilic material, has greatly improved the safe sounding of even elongated and kinked arteries.

The Terumo guidewire, Radiofocus (Fig. 8.18), made of superelastic alloy core, eliminates kinking and coil separation, and features very smooth and remarkably high compatibility due to its polyurethane outer layer, in addition to superb torque control. Thanks to its hydrophilic polymer-coated surface, the guidewire becomes extremely smooth on contact with saline solution, enabling a frictionless insertion and access to remote and difficult areas. It is important to have both types of guidewire available, the safety-J guidewires of stainless steel, and Terumo's plastic-type guidewire, in different lengths. A specific tip preparation is very helpful for precise selective guiding through markedly angulated vessels.

Even the management of atherosclerotic changes within stenoses and occlusions has been lastingly improved and facilitated by the Terumo glide wire and similar products (Navyguide, among others) on the market. The rate of successfully recanalized, chronically occluded arteries could thus be considerably increased. Nevertheless, the disadvantage of occasional subintimal passage of the Terumo "Radiofocus glide wire" requires careful, fluoroscopy-guided control by the examiner.

When standard-length guidewires are used, the possibility of connecting or enlarging these should be considered. If this aspect is neglected, it might become necessary to exchange an optimally placed guidewire for a longer one, and the obstruction that may have initially been easily overcome, then becomes a serious problem.

Depending on the therapeutic concept, or if a special therapeutic field is concentrated upon, limiting to only a few guidewire types may be useful. Cerebral angiographies, transfemoral angiographies of the arm, or coronary angiographies, for example, require longer models that are frequently equipped with special "flexible gold coils". But also in the field of peripheral non-neuroangiographies, guidewires with steerable or soft gold tips may become necessary, not least to ensure radiopacity even in complex situations, or in obese patients.

8.3.3
Sheaths and Application Systems

The first combined catheter-introducer system was originated by HETTLER (1960), with the triple-way cannula. It consisted of a 16-gauge needle stylet which punched a small hole into the arterial wall. The sheath was an adapted 18-gauge blunt cannula accepting an 38≤guidewire. As soon as the guidewire had been safely placed in the vessel, the blunt cannula, surrounded by a stiffer metal cannula plus plastic sheath, was advanced into the vessel. This plastic sheath was equipped with a metallic closure mechanism, whereby the metal cannula or an inserted catheter kept the closure system open and, upon withdrawal of the latter, it was closed by a spring. After retraction of the inner cannula and stylet, either open-ended or closed catheters, with or without spiral, could be inserted, as the situation required. This system was applied almost exclusively for retrograde punctures of the femoral artery in the groin, of the brachial artery in the antecubital fossa, for puncture of arteries and veins, and for catheterizations in the framework of layer aortographies at varying levels, as well as for selective arterial angiographies, cranial and caudal cavographies, and for catheterizations of the right and left heart.

Further developments were the techniques according to DESILETS and HOFMANN (1965), the catheter sheaths by Cordis, Terumo, and other companies (Fig. 8.19). As increasingly specific instrumentation was employed in interventional radi-

ology, these introducer systems were equipped with a side-port for lavage with stop-cock and removable proximal diaphragm stopper. This was essential, for example, in aspiration thrombectomies, as it allowed the removal of the proximal link system with closure diaphragm, to clean the vessel from embolic or thrombotic material. Today, I prefer the Cordis or Terumo sheath, while I have limited the application of the Hettler instrumentation to extremely obese patients since the puncture set is longer. Analogous new introducer sets with hemostasis valves prevent blood reflux and air aspiration more reliably than the former Hettler cannula.

For contralateral access (see Fig. 8.3) to the iliac arteries for diagnostic and mainly interventional procedures, after initial guidewire positioning, the "Balkin-up-and-over" contralateral introducer system is very helpful in angioplasties or embolizations. I myself prefer to use this contralateral introducer system for interventions in French sizes 6 or 7, and a sheath length of 40 cm with a radiopaque bend close to the tip.

The maneuvers in diagnostic vascular interventions and therapeutic measures at the puncture will normally be facilitated by the use of vascular sheaths in different lengths , diameters, and proximal-valve design (Fig. 8.19). The use of these sheaths helps reduce traumatization of the arterial wall at the puncture site. Secondary tears occurring on exchange of catheters are avoided. The exchange of catheters or other instrumentation is less painful to the patient, and the removal of clots or atheromatous material only thus becomes possible. Postmortem studies after, or without, use of a sheath have demonstrated its higher reliability in reducing traumatization to the vascular wall (SÖLDNER et al. 1995). The smaller the trauma can be kept, the smaller the risk of local thrombus formation during the diagnostic or therapeutic intervention. Nevertheless, thrombus formation between the vascular wall and the sheath may occur during the intervention because of local stasis. The prophylactic administration of heparin as

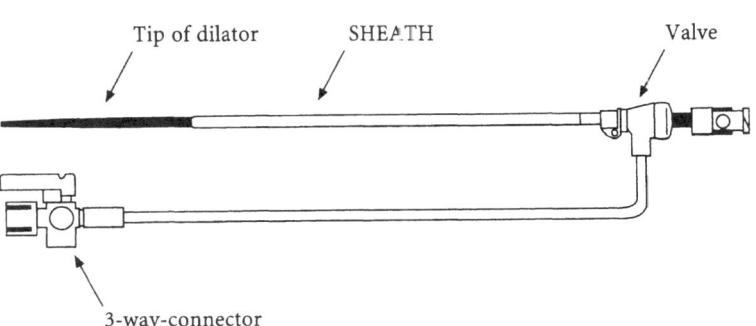

Fig. 8.19. Vascular introducer sheath

an anticoagulant has also proven beneficial in interventions using a sheath to prevent thrombi between the vascular wall and the sheath, and also at the surface of the catheter or guidewire. Without the administration of heparin, thrombi occurring on withdrawal or exchange of the catheter is one of the causes of embolism (ZEITLER 1970a,b).

The catheter-introducer sheaths have reduced local complications at the puncture site. The exchange of catheters, balloon catheters, and other instrumentation, as often as required in the individual case, for example in stent application, is possible without any tearing, involution, or indistinct puncture edges of the arterial or venous wall when using sheaths.

To document the protection of the vessel using an introducer sheath, we compared in situ specimens of the inguinal vessel after balloon catheter exchange through an introducer sheath. Histological tests showed severe intimal damage and medial tears only when no introducer sheath had been used (SÖLDNER et al. 1995). It was evident that using a sheath during angioplasty after catheter exchange in the groin arteries reduces the risk of intimal damage and local complication in the groin. Fig. 8.20a,b demonstrates the smooth puncture track achieved with a sheath, in contrast to intimal and medial tears due to an exchange of balloon catheters without sheath.

8.3.4
Catheters

Diagnostic and therapeutic catheters are produced from a variety of materials (see Table 8.5). There are catheters that are radiopaque as a whole, and others that are only radiopaque at the tip or specific parts.

Table 8.5. Catheter materials[a]

Teflon
Polyethylene
Polyvinylchoride
Polyurethane
Nylon
Polyolefin
Silicon

[a] Dilators used before catheter introduction (available in sizes 3–14 F).

As radiopaque catheters require a certain minimum wall thickness, catheters of narrow calibers of 3–5 F are being offered to an increasing extent. Theses are mainly equipped with radiopaque catheter tips, or specific metal markers to guarantee better detection under roentgen fluoroscopy. The most commonly used catheter-tip designs for selective angiography in all peripheral non-coronary vessels with specially prepared radiopacity for single use are shown in Fig. 8.21a,b.

The most common catheters used in the diagnosis of peripheral vascular disease are the pigtail catheter and the Cobra catheter, with varying bending abilities at their tip. The pigtail catheter is mainly used to deliver contrast medium into the aorta, either for abdominal aortographies or aortoarteriographies in the lower extremities, thoracic aortographies, including documentation of the supraaortic and carotid arteries, and as a starting point for visualizing the arm arteries. The pigtail catheter is also very safe and suitable for use in intravenous DSA of the aortic arch vessels, and of abdominal aorta, renal, and ilio-femoral arteries, placed into the superior vena cava or into the right atrium. For catheter angiographies of the arm arteries in transfemoral catheterization techniques, however, headhunter or

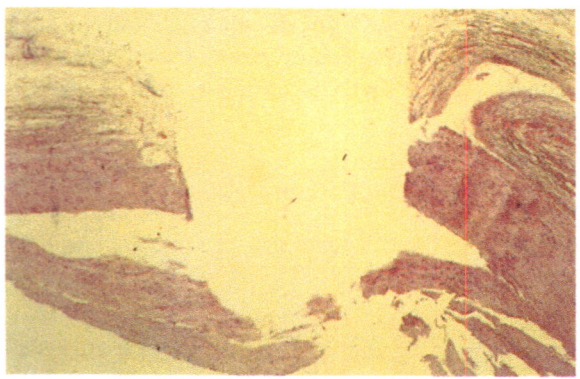
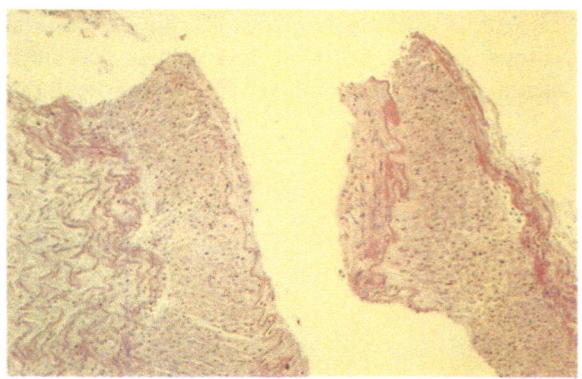

Fig. 8.20 a,b. Histologic specimen obtained from the puncture site in the femoral artery. **a** Arterial wall with intimal disruption after puncture and catheter exchange without a sheath. **b** Arterial wall with smooth puncture defect after catheter exchange with a sheath

Fig. 8.21 a,b. Angiography catheters with specially prepared tip configurations. **a** (*1*) Straight, (*2*) Pigtail, (*3*) multipurpose, (*4*) Cobra (C1, C2, C3). **b** (*5*) Shepherd-hook, (*6*) Headhunter (Simmons 1, 2, 3), (*7*) cerebral (Valavanis), first defined by OEDMAN (1959)

sidewinder catheters are employed; these are placed through the brachiocephalic artery on the right, and the subclavian artery on the left, distal to the branching point of the vertebral artery, respectively. For contralateral catheterizations in the region of the pelvic arteries, either the pigtail, sidewinder, or shepherd-hook catheter can be used. The special requirements of all diagnostic catheters are to ensure good flow despite their narrow outer diameter. The catheter has to be kink-resistant and should have a "low friction coefficient". The link for connection with the injector or syringe should be made or metal of plastic, with a Luer-Lok system. The pigtail catheter has between eight and ten side-ports in a spiraled arrangement proximal to the opening at its end, in front of the circle. In experiments, KOLLATH and SPITZ (1968) demonstrated the importance of varying side-ports at angiography. For specific purposes, a "Luer-Lok-to-Record" adapter should be kept available.

Characteristics important to the assessment of the various catheters are their trackability and pushability. When choosing the appropriate catheter for an examination or intervention, some parameters of comparison (trackability and pushability) (Fig. 8.22) may be helpful, in addition to the criteria which include catheter-tip configuration, radiopacity, composition of the surface, and a safe proximal connector. In European and international committees, clear definitions corresponding to the "DIN-Norm" (German Industrial Standards), or European and US industrial standards, are necessary.

Another catheter of particular importance in the planning of therapeutic interventions is the measuring catheter, which has clearly visible markings at defined distances (Fig. 8.23), and thereby helps in the selection of the appropriate instrumentation by exactly demonstrating vascular distances, lumina, balloon diameters, length of the required stent, and other essential criteria. The use of such a measuring catheter guarantees higher precision in the determination of longitudinal measurements than the quantitative determination of length afforded by X-ray alone. As the catheter lies in the same level of the body, the respective magnification factor is exactly defined. Situations in which measuring catheters are indispensable include the selection of endoprostheses for the therapy of av-fistulas, or aneurysms. Additional measurements using computed tomography (CT) are often very helpful.

Choosing the best suited catheter for cardiovascular and interventional radiology is as important as the surgeon's selection of the appropriate instrumentation for an operation. While initially catheters were available as individual polyethylene parts, with which the physician had to prepare the catheter himself, nowadays, pre-shaped, disposable catheters, of different materials (Table 8.6), with varying characteristics, and for most purposes, are now available. The most important criteria for diagnostic selective catheterization include: maximal flow rate, and good "memory" in shape holding. For interventions involving recanalization, however, stiffness, in combination with a soft tip, are equally as important

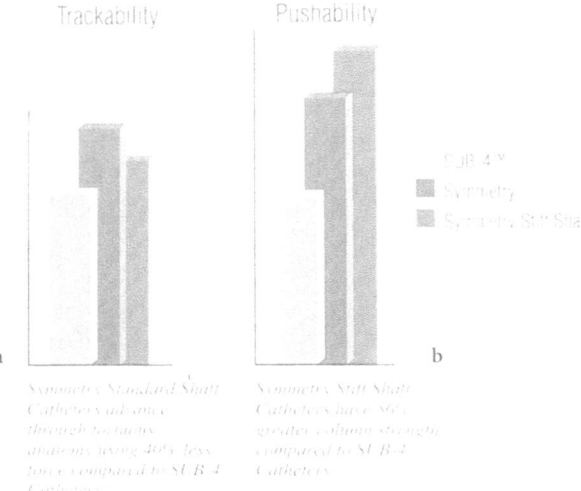

Fig. 8.22 a,b. Catheter characteristics. a Trackability, b pushability

8.3.5
Special Devices

For connection maneuvers using connecting tubes and syringes, well-fitting adapters made from metal or plastic are necessary. I myself prefer the Luer-Lok adapters. For diagnostic purposes involving hand injection, a one-way stopcock can be used, but for most diagnostic and interventional procedures, three-way stopcocks of metal or plastic have the advantage of avoiding air-injection. In addition, they enable the alternative injection of contrast agents through one port, and of saline solution through another port. In the case of pump-assisted injection, which achieves high flow rates, high-pressure stopcocks are required. In this case, as well as for changing to selective catheterization, female-to-male Luer-Loks with rotating adapters are the standard ones that I have been using. For special procedures necessitating one connection for continuous saline infusion, a second for contrast agent contact for refilling, and a third for drugs (thrombolytic or chemotherapeutic agents), a stopcock with rotating adapters and three side connections is useful to shorten the procedure. In addition, for several purposes, in particular simultaneous injection into two arteries or veins, Y-shaped connectors with two male connections are important. In the case of self-prepared catheters, different types of adapters to connect the catheter material are necessary. Special

criteria. For quick and successful selective or superselective guiding of different arteries, for diagnosis and for treatment, it is important to choose the appropriate catheter from the variety of types (Fig. 8.21a,b), including the appropriate tip configuration. For the diagnosis of peripheral vascular diseases, it is of key importance to use a catheter with the appropriate tip configuration and several side holes (Tables 8.6, 8.7).

Table 8.6. Catheter-tip configurations for "overview angiographies"

Pigtail catheter
High flow-rates
35-in. Diameter, 90-in. length
PW 10S plastic, Luer-Lok,
Pigtail tip configuration
High-strength construction
Ultra-high-flow material
Soft, kink-resistant tip
Low friction coefficient
Metal Luer-Lok or plastic-wing Luer-Lok
Ten side-ports in spiraled order

Table 8.7. Catheter-tip configurations for "overview" and semiselective angiography

Multipurpose
With tip configurations
MPA: Tip = 45° angulated
MPB: Tip = 90° angulated
Torcon NB HNB 5 (6, 7) 35, 50–100
Polyethylene P 5 (6, 7) 25–38
DSA-Royal-Flush plus catheter set
DSA-500 HLP, B S DN
Shepherd-Hook HNB 6,0 SHK 1.0

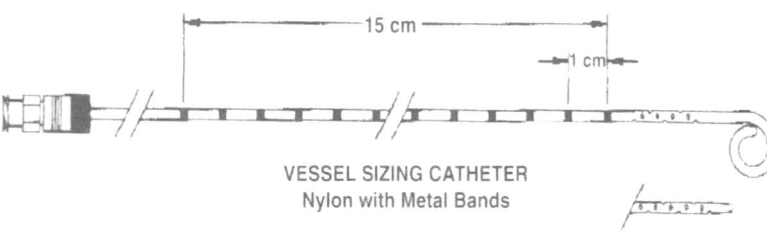

VESSEL SIZING CATHETER
Nylon with Metal Bands

Fig. 8.23. Catheter with radiopaque markers for vessel-sizing, used to determine accurate sizing of vessel and/or aneurysm lumen prior to aortic stent/graft placement. Sixteen radiopaque markers at the distal portion of the catheter are spaced 1.0 cm apart. Supplied sterile in peel-open packages, these are intended for one-time use

connecting tubes can be ordered in different lengths. In the interests of optimum radiation protection, tubes of 60–100 cm in length are recommended. This length provides the best possibility for manipulations, radiation protection, and maintenance of the aseptic condition.

Of the various catheter materials used, nylon is the most rigid; this, however, prevents a conical tapering at the end of the catheter. Therefore, the use of an introducer sheath is mandatory. Teflon catheters hold their shape extremely well, even at 37°C, in contrast to polyethylene catheters, which may lose their preshaped tip configuration when remaining in position for a longer time. For selective catheterization of the supraaortic, coronary, and visceral vessels, the use of catheters with integrated steel netting is recommended, thus affording the catheters greater stability in guiding and rotating maneuvers.

To achieve radiopacity, the catheter material can contain lead, bismuth, or barium sulphate. Another possibility is to provide the tip of the catheter, or other important markers such as, for example, the proximal and distal ends of a balloon, with gold markers which are easily visible under fluoroscopy. This helps improve maneuverability and reduce fluoroscopy times. Several indications exist whereby precise measurement of the length and diameter of the aorta and arteries, as well as of the diameter-reduction in stenoses is of great importance. In such situations, "sizing catheters" (Fig. 8.23) at the level of the respective arteries are helpful.

8.4
Contrast Media

8.4.1
Contrast Media in Various Imaging Modalities

Contrast media (cm) used in imaging diagnostics are distinguished according to the physical principle of image production: (1) CM for X-ray examinations (RCM); (2) CM used in magnetic resonance tomography (MR-CM); (3) CM used in ultrasound (US-CM).

8.4.1.1
Contrast Media for X-Ray Examinations (RCM)

For the imaging of morphological details in the living man, particularly of the inner organs – except bones and lung – we need adjuvants. The visible contrasts are caused by the varying absorption of X-rays of the different organs. The intensity of absorption depends on the atomic number of the atoms in the irradiated material and can be influenced by variations of the X-ray radiation, or by modifications of the concentration of the adjuvants. Substances of low density delivered into the body are gases (oxygen, air, and CO_2) which are described as "negative" CM. Substances with high X-ray density contain atoms with higher atomic numbers (barium, iodine, gadolinium); these are classified as "positive" CM.

Major differences (ALMÉN 1969; SPECK 1991) between the various CM exist as regards their water-solubility, chemical combination characteristics, such as ionic or non-ionic (ALMÉN 1973), and as regards their osmolarity (low-osmolar or high-osmolar CM). The high osmotic pressure of the amidotrizoate and iothalamate types of CM is the cause of most side effects (DAWSON 1988; SCHMIEDEL 1991; LAWRENCE et al. 1992; ZEITLER 1998). For this reason, the range of indications for these CM has been limited to non-vascular applications in Germany (*Bundesanzeiger* Nr. 153, 16/08/1994).

Fields of Application of X-Ray Contrast Media. CM can be administered in hollow organs for morphological and functional analysis, they can serve for the analysis of the functioning of different organs, and detect pathological vascular changes and diseases in organ systems after delivery through a vessel (SCHMIEDEL 1991; SPECK 1991). Figure 8.24 shows a simplified overview of the different tasks and indications of X-ray CM.

8.4.1.1.1
SIDE EFFECTS

Instructions for Prevention, Control, and Therapy. To prevent the occurrence of side effects (ELKE and FERSTEL 1977; PETERS and ZEITLER 1991; REIMANN et al. 1986; ANSELL 1990; LASSER et al. 1994; ZEITLER 1998), it is necessary to observe the specific CM history, including, previous CM administration, allergic reactions, chronic renal diseases, and an existing thyroid disease. An emergency bag, respirator, and oxygen are to be kept ready. The presence of an allergy, asthma, or previous adverse reactions to CM requires premedication with H_1- and H_2-receptor antagonists (DOENICKE and LORENZ 1985; REIMANN et al. 1986) and, in the case of elevated risk, an additional corticosteroid premedication (LASSER et al. 1994). Despite premedication, critical side effects may occur, for which the physician must be prepared.

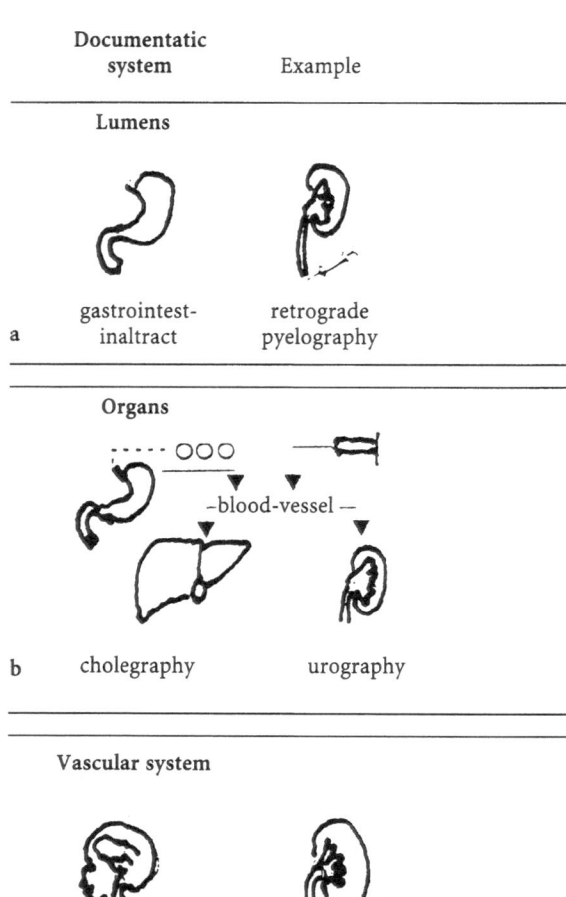

Fig. 8.24 a–c. Different CM intentions. Sites and indications used in practice to enhance anatomic strinctures or organs in normal and pathological conditions. **a** To contrast anatomical or pathological lumina: gastrointestinal tract, urogenital tract, fistula, abscess drainage, lumbar disc. **b** Transvenous parenchyma and organ function studies – parenchymal and/or capillary phase (cholegraphy, urography). **c** Angiography and cardiography to document the heart, arteries, and veins

Prophylaxis. In the case of hyperthyroidism and nodular struma (GLÖBEL and GLÖBEL 1991), a combined treatment using perchlorat and carbimazol (Thiamazol) is necessary: Perchlorat (Irenat) 3 × 300 mg per day for 1–2 days, at least 1 week prior to and 1 week following the CM examination. Thiamazol 2 × 20 mg daily, 1–2 days prior to, and up to 3 weeks following CM administration, or Carbimazol 3 × 1/2–1 tablet per day, 3 days prior to, and for 3 weeks following CM administration.

In cases of confirmed nephropathy, generous hydration before and after CM administration

(infusion of physiologic NaCl solution), and, if necessary, the administration of Dopamin, is recommended.

8.4.1.1.2
WATER-SOLUBLE, NEPHROTROPIC
CONTRAST MEDIA
We prefer and recommend monomeric non-ionic CM for intravenous and intraarterial angiography (Fig. 8.25). In special cases, dimeric CM can also be indicated. However, these are special situations: in the monomeric non-ionic CM, there is a small risk of reduced clotting time; whereas the dimeric non-ionic CM with reduced side effects can result in late allergic reactions (BEYER-ENKE and ZEITLER 1993; YOSHIKAWA 1992).

According to current knowledge based on large studies and overviews, the following can be concluded: Experience from several million patients in Europe, and from several non-European prospective multicenter studies, leads one to assume with some certainty that the side-effect rate of low-osmolar, non-ionic CM is significantly lower than that of ionic, high-osmolar CM. Irrespective of that, the side effects of ionic and non-ionic CM are the same, but only differ in frequency.

Adverse Reactions and Side Effects. The side effects that can occur after the administration of CM are classified as: frequent/mild; moderately severe and occasional; very rarely critical, life-threatening side effects/complications.

Common Side Effects. Mild and moderately severe anaphylactoid reactions, such as urticaria, nausea, vomiting, and heat sensation, occur. These can occur as typical anaphylactoid early (BUSH 1996) and late reactions (BEYER-ENKE and ZEITLER 1993; YOSHIKAWA 1992). Late reactions are those side effects that occur from 1 h up to 7 days or later after the administration of CM.

Severe and Critically Severe Anaphylactoid Side Effects. These include vertigo, bronchospasm, decrease in blood pressure, vagovagal reaction in the form of a cardiovascular collapse, and cardiac standstill.

Frequency of Adverse Reactions After Intravenous Administration of Non-ionic and Ionic CM. According to VOGEL (1986), side effects and complications in the descending urography, and after intravenous CM administration in i.v. DSA or CT, occur

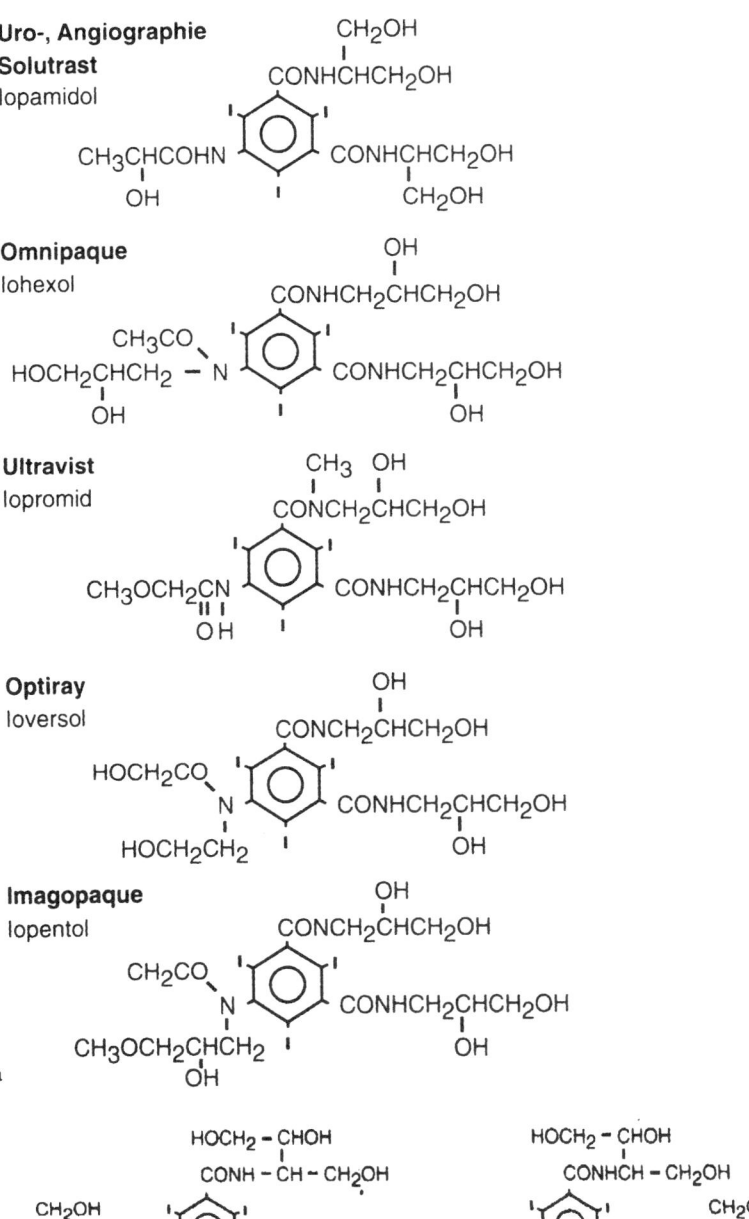

Fig. 8.25 a,b. Chemical structures of uro-angiographica. **a** *Non-ionic mono-mers:* (*1*) Iopamidol (Solutrast), (*2*) Iohexol (Omnipaque), (*3*) Iopromid (Ultravist), (*4*) Loversol (Optiray), (*5*) Iopentol (Imagopaque). **b** *Non-ionic dimers:* (*1*) Iotrolan (Isovist), (*2*) Iodixanol (Visipaque)

at a frequency of 0.008%–14%, severe side effects in 0.008%–1.8%. Lethal incidents occur at a frequency of 0.86–5.1 per 100 000 CM administrations. Prospective studies revealed a higher incidence of complications than retrospective analyses. Critical and lethal incidents occur within the first 5 min following intravenous CM administration in about 75%, a further 15% within 15 min, and 7% during the first hour following administration.

The different side effects and their frequency of occurrence after administration of ionic or non-ionic CM can be most clearly seen from KATAYAMA's study (1990) (Table 8.8).

In *patients with previous adverse reactions* to CM, the common, mild side effects occurred in 44% after use of ionic CM, and in 11% after use of non-ionic CM. Severe, rare side effects occurred in 0.73% after use of ionic CM, and in 0.18% after use of non-ionic CM (KATAYAMA 1990; YAMAGUCHI et al. 1991).

The Australian multicenter study by PALMER (1988) found severe side effects after injection of ionic CM ($n = 46\,262$) and non-ionic CM ($n = 14\,738$) in 0.1% and 0.01% of cases, respectively. These results are statistically significant.

Deaths after use of nephrotropic CM were reported in a highly varying frequency of $1:30\,000$ (SHEHADI and TONIOLO 1980) and $1:169\,000$ (KATAYAMA 1990) after intravenous CM administration (BUSH 1996). In one of 1000 CM administrations, a life-threatening complication can occur. Despite the reduction in the side-effect rate over the

Table 8.8. Adverse reactions to contrast medium (in each of the cases, one or several of the symptoms below occurred). (According to KATAYAMA 1990)

Ionic Contrast Medium (169 284 cases)

Symptoms	Incidence/cases	Incidence (%)
Nausea	7745	4.58
Urticaria	5343	3.16
Itching	5026	2.97
Heat sensation	3869	2.29
Vomiting	3111	1.84
Sneezing	2785	1.65
Flushes	1893	1.12
Coughing	975	0.58
Vascular pain	676	0.40
Palpitation	340	0.20
Dyspnea	288	0.17
Edema of the face	187	0.11
Abdominal pain	186	0.11
Abrupt blood-pressure drop[a]	175	0.10
Shaking chill	159	0.09
Hoarseness	158	0.09
Chest pain	153	0.09
Blackout[a]	30	0.02
Cardiac standstill[a]	7	0.004

Noc-ionic contrast medium (1 683 634 cases)

Nausea	1749	1.04
Heat sensation	1555	0.92
Urticaria	790	0.47
Itching	758	0.45
Vomiting	614	0.36
Sneezing	398	0.24
Flushes	271	0.16
Coughing	254	0.15
Palpitation	109	0.06
Vascular pain	80	0.05
Dyspnea[a]	63	0.04
Chest pain	47	0.03
Shaking chill	45	0.03
Abdominal pain	37	0.02
Hoarseness	31	0.02
Abrupt blood-pressure drop[a]	21	0.01
Edema of the face	15	0.01
Blackout[a]	4	0.002
Cardiac standstill	1	0.001

[a] Severe side effects.

last two decades, severe, even lethal, CM reactions cannot be completely excluded. Therefore, the protocols on the close control of patients and prevention must to be strictly observed.

8.4.1.1.3
MECHANISM OF SIDE EFFECTS

The risk of experiencing an adverse reaction to CM is between two and three times higher for allergic patients, and five times higher for patients with bronchial asthma (SHEHADI and TONIOLO 1980; BUSH 1996). In the case of previous adverse reactions to CM, the probability is between five and eleven times higher (ANSELL et al. 1980; SCHMIEDEL 1991). Thus, the major causes of side effects after intravenous or intraarterial administration of CM can be defined as: allergic reactions, elevated sensitivity to CM, or intolerance to CM. Without question, elevated sensitivity can also result from different psychological factors, such as the surrounding area, unfriendly personnel, and anxiety (LALLI 1980).

Common Anaphylactoid Reactions in Different Mono- or Polysymptomatic Appearances. These side effects occur suddenly and unexpectedly, mostly affecting patients with previous adverse reactions to CM, asthma, or allergic diseases. The definite cause is not know, and a clear identification of specific antibody formation has not been possible to date (ANSELL et al. 1980; ALMÉN 1994).

The release of histamine from mast cells and basophilic cells, initiated by the injection of CM, in contrast, could be clearly demonstrated (DOENICKE and LORENZ 1985). Moreover, CM have an influence on the coagulation, fibrinolysis, and the kinin system, and can cause the release of multiple mediate enzymes, such as histamine, bradykinin, leukotriene, and others (ANSELL 1990; ALMÉN 1994; BUSH 1996; ZEITLER 1985). In the case of typical anaphylactoid reactions, early cutaneous and bronchospastic symptoms of severe cardiopulmonary complications are observed. The occurrence of severe, even lethal reactions following the injection of CM, without any prior warning made LALLI (1980) postulate a central nervous cause, possibly even a history with very high psychiatric involvement.

Influence on the Heart and Circulatory System. CM can influence the mechanical and electrophysiologic properties of the heart, as well as central and peripheral hemodynamics. Especially under intracoronary or intracardiac administration, they cause a negative inotropy, with a drop in the velocity of the left ventricular increase in pressure and of the left ventricular blood pressure, leading to an increase of the end-diastolic filling pressure. The electrophysiologic effects are decelerations of the ventricular stimulus conduction and repolarization. Following intracoronary CM injections, there is an initial bradycardia, which may be followed by a tachycardia. In the case of patients with cardiac or pulmonary diseases, and depending on the amount of CM administered, a decrease in blood pressure, and heart failure can occur. These critical cardiac and cardiovascular side effects occur significantly less often if non-ionic CM with low osmolar pressure are used (SCHMIEDEL 1991). In cases of a severe cardiac ischemic disease and the use of ionic CM, the above-mentioned side effects occur more frequently, especially in patients with angina pectoris or acute heart attack (SEYFERTH et al. 1983). Some side effects occur because the patients have interrupted their pharmacotherapy, or changed their diet. Therefore, a small breakfast with a cup of tea in the morning before angiography is much better than a hungry and thirsty patient (WAGNER et al. 1997).

Influence on Renal Function. The majority of CM induced impairments of renal function do not manifest themselves through clinical symptoms, and are spontaneously reversible (SCHERBERICH 1991). Nevertheless, a "contrast-induced nephropathy" can be anticipated, which is the case when the value of creatine in the serum is elevated by more than 25% and is higher than 2 mg/dl, compared to the previous value (JAKOBSEN et al. 1996). Within 2 weeks, the concentration of creatine in the serum, however, only exceeds 1.4 mg/dl, when the glomerular filtration rate drops below 60 ml/min (corresponding to 50% of the normal values).

The incidence of CM induced impairments of renal function in patients with normal renal function is 0.6%–5%. Of these, 10% develop clinical symptoms (i.e., 0.06%–0.5% of CM administrations (SCHERBERICH 1991). In patients with diabetic nephropathy, a symptomatic renal insufficiency can ccur in up to 75%, if these patients have not received an infusion or hemodialysis before CM administration. The nephrotoxity of non-ionic compared to ionic CM is slightly lower.

Influence on Blood Coagulation. CM – particularly when used for angiographies – lead to a retardation of blood coagulation (DAWSON 1988). Non-ionic nephrotropic CM have less anticoagulant characteristics than ionic. In the framework of angiographies and coronary angiographies, however, this "anticlotting effect" can be beneficial for the prevention of thrombotic complications. After coronary angiographies using *ionic* CM, thromboembolic complications were reported in 0.2%–1%, and myocardial infarctions in 0.2%–0.5% of cases. Under the use of *non-ionic* CM for coronary angiographies, an increase of such CM related complications has not been observed in prospective trials (SCHMIEDEL 1991).

8.4.1.1.4
CONTROL OF PATIENTS

Instructions for the close control of patients include the following:

- Prior to the administration of water-soluble CM, the patient's history must be taken, and the patient must be properly informed on the procedure and possible risks. Clear information must be obtained regarding:
  - Previous overreaction to CM, asthma, allergies, etc.
  - Possible chronic or acute renal diseases
  - Possible cardiopulmonary risks (cardiac insufficiency, pulmonary hypertension)
  - Possible hyperthyroidism, or other thyroid diseases
  - Possible signs of neurologic or psychological abnormalities.
- The CM should be administered with the patient in a lying position. It is useful to leave an intravenous in-dwelling cannula in the patient for up to 1 h. Following CM administration, the patient must be observed during the X-ray examination and for up to 1 h afterwards. The staff must be prepared for possible emergency care. In the case of emergency, oxygen apparatus and medication for the management of side effects have to be kept within easy reach of the patient. An internal organization system for cases of severe side effects (e.g., telephone number of the anesthetist or doctor on emergency call) must be available to all medical staff and easily legible.
- Following CM administration and X-ray examination, the patient must be informed about the extremely rare possibility of a late reaction (up to 7 days after the examination) (BEYER-BNKE and ZEITLER 1993). Advice regarding vehicle-driving, rest, inability to work, diet, and intake of medication needs to be given on an individual basis.

8.4.1.1.5

PROPHYLAXIS OF SIDE EFFECTS

Premedication for Prevention of Anaphylactoid Reactions.

- In cases of elevated risk (previous CM reaction, bronchial asthma, or similar):

  Corticosteroids, methylprednisolone 40 mg orally, once every 24, 12, and 2 h prior to CM administration, and/or 20 to 30 min prior to CM administration H_1- and H_2-receptor antagonists, for example Tavegil/5-ml ampule and Tagamed/2-ml ampule. Exclusive use of non-ionic, low-osmolar CM.
- In cases of mildly elevated risk (mild previous CM reaction, general allergy, allergic dermal eczema):

  Possible use of a different CM. Approximately 20–30 min prior to CM administration, H_1- and H_2-receptor antagonists, for example a 5-ml ampule of Tavegil, plus one 2-ml ampule of Tagamed. Use of non-ionic, low-osmolar CM.
- In cases of specific risks and in addition to those mentioned in the previous two points:

Corticosteroids 30 min prior to CM administration:

250 mg of Solu-Decortin H, or 100 mg of Volon A solubile (for adults)
100 mg of Solu-Decortin H, or 50 mg of Volon A solubile (for children).

Prevention of Thyreotoxicoses. A combined treatment with perchlorat and carbimazole is recommended:

- Perchlorat: 3 × 300 mg IRENAT daily, 2 days before, and up to 3 weeks after CM administration
- Carbimazole: 3 × 1 tablet daily, 2 days before, and up to 3 weeks after CM administration.

Where necessary, a prior TSH test should be carried out.

Prophylaxis in the Case of Nephropathy. This includes hydration (generous drinking) and, where necessary, infusion of physiologic NaCl solution, as well as the administration of dopamine.

8.4.1.1.6

THERAPY OF CM-INDUCED SIDE EFFECTS

If the situation arises, in addition to the immediate administration of O_2 and emergency care – (which should be conducted in a calm manner) – the patient should first of all be calmed. Before the administration of O_2, the supply of fresh air can bring the patient some initial relief. As a cannula is in place, medication can be administered immediately.

In the case of severe side effects (anaphylactic shock), immediate action is required:

1. The doctor on emergency call, or the anesthesia department, must be notified without delay, whereby the internal organization plan of the institute must be observed
2. Artificial respiration with oxygen
3. An infusion must be started with saline
4. Medicamentous treatment according to the symptoms (methylprednisolone 1000 mg = Urbason solubile forte.

8.4.1.2
Magnetic Resonance (MR) Angiography with MR-CM

The preferred CM is gadolinium-DTPA-diglumin salt (Magnevist, Schering). Side effects or complications occur extremely seldom (0.03%) (NIENDORF et al. 1991). The dose varies between 0.1 and 0.2 mmol/kg body weight. The treatment and prevention of side effects are the same as for CM used in X-ray examinations.

8.4.1.3
Ultrasound (US) Angiography with US-CM

D-Galactose in the form of specially prepared microparticles can be used. The Doppler signal may become more intense. This technique is excellent to detect av-shunts or endoleaks. Experience and training are strongly recommended to prevent false-positive findings (SCHLIEF and BAUER 1996).

References

Abrams H (1983) Angiography, 3rd edn: vol I–III. Little Brown, Boston
Almén T (1969) Contrast agent design. Some aspects on the synthesis of water-soluble contrast agents of low osmolality. J Theor Biol 24:216–226
Almén T (1973) Effects of Metrizamide and other contrast media on the isolated rabbit heart. Acta Radiol [Suppl] 335:216
Almén T (1994) The etiology of contrast medium reactions. Invest Radiol 29 [Suppl]1:37–45
Amplatz K (1960) A vascular injector with program selector. Radiology 75:955–958
Amplatz K (1963) Translumbar catheterization of the abdominal aorta. Radiology 81:927–930

Amplatz K (1971) A simple non-thrombogenic coating. Invest Radiol 6:280–289

Amplatz K (1983) Rapid film changers. In: Abrams H (ed) Angiography, 3rd edn: vol 1 Little Brown, Boston, pp 105–124

Ansell G (1990) Adverse reactions to contrast agents. Scope of problems. Invest Radiol 25:381

Ansell G, Tweedle NK, West CR, Evans P, Couch L (1980) The current status of reactions to intravenous contrast media. Invest Radiol [Suppl]15:532–539

Athanasoulis C, Pfister RC, Greene RE, Roberson GH (eds) (1982) Interventional radiology. WB Saunders, Philadelphia, pp 3–54, 253–298

Bauer KH (1943) Thorotrast und Krebsgefahr. Chirurg 15:204–207

Baum S (1983) Catheters and injectors. In: Abrams H (ed) Angiography, 3rd edn: vol 1. Little Brown, Boston, pp 187–204

Baum S, Stein GN, Kuroda KK (1966) Complications of "no-arteriography". Radiology 86:835–838

Beck A (1992) Die Geschichte der Angiographie. Verlag Schwarzwälder Chronik, Germany

Beck A (1993) Wiederaufbereitung von Kathetern. Schnetztor, Konstanz

Benninghoff A, Görtler K (1988) Lehrbuch der Anatomie des Menschen, vol II. In: Ferner H, Staubesand J (eds) Eingeweide und Kreislauf. Urban and Schwarzenberg, Munich, p 458

Berberich J, Hirsch WS (1923) Die röntgenangiographische Darstellung der Arterien und Venen am Lebenden. Munch Med Wochenschr 2:2226–2228

Berenstein C (1983) Brachiocephalic vessel: selective and superselective catheterization. Radiology 148:437–441

Beyer-Enke SA, Zeitler E (1993) Spät-Nebenwirkungen nicht-ionischer Röntgen-Kontrastmittel. Munch Med Wochenschr 135:109–111

Bleichröder F (1912) Intraarterielle Therapie. Klin Wochenschr 49:1503

Bluhbaum T, Frik K, Kalbrenner H (1928) Eine neue Anwendung der Kolloide in der Röntgendiagnostik. Fortschr Rontgenstr 37:18–29

Bohndorf K, Günther RW (1991) A new catheter configuration for selective antegrade catheterization of the superficial femoral artery: technical note. Cardiovasc Intervent Radiol 14:129–131

Brennecke R, Brown TK, Bursch J, Heintzen DM (1978) Computerized video-image processing with application to cardioangiographic Roentgen image series. In: Nagel HH (ed) Digital image processing. Springer, Berlin Heidelberg New York, p 244

Brooks B (1924) Intraarterial injection of sodium iodide. JAMA 82:1016

Bundesanzeiger No. 135, 16/08/1994. Amidotrizoate: Anwendungsgebiete, Gegenanzeigen, Nebenwirkungen etc. Bekanntmachung über die Zulassung und Registrierung von Arzneimitteln vom 18. Juli 1994

Bush WH Jr (1996) Risk factors, prophylaxis and therapy of X-ray contrast media reactions. Advances in X-ray contrast. Kluwer Academic, UK, pp 44–53

Carlin RA, Amplatz K (1970) Downstream aortography. Am J Roentgenol 109:536–540

Cope C (1986) Micropuncture angiography. Radiol Clin North Am 24:359–367

Cope C, Burke DR, Meranze S, Baum ST (1990) Atlas of interventional radiology. J.B. Lippincott, Philadelphia

Crummy AG, Strother CM, Sackett JF, et al. (1980) Computerized fluoroscopy: digital subtraction for intravenous angiocardiography and arteriography. AJR 135:1131–1141

Davidson CJ, Mark DB, Pieper KS, et al. (1988) Thrombotic and cardiovascular complications related to nonionic contrast media during cardiac catheterization. Analysis of 8517 patients. Am J Cardiol 65:1481–1484

Dawson P (1988) Nonionic contrast agents and coagulation. Invest Radiol 23 [Suppl] 29:310–317

Dembski JC, Zeitler E (1974) Translumbale und thorakale Katheterangiographie. Fortschr Rontgenstr 120:435–437

Deray G, Jacobs C (1996) Are low osmolality contrast media less nephrotoxic? Nephrol Dial Transplant 11:930–931

Desilets DT, Hofmann A (1965) A new method of percutaneous catheterization. Radiology 85:147–150

Diella JA, et al. (1982) Nephrotoxicity from angiographic contrast material. Am J Med 72:719

Doenicke A, Lorenz W (1985) Histamin-Rezeptor-Antagonisten. Springer, Berlin Heidelberg New York

Dos Santos R, Lamas AC, Pereira-Caldas J (1929a) Arteriografia da aorta e dos vasa abdominais. Med Contemp 47:93–97

Dos Santos R, Lamas A, Caldas JP (1929b) Arteriografia des membros. Med Contemp 47:1

Dos Santos R, Lamas A, Caldas JP (1931) Artériographie des membres et de l'aorte abdominales. Masson et Cie, Paris

Dotter CT, Judkins M (1964) Transluminal treatment of arteriosclerotic obstruction: description of a new technique and a preliminary report of its application. Circulation 30:654–670

Dotter CT, Judkins MP, Frische LH (1966) Safety guidespring for percutaneous cardiovascular catheterization. Am J Roentgenol 98:957–960

Dotter CT, Rösch J, Robinson M (1978) Fluoroscopic guidance in femoral artery puncture. Radiology 127:266–267

Eichstädt H, Felix R, Zeitler E (eds) (1995) Klinische Radiologie: Herz und Große Gefäße. Springer, Berlin Heidelberg New York

Elke M, Ferstel A (1974) Notfallsituationen in der Röntgendiagnostik. Erkennung und Behandlung. Thieme, Stuttgart

Elke M, Ferstel A (1977) Notfallsituationen in der Röntgendiagnostik. Erkennung und Behandlung. In: Zeitler E (ed.) Kontrastmittelzwischenfälle. Thieme, Stuttgart, pp 129–157

Farinas PL (1941) New technique for angiographic examination of the abdominal aorta and its branches. Am J Roentgennol 46:641–645

Fink U (1991) Peripheral DSA with automated stepping. Eur Radiol 13:50–55

Forssmann W (1929) Die Sondierung des rechten Herzens. Klin Wochenschr 8:2085

Franken G, Zeitler E (1978) Experience with mechanical contrast medium injection at selective coronary angiography. Cardiovasc Intervent Radiol 1:21–26

Gidlund A (1956) Development of apparatus and methods for roentgen studies in hemodynamics. Acta Radiol [Suppl] 130:1–130

Glöbel B, Glöbel H (1991) Die Schilddrüsenfunktion nach Applikation jodhaltiger Röntgenkontrastmittel. In: Peters PE, Zeitler E (eds) Röntgenkontrastmittel. Springer, Berlin Heidelberg New York, pp 70–75

Gmelin E (1986) Schleusentechnik für die translumbale Katheterangiographie. Fortschr Rontgenstr 144:523–525

Gmelin E, Arlart JP (1987) Digitale Subtraktionsangiographie. Thieme, Stuttgart

Günther RW, Thelen M (1996) Interventionelle Radiologie. Thieme, Stuttgart

Haschek E, Lindenthal DT (1896) Ein Beitrag zur praktischen Verwertung der Photographie nach Roentgen. Wien Klin Wochenschr 9:36

Heintzen PH, Bürsch JM (1978) Röntgen-video-techniques for the dynamic studies on the heart and circulation. Thieme, Stuttgart

Hettler M (1960) Die sichere Arterienpunktion als Grundlage der Extremitätenangiographie und des Arterienkatheterismus. Fortschr Rontgenstr 92:97

Hettler M (1969) Die perkutane Kathetermethode nach Hettler. Fortschr Rontgenstr 110:553–563

Hilbertz T, Fink U, Kohz P, et al. (1992) Perivision – ein neuer Standard für die periphere Angiographie. Electromedica 60(1):2–5

Hinck VC, Judkins MP, Paxton HD (1967) Simplified selective femoro-cerebral angiography. An improved method. Radiology 89:1048

Hirsch S (1924) Die peripheren Blutgefäße im Röntgenbild. Verlag von Keim and Nemnich, Frankfurt am Main

Ichikawa T (1938) Schatten der Nierenarterie, meine Methode zur röntgenologischen Darstellung der Nierenarterie. Z Urol 32:563–564

Jakobsen JA, Berg KJ, Kjaersgaard P, Kolmannskog F, Nordal KP, Nossen JO, Rootwelt K (1996) Angiography with nonionic X-ray contrast media in severe chronic renal failure: renal function and contrast retention. Nephron 73:549–556

Janker R (1954) Röntgenologische Funktionsdiagnostik. Girardet, Wuppertal-Ellerfeld

Judkins MP, Kidd HJ, Frische LH, Dotter CT (1967) Lumen-following safety-guide for catheterization of tortuous vessels. Radiology 88:1127–1130

Kadir S (1986) Diagnostic angiography. Saunders, Philadelphia

Katayama H (1990) Survey of safety of clinical contrast media. Invest Radiol 25:7–10

Kimball JP, Sansone VJ, Ditters LA, Wissel PS (1988) Red blood cell aggregation versus blood clot formation in ionic and nonionic contrast media. Invest Radiol 23[Suppl. 2]:334–339

Kollath J, Spitz P (1968) Über den Zusammenhang zwischen der Kontrastmittelverteilung und der Anordnung der Katheteröffnungen bei der Hochdruckangiographie. Radiologe 8:242–248

Lalli AF (1980) Contrast media reactions: data analysis and hypothesis. Radiology 134:1–12

Lammer J, Schreyer H (1991) Praxis der interventionellen Radiologie. Hippokrates, Stuttgart

Lasser E, Berry C, Mishkin M, et al. (1994) Pretreatment with corticosteroids to prevent adverse reactions to non-ionic contrast media. AJR 162:523–526

Lasser EC, Sandra G, Lyon CH, Berry C (1997) Reports on contrast media reactions: analysis of data from reports to the U.S. Food and Drug Administration. Radiology 203:605–610

Lawrence V, Matthai W, Hartmaier S (1992) Comparative safety of high-osmolality and low-osmolality radiographic contrast agents: report of a multidisciplinary working group. Invest Radiol 27:2–28

Lechner G, Jantsch H, Waneck R, Kretschmer G (1988) The relationship between common femoral artery, the inguinal crease, and the inguinal ligament: a guide to accurate angiographic puncture. Cardiovasc Intervent Radiol 11:165–169

Lindgren E (1953) Technique of abdominal angiography. Acta Radiol 39:205–218

Lipchik EO, Rogoff STM (1983) The abdominal aorta: arteriosclerosis and other diseases. In: Abrams H (ed) Angiography, vascular and interventional radiology, 3rd ed: vol II. Little Brown Boston

Loose KE (1951) Die Serienaortographie bei peripheren Durchblutungsstörungen. Langenbecks Arch Klin Chir 270:462–464

Loose KE, van Dongen RJAM (1976) Atlas of angiography. Thieme, Stuttgart

Mac Mahon HE, Murphy AS, Bastes MJ (1947) Endothelial-cell sarcoma of liver following Thorotrast injections. Am J Path 23:585–611

Mann S, Zeitler E (1975) Verhalten der Serumosmolarität bei hohen Kontrastmitteldosen im Rahmen der Angiographie. Fortschr Rontgenstr 122:135–137

Mc Cullogh M, Davies P, Richardson R (1989) A large trial of intravenous Conray and Niopam 300 to assess immediate and delayed reactions. Br J Radiol 62:260–265

Meany TF, Weinstein MA, Buoncore E, et al. (1980) Digital subtraction angiography of the human cardiovascular system. AJR 135:1153–1160

Mistretta CA, Ort MG, Cameron JR, Crummy AB, Moran PR (1973) Multiple image subtraction technique for enhancing low contrast periodic objects. Invest Radiol 8:43–52

Mistretta CA, Crummy AB, Strother CM (1981) Digital angiography: a prospective study. Radiology 139:273

Niendorf HP, Haustein J, Cornelius I, Alhassan A, Clauß W (1991) Safety of gadolinium-DTPA: extended clinical experience. Magn Res Med 22:222–228

Niendorf HP, Alhassan A, Haustein J, et al. (1993) Safety and risk of gadolinium-DTPA: extended clinical experience after more than 5 000 000 applications. Advances in MRI Contrast 2:12–19

Oedman (1956) Percutaneous selective angiography of the main branches of the aorta. Acta Radiol 45:1–14

Oedman P (1959) The radiopaque polythene catheter. Acta Radiol (Stockh) 52:52–56

Olbert F, Wicke L (1973) Über Komplikationen und deren Vermeidung bei der Kontrastdarstellung des arteriellen Gefäßbaumes durch Direktpunktion und bei Katheterangiographie. Radiol Clin Biol 42:134–165

Olbert F, Hanecka L (1977) Transluminale Gefässdilatation mit einem modifizierten Dilatationskatheter. Wien Klin Wochenschr 89:281–284

Ovitt TW, Christenson PC, Fisher HD, Frost MM, Nudelman S, et al. (1979) Intravenous angiography using digital video subtraction: X-ray imaging system. Am J Roentgenol 135:1141–1144

Palmer FJ (1988) The RACR survey of intravenous contrast media reactions. Final report. Australas Radiol 32:426–428

Peirce EC (1951) Percutaneous femoral artery catheterization in man with special reference to aortography. Surg Gynecol Obstet 93:56–64

Peters PE, Zeitler E (eds) (1991) Röntgenkontrastmittel-Nebenwirkungen, Prophylaxe, Therapie. Springer, Berlin Heidelberg New York

Peters PE, Zeitler E, Clauß W (eds) (1992) Qualitätssicherung bei der Anwendung von Kontrastmitteln. Springer, Berlin Heidelberg New York

Pässler HW (1957) Unsere Technik der automatischen Serienaortographie. Röntgenblätter 10:73–78

Pässler HW (1963) Abdominale Aortographie mit besonderer Berücksichtigung der bilateralen retrograden Serienaortographie ohne Katheter. Fortschr Rontgenstr 98:279

Ratschow M (1930) Uroselektan in der Vasographie unter besonderer Berücksichtigung der Varicographie. Fortschr Rontgenstr 42:37–45

Ratschow M (1937) Leistung und Bedeutung der Vasographie als Funktionsprüfung der peripheren Blutgefäße. Fortschr Rontgenstr 55:253–256

Ratschow M (1953) Die peripheren Durchblutungsstörungen. sternkopff, Dresden

Ratschow M (1959) Angiologie, Pathologie, Klinik und Therapie der peripheren Durchblutungsstörungun. Thieme, Stuttgart

Reimann H-J, Tauber R, Kramann B, Gmeinwieser J, Schmidt U, Reiser M (1986) Prämedikation mit H_1- und H_2-Rezeptorantagonisten vor intravenöser Kontrastmitteldarstellung der ableitenden Harnwege. Fortschr Rontgenstr 144:169-173

Rinast E, Gmelin E, Zwaan M (1992) A 5-F needle-sheath system for translumbar catheter angiography. Eur J Radiol 2:130-132

Robb GP, Steinberg J (1939) Visualization of the chambers of the heart, pulmonary circulation and the great blood vessels in man. Am J Roentgenol 41:1-17

Rosen RJ, McLean GK, Oleaga JA, Freiman DB, Ring EJ (1981) A new exchange guide wire for transluminal angioplasty. Radiology 140:242-243

Rothenberger K (1986) Gibt es eine Prophylaxe für Kontrastmittelzwischenfälle? Beitr Urol 4:19-27

Rückforth J, Schurmann K, Vorwerk D, Günther RW (1998) Dosis-und Konstrastmittelein sparung bei der intravenösen digitalen subtraktionsangiographie durch Bolusverfolgung. Forstschr Rontgenstr 169:383-387

Sadekni S, Srur M, Cohn DJ, Rozenblit G, Wetter EB, Sos TA (1985) Antegrade catheterization of the superficial femoral artery. Radiology 157:531-532

Schad N (1967) Die intermittierende Kontrastmittelinjektion in das Herz. Thieme, Stuttgart

Scherberich JE (1991) Nephrotoxizität von Röntgenkontrastmitteln. In: Riemann HG (eds) Digitale Radiographie. Schnetztor, Konstanz

Schild H (1994) Angiographie – angiographische Intervention. Thieme, Stuttgart

Schlief R, Bauer A (1996) Ultraschallkontrastmittel. Radiologe 36:51-57

Schlief R, Schürmann R, Niendorf HP (1991) Ultraschallkontrastmittel auf Galaktose-Basis. In: Jahrbuch der Radiologie. Biermann Verlag, Zülpich, pp 259-265

Schmiedel E (1991) Ionische oder nichtionische Röntgenkontrastmittel. In: Günther RW, Gockel HP (eds) Jahrbuch der Radiologie 1991. Biermann, Zülpich, pp 231-250

Schröder J (1993) The mechanical properties of guidewires. Part I. Stiffness and torsional strength. Cardiovasc Intervent Radiol 16:43-46

Schröder J (1993) The mechanical properties of guidewires. Part II. Kinking resistance. Cardiovasc Intervent Radiol 16:47-48

Schröder J (1993) The mechanical properties of guidewires. Part III. Sliding friction. Cardiovasc Intervent Radiol 16:93-97

Schrott KM, Behrends B, Clauß W, Kaufmann J, Lehnert J (1986) Iohexol in der Auscheidungsurographie. Fortschr Med 104:153-156

Seldinger SI (1953) Catheter replacement of the needle in percutaneous arteriography. A new technique. Acta Radiol 39:368-376

Seyferth W, Marhoff P, Zeitler E (1982) Transvenöse und arterielle digitale Videosubtraktionsangiographie (DVSA). Fortschr Rontgenstr 136:301-309

Seyferth W, Dilbat G, Zeitler E (1983) Efficacy and safety of digital subtraction angiography with special reference to contrast agents. Cardiovasc Intervent Radiol 6:265-270

Sgalitzer (1931) Über Kontrastfüllung der Gefäße. Fortschr Rontgenstr 43:103-104

Shehadi WH, Toniolo G (1980) Adverse reaction to contrast media. Radiology 137:299-302

Simmons CR, Tsao EC, Thompson JR (1973) Angiographic approach to the difficult aortic arch: a new technique for transfemoral cerebral angiography in the aged. Am J Roentgenol 119:605-610

Söldner HJ, Mittelmeier HD, Beyer-Enke S, Zeitler E (1995) The reduction of the extent of vascular lesions during angioplasty by the use of a sheath. Fortschr Rontgenstr 163:341-344

Speck U (1991) Kontrastmittel. Springer, Berlin Heidelberg New York

Speck U (1995) Röntgenkontrastmittel. In: Eichstädt H, Felix R, Zeitler E (1995) Klinische Radiologie: Herz und Große Gefäße. Springer, Berlin, Heidelberg, 111-119

Speck U, Mützel W, Weinmann HJ (1983) Chemistry, physiochemistry and pharmacology of known and new contrast media for angiography, urography and CT enhancement. In: Taenzer V, Zeitler E (eds) Contrast media in urography, angiography and computerized tomography. Thieme, Stuttgart, pp 2-10

Steinberg J (1962) Intravenous abdominal aortography and peripheral arteriography. NY State J Med 62:1186-1192

Stribley K, Wilkins RA (1987) Technique of superficial femoral artery catheterization prior to percutaneous transluminal angioplasty. J Intervent Radiol 2:99-104

Tschakert H (1989) Kontrastmittelnebenwirkungsrate bei Zweifachinjektionen – Korrelation mit Histaminplasmaspiegeln. Rontgenpraxis 42:107-111

van Sonnenberg E, Neff C, Pfister R (1987) Life-threatening hypotensive reactions to contrast media administration: comparison of pharmacologic and fluid therapy. Radiology 162:15-19

Viamonte M Jr, Stevens RC (1965) Guided angiography. AJR 94:30-39

Viamonte M Jr, Hobbs J (1967) Automatic electric injector: development to prevent electromechanical hazards of selective angiocardiography. Invest Radiol 2:262-265

Vogel M (1986) Risiken der Röntgendiagnostik. Urban and Schwarzenberg, Berlin

Wagner HJ, Evers JP, Hoppe M, Klose KJ (1997) Muß der Patient vor intravasaler Applikation eines nichtionischen Kontrastmittels nüchtern sein? Fortschr Rontgenstr 166, 5:370-375

Wagner HJ, Feeken T, Mutters R, Klose KJ (1998) Bakteriämie bei intraarterieller Angiographie, perkütaner transluminaler Angioplastie und perkutaner transhepatischer cholangio-drainage. Fortschr Röntgenstr 169:402-407

Wallace S, Madellin H, De Jongh D (1972) Systematic heparinization for angiography. Am J Roentg 116:204-209

Weinmann HJ, Brasch RC, Press WR, Wesbey GE (1984) Characteristics of gadolinium-DTPA complex: a potential NMR contrast agent. AJR 142:619-624

Wellauer J (1957) Aortographie. In: Schinz HR, Baensch WE, Frommhold W, Glauner R, Uehlinger E, Wellauer J (eds) Lehrbuch der Röntgendiagnostik, 6th edn. Thieme, Stuttgart

Wenz W, Beduhn D (1976) Extremitätenarteriographie. Springer, Berlin Heidelberg New York

Wenz W, Beduhn D, Roth FJ, von Kaick G, Czembirek H (1970) Abdominale Angiographie. Technik, Pathomorphologie, Indikationen. Rontgenpraxis 23:97-124

Wenz W, van Kaick G, Roth FJ (1974) Abdominal angiography. Springer, Berlin Heidelberg New York

White RI Jr (1976) Fundamentals of vascular radiology. Lea and Febiger, Philadelphia

Williams PL, Warwick R (eds) (1980) Femoral artery anatomy. In: Gray's anatomy, 36th edn. W.B. Saunders, Philadelphia, pp 723–725

Wolf GL (1998) Safety of ionic and non-ionic contrast media. Radiology 206:560–561

Wolf GL, Arenson RL, Cross AP (1989) A prospective trial of ionic vs nonionic contrast agents in routine clinical practice. AJR 152:939–944

Yamaguchi K, Katayama H, Takashima T, Kozuka T, Seez P, Matshura K (1991) Prediction of severe adverse reactions to ionic and non-ionic contrast media in Japan: evaluation of pretesting. Radiology 178:363–367

Yoshikawa H (1992) Late adverse reactions to non-ionic contrast media. Radiology 183:737–740

Zeitler E (1970a) Probleme der Thrombusbildung bei Katheterangiographie. Aktuelle Probleme in der Angiologie 10:11–19

Zeitler E (1970b) Die Gefäßthrombosen nach Katheterangiographie. Aktuelle Probleme in der Angiologie, vol 10. Huber, Bern

Zeitler E (1974) Aorto-arteriographie. In: Heberer G, Rau G, Schoop W (eds) Angiologie. Founded by M. Ratschow, 2nd edn. Thieme, Stuttgart, pp 243–302

Zeitler E (1975) Die selektive Katheterangiographie der Arteria femoralis superficialis: Technik, Komplikationen und Möglichkeiten der Differentialdiagnose und -therapie. Electromedica 5:167–178

Zeitler E (ed) (1977) Kontrastmittel-Zwischenfälle (Symposium Berlin 1977). Schering, Berlin

Zeitler E (ed) (1985) Klinische Pharmakologie der Kontrastmittel. Schnetztor, Konstanz

Zeitler E (1998) Kontrastmittel in der bildgebenden Diagnostik. In: Unerwünschte Arzneimittelwirkungen. Fischer, Stuttgart

Ziedses des Plantes BG (1935) Eine röntgenologische Methode zur separaten Abbildung bestimmter Teile des Objekts. Fortschr Röntgenstr 52:69–74

8.4.1.4
CO_2 Angiography

K. Detmar

Digital subtraction angiography (DAS) with iodinated intraarterial contrast agents still represents the gold standard in vascular imaging, but for a number of patients even the nonionic contrast agent carries severe risks:

- Adverse reactions due to hypersensitivity
- Nephrotoxic effects, particularly in patients with renal dysfunction
- Decompensation in patients with hyperthyroidism.

The prevalence of severe and very severe adverse reactions range between 0.12% (Caro et al. 1991) and 0.04% (Katayama et al. 1990) for nonionic contrast agents. Therefore, carbon dioxide (CO_2) was explored as an alternative contast agent in DSA.

8.4.1.4.1
HISTORIC REVIEW

CO_2 was routinely used in the 1950s and 1960s in pneumoradiography of the heart (Scatliff et al. 1959). Animal studies were performed to evaluate the toxicity, side effects, physiology, and elimination of the intravasal CO_2. Angiography with CO_2 used as a contrast agent was evaluated by Grosse-Brockhoff et al. in 1959 and DSA by Hawkins in 1982.

Injection of CO_2 was previously carried out by hand or mechanical injectors. In the last decade dedicated CO_2 gas injectors have been developed (Seeger et al. 1993; Schmitz-Rode et al. 1993; Zwaan 1997).

8.4.1.4.2
PHYSICAL, CHEMICAL, AND PATHOPHYSIOLOGICAL EFFECTS OF CO_2 ADMINISTRATION

In vitro experiments evaluated the absorption capacity of 66 cc CO_2 per 100 cc blood (Hess and Hartmann 1959). In animal studies up to 7.5 cc/kg CO_2 intraarterially caused no serious side effects (Grosse-Brockhoff et al. 1957). More recent studies (Zwaan 1997) showed increasing systemic partial pressure of CO_2 (12 mmHg) in the first 2 min after injection of 1.66 cc/kg, and a decrease of pH of 0.033, not exceeding normal values. CO_2 is normally completely cleared by the lung.

CO_2 is compressible and needs a special injection technique. The main difference compared to liquid contrast media is that CO_2 needs to displace the blood in a vessel for a couple of seconds to give contrast in DSA. Application of large amounts of CO_2 (more than 200 cc) leads to pain due to ischemia and local acidosis. Injection of CO_2 directly into the carotid arteries of rats caused neurologic deficits and cerebral infarctions (Coffey et al. 1984).

8.4.1.4.3
TECHNIQUE AND APPLICATION

We used a modern standard DSA unit (Siemens Polytron) without any changes in hardware and software. Medical CO_2 was applied using a standard mechanical injector, sterile tubes, filters, and special three-way stopcocks, which completely seperate the CO_2 tank from the patient. Pressure of the CO_2 in the injector was at equilibrium with arterial pressure. Injection volumes and flow for patients with arteriosclerosis are given in Table 8.9. A delay of 2 min between two series is important. Glucagon (1 mg) is necessary for the imaging of the abdomen and pelvis.

8.4.1.4.4
RESULTS

In all cases ($n = 32$) image quality was acceptable, good, or excellent. Comparison with "conventional" DSA (selective application of 10 cc nonionic contrast agent) showed better visualization of small vessels and collaterals in iodinated contrast agent (Figs. 8.26, 8.27). Staging of stenoses and occlusions showed no significant differences. Angiograms of the foot require special techniques (elevation of the foot, large CO$_2$ bolus, image averaging). In a study of 128 angiograms SEEGER et al. (1993) found consistency between CO$_2$ and standard angiograms in 95%; the image quality was graded good or exellent in 91%.

8.4.1.4.5
SIDE EFFECTS

No side-effects were noticed with up to 100 cc of gas injection into the abdominal aorta. Selective injection in the femoral artery showed mild paresthesia and pain when the injected volume of CO$_2$ exceeded 60 cc and more than 80 cc caused distinct pain. There were no cases of tachycardia, tachypnea, nausea, or severe reactions to CO$_2$.

8.4.1.4.6
INDICATIONS

CO$_2$ as an arterial contrast agent is limited to the abdomen and lower limbs. Experience in upper limbs is limited and carries some risk of cerebral iscemia (EHRMAN et al. 1994). Indications for CO$_2$ angiography arise in cases where iodinated contrast media are contraindicated. Due to the diagnostic value of magnetic resonance angiography and color Doppler sonography we recommend CO$_2$ angiography for therapeutic intravascular procedures (percutaneous transluminal angiography) and angioscopy.

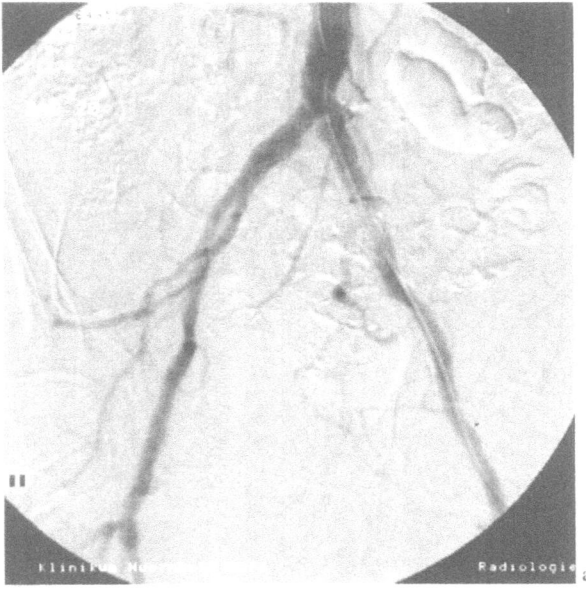

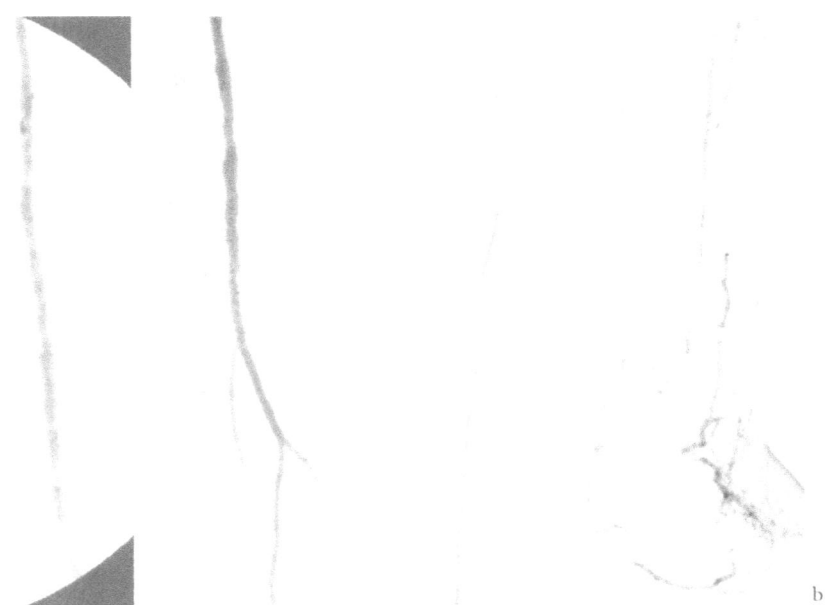

Fig. 8.26 a,b. Occlusion of the superficial femoral artery in the distal thigh. Comparision of CO$_2$ angiogram (a) and conventional DSA with iodinated contrast medium. The diagnostic value of both techniques is comparable except for the increased visualization of small vessels in (b)

158   W. Krause

Table 8.9. Injection parameters in CO_2 angiography

Region	Injection volume (cc)	Injection velocity (cc/s)	Postprocessing
Abdominal aorta	80	50	–
Iliac artery	20	15	Valuable
Femoral artery	35	12	Valuable
Popliteal artery	45	10	Valuable
Lower leg	55	10	Necessary
Foot	60–70	10	Necessary

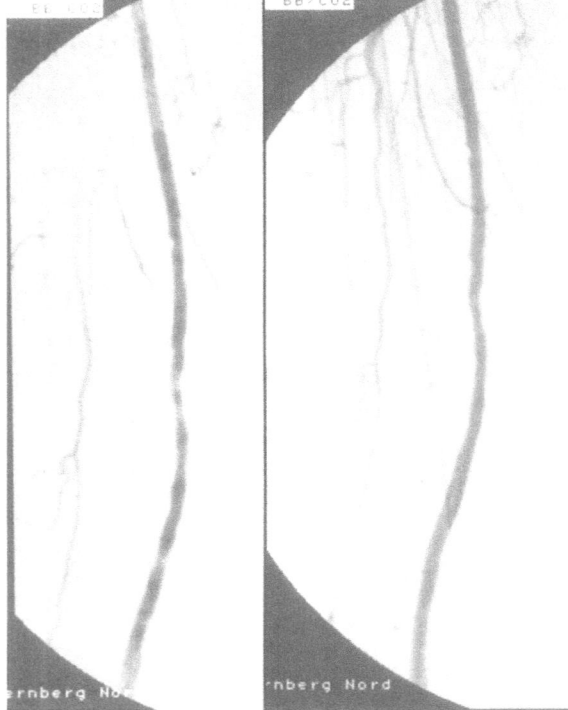

Fig. 8.27. Angiogram of thigh, lower leg, and ankle in a patient with multiple arteriosclerotic stenoses (*arrows*)

References

Caro JJ, Trindade E, McGregor M (1991) The risks of death and of severe nonfatal reactions with high- vs low-osmolality contrast media: a metaanalysis. AJR Am J Roentgenol 156: 825–832

Coffey R, Quisling RG, Mickle JP, Hawkins IF Jr, Ballinger WB (1984) The cerebrovascular effects of intraarterial CO_2 in quantities required for diagnostic imaging. Radiology 151:405–410

Ehrman K, Taber TE, Gaylord GM, et al. (1994) Comparison of diagnostic accuracy with carbon dioxide versus iodinated contrast material in the imaging of hemodialysis access fistulas. J Vasc Intervent Radiol 15:771–779

Grosse-Brockhoff F, Koch D, Loogen F, Rotthoff G, Vieten H, Willmann KH (1957) Kohlendioxyd als Kontrastmittel für die Röntgendarstellung des Herzens und der Gefäße. RÖFO 86:285–291

Hawkins IF (1982) Carbon dioxide digital subtraction arteriography. AJR Am J Roentgenol 139:9–24

Hess H, Hartmann KH (1959) Der Einfluß von intraarteriellen Gasinsufflationen auf den Blutstrom in den Extremitäten. Med Klin 34:1439–1496

Katayama MD, Yamaguchi K, Kozuka T, Takashima T, Seez P, Matsuura K (1990) Adverse reactions to ionic and nonionic contrast media. Radiology 175:621–628

Seeger JM, Self S, Harward TRS, Flynn T, Hawkins IF Jr (1993) Carbon dioxide gas as an arterial contrast agent. Ann Surg 217:688–698

Schmitz-Rode T, Alzen G, Günther RW, Pott H (1993) CO2 spray mini-injector for digital subtraction angiography vs PC-controlled injection system: experiments in dogs. Cardiovasc Intervent Radiol 16:297–302

Scatliff JH, Kummer AJ, Janzen AH (1959) The diagnosis of pericardial effusion with intracardiac carbon dioxide. Radiology 73:871–874

Zwaan M (1997) Angiographie mit Kohlendioxid. Conscientia diagnostica (Byk Gulden). Schnetztor, Constance

8.4.2
Tailored Contrast Agents for Angiography and Intervention

W. Krause

8.4.2.1
Introduction

In radiography, information is derived from local variations in the X-ray attenuation observed for the areas of interest compared to surrounding tissue material. Accordingly, radiological contrast is defined as the relative extent of variation in X-ray attenuation or image intensity for a particular anatomical detail. Unfortunately, blood, the vessel wall, and neighboring soft tissue do not differ significantly in their X-ray attenuation coefficients. As a consequence, blood vessels cannot be clearly differentiated from their surrounding soft tissue and for any delineation of vessels the injection of contrast material is mandatory. For angiography, DSA, or computed tomography angiography (CTA) techniques, contrast enhancement therefore is a prerequisite to visualize blood vessels. For other imaging modalities, such as ultrasound (US) or magnetic resonance imaging (MRI), there are non-contrast alternatives making use of either low echo-genicity of blood or the movement of erythrocytes in color Doppler techniques or relying on blood flow in MR angiography which result in significant contrast.

8.4.2.2
Chemical and Physicochemical Features

In radiographic angiography, contrast agents are injected to produce either positive or negative contrast. For positive or negative contrast, the attenuation of the agent has to be significantly different, i.e., greater or lower than that of the blood vessel. The first type includes all elements with an atomic weight significantly greater than that of carbon and oxygen. In the past, various elements have been tried for angiography, such as strontium bromide or oxide, sodium iodide, and bismuth salts (HASCHEK and LINDENTHIAL 1896; OSBORNE et al. 1923). At present, exclusively organically bound iodine is used. However, there are first attempts to utilize metal ions, such as the lanthanides gadolinium and ytterbium "masked" by highly tolerable chelates (ZWICKER et al. 1993) or the noble gas xenon (VAN ROST et al. 1996). Negative contrast is possible by decreasing the density of a carbon and oxygen containing compound relative to the density of blood. This approach is utilized for carbon dioxide angiography (HAWKINS and CARIDI 1995). Since the vast majority of all angiographic procedures are performed with iodinated contrast agents, the focus of this section shall be put on this well-established class of compounds.

Iodinated contrast agents have to be administered at extremely high doses and injection rates because the concentration of iodine in blood necessary to achieve in CT a density difference of 30 Hounsfield units (HU) relative to the surrounding tissue has to be approximately 1 mg/ml and for suffcient contrast in projection radiography up to 10–370 mg/ml are necessary, depending on several parameters such as location and diameter of the vessel and technique. Accordingly, the amounts of contrast agent which have to be administered in radiography or in interventional procedures are at the upper end of doses used in all areas of medicine. Consequently, tolerance is the main feature of iodinated contrast agents.

In interventional radiology, contrast agents are used to locate catheters, for therapy control in thrombolysis, and dilatation or embolization procedures, in angioplasty, and for stent and filter implantation. The use of contrast media (CM) in interventional radiology requires the following special characteristics to be take into consideration: First, the doses administered are normally much higher than those injected in diagnostic procedures and repeated administrations during a prolonged period of time are rather common. Second, the patients are normally highly compromised and, third, compatibility – avoiding both pharmacological interaction and precipitation – with a number of coadministered drugs has to be guaranteed.

The presently available X-ray contrast agents are derivatives of triiodobenzenes either of one (monomers) or of two ring systems (dimers), each of them containing three iodine atoms (Fig. 8.28). The remaining positions in the molecule are needed for highly hydrophilic groups, mainly hydroxyl groups, which make the compound water-soluble and which are supposed to shield the iodine atoms from any interaction with biomacromolecules. Monomers containing one carboxyl groups (ionic monomers) were synthesized first in the early 1950s and 1960s (LANGECKER et al. 1954). Exampes are diatrizoate (Angiografin Schering AG, Berlin, Germany), iothalamate (Conray Mallinckrodt, St. Louis, Mo., USA), ioxithalamate (Telebrix Guerbet, Roissy, France), iodamide (Uromiro Bracco, Milan, Italy), ioglicate (Rayvist Schering AG, Berlin, Germany), and metrizoate (Isopaque Nycomed, Oslo, Norway). Later, the ionic carboxyl groups was successfully converted into a "non-ionic" amide derivative. The first compound available was metrizamide (Amipaque Nycomed, Oslo, Norway). The disadvantage of this first non-ionic contrast agent was its chemical instability so that it had to be stored and shipped in a freeze-dried form. It was followed by the ready-to-use preparation of iopamidol (Solutrast, Isovue, Niopam Bracco, Milan, Italy), iohexol (Omnipaque Nycomed, Oslo, Norway), iopromide (Ultravist Schering AG, Berlin, Germany), ioversol (Optiray Mallinckrodt, St. Louis, Mo., USA), iopentol (Imagopaque Nycomed, Oslo, Norway), iomeprol (Iomeron Bracco, Milan, Italy), iobitridol (Xenetix Guerbet Roissy, France) and ioxilan (Oxilan Cook, Bloomington, Ill., USA). At present, four different chemical classes are available: ionic and non-ionic monomers and ionic and non-ionic dimers. Examples of dimers are the ionic ioxaglate (Hexabrix Guerbet, Roissy, France) and the non-

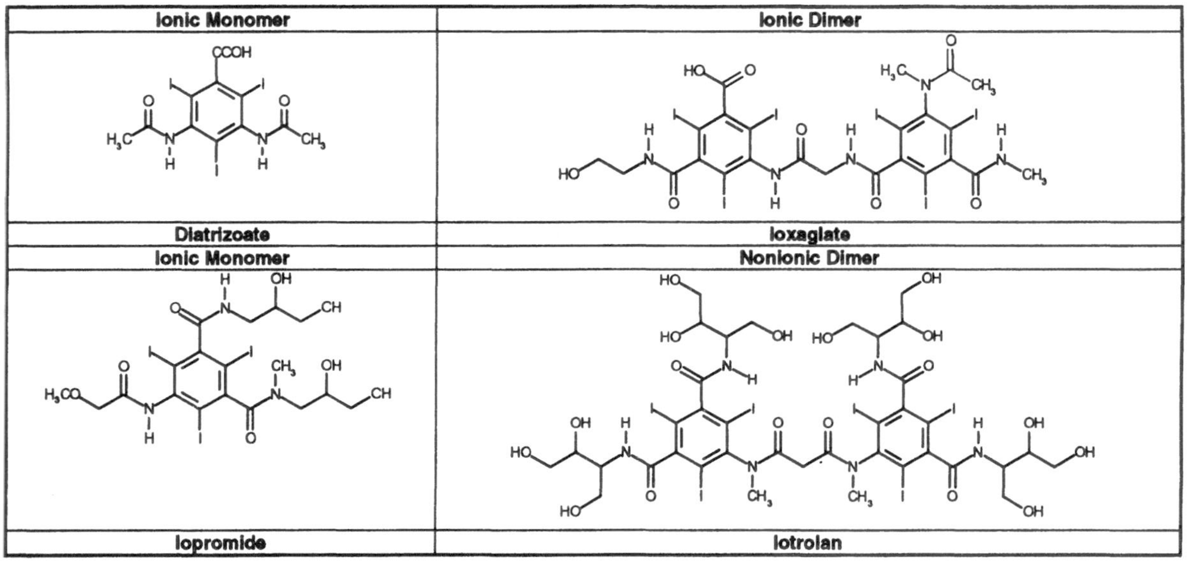

Ionic Monomer	Ionic Dimer
   Diatrizoate	 Ioxaglate
Ionic Monomer	Nonionic Dimer
   Iopromide	 Iotrolan

Fig. 8.28. Structures of representative iodinated contrast agents out of the four classes, ionic and non-ionic monomers and dimers

ionic iotrolan (Isovist Schering AG, Berlin, Germany), and iodixanol (Visipaque Nycomed, Oslo, Norway). When stored in the dark, the stability of CM preparation is extremely high so that maximal shelf-lives of up to 5 years can be achieved. The tolerability of iodinated contrast agents depends on two major physicochemical features. These are the presence or absence of electrical charge and the osmolality of the preparation. For ionic monomers, an electrical charge automatically also results in high osmolality since, at the same iodine concentration, the number of independent molecules in the solution is double that of non-ionic monomers. Osmolalities of CM preparations at a concentration of 300 mg iodine per milliliter range from isotonicity (300 mosmol/kg) for the non-ionic dimers via 500–800 mosmol/kg for the ionic dimer ioxaglate and the class of non-ionic monomers, to 1500–2000 mosmol/kg for the ionic monomers KRAUSE et al. 1993. Viscosities for the same concentration range from approximately 4–8 mPa·s. Viscosity determines the "motility" of a preparation and thereby significantly influences the pressure against which the solution has to be injected and, particularly when thin catheters are used, the delivery rate. Figure 8.29 demonstrates the differences in flow through 4- and 5-F catheters of a number of monomeric contrast agents as a function of the pressure. In general, flow rate depends on the diameter, the length, and the material out of which the catheter is made, and on the viscosity and temperature of the CM. Increasing the temperature significantly reduces viscosity. As

a consequence, CM are normally injected at 37°C. Osmolality and viscosity are, however, not only influenced by general molecular features such as the monomeric or dimeric structure, but also to a significant extent by the possibility of forming intermolecular bridges and thereby reducing the number of "free" independent molecules in the solutions. The greater the number and stability of these bridges, the lower the osmolality of the preparation. This even goes so far that non-ionic monomers can finally achieve isotonicity. However, the inevitable drawback of this advantage is that bridging is not only possible between the contrast agent molecules themselves but also between them and biomacromolecules. As an effect, interaction with the organism might start to take place resulting in adverse

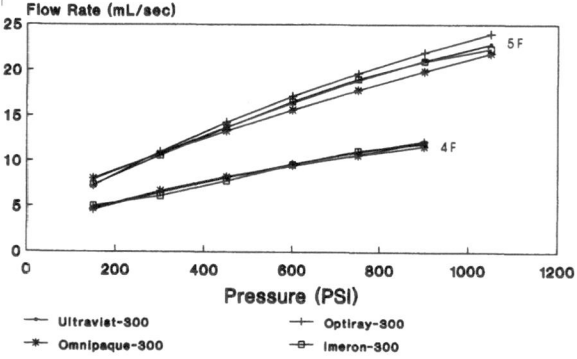

Fig. 8.29. Flow rate in 4-F and 5-F catheters (Nylex 4 and 5, Cordis) at a concentration of 300 mg iodine per milliliter as a function of pressure

events. Osmolality-related effects are expected to become significant at osmolalities starting from approximately 600 mosmol/kg. Minor factors determining tolerability are the size of the molecule and additives to the formulation. Any other – and so far unknown – factors are summarized under the term "chemotoxicity".

8.4.2.3
Pharmacokinetics

The pharmacokinetics of iodinated contrast agents used for angiography are practically identical for all types of compounds. After intravenous or intraarterial injection iodine concentrations in the blood decline biphasically with half-lives of 3–10 min and 1–2 h, respectively. Due to their extremely high hydrophilicity, the compounds are distributed exclusively in the extracellular space volume; they are not able to pass membranes such as the blood–brain barrier, only small proportions cross the placental barriers or are excreted into milk and, following oral administration, less than 5% is absorbed from the gastrointestinal tract. Iodinated contrast agents are not metabolized. Their excretion is mainly (>95%) by renal elimination (glomerular filtration). Accordingly, any renal impairment will inevitably result in prolonged retention in the body. However, by hemodialysis the compounds can effectively be cleared from the organism.

8.4.2.4
Classification of Adverse Reactions

CM side effects are extraordinarily rare and can be classified according to a variety of criteria. These include the severity (mild, moderate, severe, fatal), the time of onset (immediate, delayed), the target organ (heart, kidneys, skin, etc.), the mechanism of action (caused by electrical charge, osmolality, interactions with biological macromolecules, etc.), or the incidence (frequent, rare). Mild effects include sensations of heat or nausea, vomiting, urticaria, and pain at the injection site. Moderate adverse reactions include severe forms of the aforementioned effects and edema or bronchospasm. Severe reactions are hypotension, convulsion, shock, and cardiac arrest. Most adverse reactions are of the immediate type. Delayed effects, however, are a topic of increasing interest stimulated by the introduction of the new non-ionic dimeric contrast agents. Adverse effects

caused by the high osmolality of the preparation are at present the best understood type of side effects. They are dose-dependent and can easily be avoided by the use of low-osmolar compounds. Less well understood are the interactions with biological macromolecules which are considered the first step of molecule-specific toxicity. These interactions are mediated by ionic charge, hydrogen bonding (hydrophilic interreraction) and hydrophobic interaction between less hydrophilic parts of the contrast agent molecule and the macromolecules. To avoid these interactions, molecules displaying low protein binding have been selected. The incidence of side effects reported for angiographic procedures covers a wide range depending on indications/techniques, dosage, patients, and contrast agents.

General risk factors for the use of iodinated contrast agents include hypersensitivity to CM, allergy, hyperthyroidism, severe cardiovascular disease, reduced general condition, renal and hepatic insufficiency, diabetes, pulmonary disease, cerebral injury, paraproteinemia, pheochromocytoma, sickle cell anaemia, old age (>65 years), and extreme anxiety in the patient.

8.4.2.5
Characteristics of Adverse Reactions

In the following section, organ-specific tolerance will be dealt with, starting with the brain. Neurologic adverse reactions provoked by intravascular iodinated contrast agents are mainly due to disturbance of the blood–brain barrier. As a result, EEG changes and normally mild, fully reversible functional deficits have been reported. These effects are primarily osmolality-related. As could be demonstrated in animal experiments and was also seen in clinical trials, low osmolar or isotonic contrast agents exhibit only minimal effects (WILSON et al. 1991). Additionally, changes of the cerebral blood flow (both vasodilatation and vasoconstriction) have been reported (NAKSTAD 1989; DU BOULAY and WALLIS 1986). Clinical studies have shown that the overall risk of cerebral angiography for transient neurologic deficits is 0.5%–5.5% and for permanent deficits is 0%–1% of all cases (BIEN 1995). The increasing application of digital subtraction angiography (DSA) and the use of low-osmolar CM has considerably reduced the incidence. Table 8.10 gives an example of the high tolerance of iopromide in cerebral angiography.

Electrophysiological adverse reactions have primarily been observed after intracoronary or intracardiac injection of iodinated CM. The effects reported include bradycardia, atrioventricular (AV) conduction disturbances, QT prolongation, and ST segment and T-wave changes. Their extent is directly related to osmolality (PIAO et al. 1988; MISSRI and JERESATY 1990). The negatively charged carboxylic group of ionic monomeric or dimeric contrast agents is able to bind calcium present in blood resulting in ventricular fibrillation in approximately 0.5% of all cardiac angiographic procedures (JOHNSON et al. 1989). Hemodynamic side effects of contrast media include myocardial depression, decrease in blood pressure and contractility and an increase in left ventricular end diastolic pressure (HIRSHFELD et al. 1983; FELDMAN et al. 1988; HIGGINS 1985; BASHORE et al. 1988). This type of action could possibly pose a problem for patients with pre-existing ischemia or cardiac insufficiency. Since non-ionic low-osmolar contrast agents do not exhibit these effects to the same extent, they should be preferred (WISNESKI et al. 1989; KLINKE et al. 1989). Another, osmolality-related effect is pain at the injection site and vasodilatation resulting in a sensation of warmth. Low-osmolar or isotonic agents do not exhibit this effect or only to a minor extent (HAGEN and KLINK 1983; BARRETT et al. 1992). This could be shown both in animal experiments (KRAUSE 1994) and in clinical trials. Table 8.11 gives a summary of side effects reported during coronary angiography.

In interventional radiology, especially in percutaneous transluminal coronary angioplasty, but also in other procedures, such as stent implantation, effects on the blood-clotting system are of special interest. Although the better tolerance of non-ionic contrast agents regarding cardiovascular, renal, and systemic effects has generally been accepted, the influence on blood coagulation has remained a topic of controversy since the publication of a work by ROBERTSON (1987) indicating a higher probability of clot formation in syringes containing blood and non-ionic agents as compared to ionic compounds. Additional in vitro studies confirmed the stronger anticoagulant effect of ionic CM (GERTZ 1989; STORMORKEN and SKALPE 1986). In contrast, thromboembolic events in clinical practice have been reported both for ionic and for non-ionic contrast agents with similar incidences (HILL and GRABOWSKI 1992; DAWSON et al. 1993). Both classes of agents, ionic and non-ionic, exhibit anticoagulant and antiplatelet activities (SCHRADER 1996; GABRIEL et al. 1991; DAWSON et al. 1986; AU 1991; DAVIDSON et al. 1990; HWANG et al. 1989). However, the quality and extent of interaction is different. They include activation of the contact system, effects on platelet adhesion, aggregation and activation, thrombin generation, prolongation of clotting time, injury to the vascular endothelium, and reduction in fibrinolysis. While non-ionic substances exhibit only a minor influence, the effect of ionic agents is much more explicit. Non-ionic CM are less anticoagulant than ionic CM (ENGELHART et al. 1988; RAININKO and RIHELIÄ 1990; STRICKLAND et al. 1992; STORMORKEN et al. 1986; HOFFMEISTER and HELLER 1996; GABRIEL et al. 1991) and have been reported to primarily inhibit fibrin polymerization. In order to avoid thromboembolic side effects, prolonged contact time of blood and CM should be avoided. If an additional anticoagulant property of

Table 8.10. Tolerance of high-dose iopromide in cerebral arteriography. Summary of two randomized double-blind studies (BERGELSON et al. 1994) comparing total doses of 10–256 ml iopromide-300 ($n = 87$) with 15–207 ml iohexol-300 ($n = 39$), and 24–204 ml iopamidol-300 ($n = 47$)

Adverse reaction	Iopromide $n = 87$ (%)	Pooled comparators $n = 86$ (%)
One or more reactions	18 (21)	38 (44)
Headache, confusion, somnolence, paresthesia, dizziness	8 (9)	18 (21)
Abnormal vision, visual field defect, speech disorder	10 (12)	20 (23)

Table 8.11. Number of patients with side effects following high-dose iopromide in coronary arteriography/left ventriculography. Summary of two randomized double-blind studies (BERGELSON et al. 1994; DYET et al. 1990) comparing total doses of 41–270 ml iopromide-370 ($n = 80$) with 124–246 ml iopamidol-370 ($n = 21$), and 43–280 ml iohexol-350 ($n = 60$)

Side-effect (SE)	Iopromide-370 $n = 80$ (%)	Pooled comparators $n = 81$ (%)
One or more SE	32 (40)	35 (43)
Pain at injection site, hemorrhage, neck pain	4 (5)	1 (1)
Disturbance of cardiovascular functions	11 (14)	22 (27)
Gastrointestinal side effects	7 (9)	4 (5)
Headache, paresthesia	9 (11)	6 (7)
Dyspnea	1 (1)	1 (1)
Urogenital disturbance	7 (9)	4 (5)
	38 (49)	38 (46)

non-ionic CM is desired, heparin at a concentration of 5 IU/ml might be added directly to the preparation. Thromboembolic effects during angiography can be provoked by various other factors including length of procedure and catheterization time, intensity of vascular disease, syringe and catheter material, and insufficient flushing. Especially careful flushing probably has a great impact both on avoiding thromboembolic events and on overall safety. Compared to the abovementioned procedural factors, the choice of the particular contrast agent is most likely negligible.

Adverse renal reactions cover a broad range varying from no effect via transient laboratory parameter changes to the requirement of hemodialysis. The incidence of kidney damage induced by iodinated contrast agents is, however, highly controversial and essentially not exactly known. Estimates range from 0% to 10% (BYRD and SHERMAN 1979; PORT et al. 1974) and even rates of up to 30% are claimed by some investigators (MASON et al. 1985; D'ELIA et al. 1982; TEMEL et al. 1981). Non-ionic low-osmolar contrast agents are reported to be better tolerated than ionic monomers (HILL et al. 1991). Pre-existing renal insufficiency, diabetes, and dehydration have been identified as risk factors for renal damage (RICH and CRECELIUS 1990). The clinical signs of renal nephropathy induced by CM include serum creatinine increases within 24 h which reach peak values at 3 days, and oliguria. Within 10 days polyuria develops and creatinine values normalize. In rare cases, irreversible renal damage might result in the need for chronic hemodialysis. The mechanism of renal damage induced by iodinated contrast agents is still under debate. At present, the reason for CM-related nephropathy accepted most widely

seems to be a direct effect of the agent on the kidney by disturbing the tubular regulation mechanisms and, probably, the production of vasoactive substances (MORCOS et al. 1995). After CM injection, renal blood flow increases steeply followed by a prolonged decrease. The extent of blood flow fluctuations is greater the nearer the injection site is to the kidney and finds its maximum following administration into renal arteries. Prophylaxis against side effects comprises adequate hydration of the patient and discontinuation of comedication such as biguanides (DACHMAN 1995). Non-ionic contrast agents seem to be better tolerated than ionic compounds. As an example, data for the non-ionic monomers, iopromide, and iopamidol are summarized in Fig. 8.30.

Recently, a special type of adverse reactions, delayed allergy-like events, has gained considerable attention. The clinical signs reported include anaphylactic shock, hypotension in association with an anaphylactic reaction, angioedema, bronchospasm, dyspnea, laryngeal spasm or edema, glottis edema and skin reactions, such as exanthema, pruritis, itching, rash, and urticaria. Although the incidence reported in the literature ranges from 0.4% to 18%, it is at present assumed that the incidence is actually rather low. However, for the new non-ionic dimers, iotrolan and iodixanol, this type of side effect has been observed twice as often as for non-ionic monomers. At present, the pathomechanism of these adverse effects remains unknown and specific risk factors could not be identified. The hypotheses put forward have included the involvement of antibodies or the contact system influencing the rate of kallikrein production and the activation of T cells (EXPERT COMMITTEE ON MECHANISM 1996).

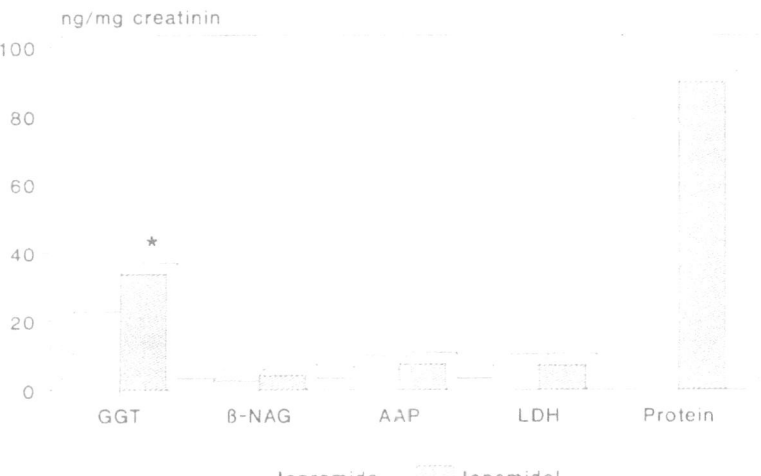

Fig. 8.30. Enzymuria and proteinuria in patients (NEWHOOSE et al. 1994) following i.v. injection of iopromide and iopamidol ($n = 40$ each). The asterisk indicates a statitistically significant difference ($p < 0.05$)

Particularly for high-volume use of contrast agents in interventional radiology, compatibility with coadministered drugs must not pose any problems. In this context, compatibility explicitly refers to effects on the solubility of both drug and contrast agent. However, effects on the pharmacological activity, especially of anticoagulant or thrombolytic drugs are also important. Table 8.12 summarizes compatibility (solubility) experiments with different drugs and contrast agents. Iopromide could be shown to exhibit the lowest degree of interaction. Figure 8.31 summarizes the results of studies investigating the inhibitory effects of contrast agents on the thrombolytics, tPA, urokinase, and streptokinase (KRAUSE and NIEHUES 1996). The conclusions to be drawn from these data are: Firstly, streptokinase is more influenced than urokinase or tPA and, secondly, the concentrations and doses of contrast agents normally used in interventional radiology are high enough to decrease the efficacy of the commonly used thrombolytics considerably. Ethyl alcohol is a widely used agent for tissue ablation and embolization. Often, in order to visualize the distribution of ethanol in the tissue, contrast material is added to the alcohol before injection. For optimum visualization, a high solubility in ethanol of the contrast agent is needed. Iopromide, again, exhibited better solubility than any of the other agents investigated.

To assist the radiologist in the decision of when to use non-ionic low-osmolar contrast agents, several guidelines have been issued in the past (RITCHIE et al. 1993; BETTMANN 1989; BENNESS 1988). In general, non-ionic contrast agents were recommended for patients at high risk of hemodynamic complica-

tions, for painful examinations and patients with marked anxiety, children and elderly patients, patients with hyperosmolar states (dehydration), renal failure, prior reactions, and strong allergic diathesis or asthma. Meanwhile, the use of non-ionic contrast agents has gained general acceptance. In summary, although ionic and non-ionic contrast agents seem to exhibit the same type of side effects, their severity is clearly different. Ionic CM elicit a between three and ten times higher risk of provoking adverse reactions than low osmolarity. Non-ionic triiodinated (monomeric) CM currently represent the state of the art with the largest choice of concentrations and vial sizes.

8.4.2.6
Future Developments

Future developments may concern both the contrast agents and the X-ray technology. The number of publications using monochromatic X-rays obtained from synchrotron facilities is increasing considerably. The brightness of synchrotron radiation is much greater than that of conventional multi-wavelength sources even after monochromatization using Bragg diffraction. Monochromatic X-rays with a wavelength immediately above the K-edge of iodine (33.2 keV) offer a maximal difference in attenuation between iodinated contrast agents and tissues. If a dual-wavelength procedure is used operating shortly below and above the K-edge of iodine and subtracting the two images, the resulting pictures offer tremendous increases in contrast sensitivity and spatial resolution compared with conventional DSA tech-

Table 8.12. Compatibility of contrast media with coadministered drugs

Drug	Diatrizoate	Ioxaglate	Iopromide	Iotrolan
Ampicillin				
Atropine				
Cimetidine		↓↓		
Diazepam				
Epinephrine				
Ethanol	↓	↓		↓
Gentamycin				
Hydrocortisone				
Lidocain				
Nitroglycerol	↓	↓		↓
Papaverine	↓↓	↓↓		
Pheniramine				
Protamine	↓↓	↓↓		
Tolazoline				

↓, Transient changes in solubility as characterized by the formation of a suspension;
↓↓, long-lasting precipitation of drug and/or contrast agent.

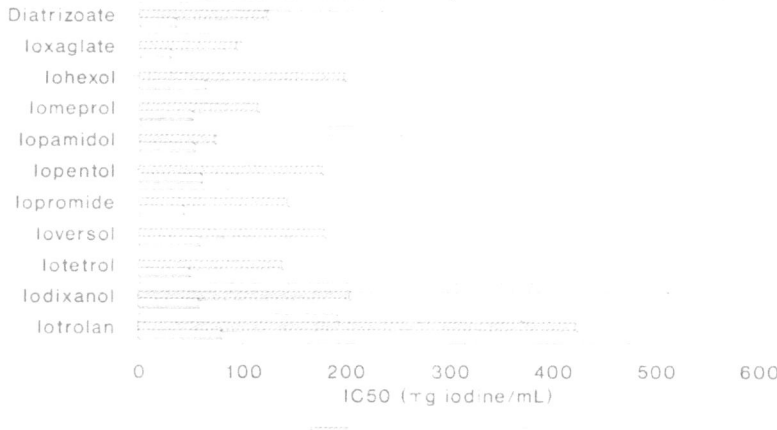

Fig. 8.31. Inhibitory effects of different contrast agents on the activity of tPA, urokinase, and streptokinase

niques. Other advantages of monochromatic X-rays are that beam-hardening artifacts are eliminated and that the energy can be optimized for the size of a patient. Using a synchrotron facility, the feasibility of monochromatic radiation in cardioangiography has already been demonstrated in patients (DIX 1995) and in animal studies. Vessels of diameters below 50 μm could be delineated in the heart of dogs (MORI et al. 1996). On the other hand, the radiation dose at the skin surface is not higher than that obtained for other radiological procedures. MORI et al. reported a dose of 0.48 mSv per image for angiograms of the canine coronary, vertebral, and internal carotid arteries. On the side of the detector, a high-definition TV system is required in order to make use of the high resolution obtained by this technique. The newest development shows single- and dual-energy CT with monochromatic synchro-tron X-rays (DILMANIAN et al. 1997) operating with a 19.5-cm field of view for symmetric and approxi-mately 36-cm field for asymmetric scanning. The use of dual-energy techniques seems to be possible. The next step will be to become independent of the need to use radiation from a synchrotron facility, but rather to develop small stand-alone units approach-ing the size of conventional CT machines (BACAL et al. 1996; SNIGIREV et al. 1996).

Other technical progress is directed towards phase-contrast imaging using polychromatic hard X-rays (WILKINS et al. 1996; MOMOSE et al. 1996). The underlying principle of this technique is that, in contrast to conventional X-rays which are hardly attenuated by carbon, nitrogen or, oxygen atoms, the X-ray phase-shift cross sections of these elements is nearly a thousand times greater than their X-ray absorption cross sections. As a consequence, tissues

can be better differentiated from each other ac-cording to differences in the phase-shift cross sec-tions. The role of contrast agents using this modality is not yet clearly defined. At present, this technique needs monochromatic X-rays from a synchrotron source.

Regarding progress in contrast agents, there are several pathways to follow. The first is to further improve tolerance. The topics to be addressed here are general, renal, and cardiovascular tolerability, neural tolerance, and delayed reactions. Since there does not seem to be much room for improvement of the presently available iodinated contrast agents, in-terest has been focussed on using metal chelates. However, the concentrations achievable with these compounds are still too low to allow their general use. The highest gadolinium concentration available is 1 M which is equivalent to 157 mg gadolinium per milliliter. Assuming a 1.5 times better attenuation coefficients for gadolinium than for iodine, 157 mg/ml is equivalent to approximately 200 mg iodine per milliliter. This concentration should be sufficient for DSA techniques.

Extensive research efforts are presently directed towards finding compounds with diminished or even without extravasation. The currently available con-trast agents leave the intravascular space volume within seconds after the injection (Fig. 8.32). As a result, there is a rapid decrease in enhancement. Repeated re-injections are therefore necessary. This is especially the case during interventional procedures where a prolonged delineation of ves-sels would constitute a significant progress. Non-extravasating or blood-pool contrast agents would be particularly useful for CT angiography. Polymers on the basis of dextran or polylysine to which

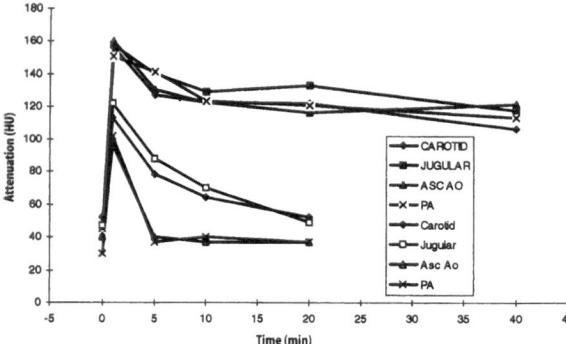

Fig. 8.32. Computed tomography enhancement of different arteries in monkeys after i.v. injection of iopromide-containing liposomes (*filled characters*; *top curves*) or after iopromide-300 (*empty characters, bottom curves*) at a dose of 300 mg iodine/kg. Data are means of five animals for the liposomes. One of the animals additionally received iopromide-300. ASCAO ascending aorta, PA pulmonary artery

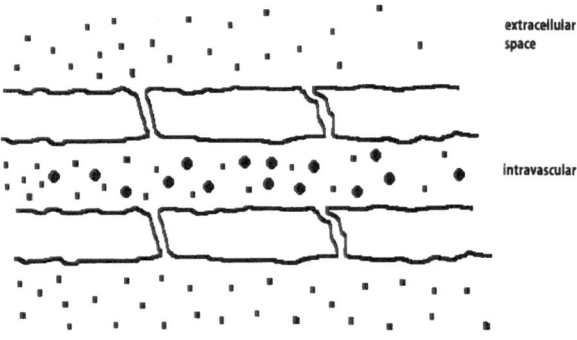

Fig. 8.33. Long intravascular circulation of "blood-pool" contrast agents followed by "extravasation" at sites of disturbed vascular endothelium such as inflammation or tumors

triiodobenzenes are coupled have been synthestized. The size of these molecules is too big to allow them to pass through the endothelial gaps into the extravascular space volume. However, so far none of these compounds has reached the stage of clinical testing. The problem found in animal experiments which is still to be solved is the improvement of tolerance and the retention of these compounds in the body. An alternative to polymers are specially designed liposomes which contain the contrast-giving substances (common contrast agents) within their encapsulation volume. Figure 8.33 gives, as an example, the time-density curves of iopromide-containing liposomes after intravenous injection into monkeys. A plateau-like enhancement of 60–80 HU can be achieved for a prolonged period of time. Contrast agents which do not leave the vessel system rapidly would primarily have the advantage of a clearer delineation of fine vascular structures and of prolongation of the residence time, allowing a more precise visualization. It remains to be seen whether any of these compounds will become clinically available in the future.

References

Au PK (1991) Non-ionic contast media and intracatheter clot formation during use of a perfusion balloon catheter. Catheterization Cardiovasc Diagn 22:235–236

Bacal M, Gaudin C, Bourdier A, Bruneteau J, Buzzi JM, Golovanivsky KS, Hay L, Rouillé C (1996) A compact radiological X-ray source. Nature 384:421

Barrett BJ, Parfrey PS, Vavasour HM (1992) A comparison of nonionic, low-osmolality radiocontrast agents with ionic, high-osmolality agents during cardiac catheterization. N Eng J Med 326:431–436

Bashore TM, Davidson CJ, Mark DB (1988) Iopamidol use in the cardiac catheterization laboratory: a retrospective analysis of 3313 patients. Cardio 5:4–10

Benness GT (1988) Guidelines revisited. Australas Radiol 32:424–425

Bergelson B, Bettmann MA, Wexler L, Wilson R, Dyet J (1994) Comparison of iopromide with iohexol and iopamidol in coronary arteriography and left ventriculography. Invest Radiol 29:S107–S111

Bettmann MA (1989) Guidelines for use of low-osmolality contrast agents. Radiology 172:901–903

Bien S (1995) Iotrolan, a non-ionic dimeric contrast agent in cerebral angiography. Eur Radiol 5:S45–S48

Byrd L, Sherman RL (1979) Radiocontrast-induced acute renal failure. A clinical and pathophysiologic review. Medicine (Baltimore) 58:270–279

D'Elia JA, Glenson RE, Arday W, Malarick C, Godfrey K, Warran J (1982) Nephrotoxicity from angiographic contrast material. A prospective study. Am J Med 72:719–725

Dachman AH (1995) New contraindication to intravascular iodinated contrast material (Letter). Radiology 197:545

Davidson CJ, Mark DB, Pieper KS (1990) Thrombotic and cardiovascular complications related to non-ionic contrast media during cardiac catheterization: analysis of 8517 patients. Am J Cardiol 65:1481–1484

Dawson P, Hewitt P, Mackie IJ (1986) Contrast, coagulation, and fibrinolysis. Invest Radiol 21:248–252

Dawson P, Cousins C, Bradshaw A (1993) The clotting issue. Etiologic factors in thromboembolism. II. Clinical considerations. Invest Radiol 28(Suppl):S31–S36

Dilmanian FA, Wu XY, Parsons EC, Ren B, Kress J, Button TM, Chapman LD, Coderre JA, Gironi F, Greenberg D, Krus DJ, Liang Z, Marcovici S, Petersen MJ, Roque CT, Shleifer M, Slatkin DN, Thomlinson WC, Yamamoto K, Zhong Z (1997) Single- and dual-energy CT with monochromatic synchrotron x-rays. Phys Med Biol 42:371–387

Dix WR (1995) Intravenous coronary angiography with synchrotron radiation. Prog Biophys Mol Biol 63:159–191

Du Boulay GH, Wallis A (1986) Cerebral arterial constriction due to contrast media. Acta Radiol Suppl (Stockh) 369: 518–520

Dyet JF, Carter EC, Hartley WC (1990) Comparison of iopromide and iopamidol in left ventricular angiography and coronary angiography. Br J Radiol 63:700–705

Engelhart JA, Smith DC, Maloney MD, Westengard JC, Bull BS (1988) A technique for estimating the probability of clots in blood/contrast agent mixtures. Invest Radiol 23:923-927

Expert Meeting on Mechanism (1996) Delayed allergy-like reactions to X-ray contrast media. Insert in Eur Radiol 5(5)

Feldman RL, Jalowiec DA, Hill JA, Lambert CR (1988) contrast-media related complications during cardiac catheterization using Hexabrix or Renografin in high risk patients. Am J Cardiol 61:1334-1337

Gabriel DA, Jones MR, Reece NS (1991) Platelet and fibrin modification by radiographic contrast media. Circ Res 68:881-887

Gertz EW (1989) Thromboembolic events and non-ionic contrast. Diagn Imag 11:106-109

Grollman JH Jr, Liu CK, Astone RA, Lurie MD (1988) Thromboembolic complications in coronary angiography associated with the use of non-ionic contrast medium. Catheterization Cardiovasc Diagn 14:159-164

Hagen B, Klink G (1983) Contrast media and pain: hypotheses on the genesis of pain occurring on intra-arterial administration of contrast media. In: Taenzer V, Zeitler E (eds) Contrast media in urography, angiography and computerized tomography. Thieme, Stuttgart, pp 50-56

Hasckek E, Lindenthal TO (1896) Ein Beitrag zur praktischen Verwertung der Photographie nach Röntgen. Wien Klin Wochenschr 9:63-64

Hawkins IF Jr, Caridi JG (1995) CO2 digital subtraction arteriography – advantages and current solutions for delivery and imaging. Cardiovasc Intervent Radiol 18:150-152

Higgins CB (1985) Cardiotolerance of iohexol, a survey of experimental evidence. Invest Radiol 20:565-569

Hill JA, Grabowski EF (1992) Relationship of anticoagulation and radiographic contrast agents to thrombosis during coronary angiography and angioplasty: are there real concerns? Catheterization Cardiovasc Diagn 25:200-208

Hill JA, Winniford M, Van Fossen DB (1991) Nephrotoxicity following cardiac angiography: a randomized double-blind multicenter trial of ionic and non-ionic contrast media in 1194 patients. Circulation 84(Suppl 2):333

Hirshfeld JW Jr, Laskey W, Martin JL, Groh WC, Untereker W, Wolf GL (1983) Hemodynamic changes induced by cardiac angiography with ioxaglate: comparison with diatrizoate. Am J Cardiol 2:954-957

Hoffmeister HM, Heller W (1996) Radiographic contrast media and the coagulation and complement systems. Invest Radiol 31:591-595

Hwang MH, EN Piano A, Murdock DK (1989) The potential risk of thrombosis during coronary angiography using non-ionic contrast media. Catheterization Cardiovasc Diagn 16:209-213

Johnson LW, Lozner EC, Johnson S (1989) Coronary arteriography 1984-1987: a report of the Registry of the Society for Cardiac Angiography and Intervention. I. Results and complications. Catheterization Cardiovasc Diagn 17:5-10

Klinke WP, Grace M, Miller R, Naqvi SZ, Roth D, Roy L (1989) A multicenter randomized trial of ionic (ioxaglate) and nonionic (iopamidol) low-osmolality contrast agents in cardiac angiography. Clin Cardiol 12:689-696

Krause W (1994) Preclinical characterization of iopromide. Invest Radiol 29(Suppl 1):S21-S32

Krause W, Niehues D (1996) Biochemical characterization of X-ray contrast media. Invest Radiol 31:30-42

Krause W, Miklautz H, Kollenkirchen U, Heimann G (1994) Physicochemical parameters of X-ray contrast media. Invest Radiol 29:72-80

Langecker H, Harwart A, Junkmann K (1954) 3,5-Diacetylamino-2,4,6-trijodbenzoesäure als Röntgenkontrastmittel. Naunyn Schmiedebergs Arch Exp Pathol 222:584-590

Mason RA, Arbeit LA, Givon F (1985) Renal dysfunction after arteriography. JAMA 253:1001-1004

Missri J, Jeresaty RM (1990) Ventricular fibrillation during coronary angiography: reduced incidence with non-ionic contrast media. Catheterization Cardiovasc Diagn 19:4-7

Momose A, Takeda T, Itai Y, Hirano K (1996) Phase-contrast X-ray computed tomography for observing biological soft tissues. Nature [Medicine] 2:473-475

Morcos SK, Brown PWG, Oldroyd S, El Nahs AM, Haylor J (1995) Relationship between the diuretic effect of radiocontrast media and their ability to increase renal vascular resistance. Br J Radiol 68:850-853

Mori H, Hyodo K, Tanaka E, Uddin-Mohammed M, Yamakawa A, Shirozaki Y, Nakazawa H, Tanaka Y, Sekka T, Iwata Y, Handa S, Umetani K, Ueki H, Yokoyama T, Tanioka K, Kubota M, Hosaka H, Ishikawa N, Ando M (1996) Small-vessel radiography in situ with monochromatic synchrotron radiation. Radiology 201:173-177

Nakstad PH (1989) The reaction of cerebral arteries to non-ionic contrast media during cerebral angiography. Neuroradiology 31:247-249

Newhouse JH, Landman J, Lang E, Amis ES, Goldman S, Khazan R, Leder R, Hedgcock M (1994) Efficacy and safety of iopromide for excretory urography. Invest Radiol 29:S68-S73

Osborne ED, Sutherland CG, Scholl AF, Rowntree LG (1923) Roentgenography of urinary tract during excretion of sodium iodide. JAMA 80:368-373

Piao ZE, Murdock DK, Hwang MH, Raymond RM, Scanlon PJ (1988) Contrast media induced ventricular fibrillation: a comparison of Hypaque-76, Hexabrix and Omnipaque. Invest Radiol 23:466-470

Port KF, Wagoner RD, Fulter RE (1974) Acute renal failure after angiography. Am J Radiol 121:544-550

Raininko R, Rihelä M (1990) Blood clot formation in angiographic catheters – in vitro tests with various contrast media. Acta Radio 31:217-220

Rich MW, Crecelius CA (1990) Incidence, risk factors, and clinical course of acute renal insufficiency after cording catheterization in patients 70 years of age or older. A prospective study. Arch Intern Med 150:1237-1242

Ritchie JL, Nissen SE, Douglas JS et al. (1993) Use of nonionic or low osmolar contrast agents in cardiovascular procedures. J Am Coll Cardial 21:269-273

Robertson HJF (1987) Blood clot formation in angiographic syringes containing non-ionic contrast media. Radiology 162:621-622

Schräder R (1996) Thrombogenic potential of non-ionic contrast media – fact or fiction? Eur J Radiol 23(Suppl 1):S10-S13

Snigirev A, Kohn V, Snigireva I, Lengeler B (1996) A compound refractive lens for focusing high-energy X-rays. Nature 384:49-51

Stormorken H, Skalpe IO (1986) Effect of various contrast media on coagulation, fibrinolysis and platelet function: an in vitro and in vivo study. Invest Radiol 21:348-354

Stormorken H, Skalpe IO, Testart MC (1986) Effect of various contrast media on coagulation, fibrinolysis, and platelet function: an in vitro and in vivo study. Invest Radiol 21:348-354

Strickland NH, Rampling MW, Dawson P, Martin G (1992) Contrast-media induced effects on blood rheology and their importance in angiography. Clin Radiol 45:240-242

Ternel JL, Marcer R, Onaindia JM, Serano A, Quereda C, Ortuno J (1981) Renal function impairment caused by intravenous urography. Arch Intern Med 72:719-725

Van Rost D, Schramm J, Soymosi L, Hartmann A (1996) Presence and removal of arteriovenous malformation: impact of regional cerebral blood flow, as assessed with xenon/CT. Acta Neurol Scand Suppl 166:136–138

Wilkins SW, Gureyev TE, Gao D, Pogany A, Stevenson AW (1996) Phase-contrast imaging using polychromatic hard X-rays. Nature 384:335–338

Wilson AJ, Evill CA, Sage MR (1991) Effects of nonionic contrast media on the blood-brain barrier. Osmolality versus chemotoxicity. Invest Radiol 26:1091–1094

Wisneski JA, Gertz EW, Dahlgren M, Muslin A (1989) Comparison of low-osmolality ionic (ioxaglate) versus nonionic (iopamidol) contrast media in cardiac angiography. Am J Cardiol 63:489–495

Zwicker C, Langer M, Urich V, Felix R (1993) CT contrast administration of iodine, gadolinium and ytterbium. In-vitro studies and animal experiments. ROFO 158:255–259

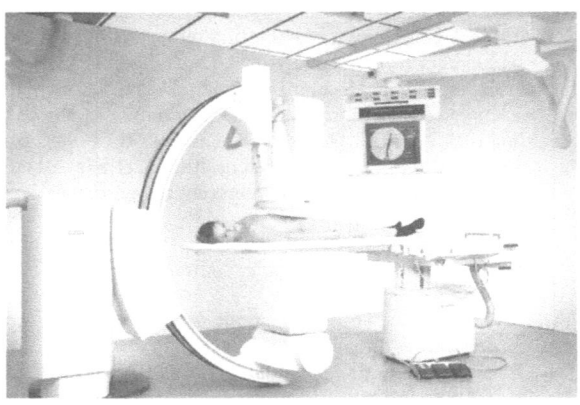

Fig. 8.34. Angiography system Angiostar Plus (Siemens, Erlangen, Germany)

8.5
Imaging Equipment

E. Ammann

8.5.1
The Imaging System

X-ray source, imaging detector, image presentation, and patient positioning are key issues in this section (Rosenbusch et al. 1995). Figure 8.34 shows an example of a special procedure room and Fig. 8.35 the room lay out. The principle scheme of how the system works is provided in Fig. 8.36.

The imaging system is a so-called closed loop or feed back system for both modes of operation: fluoroscopy to navigate catheters and recording of images as documentation, for clinical discussion and reviewing images. The X-ray source consists of the X-ray tube, the tube housing assembly, positive beam limitation and filtration, the X-ray generator with its control functions, and feedback systems for dose rate and exposure time.

The imaging detector depends on the purpose of the system because there are only a few systems dedicated to peripheral angiography. Most systems are tilting tables for radiography and fluoroscopy R/F tables; see Fig. 8.42) or special procedure rooms (see Figs. 8.34 and 8.40) with special components for peripheral angiography. Film-screen combination in cassettes or in film changers (see Sect. 8.5.2) were commonly applied where the quality of the image intensifier (II) and the digital imaging system was insufficient.

R/F tables with the table top in a horizontal position apply II systems with a spot film device (see Sect.

8.5.3). In addition, an AOT or a PUCK film changer (Siemens-Elema, Solna, Sweden) was positioned underneath the table top for peripheral angiography. Most special procedure rooms operate a C-arm system with a horizontal table top mounted on the floor (see Figs. 8.34 and 8.40) or suspended from the ceiling.

One end of the C-arm carries the X-ray tube housing assembly and the collimator. The II with the TV camera is installed on the other end of the C-arm. A PUCK film changer may be mounted on this end of the C-arm to be moved in front of the II for recording on film if the image processing system is not state-of-the-art with regard to image acquisition with a 1024 matrix. High resolution imaging systems including II, TV cameras, analog digital conversion (AD) and processing, display monitors, and archiving have reduced the application of film in daily routine. Several characteristics of a system depend on each other and will restrict application by their nature. These will be discussed in the following sections.

8.5.1.1
Shifting the Patient During Peripheral Angiography

A floating table top with a stepping device (see Sect. 8.5.5) is necessary. The connection to the injector for contrast media needs special attention for smooth operation because the connections to the injector head mounted on the table top will move or the catheter itself will move with the patient if the injector stands on the floor. The X-ray tube and image receptor remain in a fixed place. If a film changer is still used it should be besides the II used for fluoroscopy.

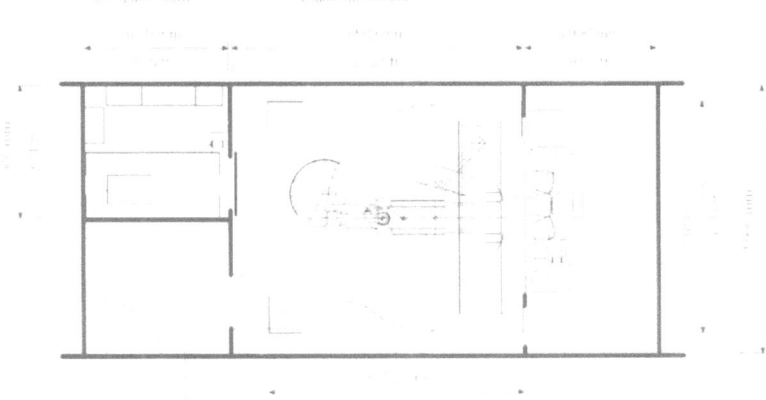

Fig. 8.35. Room layout for a general angiography system

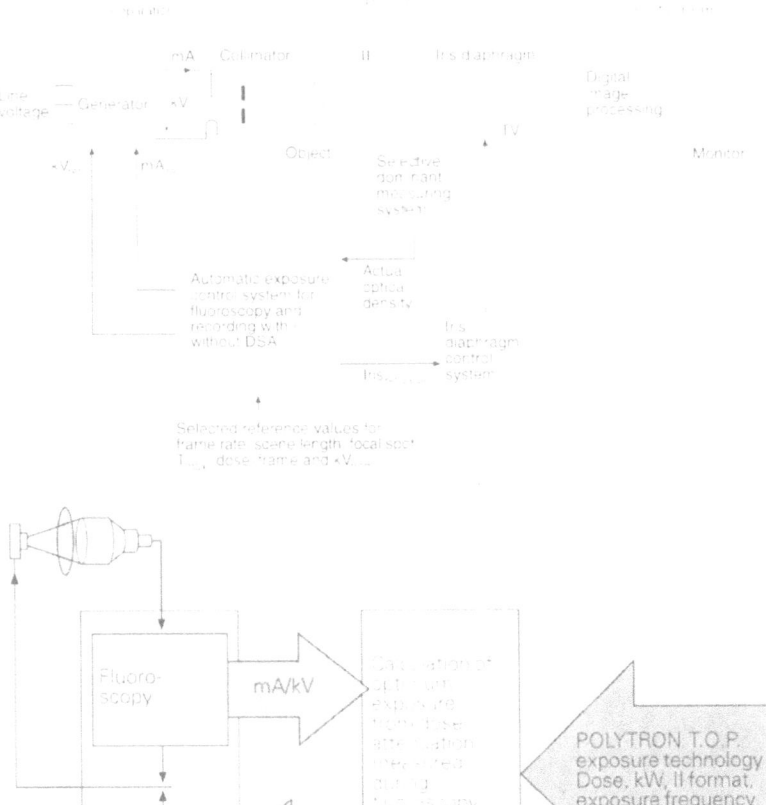

Fig. 8.36. Principle scheme (**a**) and automatic exposure control (**b**). *DSA*, digital subtraction angiography; *TOP*, time optimized process

8.5.1.2
Stationary Patient During Peripheral Angiography and Shifting Imaging Equipment

This is more comfortable for both the patient and the medical team as all critical parts, including the injector, remain in place during the examination. A system for diagnosis and intervention needs to provide instant images and appropriate means of radiation protection, particularly for the medical team.

Healthcare economics force many institutions to study and treat peripheral vessels in multi-purpose rooms as there are not enough patients for imaging equipment dedicated to peripheral angiography alone. The amount of contrast media necessary varies with different imaging equipment. Peri-scanning and Perivision (Siemens, Erlangen, Germany) (see SECT. 8.5.5) will bring the cost of contrast media down.

8.5.1.3
Some Criteria for Imaging Equipment to be Considered

- Free access to the patient during any procedure (Fig. 8.37), especially from the patient's right- and left-hand side and in unexpected emergencies.
- Examination parameters easy to control both from the bedside, as well as in the control room. Auto-calibration (Fig. 8.38), on-line display of calculated values (i.e., quantitative evaluation of the size of a vessel), and adjustment of X-ray field size without radiation (WAGGERSHAUSER 1996) (i.e., CARE, combined application to reduce exposure; Fig. 8.39).
- Dose reduction (BRASSEL 1992; HERRMANN et al. 1994) with variable filters, digital pulsed fluoroscopy (3–15 p/s), high contrast and high resolution monitors with 1-k or 2-k matrix (MERTELMEIER and KUHN 1996).
- Image receptor size of 30–40 cm.
- On-line subtraction with and without landmarking which shows some anatomical background.
- Turn-key operation should be possible, especially in emergency situations using actual date and time in addition to patient identification.
- Fluoroscopy should be possible during post-processing in the control room without an additional work station.
- Roadmap (see Fig. 8.41) with maximum opacification.
- Indication and recording of the dose area product for each procedure (take care to note whether values are compared between different systems since they are indicated either in $Gycm^2$ or $cGycm^2$).
- Digital images should be transferable in Dicom standard (MORNEBURG 1995) to a network, i.e., Sienet (Siemens, Erlangen, Germany) work station (HRUBY et al. 1994; DE SILVA 1996), digital archive, or laser camera.
- Injector interface to the X-ray system.
- Automatic protection to avoid collisions during positioning and operation.
- Patient positioning should provide a longitudinal range of the table top of more than 120 cm. A swivel range of the table top of at least +/- 30 degrees is helpful when angiographies of the

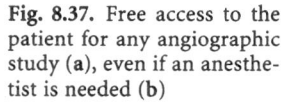

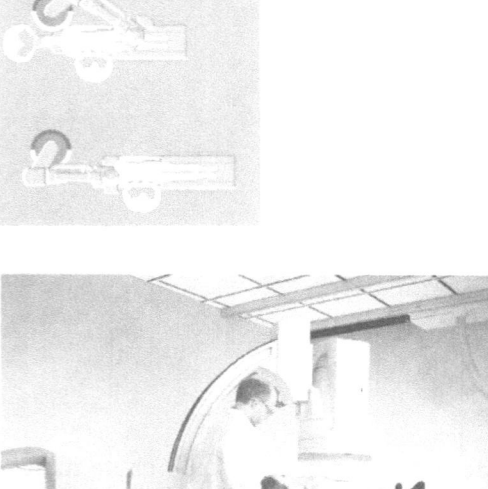

Fig. 8.37. Free access to the patient for any angiographic study (**a**), even if an anesthetist is needed (**b**)

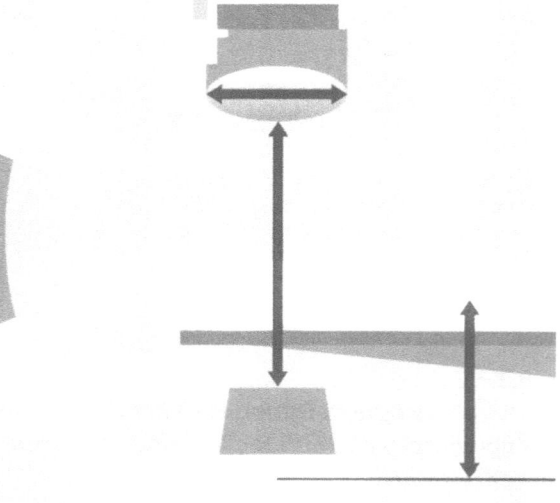

Fig. 8.38. Auto-calibration supports the calibration process for actual values of distances

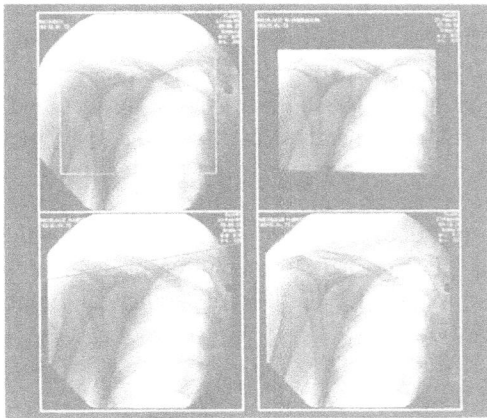

Fig. 8.39. Collimation of the X-ray beam is set without radiation automatically to the position of an electronic shutter marked on the TV monitor

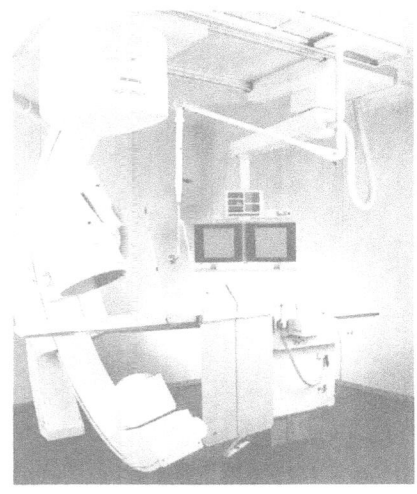

Fig. 8.40. Radiation protection for the medical team (Multistar T.O.P., Siemens)

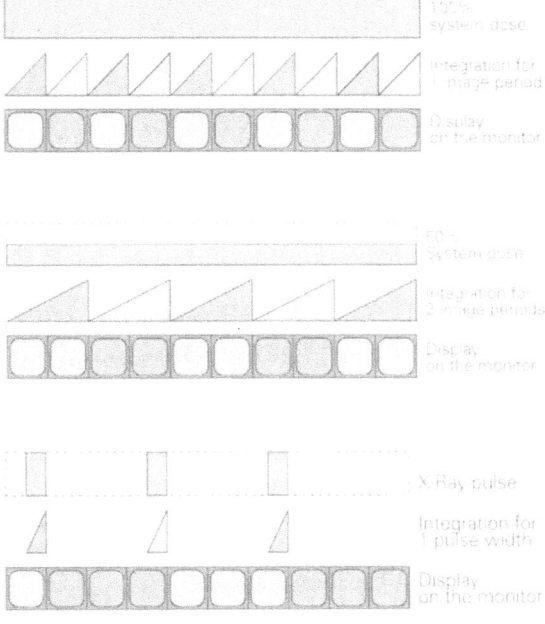

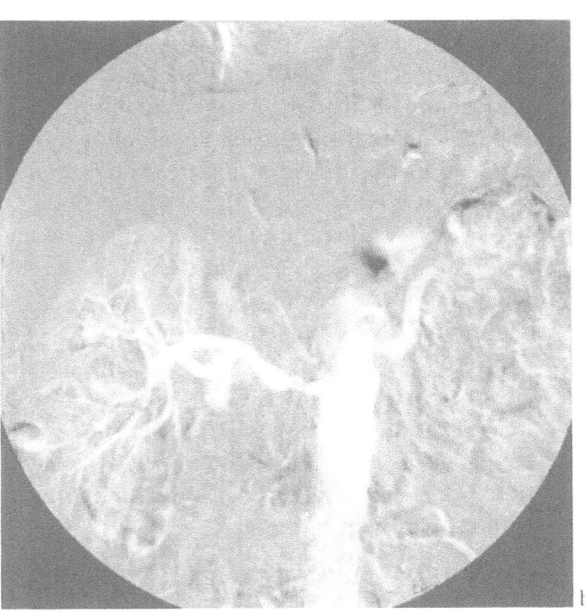

Fig. 8.41 a,b. Fluoroscopy. Continuously (a) Supervision for dose reduction without compromising image quality for slow moving objects (b), pulsed fluoroscopy for fast moving objects (c), and Roadmapping (d), the classic guiding tool for applications on non-moving vessels, i.e., skull extremities. (Courtesy of J. Seissl, Siemens, Erlangen, Germany. The reproduction shows a mediocre image quality compared to the original monitor image)

upper extremities are performed, or in case of emergencies to provide even better access to the patient.

– TV monitors should be ceiling-suspended, positioned in the foot range of the patient and swiveled to a comfortable position for the radiologist (see Figs. 8.34 and 8.40).

– A ceiling-mounted spotlight is very useful in a special procedures room.

– Additional radiation protection gear for the medical team (Fig. 8.40) (see also Sect. 8.6).

– A so-called combi-lab should be considered if other applications need to be performed in the same room (up to 30 frames per second for cardiac imaging or a tiltable table top (see Fig. 8.42) for neuroradiological applications like myelograms).

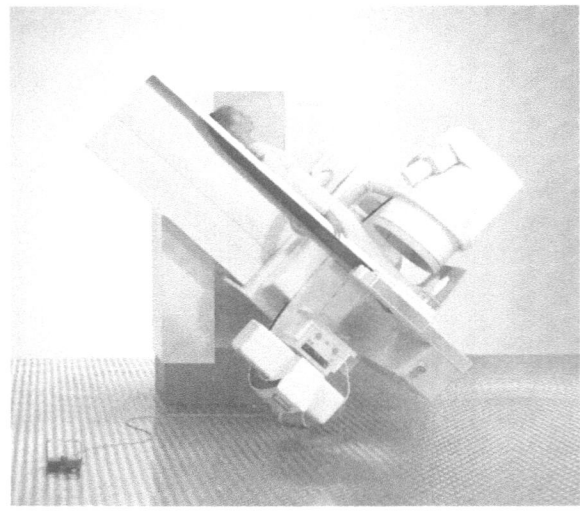

Fig. 8.42. Radiography and Fluoroscopy (R/F) table Polystar with a 40-cm image intensifier for fluoroscopy and digital spot filming. Angiographic and interventional procedures can also be performed

- The collimator and TV camera should automatically rotate so that the image remains correctly collimated and displayed on the monitor if the C-arm can be positioned at different angles on the right- or left-hand side of the patient.
- Free access to the head of the patient for an anesthetist is necessary if indicated (i.e., cerebral angiography; see Fig. 8.37b).
- The controls for II movement along the axis of the central X-ray beam is essential to bring the II as close as possible to the patient or further away for magnification techniques. This control function should be positioned directly at the II and an additional one should be on hand for a remote controlled operation.

8.5.1.4
X-Ray Tube

Filament wear, condensed metal vapor on the tube window, the condition of vacuum (arcing) and bearings influence the lifetime of a X-ray tube. It should be expected to last for the examination of about 1500 patients in a special-procedures room. Regulations determine maximum values of radiation leakage.

The delay time to switch back and forth from fluoroscopy mode to recording mode depends mainly on the inertia of the filament temperature. High speed starters or other system parameters in a spot film device, film changer, or digital imaging system may

increase the delay time. Less than 1.5 s should be expected. A focal spot (STANDARD IEC 1993) of 0.6 at 40 kW and 1.0 at 80 kW with a 12-degree anode angle for up to 40-cm field size should be installed. The heat storage capacity (STANDARD IEC 1989) of about 1.0 MJ is necessary to provide uninterrupted examinations at high patient throughput.

Auto-focus is a state-of-the-art is mode which automatically provides the smallest focal spot depending on contrast, patient transparency, and temporal resolution.

8.5.1.5
X-Ray Generator and Automatic Exposure Control System (AEC)

High frequency generators (AMMANN 1994) of up to 80-kW output with independent closed loop control systems for kilovolt (contrast), Milliampere (intensity), and Milliampere second or exposure time are applied. The continuous output should be at least 1 kW to perform uninterrupted interventional procedures.

8.5.1.6
The AEC System

This system, like the Angiomatic (Siemens, Erlangen, Germany) (see Fig. 8.37b), should provide a closed loop system for dose rate and optional selection of the measuring fields depending on the position of the dominant area of the extremities. The sensor will be an ionization chamber in the spot film device (see Sect. 8.5.3) and on the AOT film changer or a semiconductor behind the film screen combination in the PUCK film changer.

The exposure time should not exceed 100 ms as a displacement velocity of 2 mm/s in peripheral vessels due to pain or uncooperative patients needs to be considered.

Older systems without a digital system may still be in use. They were equipped with a Kilovolt (or Milliampere second) reduction device. The exposure Kilovolt value was reduced step by step to adapt image contrast and to avoid overexposure in peripheral film changer angiography depending on the anatomical position between pelvis and foot. This reduction of the kilovolt value was pre-set for each step by the technician. Today, a good AEC system (i.e., Angiomatic) does this automatically during the procedure, maintaining an optimum contrast. The K-edge for iodine is 33.2 keV (ARNOLD and EISENBERG

1979); therefore, values of around 63 kV are applied to achieve a good iodine contrast for the image. Peripheral angiography systems are usually equipped with an II-TV system providing fluoroscopy to visually control the navigation of the guidewire and catheter. A dose rate control circuitry as part of the AEC system (see Fig. 8.36) provides an instant image at a desired and pre-set contrast level. A last image hold (LIH) function reduces dose to the patient and medical staff. A further reduction in dose is highly recommended by applying Supervision (Siemens, Erlangen, Germany) (see Sect. 8.5.5) and/or digital pulsed fluoroscopy with a pulse rate of 3–15 X-ray pulses per second (Fig. 8.41).

A Remote-Diagnostics Capability. within the X-ray system is highly recommended. It increases up-time and reduces maintenance and service costs.

8.5.2
Film Changer

Due to the outstanding quality of digital imaging systems, i.e., POLYTRON (Siemens, Erlangen, Germany) which was developed in 1987, practically no film changers have been sold and installed in Europe in previous years. However, an image recorded on a film-screen combination is still superior to any digital image with regard to spatial resolution only. The silver halide crystal suspended in gelatin produces 10^9 atoms of silver in a grain of less than 1 mm in diameter when a few light photons have been absorbed (WAYRYNEN 1979).

The spatial resolution in a film changer system is therefore limited by the speed of the screen (unsharpness of film-screen combination), exposure time of the generator (motion blurring), and by the focal spot size in combination with the geometry of patient positioning and source image distance (SID/magnification factor) leading to the unsharpness of the geometry.

A long-leg cassette changer may be applied in special procedure rooms for peripheral angiography only (ZEITLER 1995). The film size measures 4×35 cm in length by 35 cm in width. The typical dose per image is 1.75 µGy and for the hole runoff 7 µGy. An optical film subtraction technique could be applied; however, this was not necessary if enough contrast medium had been injected.

General R/F rooms are used in many institutions to perform diagnostic peripheral angiography. The so-called AOT with a film magazine for 35×35 cm cut films is operated at one or two frames per second for peripheral studies. It has also been applied for general angiography, including cardiac imaging at frame rates of up to six per second, but, has been out of production for several years. Today, a highresolution digital imaging system is state-of-the-art.

The PUCK film changer (Siemens–Elema, Erlangen, Germany) (two frames per second and later four frames per second) was later integrated into remote controlled R/F tables for peripheral diagnostic studies. The C-arm was introduced in special procedure rooms in 1977 (i.e., Angioscop, Siemens-Elema, Solna, Sweden) (ROSENBUSCH et al. 1995). The PUCK 90M changer uses 35-cm cut films in the magazine and since 1991 can easily be moved by remote control in front of the II and be operated above or below the patient in a see-through technique. The see-through technique enables viewing of the runoff even before the films are developed. In changing the system from fluoroscopy to PUCK operation, the SID should be maintained. These are important features to reduce examination time; however, not all manufacturers provide them.

A remote controlled shift of the PUCK in and out of the central beam axis is highly recommended for a smooth examination. Some manufacturers provide only manual handling of the PUCK positioning. It can be dangerous to the patient and should be avoided.

The theoretical spatial resolution due to geometric unsharpness alone can be up to 3.5 line pairs (lp)/mm with a large focal spot (STANDARD IEC 1993) of 1.0, and up to 6.0 lp/mm with a small focal spot of 0.6 in a film changer system. A typical dose value per image in a film changer is 1.75 µGy, for the hole runoff about 18 µGy.

Any R/F system with a film changer requires a stepping device for the table top. It needs to be programmed before the start of a peripheral angiography. The speed of the injected contrast medium varies depending on the condition of the vessels. If not properly predicted and programmed the study has to be repeated, meaning additional contrast medium and radiation exposure.

A publication (LEVY 1993) favoring a C-arm with II and PUCK changer indicated that the PUCK was preferred for some studies of pulmonary and renal angiography and gastrointestinal bleeding. A state-of-the-art digital imaging system with the capability of acquiring, processing, and displaying images in a 1024 matrix (i.e., Polytron, which has been on the market since 1987), will certainly have an impact on Levy's conclusion.

Capital investment should be directed rather to non-invasive technologies such as Magnetic resonance angiography (MRA) and new ultrasound image acquisition and presentation techniques (SieScape, Siemens, Erlangen, Germany) than to film changers for diagnostic indications. Interventional procedures require digital angiography and digital subtraction angiography (DSA), including dose reduction means like CARE (see Fig. 8.44) with Perivision (see Fig. 8.46) and adaptive filter capability (see Fig. 8.43).

8.5.3
Image Intensifier and Spot Film Device

X-ray systems with an II and a spot film device are designed as tilting tables with the X-ray tube installed either underneath or above the table top. A multi-purpose remotely controlled R/F table is shown in Fig. 8.42.

Lymphography and phlebography (ALBERS and SCHEEL 1994; SIGMUND and GROOTHOFF 1996) are usually performed on an R/F table with a spot film device. Cassettes are used if digital angiography (DA) or DSA are not available. The cassette is loaded with a film-screen combination or a reusable storage phosphor screen. There are several different terms in use for them such as computed radiography (CR) based on the so-called Fuji system (KATO et al. 1985) or digital luminescence radiography (DLR). This technique is an alternative to DA (see Sect. 8.5.4). Both provide the advantage that all acquired images are digitally archived and therefore provide improved communication capabilities besides being cost effective.

The optical density in a DLR system is strictly linear and proportional to the logarithm of radiation dose. This is a superior property compared to the optical film density (OFD) of a film-screen combination. Its γ value varies from zero at low radiation dose and the fog area to the useful range between 0.3 and 2.5 in OFD. Above that range, the γ value decreases again to zero and becomes a negative value at even higher dose values. The reference dose value set for the AEC system is determined by the speed of the screens and the film processing equipment. An average OFD = 1.0 is recommended to be achieved by the set reference dose value. For DLR systems, the reference dose level should be set as low as possible accepting a specific noise level in the image. Underexposed images contain a higher noise level but may still be acceptable for diagnosis. Overexposed images contain less noise, however, overradiate the patient without improving diagnostic information. Therefore, all DLR applications in a spot film device should be performed with the automatic exposure control system.

The spot film device has to be equipped with an AEC system. The X-ray generator should provide an automatic kilovolt setting (see Fig. 8.36) out of the information on patient transparency during fluoroscopy to achieve the best contrast in the image (i.e., Polymatic).

Image quality can be further improved by using a high-line stationary grid designed in carbon fiber technology (AICHINGER et al. 1992). Spot film

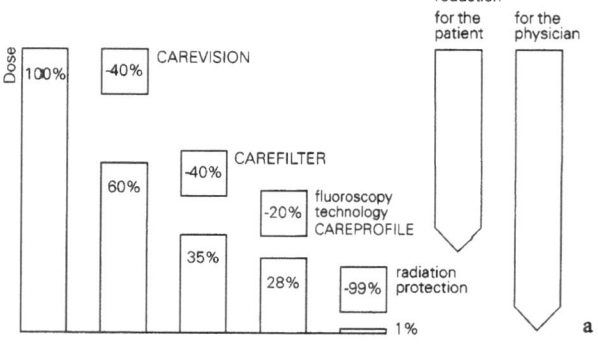

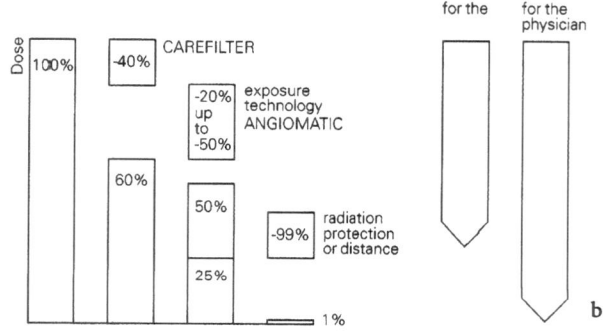

Fig. 8.44. Achievable reduction in radiation exposure by applying all available means in fluoroscopy (a) and recording (b). II, image intensifier

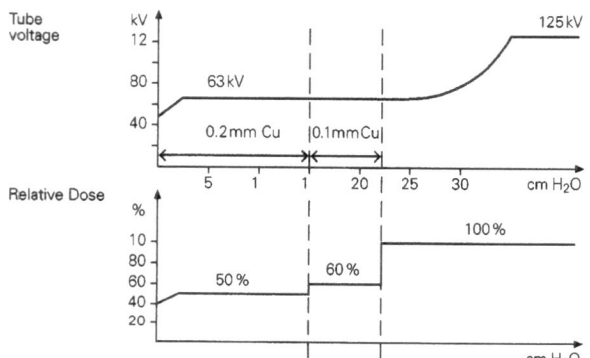

Fig. 8.43. Adaptive dose filter to reduce dose as part of CARE (combined applications to reduce exposure)

devices operate with a 30-cm II (a smaller or larger II is quite common) with zoom capability (see Table 8.13). The TV system should present the images on a high contrast and high resolution Siemomed monitor (Siemens, Erlangen, Germany) (MERTELMEIER and KUHN 1996).

8.5.3.1
The Entrance Dose Rate to the Image Intersifier

This should always be adjusted to the manufacturer's specification. It normally allows a range so that the physician can select dose rate and/or dose per image in accordance with the medical indication. Values should be recorded during acceptance testing and handed out to the user. These values should be verified at least once a year, recorded and compared with the original values. Deviations should be corrected by service engineers authorized by the manufacturer. If only higher dose levels provide acceptable image quality specific parts like the II, TV system, monitors, etc., need to be replaced, even if they are still working. (See also Sect. 8.6.)

8.5.3.2
Zoom Operation

Zoom operation in accordance with the as-low-as-reasonably-achievable (ALARA) principle (ICRP REPORT 1977) means that the II input size will be adapted to the physical size of the object examined. It is important that the entrance dose (cGycm^2) to the patient and the noise level (signal-to-noise ratio) stay constant in order to achieve the appropriate image quality. This requires a constant number of photons per mm^2 (i.e., 250) leading to different dose rates at the II input screen as shown in Table 8.13. If the dose rate is not automatically properly adjusted the patient receives a higher entrance exposure unnecessarily, or the image contains more noise.

8.5.4
Digital Subtraction Angiography and Digital Angiography

Contrast agents containing iodine (K-edge at 33.2 keV) enhances the contrast in vessels. As they are important for diagnosis or intervention, morphological details superimposed onto the vessels can be eliminated from the image by subtraction of a mask image from an image where vessels are filled with contrast medium. This technique, known as DSA (KRESTEL 1990; ROSENBUSCH et al. 1995), provides several advantages to the patient and to the medical staff. Intraarterial injection of contrast medium in a DSA application requires less contrast medium than film angiography. Also, immediate display of the image shortens examination time.

The X-ray generator needs to keep the kV value within far less then 1 kV to avoid subtraction artifacts (AMMANN 1994), which should not be confused with landmarking; this means, filling in anatomical/morphological information for better orientation in a subtracted image showing only the vascular structure.

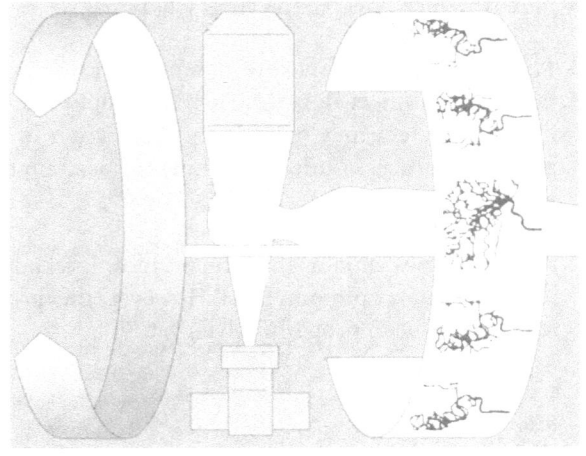

Fig. 8.45. Rotational angiography with Dynavision

Table 8.13. Dose rate and spatial resolution as a function of the image intensifier (II) zoom format for a constant number of photons (i.e., 250) per mm^2

II input screen diameter in cm	40	28	20	14 (17)
II input screen area in cm^2	1.200	600	300	150
II input screen dose rate in µG/s	0.15	0.3	0.6	1.2
Spatial resolution in line pairs/mm	1.8	2.6	3.6	4.8
Magnification factor M = 1.4, 1024 Matrix, focus 0.6				(4.2)

8.5.4.1
Overlay Fading

This has been provided in fluoroscopy operation. Anatomical background information or a reference scene can be faded in or out for optimum viewing using digital images over live fluoroscopy. This reduces the amount of contrast medium, radiation, and examination time.

8.5.4.2
Matrix Size

The image should be acquired with a matrix size of 1024 × 1024 pixels and converted in an analog digital device (AD converter) with at least 10-bit depth equivalent to 1024 gray levels. Pulsed X-ray operation for recording and even in fluoroscopy (see Fig. 8.41c) should be possible for peripheral diagnostic and interventional procedures. Between, three and 15 frames per second are necessary in fluoroscopy. The DSA operation has the advantage of recording up to six frames per second instead of the four frames per second with the PUCK film changer. To improve image quality, image integration techniques reduce noise in the subtracted image.

Pixel Shift. corrects most of the motion artifacts in the image (BURR et al. 1990). This can be done manually or a system may provide this correction in an automatic process (auto pixel shift) to speed up the whole procedure.

Auto Window. should adjust the window level automatically to an optimum level. However, this problem has not been properly solved yet.

8.5.4.3
Siemomed Monitor (Siemens, Erlangen, Germany)

This TV monitor (MERTELMEIER and KUHN 1996) with a diagonal measure of 54 cm, a light intensity of 500 cd/m², and with a 120-Hz repetition rate to avoid flicker and jitter should be used in DSA applications. Brightness and contrast should be automatically controlled by a sensor for the room light intensity. Acquisition of 1024 × 1024 matrix including postprocessing and display of this matrix size for fluoroscopy and recording is standard. A reference image or even scene during the intervention can be displayed on one single monitor in split screen tech-

nique instead of using a second monitor. Alternatively, overlay fading and Roadmap (Fig. 8.41d) modes are useful.

8.5.4.4
The AEC System

This system has to provide an easy operation in an automatic mode (AMMANN 1994), like the Digimatic or Angiomatic, to achieve an error-free optimum in image quality. The automatic exposure control system has to operate without any test exposures because regular fluoroscopy to navigate the catheter holds all the information needed for a DSA study.

Quantitative Analysis. and post processing methods improve the information content of images for the physician. Measurement of distances, angles, and grade of stenosis can be performed, preferably in an auto calibration mode (see Fig. 8.38).

The Measuring Fields. should be displayed on the monitor for a short period of time only to control their position if they are changed to match the dominant area of the object.

Scene Compare. This is very convenient to compare a dynamic pre- and post-dilatation study side-by-side on the very same monitor.

8.5.4.5
Dose Considerations (see also Sect. 8.6)

Additional filtration of the X-ray beam with copper (Fig. 8.43) reduces radiation exposure by up to 50% if applied as a so-called adaptive dose filter (ADF.)

Wedge-shaped filters and finger filters are applied in the collimation system for peripheral DSA or DA to attenuate direct radiation at the edge of the body and between patient's legs. They are automatically adjusted depending on the position of the Multistar time optimized process (T.O.P.) X-ray system (Siemens, Erlangen, Germany) (HERRMANN et al. 1994).

DSA in a generic procedure without special means to reduce radiation exposure require about 150 μGy (up to 200 μGy) per study. Many DSA systems operate on radiation dose rate levels which are not in accordance with the ALARA principle (ICRP REPORT 1977). Ignorance or economic reasons are the cause of this because out-dated components in a DSA system would need a better replacement. Therefore, there is the need to reduce radiation exposure (VANO et al. 1995) to the patient and medical staff by several means such as CARE shown in Fig. 8.44.

Particularly during interventional procedures erythema occurred. The Siemens CARE Watch with Diamentor indicates, in the examination room, the skin dose exposure rate in mGy/min during fluoroscopy and the accumulated skin dose as a percentage of a configured limit skin dose level of, i.e., 2 Gy. At increasing skin dose values, the physician can take several measures to reduce the dose rate (i.e., 3 pulses/s) and he can change the direction of the projection. This feature is especially important when children and young adults are examined to reduce the risk of carcinoma induced by excessive radiation. A print-out of every examination, such as a DSA-Log, should be installed in every system.

8.5.4.6
Digital Angiography

DA applies to the same operation but without subtraction. As IIs and digital imaging systems produce good image contrast with sufficient spatial resolution for most indications, the method of acquiring DA images is an alternative for selected studies only if on-line digital subtraction images are not available. Another indication is in areas with severe motion artifacts, as in cardiology.

8.5.5
Shifting of Patient or Stationary Patient and Modes of Operation

The stationary patient (FINK et al. 1990; PEENE et al. 1991) on the table top with a shifting imaging system has several advantages: Positioning can be achieved to less than 1-mm accuracy. The injector for the contrast medium and the catheter remain stationary during the whole procedure. The size of each step can be selected individually with on-line viewing of the flow of contrast medium. The physician has access to both sides of the patient.

A long-leg display (see Fig. 8.46c) should be available within 10 s. The collimator leaves (see Fig. 8.39) and filters (see Fig. 8.43) should be adjusted for every step on a last image hold image without radiation (WAGGERSHAUSER 1996). This reduces radiation exposure to the patient and medical staff. The position of the TV camera and the collimator depend on the

position of the C-arm. They should rotate automatically into the correct position to provide appropriate patient position on the TV monitor for the medical staff.

8.5.5.1
Modes of Operation

To retrieve diagnostic information on vessel structures, non-invasive methods should be considered before applying X-rays: ultrasound in panoramic view (SieScape) or MRA. These methods should also be considered for follow-up studies instead of X-rays.

Interventions require immediate access to good images; therefore, angiography is indicated. Table 8.14 shows a comparison of different examination techniques with X-rays in angiography.

Fluoroscopy is one specific mode for angiography. Edge enhancement is sometimes applied; however, there is the risk of artifacts. Digital pulsed

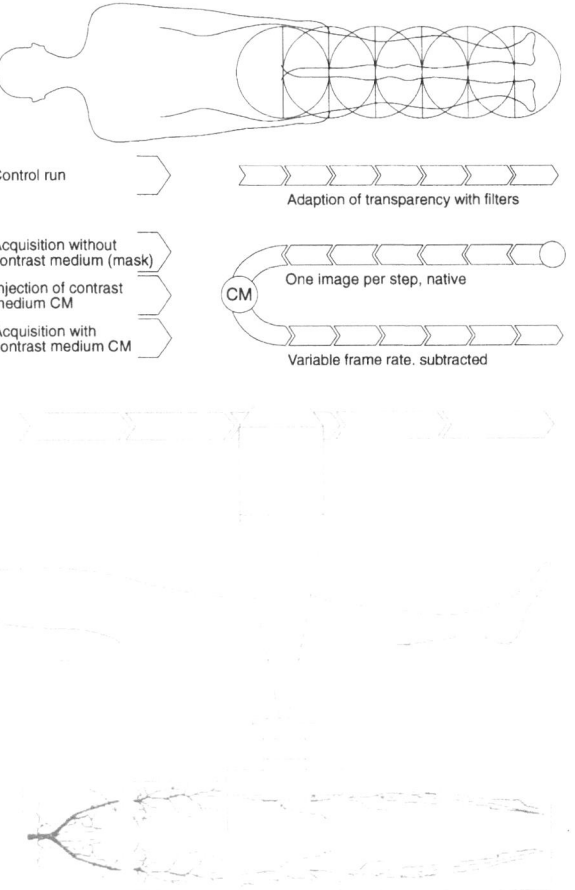

Fig. 8.46 a–c. Perivision. a Examination steps, b stepping imaging system in automatic exposure control mode without any test exposures necessary, and c "long-leg" display

Table 8.14. Comparison of different examination techniques using X-rays

Criteria	Perivision	DSA	DA	Filmchanger
Diagnostic information on vessels	+	+	O	O
Amount of contrast medium per study	+	O	O	O
Examination time per study	+	+	O	-
Immediate access to images	O	O	O	-

DSA, digital subtraction angiography; DA, digital angiography.
+, Superior; O, acceptable; -, inferior.

fluoroscopy with gap filling is known from cardiological procedures to reduce the dose to both patient and operator.

Roadmapping (see Fig. 8.41d) is the classic guiding tool if a vessel does not move (skull and extremities). Contrast medium is injected for a short test and the acquired image is stored as a mask. This mask is then subtracted from the ongoing live fluoro-image. The image on the TV monitor shows the vessel tree – normally displayed in white – and the advancing guidewire in black. Another alternative to Roadmapping is overlay fading.

For very slow moving vessels, Supervision (Siemens, Erlangen, Germany) (BRASSEL et al. 1992), shown in Fig. 8.41 can reduce radiation exposure by up to 50% and, combined with filtering the X-ray beam, by up to 70% without sacrificing image quality. Supervision integrates two TV images acquired at half the dose rate in fluoroscopy.

Rotational angiography, like Dynavision (Siemens, Erlangen, Germany) (MORNEBURG 1995) shown in Fig. 8.45, is the method used to look around the vessel lesion to determine the best projection for treatment. Dynavision provides DSA studies with one single injection of contrast medium, thus speeding up examination time.

Perivision (Siemens, Erlangen, Germany) (FINK et al. 1990) was designed for the stationary patient and a stepping imaging system (Fig. 8.46). Only one single injection of contrast medium is necessary to monitor the flow of contrast medium in an on-line DSA image. This reduces the amount of contrast medium. Subtracted Perivision images are assembled to a long-leg display without a separate workstation using the maximum opacification Auto Max Fill shown in Fig. 8.47. Perivision does not need a manually operated kV-reduction device. It requires less than half the examination time of any other method, can apply variable frame rates, and uses low radiation levels.

Bolus chasing and Peri-scanning (PEENE et al. 1991) are other methods of acquiring images. How-

ever, dose requirements in both systems are quite different and significant because there are many images necessary to chase the bolus of the contrast medium in the vessels. The bolus-chasing mode runs on a rather high radiation level compared to the Siemens Peri-scanning mode requiring about 30 μGy. The patient is shifted continuously through the X-ray beam of the imaging system in the bolus-chasing mode acquiring DA images which can later be subtracted if mask images have been acquired in advance. In the Peri-scanning mode of a Multistar T.O.P., however, the imaging system is shifted along the peripheral extremities of the stationary patient. Both modes are inferior to Perivision (Fig. 8.46).

The longitudinal range of the table top should be at least 120 cm. This allows a flexible positioning of the patient with free access. It should be possible to examine a patient from top to toe since most angiography equipment is also used for general angiography. Angiographies of the upper extremities are easier to perform if the table can be swiveled a few degrees to the left or to the right. Swiveling the table may also be helpful in cases of emergency.

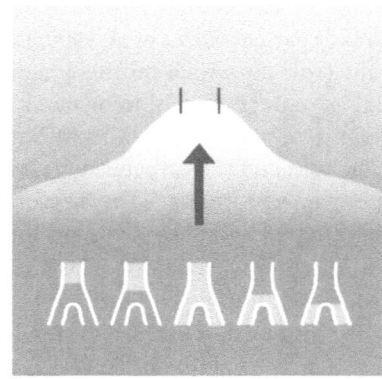

Fig. 8.47 a,b. Auto Max Fill provides the digital subtraction angiography image with maximum opacification for every step. Each image is automatically added to the "long-leg" display of Perivision

8.5.6
Spatial Resolution and Contrast

Can a vessel with a diameter smaller than the pixel size of the digital system be imaged? The answer is definitely "yes" if there is enough contrast in the vessel. However, such small vessels are not correctly reproduced. The limitation to measure the size of a vessel is given by the line spread function of the total imaging system (focal spot, geometry, distortion, AD conversion, etc.). With a 1024-matrix imaging system (real acquisition, processing, and display such as the Polytron which has been on the market since 1987) a vessel of one third of a millimeter in diameter can only be measured under almost ideal conditions (see Table 8.13). This is about equivalent to an image acquired with a film changer if normal examination conditions with a patient are applied. However, digital images acquired with an II-TV system can provide more contrast.

8.5.6.1
Spatial Resolution

The spatial resolution (HIGH 1994) is influenced by the real focal spot size, the geometric magnification, the II input size, the TV system resolution, and the matrix size. High contrast spatial resolution in line pairs per mm (lp/mm) due to the focal spot can be approximated by

where F is the measured focal spot size in mm and m is the geometric magnification. An example shows for a nominal focus of 0.6 and a magnification of 1.4 that the spatial resolution $R_F = 2.9 \, lp/mm$. This represents the dimension of a lead strip of 0.17 mm.

The spatial resolution of the display matrix in lp/mm can be calculated to

where M is the matrix size, m the geometric magnification, and D the useful II input diameter in mm. As an example of a 1024-matrix size and the same magnification of 1.4 as above, the highest spatial resolution can be achieved with a D = 14-cm zoom format of the II to $R_D = 5.12 \, lp/mm$.

The spatial resolution of the TV chain in the vertical direction in lp/mm can be calculated to

where S is the nominal number of TV scan lines (525/1049 in 60-Hz systems and 625/1249 in 50-Hz systems), a is the fraction of scan lines active in image formation ($\approx$0.91), K is the Kell factor ($\approx$ 0.7), m the geometric magnification, and D the useful II input diameter in mm. Taking the above example of a 50-Hz high resolution TV system with 1249 lines and m of 1.4 and D of 14 cm, the highest spatial resolution can be achieved to $R_{TV} = 3.98 \, lp/mm$.

Comparing $R_F = 2.9 \, lp/mm$, $R_D = 5.12 \, lp/mm$, and $R_{TV} = 3.98 \, lp/mm$, it is obvious that the focus is the limiting factor and, therefore, the spatial resolution in an image of the film changer will not show a better result than that of a state-of-the-art digital system available since 1987. However, a spatial resolution of $R_F = 5 \, lp/mm$ can be achieved on film with a 0.2 focus and a magnification of 2.0 if there is sufficient contrast in a vessel.

8.5.6.2
Contrast

Contrast (MORNEBURG 1995) depends on the iodine concentration and many other system and object parameters.

Contrast at low spatial frequencies of an II is influenced by veiling glare. A typical value is 20:1 measured with the International Commission on Radiation Units and Measurements (ICRU) radiation and a lead disk on the II input screen. The disk area should be 10% of the II input area used.

The low contrast performance of a properly adjusted system is determined by acquiring images of larger vessels of different sizes and iodine concentrations. The relationship between these parameters can be expressed by the following equation: "Contrast times object diameter times square root of dose is constant". Reproducibility of X-ray tube voltage (kV) is of the utmost importance to avoid structural artifacts in a digitally subtracted image (AMMANN 1994).

8.5.6.3
Windowing

Windowing is used to narrow down the range of contrast provided to emphasize more clearly details with low contrast. The average human eye is capable of perceiving about 35 gray levels only; however, a digital system operating at 10 (12) bits depth provides 2048 (4096) gray levels. A narrow window is set at a specific gray level (called center) and amplified to the full range of luminance at the TV monitor from black to white. All other gray levels beyond the window are shown either white for above the window or black for below the window. This feature makes digital technology superior to film.

8.5.7
Cine and Telecommunication

8.5.7.1
Cine

Filming in cine mode requires a cine camera (ARRI Munich, Germany), a control unit, special film processing units, a cine projector for viewing, and archiving space for the film rolls. In daily routine, cine film is used only in some diagnostic applications in cardiology with a frame rate of up to 30 images per second for adults and up to 60 frames per second in pediatric cardiology.

Interventions require an instant image sequence. This can be provided only in the digital cine mode. The image quality of digital cine is sufficient nowadays even for many diagnostic procedures. In particular, so-called combi labs will provide a digital cine mode. A typical value of 220 nGy per image at the II input screen (17 cm) is a standard adjustment at 80 kV. There should also be a low dose mode with 100 nGy per image available. Several advantages are offered by this mode if a somewhat noisier image can be accepted: (a) Patient dose is reduced to 50% of the standard settings; (b) as only half the tube load is required, a smaller focus can be selected providing a higher spatial resolution; (c) a 0.2-mm Cu filter in the primary beam will reduce patient dose to 25% compared to standard cine. However, this filter requires more tube output (large focal spot).

8.5.7.2
Telecommunication

The biggest advantage of a digital system is the instant availability of examination results. Most postprocessing functions are displayed on-line in the examination room and no longer require separate workstations (depending on the manufacturer). This reduces the procedure time and the medical risk to the patient because the catheter will remain in the vessel for a shorter period of time and even less con-

trast medium is necessary. Interventional treatment may be started immediately after the diagnostic procedure. Consulting an expert becomes easy with worldwide telecommunication capabilities. Archiving and retrieval of digital images and reports in a picture archiving and communication system (PACS) environment (HRUBY et al. 1994; DE SILVA 1996) are far less expensive and faster to hand than images on films and reports on paper.

The international radiological community has agreed upon the standardization of digital imaging technologies. They started with the so-called ACR/NEMA (American College of Radiology and the National Electrical Manufacturers Association) proposal some years ago which has been developed to version three and is known today under the name DICOM (digital imaging and communication) standard (MORNEBURG 1995). Digital images, including peripheral angiography, have been successfully used in a PACS system, such as Sienet, on a daily basis since 1992 (ROSENBUSCH et al. 1995). This further enhances the quality of diagnosis and treatment for the patient.

References

Aichinger H, Staudt F, Kuhn H (1992) Multiline grids for imaging in diagnostic radiology – a physical and clinical assessment. Electromedica 60:74–81

Albers G, Scheel A (1994) Practical experience with a universal R/F workstation. Electromedica 62:37–41

Ammann E (1994) X-Ray generators and AEC design. In: Seibert JA, Barnes GT, Gould RG (eds) Specification, acceptance testing and quality control of diagnostic X-ray imaging equipment. AAPM monograph no. 20, American Association of Physicists in Medicine, pp 233-265

Arnold BA, Eisenberg H (1979) Imaging techniques in angiography. In: Haus AG (ed) The physics of medical imaging: recording system measurements and techniques. AAPM monograph no. 3, American Association of Physicists in Medicine, pp 465-482

Brassel F, Becker H, Herde K (1992) Supervision – a new technique for reducing the dose in endovascular neuroradiological interventions. Electromedica 60:82–88

Buur LM, Wilson DL, Faul DD (1990) Registration of digital subtraction peripheral angiography images. Proceedings of the 16th Annual North East Bioengineering Conference, 26–27 March 1990, State College, PA, USA, pp 69–70

De Silva M (1996) Design and implementation of the first filmless children's hospital. Electromedica 64:44–47

Fink U, Heywang SH, Berger H, et al. (1990) First clinical results with digital peripheral angiography and stepping. Electromedica 58:2–8

Herrmann K, Waggershauser T, Reiser M (1994) Multistar T.O.P. – initial experiences. Electromedica 62:56–58

High M (1994) Digital fluoro acceptance testing – the AAPM approach. In: Seibert JA, Barnes GT, Gould RG (eds) Specification, acceptance testing and quality control of diagnostic X-ray imaging equipment. AAPM monograph no. 20, American Association of Physicists in Medicine, pp 709–730

Hruby W, Urban M, Mosser H, et al. (1994) Image management systems: contributing to the improvement of the cost–benefit ratio. Electromedica 62:51–55

ICRP Report No. 26 (1977) The International Commission on Radiation Protection defines ALARA: as low as reasonably achievable. International Commission on Radiation Detection, Pergamon, Oxford, p 74

Kato H, Miyahara J, Takano M (1985) Computed radiography with scanning–laser–stimulated luminescense. In: Doi K, Lanzl L, Lin PP (eds) Recent developments in digital imaging. AAPM monograph no. 12, The American Association of Physicists in Medicine, pp 237–255

Krestel E (ed) (1990) Imaging systems for medical diagnostics. Siemens AG, Berlin Munich

Levy JM (1993) C-arm film changers add diagnostic flexibility. Diagnostic Imaging 9:86–95

Mertelmeier T, Kuhn H (1996) High-resolution monitors. Electromedica 64:30–31

Morneburg H (ed) (1995) Bildgebende Systeme für die medizinische Diagnostik, 3. Aufl. Siemens AG Publicis MCD Verlag, for DICOM: pp 686–696; for DYNAVISION: p 398; for comparison: pp 131, 305

Peene P, Wilms G, Baert AL, Estievenart S (1991) Low dose digital peripheral angiography with continuous C-arm movement. Electromedica 59:110–114

Rosenbusch G, Oudkerk M, Ammann E (eds) (1995) Radiology in medical diagnostics – evolution of X-ray applications 1895–1995. Blackwell Science, Oxford

Sigmund G, Groothoff BM (1996) Digital fluoroscopy – a workhorse in the standard range. Electromedica 64:40–43

Standard IEC 613 (1989) Electrical, thermal and loading characteristics of rotating anode X-ray tubes for medical diagnosis, 2nd edn. 1989–04

Standard IEC 336 (1993) X-Ray tube assemblies for medical diagnosis – characteristics for focal spots, 3rd edn. 1993–08

Vano E, Gonzalez L, Fernandez JM, Guibelalde E (1995) Patient dose values in interventional radiology. Br J Radiol 68:1215–1220

Waggershauser T (1996) Dose reduction through radiation – free collimator positioning. Electromedica 64:20–22

Wayrynen R (1979) The photographic process. In: Haus AG (ed) The physics of medical imaging: recording system measurements and techniques. AAPM monograph no. 3, American Association of Physicists in Medicine, pp 1–15

Zeitler E (1995) Peripherel vessels. In: Rosenbusch G, Oudkerk M, Ammann E (eds) Radiology in medical diagnostics – evolution of X-ray applications 1895–1995. Blackwell Science, Oxford, pp 236–247

8.5.8
Differences Between Digital Subtraction und Digital Dynamic Angiography

8.5.8.1
Introduction

Despite considerable progress in non-invasive vascular diagnosis (color-coded duplex sonography, MR and CT angiography), angiographic visualization of the pelvic and leg vessels is still today irreplaceable for planning therapy for patients with arterial occlusive disease. A variety of angiographic procedures are employed for this. Both DSA and dynamic digital angiography (DDA) are preferred to conventional film-screen imaging (KATZEN 1995).

The aim of the following investigation is to establish an optimum diagnostic strategy on the basis of random comparison of both digital procedures. The criteria of evaluation were as follows: image quality, radiation exposure, amount of contrast medium substance required, and length of the examination.

8.5.8.2
Materials and Methods

One hundred patients with peripheral occlusive disease (Table 8.15) in stages IIa–IV according to the Fontaine classification were subjected to randomly selected pelvic and leg angiography consisting either of a combination of DDA and lower leg/foot DSA (group 1, $n = 50$) or of complete segmental DSA in four steps (group 2, $n = 50$).

The angiographies for both procedures were carried out using the General Electric DSA system Advantx-DX. The image amplifier measured 40 cm in diameter. We employed an image matrix of 512 × 512 pixles, straight 4-F angiography catheters, and non-ionic contrast medium with an iodine concentration of 300 mg/ml.

During DDA, the examiner followed the contrast bolus by manual table shifting (bolus chasing). Six images per second were obtained digitally and non-subtracted by this method. For the visualization of the arteries from the aortic bifurcation to the P3 segment of the popliteal artery, we required 80 ml of contrast medium. Subsequently, without changing catheter location, an additional DSA of the lower leg und foot was carried out using an average of 30 ml of contrast medium. Flow rate totaled 10 ml/s for each.

The DSA for group 2 was done in four steps with sequential dosing of contrast medium in amounts of 20, 20, 25, and 30 ml, respectively, with a flow rate of 10 ml/s. Image frequency was 2/s.

During the angiography procedures, we registered the exposure dose (mean dose product, MDP) separately for the catheterization, the standard pelvic-leg angiography, and the supplementary examinations (Diamentor M 2, manufactured by PTW, Freiburg, Germany). Catheter placement time was designated as the period extending from introduction of the catheter above the bifurcation of the aorta to its removal.

The quality comparison of the groups was based only on the pelvic, thigh, and knee regions; the lower leg and foot examinations were carried out by DSA for both groups, thus ruling out the possibility of comparison. In preliminary examinations, we had established that under our conditions, distal arteries of the lower leg were regularly insufficiently visualized under DDA. For evaluation of the visualization quality, we sorted the angiography images, separated into the above-mentioned stages, according to the following three categories: (1) Very good: optimal and sharp vascular image; (2) good: diagnostically adequate vascular image; (3) inadequate: lacking definition of the vessels.

In cases of arterial occlusion, we additionally registered the number of visualized collaterals down to the last visible ramification.

Statistical data analyses were carried out by means of a bilateral *t*-test for diverse variables with the help of the SPSS computer program of the Institute of Medical Informatics of the Technical University of Dresden (Prof. R. KOCH).

8.5.8.3
Results

Comparison of patients according to age, height, and weight indicated no significant differences (see Table 8.15). Analysis of image quality for DDA demonstrated at least diagnostically adequate visualization of pelvic and thigh blood vessels in all patients and of the knee area in 46 patients (92%). Angiography of the pelvic region in 16 patients (32%) and thigh region in 14 patients (28%) was evaluated as very good. Only in the knee region was visualization inadequate in 8% of the patients (Fig. 8.48).

Image quality attained by DSA was better in all regions examined (Fig. 8.49). We observed arterial occlusions in 38 patients of group 1 and 36 of group 2. While in the majority of cases (63.2%) collaterals could be identified via DDA only down to the second ramification, after DSA we recognized most frequently the third collateral ramification and, more rarely (2.8%), the fourth collateral ramification (Fig. 8.50).

Following primarily dynamic angiography, we required a total of 15 additional series in the pelvic as well as the knee areas (Table 8.16).

The average amount of contrast medium was increased by use of DDA by 13 ml to a total of 108 ml. This difference was statistically significant. The mean catheter placement time was 9.39 min for group 1 (DDA) and 12.65 min for group 2 (DSA). The difference of 3.2 min is significant (Table 8.17).

Table 8.15. One hundred patients with peripheral occlusive disease were subjected to randomly selected DSA and DDA

	Group 1 (DDA)	Group 2 (DSA)	Total
Female	14	17	31
Male	36	33	69
Number	50	50	100
Mean age (years)	67.4	67.8	67.6
Mean weight (kg)	72.1	69.4	70.9
Mean height (cm)	170.0	168.5	169.3

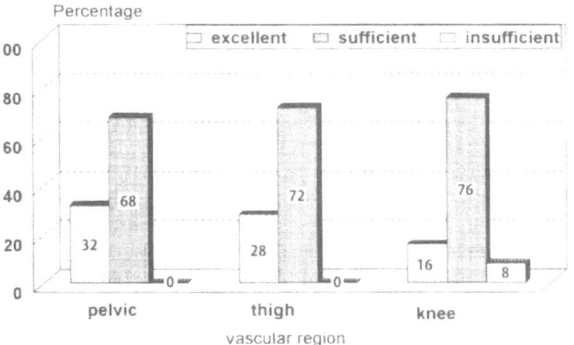

Fig. 8.48. Image quality of digital dynamic angiography

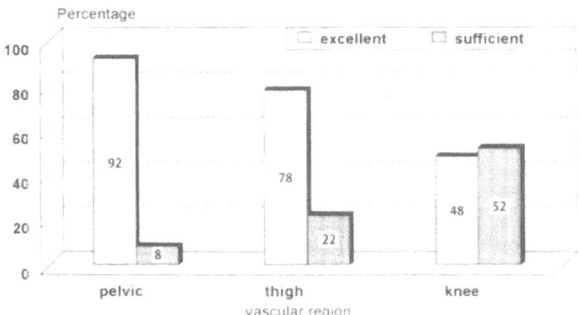

Fig. 8.49. Image quality of digital subtraction angiography

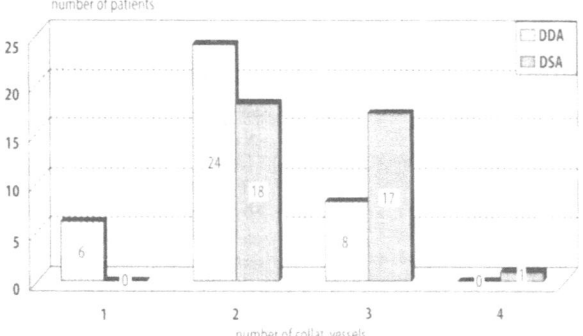

Fig. 8.50. Number of represented collateral vessels in cases of vessel occlusion. *DDA,* digital dynamic angiography; *DSA,* digital subtraction angiography

Table 8.16. Supplementary sequences in DSA technique

Region	Group 1 (DDA)	Group 2 (DSA)	Total	MDP (Gy/cm^2) Mean value
Pelvic	7	4	11	27.4
Thigh	2	–	2	4.6
Knee/lower leg	6	5	11	2.0
Total	15	9	24	

MDP, mean dose product.

In the comparison between DSA and DDA, the reduction in average MDP during the standard series totaled $29.4\,Gy/cm^2$. The MDP for the entire examination (catheterization, standard series, additional series) could be reduced under DDA by an average of $29.6\,Gy/cm^2$ (Fig. 8.51). The dose differences were likewise statistically significant ($p < 0.001$).

8.5.8.4
Discussion

Pelvic-leg angiography makes an essential contribution to determining the choice of therapy for peripheral arterial occlusive disease. Besides the quality of vessel visualization, the efficiency of the angiographic procedure utilized is important. Non-subtracted digital angiography is a suitable method for evaluating patients with peripheral vascular disease (PICUS et al. 1991).

Because of the high contrast resolution being generally free of superimpositions, DSA with arterial application of contrast medium results in better visualization of peripheral vessels and collateral arteries than non-subtracted digital angiography. For this reason, the DSA demonstrated superior quality in all regions of the procedure. In this respect, our differentiation between "very good" and "good" is unimportant for practical purposes. The 8% insufficiency of vessel visualization in the knee area by means of DDA is primarily due to unequal flow in both legs. In the comparison, this result was relativized because additional exposures of the knee area were necessary in the DSA group. A slightly varying number of additional series (in differing angulations) were required for the pelvic area in order to come to a conclusion relevant to therapy.

According to our observations, visualization of vascular occlusions over longer segments generally succeeds better using the non-subtracted technique. The examiner can distribute the exposure segments to greater advantage, depending on the flow speed of the contrast medium.

Although the practically relevant qualitative difference is small, an important finding is the reduction of radiation exposure under application of DDA by $29.6\,Gy/cm^2$ as against subtracted angiography. The difference results from the necessarily higher dose required by DSA, which is primarily determined by the masking, and by a dose necessary for fluoroscopic focusing on the segments to be visu-

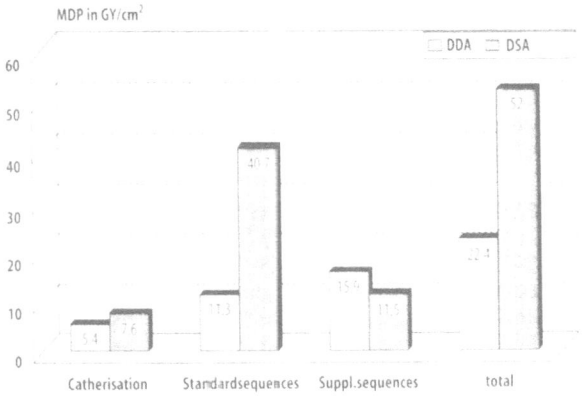

Fig. 8.51. Mean dose product (*MDP*) comparison between digital subtraction angiography (*DSA*) and digital dynamic angiography (*DDA*)

Table 8.17. Average amount of contrast medium (ACM)/time of examination

	Group 1	Group 2	p value (t-test)
ACM standard examination	108.5 ml +/- 4.54 min	95.10 ml +/- 10.76 min	<0.001
ACM supplementary sequences	27.5 ml +/- 10.61 min	29.37 ml +/- 11.95 min	0.630
ACM total	118.5 ml +/- 14.04 min	105.30 ml +/- 16.82 min	<0.001
Time of examination	9.4 ml +/- 3.9 min	12.65 ml +/- 3.63 min	<0.001

alized. In a study comparing a stepwise DSA similar to our procedure with subtracted stage shifting, HILBERTZ also arrived at considerable differences in radiation exposure unfavorable to DSA (HILBERTZ et al. 1991).

For the purposes of comparison, the length of the examination was defined by us in terms of catheter emplacement time. Also in this parameter, we established a significant difference: the DDA could be carried out with a marked reduction in examination time of 3.2 min as compared to DSA.

Consumption of contrast medium is lower during DSA than DDA. Taking the additional series into consideration, this means an average difference of 13 ml. We attribute this to the higher number of additional sequences required for DDA. We consider the dose reduction in combination with low time saving as a more decisive factor than the slightly higher amount of contrast medium required.

8.5.8.5
Conclusion

DDA is an acceptable alternative to DSA. We prefer digital bolus chasing as far as the knee and immediately subsequent DSA of the lower leg and foot for visualization of the arteries from the aortic bifurcation up to the foot. Compared to complete DSA, this procedure is recommended particularly in view of the reduced radiation dose. If diagnostic uncertainties remain, angularized sequences or selective exposures via DSA technique should be undertaken.

References

Hilbertz T, Fink U, Beck R, Berger H, Erbenwein U (1991) Digitale periphere Angiografie mit Schrittverschiebung und Substraktion – Vergleich mit Standardverfahren. ROFO 151:228–234
Katzen BT (1995) Current status of digital angiography in vascular imaging. Radiol Clin North Am 33:1–14
Picus D, Hicks ME, Darcy MD, Kleinhoffer MA (1991) Comparison of nonsubtracted digital angiography and conventional screen-film angiography for the evaluation of patients with peripheral vascular disease. J Vasc Intervent Radiol 2:359–364

8.6
Radiation and Radiation Protection

T. SCHMIDT and M. WUCHERER

8.6.1
Introduction

Angiographic examinations and interventional measures play only a minor role as regards their frequency of performance within the spectrum of diagnostics (<2%). However, the doses applied in this framework are high, which is of importance for the radiation protection of both the patient and personnel. This chapter, however, will only investigate radiation exposure to the patients.

Thanks to the introduction of film-foil systems with increasing sensitivity and refined image intensifiers, patient exposure has been almost continuously reduced over the past few decades. In general, so-called acute or deterministic radiation damage does not occur in diagnostic radiology. Only the risk of late stochastic somatic injuries due to radiological diagnostic measures is under discussion. However, the new minimally-invasive interventions sometimes require long fluoroscopy times and many images. This has led in some cases to acute skin reactions. Although even in the future general diagnostic radiology will only have to consider the risk of stochastic radiation damage, the risk of deterministic damage due to interventional measures cannot be entirely ruled out.

8.6.2
Frequency of Performance

Dependent on the health-care level, the number of examinations and/or interventions per inhabitant varies considerably in different countries. As an example of interventions, Fig. 8.52 shows a comparison between different countries over several years. As can be seen, the number of interventions per capita of the population in the United States is higher than that of Germany by about 3 years. For comparison purposes, the coronary interventions, percutaneous transluminal coronary angioplasty (PTCA), performed by cardiologists have been added. Also, the rate of increase is related to the health-care level in the various countries, with either increasing, decreasing, or stagnating figures. Table 8.18 shows the number of angiographic ex-

Table 8.18. Normalized frequencies of angiographic examinations in different countries, according to UNSCEAR (1993)

Health care level	Examinations per 1000 population
I	0.2–18
II	0.1–3
III	0–0.3
IV	$\approx 10^{-4}$

Typical countries: level I, France, Germany, USA; level II, Brazil, Turkey; level III, Ghana, Thailand; level IV, Nigeria, Rwanda.

Table 8.19. Mean number of examinations per patient, according to KICKEN (1996)

Examination	Number
Arteriography (i.a.)	1.9
DSA Arteriography (i.v.)	1.5
Phlebography (i.v.)	2.1
Interventional radiology	1.2

Table 8.20. Possible quantities to describe the radiation exposure

Dose Parameters	Symbol
Fluoroscopic time and number of frames	t
Entrance or surface dose	K_E/K_s
Dose area product	DAP
Organ dose	D_F
Effective dose	E

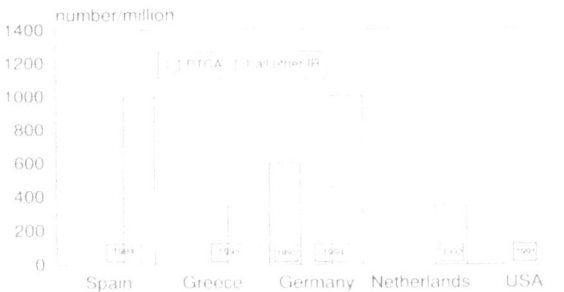

Fig. 8.52. Frequency of interventional radiology (*IR*) procedures in different countries. *PTCA*, percutaneous transluminal coronary angioplasty

aminations according to data provided by the United Nations (UNSCEAR 1993). The number of examinations per patient has been compiled in Table 8.19 according to KICKEN (1996).

8.6.3
Exposure

To quantify radiation exposure to the patient, more or less appropriate dose parameters are used (Table 8.20). In angiographic interventional measures, the entrance or surface dose deserves special attention due to the possibility of acute skin reaction. A first rough clue for the assessment of radiation exposure to the patient are fluoroscopy time and the number of frames. Table 8.21 gives an overview of the duration and number of frames for some angiographic examinations.

Interventional measures involve considerably higher fluoroscopy times and image numbers. Figure 8.53 shows the mean fluoroscopy (not examination) times and the mean number of images required for four selected interventional techniques on the basis of a large sample of patients. Based on the assumption that five frames correspond to 1 min of fluoroscopy time as regards radiation exposure, the ordinate graduation was chosen. Although in percutaneous transluminal angiography (PTA) the aspects fluoroscopy and number of frames contribute nearly equivalently to the exposure, in transjugular intrahepatic portosystemic stent shunting (TIPSS) the dose is predominant because of the long fluoroscopy time.

Figure 8.54 shows the distribution of fluoroscopy times for interventions with a mean value of 14 min. The share of examinations exceeding 30 min is about 10%. Table 8.22 and Fig. 8.55 demonstrate that radiation exposure generally tends to be higher in interventions than in angiographic measures. At dose rates to the skin of between 0.02 Gy/min (normal mode) up to 0.2 Gy/min (high-level mode), skin reactions (at least temporary ones) cannot be excluded if fluoroscopy times exceed 30 min.

Table 8.21. Mean fluoroscopic time and number of frames per examination from KICKEN (1996) and own evaluations

Angiographic examinations	Fluoroscopic time	Frames
i.a. Arteriography (extremities)	6 min	85
i.a. Arteriography (abdominal)	7 min	35
i.v. DSA arterography (abdominal)	1.5 min	60

DSA, digital subtraction angiography.

Table 8.22. Entrance dose, dose area product (DAP), and effective dose from literary and own evaluations (mean values of different publications)

Region measured	Number of works published	K_{skin} mGy	DAP $Gy \times cm^2$	$H_E{}^a$/E[a] mSv
Cerebral	19	27–300	7–80	4–20
Abdominal	5		30	6–20
Extremities	8	25–90	13–70	4–12
Thoracic	2			4–5

[a] As a consequence of different specification in literature.

A considerably better determination of patient exposure is possible with the entrance dose and the dose area product (DAP) than with fluoroscopy time and number of frames. The entrance dose, therefore, deserves special attention, especially in interventional measures involving the risk of skin reactions. The entrance dose released in angiographic measures is difficult to determine for several skin areas due to the variation of the angulation of the C-arm of the X-ray unit around the patient and the movements of the patient support relative to the tube. Most publications refer to the maximum dose measured to the patient. Table 8.22 shows mean values of skin doses in angiographic measures based on evaluations of the literature and own experience.

It seems that skin reactions can be excluded in all probability. This is, however, not the case for interventional measures. Table 8.23 shows own values based on conclusions from varying literature, and from two studies in particular carried out by the Deutsche Röntgengesellschaft (German Radiology Society) (ZEITLER 1995) and the Commission of the European Communities (CEC) (SCHMIDT et al. 1993–1995). Even though the mean values are still below the threshold limits for skin reactions, their occurrence cannot be excluded in individual cases. It is therefore of great importance to obtain information on the dose used during the examination in order to be able to reduce the dose by angulation or shifting of the patient, if necessary, and to reduce the maximum values (see also Sect. 8.5).

In all cases of vascular radiology, a highly absorbed dose has to be expected compared to classical X-ray exposures. To determine the former, the DAP, the organ doses and, possibly, the effective dose are suited. The DAP can be measured most easily. The effective dose can then be estimated, at least roughly, on the basis of the DAP. The DAP values summarized from the literature can also be found in Tables 8.22 and 8.23. As anticipated, the values of the area exposure product of interventional measures are higher.

With the help of conversion factors given in the publication by the National Radiological Protection Board (HART et al. 1994), the effective dose can be estimated from the DAP for different localizations of the body. Using PTA as an example, the different intervention localizations are given in Fig. 8.55. A comparison between angiography and interventions (Tables 8.22, 8.23) again reveals significantly higher values of the effective doses of interventions.

Table 8.23. Entrance dose, dose area product (DAP), and effective dose

Type of intervention	K_{skin} mGy	DAP $Gy \times cm^2$	E mSv
PTA	400	70	10
Lysis		110	
Embolization		180	25
TIPSS	1200 (to 5000)	220	50

E, effective dose; PTA, percutaneous transluminal angioplasty; TIPSS, transjugular intrahepatic portosystemic stent shunting.

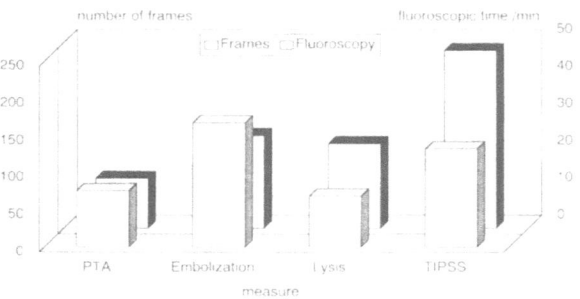

Fig. 8.53. Distribution of fluoroscopic time of interventions in radiology. *PTA*, percutaneous transluminal angioplasty; *TIPSS*, transjugular intrahepatic portosystemic stent shunting

8.6.4
Consideration of the Radiation Risks

8.6.4.1
Deterministic Effects

Tables 8.24 and 8.25 (according to WAGNER 1995) show the threshold doses for various deterministic effects. For the purposes of this section, mainly the threshold dose for the formation of erythema and other radiation-induced skin reactions is of interest. Skin reactions can in general be avoided if the dose to the skin does not exceed 2 Gy. Therefore, a much valued aspect of modern X-ray units is their facility to display the threshold doses for skin reactions as a percentage during angiographies and radiological interventions. In practice, interventions involving such relatively high exposure rates are the exception. If they are, however, inevitable, the physician has the possibility to protect the skin by varying the entrance point.

8.6.4.2
Stochastic Radiation Effects

In radiological diagnostics, attempts have always been made to determine the risk of late stochastic somatic effects due to radiation exposure. A correlation between exposure (effective dose) and such a risk can only be established, however, if a conversion coefficient for each individual patient (age and sex)

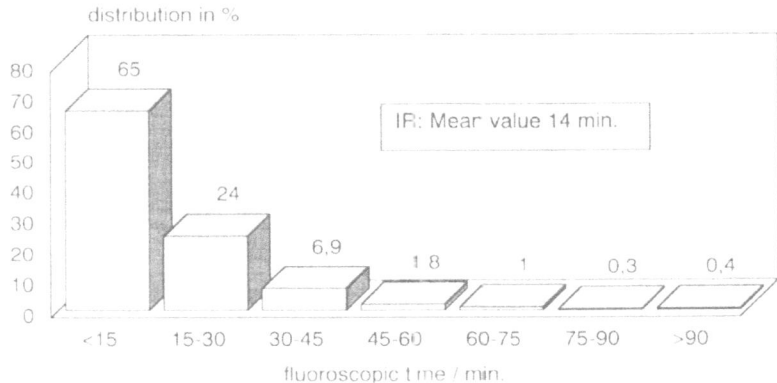

Fig. 8.54. Mean values of four types of interventional radiology (*IR*)

Table 8.24. Potential skin effects of fluoroscopy (WAGNER, 1995)

Effect	Single-dose threshold (Gy)	Onset	Peak
Early transient erythema	2	Hours	~24 h
Main erythema	6	10 days	~2 weeks
Temporary epilation	3	~3 weeks	...
Permanent epilation	7	~3 weeks	...
Dry desquamation	10	~4 weeks	~5 weeks
Moist desquamation	15	~4 weeks	~5 weeks
Secondary ulceration	20	>6 weeks	...
Late erythema	15	~6–10 weeks	...
Dermal necrosis (first phase)	18	>10 weeks	...
Dermal atrophy (first phase)	10	>14 weeks	...
Dermal atrophy (second phase)	10	>1 year	...
Telangiectasia	12	>1 year	...
Dermal necrosis (late phase)	>15?	>1 year	...
Skin cancer	Not known	>5 years	...

..., indicate no peak value for that effect.

Table 8.25. Other potential of fluoroscopy

Effect	Single-dose threshold (Gy)	Onset
Cataract (not vision impairing)	1	>1 y
Cataract (vision impairing)	5	>1 y
Parotid gland function (saliva)	>2	Prompt
Parotiditis	2–10	Prompt
Parotid gland tumors	Not known	>5 y
Bone growth deficit	6 (3 soft-tissue dose?)	May not be detected until after puberty
Bone necrosis	Very high	>6 mo
Behavioral maldevelopment	~0.5	
Central nervous system tumors	Not known	>5 y

is known. Conversion coefficients, however, have been published in the International Commission on Radiological Protection recommendations without consideration of the individual age and sex of the patient, but rather on the basis of the anticipated normal life-expectancy of irradiated and non-irradiated individuals of the population (e.g., Japan, USA). The age distribution of the patients compared to the entire population shows distinct differences, as demonstrated in Fig. 8.56 by the example of PTA: The mean age of the population of Germany was 40 years, whereas the mean age of patients undergoing PTA was 65.

The risk coefficients in Table 8.26 have been derived on the basis of the patient's age. As can be seen, consideration of the patient's age already reduces the risk coefficient by half, or even down to one third, depending on the age distribution of the patients undergoing different types of intervention. Further considerations for determining the real risk would be to compare the life-expectancy of the affected group of the population to that of the general population.

Despite the relatively high doses used in angiographic and interventional measures, a comparison of their risks and benefits always has to take the high efficacy of diagnostic and interventional measures into consideration. Not only as a result of careful patient selection will the benefit in general outweigh the associated risk, which is also present in other measures and therapies, such as in the thorax.

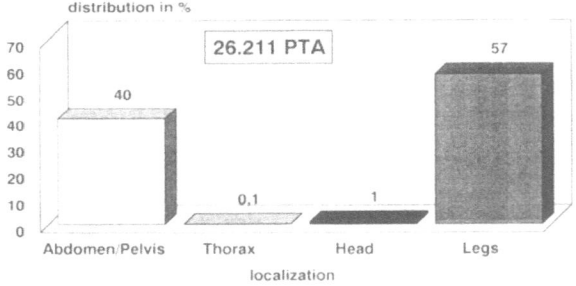

Fig. 8.55. Localizations of angioplasties in Germany between 1990 and 1994

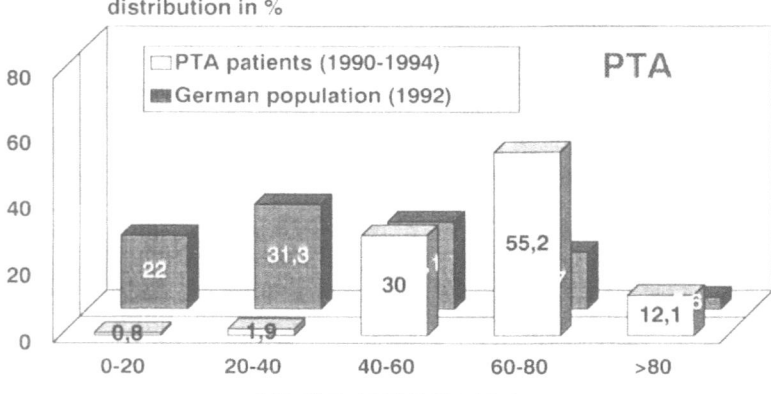

Fig. 8.56. Age distribution of percutaneous transluminal angioplasty (*PTA*) patients and of the population in Germany

Table 8.26. Risk coefficient patients for some interventional procedures

Procedure	Probability of fatal cancer %/Sv
Normal population	5 (see IECP 1993)
PTA	1.5
PTCA	2.1
Embolization	3.0

PTA, percutaneous transluminal angioplasty; PTCA, percutaneous transluminal coronary angioplasty.

References

Hart D, Jones DG, Wall BF (1994) Estimation of effective dose in diagnostic radiology from entrance surface dose and dose-area product measurements. HMSO, London

ICRP (1993) Recommendations of the International Commission on Radiological Protection 1990. Pergamon, Oxford (ICRP 60)

Kicken PJH (1996) Radiation dosimetry in vascular radiology, organ and effective dose to patients and staff, Dutuwyse, Universitaire Pers Maastricht, Maastricht

Schmidt T, Maccia C, Neofotistou V, Padovani R, Vano-Carruana E (1993–1995) Evaluation of dose in risk due to interventional radiology techniques. EC, Brussels (EC Final report contract: FI3PCT930070)

Unscear (1993) United Nations Scientific Committee on the Effects of Atomic Radiation. Sources and effects of ionizing radiation. Report to the General Assembly, with Scientific Annexes. United Nations, New York

Wagner LK (1995) Biologic effects of high x-ray doses RSNA, Syllabus: A categroical course in physics, Physical and technical aspects of angio-graphy and interventional radiology 1995, 167–170

Zeitler E (1995) Arbeitsgemeinschaft für Interventionelle Radiologie. Jahresbericht der Deutschen Röntgengesellschaft 43:64–65

8.7
Complications of Angiography

E. ZEITLER

The incidence of complications requiring direct therapy at and after angiography has been reported by HESSEL and ADAMS (1981) as: 1.7% after femoral, 2.9% after translumbar, 3.3% after axillary, and 7% after brachial arteriotomy catheterization. The mortality rate described in the same survey by HESSEL and ADAMS was 0.03%. The lethal cases among these 0.03% resulted, in particular, from arterial dissection and ruptured aneurysm (27%), vasovageal reactions, cardiac (17%) and neurologic (7%) complications, renal failure (7%), pulmonary embolization (3%), and non-specified causes. In departments where more than 800 arteriograms were obtained annually, the rate of non-fatal complications was significantly lower than in departments with less than 800 arteriograms per year.

The above incidence of complications after diagnostic angiographies was the result of a questionnaire analyzing angiographies carried out between July 1974 and June 1975. According to the data gathered from 514 hospitals (of 2066) in the United States and a total of 118591 angiographic examinations, statistically significant complication and death rates after femoral access and catheterization were the lowest (HESSEL 1983). Cholesterol crystal embolization was observed in the past when stiffer guidewires and catheters were used (FINE et al. 1987). These can be reduced by using glidewires (Terumo) and soft-tip catheters in patients with extreme atherosclerosis.

Meanwhile, since 1975, more than 20 years having elapsed, several things have changed: Less toxic CM which permit painless angiography have come onto the market. The reduction of side effects has been achieved due to the low osmolality of the ionic dimeric CM ioxaglinate (Hexabrix), and the non-ionic monomeric CM (Iohexol, Iopamidol, Iopromide and others; see Sect. 8.4). These have reduced moderate and severe side effects to 3%, as well as the death rate (GMELIN and ARLART 1987; SAINT-GEORGES and AUBE 1985; WAUGH and SACHARIAS 1992). General anesthesia in adults is unnecessary nowadays in nearly all cases; only children, patients with acute trauma, and psychiatric patients still require general anesthesia if angiography is indicated (SIGSTEDT and LUNDERQUIST 1978; WAGNER 1993). General premedication using H_1-and H_2-receptor antagonists and/or corticosteroids in patients with previous side effects, asthma, or other allergic diseases has reduced idiosyncratic severe and moderate side effects.

DSA has not only led to a reduction in both the amount and the concentration of CM, with equally satisfying results, but has also helped to shorten examination times (ARLART 1997; NEUFANG and BEYER 1988). DSA has also enabled the general use of small catheters (5–3 instead of 6- and 7-F diameters). New catheter types with high flow rates and small outer diameters have reduced local complications. New catheter materials and safety guidewires have diminished the risk of thrombus formation, cholesterol crystal embolization, and dissection and rupture of aneurysms, both in normal and diseased arteries.

Additional systemic heparinization or the use of heparinized guidewires and catheters has reduced thrombotic complications (BOOKSTEIN et al. 1982; VOGEL et al. 1986; WALLACE et al. 1972; ZEITLER 1997). Postprocedural bleeding and hematomas have been reduced (and almost eliminated) by applying puncture-hole closure devices (ZEITLER 1997).

Translumbar and transaxillary angiography techniques, with their specific complications (STAAL et al. 1966), are no longer used except for rare indications where by transfemoral or transbrachial catheterization is impossible (GROLLMAN and MARCUS 1988; YANDOW et al. 1988).

In general, angiography of the peripheral arteries has progressed enormously (NEUFANG and BEYER 1988; NEUFANG et al. 1983; SAINT-GEORGES and AUBE 1985; GMELIN and ARLART 1987; ARLART 1997) thanks to:

- New, less toxic CM
- The lack of need for general anesthesia
- Digital angiography/DSA
- New, smaller soft-tip catheters
- Heparinization
- Improved postprocedural care.

With efficient patient care prior to, during, and after the procedure, adequate premedication can limit specific risks. Only the nephrotoxicity of CM has not improved to any statistically significant extent with the new CM. However, radiologists are aware of the risk of renal insufficiency in patients with nephropathy, diabetes, and dehydration and, prior to angiography, the patient's personal history gives an indication of special premedication that may need to be observed. General control of creatinine levels before angiography is very important to reduce nephrotoxic complications. If creatinine levels are elevated, postprocedural care is necessary and, in some cases, dialysis is very helpful. Nevertheless, even in the late 1990s, we still have to admit that general and local complications (Table 8.27), even if seldom, can occur (ZEITLER 1974; HESSEL and ADAMS 1981; WAGNER 1993; NEIMANN and YAO 1985; FINE et al. 1987; ALTIN et al. 1989).

8.7.1
Local Complications

After transfemoral catheterization, bleeding at the puncture site may result in surgical repair and, later on, in blood transfusion. After non-coronary diagnostic angiography, we observed a need for surgery

Table 8.27. General and local complications occurring during angiography

General Complications
  Idiosyncratic shock
  Moderate and severe allergic side effects
  Vasovagal reactions
  Acute cardiac symptoms (angina, heart infarction)
  Contrast-medium induced nephropathy
Local Complications
  Afterbleeding at the puncture site
  Pulsating hematoma/pseudoaneurysm
  Thrombotic occlusion at the puncture site and
    hemodynamic stenosis
  Peripheral embolization
  Arteriovenous fistula
  Catheter and guidewire problems (tearing off, knot
    formation, and others)
  Contrast medium paravasation
  Infection at the puncture site
  Deep venous thrombosis involving the risk of pulmonary
    embolization

in six patients out of 8400 arteriographies, with catheters of 7 and 8 F (0.07%). Earlier publications have reported a need for surgery in between 0.06% and 0.5% of cases (VOGEL et al. 1986).

Suprainguinal puncture can result in large retroperitoneal hematomas, followed by centralization, which can prove lethal unless infusion therapy and surgical repair are started early (HESSEL 1983; NEIMANN and YAO 1985). Doppler sonography is extremely effective for the early detection of local complications (BARNES et al. 1974).

Pseudoaneurysms following diagnostic angiography, in contrast to interventional procedures using 7- and 8-F catheters, were observed very seldom (ALTIN et al. 1989). They can be diagnosed with ultrasound (BARNES et al. 1974), as well as with biplane or rotating angiography. With the help of ultrasound guidance, pulsating hematomas can also be controlled by percutaneous compression. Inflammation may occur around the puncture site. Therefore, surgeons recommend performing catheterization from the nondiseased side. Infection without hematoma is extremely seldom.

Arteriovenous (av) fistulas are extremely rare (ALTIN et al. 1989); HESSEL (1983) has published an incidence of 0.01%. We observed av-fistulas after coronary and cerebral catheterization with prolonged procedure times, but not after peripheral diagnostic angiographies.

Thrombus formation at the puncture site may be followed by local thrombotic occlusion, but smaller thrombus material can also be detected around the catheter with Doppler ultrasound or angiography (FORMANEK et al. 1970; BARNES et al. 1974; OVITT et al. 1974; NEIMANN and YAO 1985). Heparinization of catheters and guidewires, as well as systemic heparinization (WALLACE et al. 1972; MILLER and MILLER 1974) has helped to reduce thrombus formation, but requires more intense aftercare to prevent bleeding.

Angiography may also be followed by thrombotic occlusion, beginning at the pre-existent stenosis, and short occlusions may become more extensive (MAY and NISSL 1969). Angiographic controls before PTA and after diagnostic intravenous or intraarterial DSA were able to demonstrate new occlusions in the iliac arteries in 8%, and in the femoropopliteal arteries in 14%. All of those patients who experienced thrombotic occlusions had pre-existent severe stenoses (BEYER-ENKE et al. 1994).

The risk of neurologic complications of the brachial plexus following axillary catheterization has been published (MOLNAR and PAUL 1972), with irreversible sensory and motoric defects in up to 9% (STAHL et al. 1966). Neurologic complications result from outside compression of the plexus, or small hematomas inside the neurologic fibrous capsule. In 30 years as an expert witness, I have seen total plexus paralysis in three patients after needle angiography with intraaxillary hematoma not followed by surgical repair. All three came from the same neurology clinic and their indication was vertebral angiography. At the Department of Diagnostic and Interventional Radiology of the Nuremberg clinic, I observed one sensory neurologic defect out of 54 catheter angiographies with transaxillary access. I insisted that the surgeon operate, whereupon he found a small hematoma in the neurologic structures. After cleaning the nerves with saline, there was no more neurologic deficit. HESSEL and ADAMS (1981) have also reported on arm amputation following plexus injury. Complications in the axillary artery, as well as in other regions, can be prevented by using a sheath that facilitates the exchange of catheters during one examination. After brachial angiography with arteriotomy or Seldinger Catheterization, thrombotic occlusion was seen in the past in 1%–7% (HESSEL 1983; VOGEL et al. 1986). Since the arrival of 3- to 5-F catheters and sheaths in the hands of experienced angiographers, and the prophylactic injection of 5000 IU of herapin, this complication has occurred very rarely in recent years (GROLLMAN and MARCUS 1988).

Complications observed following translumbar aortography, such as hematoma (YANDOW et al.

1988), or paraplegia (HESSEL 1981; ZEITLER 1974), could be enormously reduced with less toxic CM, smaller puncture needles, and, finally, because the indication has very rarely been made since DSA, brachial arteriography, and small catheters which can be applied under Doppler guidance have been available. Thus, angiography with ultrasound-guided puncture, the use of small catheter sizes, and safety floppy guidewires has become a very lowrisk diagnostic procedure providing precise information and answers to the most clinically relevant questions in peripheral vascular diseases.

8.7.2
General Complications

These in most cases, are the result of reactions to CM and are discussed in greater detail in Sect. 8.4.

References

Altin RS, Flicker S, Naidech HJ (1989) Pseudoaneurysm and arteriovenous fistula after femoral artery catheterization. Association with low femoral punctures. AJR Am J Roentgenol 152:629–631

Arlart IP (1997) Radiologische Untersuchungstechniken des Gefäßsystems – angiographisches Instrumentarium und Zubehör. In: Zeitler E (ed) Klinische Radiologie: Arterien und Venen. Springer, Berlin Heidelberg New York, pp. 111–127

Barnes RW, Petersen JL, Krugmire RB Jr, Strandness DE Jr (1974) Complications of percutaneous femoral arterial catheterization: prospective evaluation with the Doppler ultrasonic velocity detector. Am J Cardiol 33:259–261

Beyer-Enke SA, Zhai F, Zeitler E (1994) Qualität, Nutzen und Risiken der Becken-/Bein-Angiographie vor PTA. Acta Radiol 4:307–312

Bookstein JJ, Moser KM, Hougie C (1982) Coagulative intervention during angiography. Cardiovasc Intervent Radiol 5:46–56

Fine MJ, Kapoor W, Falanga S (1987) Cholesterol crystal embolization: a review of 221 cases in the English literature. Angiology 38:769–784

Formanek G, Frech RS, Amplatz K (1970) Arterial thrombus formation during clinical percutaneous catheterization. Circulation 41:833

Gmelin E, Arlart JP (1987) Digitale Subtraktionsangiographie. Thieme, Stuttgart

Grollman JH jr, Marcus R (1988) Transbrachial arteriography: techniques and complications. Cardiovasc Intervent Radiol 11:32–35

Hessel SJ (1983) Complications of angiography and other catheter procedures. In: Abrams HL (ed) Angiography, vascular and interventional radiology, 3rd edn. Little, Brown and Company, Boston, pp 1041–1056 (vol. II)

Hessel SJ, Adams DF (1981) Complications of angiography. Radiology 138:273–281

May R, Nissl R (1969) Gefäßverschlüsse nach Angiographien. Fortschr Rontgenstr 110:64–71

Miller HC, Miller GAH (1974) Experience with systemic heparinization during cardiac catheterization by brachial arteriotomy. Br Heart J 36:1122–1124

Molnar W, Paul DJ (1972) Complications of axilliary arteriotomies: an analysis of 1762 consecutive studies. Radiology 104:269–275

Neimann HL, Yao JST (1985) Angiography of vascular disease. Churchill Livingston, New York

Neufang G, Friedmann G, Peters P, Mödder U (1983) Indikationen zur intraarteriellen digitalen Subtraktionsangiographie (i.a. DSA) bei Gefäßprozessen. Fortschr Rontgenstr 139:160–167

Neufang KFR, Beyer D (1988) Digitale Subtraktionsangiographie. Springer, Berlin Heidelberg New York

Ovitt TW, Durst S, Moore R, Amplatz K (1974) Guide wire thrombogenicity and its reduction. Radiology 111:43–46

Saint-Georges G, Aube M (1985) Safety of outpatient aortography: a prospective study. AJR Am J Roentgenol 144:235–236

Sigstedt B, Lunderquist A (1978) Complications of angiographic examinations. AJR Am J Roentgenol 130:455–460

Staal A, van Voorthuisen AE, van Dijk LM (1966) Neurological complications following arterial catheterization by the axillary approach. Br J Radiol 39: 115–121

Vogel H, Bartsch L, Pientka CHR, Rejzek Th (1986) Arteriographie. In: Vogel H (ed) Risiken der Röntgendiagnostik. Urban & Schwarzenberg. Munich, pp. 29–78

Wagner HH (1993) Aortographie und Arteriogrphie peripherer Gefäße. In: Alexander K (ed) Gefäßkrankheiten. Urban & Schwarzenberg, Munichen, pp. 228–238

Wallace S, Medellin H, De Jongh D, Gianturco C (1972) Systemic heparinization for angiography. AJR Am J Roentgenol 116: 204–206

Waugh JR, Sacharias N (1992) Arteriographic complications in the DSA era. Radiology 182: 243–246

Yandow D, Wojtowycz M, Alter A et al. (1988) Detection of retroperitoneal hemorrhage after translumbar aortography by computerized tomography. Angiology 31: 655–659

Zeitler E (1974) Aortoarteriographie. In: Heberer G, Rau G, Schoop W (eds) Angiologie. Thieme, Stuttgart, pp. 243–298

Zeitler E (ed) (1997) Klinische Radiologie: Arterien und Venen. Springer, Berlin Heidelberg New York

8.8
Interpretation, Report and Documentation

E. Zeitler

The interpretation of arteriographies primarily needs to answer the questions raised by the referring physician as precisely as possible. Vascular surgeons require angiographic findings to assess local (angiographic) operability (Vollmar 1975), and to plan surgery. The majority of obliterative lesions are of a segmental nature, a fact on which reconstructive vascular surgery (van Dongen 1970) and percutaneous angioplasty (Dotter et al. 1983) are based.

In addition, angiography can become necessary if an operation involving general anesthesia is contraindicated due to other diseases or conditions which may have an influence (e.g., severe diabetes, critical disorders of the coronary or cerebral circulation, or old age), in order to assess the chances of an interventional radiologic or minimally invasive surgical intervention (endoluminal surgery), under local anesthesia. The objective *interpretation* has first to confirm, or disprove, the clinical diagnosis (Bollinger 1979; Schoop 1988; Alexander 1994). Such diagnoses in the region of the lower extremities are discussed in more detail in the following sections.

8.8.1
Acute Arterial Thromboembolic Disease

According to Mathias (1997), this situation requires the following documentation: Where is/are the arterial occlusion(s) located, how long are they, and do multiple arterial occlusions due to their location indicate an embolism having occurred? The morphologic condition of the arteries in a proximal direction to the heart in relation to the occlusion (inflow arteries), and in a distal direction from the heart (run-off arteries) has to be evaluated. An analysis of the shape of the end of the occlusion (concave or convex), and its location may suggest embolism, or an acute thrombotic occlusion that has developed from a pre-existent arteriosclerotic stenosis. In addition, the source of embolism needs to be identified as precisely as possible on the basis of angiographic and clinical findings. Possible sources include aneurysms in the region of the aorta or inflow arteries, local thrombotic changes, indications from clinical or other examinations suggesting ventricular or atrial cardiac thrombi, or, in the case of existent deep venous thrombosis of the leg, the possibility of paradoxical embolism.

8.8.2
Chronic Peripheral Occlusive Vascular Disease (POVD)

Firstly, such lesions require objective confirmation of the type of obliteration (pelvic, upper leg, lower leg, or peripheral pedal occlusion or stenosis). Moreover, the location of isolated or multiple occlusions and stenoses needs to be defined. It is then important to precisely determine their anatomic relationship to vascular bifurcations, such as the aortic, femoral, or popliteal bifurcation. In the analysis of occlusions (see Chap. 25, Fig. 25.6), it needs to be determined whether or not important collateral pathways exist and, if so, which type. In the case of a longer existing collateral circulation, the collateral arteries which distally join the main artery often develop stenoses with poststenotic dilatation ("sinus phenomenon"; ZEITLER 1974).

Isolated or multiple occlusions need to be precisely determined as regards their length and anatomic relationship to neighboring arteries (e.g., renal artery, hypogastric artery, etc.; skeleton-projectional: knee joint, ankle joint, or similar). While their extension in a proximal direction is unproblematic, their extension in a distal direction requires sufficiently long imaging series, as inflow from the collateral circulation can take place at varying distances from the proximal end of the occlusion. The exact definition of non-occluding luminal narrowings – stenoses – provides better information if performed on two or more levels. The difficulty lies in determing the precise percentage of the degree of stenosis, without quantitative measurement. Moreover, detecting fresh thrombotic areas inside the stenosis or occlusion is difficult. This, however, can be of importance since fresh thrombi are amenable to thrombolysis, either pharmacological or mechanic, while, on the other hand, they involve the risk of embolization following mechanical manipulation.

An attempt to characterize stenoses (see Chap. 25, Fig. 25.1) is therefore imperative. This includes information on the type of stenosis – isolated or multiple, with a smooth or verrucous (rough) surface. Also, the length of the stenosis and possible existance of atheromatous ulcers and their extension, and the documentation of existing poststenotic dilatations not only have to be documented, but also to be recorded.

Besides the standard characterizations, such as concentric/excentric, smooth/verrucous surface, singular or multiple, the lesions can be described as type A, B, or C stenotic lesions analoguous to the method used in coronarography (HAASE and REIFART 1994). Such a classification facilitates understanding in comparative analyses as follows:

- *Type A lesion (minimally complex)*: Concentric, length 1 – 2 cm; no ostial or bifurcational location; smooth surface; little or no calcification
- *Type B lesion (moderately complex)*: Excentric, length 2–5 cm; irregularities in front of or behind the stenotic lesion; existent small atheromatous ulcer; close to bifurcations (e.g., iliac bifurcation);

ostial stenosis (deep femoral; aortoiliac bifurcation) with no signs of fresh thrombus
- *Type C lesion (severely complex)*: Diffuse irregularities over long distances; segmental stenoses longer than 4 cm; bifurcational or ostial lesions with irregular surface; extensive tortuosity, e.g., critical lesions on the aortoiliac bifurcation or popliteal bifurcation.

8.8.2.1
Quantitative Measurement

In addition to a description of the quality of obliterations, stenoses and occlusions, the quantitative definition of stenoses can help in the clear definition, comparison, and selection of balloon size or specific stent characteristics. For that purpose, the prestenotic luminal diameter in an arterial segment without abnormalities, the narrowest diameter within the stenosed segment, and the poststenotic artery diameter at a site not showing a poststenotic dilatation, need to be measured. The degree of stenosis is indicated as a percentage of the prestenotic luminal diameter as follows:

Where D presten. indicates the prestenotic arterial diameter and D stenotic indicates the narrowest arterial diameter within the stenosis. This method of determining the degree of stenosis can lead to an overestimation in the case of slitshaped stenoses, whereas in cases of circular stenoses, an underestimation may occur.

To determine the degree of stenosis in relation to the area of the circle, the percentage of stenosis is calculated using the following formula:

A quantitaive determination can also be performed with densitometry. This is possible in the framework of digital angiography by means of contour marking and densimetric analysis in the relevant prestenotic segment, as well as in the stenosed area. Under- or overestimation that may occur in excentric or slitshaped stenoses can be limited with densitometry. While in the framework of coronary angiography both preprocedural and postprocedural – prior to and after PTCA – detailed documentation of the quantitative determination of the degree of stenoses are available (RAFFENBEUL, LICHTLEN 1979; REIBER et al. 1986; SERRUYS et al. 1984), such consequential systematic quantitative definitions of stenoses have not, or seldom, been carried out in the region of the peripheral arteries. The "coronary angiographic analysis system" (CAAS) (REIBER et al. 1986) has been extensively validated on more than 1700 patients who underwent several forms of nonoperative coronary revascularization. The CAAS system functions by detecting lumen borders with the edge-detection method in two orthogonal projections, and by densitometry to assess the relative area stenosis by comparing the density of contrast in the diseased and normal segments. Using the densitometry method, precise results can be obtained in a single projection, even if the cross-sectional shape is irregular. Densitometry can obtain the percentage of area stenosis, and minimal luminal cross-sectional area both as relative measurements of area stenosis, a ratio based on the relative differences in brightness. For absolute measurements, the reference diameter must be determined from the edge-detection data (STRAUSS et al. 1992).

The classification of occlusions shorter than 3 cm, 3–10 cm, and longer than 10 cm is important to determine the optimum indications for interventional radiology, thrombolysis, and vascular surgery. In the same way, it is important to define the situation of run-off vessels in calf and foot arteries. If angiography does not provide a precise answer, other methods such as ultrasound or MRA, as well as spiral CT, can be helpful undoubtedly by flow-measurement, duplex sonography and MRA can sometimes help to find run-of vessels on the calf and foot more effectively than roentgen angiography. On the other hand, the thoracic and abdominal aorta, as well as the supraaortic arteries, can be diagnosed very precisely with spiral CT or MRA without arterial catheterization.

Back in 1966, MÜNSTER et al. had angiographically demonstrated in 1713 legs that local disease is more common in young age and that combined obliterations in several areas are the result of progression with age. Table 8.28 shows the incidence of obliterations in distal, femoral, and iliac artery segments. Moreover, the location of a segmental occlusion plays an important role in the extent of collateral vessel formation (BOLLINGER 1969). Occlusions in bifurcations and multiple occlusions are unfavourable.

8.8.3
Aneurysmatic Disease

To define aneurysms, it is important to measure the length, width, and location of the ectatic and thrombosed part of the lesion. It is necessary to have a look at involved arteries near the aneurysm, such as the renal, mesenteric, or hypogastric artery, and, in the same way as with documentation of calcified parts of aneurysms, to investigate whether inflammation and symptoms of mycotic aneurysms exist. In several types of aneurysm, or polyaneurysmatic disease, similar lesions exist on both legs, or in the same area. This is most important in the diagnosis of popliteal aneurysms and polyaneurysmatic disease (BRUNNER and HUWYLER 1975; VOLLMAR and NOBBE 1976; SANDMANN and KNIEMEYER 1991; IMIG and SCHRÖDER 1995; ZEITLER 1997). It is important to document peripheral embolization and the patency of run-off vessels.

8.8.4
The Upper Extremities

In the supraaortic arteries (brachiocephalic and subclavian arteries), stenoses and occlusions must be defined very precisely in terms of diameter, localization, and extension, and the collateral circulation needs to be checked. This is particularly the case in subclavian steal syndrome, as well as in subclavian steal plus carotid recovery phenomenons. In addition, the cerebrovascular arteries in the neck need to be examined and functional angiography may be necessary. Angiography in elevated arms or after neck rotation can be especially valuable in functional angiographic studies to diagnose intermittent compression against the arteries (e.g. •• TOS).

8.8.5
The Report and Document

The report following qualified angiography should provide answers to clinical questions and additionally include all information found regarding anatomic variations and important vascular changes which define special diseases, such as compression, string sign, av-shunts, and information about good flow, pendulant flow, or stasis.

It is the angiographer's task to document all important lesions, abnormalities, and run-in and run-off vessels so that any doctors subsequently involved

Table 8.28. Incidance of arterial obliterations - agedepedent (acc. MÜNSTER et al. 1966)

Segment	20–30 years, 15 patients, 24 extremities (%)	31–40 years, 81 patients, 135 extremities (%)	41–50 years, 146 patients, 246 extremities (%)	51–60 years, 389 patients, 704 extremities (%)	61–70 years, 299 patients, 561 extremities (%)	Over 71 years, 22 patients, 43 extremities (%)	Total obliterations	Incidence of obliterations (%)
A	–	–	5	15	10		30	3.2
1	4.2	2.2	19.9	21.4	22.6	16.3	338	19.7
2	25.0	14.8	30.5	25.1	33.7	11.6	472	27.6
I	8.3	1.5	11.0	13.5	19.2	13.9	240	14.0
II	25.0	15.5	6.9	5.5	5.7	16.3	122	7.1
3	25.0	30.4	26.4	37.1	45.4	27.9	640	37.4
4	25.0	29.6	35.8	50.1	61.0	39.5	846	49.4
5	37.5	32.6	45.9	61.3	66.5	67.4	1000	58.4
6	29.2	22.2	11.0	13.8	20.0	23.2	283	16.5
7	33.3	24.4	9.8	9.6	12.6	20.9	213	12.4
8	33.3	26.0	9.8	8.1	8.6	20.9	181	10.6
9	50.0	51.1	32.5	33.9	32.1	37.2	586	34.2
10	41.7	39.3	19.1	12.6	15.5	30.2	299	17.5
11	54.2	54.8	26.8	23.1	23.5	39.5	465	27.1

Patient initials: _____ Sex: M F Age: _____   Patient I.D. # _____
Hospital: _____ Date Admitted __/__/__ Date Discharged __/__/__
Physician Performing Procedure: _____ Date of Procedure __/__/__

Instructions: Place an "X" in the appropriate box and supply other data as indicated.

1. VESSEL DILATED
   a ☐ Common iliac, rt.   j ☐ SFA, lt.   s ☐ Carotid, lt.
   b ☐ Common iliac, lt.   k ☐ Popliteal, rt.   t ☐ Subclavian, rt.
   c ☐ External iliac, rt.   l ☐ Popliteal, lt.   u ☐ Subclavian, lt.
   d ☐ External iliac, lt.   m ☐ Renal, rt.   v ☐ Vertebral, rt.
   e ☐ Common femoral, rt.   n ☐ Renal, lt.   w ☐ Vertebral, lt.
   f ☐ Common femoral, lt.   o ☐ Renal Transplant   x ☐ Vein Graft
   g ☐ Profunda femoris, rt.   p ☐ SMA   y ☐ Prosthetic Graft
   h ☐ Profunda femoris, lt.   q ☐ Celiac   z ☐ Mescaval—Shunt
   i ☐ SFA, rt.   r ☐ Carotid, rt.   zz ☐ Other

2. ETIOLOGY OF LESION
   a ☐ ASVD b ☐ Fibromuscular hyperplasia c ☐ Surgical stricture d ☐ Other, specify _____
                                               (anastomosis)

3. INDICATION(S) FOR PROCEDURE
   EXTREMITY (Ilio-Femoro-Popliteal, Calf Arteries)
   a ☐ Claudication b ☐ Rest pain c ☐ Limb salvage d ☐ Other, specify _____
   ABDOMINAL AORTA
   e ☐ Claudication f ☐ Impotence g ☐ Other, specify _____
   PROSTHETIC GRAFTS
   h ☐ Claudication i ☐ Rest Pain j ☐ Limb Salvage
   VEIN BYPASS GRAFTS
   k ☐ Claudication l ☐ Rest Pain m ☐ Limb Salvage
   ARTERIOVENOUS FISTULAS
      (HEMODYALISIS)
   n ☐ Decreased Flow o ☐ Other, specify _____
   HYPOGASTRIC p ☐ Rt. q ☐ Lt.
   r ☐ Impotence s Decreased Penile Pressures t ☐ Other, specify _____
   RENAL u ☐ Rt. v ☐ Lt.
   w ☐ Hypertension x ☐ Preservation of renal function y ☐ Renin Ratios, specify _____
   SMA
   z ☐ Mesenteric Angina aa ☐ Abdominal Bruit. bb ☐ Other, specify _____
   CELIAC AXIS
   cc ☐ Median Arcuate dd ☐ Abdominal Bruit. ee ☐ Other, specify _____
   MESO/CAVAL—PORTO/CAVAL SHUNTS
   ff ☐ Portal Hypertension gg ☐ Other, specify _____
   CAROTID hh ☐ Rt. ii ☐ Lt.
   jj ☐ Bruit. kk ☐ TIAs ll ☐ Other, specify _____
   SUBCLAVIAN mm ☐ Rt. nn ☐ Lt.
   oo ☐ Bruit. pp ☐ Absent Pulses qq ☐ Pain rr ☐ Other, specify _____
   VERTEBRAL ss ☐ Rt. tt ☐ Lt.
   uu ☐ TIAs vv ☐ Other, specify _____

4. NATURE OF LESION Length a _____ cm.
        No   Yes
   b ☐   c ☐ Calcified?   h ☐ Single i ☐ Multiple
   d ☐   e ☐ Total occlusion?   j ☐ Concentric k ☐ Eccentric
   f ☐   g ☐ Stenosis?   l ☐ _____ % lumen occluded
   m ☐   n ☐ Renal? If yes, specify: o ☐ orifice p ☐ main artery q ☐ branch

5. TYPE OF RUN-OFF
   a ☐ Excellent b ☐ Fair c ☐ Poor d ☐ None

6. RISK FACTORS a ☐ None
   b ☐ Tobacco c ☐ Hyperlipidemia d ☐ Diabetes e ☐ Hypertension

7. CHARACTERISTICS OF BALLOON Diameter a _____ mm.   Length b _____ cm.
   Manufacturer:
   c ☐ Cook d ☐ Schneider e ☐ USCI f ☐ Medi-tech g ☐ Other, specify _____

8. CHARACTERISTICS OF CATHETER, "Dotter Technique"
                   No   Yes   8   10   12
   Dotter?   a ☐ b ☐ If yes, specify French size c ☐ d ☐ e ☐ Grüntzig f ☐____
   Van Andel?   g ☐ h ☐ If yes, specify French size i ☐ j ☐ k ☐ Olbert l ☐____

9. ANGIOGRAPHIC APPEARANCE AFTER PTA
   Vessel occluded? a ☐ No b ☐ Yes
      If no, specify % lumen patency c ☐ less than 25% d ☐ 25–50%
   e ☐ 51–80% f ☐ greater than 80%

10. PRESSURES
    Pressures obtained across lesions?   a ☐ No   b ☐ Yes
    If yes, specify peak to peak systolic gradient before TA_____(mmHg)
after TA_____(mmHg)
11. INFLATION PRESSURE IN ATMOSPHERES _____ ATMS
12. TOTAL LENGTH OF BALLOON INFLATION PER AREA a____ Sec/Min b____ Sec/Min
    c____ Sec/Min d____ Sec/Min e____ Sec/Min f____ Sec/Min
13. COMPLICATIONS—Check all that apply.   a ☐ None (proceed to #13)
    b   ☐ Peripheral embolization   j ☐ Infarction of portion of kidney
    c   ☐ Occlusion of vessel dilated   k ☐ Renal failure, transient
    d   ☐ Occlusion of collateral   l ☐ Renal failure, permanent
    e   ☐ Dissection of vessel   m ☐ Large hematoma at puncture site
    f   ☐ Perforation of vessel   n ☐ False aneurysm at puncture site
    g   ☐ False aneurysm in vessel dilated o ☐ Infection at puncture site
    h   ☐ Vessel rupture   p ☐ Blood loss of ____ units
    i   ☐ Occlusion of renal branch
14. RESULTS OF COMPLICATION
    Death within 48 hours?   a ☐ No   b ☐ Yes
    Surgery necessary?   c ☐ No   d ☐ Yes   If yes,   e ☐ surgery successful, no permanent morbidity
                             f ☐ limb loss, specify _____
                             g ☐ organ loss, specify _____
15. POST-DILATATION MEDICATION   a ☐ None
    b ☐ ASA (__days)   c ☐ Persantin (__days)   d ☐ Heparin (__days)   e ☐ Coumadin (__days)
        (__weeks)   (__weeks)   (__weeks)
        (__months)   (__months)   (__months)
16. CLINICAL RESULTS
    Initial: a ☐ Excellent   b ☐ Good   c ☐ Fair   d ☐ Failure
    If renal dilatation, specify eBP before TA _____ (mmHg) eBP after TA _____ (mmHg)
        AND
    whether antihypertensive medication is   f ☐ same as before TA
                                             g ☐ less than before TA
                                             h ☐ greater than before TA

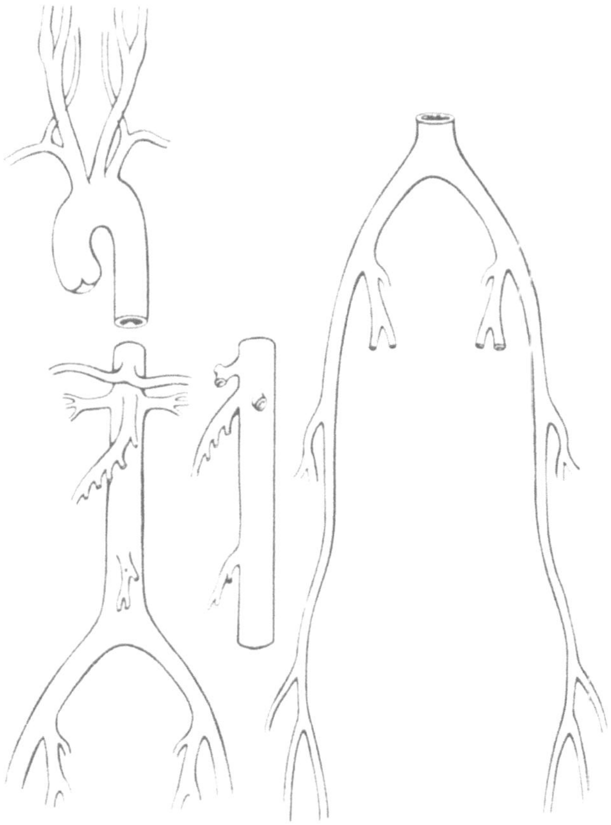

Fig. 8.57. Sample form for documenting angiographic results

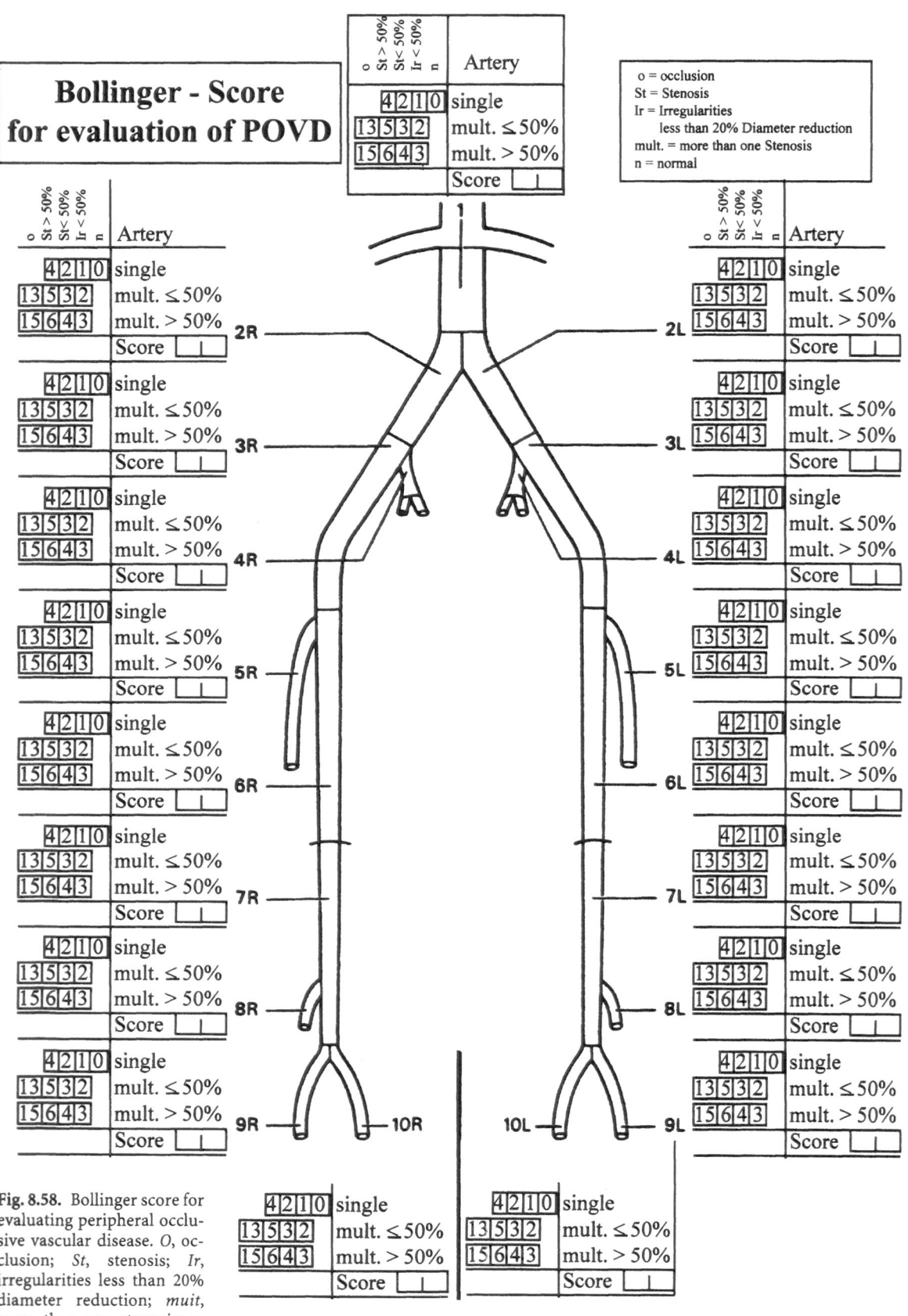

Fig. 8.58. Bollinger score for evaluating peripheral occlusive vascular disease. *O*, occlusion; *St*, stenosis; *Ir*, irregularities less than 20% diameter reduction; *muit*, more than one stenosis; *n*, normal

in the patient's treatment find all important information both in the documented angiographies (hard copies, video-, or cine-angiography), as well as in the written report.

Severe lesions need to be documented in more than one direction. Flow changes can also be documented and, prior to a final decision the result should be discussed among different specialists on the basis of hard copies, or directly during a monitor demonstration. Angiography, therefore includes optimal, informative images, combined with a written report. In special situations, such as treatment controls, comparison with previous findings becomes necessary. Thus, some clinics use drawings, computer documentation, or standard report forms (Fig. 8.57) (CASTANEDA-ZUNIGE and AMPLATZ 1983). To compare angiogaphic results before and after various treatment, or to study progression and regression, documentation using the Bollinger score (Fig. 8.58), or similar system, can be helpful (DURHAM and RUTHERFORD 1994).

Having documented and made a report of precise angiographies in combination with the clinical symptoms and laboratory data, a basis for clear indications for the various treatment modalities has been formed.

References

Alexander K (1994) Gefäßkrankheiten. Urban & Schwarzenberg, Munich

Bollinger A (1969) Durchblutungsmessungen in der klinischen Angiologie. Huber, Bern

Bollinger A (1979) Funktionelle Angiologie. Lehrbuch und Atlas. Thieme, Stuttgart

Bollinger A, Breddin K. et al. (1981) Semigmantidatioe assessment of lower -limb atherosclerosis from routine angiographic images, Atherosclerosis 38:339-346

Brunner U, Huwyler R (1975) Das arteriosklerotische femoropopliteale Aneurysma. In: Brunner U (ed) Die Kniekehle. Huber, Bern, pp. 51-59

Castaneda-Zuniga WR, Amplatz K (1983) Use of standard reporting forms. In: Castaneda-Zuniga WR (ed) Transluminal angioplasty. Thieme-Stratton, New York, pp. 45-47

Dotter CT, Grüntzig AR, Schoop W, Zeitler E (1983) Percutaneous transluminal angioplasty. Springer, Berlin Heidelberg New York

Durham JD, Rutherford RB (1994) Standards for reporting lower-extremity ischemia. In: La Berge JM, Darcy MD (eds) Peripheral vascular interventions. Syllabus, SCVIR, pp. 206-215

Haase J, Reifart N (1994) Coronary angiography. In: Lanzer P, Rösch J (eds) Vascular diagnostics. Springer, Berlin Heidelberg New York, pp. 243-266

Imig H, Schröder A (1995) Varizen, Poplitea-Aneurysmen. Steinkopff, Darmstadt, pp. 97-131

Raffenbeul W, Lichtlen PR (1979) Intravitale Morphometrie. In: Lichtlen PR (ed) Koronarangiographie. Straube, Erlangen, pp. 325-339

Mathias K (1997) Phänomenologie von Gefäßerkrankungen. In: Zeitler E (ed) Klinische Radiologie: Arterien und Venen. Springer, Berlin Heidelberg New York, pp. 129-142

Münster W, Wierny L, Porstmann W (1966) Localization and frequency of arterial obliterations of the lower extremities. Analysis of 952 aortographies. Dtsch Med Wochenschr 91:2073-2079

Reliber JH, Serruys PW, Slager CJ (1986) Quantitative coronary and left ventricular cineangiography: methodology and clinical applications. Martinus Nijhoff, Boston

Sandmann W, Kniemeyer HW (eds) (1991) Aneurysmen der großen Arterien. Huber, Bern

Schoop W (1988) Praktische Angiologie. Thieme, Stuttgart

Serruys PW, Reiber JHC, Wijns W et al. (1984) Assessment of percutaneous transluminal coronary angioplasty by quantitative coronary angiography: diameter versus densitometric area measurements. Am J Cardiol 54:482-488

Strauss BH et al. (1992) Methodologic aspects of quantitative coronary angiography (QCA) in interventional cardiology. In: Serruys PW, Strauss BH, King III SB (eds) Restenosis. Kluwer Academic, Dordrecht, pp. 11-50

Van Dongen RJ (1970) Photographic atlas of reconstructive arterial surgery. HE Stenfert Kroese, NV Leiden

Vollmar J (1975) Rekonstruktive Chirurgie der Arterien. Thieme, Stuttgart

Vollmar JF, Nobbe FP (eds) (1976) Arteriovenöse Fisteln – Dilatierende Arteriopathien (Aneurysmen). Thieme, Stuttgart

Zeitler E (1974) Aortoarteriographien. In: Heberer G, Rau G, Schoop W (eds) Angiologie. Founded by M. Ratschow. Thieme, Stuttgart, pp. 241-298

Zeitler E (1997) Angiologische Diagnostik, Angiologische Therapie. In: Zeitler E (ed) Klinische Radiologie: Arterien und Venen. Springer, Berlin Heidelberg New York, pp. 167-256

Zeitler E, Heuck FHW (1997) Aneurysmen und dilatative Angiopathie. In: Zeitler E (ed) Klinische Radiologie: Arterien und Venen. Springer, Berlin Heidelberg New York, pp. 277-312

Appendix Table 1. Conversion table

BAR	PSI	ATM	PSI	BAR	ATM
1	14.5	1.02	1	0.1	0.1
2	29.0	2.04	5	0.3	0.4
3	43.5	3.06	10	0.7	0.7
4	58.0	4.08	50	3.5	3.5
5	72.5	5.10	100	6.9	7.0
7	101.5	6.12	200	13.8	14.1
8	116.0	7.14	300	20.7	21.1
9	130.5	9.18	400	27.6	28.1
10	145.0	10.20	500	34.5	35.2
11	159.0	11.22	600	41.4	42.2
12	174.0	12.24	700	48.3	49.2
			800	55.2	56.3
			900	62.1	63.3
			1000	69.0	70.3
1 bar = 1.02 atm = 14.5 psi			1100	75.9	77.4
			1200	82.8	84.4

French	mm	Inches	Gauge	OD (mm)	OD (Inch)
0.5	0.16	0.006	27	0.41	0.016
1	0.33	0.013	26	0.46	0.018
1.5	0.49	0.019	25	0.51	0.020
1.8	0.59	0.023	24	0.56	0.022
2	0.67	0.026	23	0.64	0.025
2.5	0.82	0.032	22	0.71	0.028
3.0	1.00	0.039	21	0.81	0.032
4	1.33	0.052	20	0.97	0.038
5	1.67	0.078	19	1.07	0.042
6	2.00	0.079	18	1.27	0.050
7	2.33	0.092	17	1.50	0.059
8	2.67	0.105	16	1.65	0.065
9	3.00	0.118	15	1.83	0.072
10	3.33	0.131	14	2.11	0.083

1 Fr = 0.0131 inch = 0.33 mm
1 inch = 2.54 cm

9 CT Angiography: Spiral (Helical) CT and Electron Beam Tomography

M. Oldendorf and U. Szeimies

CONTENTS

M. Oldendorf, MD, Institut für Diagnostische und Interventionelle Radiologie, Klinikum Nürnberg-Nord, Flurstraße 17, 90340 Nürnberg, Germany
Ulrike Szeimies, MD, Institut für Radiologische Diagnostik, Kernspintomographie, Klinikum Innenstadt, Universität München, Ziemssenstraße 1, 80336 München, Germany

9.1
Basics of Spiral (Helical) CT

9.1.1
The Spiral (Helical) CT Scan Principle

In X-ray CT attenuation profiles of a transverse slice of a patient or object are measured from a multitude of angular positions. An X-ray tube, with its beam collimated to a fan defining the image plane, and a detector array run on a circular path around the patient. Typically, 360 degrees are covered to collect a complete set of data.

9.1.2
Volume Scanning

Using a spiral CT scanner a volume scanning procedure in non-planar geometry is carried out. This is done by extending the scan over many tube rotations while the patient is continuously shifted through the gantry. While the X-ray tube and detector system rotate around the patient, the data is acquired. The patient travels at a speed of one slice thickness per 360-degree rotation. The focus of the tube describes a "spiral" or "helical" path which led to these two names being commonly used for this scanning procedure (Kalender 1995).

9.1.3
Pitch

The ratio of table feed over slice thickness is commonly termed pitch and is very important for image quality, patient dose, and practical considerations. The image reconstruction of each single image uses the same hardware, algorithms, and reconstruction kernels as in conventional CT. However, an additional step in data processing, the so-called slice-, section-, or z-interpolation is necessary before image reconstruction can be started.

9.1.4
Reconstruction Increment

Of decisive importance is the possibility that the reconstruction increment, the position and spacing of successive images, can be chosen freely and retrospectively. Moreover, the computer system will be decisive in establishing how many images can be reconstructed from a given scan volume within a tolerable time.

9.1.5
Image Quality

The image quality in spiral CT is comparable to that in conventional CT in every respect due to the fact that the complete measurement system is the same in both scan modes. Differences in image quality have to be expected with respect to pixel noise due to the added processing step of z-interpolation and with respect to slice sensitivity profiles due to moving the object during the scan and the necessary z-interpolation. As a direct consequence, resolution along the z-axis, the body's longitudinal direction, will also be influenced. Furthermore, there may be subtle differences in artifact behavior, seen mostly off center. The above-mentioned differences will depend on the type of z-interpolation algorithm used. If no z-algorithm is specified, 180-degree algorithms are referred to; they are chosen as default algorithms due to their predominant use (KALENDER 1995).

9.2
Spiral (Helical) CT Angiography

CT angiography is based on a spiral or helical CT investigation using the technical equipment as mentioned above. To obtain angiographic-like pictures, different visualization tools should be applied. It seems to be useful to extract all data gained by one CT investigation. Routinely using all secondary imaging techniques will avoid misinterpretation. Moreover, it seems to be of great importance that paravasal structures, such as bones and soft tissue, can be displayed.

9.2.1
Scan Time and Length

The total scanning time depends on the scan time per slice thickness and the number of detectors that are available within the gantry. Scanning times of 0.75 and 1.0 s can be found in all scanners available on the market today (1997); multiple detectors will reduce the time by up to 50% or even more.

The choice of the scan length and the slice thickness depends directly on the region to be investigated along the z-axis and the size of the arteries. In all cases the pitch should be as small as possible, never exceeding 2.0.

9.2.2
Reconstruction Increment

The reconstruction interval, i.e., the distance at which the images are reconstructed from the raw data set, has an influence on the quality of the angiographic pictures. Theoretically, between three and five pictures for each slice thickness is best; a reconstruction increment of half the slice thickness is an optimal solution (KALENDER 1995) but can be used only in specific cases.

9.2.3
Secondary Imaging

9.2.3.1
Multiplanar Image Reconstruction

Multiplanar image reconstruction (MPR), a classical image reformatting process, is a post-processing facility which is not threshold-dependent, and which is helpful in displaying thrombosed walls of aneurysms and dissections. The relationship between vessels, bones and soft tissue is documented. No editing maneuvers are necessary (Table 9.1).

Table 9.1. Application tools: multiplanar image reconstruction (MPR)

Multiplanar Image Reconstruction
• Planar image sampling
• No editing maneuvers necessary
• Best survey
• Runs very fast
• Choice of selecting interesting level

9.2.3.2
Shaded Surface Display

Shaded surface display (SSD) is a threshold-dependent technique. In the viewing direction the first voxel along each ray with a CT value above a defined density threshold is considered. Afterwards, a surface is calculated as if the structure were illuminated by a light source, thus achieving a three-dimensional (3D) impression. Density changes within these objects are not recorded; alterations within the lumen of the vessel, e.g., thrombi, calcifications or dissections, are not visible. This method is helpful in differentiating high contrast vessels which superimpose each other, particularly in the region of the aortic arch (Table 9.2).

Table 9.2. Application tools: three-dimensional shaded surface display (SSD)

3D Shaded surface display
• Defined density threshold
• First voxel above is displayed
• Surface calculation and illumination
• 3D Impression without perspective
• 360 Projection angles in each axis
• Runs fast

9.2.3.3
Maximum Intensity Projections

Maximum intensity projections (MIP) are commonly used for displaying vessels. Arteries, as well as venous structures, are displayed. The possibility of looking at the vessels in all three spatial axes at different projection angles gives an angiographic-like impression to the viewer. Synonyms for MIP are brightest pixel projection (BPP) or brightest voxel projection (BVP) and can be used as well as MIP. For more details see Sect. 2.3.

9.2.3.4
Volume Rendering Technique

With the volume rendering technique (VRT) internal surfaces are displayed semitransparently as a result of the corresponding information (Fig. 9.1). The gray-scale values change with the surface condition of the tissue structures. VRT is used less for angiographic image post-processing than for endoscopic imaging in virtual endoscopy and bronchoscopy. For further details see Sect. 2.9.

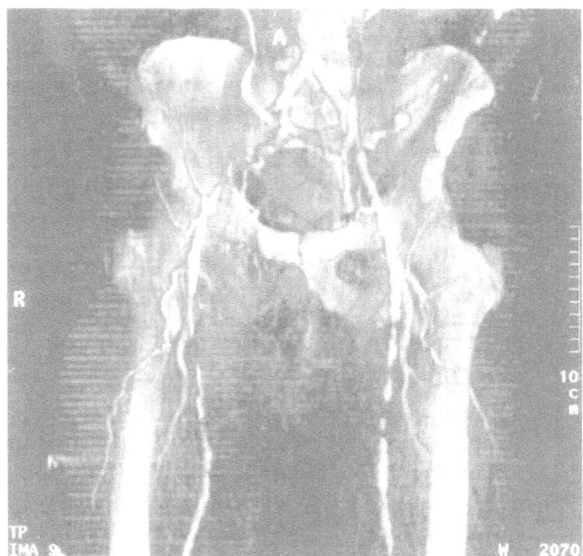

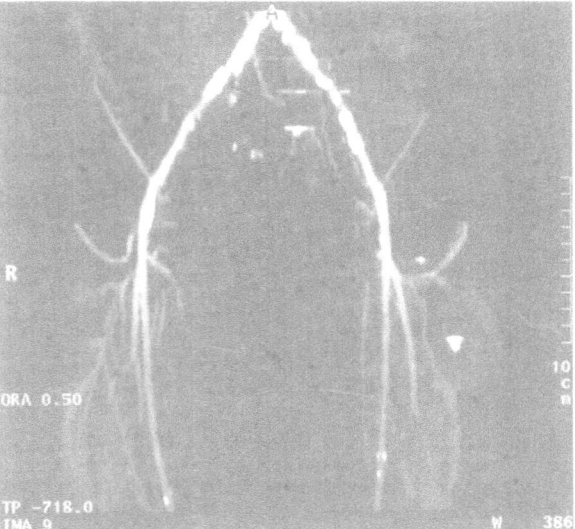

Fig. 9.1 a,b. The volume rendering technique. **a** Occlusions along the right iliacal artery and high grade stenoses along the femoral arteries; no differentiation between calcification and well-contrasted vessel is possible. **b** This decision is only possible when using the MIP technique

9.3
MIP Reconstruction

9.3.1
Principles

MIP is a two-dimensional volume rendering technique. The axial slices gained from one investigation are put together. Afterwards, a viewing direction has to be chosen. Along this viewing direction parallel rays penetrate the image and the highest CT value is displayed. Because a volume is scanned, the parallel rays cast through a volume of interest (VOI). MIP images have no information about the depth of the object. Differentiation between background and foreground is not possible on the single MIP images. The 3D impression is generated by rotating the different projection angles using a cine loop video-like technique.

9.3.2
Range of Applications

Because on a MIP image the highest CT value is displayed without giving the exact position along the projection ray – and MIP images do *not* provide depth information – complex overlying vessel structures cannot be differentiated because they join and have no exact demarcation to each other (Fig. 9.2; see Fig. 9.5). Therefore MIP images are suited to displaying the vascular anatomy and pathology

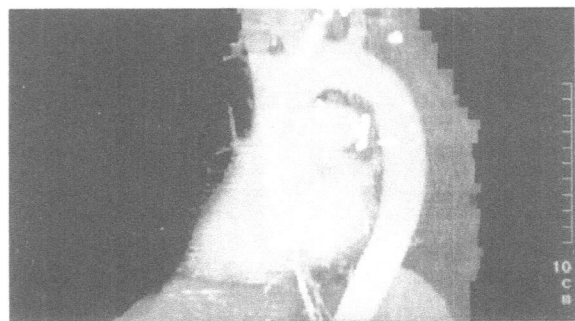

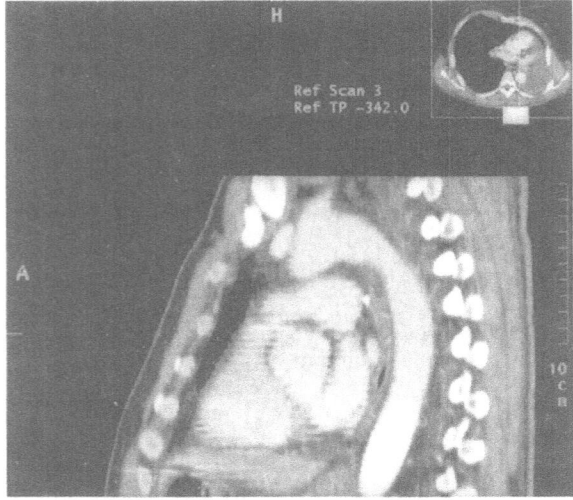

Fig. 9.2 a,b. Maximum intensity projections (MIP) VS. multiplanar image reconstruction (MPR). **a** Lateral view of the thoracic aorta descendens, displayed in MIP. **b** MPR postprocessing techniques. Complex overlying structures within the heart are only visible on the MPR image

of vessels that do not overlay: the skull base, the carotic bifurcation, the abdominal aorta and its main branches, and the iliac arteries. On the other hand, MIP is less useful in the aortic arch, its main branches, and in displaying arteriovenous malformations.

9.3.3
Editing

As mentioned above, the highest CT values are displayed within the whole scanned volume, including bones. To achieve angiographic-like images without overlying bones and soft tissue structures, editing procedures are necessary to exclude structures that might superimpose the vessels. Two different techniques to exclude structures with a high CT value can be used:

1. Cutting: A line can be drawn, circumferencing the object and excluding objects outside this area (cutting function). Disturbing structures, mostly bones or contrast-filled intestines, can be excluded. A slab-editor is useful to put together several axial slices (thin-slab editing). Using this technique it is necessary to check exactly the borderlines in order not to cut away vessel structures (Fig. 9.3b).
2. Region growing: With this method a threshold range has to be chosen above which disturbing structures are extinguished. The threshold must be low enough to exclude faint bone structures but higher than the background to avoid the insufficient display of small vessels. Afterwards, pixel seeds have to be placed on structures to be removed (bones, etc.), giving the seeds the predefined CT values. Using the seeds one must be careful along the aorta: well-contrasted vessels and calcifications along the vessel-wall situated close to vertebral structures can be extinguished. To avoid the editing of each single axial image a slab editor is also useful to put together several axial slices (thin-slab editing).

9.3.4
Background Noise

With the length of the ray passing through the edited volume of interest, the image noise also grows. The image noise is high in adipose patients and increases by using low radiation doses. Background noise also increases when organs enhance with contrast medim

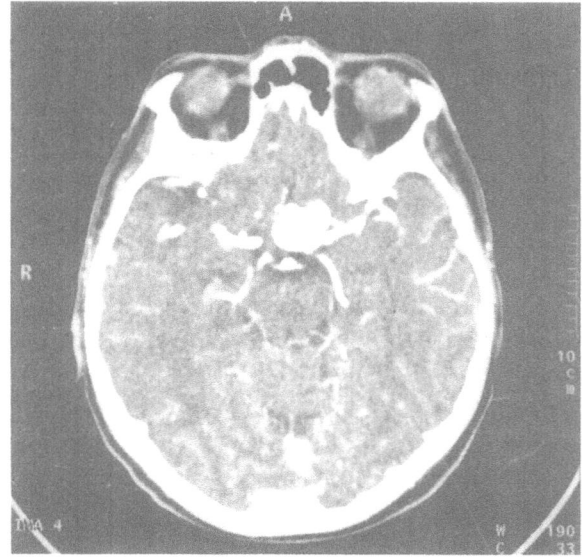

a

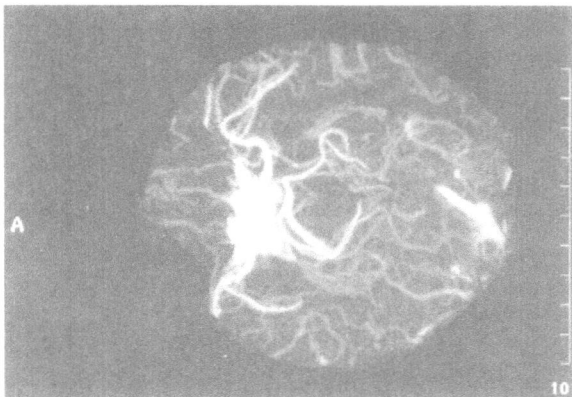

b

Fig. 9.3 a. Circle of Willis, cutting function: partly calcified aneurysm, seen in the axial image. **b** For MIP imaging bones were excluded using the cutting function. Slice thickness, 1 mm; pitch, 1.0; scan length, 60 mm; reconstruction interval, 1.0 mm

9.4
Scannning Parameters and Contrast Media

For optimizing spiral (heical) CT angiography it is necessary to adapt the scanning parameters and the amount of contrast media to the scanned region.

9.4.1
Scanning Parameters

9.4.1.1
Skull Base (Circle of Willis)

To guarantee high spatial resolution, a slice thickness of 1–2 mm and a table feed of 1–2 mm/s can be selected in the region of the skull base (circle of Willis). A total scan length of 4–8 cm is sufficient, with a pitch of 1.0–1.5 and a reconstruction interval of 1.0 mm (see Fig. 9.3).

9.4.1.2
Carotid Arteries

Carotid arteries, as well as vertebral arteries, should be displayed with their origins from the aortic arch or subclavian artery. A slice thickness of 2–3 mm is adequate and a total scan length of 15 cm will be sufficient, with a pitch of 1.5–2.0 and a reconstruction interval of 1.0–1.5 mm (Fig. 9.4).

9.4.1.3
Thoracic and Abdominal Aorta

The longer the scanned region along the z-axis, the more important the maximum heat capacity of the X-ray tube will become, as well as the capacity of the computer system.

during data acquisition. Any kind of test bolus enlarges the background noise, as well as a long delay time before the scanning begins. The noise will also increase towards the end of a spiral (helical) CT investigation.

The organs most affected include: the thyroid, kidneys, liver, spleen and – very disturbingly – the small bowel, imitating oral contrast media given before. With increasing background noise, the vessels "drown" in the background. A precontrasted vein that runs parallel to the artery will make the apparent size of the artery in the MIP images decrease due to partial volume averaging (PROKOP et al. 1997). The smaller the vessel, the greater the effect will be – an occlusion of the vessel may even be simulated (see Fig. 7) (Table 9.3).

Table 9.3. Application tools: maximum intensity projections (MIP)

Maximum intensity projections (Ray Tracing Projections)
• Angiographic-like imaging
• Highest value within a definite volume is displayed (maximum intensity)
• Editing is necessary
• Two-dimensional image impression
• 360 Projection angles in each axis

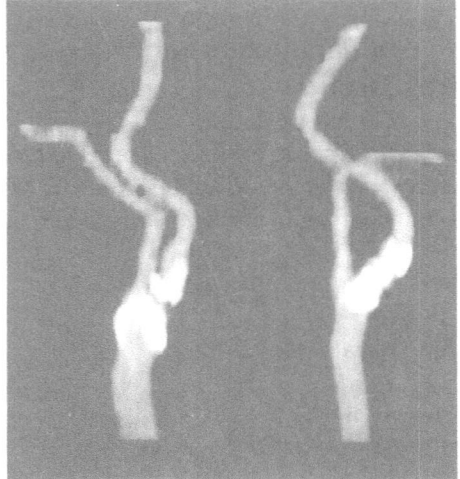

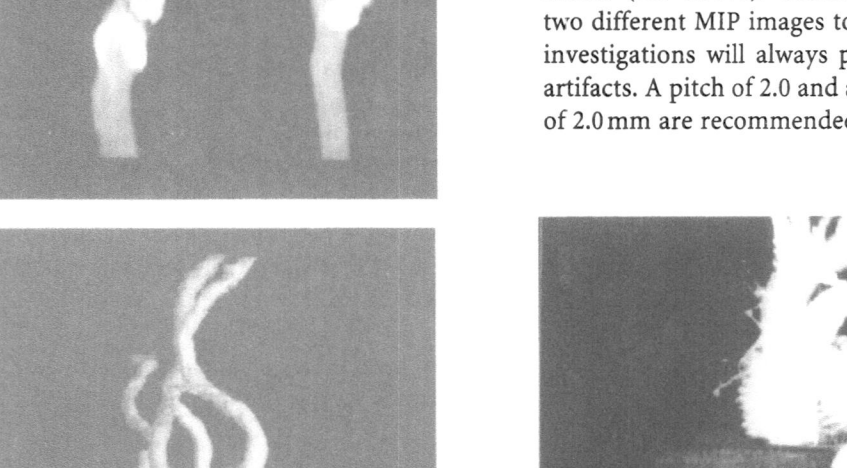

Investigating the aorta, a slice thickness of 3 mm is sufficent. The thoracic aorta must be displayed a few centimeters cranial from the aortic arch down to the diaphragm, the abdominal aorta from the diaphragm to the aortic bifurcation. In both cases 30–40 cm have to be calculated. A two-step scanning procedure cannot be recommended because of the increase in background noise caused by the contrast media (see above). Secondly, the trial of fitting two different MIP images together gained from two investigations will always produce ramps and step artifacts. A pitch of 2.0 and a reconstruction interval of 2.0 mm are recommended (Fig. 9.5) (Table 9.4).

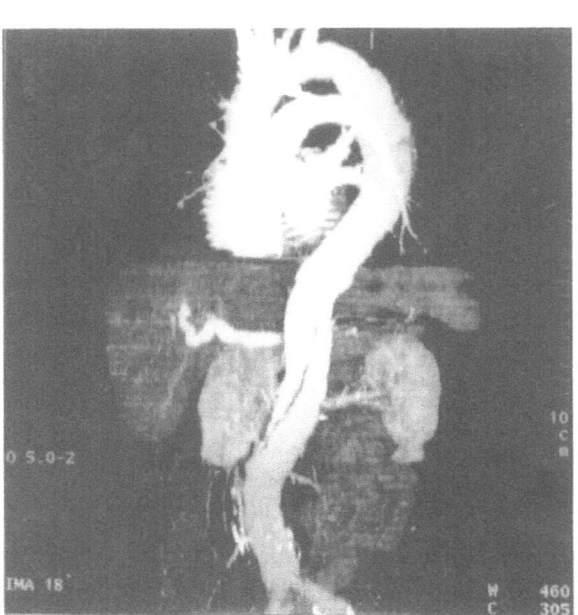

Fig. 9.4 a,b. The carotid artery. Calcified stenosis at the right internal carotid artery, partly seen on the maximum intensity projection image (a). No conclusions regarding the grade of the stenosis or the situation along the left internal carotid artery are possible. This is a three-dimensional image with no further information. Slice thickness, 2 mm; pitch, 1.0; scan length, 120 mm; reconstruction interval, 1.0 mm

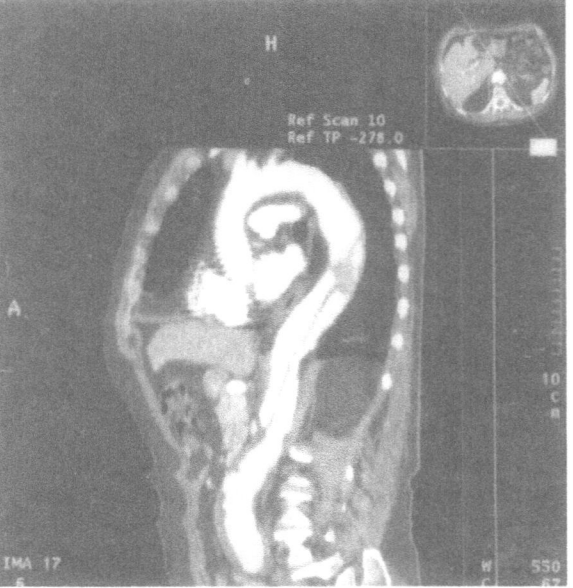

Fig. 9.5 a,b. The thoracic and abdominal aorta. Dissection along the descending aorta thoracica involving the upper parts of the abdominal aorta. The dissection is better seen in the multiplanar image reconstruction image (a) than on the maximum intensity projection (b). There is a motion artifact at the bottom of the left kidney. Covering the entire aorta a slice thickness of 3 mm and a pitch of 2.0 was used, with a reconstruction interval of 1.5 mm

Table 9.4. Secondary imaging: aortic aneurysms

Aortic Aneurysm		
• Calcifications	⟶	(MPR, MIP)
• Thrombi	⟶	(MPR)
• Dissection	⟶	(MPR)
• Cranio-caudal extend	⟶	(MIP)

MPR, multiplanar image reconstruction; MIP, maximum intensity projections.

9.4.1.4
Celiac Trunk and Superior Mesenteric Artery

Patients with tentative diagnosis of pancreatic or liver tumor require a contrast CT scan to clarify suitability for surgery. A slice thickness of 3 mm is suitable for good axial slices, having sufficient soft tissue contrast and being small enough for the angiographic evaluation. A pitch of 1.5 and a reconstruction interval of 1.5–2.0 mm are recommended.

9.4.1.5
Renal Arteries

Renal arteries run for a long distance parallel to the scan plane. Therefore, they are susceptible to misinterpretation: Step artifacts may resemble stenoses or even occlusions. Therefore, a slice thickness of 1–2 mm is recommended. The cranio-caudal extension is of less importance when looking for renal artery stenoses; 5–9 cm is optimum with a pitch of 1.0 and a reconstruction interval of 1.0 mm (Table 9.5).

Table 9.5. Secondary imaging: renovascular hypertension

Renovascular hypertension		
• Calcifications	⟶	(MPR, MIP)
• Stenosis grade II (50%–75%)	⟶	(MIP)
• Stenosis grade III (>75%)		
• Occlusion	⟶	No Decision in MPR, MIP or 3D

MPR, multiplanar image reconstruction; MIP, maximum intensity projections; 3D, three-dimensional.

9.4.1.6
Iliac Arteries and Peripheral Arteries

In iliac and peripheral arteries the recording of a long distance, such as in the aorta, is predominant. A slice thickness of 3 mm is recommended, along with a pitch of 2.0 and a reconstruction interval of 2.0 mm (Figs. 9.6, 9.7) (Table 9.6).

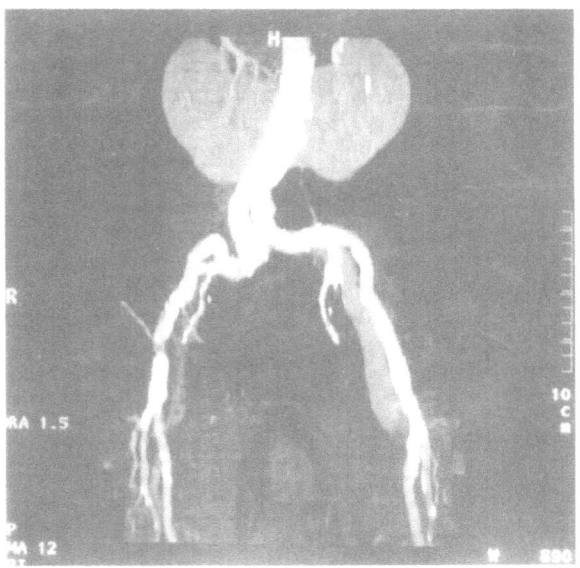

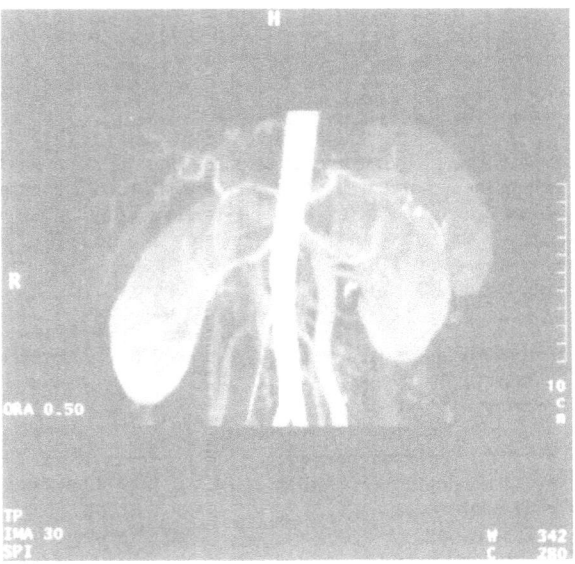

Fig. 9.6 a,b. Maximum intensity projection imaging (MIP). Using MIP, pathological structures of arteries and veins are displayed in one image. **a** High grade stenosis in the right iliac artery and arteriovenous fistula in the puncture area on the left with early filling of the left iliac vein. **b** Subtotal occlusion of the lower part of the caval vein caused by a tumor and collateralization along the ovarian vein

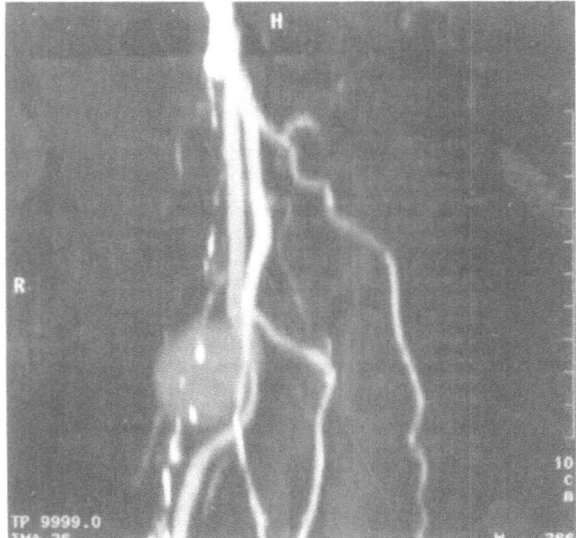

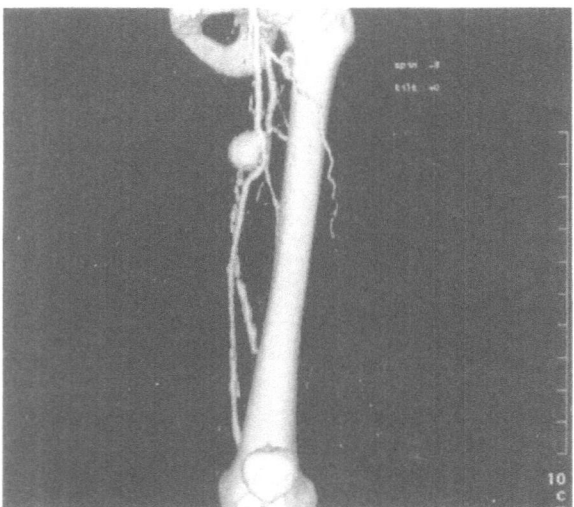

Fig. 9.7 a,b. The peripheral arteries. There is an aneurysm along the femoral artery. The anatomic situation is best seen three-dimensionally (a), with the vessel situation and calcifications shown by maximum intensity projections (b). Slice thickness, 3 mm; pitch, 2.0; scan length, 3.5 mm; reconstruction interval, 1.0 mm

Table 9.6. Secondary imaging: peripheral arterial occlusive disease

Peripheral arterial occlusive disease		
• Calcifications	⟶	(MPR, MIP)
• Thrombi	⟶	(MPR)
• Dissection	⟶	(MPR)
• Stenosis grade II <25%–>75%	⟶	(MIP)
• Stenosis Grade III (>75%)		
• Occlusion	⟶	No decision in MPR, MIP or 3D

MPR, multiplanar image reconstruction; MIP, maximum intensity projections; 3D, three-dimensional.

9.4.2
Contrast Medium Application

Homogeneous contrasting of all vessels during the scan period is of decisive importance to avoid misinterpretations. To start the application of contrast media with the beginning of the spiral (helical) CT depends on several factors: the region to be investigated, the structures (arteries and veins) that need to be displayed, and the age of the patient.

Non-ionic contrast media should preferred for better compatibility. The concentration of iodine should not be below 300 g/1000 ml to achieve sufficient contrasted vessels.

To avoid artifacts caused by the inflow of the contrast medium over a cubital vein, investigations of the thoracic region need to be scanned in a caudo-cranial direction.

9.4.2.1
Time Estimation

Estimation of the time needed for the contrast medium to reach the vessel can be used in the skull base, neck, aorta region, and iliac arteries. A scan delay of 20 s in the regions mentioned above cannot be recommended in patients with heart and circulation problems.

9.4.2.2
Test Bolus

A total of 10–20 ml of contrast medium is given at a flow rate of 4 ml/s. A region of interest (ROI) is placed right into the vessel to be investigated and test scans without table movement check the increase of density inside the vessel until a definite threshold is reached. The delay time is measured afterwards. An increase in background noise, caused by the applied contrast medium, cannot be avoided using this technique (Figs. 9.8a, 9.9).

9.4.2.3
Computer-Assisted Delay System

The best way to achieve an exact timing is by using a computer-assisted delay system, which measures the density values within a predefined ROI with an extremely low dose. By scanning every 10 s without

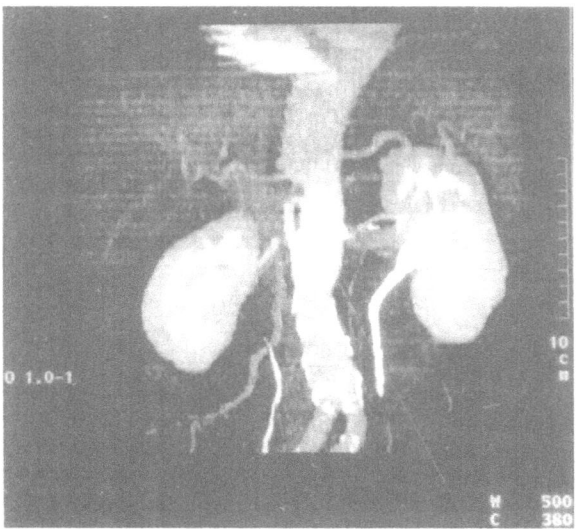

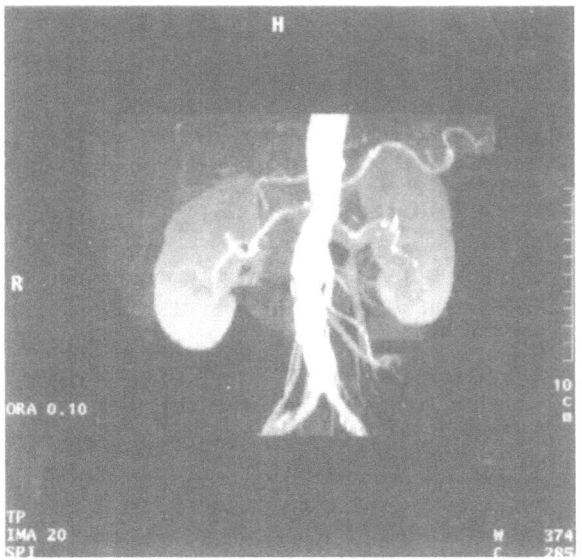

Fig. 9.8 a,b. Aortic aneurysm distal to the renal arteries with no dissection. a The overlying structures of the renal system are observed by using a test bolus. There is high background noise. b The computer-assisted delay system with no background noise and no artifacts in the renal system (patient with elongated, calcified aorta abdominalis)

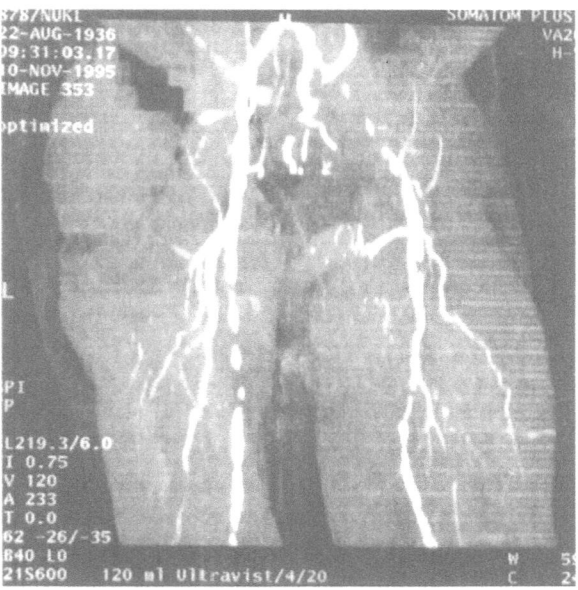

Fig. 9.9. Multiple stenoses and occlusions of the left iliac artery and right femoral artery. To achieve high vessel contrast a test bolus was given before starting the spiral scan, thus causing high background noise within the muscles

table feed, a predefined threshold should be reached. The table then moves automatically to the predefined position with an automatic start of the spiral (helical) CT (Fig. 9.6b).

9.4.2.4
Flow Rate and Total Amount

An automatic injection system is necessary for all CT angiography investigations. A flow rate of 3.5–4.0 ml/s can be recommended in all cases. The total amount of contrast media is 120 ml in patients of up to 70 kg of weight and 150 ml for adipose patients and patients taller than 180 cm (Table 9.7).

Table 9.7. Scanning parameters for CT angiography

Scan region	Slice thickness	Scan length	Pitch	Reconstruction interval	Contrast medium	Flow rate (ml/s)
Skull base (circle of Willis)	1–2 mm	40–80 mm	1.0–1.5	1.0 mm	100–120 ml	3.5–4.0
Carotid arteries	2–3 mm	120–140 mm	1.5–2.0	1.0–1.5 mm	100–120 ml	3.5–4.0
Thoracic, abdominal aorta	3 mm	300–500 mm	2.0	2.0 mm	120–150 ml	4.0
Celiac trunk superior mesenteric artery	3 mm	200–300 mm	1.5–2.0	1.0–1.5 mm	120–150 ml	4.0
Renal arteries	1–2 mm	50–90 mm	1.0	1.0 mm	100–120 ml	4.0
Iliac, peripheral arteries	3 mm	40–1400 mm	2.0	2.0 mm	120–150 ml	3.5–4.0

9.5
Radiation Dose

In conventional CT, as well as in spiral CT, the radiation dose will increase with tube current, tube voltage, scan time, and slice thickness. The same conversion factors from milliampere persecond product to dose apply in both cases.

9.5.1
Dose Reduction

Spiral (helical) CT, however, may help to limit patient dose while simultaneously increasing diagnostic information. The most important point is the possibility to use pitch values lager than 1, leading to an immediate reduction in dose as compared to contiguous single-slice scanning. Other practical reasons are: that tube currents are set to lower values due to technical limitations and the practice of taking overlapping scans in conventional CT is replaced by the ability to calculate arbitrarily overlapping images from one spiral (helical) scan.

9.6
Artifacts and Ghosts

There are a number of effects or artifacts which need to be mentioned for CT angiography. They have an effect on the single slices as well as on the secondary image reconstruction. One must differentiate between artifacts coming directly from the scanning system and those which are CT angiography-related.

9.6.1
Spiral (Helical) CT-Specific Artifacts

It is to be expected that partial volume effects are enhanced in spiral CT due to the degradation of slice sensitivity profiles (SSP), a potentially negative effect in single slices which may be observed in situations where the choice of thin slices seems to be indicated (bone imaging, skull base). In CT angiography thin slices are commonly used as well as 180-degree algorithms which both reduce this effect. The degradation of SSP will influence contrast and spatial resolution in the single slices (KALENDER 1995). For CT angiography, the use of secondary-image reconstruction tools renders this effect of less importance.

9.6.2
CT Angiography-Related Artifacts

Several effects have been observed which cannot be attributed to SSP degradation but to the interpolation in the z-axis.

9.6.2.1
Arterial Pulsation

In the MIP images the pulsation of arteries may lead to undulating, ramplike contours. This phenomenon is seen in the thoracic aorta and abdominal aorta and along the renal arteries and the superior mesenteric artery. This phenomenon can be reduced by using an image reconstruction with a 360-degree interpolation algorithm instead of a 180-degree algorithm because the data are averaged over a longer time interval (PROKOP et al. 1997) (Fig. 9.10).

9.6.3
Motion Artifacts

Insufficient breath-holding leads to a misinterpretation of smaller arteries that run along the x-axis or obliquely through the scan plane. This is important for the renal arteries: aneurysms can be diagnosed, as well as stenoses. In arteries that run along the z-axis like the aorta, this problem is not encountered.

When a patient holds his/her breath but moves during data acquisition large steps and discon-tinuities will be seen in the secondary image reconstruction. This effect will lead to a second investigation rather than to an incorrect diagnosis (see Fig. 9.5a).

9.6.4
Zoom Factor

All pictures gained from one investigation need to be reconstructed using the same zoom factor. If the ROI is too small changing the zoom factor is not permitted, otherwise there will be step-like artifacts similar to those seen in patient movement.

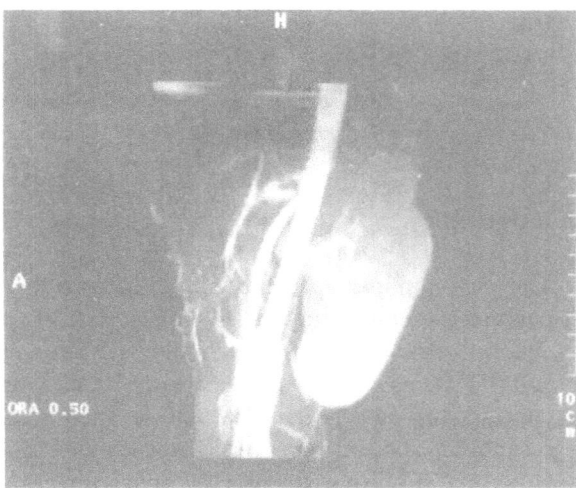

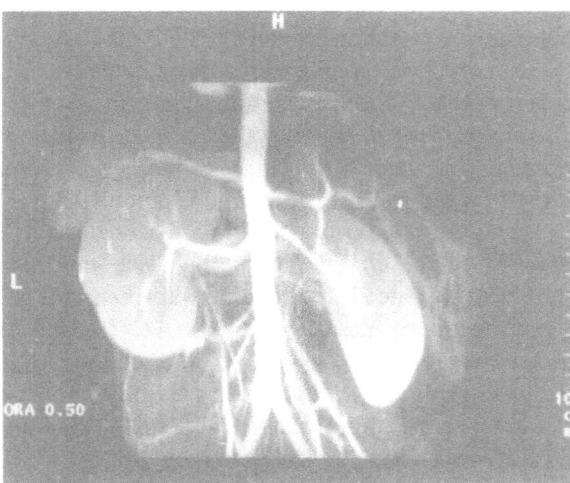

Fig. 9.10 a,b. Artifacts caused by arterial pulsation, causing ramp-like contours along the superior mesenteric artery and the distal aorta; these are best seen in the lateral view (a). A 180-degree algorithm was used

9.7
Electron Beam CT Angiography

Electron beam tomography (EBT; ultrafast CT) was developed in the early 1980s for cardiac imaging. (BOYD 1979, 1983) Scan times of 50–100 ms are good pre-conditions for CT angiography. ECG triggering in all scanners are preconditions of good cardiac imaging using axial slices for calculating coronary artery calcification. With greater software development, EBT could become a powerful CT angiography scanner.

9.7.1
Principles

The EBT scanner uses a conventional parallel tomographic acquisition system coupled with electron-beam scanning technology. This system, therefore, has no moving parts and imaging is facilitated by magnetic deflection of the electron beam prior to striking a series of four parallel but fixed tungsten targets.

9.7.2
Cardiac Imaging

For cardiac imaging all four targets can be used; the technology acquires images from an ECG trigger and scans are done prospectively at multiple time points during the cardiac cycle. Up to eight slices can be scanned without table movement, obtaining data for eight cross-sectional levels at a slice thickness of 3 mm. The interscan delay time is only 8 ms. Using contrast media, measurements of cardiac output can be taken.

9.7.3
Coronary Arteries

For scoring calcification of coronary arteries 20 contiguous slices need to be obtained through the base of the heart, including the proximal coronary arteries. Scan time should be 100 ms per image with a slice thickness of 3 mm and ECG triggering is necessary. The score is calculated according to the image and quantification analysis of JANOWITZ et al. (1991).

References and Suggested Reading

Boyd DP (1983) Computerized transmission tomography of the heart using scanning electron beams. In: Higgins CB (ed) CT of the heart and the great vessels: experimental evaluation and clinical application. Intura, Mount Kisko, NY

Boyd DP, Gould RG, Quinn JR, et al. (1979) A proposed dynamic cardiac 3-D densitometer for early detection and evaluation of heart disease. Trans Nucl Sci 26:2724–2727

Galanski M, Prokop M, Chavan A, Schafer CM, et al. (1993) Renal arterial stenoses: spiral CT angiography. Radiology 189(1):185–192

Goodman LR, Curtin JI, Mewissen MW, et al. (1995) Detection of pulmonary embolism with unresolved clinical and scintigraphic diagnosis: helical CT versus angiography. AJR Am J Roentgenol 164(6):1369–1374

Heiken JP, Brink JA, Vannier MW (1993) Spiral (helical) CT. Radiology 189(3):647–656

Janowitz WR, Agatston SA, Viamonte M (1991) Comparison of serial quantitative evaluation of calcified artery plaque by ultrafast computed tomography in persons with and without obstructive coronary artery disease. Am J Cardiol 68(1):1–6

Kalender WA (1995) Principles and performance of spiral CT. In: Goldman LW, Fowlkes BJ (eds) Medical CT and ultrasound: current technology and applications. Advanced Medical Publishing, pp 379–410

Kalender WA, Poclain A (1991) Physical performance characteristics of spiral CT scanning. Med Phys 18:910–915

Kalender WA, Wedding K, Poclain A, et al. (1994) Grundlagen der Gefäßdarstellung mit Spiral CT. Aktuel Radiol 4:287–297

Katz DA, Marks MP, Napel SA, Bracci PM, Robert SL (1995) Circle of Willis: evaluation with spiral CT angiography, MR angiography, and conventional angiography. Radiology 195(2):445–449

Napel S, Marks MP, Rubin GD, et al. (1992) CT angiography with spiral CT and maximum intensity projection. Radiology 185(6):607–610

Park JH, Chung JW, Im JG, Kim SK, et al. (1995) Takayasu arteriitis: evaluation of mural changes in the aorta and pulmonary artery with CT angiography. Radiology 196(1):89–93

Poclain A, Kalender WA, Marchal G (1992) Evaluation of section sensitivity profiles and image noise in spiral CT. Radiology 185(1):29–35

Poclain A, Kalender WA, Brink J, Vannier MA (1994) Measurement of slice sensitivity profiles in Spiral CT. Med Phys 21(1):133–140

Prokop M, Schaefer C, Kalender WA, Poclain A, Galanski M (1992) Gefäßdarstellungen mit Spiral CT. Der Weg zur CT Angiographie. Radiologe 33(12): 694–704

Prokop M, Shin HO, Schanz A (1997) Use of maximum intensity projections in CT angiography: a basic review. Radiographics 17(2):433–451

Remy-Jardin M, Remy J, Wattinne l, Giraud F (1992) Central pulmonary thromboembolism: diagnosis with spiral volumetric CT with the single breath hold technique-comparison with pulmonary angiography. Radiology 185:381–387

Rubin GD, Dake MD, Napel SA, McDonnell CH, Jeffrey RB (1993) Three dimensional spiral CT angiography of the abdomen: initial clinical experience. Radiology 186(1):147–152

Rumberger JA (1991) Ultrafast computed tomography. Curr Opin Cardiol 6:972–977

Semba CP, Rubin GD, Dake MD (1994) Three-dimensional spiral CT angiography of the abdomen. Semin Ultrasound CT MR 15(2):133–138

Steger W, Vogl TJ, Rausch M (1995) CT-Angiographie bei Karotisstenosen. Roto 162(5):373–378

Stehling MK, Lawrence JA, Weintraub JL, Ratopoulos V (1994) CT angiography: expanded clinical applications. AJR Am J Roentgenol 163(4):947–955

Van Hoe L, Marchal G, Baert AL, Gryspeerdt S (1995) Determination of scan delay in spiral CT angiography: utility of a test bolus injection. J Comput Assist Tomogr 19(2):216–220

Zeman RK, Bergman PM, Sulverman PM, et al. (1995) Diagnosis of aortic dissection: value of helical CT with multiplanar reformation and three-dimensional rendering. AJR Am J Roentgenol 164:1375–1380

9.8
Volume Rendering in CT Angiography

U. Szeimies

9.8.1
Introduction

The common perception of the clinical value of computed tomography angiography (CTA) has changed due to decisive technological advances: spiral systems with faster data aquisition, longer coverage of regions of interests, higher spatial resolution, and an improved signal-to-noise ratio. However, two-dimensional (2D) axial images do not optimally transfer the three-dimensional (3D) nature of vessel pathology. CTA with 3D image reconstruction seems to be a suitable interface between the radiologist and clinician. But it is important to understand the basic principles and image characteristics of these rendering techniques to know their possible limitations and pitfalls.

There are several algorithms for reconstructing a CTA data set. The commonly used modalities, besides the true 2D multiplanar reformation (MPR), are maximum intensity projection (MIP) and surface shaded display (SSD). Volume rendering (VR), a relatively new technique, has become more and more a viable clinical tool to increase the diagnostic utility with recent advances in computer processing and display technology (RUBIN et al. 1996) (Table 9.8).

Table 9.8. Comparison of three CTA rendering techniques

	SSD	MIP	VR
3D image	+	-	+
Evaluation of vascular interrelationship	+	-	+
Depiction of			
– calcification	-	+	+
– vessel kinking	+	-	+
– mural thrombus	-	-	+
Threshold independence	-	+	-
Intraluminal information	-	-	+
Artifacts, pseudolesions	+	-	-
Computational costs	-	-	+
Interrelationship to bones (no bone removal necessary)	+	-	+

SSD, surface shaded display; MIP, maximum intensity projection; VR, volume rendering.

9.8.2
Surface Shaded Display

Surface shaded display (SSD) was the first 3D rendering technique that was applied to medical images and was initially used for bone imaging (VANNIER et al. 1984; TOTTY and VANNIER 1984). Reconstruction with CTA data showed mixed results (DILLON et al. 1993; GALANSKI et al. 1993; REMY et al. 1994). The algorithm connects neighboring pixels with CT intensities above a preset threshold. It uses a binary classification, i.e., each voxel within a volume data set is classified as either belonging or not belonging to the object to be rendered. The shading effect is due to a simulated light source back to the observer (ADACHI and NAGAI 1995). This tissue classification in an all or none fashion results in a reduction in the original volume of data, so it requires only modest computer power and can operate rapidly. Further advantages of this algorithm are a clear depiction of 3D interrelationship with a good edge delineation.

However, for vessel imaging there are crucial, disadvantages: ignoring the fact that voxels are often mixtures of tissues and are not a truly "black or white data set" (FISHMAN and NEY 1993) the diagnostic impact is limited: there is no intraluminal information, calcifications are not distinguishable from the lumen and the mural thrombus can hardly be visualized. The algorithm is very sensitive to changes in threshold, so it yields over-or underestimations of stenoses (BLUEMKE and CHAMBERS 1995) and the depiction of narrow vessels is inaccurate (Fig. 9.11c).

9.8.3
Maximum Intensity Projection

MIP has until now been the most popular method of creating 3D CTA (MARKS et al. 1993; NAPEL et al. 1992), because it renders angiogram-like images. The algorithm selects only the voxel with the maximum intensity (highest CT number) along each ray through the volume. Like in SSD there is a reduction of image data to about 10%, so it is a computationally fast technique. Preserving attenuation information it yields acceptable results even in cases in which SSD fails (PROKOP et al. 1997). The advantages of this rendering technique are a good depiction of small vessels, a good differentiation between vascular and non vascular structures, and the visualization of mural calcium (Fig. 9.11b). It has only a few variables and is independent of

thresholds, so it is a reliable and objective method of vessel imaging.

However, in selecting only the highest intensity, there is the need to remove boney structures which can be time-consuming when working with larger data sets. Editing modalities such as region growing algorithms or cutting functions made this more comfortable (PROKOP et al. 1997), but the "intelligent" and reliable bone removal algorithm is not yet a part of the workstations routinely used. Varying degrees of obliquity are necessary to project vessels from each other since MIP is incapable of distinguishing overlying vessels. It fails to properly convey the relationship of vessels to viscera and is deficient in data beyond the vasculature (JOHNSON et al. 1996a). Many images in different projections are needed to understand the 3D structure because it delivers no spatial information. Vascular calcification obscures the lumen, so that evaluation of the true dimension of calcified stenoses is difficult. However, because of its easy handling, low computational effort, and threshold independence MIP is suited to displaying relatively simple anatomic situations (PROKOP et al. 1997). SSD, with its artifacts which are fatal for vessel evaluation, should only be used for the sake of 3D visualization.

9.8.4
Volume Rendering

With recent advances in computer processing combined with powerful workstations, VR is becoming more and more a versatile tool for vessel imaging. Unlike the algorithms of SSD and MIP, VR computes the entire volume of the spiral CT data set. It combines the advantages of SSD and MIP with a clear 3D appearance and a digital subtraction angiography (DSA)-like accuracy in the depiction of vascular structures (JOHNSON et al. 1996a).

The VR algorithm sums the weighted contributions of all voxels along a ray through the data volume so each pixel is displayed. In a first step of volume formation a contiguous set of slices is stacked on top of the other pixel with the use of bicubic interpolation, so that the new slices have an interslice spacing equal to the pixel size. The result is a volume of data containing cubic voxels with interpolated Hounsfield densities (NEY et al. 1990).

In a next step a voxel-intensity histogram is generated. The number of voxels incorporated, as well as voxel opacity, brightness, and gray scale can be adjusted (JOHNSON et al. 1996b). Different tissue

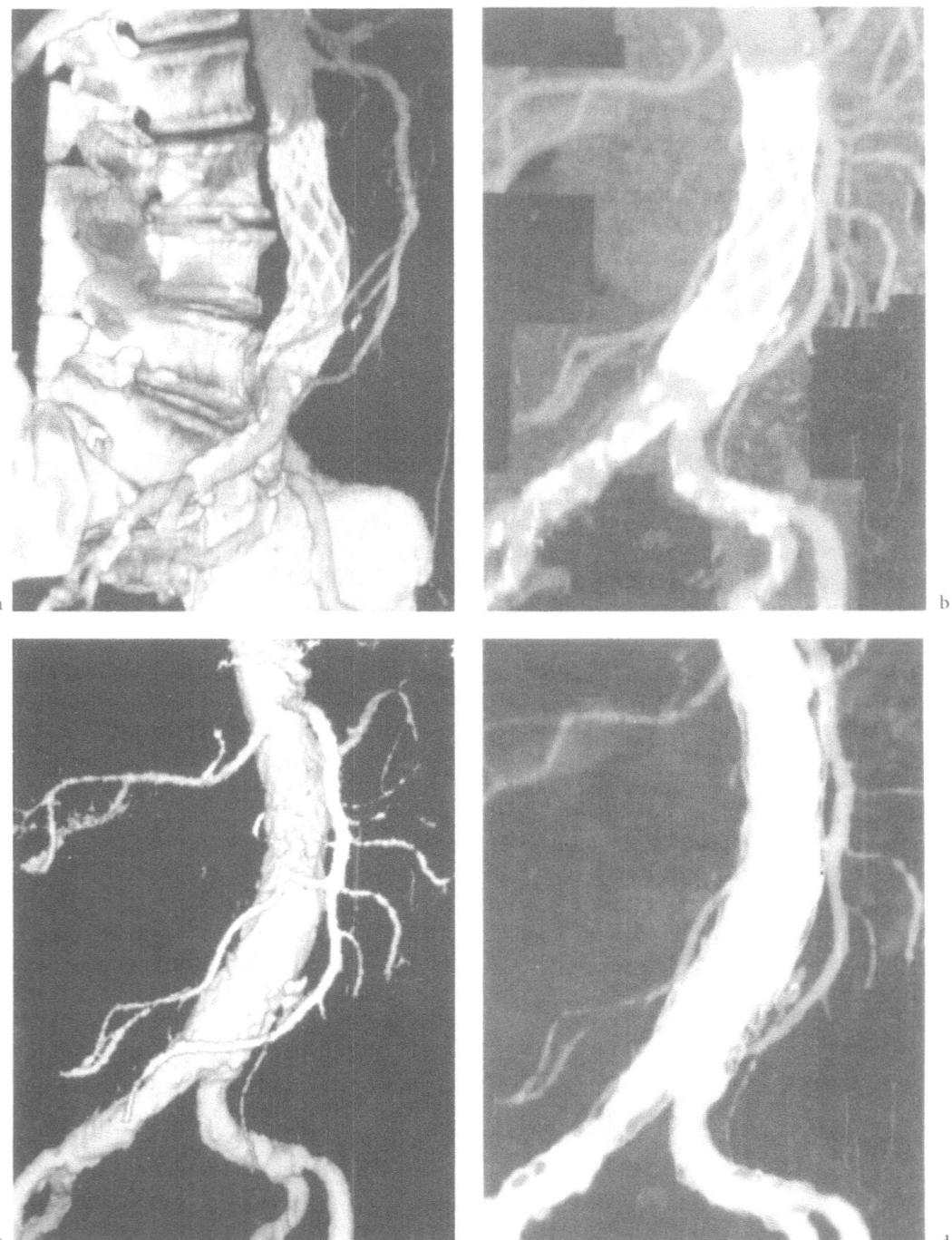

Fig. 9.11 a–d. 67-year-old male patient with an excluded 5-cm diameter aortic aneurysm. A Dacron-covered nitinol stent was placed percutaneously in the infrarenal aorta. Follow-up computed tomography angiography (CTA) was performed 6 months after intervention. a Volume-rendered CTA image shows the simultaneous display of the stented aorta and the spine. For stent evaluation (i.e., loosening of the stent struts, angulation, deformation) and patency control volume rendering has the potential to replace follow-up intraarterial digital subtraction angiography (DSA). b–d Same frontal viewing angle with three different reconstruction techniques after bone segmentation. (b) Maximum intensity projection shows a clear depiction of the metal stent and calcified plaques of the iliac arteries. However, different orientations are necessary to gain a three-dimensional (3D) conception. Overlying vessels (branches of the superior mesenteric artery) cannot be differentiated from the stented aorta. (c) Surface shaded display provides a good 3D image, but stents or calcifications are not distinguishable from the enhanced lumen. Depending on the selected preset, pseudostenoses of small vessels can occur. (d) Volume-rendered image with a different preset than (a). The metal stent struts are transparently displayed and the contrast column is set opaque. The slight narrowing of the right common iliac artery corresponded with i.a. DSA findings

types were defined by assigning opacity values to a voxel according to the density (HU ranges). In the binary (surface-based) classification (SSD) the voxel is assigned 100% or 0%. This means the tissue is assumed to consist of 100% or 0% of the given material. In the percentage-based classification it is assumed that each voxel can contain more than one tissue type, so this is a closer approximation of the true voxel content (FISHMAN EK NEY 1993). In the human body there are four major materials: air, fat, soft tissue, and bone. However, more than two mixtures are rare. If the voxel contains less than 100% of the material the opacity is scaled by the appropriate precentage; if there is a mixture the opacity value is the sum of the weighted opacity values (NEY et al. 1990).

The method of calculating the percentage contents of a voxel is a probabilistic classification with a trapezoidal approximation that closely models the actual volume averaging in CT voxels. The result is a more accurate image with superior quality because of less computer-generated artifacts (FISHMAN and NEY 1993).

Number and attenuation of the incorporated voxels and image contrast can be influenced by changing window level and window width. Window level dictates the number and attenuation of voxels integrated into the final image. An increase of the level results in an exclusion of voxels with lower attenuation, only high-contrast structures (vessels, bones) are displayed. A decrease of window level yields an image which includes structures with lower attenuation (viscera). Window width controls contrast; an increase results in an increase of the gray scale with an decrease of image contrast and vice versa (JOHNSON et al. 1996).

Multiple rays are projected from the front to the back of the volume data set. The final display yields the accumulated image of all structures through which the ray passes. The visualization of volume data can simultaneously display superficial and deep structures. It is possible to gain intraluminal information: intimal dissections, flaps, thrombus, calcified plaques, degree of stenosis, subtle intravascular filling defects (KUSZYK et al. 1995), and outlets of major branches. Altering the opacities, VR has the ability to view through calcified plaque and metal stent to evaluate vessel patency. With additional shading effects there is an excellent 3D appearance with the advantage of being able to evaluate extraluminal information. Particularly in terms of interpreting complex vascular interrelationships to viscera and visualization of multiple overlapping

vessels VR is superior to other rendering techniques.

Correct rate and timing of contrast infusion is important for an optimal CTA examination. However, manipulating opacity and window width and level can improve image quality of non-optimal contrast-enhanced vasculature. With real-time interactive VR (JOHNSON et al. 1996b), 3D imaging of vessel pathology is possible at any viewing angle within seconds. With the use of interactive cutting functions time consuming data segmentation can often be avoided (Fig. 9.12).

However, within this complex algorithm with hundreds of variables compared to MIP rendering there are some drawbacks: more computer power is required with higher computational costs because of the use of the entire volume data set (HEATH et al. 1995). Very transparent image displays may not clearly define discrete surfaces, which could hinder exact measurement. Because of the variety of different adjustments of opacities, HU classification ranges and window width and level VR is an operator-dependent modality and image quality strongly depends on the user's experience. However, in clinical routine the workstations have fixed presets, so individual adjustments are only required in case of insufficient image quality.

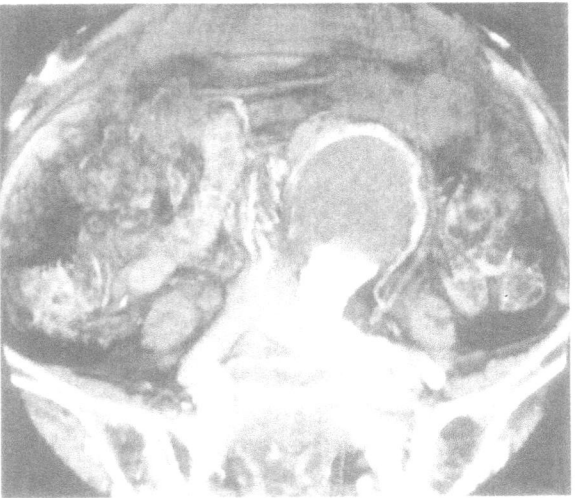

Fig. 9.12. Computed tomography angiography with volume rendering of a 7-cm diameter infrarenal aortic aneurysm. With interactive cutting functions in any orientation prompt evaluation of vessel pathology is possible without the need for bone segmentation. An oblique-axial view depicts the thrombosed aneurysmal sac with a calcified wall. The dorsal portion of the aneurysm shows the perfused lumen with its iliac bifurcation. Right of the aneurysm the non-enhanced inferior vena cava and iliac veins are observed

Exploiting the maximum diagnostic value of volumetric CT data, set VR holds various possibilities. As with MIP reformation, imaging of all main vessel regions is possible. As a bad scanning technique produces equally bad 3D images, a good compromise between image quality, aquisition time, and dose should be chosen. In recent studies the recommended collimation varies between 1 mm and 4 mm with a reconstruction interval of 1 mm–2 mm and a pitch factor of 1.0–2.0 (Davros et al. 1997; Brink et al. 1995; Ney et al. 1991; Prokop et al. 1997) according to the region of interest. For example, a reasonable compromise between image quality and coverage in scanning abdominal aortic aneurysms can be a slice thickness of 3 mm, interscan spacing of 1 mm, and a pitch factor of 1.5 (Szeimies et al. 1996) (Fig. 9.13). In depicting small, peripheral vessels the quality of volume-rendered images is strongly dependent on optimal vessel contrast and appropriate scanning protocol. With a collimation of 2 mm good visualization of segmental renal arteries is possible. However, the exact evaluation of pathologic changes in peripheral small arteries is still the domain of intraarterial DSA.

9.8.5
Volume Rendering of Aortic Aneurysms

Visualization of different enhanced structures enables VR for optimal evaluation of aortic aneurysms. It enables the simultaneous display of calcified plaques, mural thrombus, and enhanced vessel lumen. An additional advantage in comparison to MIP lies in the 3D imaging of vessels and the interrelationsship to boney structures. With only a few steps clear depiction of vessel kinking and coiling is possible. Evaluation of the distal neck, proximal extent, and visceral branches facilitates the decision of whether to proceed with open surgery or endoluminal exclusion of the aneurysm. Additional measurement programs can determine the aortoiliac quantification-like mean diameter, overall path length, and branch angulation (Fig. 9.14). However, i.a. DSA with a callibration catheter is still advisable for the precise preinterventional planning of transfemoral-placed endoluminal grafts. In occlusive disease 3D-CTA with VR can help to decide whether angioplasty or reconstruction is advisable with its clear depiction of calcified plaques and

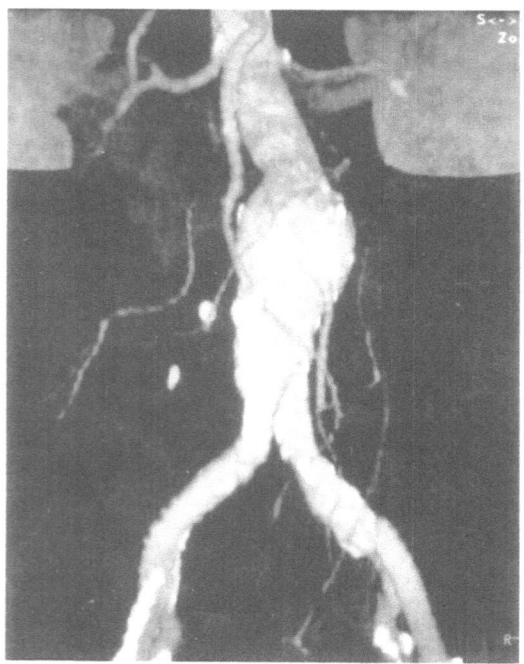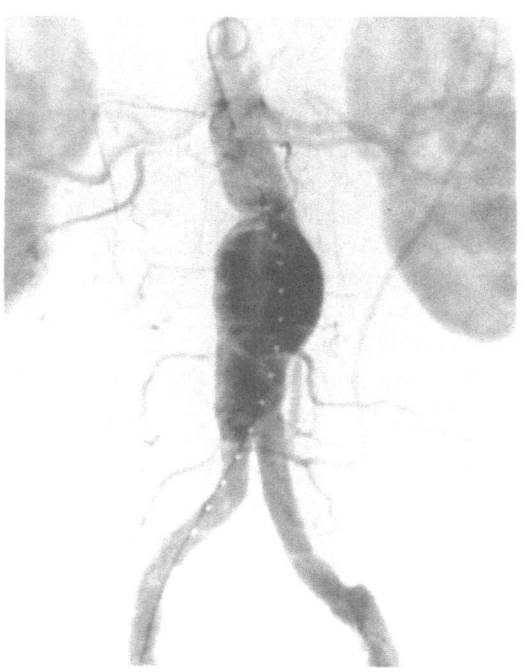

Fig. 9.13 a,b. Comparison of an abdominal aortic aneurysm with volume-rendering computed tomography angiography (CTA) (a) and i.a. digital subtraction angiography (b). The patient was scanned with 150 mA and 120 kV. According to the CTA protocol a collimation of 3 mm and a pitch of 1.5 with a spacing interval of 1 mm was used. Contrast media (130 ml) was applied with power injection at a flow of 3.2 ml/s and a scanning delay of 25 s, determined using the bolus tracking program. Examination time for the patient was 56 s. Three-dimensional image reconstruction with volume rendering was performed in 6 min. For the sake of a prompt vessel evaluation the bones were removed with volume sculpting; however, small vessels adjacent to the spine (lumbar arteries) can be cut away. The serrated contours are due to pulsating artifacts. Note the visualization of the inferior mesenteric artery origin and the calcified plaque

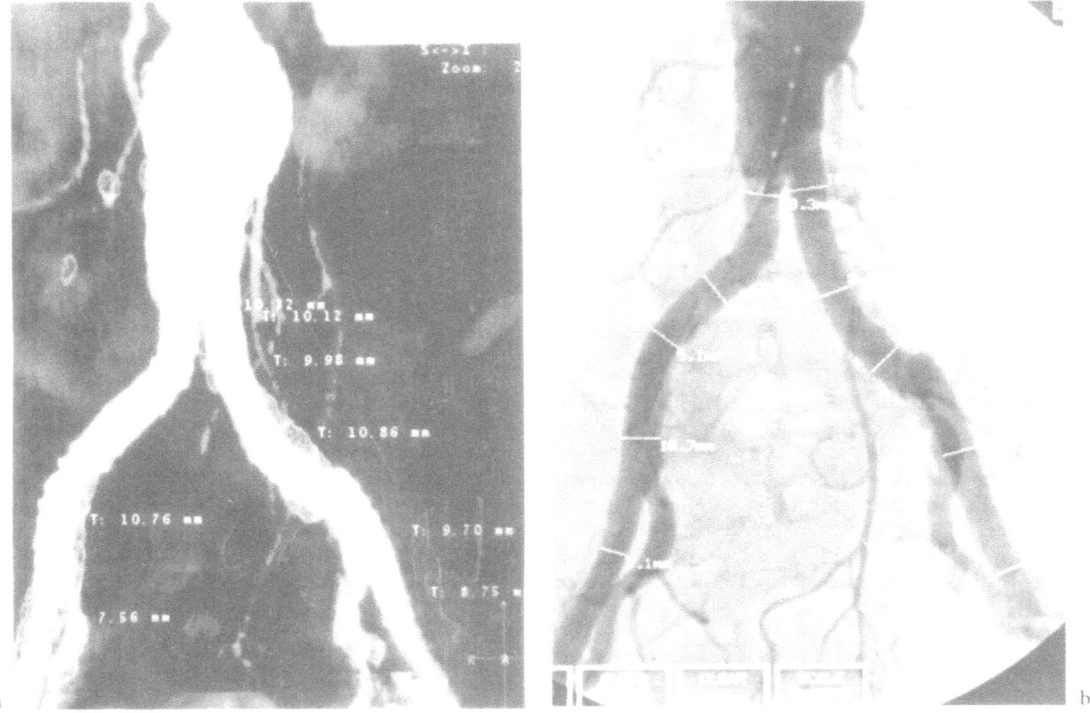

Fig. 9.14 a. Iliac quantification with computed tomography angiography measurement. With volume rendering only the enhanced lumen is displayed. The mural calcium of the common iliac arteries is transparently displayed. **b** The corresponding i.a. digital subtraction angiography performed with a 5-F callibration catheter

thrombus. Another advantage is the assessment of vascular stents. Dislocation, angulation, deformity, desintegration of stent struts, and an early leakage can be detected. Patency control of a stented contrast-enhanced vessel is possible with the ability of VR to render a transparent image of the metal structures (Fig. 9.11d).

3D-CTA with VR is a fast and accurate method of determining vessel anatomy and pathology. As speed and cost of computer processing hardware improves the more rapid rendering of SSD and MIP will become less of an advantage (JOHNSON et al. 1996b). However, like with all 3D reconstruction modalities, combined evaluation of the 2D axial slices of the original data set with the rendered images provides maximum data information. This also reduces the probability of misinterpreting rendering artifacts. The routine use of VR promises to improve patient outcomes and to decrease medical cost as diagnosis can be made more confidently with CTA.

References

Adachi H, Nagai J (1995) Three dimensional CT angiography. Little, Brown, Boston

Bluemke DA, Chambers TP (1995) Spiral CT angiography: an alternative to conventional angiography. Radiology 195:317–319

Brink JA, Lim JT, Wang G, Heiken JP, Deyoe LA, Vannier MW (1995) Technical optimization of spiral CT for depiction of renal artery stenosis: in vitro analysis. Radiology 194:157–163

Davros WJ, Obuchowski NA, Berman PM, Zeman RK (1997) A phantom study: evaluation of renal artery stenosis using helical CT and 3d reconstructions. J Comput Assist Tomogr 21 (1): 156–161

Dillon EH, Van Leeuven MS, Fernandez MA, Mail WP (1993) Spiral CT angiography. AJR Am J Roentgenol 160:1273–1278

Fishman EK, Ney DR (1993) Advanced computer applications in radiology: clinical applications. Radiographics 13:463–475

Galanski M, Prokop M, Chavan A, Schaefer CM, Jandeleit K, Nischelsky JE (1993) Renal artery stenosis: spiral CT angiography. Radiology 189:185–192

Heath DG, Soyer PA, Kuszyk BS, Bliss DF, Calhoun PS, Bluemke DA, Choti MA, Fishman EK (1995) Three-dimensional spiral CT during arterial portography: comparison of three rendering techniques. Radiographics 15:1001–1011

Johnson PT, Heath DG, Kuszyk BS, Fishman EK (1996a) CT angiography with volume rendering: advantages and application in splanchnic vascular imaging. Radiology 200:564–568

Johnson PT, Heath DG, Bliss DF, Cabral B, Fishman EK (1996b) Three-dimensional CT: real time interactive volume rendering. AJR Am J Roentgenol 167:581–583

Kuszyk BS, Heath DG, Ney DR, Bluemke DA, Urban BA, Chambers TP, Fishman EK (1995) CT angiography with volume rendering: imaging findings. AJR Am J Roentgenol 165:445–448

Marks MP, Napel S, Jordan JE, Enzmann DR (1993) Diagnosis of carotid artery disease: preliminary experience with maximum-intensity-projection spiral CT angiography. AJR Am J Roentgenol 160:1267–1271

Napel S, Marks MP, Rubin GD, Dake MD, McDonnell CH, Song SM, Enzman DR, Jeffrey RB(1992) CT angiography with spiral CT and maximum intensity projection. Radiology 185:607–610

Ney DR, Fishman EK, Magid D, Drebin RA (1990) Volumetric rendering of computed tomography data: principles and techniques. IEEE Comput Graphics Appl 3:24–32

Ney DR, Fishmann EK, Magid D, Robertson DD, Kawashima A (1991) Three-dimensional volumetric display of CT data: effect of scan parameters upon image quality. J Comput Assist Tomogr 15 (5):875–885

Prokop M, Hoen OS, Schanz A, Schaefer-Prokop CM (1997) Use of maximum intensity projections in CT angiography: a basic review. Radiographics 17:433–451

Remy J, Remy-Jardin M, Giraud F, Wattinne L (1994) Angioarchitecture of pulmonary arteriovenous malformations: clinical utility of three-dimensional helical CT. Radiology 191:657–664

Rubin GD, Napel S, Leung AN (1996) Volumetric analysis of volumetric data: achieving a paradigm shift. Radiology 200:312–317

Szeimies U, Kueffer G, Steckmeier B, Scheck R, Pfluger T, Hahn K (1996) Comparison of three rendering techniques in spiral CT angiography: surface-shaded display, maximum intensity projection, and 3D volume-rendering technique. Radiology 201(P):419

Totty WG, Vannier MW (1984) Complex musculoskeletal anatomy: analysis using three-dimensional surface reconstruction. Radiology 150:173–177

Vannier MW, Marsh JL, Warren JO (1984) Three-dimensional CT reconstruction images for craniofacial surgery planning and evaluation. Radiology 150:179–184

10 Ultrasound Angiography

S.A. Beyer-Enke and M. Mück-Weymann

CONTENTS

PRIV.-DOZ. S.A. BEYER-ENKE, MD, Institut für Diagnostische und Interventionelle Radiologie, Klinikum Nord, Flurstraße 17, 90340 Nuremberg, Germany
MICHAEL MÜCK-WEYMANN, MD, Klinik und Poliklinik für Psychotherapie und Psychosomatische Medizin, Technische Universität Dresden, Fetscherstraße 74, 01307 Dresden, Germany

A new era in diagnostic imaging began with the development of the first real-time sonograph, the VIDOSON, by Krause and Soldner of Siemens Inc., Germany, in 1965. Based on a long series of individual physical, technological, and medical discoveries in the field of ultrasonographic applications since the end of the nineteenth century the engineers succeeded in providing a revolutionary, noninvasive, real-time imaging procedure first to gynecologists and shortly thereafter to both internists and radiologists. Aside from imaging, the introduction of the ultrasonic Doppler technique in the 1960s also made a noninvasive, on-line evaluation of functional parameters possible, i.e., the blood flow characteristics in vessels. With recent technological advances which provide a combination of sectional imaging of tissue with the spectral Doppler and, later on, the color-coded Doppler, it is today possible to provide a sectional display of the inner organs. In addition, dynamic processes like the flow of blood in the veins and arteries can be color-coded, displayed simultaneously with the sectional two-dimensional (2D) image, and evaluated quantitatively or semi-quantitatively with the spectral Doppler. The physical and technical principles of this method, as well as several important pathophysiological models, will be summarized and verified with findings from clinical practice.

10.1 B-Scanning

Similar to radar technology methods, ultrasound images of the inner body are formed through the scattering and reflection of ultrasonic waves on the walls and tissue structures of the body's organs. The piezoelectric effect is used for both the production of sound waves and for the transformation of the reflected sound wave echos into electrical signals. The piezoelectric effect explains the method by which the application of a certain voltage to specific crystals leads to a rhythmic deformation of the crystalline structure. The sound wave generated by these deformations penetrates the body surface, is reflected by the organs and tissue, and recurs to the crystal as an echo to produce an electric echo signal. These reflections are generated when the sound passes through sections of different acoustic impedance. When measuring the travel time of an ultrasound signal, the origin of a received reflection can be clearly identified, while the brightness of the image codes the quantity of difference of impedance. Storage of the individual contiguous lines attained through this pulse-echo procedure leads to a 2D sectional image. Ultrasound characterizes a bandwidth of wavelengths with frequencies over 2 kHz. The average propagation velocity of ultrasound waves in biological materials in 1540 cm/s. For medical applications frequencies ranging between 2 MHz and 100 MHz are used, while the oscillation frequency depends on the geometry and technology of the crystals used. Typically used transducer frequencies are 2.25 MHz (for cardiologic and transcranial applications), 3.5 MHz, and 5.0 MHz (for abdominal, obstetric, and gynecological applications), as well as 7.5 MHz or 10.0 MHz (for smaller applications). Some special applications such as intraluminal or dermatological imaging use frequencies up to 100 MHz.

The following applies to all ultrasound techniques: the higher the transmitter frequency the lower the penetration depth, and the lower the wavelength (i.e., the higher the frequency) the higher the resolution. While resolution signifies the minimum distance between two point-shaped objects which can be discriminated from one another, higher resolution normally deals with more information about the tissues and leads to a clearer diagnosis. Therefore most ultrasound applications require a compromise between the desired resolution and anatomical conditions. Referring to the formula $\lambda = c/f$, where λ is the wavelength, f is the frequency, and c is the propagation velocity, for transducers using a frequency of the bandwidth between 2 MHz and 100 MHz wavelengths range between 0.7 mm and 0.015 mm. There is a significant difference between the resolution axial to the direction of spreading of the sound waves, and the lateral resolution. The axial resolution depends on the pulse length of the transmitted sound and is approximately two wavelengths (e.g., 0.6 mm in a 5-MHz transducer). The lateral resolution depends to the form of the shape of the complex sound field and is approximately four or five wavelengths (e.g., 1.4 mm in a 5-MHz transducer). Therefore, two points lying one behind the other (relative to the spreading direction) can be more clearly distinguished than two points lying side by side.

Depending on the absorbtion characteristics of the tissue (transmission frequency and image depth) sound waves are attenuated. Echoes of more deeply seated targets are more attenuated on their way back to the transducer than those near the transducer. To compensate this effect, the reflected signal is amplified as a function of the travel time (time gain compensation, TGC): echoes from deeper structures are handled with a higher amplification by the receiver.

10.2
The Doppler Effect

At the beginning of the nineteenth century, Johann Christian Doppler, a physicist, observed a blue-shift (i.e., toward the shorter wavelengths) in the light of stars which were moving relatively towards the earth. Everyone is familiar with the analog phenomenon which is observed with sound waves: The sound of a car's engine which is travelling towards us at high speed is heard at a higher frequency than if the car were travelling away from us. This Doppler effect is also seen in the scattering of ultrasound waves by the red blood cells: Scattering echoes from the erythrocytes travelling towards the probe have a higher frequency in relation to the transmitted frequency. This frequency shift is proportional to the rate and direction of the blood cell velocity. The frequency shift Δf of the echo signal scattered by the erythrocytes, as compared to the transmitted frequency f, is described by the Doppler formula:

$$\Delta f = \frac{f}{c} * v * \cos \Theta$$

The frequency shift Δf (i.e., the Doppler frequency) is a direct parameter for the measurement of the flow velocity v. For a given magnitude of v, Δf will be larger with a higher transmitted frequency. Since the detection of Δf has an upper and a lower limit due to technical limitations, e.g., the signal-to-noise ratio, the Doppler formula reveals the following relationships: For the detection of high velocities it is recommended that a lower transmission frequency f be selected, whereas f should be selected as high as possible for low velocities.

Δf is also dependent on the angle of insonation, θ: Δf is at its highest when the incident sound beam is parallel to the vessel's axis. For a perpendicular incidence of sound wave insonation, the cosine of θ is equal to 0 and no Doppler signal can be registered.

To detect the velocity *v* from the Doppler frequency Δ*f*, the angle of incidence θ must be measured in the 2D image and an angle correction must be performed.

The echoes from the blood, however, are a factor of 100–1000 times weaker than the echoes from the body's organs which provide the sectional image. Therefore, the development of highly sensitive detectors and high-efficiency processing units was mandatory for visualizing blood flow. Today low flow in very small vessels down to 0.1 mm can be visualized (Figs. 10.1, 10.2).

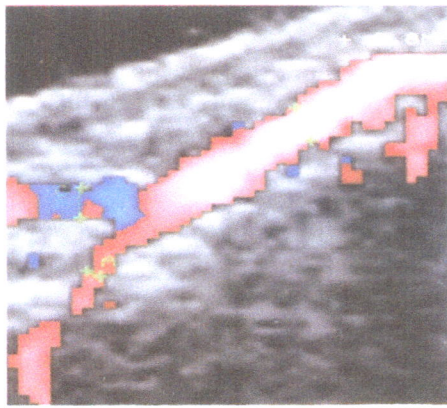

Fig. 10.1. Blood flow in a finger artery (size down to 0.1 mm)

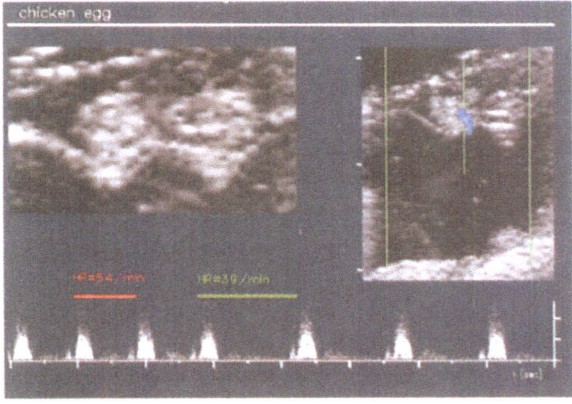

Fig. 10.2. Cardiac blood flow in a chicken embryo

10.3
Spectral Doppler vs. Color Flow Imaging

The two Doppler techniques, the spectral Doppler and the color-coded Doppler, differ, among other things, in their method of presenting the information obtained for measuring flow velocity. In the cases of the continuous-wave Doppler (CW Doppler) and the pulsed-wave Doppler (PW Doppler), the vessel is cut by a single sound beam. The flow velocities are detected only along this sound beam direction and displayed in a spectral distribution using a fast Fourier transformation. With the CW Doppler mode, this measurement is carried out over the entire depth of the sound beam, whereas only echo signals from a sample volume in a user-selected depth are analyzed with the PW Doppler mode. In the case of the color Doppler, also known as color flow imaging, the blood flow is detected from a multitude of sample volumes distributed over the entire 2D image, or a part of it, using autocorrelation or related algorithms, and displayed as a color-coded image.

CW and PW Dopplers differ in their mode of signal acquisition, although their signal processing and spectral presentation of the results are quite similar. Under CW operation, two separate crystals are used in the probe, one of which continuously transmits while the other simultaneously receives the incoming echo signals. Due to this continous operation, it is impossible to assign an echo's point of origin. On the other hand, this procedure has the advantage of being able to analyze even very high flow velocities unambiguously. PW Doppler meets the requirements for measuring flow velocities in relationship to a certain area of interest. One common crystal is used in the probe for both receiving and transmitting signals and it transmits sequences of short pulses into the body as required for 2D imaging. After the pulse travel time to the selected sample site and back, the sample gate is opened for a short period of time to receive the echoes. The travel time determines the shortest possible time interval between two successive transmission pulses. The pulse repetition frequency for the transmitted pulses cannot be selected at a value higher than (1/travel time) without risking the loss of unambiguous depth assignment.

10.4
Aliasing

The aliasing effect determines the upper limit of flow velocity which can be measured unambiguously in both pulsed-spectral and color Dopplers. In the Doppler spectrum, aliasing can be recognized by the fact that positive frequencies above the cutoff frequency (i.e., the so-called Nyquist frequency) reappear as negative frequencies at the lower end of the spectrum. Shifting of the reference axis for the direction of flow can extend the measuring range from one direction up to twice the cutoff frequency. Doppler frequencies over twice the Nyquist frequency cannot be detected unambiguously at all. In the color image, aliasing appears as a red color within the blue or vice versa. The appeearence of the aliasing shown on the left side of Fig. 10.3 is very different from the appeearence caused by changes in flow direction as shown in the middle of the same figure. During (virtual) changes in flow direction, color may be coded as red behind blue.

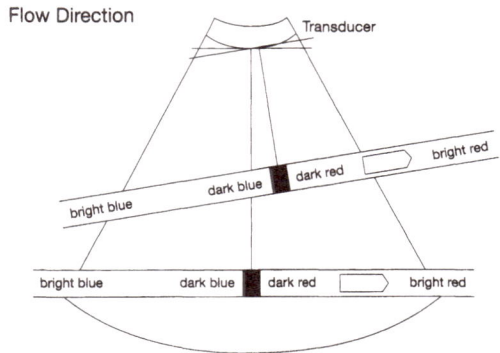

Fig. 10.4. Angle dependency of flow direction and color-coding

10.5
Flow Direction and Color Coding

While spectral PW Doppler is used to measure the temporal course of velocity distribution in a pre-selected sample site, the color Doppler technique analyzes the flow velocity in many sample volumes distributed over the entire sectional image or some part of it. The result is the spatial distribution of one local value, the mean velocity, and its direction in the perfused vessel in a temporal sequence determined by the frame rate. The relationship between color-coding and direction of the blood flow becomes clear from the diagram with a curved array (Fig. 10.4). In the diagram, flow toward the transducer is coded blue, whereas flow away from the transducer is coded red. A vessel running parallel to the tangent at the center of the arc of the transducer's surface re-veals a colorless (black) region exactly in the center of the image. The vessel at this point is hit at a right angle by the sound waves and, since the cosine of 90 degrees is zero, the Doppler signal is also zero. To the

left of this point, the blood demonstrates a relative flow towards the transducer and the display in the color image is therefore coded blue. To the right, the relative flow is away from the transducer and the color image is therefore red. A second vessel runs from the lower left to the upper right of the image and is parallel to the second tangent located in the right of the transducer center. For this reason, the color change point is shifted to the right. Differences in color saturation indicate various velocities: The lighter the color, the faster the velocity.

10.6
Power Doppler Imaging

Color Doppler yields flow information about flow direction and mean velocity over the entire sectional image or some part of it. From a diagnostic point of view, the accuracy of velocities and direction is the advantage of this technique, e.g., for detection of flow dynamics and flow turbulences. Limitations of the conventional color Doppler may be – sometimes – the aliasing effect, angle dependency, and a lack of low flow sensitivity.

Power Doppler is a not really a new imaging mo-dality, but its sensitivity for detecting flow has been improved in recent years. So today the power mode is especially used to visualize low flow, particularly in very small vessels.

The higher sensitivity of the power mode is real-ized by using only the amplitude of the Doppler sig-nal and not the Doppler frequencies. Although the ultrasound beam profile is usually slightly divergent, and blood flow is not strictly laminar even in intact vessels, the power mode Doppler is virtually inde-pendent of Doppler angle. Therefore, an angiogram-like image can be presented (Fig. 10.5). However, on

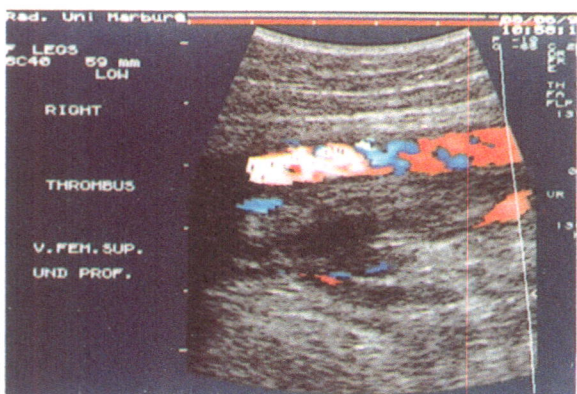

Fig. 10.3. Blood flow in a superficial femoral artery demon-strating aliasing and changes of flow direction (see text for details)

the other hand, using very high persistence (i.e., higher sampling rate for one image than with the conventional color Doppler technique) the power mode is very sensitive to moving artifacts. Therefore, the conventional color Doppler is today the standard method used, and the power Doppler can sometimes help in low flow diagnosis.

10.7
Qualitative Diagnostics

Arteries near the surface can be shown directly by duplex or color-coded ultrasound angiography. Every artery which is hidden behind bony or gas-filled structures must be assessed by functional means in central or peripheral parts of that vessel or with continuous wave assessment proximal or distal to the hidden vessel parts. B-scanning shows the vessel wall, the lumen, and the surrounding structures. The color-coded mode is the equivalent of moving blood particles. Spectrum analysis is the functional parameter. The vessel wall consists of intima, tunica media, and the adventitial layer. The equivalent in the external ultrasound are seven echo zones (DE GROOT and BANGA 1994). The far wall (echo zones 5 and 6) is the edge of the intima media complex and corresponds to the histologic specimen (Fig. 10.6). The leading and far edges (transducer near vessel walls) are gain-dependent.

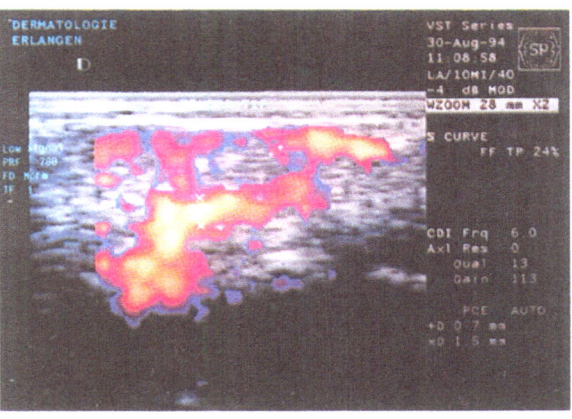

Fig. 10.5. Vessels of the finger tip shown in an angio-like power Doppler mode

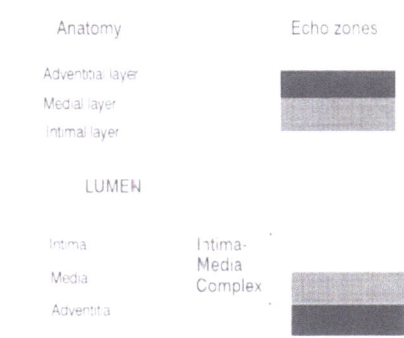

Fig. 10.6. Correlation of ultrasound anatomy and histopathology (modified from DE GROOT and BANGA 1994)

10.7.1
Carotid/Vertebral Arteries

10.7.1.1
Examination Method

The carotid arteries are examined with the window through the jugular vein. The first examination is in a longitudinal fashion to see the normal anatomy. Thereafter transversal slices are performed to examine the carotid bulb. The first pathology to describe are the types of morphological changes. At last a spectrum is derived regarding stenosis and the proximal internal carotid artery.

The vertebral artery is seen only in part due to the overlying boney structures. The artery can be visualized from a view parallel to the thyroid. The functional measurement is most important because of the incomplete visualization.

10.7.1.2
Morphology

The first step in the interpretation of carotid artery disease is the correct anatomical orientation. The bifurcation lies variable submandibular, which means that in short necks the distance to the mandibula may only be 2 cm. However, the transversal slice always shows the correct location. A total of 49% of internal carotid arteries lie dorsolateral (Table 10.1). Because the bifurcation acts as a flow divider the carotid bulb has a low flow area at the dorsal part. This area can be visualized in the color-coded mode as a blue-coded zone at the systole (BHARADVAJ et al. 1984). The disappearance of this sign is an early symptom of atherosclerosis except in 6% of all patients in which the dilatation of the bulb is missing (Fig. 10.7a–c).

Table 10.1. Location of the internal carotid artery in relation to the external carotid artery

Artery location (anatomic variations)	(%)
Dorsolateral	49
Dorsal	21
Dorsomedial	18
Ventromedial	9
Medial	3

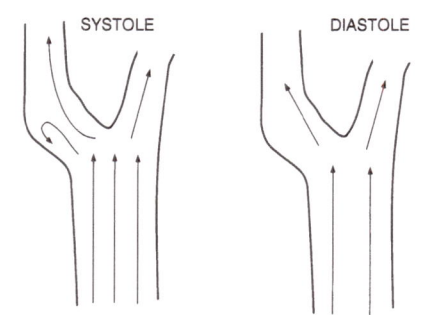

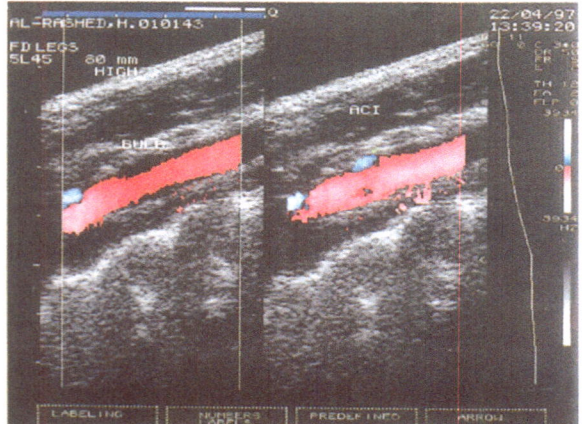

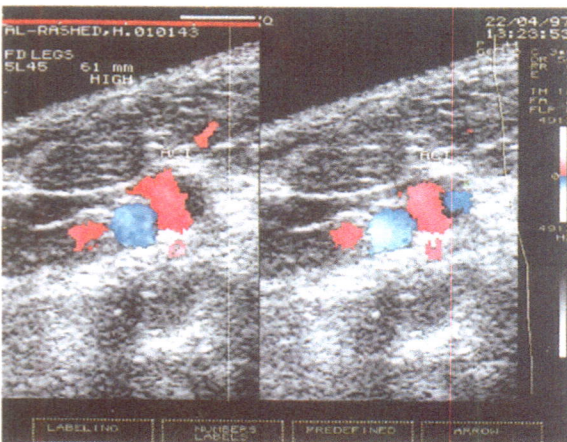

Fig. 10.7. a Flow pattern in the carotid bifurcation (according to BHARADVAJ et al. 1982). **b** Color-coded duplex imaging of the carotid bulb in sytole (*right half*) and diastole (*left half*). Secondary flow marked with a *green arrow* (*blue signal*). **c** Same image in transverse slice

The common carotid artery measures 65–70 mm. In longitudinal studies differences of 0.1 mm are within the reproducible range. The thickness of the carotid wall is 1–1.5 mm.

Two descriptions of pathology are important for the indication to surgery: the narrowing of the vessel and the configuration of the plaque.

Measuring the narrowing of the vessel lumen was a matter long discussed by the North American Symptomatic Endarterectomy Trial (NASCET) since the study found a rate of 13.1% of fatal stroke following medical treatment compared to 2.5% in the surgery group if the stenosis was higher than 70% (NASCET 1991). The problem was where to measure the stenosis (FOX 1993). One method of measurement using the unaffected apical lumen is easy to perform (Fig. 10.8). But divisor and divident of the measurement ratio are highly variable (HUSTON et al. 1993). Precisely for this problem additional functional results are useful because they permit a stenosis ratio by different means. The peak systolic flow increases with the degree of stenosis. The correlation is not a linear one. Stenosis of more than 95% leads to a flow decrease. In cases of total occlusion heavily calcified plaques must be ruled out and collaterals such as the ipsilateral vertebral artery or a retrograde flow in the external carotid artery must be shown. Accordingly, sensitivity shows a high variance depending on the degree of stenosis and number of patients.

It is important to achieve a standardized description of the vessel wall alterations which can be visualized: (a) echolucent, calcified, (b) regular surface,

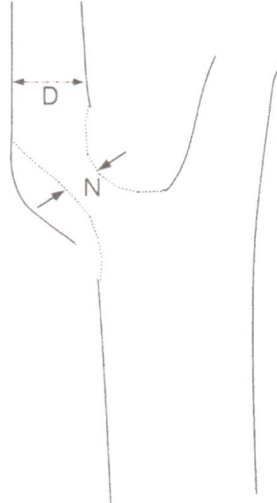

Fig. 10.8. Calculation of internal carotid stenosis: $(1-N/D) \times 100$ (FOX 1993)

irregular contour, ulceration, and (c) structure homogeneous, inhomogeneous.

A classification into four different types has been introduced. The predominant factor is echolucency (GRAY-WEALE et al. 1988). These classifications do not correlate with symptoms or add to the sensitivity of predicting symptoms (HOLDSWORTH et al. 1995). Another study has had results which show that lesion 1 and higher degree stenosis (80%–99%) have a higher incidence of infarction areas in computed tomography (GEROULAKOS et al. 1994). Unfortunately the latter study had far fewer patients which makes the comparison problematic. Another way of differentiating carotid plaques is to divide the pixel of the ultrasound image into small separate velocity vectors drawn against the time of a heart cycle. From this maneuver numerous movement directions result. If they move synchronous and parallel in the course of some heart cycles the plaques can be assessed as stable (HENNERICI 1995). If the pattern of the vectors is irregular this sign of instability may be a warning of the possibility of embolization (MEAIRS et al. 1995). It may prove to be an indication for surgery (Fig. 10.9).

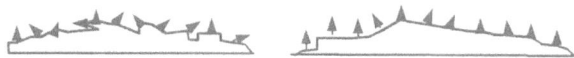

Fig. 10.9. Plaque morphology and different velocity vectors (according to HENNERICI 1995)

Lesions are always heterogeneous regardless of severity (POLAK et al. 1993). Irregularity increases with the degree of stenosis. More irregular, inhomogeneous, or calcified lesions are predictors of permanent neurological deficiencies.

10.7.2
Peripheral Arteries

10.7.2.1
Examination Method

Anamnesis, pulse, and ankle/brachial index are important and easy tests to perform. From these a diagnosis with 90% accuracy is possible. Color-coded duplex ultrasound can confirm that diagnosis and show where the lesion lies and what sort of lesion it is. With this information the puncture site for angiography and the direction can be chosen in the event of performing angioplasty in one session.

Aortic branches and iliac vessels are examined with a 3–3.5-MHz scanner, whereas femoral arteries and tibial vessels are visualized with a 5-MHz scanner. If the femoral pulses are good it is sufficient to take a Doppler spectrum in the common femoral artery. If it is triphasic with a normal velocity no further examination is needed in the iliac arteries. The arteries are examined thoroughly from groin to ankle.

10.7.2.2
Morphology

Criteria for stenosis and occlusions are shown in Table 10.2. Highly calcified stenosis where the shade hides the obliterated lumen are problematic. Different angles permit visualization of the whole vessel. Atherosclerotic lesions are probable if vessel walls are irregular with high signals and calcification. If such lesions are not present other causes may be responsible i.e., dissections, embolies, etc. An example of a dissection is shown in Fig. 10.10a,b. Ante- and retrograde flow are typical of this lesion. An embolus following iliac angioplasty is depicted in Fig. 10.11a,b. The thrombus can be clearly visualized with color-coded sonography. An aortic aneurysm is shown in Fig. 10.12 The dilated vessel is seen as well as the thrombosed parts of the aorta.

10.7.3
Mesenteric Vessels

Mesenteric Vessels can be depicted clearly. The superior mesenteric artery and splenic vein are shown in Figure 10 13a,b. The arterial vessels can be seen up to their second or third branches. Thrombo-

Table 10.2. Criteria for stenosis and occlusion in color-coded duplex ultrasound

Stenosis	Occlusion
Reduction of color-coded lumen	No color signal
Wall thickening	Proximal collateral vessel (obligatory)
Flow acceleration (color change)	Distal collateral vessel (optional)
Flow deceleration behind lesion	As stenosis

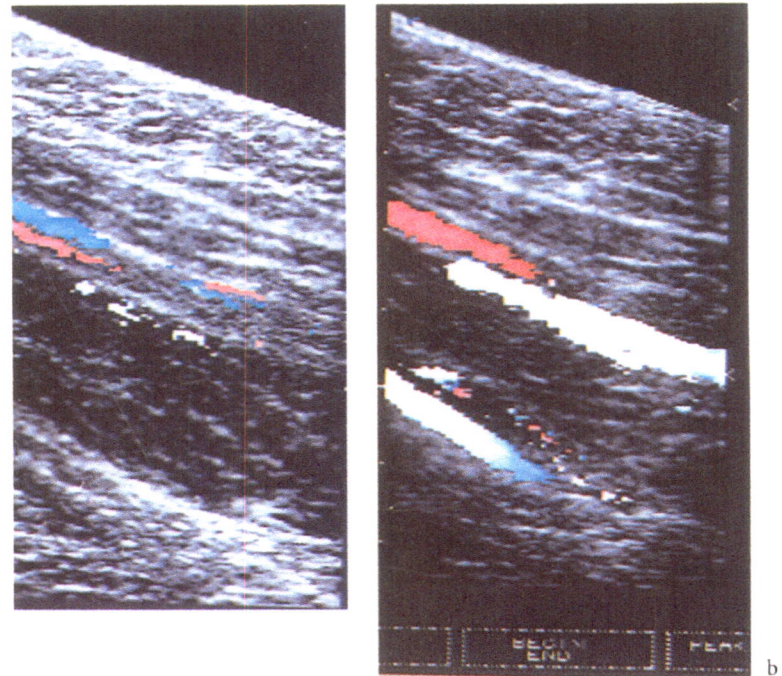

Fig. 10.10 a,b. Dissection of the superficial femoral artery in a 19-year-old girl after a horseshoe accident (*double signal sign*)

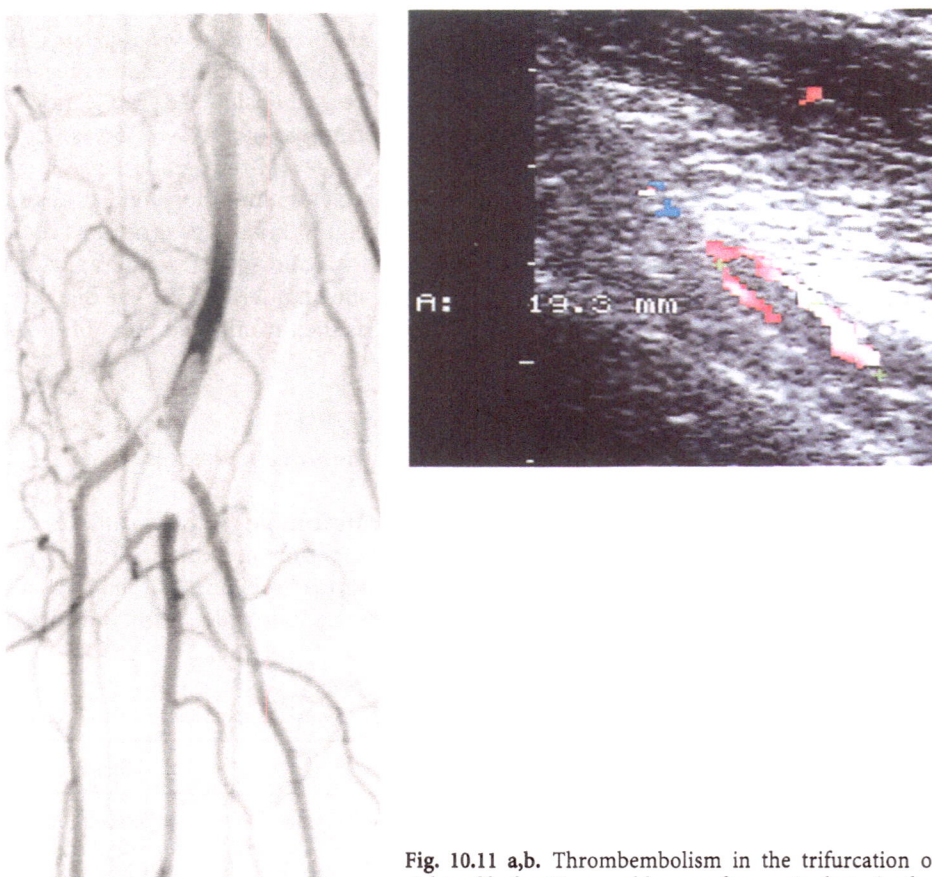

Fig. 10.11 a,b. Thrombembolism in the trifurcation of the right calf of a 56-year-old man after angioplasty in the iliac artery. **a** Angiography, **b** color-coded duplex sonography

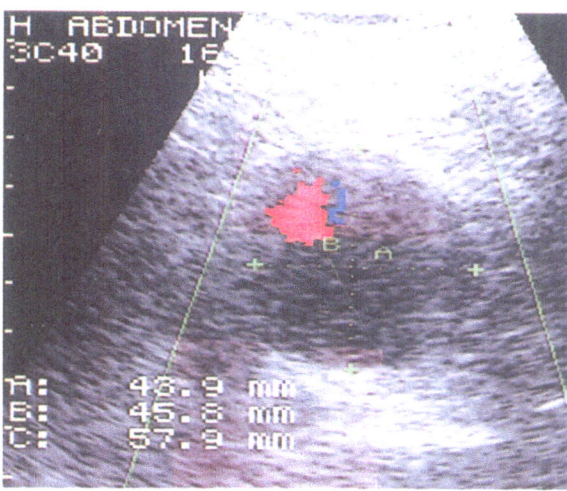

Fig. 10.12. Aortic aneurysm in a transverse slice. Note the dilated lumen with thick thrombotic ring

sis of the portal vein has a typical image (Fig. 10.14a,b). Immediately dorsal to the hepatic artery the echolucent vein can be seen.

10.7.4
Veins

10.7.4.1
Examination Method

The examination starts in the groin. Spectral analysis is derived over the vena iliaca externa with and without the Valsalva maneuver to see if the iliac vessels are patent. Then the vena femoralis communis and bifurcation are judged morphologically (Fig. 10.15a,b). The first figure shows a complete obstruction, while the second shows a stenotic lesion. The vessels are dilated and their margins are blurred. The next area is the distal superficial femoral vein and the popliteal vein. The vessels are examined longitudinally and transversally (Table 10.3). The tibial veins must be examined thoroughly. If the visualization is insufficient slight pressure can be used at the tarsal feet. Tubular anechoic structures are suspicious. Evident is the demonstration of anechoic tubular structures with a distal and/or proximal signal. Collateral vessels and echoic thrombi or irregular recanalization are hints of old thrombosis.

Vein examinations can be performed with continuous wave (CW), conventional, or color-coded Doppler (CCD) systems. The most elegant way is of

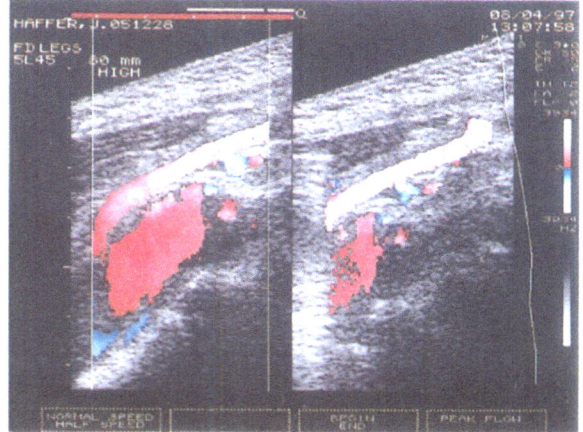

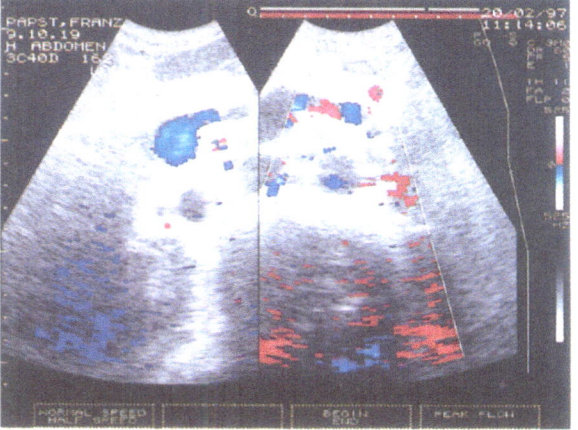

Fig. 10.13. a Superior mesenteric artery in longitudinal slice. **b** Splenic vein and confluens in a transverse slice

course the CCD mode. The first step is the interpretation of the color-filled lumen. Images are to be performed as longitudinal and transversal slices. If the color signal is absent additional information consists of perivascular edema and echogenicity of the lumen filling (Table 10.3). If there is no marginal

Table 10.3. Ultrasound criteria for deep vein thrombosis by color-coded duplex sonography

Signs

1. No color signal form the vein lumen in two projections
2. Only marginal color signal from the lumen
3. No Doppler signal in (1)
4. Reduced compressibility of the vein (*cave* embolization)
5. Tubular structure of low echogenicity beneath tibial artery
6. No flow lowering with Valsalva maneuver in common femoral vein
7. Perivascular edema
8. Loss of distinction of the vessel wall

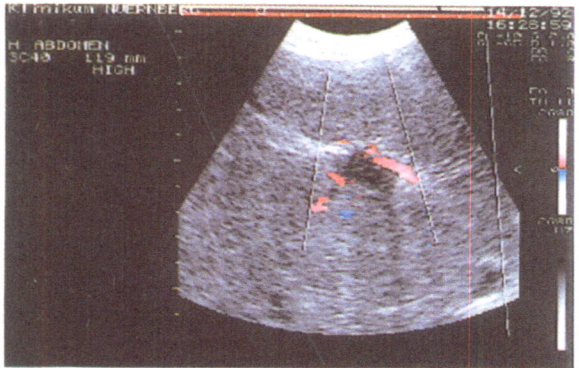

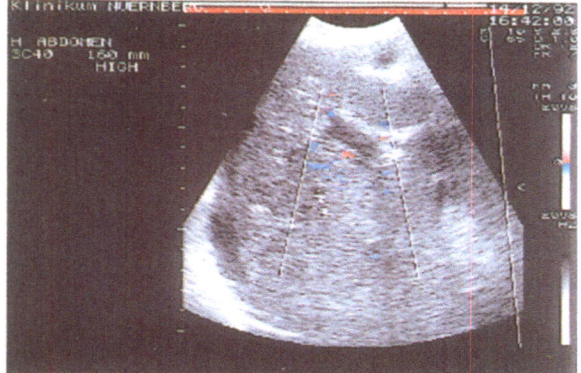

Fig. 10.14 a,b. Thrombosis of the portal vein (echolucent structure below the hepatic artery, *red signal*). Transverse and oblique projections

flow (floating thrombus), compression with the transducer reveals whether the thrombus is already rigid (old). Age determination by tissue characterization is possible in about 90% of thromboses (PARSONS et al. 1993).

10.8
Quantitative and Functional Measurements

10.8.1
Carotid Arteries

The signal in the external carotid artery is, under normal circumstances, a high impedance signal. This means that there is a low diastolic flow. In the internal artery there is a low peripheral resistance which causes a higher diastolic flow. In stenotic vessels turbulences and flow accelerations can be found. This depends on the location and distance from the stenosis. The common carotid artery shows the combination of both vessels. The low resistant flow can be used to monitor brain edema. The flow

pattern of a patient after suicidal strangulation and the result following therapy are shown Fig. 10.16a–c. The images were taken just after admission (a) and after antiedematous therapy (b,c).

The vertebral artery can be visualized only partially because it is overlayed by boney structures. Windows are parallel and sagittal in direction to the cervical spine. At least two segments should be observed. Another window is behind the mastoid where the atlas kink is visible. Systolic flow should be only a little lower than in the internal carotid artery (60 cm/s ± 10/systoic vs. 80 cm/s ± 15). The subclavian steal syndrome shows a retrograde flow which can be reduced by compressing the upper arm beyond the systolic pressure.

Wave velocities increase almost linear from the aortic arch to the feet (McDONALD 1968). The increase to the carotids is just the half. The three-dimensional velocity profiles of the vessel walls have great irregularities (RENEMAN et al. 1985; HOEKS

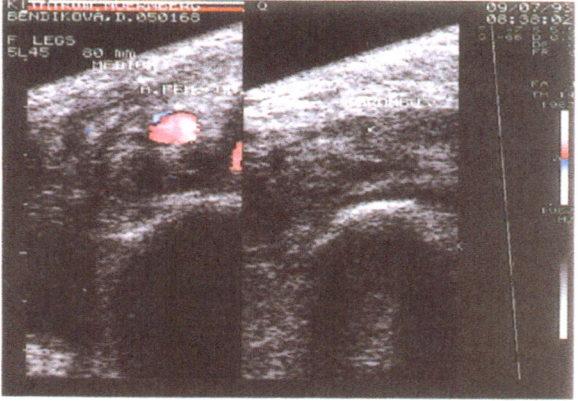

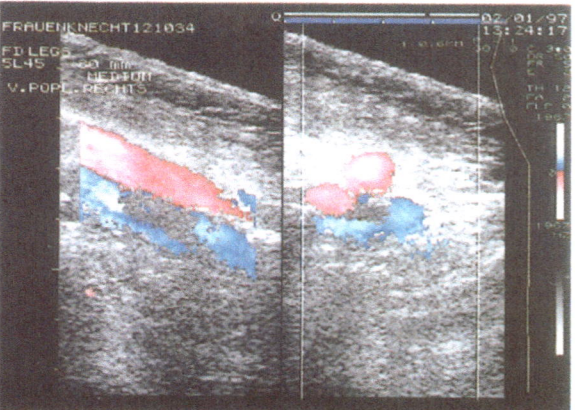

Fig. 10.15. a Complete obstruction of the common femoral artery with perivascular edema: acute deep vein thrombosis. **b** Thrombus in the femoral bifurcation with beginning of revascularization

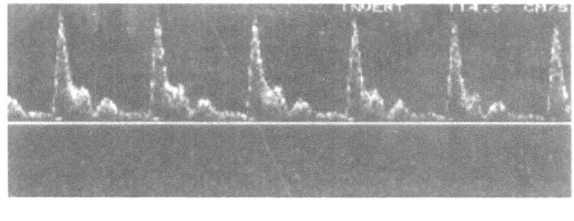
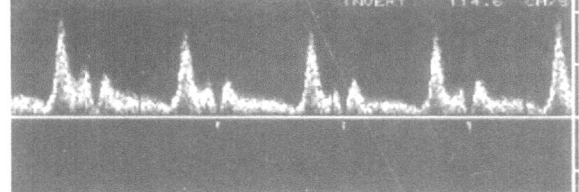
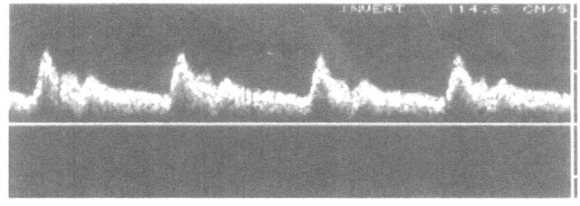

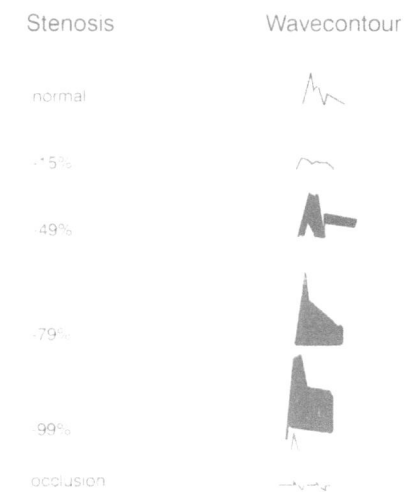

Fig. 10.17. Carotid artery stenosis and velocity wave contour (modified from BEACH and PHILLIPS 1992)

Fig. 10.16. a Signal over the internal carotid artery in a patient following suicidal strangulation and consecutive brain edema. 10.16 **b,c** Increasing diastolic flow with reduction of edema under therapy

et al. 1995). Flow disturbance and wall distensibility must be considered for diagnosis, otherwise 30%–43% of minor lesions would have been missed. Wall displacement is quite different between the anterior and posterior walls. From these observations the shear rate has been calculated to about 800 s^{-1} for the anterior wall and 650 s^{-1} for the posterior wall.

The Doppler waveform is characteristic if taken at the point of stenosis or occlusion (Fig. 10.17). Highly significant are the alterations in blood flow distal to the stenosis (JOHNSTON et al. 1992). Distortion of flow is higher in 65% of stenoses than in 75% of graded ones. In the latter the jet stream flow is predominant. Energy conversion of pressure, velocity, and heat show a typical pattern (RODBARD 1966). Pressure has an asymmetric U-function with the deepest point in the stenosis where the velocity is at its highest point. Heat increases from that area steadily. The flow velocity profiles can be displayed three-dimensionally to clarify the ultrasound recordings (SHEHADA et al. 1993).

Flow measurements are reproducible and have significant correlations ($r = 0.68$). They may be used wherever applicable, for instance in arteriovenous malformations (PAULSON et al. 1997).

10.8.2
Liver

The hepatic artery has a substantial variability regarding its functional parameters (PAULSON et al. 1996).

After ingestion of contrast medium the resistive index in the hepatic artery (propria) shows a marked increase from 0.65 ± 0.05 to 0.73 ± 0.06 after 15 min (PLATT et al. 1996). The diastolic flow decreases to zero. The flow in the vena porta increases from 940 ml/min ± 140 to 1.110 ml/min ± 210.

10.8.3
Peripheral Arteries

In the arteries the functional measurement plays an important role. Under normal conditions the waveform contour shows typical alteration, for instance in different body positions (Fig. 10.18a,b). With the feet lowered at 10 degrees the peripheral resistance increases and a pentaphasic flow pattern can be observed (a). An artificially increased peripheral resistance results in a deep diastolic backflow (b). Peak systolic values are changed before, during, and after the stenosis/occlusion. Furthermore, reproducible values are available without any problem so that longitudinal observations are possible (Fig. 10.19). The flow changes can be observed proximal and distal to the lesion depending on whether the examination is performed in rest or following exercise.

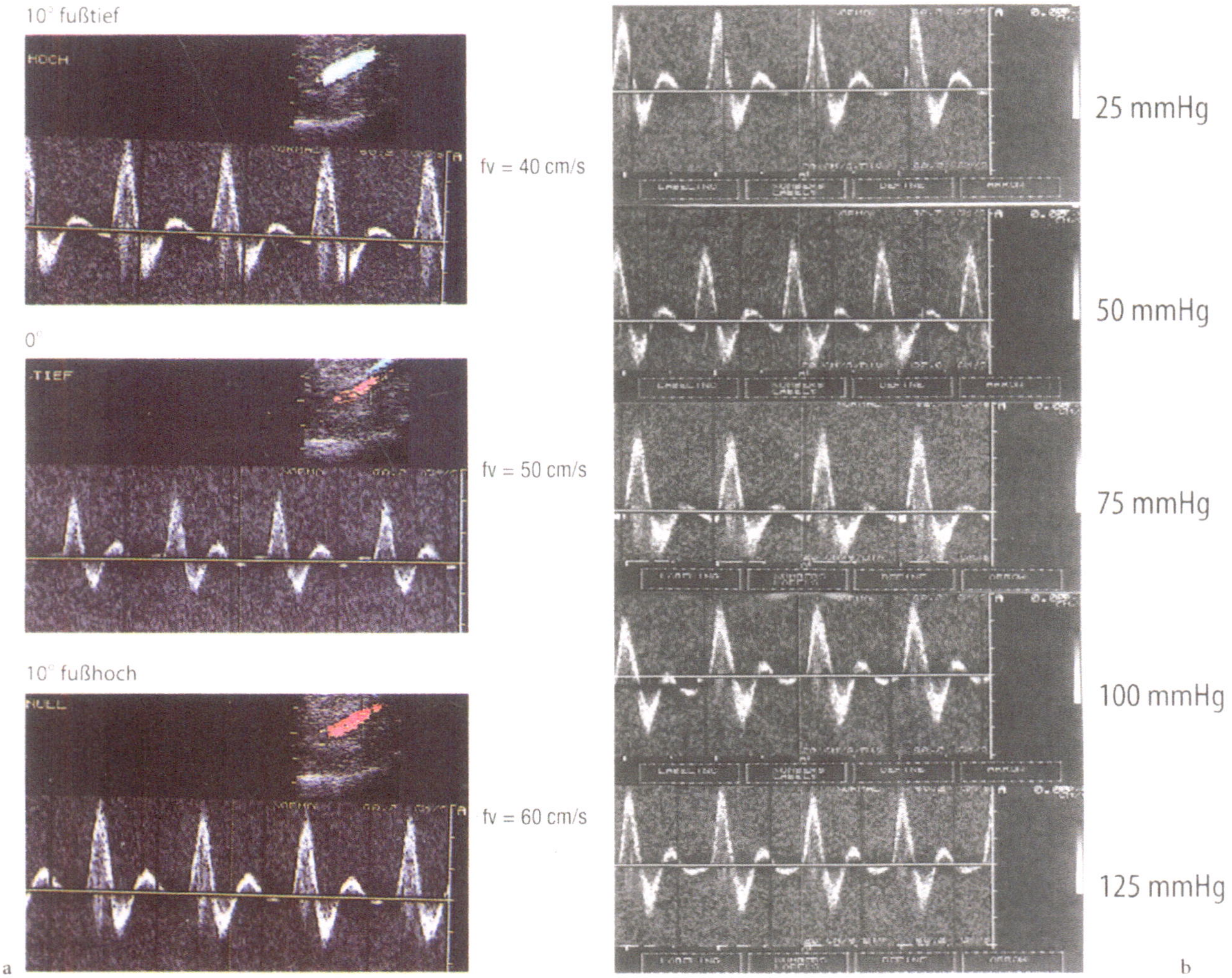

Fig. 10.18. a Velocity wave patterns in young healthy volunteers depending on body position (resting position: lowered 10 degrees, horizontal, and raised 10 degrees. **b** Velocity wave patterns in young healthy volunteers; measurements on the surperificial femoral artery with artificially increased peripheral resistance (sphygmomanometer). Fv, Maximum systolic velocity

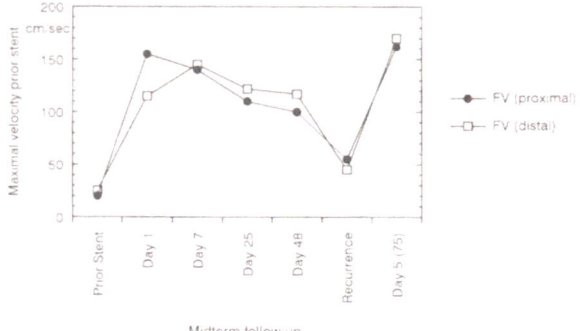

ig. 10.19. Follow-up in a patient with occlusion of the superficial femoral artery; measurements after two treatments Proximal to the lesion in rest (*black dots*), distal after exercise (*open squares*)

10.8.4
Veins

Regular breathing of the patient is important for the diagnosis of the veins. If the examination is performed while breath-holding there is nearly no flow in the vessels. The Valsalva maneuver can be used to assess the competence of the vena saphena magna with the color-coded duplex ultrasound. While pressing, there is a dilatation of the saphena origin but no flow. In case of incompetence the examination yields a peripheral backflow just as in the accompanying arteries.

10.9
Significance of Disease in Arteries and Veins

10.9.1
Carotid Arteries

Duplex ultrasound is sufficient in about 90% of cases as an indication for endarterectomy. Of chief importance is the correct diagnosis of the 70%–99% stenosis. Regarding peak and end diastolic stenosis, there are clear cut offs for differentiation (MONETA et al. 1993). Depending on stenosis grading and techniques used, sensitivities vary between 50% and 99% (Table 10.4).

Regarding low grade stenosis (<30%) the receiver operator characteristics (ROC) analysis, the main peak velocity has its highest accuracy for a cutoff of 1.2 m/s (FAUGHT et al. 1994). For high degree stenosis (>70%) this value is 2.1 m/s. With these ROC levels the accuracy of color flow duplex scanning is 89% for low grade lesions (<30%) and 97% for middle grade stenosis (30%–70%) and 95% for high degrees, respectively.

Inconsistent visualization near and opposite the vessel wall of the carotid bulb can occur in up to 10% of cases performed in B-mode at different visits (CROUSE and THOMPSON 1993).

In studies comparing magnetic resonance imaging (MRI), Doppler, and digital subtraction angiography (DSA), Doppler had a slightly higher coincidence (78% vs. 76%) than DSA (BUIJS et al. 1993). Compression of the superficial temporal artery (tap Maneuver) is not always reliable in identifying the external carotid artery (ECA) (KLIEWER et al. 1996).

10.9.2
Mesenteric Vessels

In 92% of cases a vascularity can be depicted in angiographically hypervascular liver tumors (LENCIONI et al. 1996). In angiographically silent tumors none could be visualized by Doppler methods. If the power Doppler signal is more pronounced than the signal in the color Doppler mode the probability of a malignant lesion is twice as high compared to other lesions. (CHOI et al. 1996). Vessel patterns typical for tumors do not exist.

Because of the broad ultrasound window the vena porta is always assessable. With a sensitivity of 93% and a specificity of 99% this vessel is diagnostically without any problem (BACH et al. 1996). The clinical importance is to a lesser extent the relatively rare thrombosis of the portal vein.

Doppler ultrasound is an effective tool to control stenosis or occlusions in transjugular portosystemic shunts (TIPS). Occlusion were shown in 96% of cases and ruled out in 99% (FELDSTEIN et al. 1996). A threshold of 0.5 m/s permits detection of 78% of stenotic parts in the stent and had a negative predictive value of 99%.

In mesenteric arteries stenosis can be shown directly and following lowering of the peripheral resistance. In normal controls the velocity in the superior mesenteric artery is maximally 150 cm/s which increases to 200 cm following meal-times (VOLTEAS et al. 1993). Patients with stenosis higher than 50% have systolic values of over 200 cm/s. The values increase to more than 300 cm/s following meal-times.

10.9.3
Peripheral Arteries

Up until now measurements to diagnose vascular arterial lesions have been possible with a normal bidirectional Doppler. In model stenosis correlations reach 0.98 for maximal peak, mean, and average velocities. Problems occurred in differentiating high degree stenosis from occlusions. Furthermore, it was difficult to estimate lesion length and to recognize a multivessel disease. With the color-coded duplex, however, ultrasound sensitivities between 80% and 98% and specificities ranging from 93% and 100% are possible (COSSMAN et al. 1989; MONETA

Table 10.4. Correlation of exact description of arterial lesions by color-coded duplex ultrasound (measurements according to the BOLLINGER Score; BOLLINGER et al. 1981)

Deep femoral artery	Superficial femoral artery	Popliteal artery	Anterior tibial artery	Peroneal artery	Posterior tibial artery
38%	69%	46%	23%	23%	31%

et al. 1992) (Table 10.4). What is lacking is the right graduation of stenosis. If the duplex mapping is compared with BOLLINGER's classification of different lesions (BOLLINGER et al. 1981) at one time the correlation is not as good (Table 10.5). If it is used for deciding therapy results are much better (Table 10.6). Stenoses in the femoropopliteal arteries can be shown clearly (Fig. 10.20a,b). Results after angioplasty are obvious. Complications like dissections are better visualized than with angiography (Fig. 10.21a–d). Nevertheless, duplex scanning is an alternative to angiography and should be used first (LONDON et al. 1996). Ultrasound overestimates lesions by up to 50% and underestimates higher lesions.

10.9.4
Veins

The first publications for B-mode ultrasound plebography showed sensitivities of 94%–100% with specificities of 92%–100% (SULLIVAN et al. 1984; AITKEN and GODDEN 1987). Newer publications have sensitivities as low as 76% and specifities of 88% (LANGHOLZ and HEIDRICH 1991). The conventional duplex ultrasound lies around 90% for both parameters (Table 10.7).

Publications about color-coded duplex ultrasound show increasing values for sensitivity and specifity over recent years of up to 96%–98%, a development in complete contrast to diagnosis with the B-mode. Most important is the prevalence of thrombosis and the presence of symptoms (ROSE

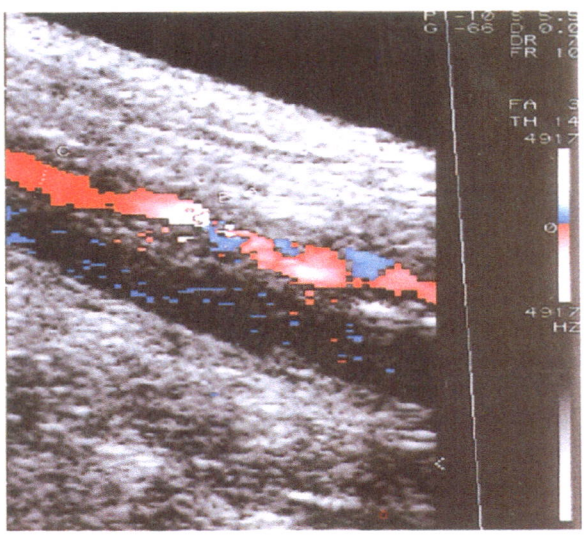

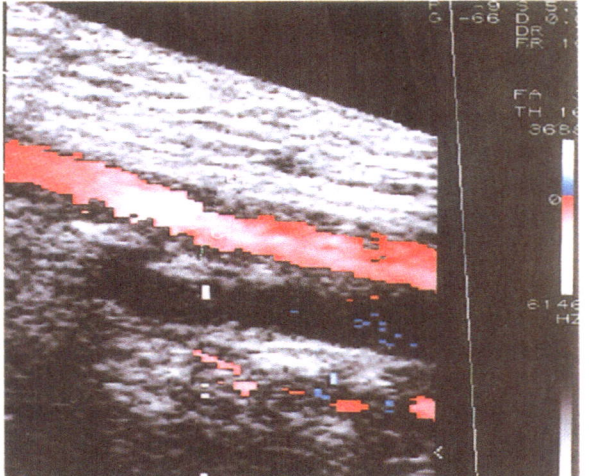

Fig. 10.20. a Stenosis of the superficial femoral artery; **b** follwoing angioplasty

Table 10.5. Sensitivities of duplex ultrasound in detecting lesions of the internal carotid artery

Ref	Stenosis <50%	Stenosis >50%	Occlusions	Technique
DAISS et al. 1984	50%	85%	87%	DS
MOORE et al. 1988	94%	98%	100%	DS
POLAK et al. 1992	91%	85%	100%	CCDS
DERDEYN et al. 1995	99%	100%	98%	CCDS

DS, duplex sonography; CCDS, color-coded duplex sonography.

Table 10.6. Sensitivity, specifity and accuracy of color coded duplex sonography regarding the therapy planned to be performed in the lesion (surgery, angioplasty, conservativ)

	Superficial femoral artery	Popliteal artery	Tibial artery
Sensitivity	90%	50%	25%
Specifity	100%	100%	84%
Accuracy	92%	92%	72%

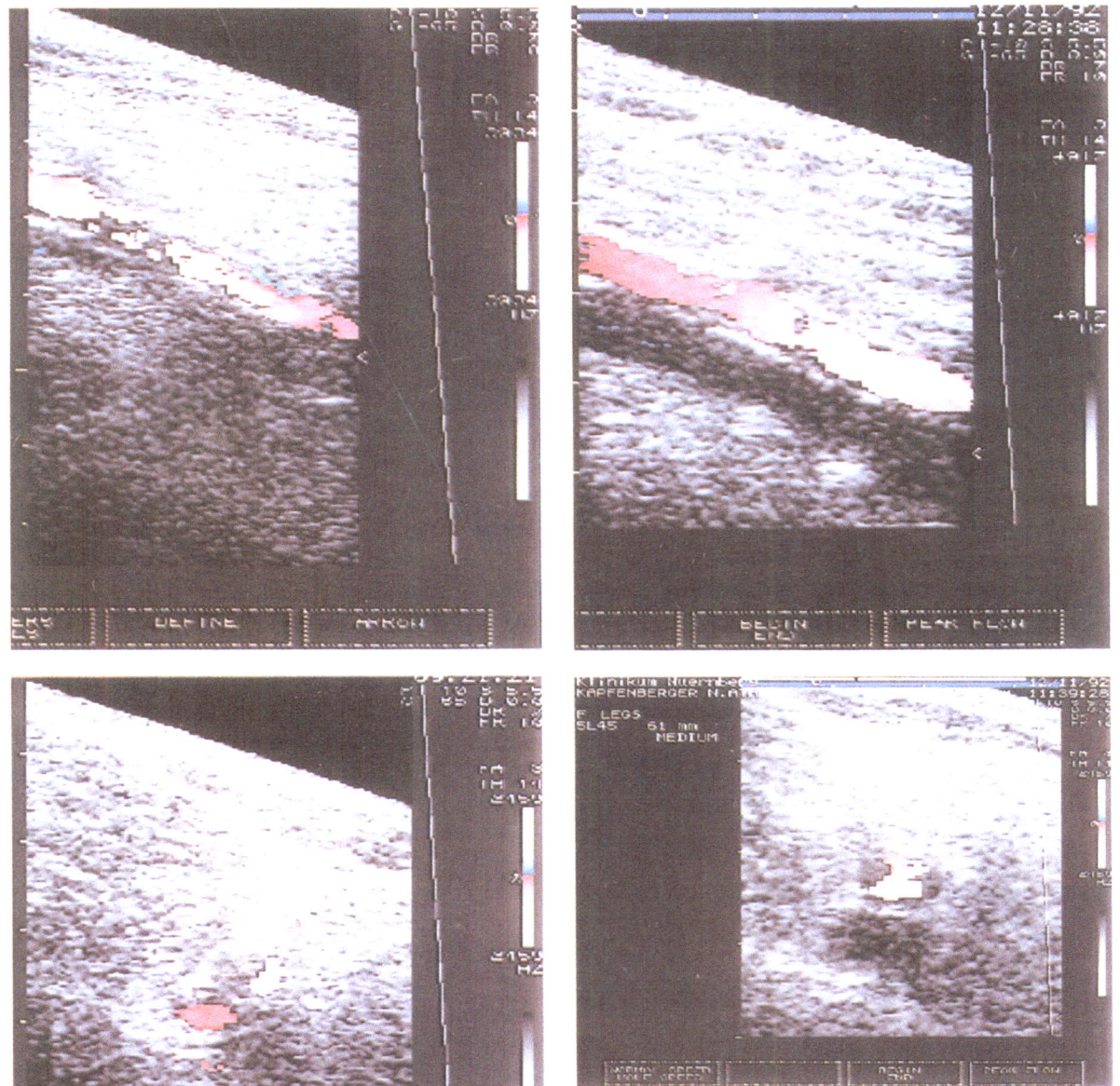

Fig. 10.21. a Stenosis of the superficial femoral artery; **b** transverse slice; **c** following angioplasty; **d** lumen dilated, dissection in the transverse slice

Table 10.7. Sensitivities (range) of B-mode, duplex and color coded duplex ultrasound (CCDS) phlebography (mod. from NEUERBURG-HEUSLER and HENNERICI 1995)

Iliac vein	Common femoral vein	Superficial femoral vein	Popliteal vein	Tibial vein	Technique
78%	100%	95%–100%	95%–98%	60%–89%	B-mode
93%–100%	100%	93%–100%	90%–100%	62%–93%	Duplex
95%–100%	95%–100%	95%–99%	97%–100%	72%–95%	CCDS

et al. 1990). Another important requirement is technical adequacy of the examination; if this is present, accuracy reaches 98% even in the calf.

Without doubt, in iliac vessels, in the vena profunda femoris, and in the muscular veins of the calf the CCD mode is superior to phlebography. In the tibial veins phlebography is more sensitive. Nevertheless, thrombosis can be detected (Fig. 10.22). Calf vessels have anatomic variants, a low flow, and are hidden behind boney or fascial structures. Sensitivity of 88% with a specificity of 96% is possible in calf venous thrombosis with compression ultrasound (YUCEL et al. 1991).

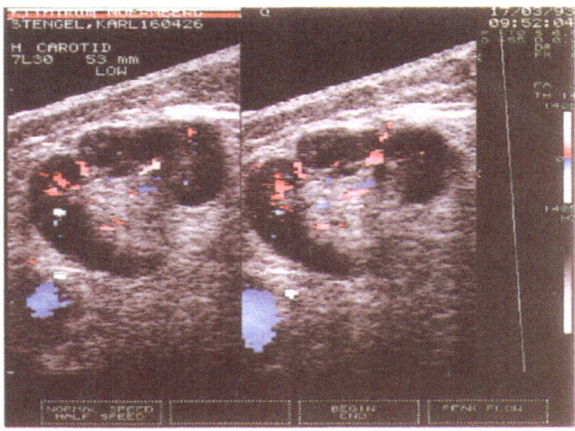

Fig. 10.23. Enlarged groin lymphoma with hyperperfusion in a patient with malignant melanoma

10.9.5
Tumors

Typically patterns in power Doppler ultrasound are vessels which penetrate and lie. In breast carcinoma a sensitivity of 68% with a specificity of 95% is achievable (RAZA and BAUM 1997). An interesting attempt is to count the number of vessels (COSGROVE et al. 1993). Malignant lesions have a higher subjective number with 2.2 compared to 0.2 and 0.05 in benign lesions. Occupied lymph nodes are impressive (Fig. 10.23). Hilar vessels and hypervascularity in the peripheral parts are clearly seen. Also, vessel density and area are higher in carcinoma. Following application of microbubbles, carcinomas had a greater and longer enhancement than benign lesions (KEDAR et al. 1996). Vessels had a higher tortuosity. The time to peak was shorter in carcinomas.

In prostate cancer the gray scale and Doppler are positive in 80% (RIFKIN et al. 1993). Doppler ultrasound alone has a positive finding in only 7%. The parameters are morphological.

In patients with chronic renal failure renal cell carcinomas occur in about 2%. Angiography is often not positive. Doppler ultrasound can, in up to 50% of cases, result in positive diagnosis when angiography is negative (TAKASE et al. 1994).

For tumors a high grade flow is used as a sign of malignancy. This sign is not very reliable because it is also found in inflammatory diseases. For prostate cancer NEWMAN et al. (1995) found a sensitivity of 49% with a specificity of 93%. For liver metastases the sensitivity was 100% with a specificity of 57% (LEEN et al. 1995). In testes 95% of tumors larger than 1.6 cm were hypervascular (HORSTMAN et al. 1992). Peak systolic velocities ranged from 8.4 cm/s to 65 cm/s (mean 9.8 cm/s). Their collective results were rather inhomogeneous. Beneath seminomas and teratomas they examined lymphomas and leukemic infiltrations.

ROC analysis of perfusion velocities in tumors showed a velocity of 0.4 m/s is a good threshold for distinguishing malignant and benign tumors (DOCK et al. 1991). The accuracy remains at about 70%.

Tumors deriving from vascular structures are easy to examine and check therapeutic results. (Fig. 10.24a–c). The vascularity is clearly seen and reduced perfusion following therapy is obvious.

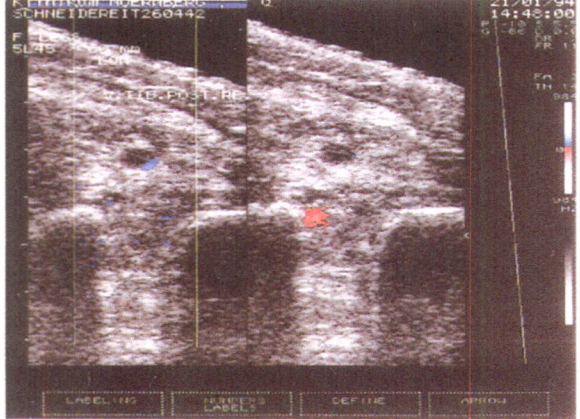

Fig. 10.22. Thrombosis in posterior tibial artery and vein (marginal flow signal)

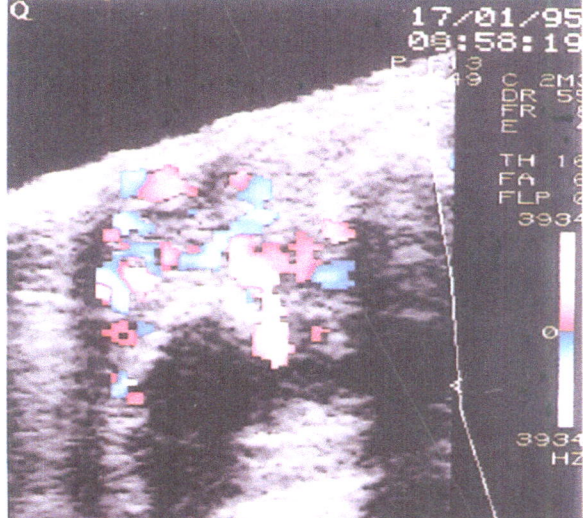

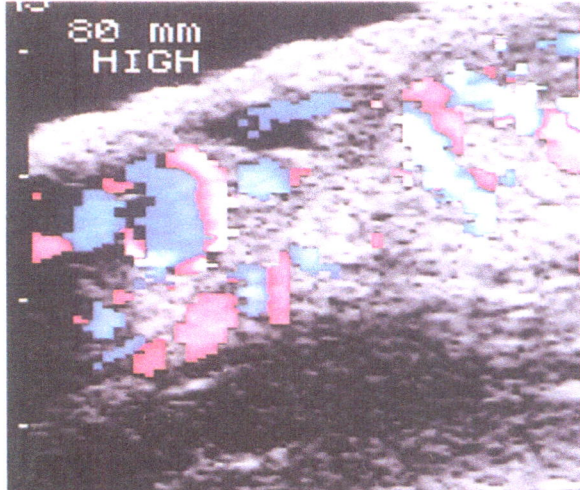

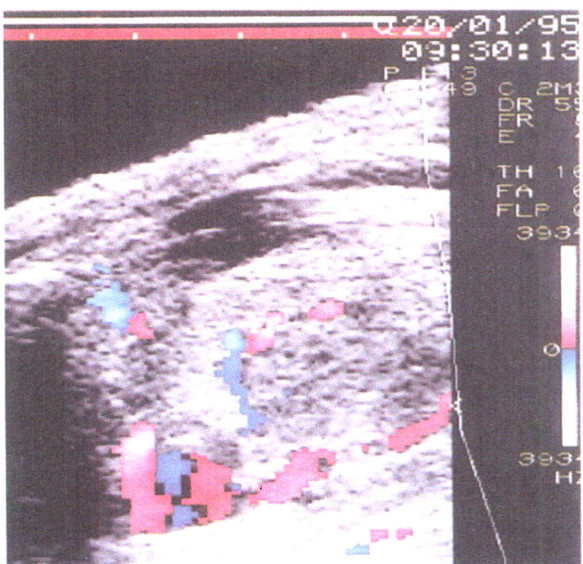

10.9.6
Other Organs

10.9.6.1
Vasogenic Impotence, Varicoceles, and Testicular Torsion

The correlation between pharmacocavernoso-graphy-metry is as high as 0.93 (MERCKX et al. 1992). Parameters included the resistance index in the cavernosal draining vein and change of cavernosal volume.

Measurements in the deep penis artery show an increase from 8–20 cm/s (V_{max}) to 35–45 cm/s after application of papaverin. With a sensitivity of 85% and a specificity of 33% these measurements are suitable for screening. Since this substance is no longer available in Germany prostaglandines need to be evaluated. For this substance an injection into both corpora cavernosa is important. The peak systolic value should be higher than 25 cm/s (BAEK et al. 1996). The end diastolic value is normal when it is lower than 5 cm/s (venogenic impotence).

The venous backflow can be visualized without any problem; 2 mm is the maximum limit of a normal pampiniform vein. The sensitivity of color Doppler ultrasound is 93% (PETROS et al. 1991). After surgery 64% of patients still showed an increased flow on the operated side (CVITANIC et al. 1993). Clinical improvement (sperm rate, partner's pregnancy) was shown in 58%. These results justify the examination.

Shunt-type configuration of the veins led to a high prevalence of postoperative varicoceles. In an animal model with graded torsion, flow decreased to a venous waveform and was completely absent after the first 180 degrees.

For this entity color-coded duplex ultrasound is the diagnostic tool of choice. Sensitivity is 86% and accuracy lies at 97% (BURKS et al. 1990). Only the criterion of an arterial flow in the testicular artery was missing. The high accuracy is afforded by the high prevalence of inflammatory diseases which otherwise lead to comparable clinical signs. These lead mostly to increased perfusion.

Fig. 10.24. a Arteriovenous malformation on the hand of a young man. **b,c** Following embolization: defects centrally in the tumor; **b** longitudinal slice; **c** transverse slice

10.10
Screening/Follow-Up with Ultrasound Angiography

10.10.1
Carotid Arteries

Ultrasonic biopsy is a valuable screening method if it is considered that near and far wall interfaces are not identical with the intima, media, and adventitial layers (Table 10.8; BELCARO et al. 1991). The ten-point scoring system is able to survey greater populations. Follow-up studies show that plaque progression results in increasing vessel diameter, whereas unchanged plaques also correlates with an unchanged diameter (STEINKE and HENNERICI 1994).

NASCET demonstrated a benefit for patients with internal carotid artery stenosis (ipsilateral) of more than 70% (NASCET 1991). Asymptomatic patients seem to profit with even lower grade stenosis, whereby men and women or patients both younger or older than 68 years of age do not profit similarily (ACAS 1995).

The threshold in Doppler ultrasound is the criterion for further diagnostics. Studies which imply a high false positive rate (high sensitivity) has the disadvantage of risking an unnecessary examination or operation (DERDEYN et al. 1995).

10.10.1.1
High Intensity Transient Signals

High intensity transient signals (HITS) are detected in transcranial Doppler from microemboli. Their diameter ranges from 20 to 150 μm. Air injections require smaller volumes (0.1–5 μl) than atherosclerotic material (0.1 ml). The signal is of short duration

Table 10.8. Criteria for ultrasonic biopsy (modified from BELCARO et al. 1991)

Class	Ultrasound criteria	Scoring points
A	Normal ultrasound layering, clear separation, no disruption of intimal interface for at least 5 cm	0
B	Interface disruption	2
C	Intima media complex granulation	4
D	Plaque: wall thickening, increased density	6
E	Plaque and stenosis	8
F	E and symptoms	10

at high frequency and can be detected automatically (MARKUS and TEGELER 1995). Their clinical importance is the evidence of an emboli source which must be diagnosed and cured.

10.10.2
Peripheral Arteries

If the velocity ratios were used for stenosis estimation three out of six patients developed an occlusion after a median of 28 weeks (WHYMAN et al. 1993). Two out of three patients with minor stenosis showed no change in their lesion. In our paper the incidence of de novo occlusions varied between 8% (iliac) and 14% (femoropopliteal) (BEYER-ENKE et al. 1994). In the literature the extremes lie between 1.7% and 20% (GALLINO et al. 1983; MAY and NISSL 1969). For these inconsistencies Doppler is indicated for screening exams. For follow-up after stent application the color-coded Doppler is a reliable tool (Fig. 10.25a,b). Stenosis can be seen clearly. Results following therapy are impressive.

10.10.3
Veins

Long-term studies show that in 53% of patients vein segments are reopened after 30–90 days (STRANDNESS et al. 1983). Some publications using B-mode ultrasound have very bad results (GINSBERG et al. 1991). Sensitivities of 50% for femoral thrombosis and 12.5% for calf vein are hints at systematic errors. The reasons thus far is unclear. The diameter of the vein decreases mostly in the first 3 months (MURPHY and CRONAN 1990). The reduction is about 40% (superficial and popliteal vein). Echogenicity increases slightly from month 1 to month 2. The difference is not significant.

10.10.4
Renal Artery

10.10.4.1
Artery Stenosis

The renal artery can be well visualized only in young healthy volunteers. The technical success rate in patients is 33% (DESBERG et al. 1990). If the arteries can be visualized a significant difference in peak systolic velocity can be shown proximal and distal to the

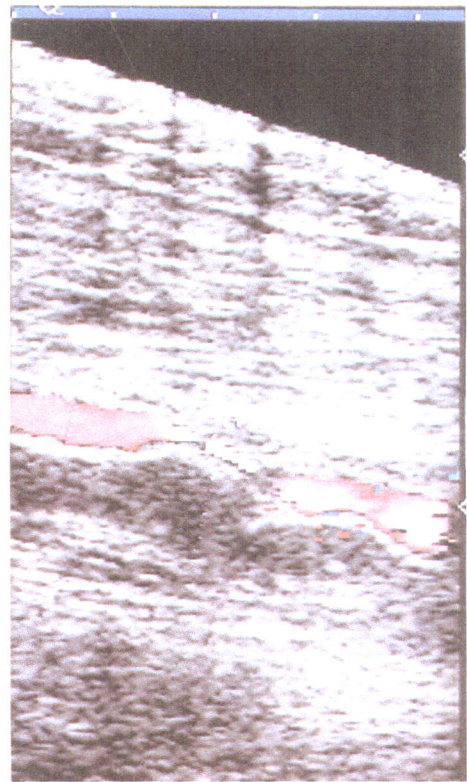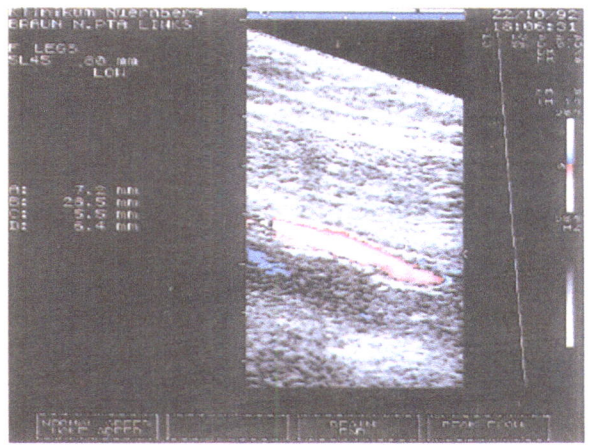

Fig. 10.25. a Stent stenosis in the superficial femoral artery; **b** after angioplasty

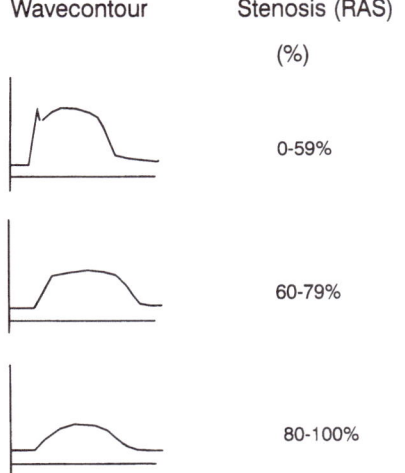

Wavecontour	Stenosis (RAS) (%)
	0-59%
	60-79%
	80-100%

Fig. 10.26. Renal artery stenosis (*RAS*) and velocity wave contour (modified from STAVROS et al. 1992)

1992). In up to 60% of stenoses the result was equivocal. For higher stenoses degrees differences were observed.

Absence of the early systolic rise seems to be a parameter to detect stenosis above 60% (Fig. 10.26). Sensitivity and specificity were higher then 95% (STAVROS et al. 1992).

The results are not homogeneous. Other authors are not able to reproduce such positive results (KLIEWER et al. 1993). They found a reduced acceleration time in patients with severe stenosis (2.99 m/s^2 vs 1.33 m/s^2). Recent data confirms these results (HALPERN et al. 1995). Early systolic acceleration may be absent in young healthy patients and a threshold of 3 m/s^2 may result in many false positive findings.

10.10.4.2
Inflammatory Diseases

Recent observations show that the resistive index (peak systolic shift–diastolic shift/peak value) is a reliable parameter for stable or improving prognosis (PLATT et al. 1997). Doppler values are of higher prognostic value than complement (C3, C4) or DNA

stenosis for grades higher than 70% compared to normal or lower than 50% (>65 cm/s vs <65 cm/s proximally and >40 cm/s vs. <65 cm/s distally).

So the indirect measurement in the hilus or peripherally is methodologically easier. Because the resistive index (Pourcelot) was not diagnostic an acceleration index was created (LAFORTUNE et al.

antibodies. In patients with worsened outcomes the resistive index was 0.78 ± 0.016 compared to 0.64 ± 0.13 in improved cases.

10.11
Intravascular Ultrasound

10.11.1
Technique

All instruments used for intravascular ultrasound (IVUS) are composed of a piezoelectric element and a mechanical or electronic mirror construction.

Two different systems are commercially available. Most systems are catheter-based with rotating elements (rotating mirror) and electronically switched-phase array catheter tips are used. The shaft diameters vary between 2.9 and 9.2 F depending on the anatomical structure under investigation. Sound frequencies range from 12.5 MHz to 40 MHz (Table 10.9). Axial resolution is always superior to the lateral resolution and increases with higher frequencies. At 20 MHz the axial resolution varies between 0.15 and 0.2 mm. Lateral resolution is in the range of 0.4–0.6 mm. Unfortunately, the penetration depth decreases with higher frequencies. The penetration depth at 12 MHz is 25 mm and 5 mm at 40 MHz. With higher frequencies even blood has a definite echogenicity. It may be important to flush the vessel with saline to demonstrate the intimal border or flaps.

The second type are guide-wire mounted crystals. Their great advantage is that they can be used with normal catheter systems.

Most systems have a forward view angle of about 30 degrees, so that catheter tip and shown vessel wall are not precisely identical. A concentric intraluminal positioning of the instrument is important. Otherwise, as with non-orthogonal positioning, distortion of the images may occur presenting an oval lumen aspect. For this reason clear documentation of the catheter (wire) position is obligatory.

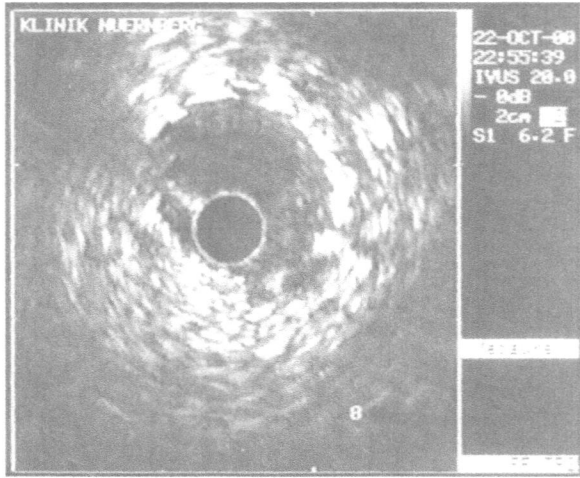

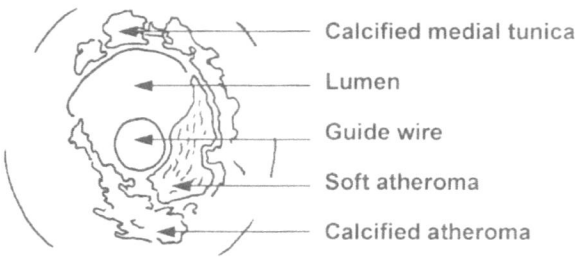

Fig. 10.27. Intravascular ultrasound image with central catheter. Atheroma at 6–9 o'clock. Thrombus at 2–6 o'clock

For exact reconstruction a stepwise movement of the instrument is crucial, either motor-driven or by marking at the catheter sheath. Documentation by radiography is helpful to define the position of the instrument. Orientation in the second dimension can be seen in a two-plane contrast image or by rotating the system.

10.11.2
Clinical Use

Intravascular ultrasound permits a transversal slice technique for assessing the vessel lumina. Correlation coefficients for the true lumen is as high as $r </= 0.99$ compared to histologic specimens. Due to the leading-edge phenomenon the intima media complex can be measured with a high degree of reproducibility. Elastic arteries can be distinguished from muscular type. The latter have a tunica media with a low echogenicity. Thrombus and soft atheroma are also hypoechoic and difficult to differentiate. Homogeneous reflections are more typical for thrombotic material (Fig. 10.27). Plaques and dense atheroma are hyperechogenic

Table 10.9. Frequency and anatomical structure (examples)

MHz	Vessel
12.5	Hepatic ducts, aorta
20	Femoropopliteal and iliac arteries
30	Coronary arteries

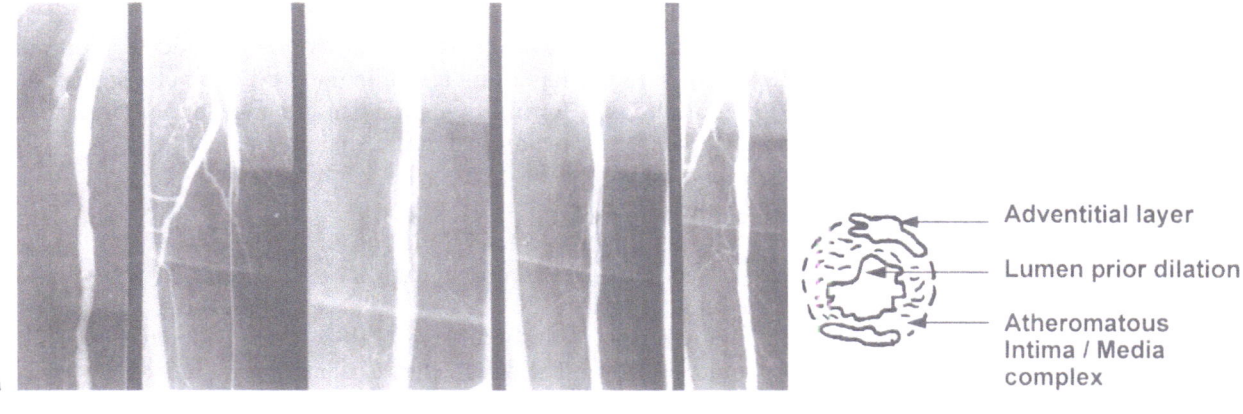

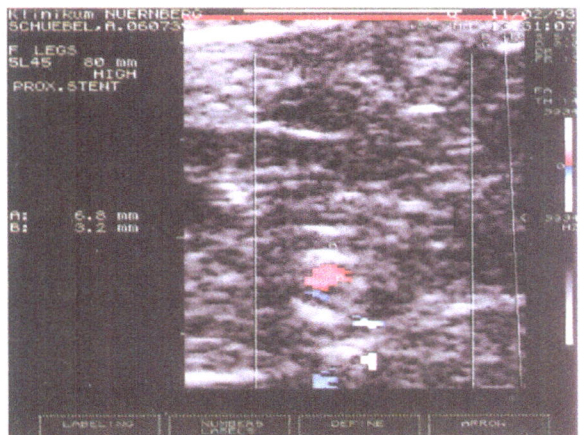

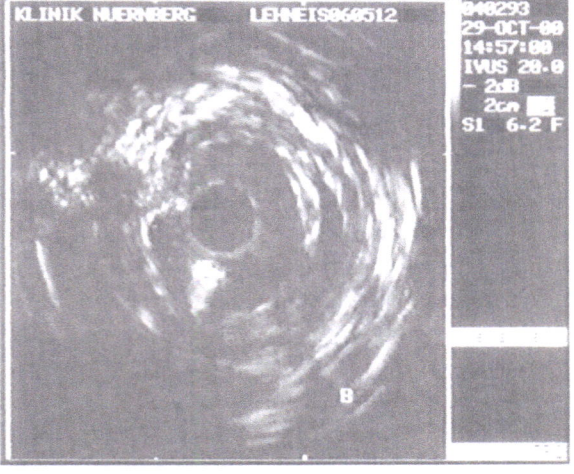

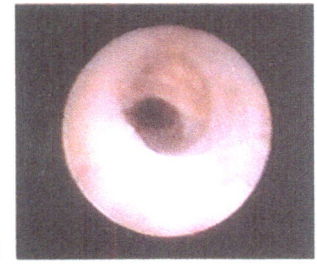

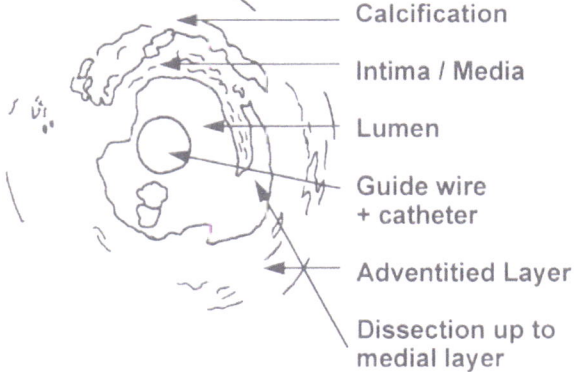

Fig. 10.28. a Conventional radiographic image: native, following primary angioplasty followed by atherectomy, before and following secondary definite angioplasty. **b** Color-coded Doppler ultrasound; transverse slice prior to therapy. **c** Angioscopy. Superficial femoral artery prior to therapy (proximal stenosis). **d** Intravascular ultrasound. Same vessel following therapy in the mid superficial femoral artery (submedial dissection)

and their surface structure can be demonstrated even if underlying structures are invisible due to total reflection of sound waves. Calcifications in the atheroma can be identified as very echogenic structures even if they are invisible in the angiographic image. A comparison of four diagnostic images are shown on Fig. 10.28a–d. The configuration of the lesion can be identified as a circular smooth or an irregular, complicated calcified atheroma, which would influence the decision of therapeutic procedure.

Refering to the interpretation of IVUS images, valuable criteria includes the definition of the vessel wall area. This is the outer border of the tunica media, which is slightly echolucent (external elastic membrane, EEM). The adventitial layer is hyperechoic. In the atherosclerotic process the media shows an atrophy and becomes irregular and smaller. From this area the luminal area is subtracted. The result is the plaque area. Clinical data has shown that angioplasty results in dilation of the EEM border, which correlates with the vessel diameter. The plaque area remains nearly unchanged following angioplasty.

In the development of atherosclerosis the thickness of the vessel wall increases as the lumen narrows. This phenomenon is known as the GLAGOV theory (GLAGOV et al. 1987). The compensatory enlargement of the vessel leads to the consequence that 40% of the lumen has to be occupied by plaque until the lumina are narrowed. These changes are visible when examined by IVUS. According to this hypothesis, an inadequate remodeling could be the reason for the development of focal stenosis (MINTZ et al. 1997).

A number of experimental and clinical studies using IVUS demonstrate that the late lumen loss is due to vessel constriction rather than an increase in plaque volumina. Measurements were made by

cross-sectional area inside the EEM (MINTZ et al. 1996). Understanding arterial remodeling is the most important fact or in the prevention of restenosis following angioplasty and its prevention, for instance, by internal or external radiation.

10.11.2.1
Balloon Angioplasty

Ideal tools are IVUS-assisted balloons (Fig. 10.29). The direct effect of dilatation is immediately visible. From this investigation we know that deflation following the first balloon angioplasty is followed by an elastic recoil of nearly 50% (ISNER et al. 1992). The second inflation results in an additional diameter of the lumen of up to 40%. Ultrasound angioplasty has been performed instead of angiography. In these cases IVUS was the only imaging modality. In normal cases the diameter of the angioplasty balloon is chosen to match the proximal unaffected lumen in order to prevent overdilation. According to the Glagov phenomenon it has been

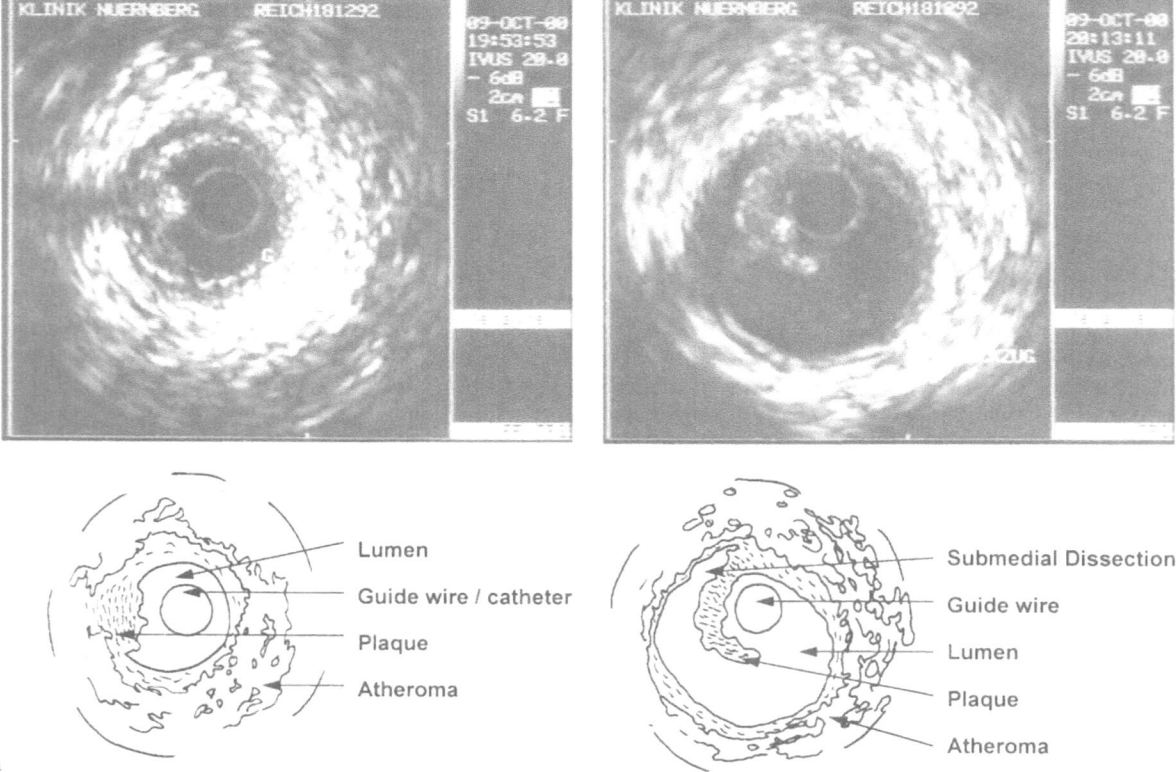

a   b

Fig. 10.29. a Intravascular ultrasound; external iliac artery prior to angioplasty with high degree of stenosis. **b** Same vessel following angioplasty; submedial dissection and flap (9–12 o'clock)

hypothesized that in arterial segments with remodeling an overdilation may result in an improved luminal dimension. In this CLOUT trial no increase in dissections or complications was recognized (STONE et al. 1997).

The judgement of the vessel wall following angioplasty is very important (Fig. 10.28a,b). Dissections can be classified according the angiographic scheme (Table 10.10).

This classification was modified for specific IVUS criteria. They differ according to dilation of the normal vessel wall, flaps, and depth of dissection (Table 10.11) (GERBER et al. 1992). The lumen gain is mainly due to dilation of the whole vessel. The plaque area decreases only to a small extent (VAN DER LUGT et al. 1997). Ruptures mainly occur in the plaque and to a smaller extent in the media (26% vs. 17%). Dissection can be observed in 57%. Because the classification of residual stenosis is superior to angiography this could be of predictive value of early outcome following angioplasty. This advantage cannot be overcome even by two-plane angiography.

Table 10.10. Dissections following angioplasty (DORROS et al. 1983)

Type	Criteria
A	Small radiolucent area in vessel lumen
B	Linear, nonpersisting extravasation
C	Extraluminal, persisting exstravasation
D	Irregular filling defect
E	Lumen defect and flow reduction
F	Total occlusion

Table 10.11. IVUS classification of morphology following angioplasty (GERBER et al. 1992)

Plaque	Type	Criteria	(%)
Concentric	1	Wall distension	4
	2	Intimal disruption	2
	3	Disruption intima/media	17
	4a	Subintimal dissection/flap	4
	4b	Submedial dissection/flap	4
Excentric	5	Circular dissection	31
	6	Dissection of normal vessel wall	13
	7a	Subintimal dissection/flap	29
	7b	Submedial dissection/flap	29

10.11.2.2
Stents

Stents are ideal for observation and follow-up because the struts are clearly visible due to their high echogenicity. The earliest application was to measure the diameter of the adjacent normal lumen to determine the exact size of the stent. Furthermore, adequate length to cover the whole lesion was investigated. It is important that no struts of the stent are intraluminal due to thrombotic complications. In our collective study there was a patient whose stent in the femoral artery was extracted percutaneously. Parts of it remained in the vessel lumen. Although these parts had no contact to the vessel wall the artery remained open, probably because the patient was under coumarin.

Many of the recent insights come from cardiology research. From this point of view there may be crucial differences to other parts of the body.

Nevertheless, many of the insights are comparable to other vessel regions. Longitudinal studies have shown that narrowing of the stent lumina are due only to neointimal formation (MUDRA et al. 1997). No compression of the stent was noted. No relevant progression of disease in the adjacent arterial segment was demonstrable. The neointima formation was uniformly distributed over the whole stent (HOFFMANN et al. 1996). There was no difference between overlapping and non-overlapping stents. Also, at the articulation of the Palmaz-Schatz stent there was no greater neointimal tissue formation.

The result that late lumen loss is due to arterial remodeling makes stent placement attractive again. If "bigger is better", stents are the ideal tool to achieve adequate lumina.

10.11.2.3
Limitations

IVUS discriminates thrombotic material poorly. Some important factors for restenosis like oxidant stress or functional parameters cannot be made visible by IVUS. The vessel wall is only demonstrable in arterial segments which can be catheterized. Occluded and distal segments are invisible, as well as collaterals. Catheter-based systems require an exchange of diagnostic and therapeutic instruments with a low risk of embolization.

In some studies only 79% of the images are of diagnostic quality. Ultrasound examinations are

generally highly dependent on the skill of the
researcher.

References

ACAS (1995) Executive Committee of the Asymptomatic Carotid Atherosclerotic Study. Endarterectomy for asymptomatic carotid artery stenosis. JAMA 273: 1421–1428

Aitken AGF, Godden DJ (1987) Real-time ultrasound of deep vein thrombosis. Clin Radiol 38:309–313

Bach AM, Hann LE, Brown KT, et al. (1996) Portal vein evaluation: comparison to angiography combined with CT arterial portography. Radiology 201:149–154

Baek S, Kim HY, Choi H, Chung WS (1996) Diagnostic value of double injection of a vasoactive drug in penile Doppler US. Radiology 201(p):337

Beach KW, Phillips DJ (1992) Sensitivity and precision of fast Fourier transform spectral waveform analysis in mild carotid atherosclerotic disease. In: Labs KH, Jäger KA, Fitzgerald DE, et al. (eds) Diagnostic vascular ultrasound. Arnold, London pp 57–68

Belcaro G, Barsotti A, Nicolaides AN (1991) Ultrasonic biopsy- a non-invasive screening technique to evaluate the cardiovascular risk and to follow up the progression and the regression of arteriosclerosis. VASA 20:40–50

Beyer-Enke SA, Söldner J, Zeitler E (1993) Genauigkeit der Farbduplexsonographie zur Diagnostik der pAVK des Beines vor PTA. Ultraschalldiagnostik 1993, Oct. 10–12, Innsbruck

Beyer-Enke SA, Zhai R, Zeitler E (1994) Qualität, Nutzen und Risiken der Becken/Bein-Angiographie vor PTA. Aktud Radiol 4:307–312

Bharadvaj BK, Mabon RF, Giddens DP (1982) Steady flow in a model of the human carotid bifurcation. J Biomech 15:349–362

Bollinger A, Breddin K, Hess H, et al. (1981) Semiquantitative assessment of lower limb atherosclerosis from routine angiographic images. Atherosclerosis 38:339–346

Bude RO, Kennelly MJ, Adler RS, Rubin JM (1994) Nonpulsatile arterial waveforms: experimental study during graded testicular torsion in an animal model. Radiology 193(p):336

Buijs PC, Klop RBJ, Eikelboom BC, et al. (1993) Carotid bifurcation imaging. Eur J Vasc Surg 7:245–251

Burks DD, Markey BJ, Burkhard TK, et al. (1990) Suspected testicular torsion and ischemia: evaluation with color Doppler sonography. Radiology 175:815–821

Choi BI, Kim HY, Han JK, et al. (1996) Power versus conventional color Doppler sonography. Radiology 200:55–58

Cosgrove DO, Kedar RP, Bamber JC, et al. (1993) Breast diseases: color Doppler US in differential diagnosis. Radiology 189:99–104

Cossman DV, Ellison JE, Wagner WH, et al. (1989) Comparison of contrast arteriography to arterial mapping with color flow duplex imaging in the lower extremities. J Vasc Surg 10:522–529

Crouse JR, Thompson CJ (1993) An evaluation of methods for imagimg and quantifying coronary and carotid lumen stenosis and atherosclerosis. Circulation 87 Suppl 2:II17–133

Cvitanic ON, Cronan JJ, Sigman M, Landau ST (1993) Varicoceles: Postoperative Prevalence – a prospective

study with color doppler US. Radiology 187:711–714

Daiss W, Diener HC, Thron A, et al. (1984) Diagnosis of stenosis and occlusion of extracranial arteries. Dtsch Med Wochenschr 109:1595–1599

De Groot MR, Banga JD (1994) Non invasive ultrasound measurement of intimamedia thickness. Eur J Vasc Surg 8:257–263

Derdeyn CP, Powers WJ, Moran CJ, et al. (1995) Role of Doppler US in screening for carotid atherosclerotic disease. Radiology 197:635–643

Desberg AL, Paushter DM, Lammert GK, et al. (1990) Renal artery stenosis: evaluation with color Doppler flow imaging. Radiology 177:749–753

Dock W, Grabenwöger F, Metz V, et al. (1991) Tumor vascularization: assessment with duplex sonography. Radiology 181:241–244

Dorros G, Cowley MJ, Simpson J, et al. (1983) Percutaneous transluminal angioplasty: report of complications from the National Heart, Lung and Blood Institute PTCA Registry. Circulation 67:723–730

Faught WE, Mattos MA, van Bemmelen PS, et al. (1994) Color flow duplex scanning. J Vasc Surg 19:818–828

Feldstein VA, Patel MD, LaBerge JM (1996) Transjugular intrahepatic portosystemic shunts. Radiology 201:141–147

Fox AJ (1993) How to measure carotid stenosis. Radiology 186:316–318

Gallino A, Mahler F, Probst P (1983) Progression to total occlusion of lower limb artery stenoses selected for PTA. Lancet 2:59–60

Gerber T, Erbel R, Görge G, et al. (1992) A classification of morphologic effects of coronary balloon angioplasty assessed by intravascular ultrasound. Am J Cardiol 70:1546–1554

Geroulakos G, Domjan J, Nikolaides A, Stevens J, Labropoulos N, Ramaswami G, Belcaro G, Mansfield A (1994) Ultrasonic carotid artery plaque structure and the risk of cerebral infarction on computed tomography. J Vasc Surg 20:263–266

Ginsberg JS, Caco CC, Brill-Edwards PA, et al. (1991) Venous Thrombosis in Patients who have undergone Major Hip or Knee Surgery. Radiology 181:651–654

Glagov S, Weisenberg E, Zarins CK, et al. (1987) Compensatory enlargement of human atherosclerotic coronary arteries. N Engl J Med 316:1371–1375

Gray-Weale AC, Graham JC, Burnett JR, et al. (1988) Carotid artery atheroma. J Cardiovasc Surg 29:676–681

Halpern EJ, Deane CR, Needleman L, et al. (1995) Normal renal artery spectral Doppler waveform: a closer look. Radiology 196:667–673

Hennerici M (1995) Plaque morphology. 17th World Congress of the International Union of Angiology, April 3–7, London

Hoeks APG, Reneman RS (1995) Biophysical principles of vascular diagnosis. J Clin Ultrasound 23:71–76

Hoffmann R, Mintz GS, Dussaillant GR, et al. (1996) Patterns and mechanisms of in-stent restenosis. Circulation 94:1247–1254

Holdsworth RJ, McCollum PT, Bryce JS, Harrison DK (1995) Symptoms, stenosis and carotid plaque morphology. Eur J Vasc Endovasc Surg 9:80–85

Horstman WG, Melson GL, Middleton WD, Andriole GL (1992) Testicular tumors: findings with color Doppler US. Radiology 185:733–737

Huston J III, Bradley DI, Wiebers DO, et al. (1993) Carotid artery: prospective blinded comparison of two-dimensional time-of flight MR angiography with conventional angiography and duplex US. Radiology 186:339–344

Isner JM, Rosenfield K, Losordo DW, Ramaswamy K (1992) Clinical experience with intravascular ultrasound as an adjunct to percutaneous revascularisation. In: Tobis JM, Yock PG (eds) Intravascular ultrasound imaging. Churchill Livingstone, New York, pp 171–197

Johnston KW, Ojha M, Wong PKC (1992) Flow patterns in the region of modelled arterial stenoses. In: Labs KH, Jäger KA, Fitzgerald DE, et al. (eds) Diagnostic vascular ultrasound. Arnold, London, pp 57–68

Kedar RP, Cosgrove D, McCready VR, et al. (1996) Microbubble contrast agent for color Doppler US. Radiology 198:679–686

Kliewer MA, Topler RH, Caroll BA, et al. (1993) Renal Artery Stenosis: Analysis of Doppler waveform Parameters and Tardos-Parms Pattern. Radiology 189:779–787

Kliewer MA, Freed KS, Hertzberg BS, et al. (1996) Temporal artery tap. Radiology 201:481–484

LaFortune M, Patriquin H, Demeule E, et al. (1992) Renal artery stenosis: slowed systole in the downstream circulation. Radiology 184:475–478

Langholz J, Heidrich H (1991) Sonographische Diagnose der tiefen Becken-/Bein-venenthrombose. Ultraschall Med 12:176–181

Leen E, Angerson WJ, Wotherspoon H, et al. (1995) Detection of liver metastases. Radiology 195:113–116

Lencioni R, Pinto F, Armilotta N, Bartoluzzi C (1996) Assessment of tumor vascularity in hepatocellular carcinoma. Radiology 201:353–358

London NJM, Sensier S, Hartshorne T (1996) Can lower limb ultrasonography replace arteriography? Vasc Med 1:115–120

Markus HS, Tegeler CH (1995) Experimental aspects of high-intensity transient signals in the detection of emboli. JCU 23:81–87

May R, Nissl R (1969) Gefäßverschlüsse nach Angiographien. Fortschr Geb Röntgenstr 110:64–71

McDonald DA (1968) Regional pulse-wave velocity in the arterial tree. J Appl Physiol 24:73–78

Meairs S, Röther J, Neff W, Hennerici M (1995) New and future developments in cerebrovascular ultrasound, magnetic resonance angiography, an related techniques. JCU 23:139–149

Merckx LA, de Bruyne RMG, Goes E, et al. (1992) The value of dynamic color duplex scanning in the diagnosis of venogenic impotence. J Urol 148:318–320

Mintz GS, Popma JJ, Pichard AD, et al. (1996) Arterial remodeling after coronary angioplasty. Circulation 94:35–43

Mintz GS, Kent KM, Pichard AD, et al. (1997) Contribution of inadequte arterial remodeling to the development of focal coronary artery stenoses. Circulation 94:35–43

Moneta GL, Yeager RA, Antonovic R, et al. (1992) Accuracy of lower extremity arterial duplex mapping. J Vasc Surg 15:275–284

Moneta GL, Edwards JM, Chitwood RW, et al. (1993) Correlation of North American Endarterectomy Trial (NASCET) angiography definition of 70% to 99% internal carotid artery stenosis with duplex scanning. J Vasc Surg 17:152–159

Moore WS, Ziomek S, Quinones-Baldrich WJ, et al. (1988) Can clinical evaluation and noninvasive testing substitute for arteriography in the evaluation of carotid artery disease. Ann Surg 208:91–94

Mudra H, Regar E, Klauss V, et al. (1997) Serial follow up after optimized ultrasound guided deployment of Palmaz-Schatz stents. Circulation 95:363–370

Murphy TP, Cronan JJ (1990) Evolution of deer venous thrombosis: a prospective evaluation with ultrasound. Radiology 177:543–548

NASCET North American Symptomatic Carotid Endarterectomy Trial Collaborators (1991) Beneficial effect of carotid endarterectomy in symptomatic patients with high grade carotid stenosis. N Engl J Med 325:445–453

Neuerburg-Heusler C, Hennerici M, (eds) (1995) Gefäßdiagnostik mit Ultraschall, 2nd end. Thieme, Stuttgart

Newman JS, Bree RL, Rubin JM (1995) Prostate cancer: diagnosis with color Doppler sonography with histologic correlation of each biopsy site. Radiology 195:86–90

Parsons RE, Sigel B, Feleppa EJ, et al. (1993) Age determination of experimental venous thrombi by ultrasonic tissue characterization. J Vasc Surg 17:470–478

Paulson EK, Kliewer MA, Frederick MG, et al. (1996) Hepatic artery: variability in measurement of resistive index and systolic acceleration time in healthy volunteers. Radiology 200:725–729

Paulson EK, Kliewer MA, Frederick MG, et al. (1997) Doppler US measurement of portal venous flow. Radiology 202:721–724

Petros JA, Andriole GL, Middleton WE, Picus DA (1991) Correlation to testicular color doppler ultrasonography, physical examination and venography in the detection of left varicoceles in men with infertility. J Urol 145:785–788

Platt JF, Bude RO, Ellis JH, et al. (1996) Hepatic hemodynamic alterations after acministrations of oral CT contrast agents. Radiology 199:713–716

Platt JE, Rubin JM, Ellis JH (1997) Lupus nephritis: predictive value of conventional and Doppler US and comparison wit serologic and biopsy parameters. Radiology 203:82–86

Polak JF, Bajakian RL, O'Leary DH, et al. (1992) Detection of internal carotid artery stenosis. Radiology 182:35–40

Polak JF, O'Leary DH, Kronmal DA, et al. (1993) Sonographic evaluation of carotic artery atherosclerosis in the elderly. Radiology 188:363–370

Raza S, Baum JK (1997) Solid breast lesions: evaluation with power Doppler US. Radiology 203:164–168

Reneman RS, van Menode T, Nick P, et al. (1985) Flow velocity patterns in and distensibility of the carotid bulb in subjects of various ages. Circulation 71:500–509

Rifkin MD, Sudakoff GS, Alexander AA (1993) Prostate: techniques, results, and potential applications of color Doppler US scanning. Radiology 186:509–513

Rodbard S (1966) Dynamics of blood flow in stenotic vascular lesions. Am Heart J 72:698–704

Rose SC, Zwiebel WJ, Nelson BD, et al. (1990) Symptomatic lower extremity deep venous thrombosis: accuracy, limitations, and role of color duplex flow imaging in diagnosis. Radiology 175:639–644

Shehada REN, Cobbold RSC, Johnston KW, Aarnink R (1993) Three-dimensional display of calculated velocity profiles for physiological flow waveforms. J Vasc Surg 17:656–660

Smith JL, Evans DH, Fan L, et al. (1994) Processing Doppler ultrasound signals from blood-borne emboli. Ultrasound Med Biol 20:455–462

Stavros AT, Parker SH, Yakes WF, et al. (1992) Segmental Stenosis of the Renal Artery Radiology 184:487–492

Steinke W, Hennerici M (1994) Compensatory carotid artery dilatation in early atherosclerosis. Circulation 89:2578–2581

Stone GW, Hodgson JM, Goar FGS, et al. (1997) Improved procedural results of coronary angioplasty with intravascular ultrasound-guided balloon sizing. Circulation 95:2044–2052

Strandness DE, Langlois Y, Cramer M, et al. (1983) Long term sequelae of acute venous thrombosis. JAMA 250:1289–1292

Sullivan ED, Peters DJ, Cranley JJ (1984) Real-time B-mode venous ultrasound. J Vasc Surg 1:465–471

Takase K, Takahashi S, Tazawa S, et al. (1994) Renal cell carcinoma associated with chronic renal failure. Radiology 192:787–792

Van der Lugt A, Gussenhoven EJ, Mali WPTM, et al. (1997) Effect of balloon angioplasty in femoropopliteal arteries assessed by intravascular ultrasound. Eur J Vasc Endovasc Surg 13:549–556

Volteas N, Labropoulos N, Leon M, et al. (1993) Detection of superior mesenteric and coeliac artery stenosis with color flow duplex imaging. Eur J Vasc Surg 7:616–620

Westra SJ, Levy DJ, Chaloupka JC, et al. (1997) Carotid artery volume flow. Radiology 202:725–729

Whyman MR, Ruckley CV, Fowkes FGR (1993) A prospective study of the natural history of femoropopliteal stenosis using duplex ultrasound. Eur J Vasc Surg 7:444–447

Yucel EK, Fisher JS, Egglin TK, et al. (1991) Isolated calf venous thrombosis: diagnosis with compression US. Radiology 179:443–446

11 Angioscopy

A. Beck

CONTENTS

11.1
Introduction

Vascular endoscopy using rigid instruments has been known for the last 40 years and was first described by the vascular surgeon VOLLMAR (1969) at the University of Ulm in Germany. Its clinical use was obviously limited so that this new diagnostic method could not be introduced as a routine procedure. Angioscopy was reserved for the field of vascular surgery due to the large diameters of the endoscopes which need a surgical approach and the possibility of bloodless inspection of the vessel. Percutaneous inspection of the vessels was not possible in the 1950s. After the development of flexible fibreglass optics this method has been accepted in many medical specialities. Technical improvements allowed increasingly subtle visualization in all areas of angioscopic application (BECK 1993; FERRIS et al. 1985; MEHIGIAN and OLCOTT 1986). Over the last 8 years ultrathin endoscopes have been developed (AUSTER et al. 1984; BECK et al. 1992). They can be introduced into the artery and even into the vein by a transfemoral approach using angio-graphic sheath sets of common sizes without the need for vascular surgery. Several

A. BECK, Prof. Dr. Dr., Klinikum Konstanz, Institut für Röntgendiagnostik und Nuklearmedizin, 78461 Konstanz, Germany

problems needed to be solved: reduced blood-flow in the area of planned angioscopy, light intensity, documentation, rinsing of sodium chloride solution, or application of CO_2 (BECK et al. 1996) instead of liquid medium. All in all angioscopy resulted from interest to visualize angiographic (BECK 1987), sonographic (BECK et al. 1987a; 1987b), oscillographic and Doppler sonographic findings. Immediate restenosis or reocclusion following interventional procedures like percutaneous transluminal angioplasty (PTA) is not uncommon and the detection of these problems was the aim of early angioscopic research, followed by the supervision of implantation of vascular endoprostheses and the follow-up results of these stents of different types (BECK et al. 1994, 1996; CHOUX et al. 1986; LITVAK et al. 1985; SANBORN 1986).

Even in these times of modern vascular surgery and new interventional methods the thrombotic or thromboembolic occlusion of arteries has remained an insufficiently solved medical problem. For this reason percutaneous angioscopy is supported to understand the mechanisms of interventional methods like PTA, thrombus extraction, Fogarty manoeuvres and local catheter lysis.

11.2
Materials and Methods

Different types of angioendoscopes with outer diameters of 0.7–2.1 mm and working channels of 0.35–0.40 mm, combined with a conventional light source are used (Table 11.1). Six prototypes from Olympus Optical, Hamburg, with diameters of 0.9–2.1 mm, 20 single-use endoscopes from Meadox Surgimed, five endoscopes from Guerbet Medical, France (Fig. 1), and one from A.D. Krauth, Hamburg, have been used in the last 10 years. The first endoscopes in the early 1980s needed a light source like gastroscopical instruments and could be used by direct inspection. The modern angioendoscopes of the last 3 years have an integrated electronically-

Table 11.1. Different types of angioendoscopes used in our study

	Type of angioendoscopes	Outer diameter	Image quality	Catheter guided	Working channel
1	Prototype Olympus GF 15	1.5 mm	+	-	+
2	Prototype Olympus EF 10	1.0 mm	(+)	+	+
3	Prototype Olmpus JV 08	0.8 mm	(+)	+	-
4	Prototype Olympus JF 2.0	2.0 mm	++	-	+
5	Meadox Surgimed 1.9	1.9 mm	++	-	+
6	Intra med 1.9	1.9 mm	++	-	+
7	Guerbet endoscope 0.8	0.8 mm	++	-	-
8	Krauth Angioendoscope 1.3	1.3 mm	+	+	-

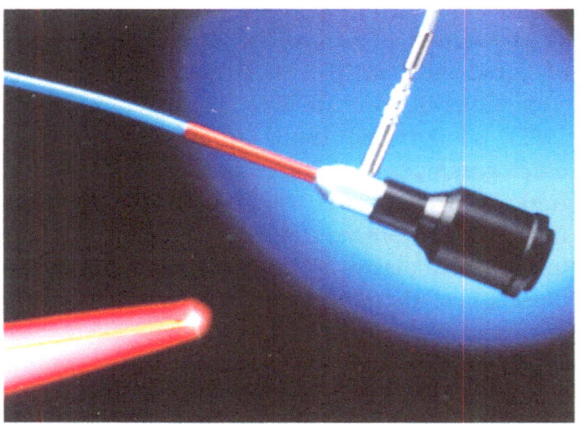

Fig. 11.1. Angioendoscope (Guerbet Medical, France) with an autodiameter of 0.9 mm

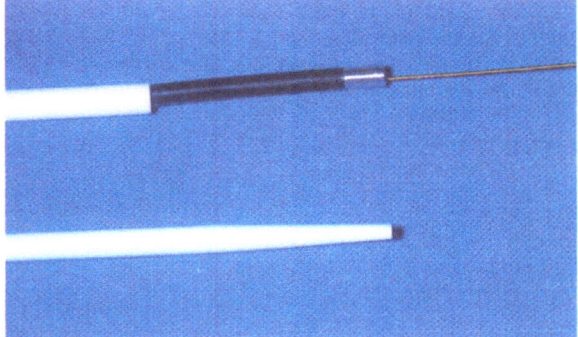

Fig. 11.2. Angioendoscope (prototype, Olympus Optical, Hamburg) within a common F-5 sheath set. A guide-wire (18 inches) is introduced into the working channel

guided light source with digital transmission of the signal on a television screen. In the past documentation consisted only in direct photography using an attached camera for single shots or, even better, using a quick-shot camera with up to four pictures/s. In the last 3 years the new angioendoscopes have been combined with a television mode, capable of storing the entire angioscopic findings during examination (Fig. 2). The disadvantage of this method is the difficulty in reproducing sharp pictures, which can be better obtained with conventional film examination using a conventional camera. For documentation we used diapositive films with 800–1000 ASA and achieved good results.

The approach for angioendoscopy is transfemoral in most cases. Necessary for all angioendoscopies is the correct positioning of a sheath set, which must be placed without bending to avoid damage to the flexible endoscopes. Different sizes from F 5 up to F 9 are used. The sheath set is normally placed into the artery under local anaesthesia (Fig. 3).

After withdrawal of the dilator the endoscope is placed into the region of interest under fluoroscopic control. This is the procedure for the distal femoral

and popliteal arteries and the trifurcation, including the crural arteries. Visualization of central arteries, i.e. renal, mesenteric and supraaortic arteries can be performed by placing a F-9 sheath set and then inserting a F-8 selective catheter into the region of interest. The tip of the selective catheter must be widened prior to the procedure by a warmed sterile needle for the passage of the angioendoscope. The endoscope is placed into the vessel after removal of the catheter using the Seldinger technique.

The main problem in angioendoscopy is achieving of a short period of bloodlessness. In the iliac artery proximal blockage of the blood stream can be achieved by a balloon-wedge catheter, which can be placed using a cross-over technique from the contralateral artery. The region of interest in the distal artery can be achieved by a second puncture distal to the blocked artery.

Total bloodlessness cannot be obtained because of multiple collaterals of muscle arteries. Nevertheless, the above-mentioned procedure is sufficient for distal femoral and popliteal arteries because the collateral blood stream is diluted by sodium chloride solution or CO_2 perfusion. Vessels tolerate total

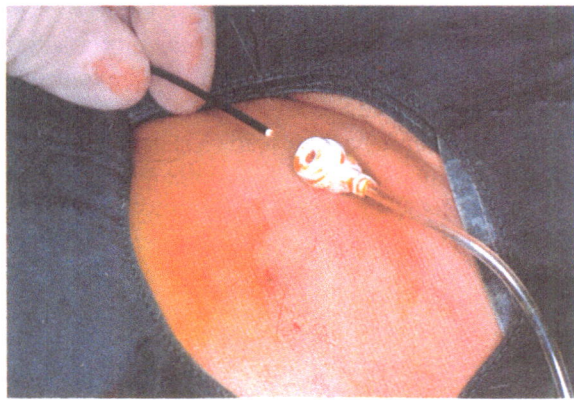

Fig. 11.3. Transfemoral insertion of an angioscope into the sheath set

blockage for a maximum of 5–8 min. Bloodlessness of the femoral and popliteal arteries can also be obtained by puncture of the femoral artery loco typico and by implantation of a sheath set. The artery is compressed manually proximal to the site of puncture. Visualization of the region of interest is possible for some seconds and does not need a second puncture. A third method of achieving bloodlessness is to block the vessel ipsilaterally using a wedge catheter and to puncture distal to the blockage. This procedure is technically easier to perform than the cross-over technique. Direct puncture of the superficial femoral artery can be difficult in some patients.

Visualization of renal, mesenteric and supraaortic arteries can be achieved by partial blockage of the proximal part of the artery using a catheter with a large outer diameter of F 9. The endoscope is inserted through this catheter and placed into the area of interest.

After approximate total blockage of a vessel a maximum of 400 ml of 0.9% sodium chloride solution is infused into the working channel of the endoscope, using a pressure of up to 300 mmHg. The infusion of sodium chloride is managed manually or even better by an infusion pump. Thus visibility is obtained for 4–8 s. Each endoscopic control needs 10–15 ml of 0.9% sodium chloride solution, so that 1–2 min of visualization can be achieved in every patient. The findings are documented by video or high-speed cameras.

We started using CO_2 in the peripheral arteries five years ago, and even in the renal and mesenteric arteries by manual infusion of CO_2 through the guiding catheter or through the working channel of the endoscope. The amount of 30 ml for each endoscopic inspection should be limited. The

maximum for the whole procedure in one patient should not exceed 300 ml. More than 200 angiographies using CO_2 were be performed with no serious problems. The quality of angioscopic pictures made using CO_2 injection is better than those using sodium chloride. In particular, the sharpness of the pictures and their three-dimensional imaging are impressive.

The performance of more than 800 angioscopies was always combined with angiographies. The basic procedure in all angioendoscopic methods is the Seldinger technique under fluoroscopic control. Endoscope placement should be performed only in angiographic procedures. All stenoses and local thromboses are first checked by angiography and then by angioendoscopy. The gold standard for the first vascular information is based on before and after intervention of percutaneous transluminal angioscopy (PTA) and local lysis angiography. Stenoses can be controlled before and after PTA as can the local thrombosis before and after local lysis. Lytic agents of up to 800 000 U of urokinase or 20 mg recombinant tissue plasminogen activator (r-PA) can be administered via the working channel of the endoscope or by the sheath set. A permanent visualization of a local catheter lysis can be obtained.

If the effect of dilatation or local lysis is not sufficient, stents can be used to keep the artery open. In our clinic we used different types of balloon-expandable and self-expandable stents. We were able to place 210 stents into different arteries and 40 could be controlled by angioendoscopy during the procedure and 40 after 6–24 months as a long-term result. Using angioendoscopy we were able to see remarkable restenoses which were hidden in the plain-film angiography. Another method for extracting thromboses or emboli has been developed: A mechanical thrombus extraction device consisting of an electric motor which moves a guide-wire and a twist drill up to 40–200 rotations/min can be used. The drill never leaves the catheter tip, so that wall lesions cannot occur. After the removal of thrombi, an angioscopic view can be obtained. Thrombotic material is sucked into the catheter, crushed by the moving screw and washed out in pieces of less than 0.1 mm. Damage to the vessel walls can be much better seen than with angiographic examination. A total of 29 patients were treated using this method and examined angioscopically. The thrombi could be extracted from the iliac artery in four cases, the femoral artery in 16 cases, the popliteal artery in three cases and the posterior tibial artery in one case. In 20 cases of arterial thrombosis we successfully extracted the thrombi completely. In four cases the thrombotic material was too old for mechanical extraction, meaning that a surgical Fogarty procedure had to be performed.

11.3
Indication for Angioscopy

Initially, only uncertain angiographic situations were indications for angioscopy. Since gaining positive experience with angioscopy in animals and reducing the diameter of endoscopes to sizes equal to 5 F, indications for angioscopy have been continuously extended. The indication for angioscopy was extended to PTA, local thrombolysis, and the differentiation of local thrombosis versus thromboembolism (Table 11.2).

Another indication for angioscopy seems to be the control of angiographically impossible recanalization situations. In these cases the dissection of a vessel can be prevented by continuous angioscopic control. Direct visualization of the new interventional techniques such as intravascular stent insertion is likely to be a major field for angioscopy, and it is especially helpful in the inspection of the

intimal layer within the stent.

Furthermore, thrombus extraction procedures using a flexible, spiral-shaped wire can be controlled impressively by angioscopy. Particularly in the field of laser angioplasty angioscopy is a developing procedure, as the effects of laser angioplasty are still incompletely explained and documented in vivo. The recanalization of long stenoses using the new method of rotation angioplasty or atherectomy could primarily be controlled by angioscopy.

11.4
Angioscopic Diagnosis of Vascular Changes

At angioscopy normal human arteries have a tubular shape with a smooth intimal surface. The vascular wall is pale pink. It can be quickly cleared of blood by flushing the angioscope with sodium chloride solution or CO_2 (Table 11.3). In contrast, this is more difficult in atherosclerotic or thrombotic vessels where blood components adhere and can only be partially removed from the vascular wall (Figs. 11.4, 11.5). A consistent feature of healthy vessels is their elasticity, which allows the endoscopes to be

Table 11.2. Current indications and diagnostic prediction of percutaneous transluminal angioscopy versus angiography

Diagnostic problem	Indication	
	Angioscopy	Angiography
Grading of atherosclerosis	++	++
Diagnosis of uncertain vascular occlusions	++	+
Differential diagnosis:		
Local thrombosis/thromboembolism	++	(+)
Inflammatory vascular changes	+	+
Actinic vascular injury	++	+
Control of PTA	++	+
Control of local lysis	++	++
Control of stents	++	+
Control of thrombus extraction	++	+
Control of rotation angioplasty	++	+

++ Unequivocal diagnostic result; + likely diagnostic result; (+) limited diagnostic result.

Table 11.3. Angioscopic findings in healthy human vessels

Angioscopic findings	Normal	Pathological
Tubular appearance, round or oval cross-section	+	-
Homogeneous pale pink colour of all vascular parts	+	-
Vascular elasticity	+	-
Little adherence of blood components during angioscopic flush	-	+
Quickly recurring blood stream after sodium flush	+	-

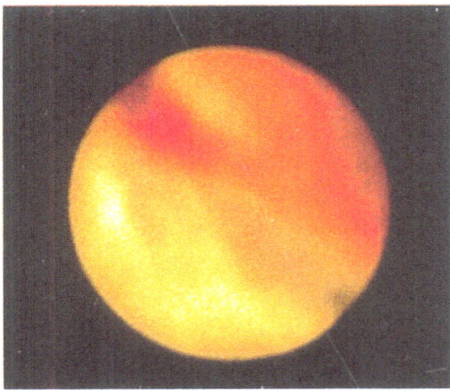

Fig. 11.4. Arteriosclerotic lesion with a high-grade slit-formed stenosis

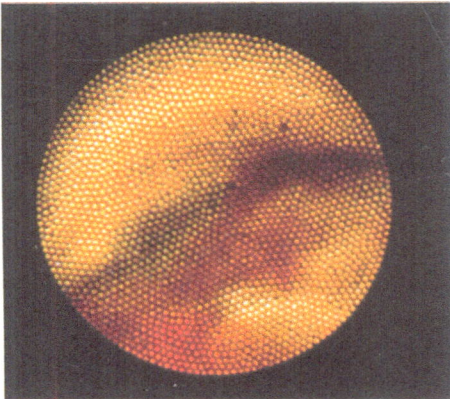

Fig. 11.5. Combined arteriosclerotic and thrombotic lesion in a 64-years-old man with angiographically diagnosed femoral stenosis

advanced without resistance. The blood flow returns more quickly in healthy vessels compared with atherosclerotic vessels, where it is markedly prolonged. Very small vessels infiltrating the vascular wall are not normally present, but these were found in some cases with inflammatory vascular changes, as well as in some patients in whom radiotherapy had damaged the vessel and caused stenosis.

Several pathological vascular features are observed by angioscopy (Table 11.4): the vessels loose their tubular appearance, which is especially evident in atheroslerotic segments, but which is also present in parts of the vessel effected by inflammation or radiation. In these cases concentric or eccentric stenoses of variable degrees and complete obliteration are regularly observed. The most consistent angioscopic feature of pathological vascular change is atherosclerotic plaques of different sizes and

Table 11.4. Angioscopic findings in atherosclerosis

Degree of atherosclerosis
  Segmental
  Generalized
Discolouration of vascular wall
  Flat
  Circular striped
  Dusky red, greyish, white
Configuration of plaques
  Eccentric
  Concentric
  Flat
  Raised, pointed
  Raised, round
  Disseminated
  Vulnerable
  Rigid
Degree of stenosis
Configuration of stenosis
  Eccentric
  Concentric
Cross-sectional appearance

shapes. Deposits on the vascular endothelium are easily recognized by angioscopy.

The degree of atherosclerosis is easily documented. Deposits can increase in size and sometimes completely cover the endothelial surface. In atherosclerotic vessels the adherence of blood components to the vascular wall is strikingly prolonged. Clearing blood components from these vascular parts using sodium chloride or CO_2 is inadequate. The characteristic elasticity of healthy vessels is markedly diminished or absent in atherosclerotic regions. Early stages of atherosclerosis show almost uniform flat deposits on otherwise healthy endothelium, while at later stages these may have any shape – at this stage eccentric stenoses are predominantly found. Radiologically concentric stenoses, often involving only one vascular segment, have been shown to be markedly more extensive and complex than previously suggested by angiography.

Local vascular thrombosis is technically difficult to detect by angioscopy (Table 11.5). Thrombotic deposits can be seen angioscopically only when the mixture of blood and sodium chloride solution or CO_2 is drained by collateral vessels, or if the residual lumen is large enough to ensure run-off of the solution. If organized, local thrombosis can be localized unequivocally and the thrombolysis can be initiated through the working channel of the angioscope. After the tip of the angioscope has been placed directly in front of the thrombus, lytic agents can be injected through the working channel of the endoscope or the sheath set.

Table 11.5. Angioscopic findings of thrombotic versus thromboembolic vascular occlusions

Angioscopic findings	Thrombosis	Thromboembolism
Reduction of blood flow, stasis	+	+
Adherence of thrombotic material	++	(+)
Prolongation of detaching wall-adherent blood components	++	(+)
Colour of thrombus: light red	++	(+)
Colour of thrombus: dark black	(+)	++
Smooth surface of thrombus	(+)	++
Rough surface of thrombus	+	(+)
Wall-adherent fibrin deposits	++	(+)

++ Unequivocal diagnostic feature; + diagnostic hint; (+) possible diagnostic feature.

The surface of a thrombus has different coloured shapes. An early thrombus, for example, is brighter than a later one, the surface of which is usually dark and may eventually become black. The nature of the surface of the thrombosis is also different; fresh thrombotic lesions are covered by fibrinous deposits that look like floating algae when flushed with angioscopic solution (Fig. 11.6).

In three patients with primary vascular stenosis (Buerger's disease, thromboangiitis obliterans) we were able to detect typical signs: Fibrinoid necrosis with infiltration of the vascular intima could be detected easily. The first sign of this disease is fibrinoid necrosis of the intima, which favours the apposition of the thrombotic material. The vascular wall appeared dusky red with cord-like connective-tissue scarring of the entire wall. The finding of a "polypoid" lining of the entire vascular intima causing stenosis was impressive (Table 11.6).

11.5
Angioscopy in Interventional Vascular Procedures

The results of vascular interventional radiology can be documented by angioscopy very easily. Angioscopy performed after dilatation of vascular stenosis has revealed several results which had not been diagnosed unequivocally before (Table 11.7).

In local lysis a striking finding was that the surface of the vascular thrombi was relatively firm and shiny (Fig. 11.7). Initial perforation of the thrombus with a guide-wire is essential and a precondition of successful lysis. This angioscopic finding underlines the fact that local lysis should be initiated directly at the thrombus as fibrinolytic agents otherwise escape through collateral vessels. A continuously developing appositional thrombus can be dissolved from

the proximal to the distal end, whereas a prominent embolus with an irregular consistency can be dissolved only protractedly or not at all (Figs. 11.8, 11.9).

Angioscopy can be performed even during stent implantation and during long-term examinations. Stent follow-up examinations should be performed expediently by angiography and angioscopy as the blood flow and positioning of the stent can easily be

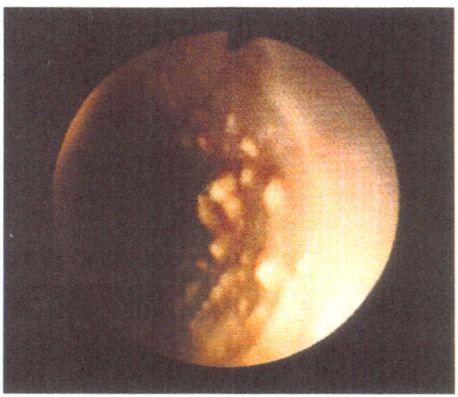

Fig. 11.6. Arteriosclerotic eccentric lesion of an angiographically normal popliteal arter

Table 11.6. Summary of angioscopic features of inflammatory vascular changes and actinic-induced alterations

"Polypoid" internal lining of the vascular lumen
Dusky red discolouration of the luminal wall
Cord-like, white vascular scarring of the whole length
Concentric long stenosis
Additional signs of atherosclerosis
Thrombotic deposits on vascular wall
Augmented adherence of blood components to vascular wall detected by angioscopic flushing
Rigidity of vascular wall (typical for actinic alteration)
Scarring limited to the radiation field (typical for actinic alteration)

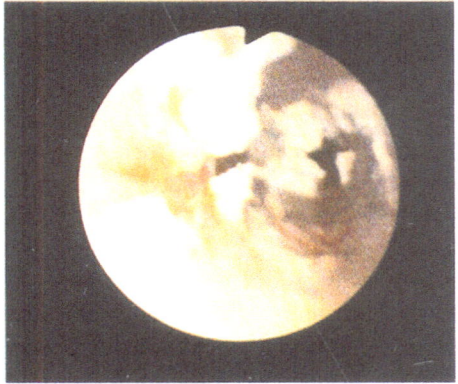

Fig. 11.7. High-grade stenosis of the femoral artery with multiple eccentric plaques

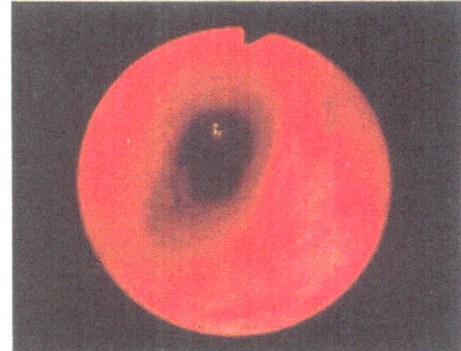

Fig. 11.8. Thrombotic occlusion of the popliteal artery with slight pathological findings. The black formation in the middle of the artery is the thrombotic lesion

Table 11.7. Summary of angioscopic vascular results after PTA

Minor ability to compress atheroma
Extension of the vascular lumen by tearing
Atherosclerotic plaques (primarily longitudinal, rarely circular tears)
Increased instability of the vascular wall when the lumen has a slit-like cross-section
Wall-adherent thrombi in tears of atheromatous plaques that have been caused by PTA
Possible embolization of prominent atherosclerotic plaques
Possible embolization of wall-adherent thrombi
Increment of blood flow after successful dilatation
Inflammatory and actinic stenoses are not as successfully dilated as stenoses of other origin

---

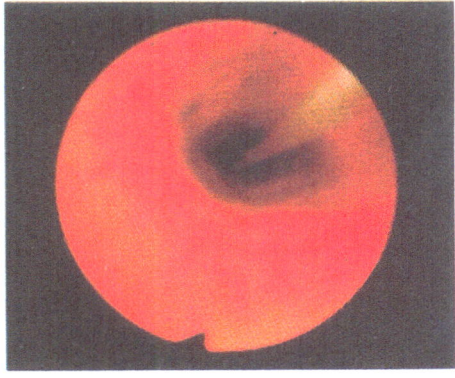

Fig. 11.9. After local catheter lysis of the same patient as in Fig. 11.8 a complete artery could be observe

controlled by angioscopy, whereas restenosis or thrombosis can be evaluated best by angiography. We were able to angioscopically control 80 implantations into different vessels of the iliac, renal, femoral, popliteal and subclavian regions (Fig. 11.10). Angioscopic long-term follow-up studies where undertaken after 3–20 months (Table 11.8); initial intimal formation covering the metal lattice could be seen. In many cases we observed the intimal hyperplasia in combination with newly grown atherosclerotic plaques in the stents (Figs. 11.11, 11.12). The grade of restenosis was not dependent on different types of stents. Covered stents had a significantly higher rate of severe restenosis in the lumen, obviously caused by the rough inner surface of the tissue.

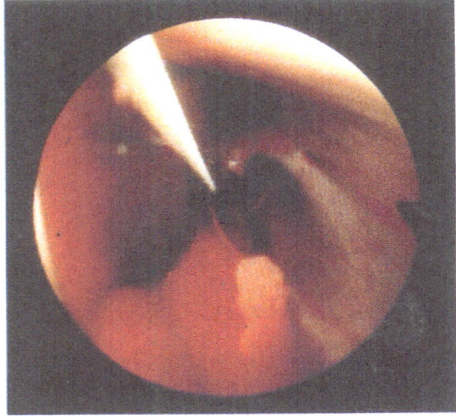

Fig. 11.10. Angioscopic view of an iliac vein which is partially occluded by thrombotic lesions. At 11 inches the guide wire can be seen

Table 11.8. Summary of the endoscopic findings of intervascular stent control

Immediate control (during stent implantation)
  Procedure of stent implantation
  Control of stent position
  Control of intravascular fastening
  Control of blood flow after stent implantation
Late control (at earliest after 3 months)
  Assessment of new intimal layer
  Assessment of recurring stenoses, especially in covered
    stents
  Assessment of thrombosis
  Control of adjacent vessel
  Control of stent position
  Assessment of blood flow

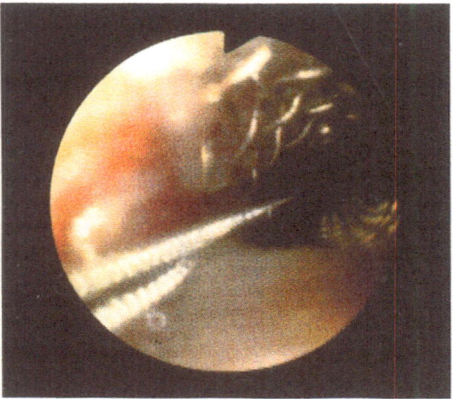

Fig. 11.11. Angioscopic control of a stent-implantation immediately after procedure. At 5 inches the guide wire can be observed

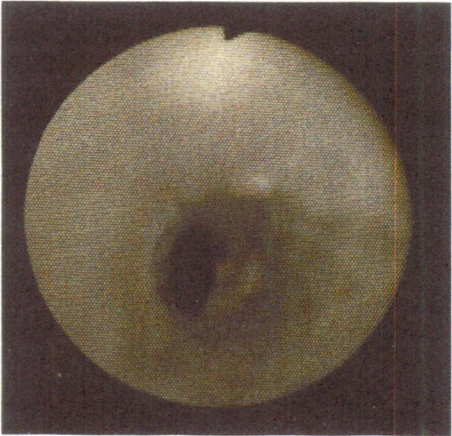

Fig. 11.12. Angioscopic control after 12 months. The metallic lattice is covered by the neo-intima with a small arteriotic plaque at 11 inches. The whole artery is brightly patent

11.6
Conclusions

With the development of angioscopes measuring less than 2 mm in diameter it has become possible to examine the vascular system by percutaneous transluminal angioscopy and to visualize regions of human arteries previously visualized only by angiography. For the introduction of this method it was necessary to achieve temporary occlusion of blood flow in the vascular region of interest. This problem has been solved and clinically tested by a technically simple method. Angioscopy permits the differentiation between local thrombosis and thromboembolism and allows precise evaluation of atherosclerosis and actinic vascular changes. Furthermore, angiographic stenoses can be distinguished angioscopically as lipidosis, sclerosis, atheroma, inflammation, or new or old thromboses. Interventional procedures such as dilatation, recanalization and local thrombolysis can be directly controlled and visualized by angioscopy. The mechanism of balloon dilatation and it's effects can be demonstrated in vivo, providing new insight into the pathophysiological mechanisms. Recurrent vascular occlusions after balloon dilatation can be shown to be due mostly to arterial wall instability induced by angioplasty.

Local catheter thrombolysis can be continuously monitored by angioscopy, and even embolization of thrombotic material can be observed during the procedure. Peripheral embolization of atherosclerotic plaques or mural thrombi can be observed angioscopically during the introduction of guidewires and catheters.

The implantation of different types of stents can be controlled under direct vision and the new intimal lining of stents can be evaluated by angioscopy. Various devices for percutaneous transluminal thrombus extraction or atherectomy can be observed easily.

Overall, percutaneous transluminal angioscopy has its place in the field of percutaneous diagnostic and interventional methods. Although angioscopy is currently not used on a routine basis, it is nonetheless of great help in difficult interventional procedures and is capable of answering specific questions that can not be answered by other diagnostic methods. Problems with difficult handling, resterilization, generally high costs and extensive technical equipment are still matters for discussion.

References and Suggested Reading

Auster M, Kadir S, Mitchel SE, Williams GM, Perler BA, Chang R, Whith RI Jr (1984) Iliac artery occlusion: management with intrathrombus streptokinase infusion and angioplasty. Radiology 153:385

Beck A (1987) Perkutane Angioskopie. Erste Erfahrungsberichte der PTA und der lokalen Lyse unter angioskopischen Bedingungen. Radiologe 27:555–559

Beck A (1993) Percutaneous transluminal angioscopy. Springer, Berlin Heidelberg New York

Beck A, Nanko N (1988) Angioskopische Kontrolle der perkutanen Gefäßendoprothese. Erfahrungsbericht über ein speziell entwickeltes transfemorales Gefäßendoprothesenmodell und dessen angioskopische Kontrolle in situ. Corvas 3:119–123

Beck A, Grosser G, Hellwig A, Papacharalampous X (1987a) Ultraschallkontrolle der Katheterdilatation. Ultraschalldiagnostik 1986. Springer, Berlin Heidelberg New York, 190–192

Beck A, Grosser G, Hellwig A, Papacharalampous X (1987b) Ultraschallgesteuerte Kontrolle der lokalen Lyse. Ultraschalldiagnostik 1986. Springer. Berlin Heidelberg New York, 193–195

Beck A, Milic S, Spagnoli AM, Mundinger A, Blum U (1989) The clinical value of percutaneous transluminal angioscopy. Angioscopical findings in primary vascular diagnosis and in interventional radiology. Clin Ter 131:93–105

Beck A, Hufnagel A, Mundinger A, Vogel T, Bruker G, Stengele O (1992) Thema: Perkutane transluminale Angioskopie. Eine neue Möglichkeit zur Kontrolle der intravasalen Verhältnisse nach Dilatationen, Rekanalisationen, lokalen Lysen und Stentimplantationen. Kassenarzt 19:36–44

Beck A, Neuss J, Heiss HW, Papacharalampous X, Mundinger A, Wenz W (1993) Der heutige Stand der perkutanen transluminalen Angioskopie: Eine neue Methode zur Kontrolle der intravasalen Situation nach Dilatation, Rekanalisation, lokaler Lyse, Stent-Implantation, mechanischer Thrombusextraktion und Atherektomie (Teil I und II). Kardiol Assist 5/3:6–12, 5/4:15–20

Beck A, Mundinger A, Papacharalampous X (1994) Die perkutane transluminale Angioskopie: Indikation, Technik und derzeitige klinische Wertigkeit. Vasa 43:78–79

Beck A, Stengele O, Bruker G, Beller K, Thieme T, Temmen R (1996) Der klinische Einsatz der CO_2-Angiographie: Zweijährige klinische Erfahrung mit Verwendung von CO_2 als peripher-arterielles Kontrastmittel. CO_2-Studie an cerebralen Gefäßen im Hundeversuch. ROFO 164:200

Block PC, Elmer D, Fallon JT (1983) Release of arteriosclerotic debris after transluminal angioplasty. Radiology 146:276

Castaneda-Zuniga WR, Amplatz K, Laerum F (1981) Mechanics of angioplasty: an experimental approach. RG 1:1–14

Chaux A, Lee ME, Blanche C, Kass RM, Sherman TC (1986) Intraoperative coronary angioscopy. J Thorac Cardiovasc Surg 92:972–976

Cortis BS, Hussein H, Khandekar CS, Pricipe J, Tkaczuk RN (1984) Angioscopy in vivo. Cathet Cardiovasc Diagn 10:493–500

Dotter CT, Rösch J, Seaman AJ (1974) Selective clot lysis with low-dose streptokinase. Radiology 11:31

Dotter CT, Buschman RW, McKinney MK, Rösch J (1983) Transluminal expandable nitinol coils stent grafting: preliminary report. Radiology 147:259–260

Duprat G Jr, Wright KC, Charnsangavej C, Wallace S,

Gianturco C (1987) Flexible balloon-expanded stent for small vessels. Radiology 162:276–280

Ferris EJ, Ledor K, Ben-Avi DD, Baker ML, Robbins KV, McCowan TC, Sharma B (1985) Percutaneous angioscopy. Radiology 157:319–322

Fischer M (1987) Möglichkeiten und Grenzen der lokalen Thrombolyse peripherer arterieller Verschlüsse. Med Klin 82:255–158

Frädrich G, Beck A, Bonzel T, Schlosser V (1987) Acute surgical intervention for complications of percutaneous transluminal angioplasty. Eur J Vasc Surg 7:197–203

Greenstone SM, Shore JM, Heringman EC, Massel TB (1966) Arterial endoscopy (arterioscopy). Arch Surg 93:811–812

Grundfest WS, Litvack F, Sherman T, Carroll R, Lee M, Chaux A (1983) Delineation of peripheral and coronary detail by intraoperative angioscopy. Radiology 148:161–166

Hess H, Mietaschk A, Ingrisch H (1982) Kombination der perkutanen transluminalen Angioplastie mit lokaler Thrombolyse. Vasa 11:282–286

Hoffmann MA, Fallon JT, Greenfield AJ (1981) Arterial pathology after percutaneous transluminal angioplasty. AJR Am J Roentgerol 137:147–156

Ito T, Hori M (1983) Vascular endoscopy for major vascular reconstruction: experimental and clinical studies. Surgery 93:391–396

Katzen BT, Rossi P, Passariello R, Simonetti G (1981) Low dose streptokinase in the treatment of arterial occlusions. AJR Am J Roentgerol 136:1171–1178

Laerum F, Castaneda-Zuniga WR, Rysavy JA, Moore R, Amplatz K (1982) The site of arterial wall rupture in transluminal angioplasty: an experimental study. Radiology 144:769–770

Litvack F, Grundfest WS, Lee ME, Foran R, Chaux A, Berci G, Rose HB, Matloff JM, Forrester JS (1985) Angioscopic visualization of blood vessels interior in animals and humans. Clin Cardiol 8:65–70

Mazieres M (1987) L'endoprothèse coronarienne: serait-elle la solution au problème des réstenoses après angioplastie coronaire? Panminerva Med 14:2517

Mehigan JT, Olcott C (1986) Video angioscopy as an alternative to intraoperative arteriography. Am J Surg 152:139–145

Miller RA (1982) Endoscopic instrumentation: evolution, physical principles and clinical aspects. Br Med Bull 42:223–226

Olcott C (1987) Clinical applications of video angioscopy. J Vasc Surg 5:664–666

Palmaz JC, Windeler SA, Garcia F, Tio FO, Sibbitt RR, Reuter SR (1986a) Arteriosclerotic rabbit aortas: expandable intraluminal grafting Radiology 160:723–725

Palmaz JC, Sibbitt RR, Tio FO, Reuter SR, Peters JE, Garcia F (1986b) Expandable intraluminal vascular graft: a feasibility study. Surgery 99:199–205

Raso AM, Carlin C, Falco E (1986) La valoracion de los troncos supraaorticos por medio de la ultrasonographia Doppler y angioscopio. Angiologia 38:306–314

Rizk G, Goodale R, Amplatz K (1973) Vascular endoscopy. Radiology 106:33–36

Sanborn TA (1986) Vascular endoscopy: current state of the art. Br Med Bull 42:270–275

Schild H, Gröninger J, Schmied W, Weilemann L, Lindner P, Wagner P, Brunier A, Thelen M, Meyer J (1987) Lokale Fibrinolysetherapie von Gefäßverschlüssen im Becken-Bein-Bereich und der oberen Extremität. ROFO 146:57–62

Schrempp K, Müller G, Günther D (1980) Komplikationen bei Angiographien. Radiologe 20:135–140

Sigwart U, Puel J, Mirkovitch V, Joffre F, Kappenberger L (1987) Intravascular stents to prevent occlusion and restenosis after transluminal angioplasty. N Engl J Med 316:701–708

Snidermah KW, Bodner LJ, Saddekni S, Srur M, Sos TA (1984) Percutaneous embolectomy by transcatheter aspiration. Radiology 150:357–361

Spears JF, Marais HJ, Serur J (1983) In vivo coronary angioscopy. J Am Coll Cardiol 5:1311–1314

Starck EE, McDermott JC, Crummy AB, Turnipseed WD, Acher CW, Burgess JH (1985) Percutaneous aspiration thromboembolectomy. Radiology 156:61–66

Tanabe T, Yokota A, Sugie S (1980) Cardiovascular endoscopy: development and clinical application. Surgery 87:375–378

Towne JB, Bernhard VM (1977) Vascular endoscopy: useful tool or interesting toy? Surgery 82:415–419

Uchida Y, Masuo M, Tomaru T, Kato A, Sugimoto T (1986) Fiberoptic observation of thrombosis and thrombolysis in isolated human coronary arteries. Am Heart J 4:690–696

Vollmar J (1969) Die Gefäßendoskopie. Ein neuer Weg der intraoperativen Gefäßdiagnostik. Endoscopy 1:141–151

Zeitler E (1982) Die perkutane Rekanalisation arterieller Obliteration mit Katheter nach Dotter (Dotter-Technik). Dtsch Med Wochenschr 97:1392–1394

Zeitler E, Schoop W, Zahnow W (1971) The treatment of occlusive arterial disease by transluminal angioplasty. Radiology 99:19–26

Zollikofer CL, Salomonowitz E, Sibley R, Chain J, Bruhlmann WR, Castaneda-Zuniga WR, Amplatz K (1984) Transluminal angioplasty evaluated by electron microscopy. Radiology 153:369–374

12 Magnetic Resonance Angiography

R. Loose, K. Detmar and U. Böttcher

At the beginning of the 1990s, the principles of magnetic resonance angiography (MRA) using time-of-flight (TOF) and phase-contrast (PC) techniques were developed and introduced in clinical practice (Ross et al. 1989; Pernicone et al. 1990; Dumoulin et al. 1990; Edelman et al. 1990). First reports of the influence of flowing blood on MR images appeared in 1978 (Singer 1978) and first clinical applications of MRA started in 1984 (Bryant et al. 1984). The new technique provided a powerful tool for the evaluation of vascular anatomy and disease. Without the use of X-rays and, in part, without the use of contrast media, the velocity and direction of blood flow in arteries and veins can be visualized (Arlart et al. 1991; Bongartz et al. 1991; Graves 1997). Many of these techniques are now available as commercial hard- and software packages. As MRA is a method which depends largely on system performance of the magnetic resonance imaging (MRI)

scanner, constant new developments, such as ultra-fast sequences, high performance gradients, echo planar imaging (EPI), moving-table systems, and phased-array coils offer ever increasing MRA applications and image quality.

12.1
Technical Considerations

MRA can essentially be performed on many MRI systems with different field strengths ranging from about 0.2 T up to 2 T and more. Nevertheless, the need for short acquisition times, high spatial resolution, good contrast, and high signal-to-noise ratios makes high-field systems preferable for MRA. Fast sequences with short echo times improve visualizations of vessels and hence fast gradients are beneficial. Adapted coils with a high signal output are helpful or even necessary to achieve the desired goals (Laub 1993).

12.2
Imaging Techniques

As the great variability of central and peripheral vascular anatomy presents special challenges for MRA, different techniques and pulse sequences are available and used:

- Flow in the arteries is often pulsatile. ECG-triggering or contrast enhancement is used to reduce ghost artifacts caused by pulsatility.
- Datasets with large volumes of interest need to be acquired.
- Arteries and veins, which are often located close together, need to be distinguished.

The ability to image the large superior–inferior extent of the peripheral vessels with coronal or sagittal inflow MRA is limited by the long T_1 relaxation time of blood and the saturation of the blood signal. Table 12.1 summarizes the advantages and disadvantages of the three main techniques used today.

R. Loose, MD, PhD, K. Detmar, MD, Institut für Diagnostische und Interventionelle Radiologie, Klinikum Nord, Flurstraße 17, D-90340 Nürnberg, Germany
U. Böttcher, PhD, Siemens AG, Medizinische Technik, Med MRA, Henkestraße 127, D-91052 Erlangen, Germany

12.2.1
Two-/Three-Dimensional Time-of-Flight MRA

The TOF technique is based on the physical principle that non-saturated, fully relaxed spins flowing into a measuring volume generate high signal intensities (Hausmann 1996). In contrast, stationary spins are partially saturated and transmit a lower signal intensity. The effective contrast is a function of the repetition time, TR, the flip angle, and the velocity of the blood flowing into the measured volume. Figure 12.1 shows the principle of TOF-MRA.

Differentiation between reverse flow directions (arteries and veins) can be achieved by saturation pulses, which have to be applied parallel to the imaging plane. Flow-induced phase effects which may destroy the MR signal are reduced by a flow compensation of the sequence, short echo times, and small voxels.

The pulsatile nature of blood flow generates different problems in peripheral MRA. The high flow during the systolic period can generate ghost artifacts in two-dimensional (2D) TOF. Reduced, or even reverse, flow in the diastolic phase can lead to saturation problems with reduced signal intensities. Both problems can be overcome by ECG-triggered 2D TOF measurements. Acquisition at the moment of maximum systolic flow minimizes ghost artifacts and yields high vascular contrasts. Several lines of data can be measured during one cardiac cycle, and hence only a few heart beats are necessary to acquire one full slice. The final dataset after a 2D TOF acquisition is a three-dimensional (3D) dataset, and

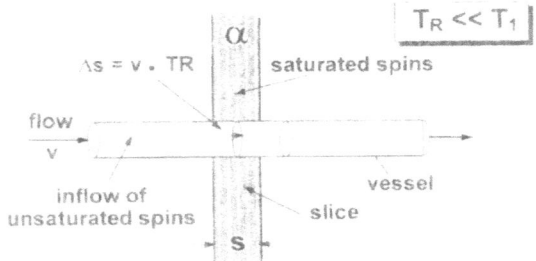

Fig. 12.1. Stationary spins in the slice with thickness s will be partially or fully saturated (low signal) whereas inflowing unsaturated spins contribute with a high signal intensity. TR=repetition time, α=flip angle, v=velocity of blood, Δs=distance of travelling spins during repetition time TR.

hence projections with different orientations can be postprocessed.

12.2.2
Two-/Three-Dimensional Phase-Contrast MRA

The basic idea of PC-MRA is that spins moving along a magnetic field gradient acquire a phase shift in the transverse magnetization which depends on the velocity of blood flow. A subtraction of two datasets with opposite bipolar gradient pulses eliminates the contribution of stationary tissue and shows only signals of flowing spins (Hausmann 1996). A sequence with an appropriate velocity encoding value (VENC)

Table 12.1. Advantages and disadvantages of the principal three techniques

Technique	Advantages	Disadvantages
ECG-triggered 2D TOF, axial	Good vessel contrast Reduced ghost artifacts Contrast agent not required Traveling saturation bands can be used 3D data set available	Requires good ECG signal Saturation on in-plane flow Long acquisition times
Contrast-enhanced MRA, coronal	Excellent vessel contrast Large imaged volume Best estimate of stenosis Fastest acquisition No need for ECG 3D data set available	Expense of contrast material Injection timing is critical Acquisition must be completed during first passage of the contrast agent
ECG-triggered 2D PCA, thick coronal slice	Large imaged volume Short acquisition time Velocity information available over full heart cycle	Single view, only 2D information Requires ECG signal Prior knowledge of the flow velocity might be necessary
3D PCA	Large imaged volume No background signal Independence of flow direction	Long acquisition time No imaging of thrombi and vessel-wall Prior knowledge about the flow velocity is necessary

2/3D, two-/three-dimensional; TOF, time of flight; MRA, magnetic resonance angiography; PCA, phase-contrast angiography.

has to be selected since PC-MRA can only visualize flow in a specific range of velocities. The pulsatile nature of arterial flow requires a triggering of the 2D PC-MRA measurements. Large volumes can be imaged in a relatively short time, achieving an overview of the region of interest.

For peripheral PC-MRA, sequences which encode the flow in readout direction (normally head to feet) with different VENCs (multi-VENC sequences) can be used to visualize blood flow with very different velocities within one measurement.

12.2.3
Contrast-Enhanced MRA

The technique of contrast-enhanced MRA (CE-MRA) is gaining more and more attention nowadays (MARCHAL et al. 1996). In non-contrast-enhanced TOF-MRA examinations, due to repetitive radio frequency (RF) excitation pulses, the signal intensity of inflowing blood decreases rapidly to the amplitude of the surrounding tissue ("saturation"). Despite repetitive RF pulses, the signal in blood vessels after gadolinium-diethylenetriaminopentoacetic acid (Gd-DTPA) injection remains higher than in surrounding tissue, as one of the primary effects of Gd-chelates (e.g., Gd-DTPA) is a shortening of the T_1 relaxation time. A T_1 reduction from 1200 ms to 300 ms was observed with a dose of 0.3 mmol/kg Gd-DTPA (TU et al. 1994).

One disadvantage of Gd-DTPA-based contrast agents is the relatively short time they remain in the arteries and veins. In addition, following initial passage, one observes a mixed contrast enhancement between arteries and veins and, after about 30 s–1 min, fast parenchymal contrast (e.g., liver, spleen, kidneys). Figure 12.2 shows the timing of CE-MRA and the acquisition window.

Blood pool agents, which selectively remain in the blood vessels for a longer time, are not yet available for clinical use (LAUFFER et al. 1998). The CE-MRA technique uses very fast 3D sequences to acquire heavily T_1-weighted images during the presence of a contrast agent in the blood, whereby the T_1 of the blood is reduced below the T_1 of any other tissue. This technique is very fast and can use large fields of view without any saturation problems. This also leads to a good estimation of stenosis. Optimal CE-MRA results can be obtained with MR scanners fast enough to complete data acquisition during the first passage of contrast bolus. This technique can be provided with ultrafast sequences which require high field systems

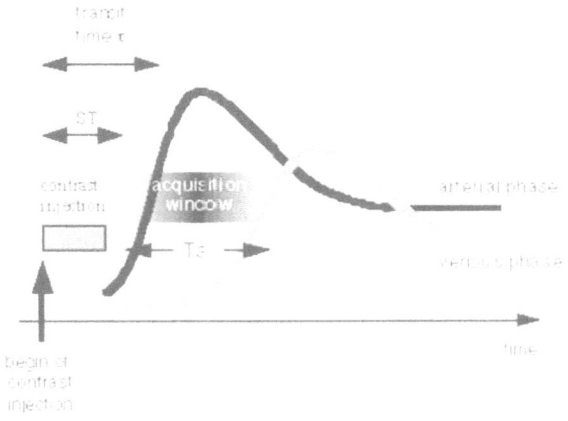

Fig. 12.2. Timing issues in contrast-enhanced magnetic resonance angiography. The acquisition window of the scan has to cover the peak of the arterial phase. Scan time, Ts, and transit time, τ, need to be adjusted carefully for optimal results

(>1 T), high performance gradients (>20 milliTesla/m), and fast gradient rise times (<0.3 ms).

As may of the presently installed scanners need MRA acquisition times of over 1 min, the mean contrast during data acquisition is significantly lower than the peak contrast. For a given TR and T_1 of blood, an optimal MRA signal is obtained at the Ernst angle (MARCHAL et al. 1996). Furthermore, MRA image quality is influenced by the time of maximal vascular contrast and the k-space sampling scheme. Generally, maximal intravascular contrast should be reached during sampling of the central lines of k-space. The duration of the acquisition window, Ts, and the transit time, τ, of the contrast agent determine the timing of the scan. A high contrast-agent concentration in the vessel of interest should be achieved for a duration of half the acquisition window and this period should be around the middle of the scan time. The contrast agent should be injected for a time Ts/2. With a time scale beginning with the contrast injection, the scan should be started at a time ST:

$$ST = \tau - Ts/4$$

after the beginning of contrast injection.

12.2.4
Postprocessing and Viewing Techniques

Generally, all MRA techniques are capable of acquiring a 3D dataset, either as a 3D volume or a series of contiguous 2D slices. As in CT imaging, one can review a series of 2D slices step by step or perform multiplanar reconstructions. A 2D projection of a 3D dataset, where all voxels contribute with image information, cannot be visualized. Thus, to obtain such a 2D projection of the vascular anatomy of 3D data, one needs to extract the unique structure of all blood vessels slice by slice and erase all other image information. This procedure assumes that the vascular signal is higher than a certain threshold which is used to suppress the background. With these datasets of "bright blood images", one can perform maximum intensity projections (MIP) (LAUB 1996). Figure 12.3 shows the principle of generating a 2D MIP out of a 3D dataset, Multiple MIPs with small increments of the viewing angle can be displayed as a contiguously rotating object in a cine-loop. Figure 12.4a shows a single slice of a dataset with "bright" vessels, while Fig. 12.4b shows one MIP image of the entire volume.

The MIP algorithm works well as long as the vessel in the 3D dataset have sufficient contrast. Small vessels with only a few voxels of volume and insufficient contrast remain below the discrimination threshold. If the threshold is lowered too much, artifacts and noise from the surrounding tissue increase. The visualization of small vessels can be improved if not the entire 3D volume, but only a smaller region of interest is processed ("targeted MIP").

In the case of ambiguous MIP results, it is strongly recommended that source images be reviewed (Fig. 12.4). The degree of stenoses and the

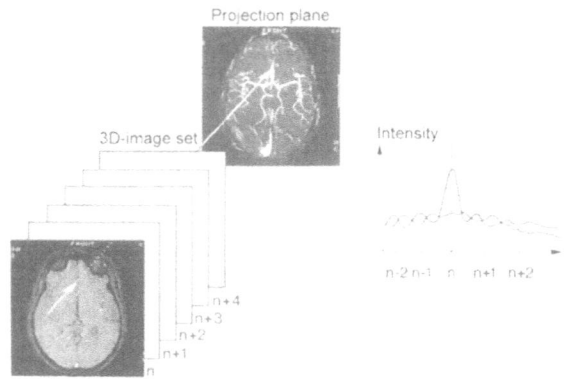

Fig. 12.3. The principle of generating a two-dimensional maximum intensity projection out of a three-dimensional dataset

diameter of vessels is often misinterpreted. Generally speaking, a patent vessel in a MIP image is also patent in reality, whereas not all "occlusions" in MIP images are true. One of the reasons for this are curved vessels, which leave the MIP target volume for a short distance.

12.3
Indications, Contraindications, and Risks

If an indication is given to visualize vascular anatomy or pathology, the investigator must choose among

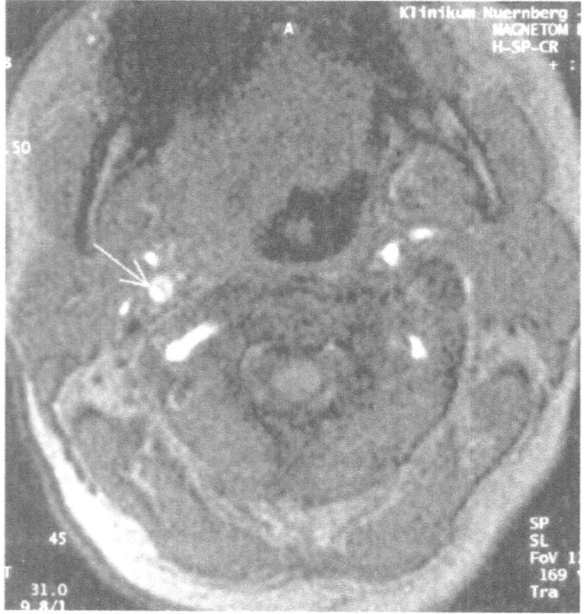
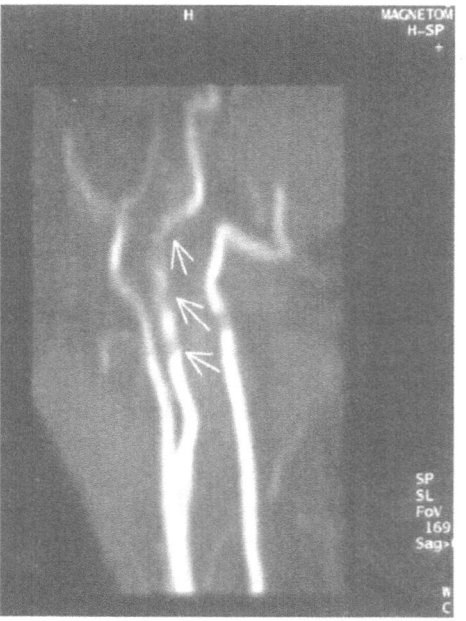

Fig. 12.4 a,b. a Tree-dimensional (3D) time-of-flight (TOF) angiography. Repetition time (TR) 35msec, echo time (TE) 10msec, flip angle 25 degrees, time of acquisition (TA) 6.4min. One single transverse image (a) of the dataset shows a direction in the internal carotid artery. The arrow points to the dissection membrane. Only the smaller section of the vessel (bright) is patent. **b** Maximum-intensity-projection (MIP) of the right carotid artery shows signal loss and narrowing (arrows) of the vessel, but the dissection cannot be seen in the MIP image

procedures which differ in X-ray irradiation, cost, availability, invasiveness, and contrast side effect. Generally, indications for MRA result from limitations and contraindications of alternative methods such as digital subtraction angiography (DSA), CT angiography (CTA), and Doppler ultrasound. MRA should be preferred if the vascular anatomy or pathology is of additional interest when soft tissues or parenchymal organs need to be visualized (e.g., thoracic or abdominal malignancies). MRA should be chosen for all examinations where the age of the patient suggests a radiationless procedure. Further important indications include a history of adverse reactions to iodine contrast, hyperthyroidism, and renal failure.

MRA and, in general, MRI are safe and well established procedures with only few absolute, and some relative, contraindications. Absolute contraindications include cardiac pacemakers, other electronic implants such as drug pumps or neurostimulators, neurosurgical metal clips of unknown compound, and ferromagnetic foreign bodies of critical location or size. Relative contraindications may arise from non-ferromagnetic metal implants at various locations. Hence, the decision to perform a MRA examination has to be made by the physician according to each individual case. Risks may arise from mechanical forces caused by the static magnetic field or from induced voltages either by the switched gradients or the RF field. Generally speaking, modern clips and stents used in vascular surgery and interventional radiology produce only small interference with MRI and MRA, which can be noticed as signal void close to the clip or stent and inside the stent. Many old, and some new, endovascular coils still contain ferromagnetic compounds which cause a strong signal void of some centimeters in the target volume. Further relative contraindications include patients with claustrophobia and patients unable to remain in a motionless position during the time necessary for data acquisition.

12.4
Time and Costs

With modern MR scanners, a complete MRA examination with all relevant sequences may be completed in about 30 min. If MRA is performed after a conventional MRI examination, additional time consumption is only about 15 min.

An estimate of the costs of MRA compared to DSA (Boos et al. 1997) demonstrated that the price of MRA is about three times lower than DSA with non-ionic

contrast material. The costs of MRA strongly depend on the imaging technique. Whereas TOF-MRA and PC-MRA need no additional contrast, the price of CE-MRA is dose-dependent with scan protocols using single, double, or triple doses of Gd-DTPA. CTA may be performed with less costs compared to MRA, but is limited in its application to certain anatomic regions.

12.5
Future Aspects of MRA

Conventional X-ray angiography and DSA have been the gold standard for the evaluation of vascular disease over the last decades. Whereas the number of interventional angiographic procedures is increasing, more and more diagnostic examinations are performed with color-coded Doppler sonogra-phy (CCDS), CTA, and MRA. MRA has the greatest potential to visualize the entire vascular anatomy and pathology of the human body without irradiation and, in part, without contrast media. If MRA examinations are performed using i.v. gadolinium contrast, the volume is much lower compared to iodine contrast and the risk of adverse reactions is low. In the case of contraindications to iodine contrast, Gd-DTPA has already been used for arterial DSA (SCHILD et al. 1994). With high-speed imaging gradients, it is possible to achieve sequence repetition times of 4 ms or less (ALLEY et al. 1998). Hence, high-resolution images ($512 \times 512 \times 64$) can be obtained in under 30 s. The long extension of peripheral vessels can be visualized with new mobile patient platforms (Ho et al. 1997) (e.g., "MobiTrak", Philips, Eindhoven). The development of new contrast materials, which remain in the endovascular system for longer than conventional gadolinium compounds, will improve the visualization of vascular anatomy even with "standard" scanners (LAUFFER et al. 1998).

12.6
Clinical Applications of MRA

12.6.1
Thoracoabdominal Aorta

12.6.1.1
Technique

The thoracoabdominal aorta, including its side branches, is almost exclusively depictable by means of the body-coil or array coils. The spatial resolution of MRA is, as a consequence, restricted. Pixel sizes of up to 2 mm and slice thicknesses of up to 4 mm are usual.

The above-mentioned sequences are varyingly suited for the diagnostic evaluation of pathologic conditions of the aorta. For some time now, due to the optimum visualization in each flow direction and flow speed, the short examination time, and the low rate of artifacts at breath-holding, CE-MRA using gadolinium has been favored, despite the cost of contrast material. Phase-contrast angiography (PCA) and TOF techniques (WANNER et al. 1991; WEGMÜLLER and VOCK 1993) offer the advantage of better differentiation between true and false lumina in the imaging of dissections, flapping tissue fragments, in the blood stream, turbulent flow, and regurgitations. Specific techniques, such as ECG-triggered segmental gradient-recalled echo (GRE) sequences used in cardiac diagnostics, enable the visualization of moving small flapping tissue fragments, mural structures of dissections, and anomalies of the heart valves, as well as the documentation of the direction of the blood flow in relation to the cardiac cycle (SEELOS et al. 1994; WILLIAMS et al. 1994).

In practice, the assessment of acute symptomatic aneurysms is in general restricted to spiral CT, transesophageal sonography, and CE-MRA with fast sequences (SOMMER et al. 1995). In subacute cases, the 2D TOF technique can be employed distal of the aortic arch, but has also been largely replaced by CE-MRA (Fig. 12.5a,b). Due to its susceptibility to breath-related artifacts, the subdiaphragmal applicability of PCA is limited. Particularly critical points are the ramifications of the carotid arteries from the aortic arch: Because of the pulsatility of the aortic arch and respiratory movements, CE-MRA in the breath-hold technique has proven to be superior. Alternatively, 3D TOF techniques are used (KUMAR et al. 1996). Experience in this vascular territory, however, is significantly less than that in the region of the carotid bifurcation and intracranial vessels.

Variations in vascular anatomy are clearly visualized by MIPs of CE-MRA (BOGAERT et al. 1992), particular in the case of tumors or vascular malformations.

Stenoses can be detected in all techniques. Poststenotic signal deletion leads to overestimation of the length of stenoses, as well as the degree

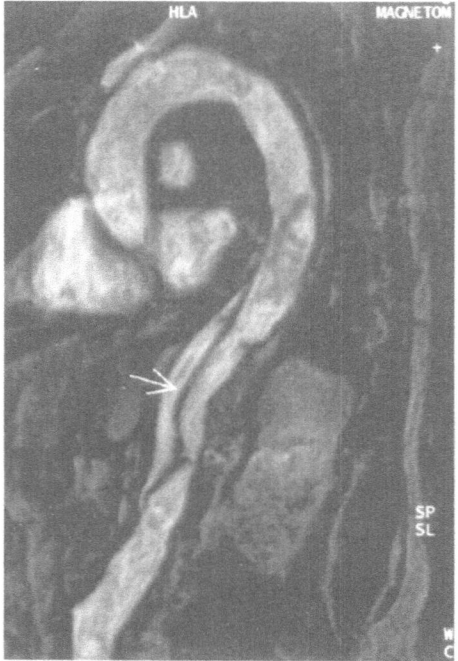
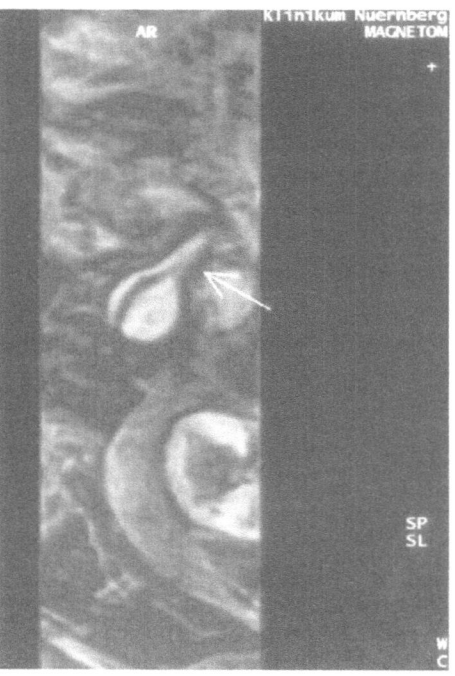

Fig. 12.5 a,b. Fast imaging with steady precession three-dimensional gradient-recalled echo (FISP), 6.9/3.0/25 (TR/TE/flip angle; single-dose contrast-enhanced magnetic resonance angiography, non-breath-hold technique; time of acquisition 2.19 min). Patient with abdominal pain. **a** 2.5-mm Coronal oblique single slice shows a dissection in the descending aorta. **b** Axial reformatting shows the dissection entering the superior mesenteric artery, causing the clinical signs of acute abdomen. Maximum intensity projection postprocessing gives no further information, but would hide the dissection membrane

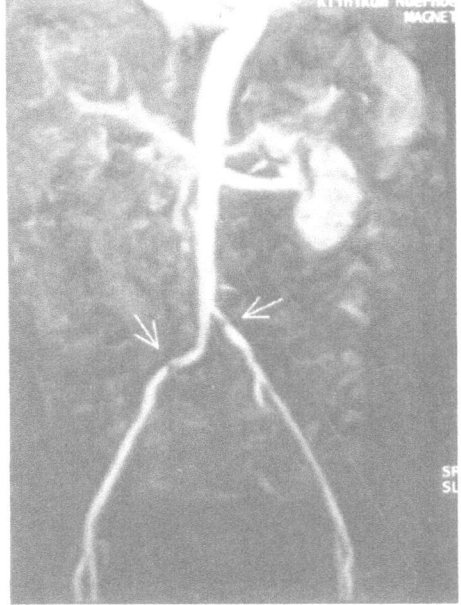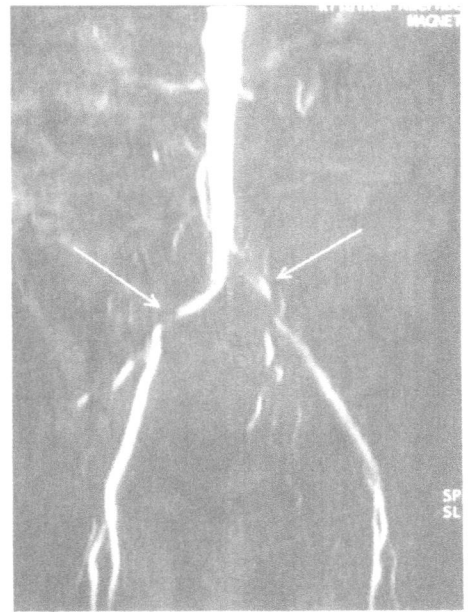

Fig. 12.6 a,b. Comparision between time-of-flight (TOF)-magnetic resonance angiography (MRA) [ECG-triggered TOF; 608/10/ 70; time of acquisition (TA) 12.50 min] in (b), and contrast-enhanced MRA (10.2/2.9/30; TA 2.35 min; 0.1 mMol/kg gadolinium) in (a). TOF-MRA shows wide extinction of signal in the whole left common iliac artery (CIA) and 2 cm signal loss in the right CIA. Both could be misinterpreted as an occlusion. CE-MRA (a) shows high-grade, short stenoses in both vessels

of stenosis, due to the accelerated flow in the constricted lumen (Fig. 12.6a,b). Extremely short stenoses (<2 mm) are only visualized insufficiently because of the thickness of the single slices. All in all, CE-MRA has considerable advantages (BONGARTZ et al. 1997; PRINCE et al. 1997). Depending on the clinical problem, the combination of CE-MRA and a TOF and ECG-triggered GRE sequence, respectively, have yielded reliable results.

12.6.2
Side Branches of the Aorta

12.6.2.1
Supraaortal Arteries

In this vascular region, the interest focuses on the identification of stenoses, dissections or occlusions, tumor-related compression of vessels (Fig. 12.7a,b), and variations of the ramification. Due to the pulsatility within the aortic arch and respiratory motion, visualization using 2D and 3D PCA and TOF techniques becomes more difficult, but is feasible (LEWIN et al. 1991; KUMAR 1996). These, however, have nearly been replaced by CE-MRA (Fig. 12.8a,b) because of their susceptibility to artifacts (PRINCE et

al. 1997). Up to now, the visualization of collateral vessels in all of the MR techniques is still inferior to arterial DSA. Reasons for the increasing importance of CE-MRA include limited applicability of color-coded duplex sonography in the deep vascular region, good correlation to i.a. DSA, and costs comparable to DSA.

12.6.2.2
Renal Arteries

Due to their high clinical incidence, renal artery stenoses are a major field of clarification with MRA techniques, besides DSA and color-coded duplex sonography. The almost right-angled branching of the renal arteries prevents the use of conventional axial 2D TOF techniques, whereas 3D PCA has numerous advantages (DUDA et al. 1996; VOCK et al. 1991; GEDROYC et al. 1995). All non-breath-hold techniques suffer from respiratory movement of the kidneys. In particular, the signal from peripheral parts of the renal artery is blurred and small vessels, such as polar arteries, cannot be visualized satisfactorily. For this reason, 3D TOF techniques, improved by TONE (tilted optimized nonsaturating excitation) pulse, were developed (RODITI et al. 1994). The cor-

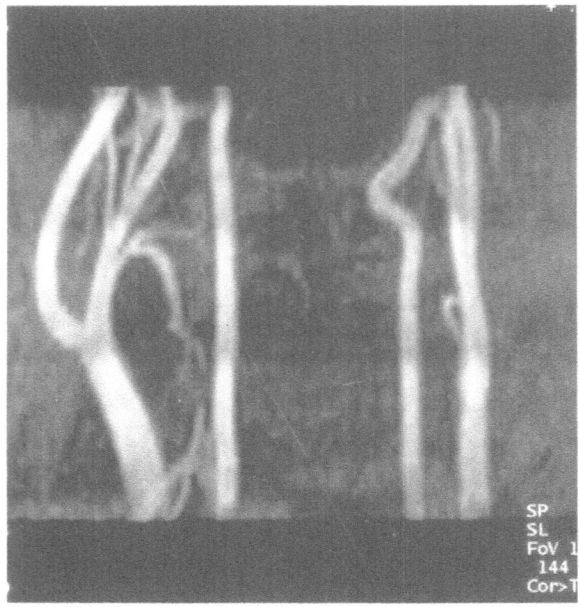 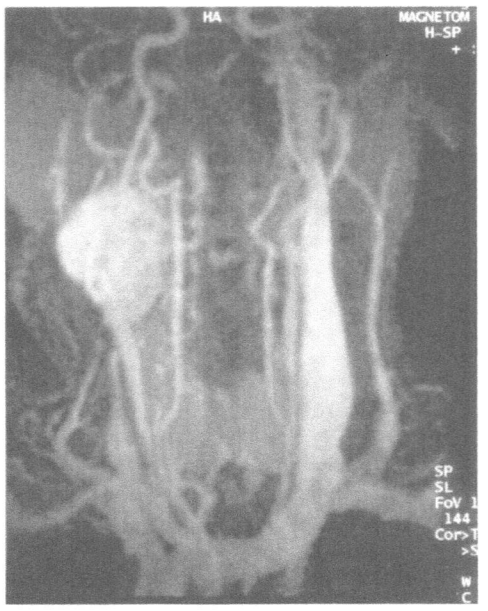

Fig. 12.7 a,b. Comparision of three-dimensional (3D) multislab time-of-flight (TOF) image (35/10/25; time of acquisition, 6:4 min) (a) and FISP 3D contrast-enhanced magnetic resonance angiography (MRA) (b) (same technique as in Fig. 12.6). a TOF-MRA shows lateralizatoin of carotid artery and cranialization of the upper thyroidal artery. b Contrast enhanced (CE-)MRA shows an enhancing, large tumor in the carotid bifurcation (glomus caroticum tumor) with compression of right jugular vein

relation to "conventional" i.a. DSA is diagnostically satisfactory (BORELLO et al. 1995; HANY et al. 1997). Competing with duplex sonography, MRA is also used in the diagnosis of stenoses/thromboses of kidney transplants (BRICHAUX et al. 1995), anatomical variations, and vascular malformations (Fig. 12.9). Factors having a negative influence on the visualization of renal arteries include: obesity, tachypnea, and multiple stenoses of the abdominal aorta and renal arteries. In such situations, CE-MRA (Fig. 12.10) offers considerable advantages and a better correlation with i.a. DSA (PRINCE et al. 1997; HANY et al. 1997; HOLLAND et al. 1996).

12.6.2.3
Visceral Arteries

Due to its course, which mainly follows the longitudinal body axis, the superior mesenteric artery is the only vessel depictable using the TOF technique. Natural respiratory movements and pulsatility, however, render visualization in the TOF and PC technique more difficult. Due to the divergent and partly tortuous course of the vessels of the celiac trunk, CE-MRA is the preferred modality (PRINCE et al. 1995, 1997; STEHLING et al. 1997). Current indica-

tions include vascular malformations and aneurysms, mesenterial ischemia (MEANEY et al. 1997), and screening of suspected vascular variations (Fig. 12.11a–c) prior to abdominal surgery. Experience gained in this field to date, however, is limited.

12.6.2.4
Iliac Arteries

The external iliac vessels are, in principle, amenable to all the above-mentioned techniques. The 2D TOF technique is the method of choice for demonstrating excentric stenoses, atheromas, and extraluminal processes (e.g., extrinsic tumors, pelvic spur), when axial images are analyzed. These situations always require the consideration of the relative overstaging of vascular stenoses, and the lacking depiction of vascular segments in the case of elongation, coiling, and kinking. Additional CE-MRA ensures higher reliability. The combination of both techniques (SNIDOW et al. 1995) is at least equal to the determination of the degree of stenosis with i.a. DSA, with a sensitivity/specificity of over 95% (LAISSY et al. 1995; SNIDOW et al. 1996). The curved course of the external iliac vessels in the small pelvis requires CE-MRA (Fig. 12.12a,b). The overlying intestinal structures

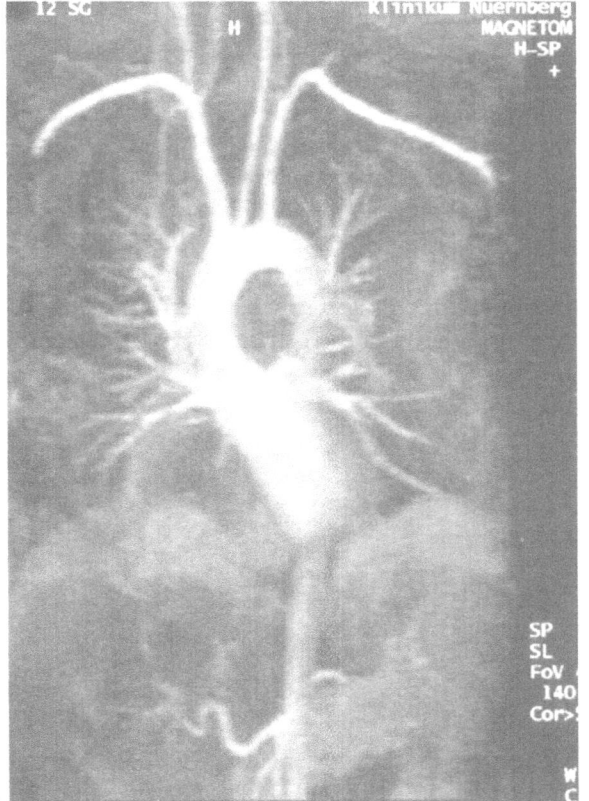
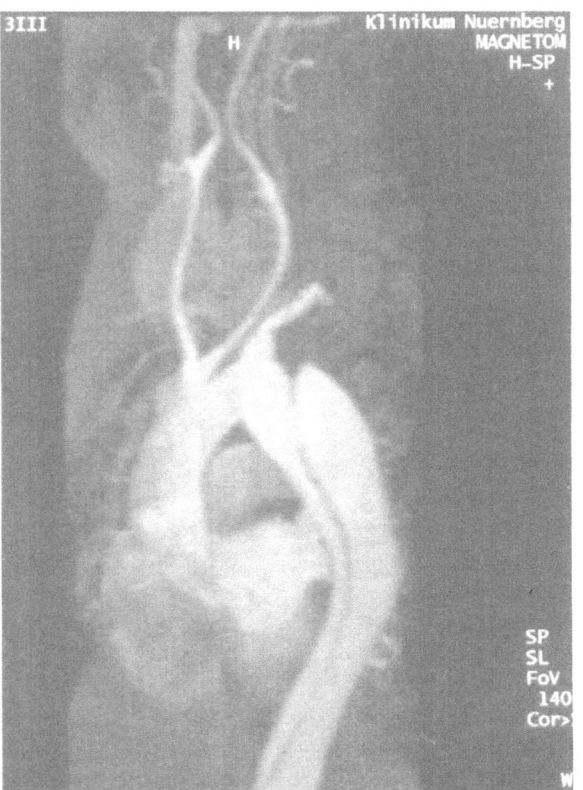
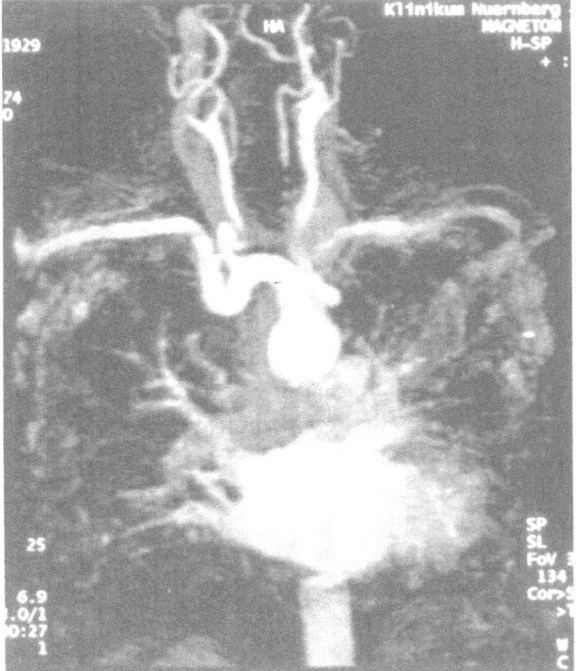

Fig. 12.8 a–c. Normal vascular anatomy of the aortic arch and supraaortal vessels. **a** Fast imaging with steady precession three-dimensional gradient recalled echo (6.7/2.8/30; time of acquisition 32 sec); breath-hold technique, single-dose contrast enhanced magnetic resonance angiography, subvolume sagittal-oblique maximum intensity projection MIP. **b** Same technique in a 42-year-old female patient. Dissecting aneurysm of the descending aorta. Variation of vascular anatomy: Common origin of both carotid arteries. **c** Same technique with reduced acquisition time in a 63-year-old female patient, subvolume maximum intensity projection. Kinking of both carotid arteries and stenosis of subclavian artery on the left side

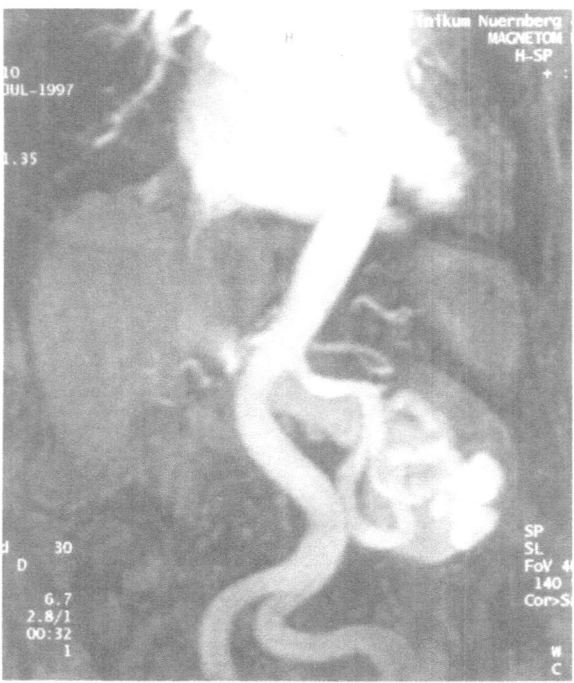

Fig. 12.9. Female patient (52 years) with arteriovenous (av)-malformation of the left kidney. Contrast-enhanced magnetic resonance angiography (6.7/2.8/30; time of acquisition, 32 s). Breath-hold technique, double dose of contrast medium. Coronal – oblique orientation; the right kidney is outside the maximum intensity projection volume. Early contrast enhancement of the wide left renal vein due to av-shunts of the malformation

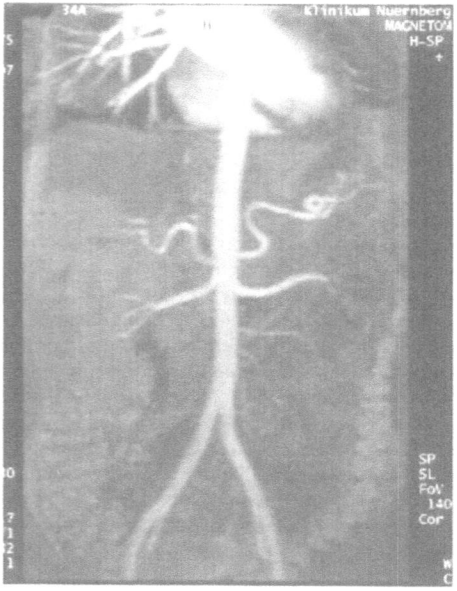

Fig. 12.10. Single-dose breath-hold contrast-enhanced magnetic resonance angiography (6.7/2.8/30; time of acquisition, 32 s). Normal visualization of both renal arteries, coiling of splenic artery

necessitate good suppression of background signal, which can be achieved with ECG-triggered TOF sequences, echo time (TE), or PCA.

Indications include occlusive vascular disease in the pelvis and aortoiliac aneurysms, both for primary diagnosis and as follow-up controls after percutaneous transluminal angioplasty (PTA) (LAISSY et al. 1995), stent implantation, or bypass surgery. Additional indications include arteriovenous (av)-malformations, av-fistulas, and neoplasias with distinct vascularity in the pelvis, and also as a control method following interventions, e.g., embolization and grafts (PRINCE et al. 1997).

12.6.3
Leg Arteries

12.6.3.1
Technique

Visualization of the peripheral arteries using TOF and PC techniques is easy, as long as uncontrolled movements of the extremities are avoided by safe positioning of the patient, and possibly fixation. The examination is normally performed with the body coil, in complex situations using extremity or wrap-around coils producing more intense signals. Using CE-MRA, the exact bolus timing is highly important. According to the heart rate and proximally existing stenoses or occlusions, the transit time of the contrast bolus varies. The estimation of the transit time is possible by means of bolus tracking. The contrast timing is especially complicated in the periphery, as the arterial flow not only depends on the heart rate, but also on the pathology of the vascular segments and peripheral resistance.

Visualization of the leg arteries, from the pelvis to the feet, requires at least two or three single examinations due to the limited field of view. Thus, the complete examination is still time consuming, and the costs of CE-MRA, due to the required repeated contrast-medium injections, are high. Moving-bed examinations are under evaluation (Ho et al. 1997) to image all leg arteries during continuous infusion of contrast material.

The documentation of collateral vessels and of the peripheral arteries in the foot is still inferior to i.a. DSA. TOF imaging of curved vessels suffers from saturation of inflowing spins (MARCHAL et al. 1990). Moreover, there are problems in the detection of fresh thrombi with the TOF technique (REISER and SEMMLER 1997). One advantage of MRA is its reliable

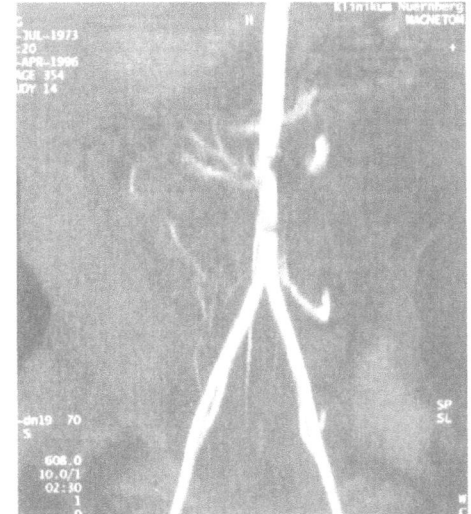
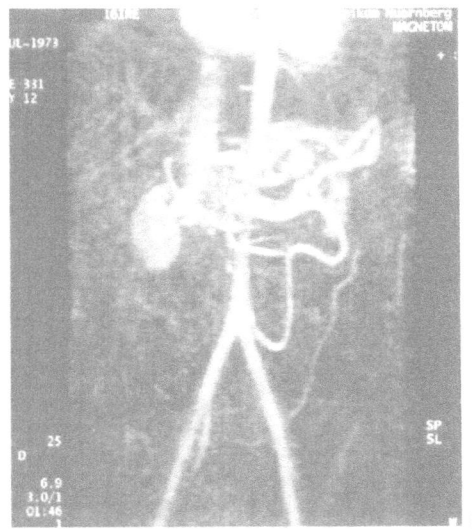

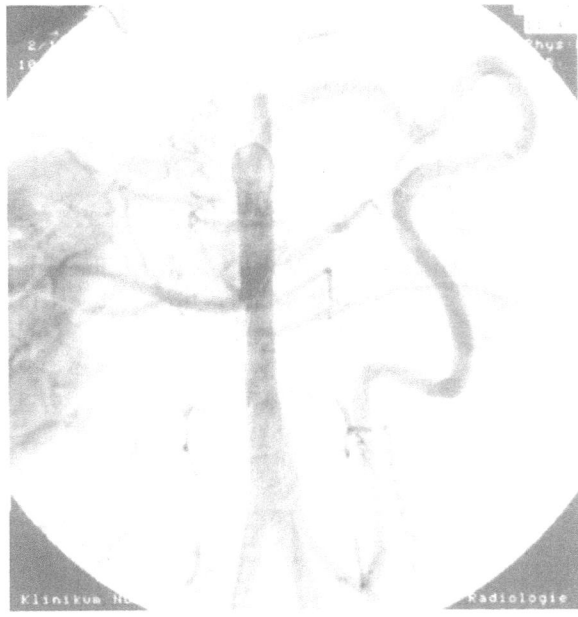

Fig. 12.11. a Time-of-flight magnetic resonance angiography (TOF-MRA), and **b** contrast-enhanced MRA, (same technique as in Fig. 12.6), and i.a. digital subtraction angiography (DSA). Patient with fibromuscular dysplasia. Occlusion of mesenteric trunk, anastomosis of Riolan; good correlation with i.a. DSA. TOF-MRA (**b**) shows only a short part of the anastomosis due to the reverse flow direction into the upper abdomen. A stent in the left renal artery is causing signal extinction in the left aortic rim

documentation of vessels suited for bypass following vascular occlusion (VOSSHENRICH et al. 1994).

Studies in peripheral occlusive vascular disease have revealed an accuracy with MRA of 43% (McCAULEY et al. 1994), 66% (KRUG et al. 1995; VOSSHENRICH et al. 1996), and 80% (BAUMGARTNER et al. 1993; CAMBRIA 1995), whereby the potential overstaging of stenoses using TOF-MRA requires special attention (VOSSHENRICH et al. 1996).

Considering current demands for the high performance of the different modalities used, the examination of local processes is justifiable, unless a diagnosis can also be achieved by color-coded duplex sonography. Such situations include:

- Postoperative control of bypasses
- Control of interventional procedures, such as angioplasty (Fig. 12.13), i.a. or i.v. lysis therapies, or embolization
- Visualization of inflammatory processes requiring the additional documentation of soft-tissue structures and bone marrow, especially gangrene
- Visualization of av-fistulas, aneurysms, dissections, and av-malformations.

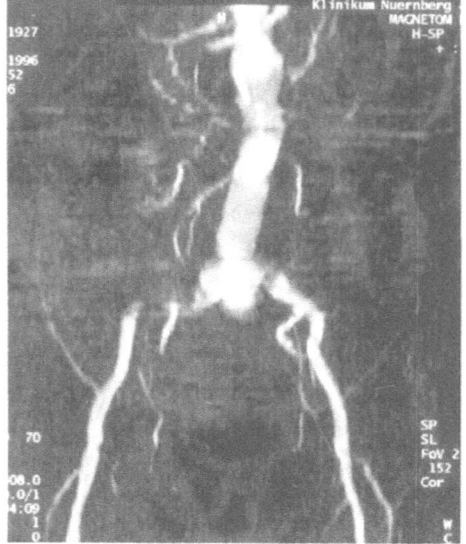
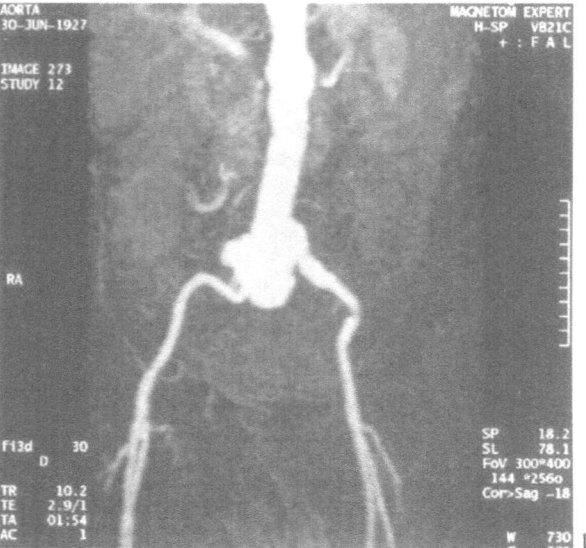

Fig. 12.12. a Time-of-flight magnetic resonance angiography (TOF-MRA) (608/10/70; ECG-triggered; time of acquisition, 16:30 min). Patient (69 years) with tubing of the infrarenal aorta. Signal extinction of the right common iliac artery. Comparison with contrast-enhanced (CE)-MRA shows that this is caused by the blood flow in an upward direction of the elongated iliac artery. CE-MRA clearly shows an aneurysm of the aortic bifurcation. The poorer visualization in (**a**) is caused by turbulence of the blood flow in the aneurysm

12.6.4
Arm Arteries

12.6.4.1
Technique

The body-coil and, in complex situations, also wrap-around coils are used. PC-, TOF-, and CE-MRA are employed according to the indication. Disturbing breath or flow artifacts from the thorax can be avoided using wide presaturation pulses. In dialysis shunts, the arterial and venous leg, including possible stenoses, can be depicted using PCA. The differentiation of slow flow from thromboses is mostly possible by evaluating the phase images (REISER and SEMMLER 1997). Complementary evaluation of blood flow is possible using ECG-triggered PC-RACE sequences. Indications include:

- Diagnosis of shunt dysfunction in dialysis patients
- Av-malformation
- Tumor invasion into major vessels, particularly Pancoast's tumors.

The diagnosis of peripheral occlusive vascular disease is of secondary interest.

Particularly in the region of the upper extremities, color-coded duplex sonography is an established clinical standard methodology, such that

MRA techniques are reserved mostly for the visualization of complex vascular structures in the case of av-malformations or tumor invasion. The diagnosis of shunt disfunctions, in contrast, has met with increasing interest (WALDMANN et al. 1996; PRINCE et al. 1997).

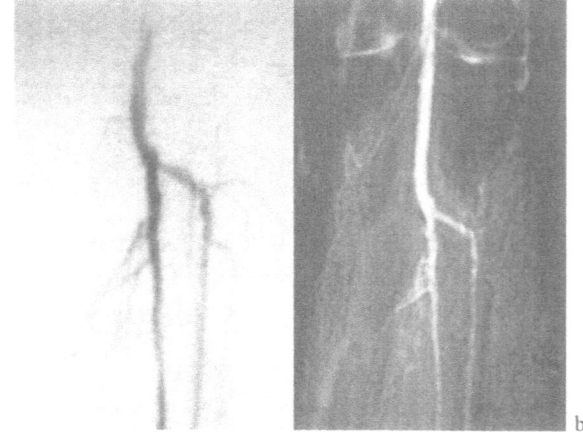

Fig. 12.13. ZEITLER and HEUCK. I.a. (DSA) (**a**) and contrast-enhanced magnetic resonance angiography (**b**) (6.7/2.8/30; single-dose contrast medium; extremity coil). Occlusion of the posterior tibial artery, low-grade stenoses of anterior tibial artery. Corresponding information with both techniques, but better visualization of small vessels in i.a. DSA

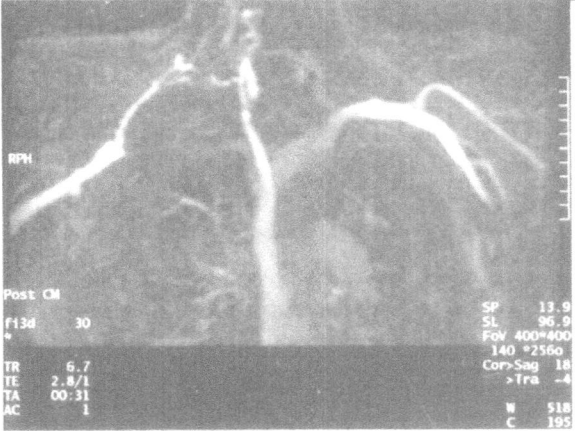

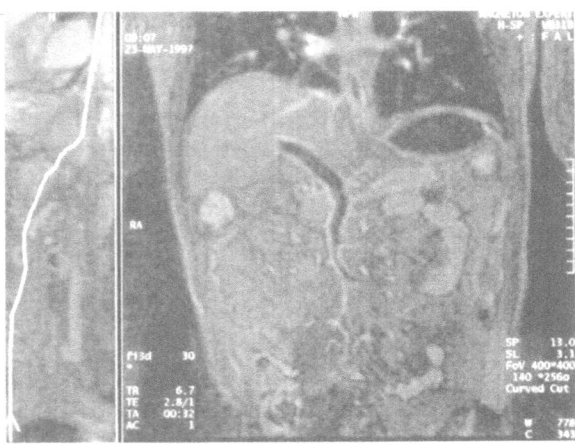

Fig. 12.14. Contrast-enhanced magnetic resonance venography with 1:10 diluted contrast medium injected in a forearm vein on both sides (6.7/2.8/70; breath-hold technique). Occlusion of the right subclavian vein with cervical collateral flow into the right jugular vein. Normal veins on the left side. Signal loss in the left brachiocephalic vein due to non-contrasted inflow from the left jugular vein

Fig. 12.15 a,b. Contrast-enhanced magnetic resonance venography of portal vein thrombosis (6.7/2.8/30; double-dose contrast medium breath-hold technique). Curved cut following the anatomical course of the portal vein (**b**) based on sagittal reformatted images (**a**). Wide thrombus (*dark*) in the portal vein

12.6.5
Veins

Venous vessels can be documented in all the above-mentioned techniques with MR venography (MRV) (ALART et al. 1991; DAVIS et al. 1995; SIEWERT et al. 1992). Using TOF techniques, the arterial flow is excluded from the visualization by traveling saturation impulses. Using PCA, a low flow velocity according to the venous system needs to be selected (<15 cm/sec). Signals from arterial vessels, however, can not always be eliminated due to velocity overfolding (REISER and SEMMLER 1997). CE-MRA has also proven reliable for the documentation of veins. Its quick performance using the breath-hold technique and independence from the flow direction are essential advantages over non-contrast-enhanced techniques. Direct MRV can be performed with 1:10 diluted contrast medium (Fig. 12.14). The practical importance of MRV, however, is discussed controversially.

In the upper and lower extremities, both TOF- ad PC-MRV provide good results at acceptable acquisition times. The overview of a vascular segment of up to 50 cm in length is a particular advantage compared to color-coded duplex sonography in the case of anatomical variations and malformations. A disadvantage, however, is the unavoidable overlying of the superficial venous system, and the lack of functional aspects (e.g., breath modulation, compressibility). TOF-MRV, moreover, bears the risk of false interpretation of hyperintensive thrombi (DEBATIN 1995).

All in all, the use of MRV in the extremities is restricted to complex situations, since duplex sonography enables reliable interpretations.

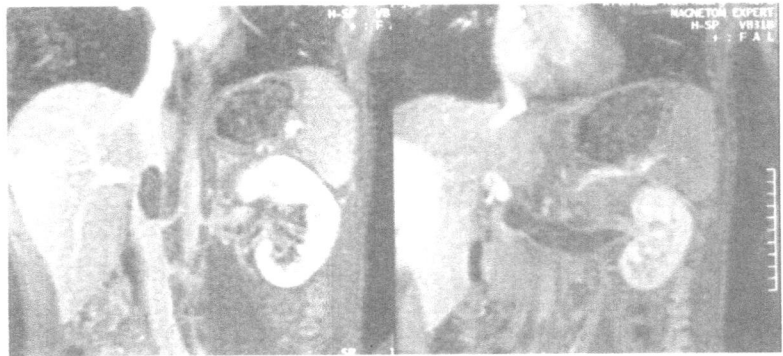

Fig. 12.16. Coronal oblique single slices (same parameters as in Fig. 12.16) of the left renal vein (**b**) with thrombotic occlusion. Extension of the thrombus into the caval vein (**a**). Patient with testicular teratocarcinoma. Tumor cells were found within the surgically removed thrombus

12.6.5.1
Portal System

As this venous system can only be visualized indirectly by i.a. DSA or transhepatic puncture, there is a chance for MRV (ARLART et al. 1991). Because of the flow in oblique orientation to the liver, angulated, axial TOF sequences are suited. PC sequences are normally performed in coronal orientation. CE-MRV has steadily increased in importance due to its quick practicability in breath-hold technique, but so far requires the double-dose or even triple-dose technique (PRINCE 1996), and a precise bolus timing. Indications include: thromboses of the portal vein (Fig. 12.15a,b), and segmental thromboses of the liver veins (SILVERMAN et al. 1991; LEWIS et al. 1993), as well as for documentation of portosystemic collaterals and varices in the case of portal hypertension (ARLART et al. 1991; JOHNSON et al. 1991), and the checking of surgically created portosystemic shunts. Transluminal intrahepatic portosystemic stent shunts (TIPSS) can only be assessed with certain limitations due to the paramagnetic properties of the stents (DAVIS et al. 1995). Hepatofugal flow in the portal vein can be clearly identified with the TOF and PC techniques. Spontaneous shunts, e.g., hepatorenal shunts, can be documented with high sensitivity (HUGES et al. 1995).

12.6.5.2
Abdominal Veins

Thromboses of the vena cava and the renal and splenic veins can be reliably documented using MRV (ARLART et al. 1991; DAVIS et al. 1995). TOF-MRA is preferable as it allows the documentation of the anatomic course of a thrombosed vessel. PCA and CE-MRA show a near total signal loss in the thrombosed area (Fig. 12.16a,b). Further indications include av-malformations, venous anomalies, and external venous compression through tumors, arterial variations, or aortic aneurysms (GUHL et al. 1995). The identification of thrombi of the renal veins is of key importance in the staging of kidney carcinomas (DAVIS et al. 1995).

References

Alley MT, Shifrin RY, Pelc NJ, Herfkens RJ (1998) Ultrafast contrast-enhanced three-dimensional MR angiography: state of the art. Radiographics 18:273-285

Alart IP, Guhl L, Fauser L, Edelman RR, Kim D, Laub G (1991) MR-Angiographie (MRA) der Abdominalvenen. Radiologe 31:192-201

Baumgartner I, Maier SE, Koch M, Schneider E, von Schulthess GK, Bollinger AC (1993) Magnetresonanzarteriographie, Duplexsonographie und konventionelle Arteriographie zur Beurteilung der peripheren arteriellen Verschlußkrankheit. Fortschr Rontgenstr 159:167-173

Bogaert J, Verschakelen JA, Smet MH, Baert AL (1992) Pictorial essay: right aortic arch. J Belge Radiol 75:406-409

Bongartz G, Boos M, Winter K, Brändli M, Scheffler K (1997) MR-Angiographie der Thorakalgefäße. Radiologe 37:529-538

Boos M, Scheffler K, Ott HW, Radü EW, Bongartz G (1997) Konventionelle MRA und CE-MRA der extrakraniellen Gefäßabschnitte. Radiologe 37:515-528

Borrello JA, Li D, Veseley TM, Vining EP, Brown JJ, Haacke EM (1995) Renal arteries: clinical comparison of three-dimensional time-of-flight MR angiographic sequences and radiographic angiography. Radiology 197:793-799

Brichaux J-C, Grenier N, Douws C, Degrèze P, Paulussière J, Trillaud H, Morel D, Potaux L (1995) Time-of-flight MR angiography of kidney transplants. Eur. Radiol 5:406-413

Bryant DJ, Payne JA, Firmin DN, Longmore DB (1984) Measurement of flow with NMR imaging using a gradient pulse and phase difference technique. JCAT 8:588-593

Cambria RP, Kaufman JA, Litalien GJ, Gertler JP, LaMuraglia GM, Brewster DC, Geller S, Atamian S, Waltman AC, Abbott WM (1997) Magnetic resonance angiography in the management of lower extremity arterial occlusive disease. A prospective study. J vasc Surg 25:380-389

Davis CP, Debatin JF, Fuchs WA (1995) MR-Venographie des Abdomens. Schweiz Med Wochenschr 125:639-648

Duda SH, Schick F, Teufl F, Müller-Schimpfle M, Erley C, Schneider W, Miller S, Claussen CD (1996) Phase contrast MR angiography for detection of arteriosclerotic renal artery stenosis. Acta Radiol (Denmark) 38:287-291

Dumoulin CL, Yucel EK, Vock P et al. (1990) Two- and three-dimensional phase contrast MR angiography of the abdomen. J Comput Assist Tomogr 14:779-784

Edelman RR, Wentz KU, Mattle H, et al. (1989) Projection arteriography and venography: initial clinical results with MR. Radiology 153:351

Edelman RR, Mattle HP, Atkinson DJ, Hoogewoud HM (1990) MR Angiography. AJR 154:937-946

Edelman RR, Mattle HP, Wallner B, et al. (1990) Extracranial carotid arteries: evaluation with „black-blood" MR angiography. Radiology 177:45-50

Gedroyc WMW, Neerhut P, Negus R, Palmer A, Al Cutobi A, Taube D, Hulme B (1995) Magnetic resonance angiography of renal artery stenosis. Clin Radiol 50:436-439

Graves MJ (1997) Magnetic resonance angiography. Br J Radiol 70:6-28

Guhl L, Alart IP (1996) The splenoportal venous system. In Alart IP, Bongartz GM, Marchal G (eds) Magnetic resonance angiography. Springer, Berlin Heidelberg New York

Hany TF, Pfammatter T, Schmidt M, Leung DA, Debatin JF (1997) Wertigkeit der Kontrastverstärkten 3D-MR Angiographie der Nierenarterien. Radiologe 37:574-553

Hausmann R (1996) Imaging techniques of magnetic resonance angiography. In: Arlart IP, Bongartz GM, Marchal G (eds) Magnetic resonance angiography. Springer, Berlin Heidelberg New York, pp 35-47

Ho KY, Leiner T, de Haan MW, Kessels AGH, Kitslaar PJ, van Engelshoven JM (1997) Moving bed infusion tracking technique: a new MR angiography technique for imaging the peripheral arteries. RSNA 1997 Abstract book. Radiology 205:301

Holland GA, Dougherty L, Capenter JP, et al. (1996) Breath-hold ultrafast three-dimensional gadolinium-enhancesd MR angiography of the aorta and the renal and other visceral abdominal arteries. Am J Roentgenol 166: 971-981

Huges LA, Hartnell GG, Finn JP (1995) Time-of-flight MR angiography of the portal venous system: value compared with other imaging procedures. Am J Roentgenol 166:375-378

Johnson ED, Ehmann RL, Rakela J, et al. (1991) MR angiography in portal hypertension detection of varices and imaging techniques. J Comput Assist Tomogr 15:578-584

Krug B, Kugel H, Harnischmacher U, et al. (1995) Peripheres arterielles Verschlußleiden: Vergleich der diagnostische Wertigkeit von MRA und DSA. Fortschr Rontgenstr 162:112-119

Kumar S, Roy S, Radhakrishnan S, et al. (1996) Three dimensional time-of-flight MR angiography of the arc of aorta and its major branches: a compatative study with contrast angiography. Clin Radiol 51:18-21

Laissy JP, Limot O, Henry-Fuegas M, et al. (1995) Iliac artery patency before and immediately after percutaneous transluminal angioplasty: assessment with time-of-flight MR angiography. Radiology 197:445-449

Laub G (1993) Grundlagen der MR-Angiographie. Radiologe 33:81-86

Laub G (1996) Postprocessing techniques. In: Arlart IP, Bongartz GM, Marchal G (eds) Magnetic resonance angiography. Springer, Berlin Heidelberg New York, pp 57-61

Lauffer RB, Parmelee DJ, Dunham SU, Ouellet HS, Dolan RP, Witte S, McMurry TJ, Walovich RC (1998) MS-325: Albumin-targeted contrast agent for MR angiography. Radiology 207:529-538

Lewin JS, Laub G, Hausmann R, et al. (1991) Three-dimensional time of flight MR angiography: applications in the abdomen and thorax. Radiology 179:261

Lewis WD, Finn JP, Jenkins RL, et al. (1993) Use of magnetic resonance angiography in the pretransplant evaluation of portal vein pathology. Transplantation 56:64-68

Marchal G, Bosmans H, Van Hecke P, Speck U, Aerts P, Vanhoenacker P, Baert AL (1990) MR angiography with gadopenteate dimeglumine-polylysine: evaluation in rabbits. Am J Roentgenol 155:407-411

Marchal G, Bosmans H, Van Hecke P, et al. (1991) Experimental Gd-DPTA polylysine enhanced MR angiography: sequence optimization. JCAT 15:711

Marchal G, Bosmans H, Wilms G (1996) Contrast-enhanced magnetic resonance angiography. In: Arlart IP, Bongartz GM, Marchal G (eds) Magnetic resonance angiography. Springer, Berlin Heidelberg New York, pp 93-106

Mayo-Smith WW, Saini S, Slater G, et al. (1995) MR contrast material for vascular enhancement: value of superparamagnetic iron oxide. AJR 166:73-77

McCauley TR, Monib A, Dickey KW, et al. (1994) Peripheral vascular occlusive disease: accuracy and reliability of time-of-flight MR angiography. Radiology 192:351-357

Meaney JFM, Prince MR, Nostrant TT, Stanley JC (1997) Gadolinium-enhanced MR Angiography of visceral arteries in patients with suspected chronic mesenteric ischemia. JMRI 7:171-76

Pernicone JR, Siebert JE, Potchen EJ (1990) Three-dimensional phase contrast MR angigraphy in the head and neck: preliminary report. AJR 155:167-176

Petersen MJ, Cambria RP, Kaufman JA, La Muraglia GM, Gertler JP, Brewster DC, Geller SC, Waltman AC, L'Italien

GJ, Abbott WM (1995) Magnetic resonance angiography in the preoperative evaluation of aortic aneurysms. J Vasc Surg (United States) 21(6):891-898

Prince MR, Yucel EK, Kaufman JA, et al. (1993) Dynamic gadolinium-enhanced three-dimensional abdominal arteriography. J Magn Res Imaging 3:877-881

Prince MR, Narasimham DL, Stenley JC, et al. (1995) Breathhold Gadolinium-enhanced MR angiography of the abdominal aorta and ist major branches. Radiology 197:785-792

Prince MR, Grist TM, Debatin JF (1997) 3D Kontrast angiography. Springer, Berlin Heidelberg New York

Reiser M, Semmler W (1997) Magnetresonanztomographie. Springer, Berlin Heidelberg New York

Roditi GH, Smith FW, Redpath TW (1994) Evaluation of tilted, optimized, non-saturating excitation pulses in 3D magnetic resonace angiography of the abdominal aorta and major branches in volunteers. Br J Radiol 67:11-13

Ross JS, Masaryk TJ, Modic MT (1989) Magnetic resonance angiography of external carotid arteries and intracranial vessels: a review. Neurology 39:1369-1376

Schild HH, Weber W, Boeck E, Mildenberger P, Strunk H, Düber Ch, Grebe P, Schadmand-Fischer S, Thelen M (1994) Gadolinium-DTPA (Magnevist®) als Kontrastmittel für die arterielle DSA Fortschr Rontgenstr 160(3):218-221

Seelos KC, von Smekal A, Steinborn M, Gieseke J, Kaas P, Urban J, Redel DA, Reiser M (1994) MR-Angiographie des Herzens und der thorakalen Gefäße. Radiologe 34:454-461

Siewert B, Kaiser BA, Layer G, Traber F, Kania U, Hartlapp J (1992) MR-Venographie bei tiefen Bein- und Beckenvenenthrombosen. Vergleich von 2D-Einzelschichtbildern und 3D-MIP-Rekonstruktionen mit der Phlebographie. Fortschr Rontgenstr 156:549-554

Silverman PM, Patt RH, Garras BS, et al. (1991) MR imaging of the portal venous system: value of gradient echo imaging as an adjunct to spin-echo imaging. Am J Roentgenol 157:297-302

Singer JR (1978) NMR diffusion and flow measurements and an introduction to spinphase graphing. J Phys E 11:281-291

Snidow JJ, Aisen AM, Harris VJ, et al. (1995) Iliac artery MR angiography: a comparison of three-dimensional gadolinium-enhanced and two-dimensional time-of-flight techniques. Radiology 196:371-378

Snidow JJ, Johnson MS, Haris VJ, et al. (1996) Three-dimensional gadolinium-enhanced MR angiography for aortoiliac inflow assessment plus renal artery screening in a single breath hold. Radiology 198:725-732

Sommer T, Fehske W, v Smekal A, Holzknecht N, Gieseke J, Keller E, Wörtz P, Steudel A, Schild H (1995) Spiral-CT, multiplane transoesophageale Echocardiographie und Magnetresonanztomographie in der Diagnostik thorakaler Aortendissektionen. Fortschr Rontgenstr 162:104-111

Stehling MK, Holzknecht N, Laub G (1997) Gadolinium-verstärkte Magnetresonazangiographie der Abdominal-gefäße. Radiologe 37:539-546

Tu R, Kennel T, Tursk P (1994) Preliminary assessment of gadolinium-enhanced magnetic resonance angiography. Acad Radiol 1:47-55

Vock P, Terrier F, Wegmüller H, et al. (1991) Magnetic resonance angiography of abdominal vessels: early experience using the three-dimensional phase-contrast technique. Br J Radiol 64:10-16

Vosshenrich R, Fischer U, Grabbe E (1994) MR Angiographie der peripheren Gefäße. Radiologe 34:447-42

Vosshenrich R, Fischer U, Funke M, Grabbe E (1996) 2D-time of flight-MR-Angiographie der peripheren Gefäße.

Experimentelle und klinische Studien zur Wertigkeit der Methode bei AVK. Fortschr Rontgenstr 164:25–30

Waldman GJ, Patynama PM, Chang PC, et al. (1996) Magnetic resonance angiography of dialysis shunts: initial results. Magn Reson Imaging 14(2):197–200

Wanner B, Edelman RR, Kim D, Finn JP (1991) Darstellung thorakaler und abdomineller Aortenaneurymen mit MR-Angiographie. Fortsch Rontgenstr 154:11

Wegmüller H, Vock P (1993) MR-Angiographie des Abdomens. Radiologe 33:81

Williams DM, Joshi A, Dake MD, Deeb GM, Miller DC, Abrams GD (1994) Aortic Cobwebs: an anatomic marker identifying the false lumen in aortic dissection-imaging and pathologic correlation. Radiology 190:167

Zeitler E (ed) (1984) Klinische Radiologie: Arterien und Venen Springer, Berlin Heidelberg New York

13 Phlebography and Lymphography

E.-I. Richter

13.1
Phlebography

Phlebography is defined as a specific radiological diagnostic method which is closely connected to the development of injectable contrast medium (CM) and therefore relatively young. The first to describe it were Berberich and Hirsch (1923), who conducted systematic experiments on living persons. The examination consists, firstly, of morphological assessment but also of functional phleboscopic assessment of the venous system of a certain body region. With this method it is possible to recognize, describe, and evaluate venous changes.

E.-Iris Richter, MD; Department of Röntgendiagnostik, Klinikum Nürnberg Nord, Flurstraße 17, 90340 Nürnberg, Germany; *address for correspondence:* Heynestr. 41, Nuremberg, Germany

13.1.1
Equipment

As equipment for the ascending phlebography of the lower extremities, a tiltable target X-ray apparatus is used, the pedestal of which can be adjusted to a higher position in order to cover the foot or malleolus veins. The X-ray tube may be arranged as an upper table tube or a lower table tube. All X-ray devices today are combined with an image-intensifying television chain. At the sides of the table there are adjustable handles for the support and safety of the patient. The table itself can be moved horizontally and vertically. The examination is documented, partly with time lapse, on cassette formats of 35 × 35 cm or 35 × 43 cm with the possibility of subdivision. On average, between four and six radiograms are made. The crural and genual regions are visualized generally in two layers. It takes 10–20 min from puncture to radiogram of the extremity. The time of fluoroscopy ranges from 30–60 s. Depending on the weight of the patient, the area dose product varies between 400 and 1000 cGY cm^2.

13.1.2
Technique

For ascending phlebography of the lower extremities, the 60-degree (Fig. 13.1) positioning of the patient has gained wider acceptance than horizontal positioning. The leg to be examined should bear as little weight as possible. This is ensured by an additional block of wood on which the leg not examined, the pivot leg, can stand firmly during the whole course of the examination.

Before examination, a warm footbath or a fomentation is desirable to make it easier to find a vein that can be punctured, if inspection indicates such a necessity.

Before application of a supramalleolar tight tourniquet the leg, in case of a marked superficial varicosis, is bound with an elastic 8-cm wide bandage

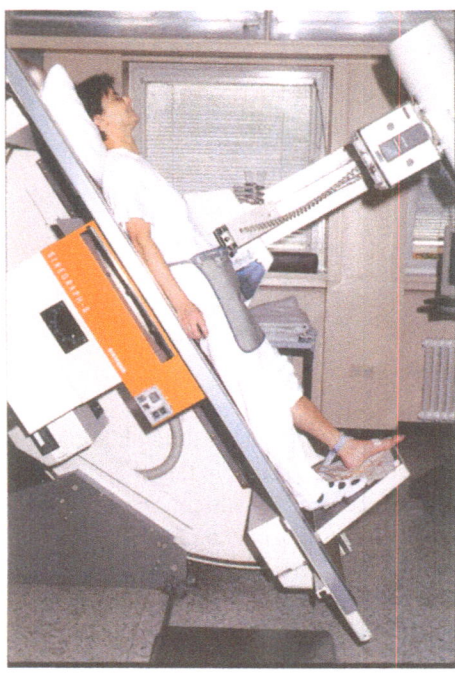

Fig. 13.1. Tiltable target fluoroscopy equipment with television chain; patient in oblique position

under light pressure. For preoperative phlebograms it is additionally necessary to apply a measuring device to the exterior of the extremity; this may be, for example, a metal chain with marked intervals. Also, the extent of an ulcus cruris is marked on the bandage or the skin. The dorsal foot vein is then punctured with an 18-G Butterfly or a Venofix needle. With the help of a connecting extension tube, CM is manually applied in full view and while the malleolar block is continued (Fig. 13.2).

The radiological documentation is a standardized procedure: First of all, the lower leg needs to be visualized in an anteroposterior projection with slight exterior rotation. The caudal limitation of the picture is the foot or the malleolus. In the following step of the examination, the knee joint cleft is in the center ray. Transitions of the radiograms are always overlapping. With the third exposure, the superficial femoral vein is visualized. The infrainguinal region, including the cross (Fig. 13.3), and also the common femoral vein are X-rayed on a supplementary cassette (24 × 30 cm). If the pelvic veins and the inflow of the vena cava inferior are contrasted, their documentation will suffice on the 24 × 30 cm format. Depending on the findings and the problem that is looked for in the lower leg region, the final documentation will proceed in interior and exterior

rotations as well as in a lateral projection. The diagnosis may suggest this kind of procedure at the very beginning; in this case, the pelvic region should be exposed at the end. This has the additional advantage of transporting CM by means of a passive muscle pump of the sura from the crural veins centripetally. In such a way the moistening time of the CM at the endothelium of the vein wall is reduced.

Orthostatic leg phlebography is indicated in the following cases:

- Suspected acute phlebothrombosis
- Preoperatively in case of varicosis, in order to assess subfascial veins and the perforating veins
- To assess the superficial venous system, but not for verification of a superficial thrombophlebitis
- To diagnose venous insufficiency (Fig. 13.4)

13.1.3
Phlebography of Leg and Pelvic Veins

In ascending phlebography of the lower extremities, the deep leg and pelvic veins, including the muscular vessels, are visualized. At the same time, by means of Valsalva's maneuver it is possible to show insufficient perforating veins. Also, insufficient transfascial connections can be objectified in order to exclude a

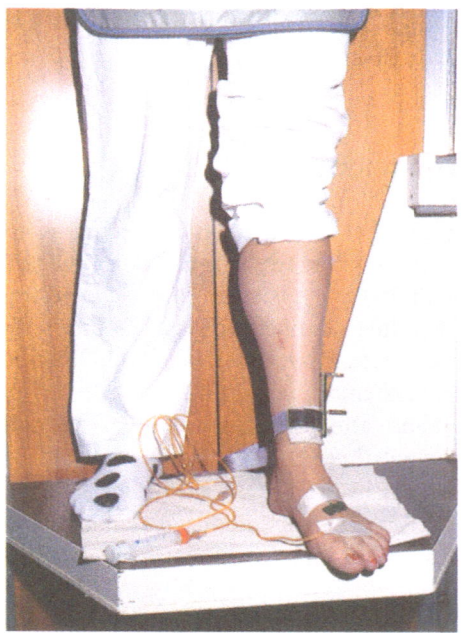

Fig. 13.2. Supramalleolar stasis. The Butterfly needle in site has been connected to an extension tube

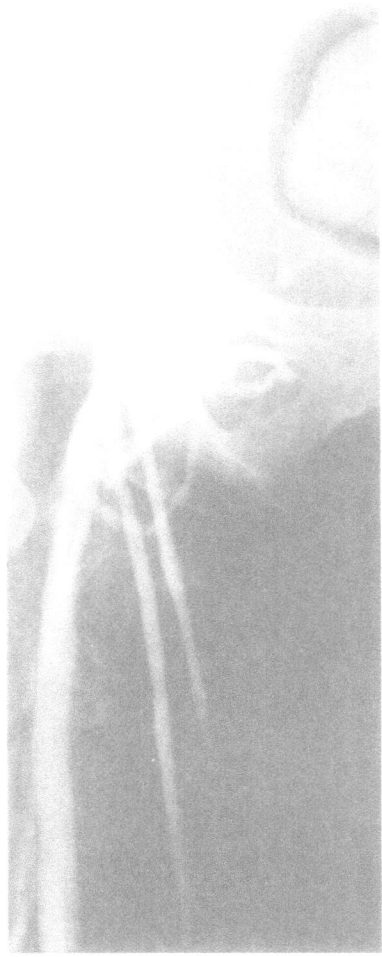

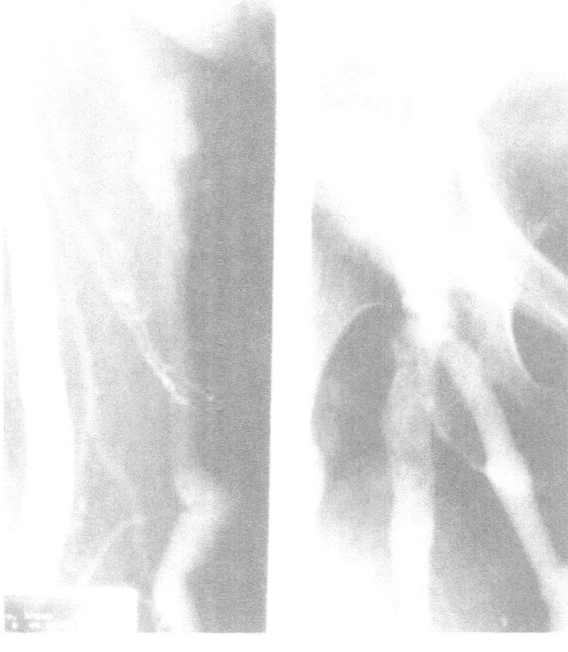

Fig. 13.4. Insufficiency of the vena saphena magna. Moreover, inflow phenomenon of the superficial femoral vein via the deep femoral vein. Lateral compression of the right external iliac vein by the crossing artery

Fig. 13.3. Infrainguinal region with doubling of the vena saphena magna with isolated inflow. Condition after occlusion of the pelvic veins and additional collateral circulation via the pudendal circulation

stem varicosis of the saphena magna (Fig. 13.5) or parva (HACH and HACH-WUNDERLE 1996).

Radiological symptoms of perforation insufficiency include the following:

– Flow reversal
– Horizontal progression
– Dilatation
– Valvular insufficiency
– Unpaired
– Syphonlike opening
– Dow's sign

Varicography is carried out with a specific target question concerning the leg veins. Also, Pelvic vein phlebography is also carried out with a specific target question in mind. (Fig. 13.6)

The use of digital techniques has the advantage that, for example, the pelvic veins can be better visualized with lesser CM, that osseous overlap does not interfere because of subtraction, and that the cassette does not have to be changed. The injection is made into the femoral veins after direct puncture. Both sides are depicted simultaneously. If there is vascular occlusion on one side, unilateral radiological examination is recommended in order to assess collateral circulation.

13.1.4
Sources of Error

If the CM flows into the great saphenous vein or into the proximal section of the marginal tibial vein,

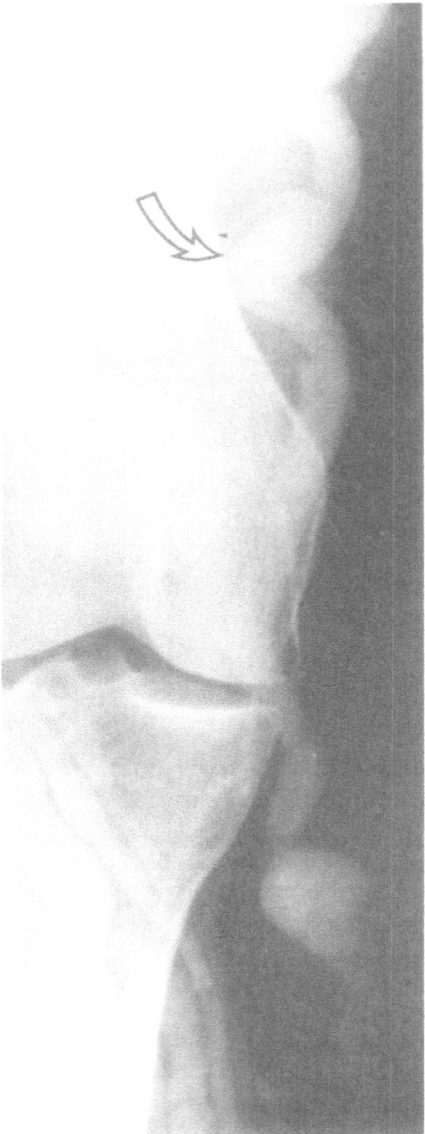

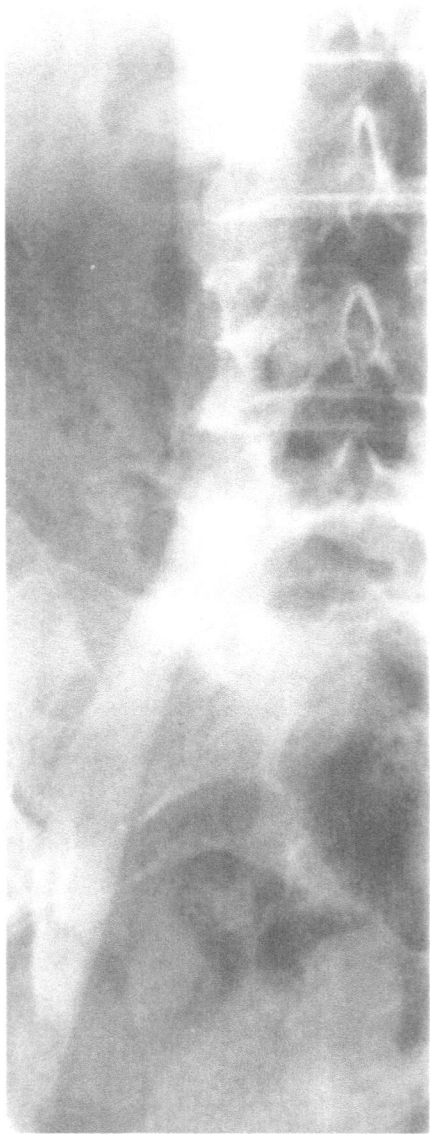

Fig. 13.5. Truncal varicosis of the vena saphena magna with marked tortuosity

Fig. 13.6. Visualization of the inferior vena cava by ascending phlebography of the right lower extremity

drainage along the deep vessels is retarded. The deep veins may then be only incompletely, or not at all, visible so that there is the danger of an incorrect diagnosis of deep thrombosis.

If the tourniquets are applied too high, a similar effect will ensue. If the block in the region of the malleolus is too tight, the depiction of individual conduction veins will be missing. If the cuff is inadequate or missing altogether, all crural veins will be depicted. Because of the overlay of both systems, this will lead to difficulties in vascular evaluation.

Depending on the size of the leg, the medial soft tissues may not be covered by the rays, or they may

lie outside of the format frame, so that incomplete stem varicosis of the great saphenous vein may be overlooked. It is possible to confuse it with stem varicosis of the small saphenous vein, when the Vv. gastrocnemiae, which join together with a common stem above the knee joint cleft (2–3 cm) are enlarged in fusiform shape and show regressive changes at the valves.

Sometimes, in the presence of deep leg vein thrombosis, due to heightened pressure or volume load, phlebectasia of the great saphenous vein is be confused with a stem varicosis as a collateral function.

Varicography may involve longer CM contact to the venous wall, which may lead to thrombophlebitis. Therefore, this examination should only be carried out directly before operation (JÄGER 1980; HACH and HACH-WUNDERLE 1996).

13.1.5
Phlebography of Arm and Shoulder Veins

In contrast to venous disease of the lower extremities, thrombosis of the arm and shoulder region seldom occurs; it makes up 1%–2% of all venous diseases (MAAS et al. 1995).

Indication for phlebography is given in the following cases:

- Tumor compression or infiltration (Fig. 13.7)
- Constriction with hemodynamic effects (stenosis, thoracic outlet syndrome)
- Presumption of a thrombosis induced by a catheter (vena cava or Hickman catheter)
- Necessity for preoperative visualization of the venous anatomy before dialysis shunts
- To evaluate the prognosis of mediastinal and bronchial tumors
- Follow-up after a lysotherapy

Depending on the clinical specific target question, the CM is applied from the dorsum of the hand or from the medial cubital vein.

For the puncture of the vein (21-G Butterfly or Venofix), the tourniquet is applied above the place to be punctured. The CM injection can be administered automatically with a pressure excertion of 8–10 ml/s or manually with a 10-ml injection syringe. In both cases, a connection line (PVC 1200 PSI) is interposed for protection from the X-rays.

One can successfully document not only the arm veins, the axillary vein (Fig. 13.8), and the subclavian vein, but also at the same time the vena cava cranialis.

For the mediastinal phlebogram, the CM is applied to both intermedian cubital veins simultaneously. The connection lines are fastened to a Y-connector. The flow rate of the CM is not affected by this.

It stays with 8–10 ml in the low pressure region. Only the amount of CM in the injector rises to 20–30 ml.

For documentation of mediastinal phlebograms, 35 × 35 cassettes can be used as long as one works with an image-intensifying television chain.

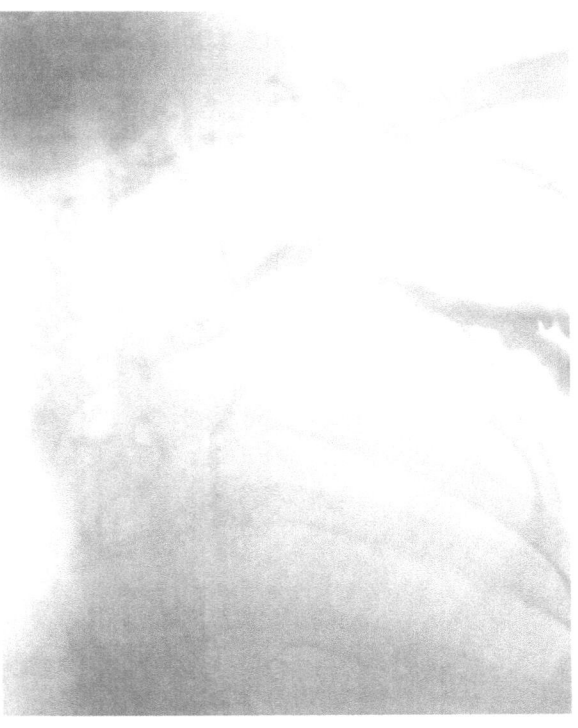

Fig. 13.7. Tumor compression of an anonymous vein where a stent was implanted. Collateral circulation due to a nearly completely occluded superficial vena cava. Examination performed using digital technique

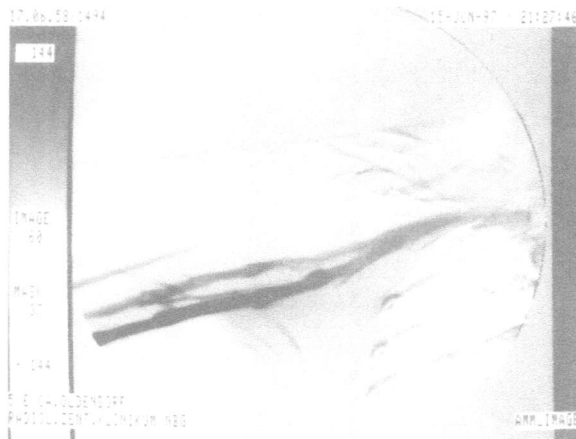

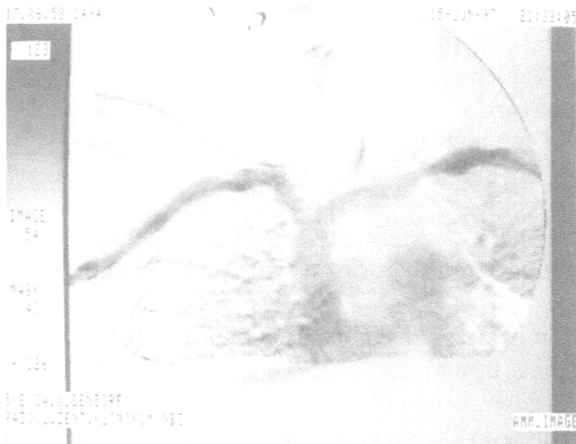

Fig. 13.9. Digital phlebogram of the mediastinum

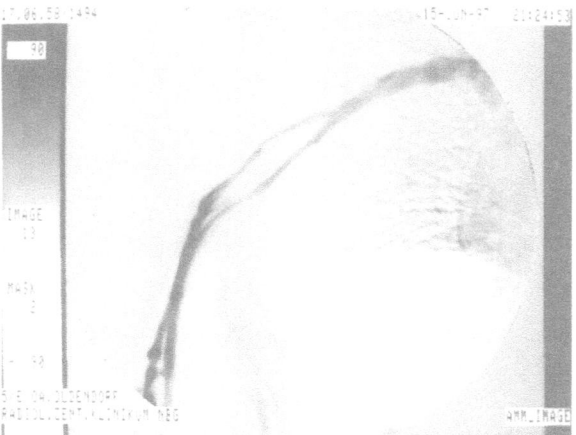

Fig. 13..8. Digital visualization of the axillary veins under abduction and adduction

The digital technique has proven to be of particular advantage for arm–shoulder phlebography and for mediastinum. Often, one needs to go through the procedure only once in terms of the vena cava cranialis and the subclavian veins. This saves time and also additional CM (Fig. 13.9). By means of follow-up picture processing at the console, the radiological findings can be emphasized without interfering shadows or overlays. Digital arm phlebography is realized in layers, the veins being flushed out after every turn with physiological NaCl solution. In contrast to the muscular pump of the lower extremities, the arm veins are not emptied in this way. For a new picture series, the mask should be free of CM. In such a way good one-line pictures are possible, so that there is no need for the follow-up processing phase, which may impair the clarity and precision of the documentation.

Thromboses of the arm and shoulder girdle form directly under external impact and are localized at the place of impact. Also, indirect trauma (for example myorrhexis) can lead to thrombosis in the same area. The traumatically induced thrombosis of the arm veins and the subclavian vein is called thrombosis *par effort* (Fig. 13.10).

At the end of the nineteenth century, Paget and Von Schroetter described the isolated occlusion of the axillary vein and/or the subclavian vein primarily in the right shoulder–arm region. Thrombophlebitis of the arm veins is caused by direct damage to the venous wall after intravenous injections with hypertonic agents. Acute arm vein thromboses do not produce fulminant pulmonary embolism. The hydrostatic load of the arm veins is low and their caliber is too small. Chronic stasis does not normally happen in the arm. This is enough reason in conventional therapy not to bind pressure bandages as tightly as in the lower extremitites. The special case of chronic stasis develops after breast operations in the form of a pervenous callus with light venous congestion without thrombotic occlusion. The venous valve system remains intact (MAY and NISSL 1959).

13.1.6
Complications and Possible Dangers of Phlebography

The veins with their valve system are very sensitive. Therefore, incidents during diagnostics can become significant when the actual, presumed basic disease is relatively harmless in comparison to expected therapeutic consequences. Injuries during venous puncture in the form of hematomas are basically

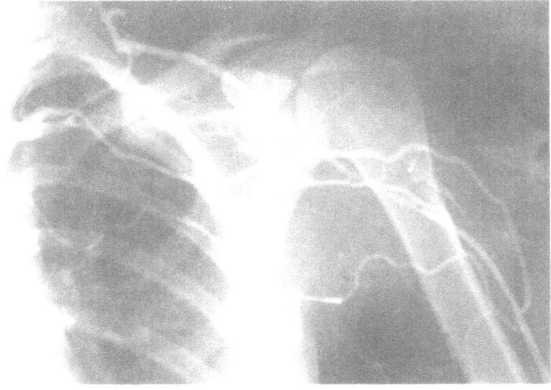

Fig. 13.10. *Par effort* thrombosis of the left subclavian vein in a 15-year-old girl due to unilateral stress to that arm during a visit to the cinema

harmless. They cause the tissue pressure to rise in the region of the puncture, so that bleeding will stop. Secondary bleeding from a punctured vessel is only of a higher degree if the vessel is not surrounded with healthy connective tissue.

Low paravasal CM injections cause local pain even with today's modern CM; this pain will soon subside with no further consequences. In case of extended paravasion, thrombotic phlegmasia cerulea dolens can develop as a result. Generalized pain in phlebography is not known to exist.

Other local CM injuries include deep vein thrombosis, a superficial venous inflammation especially in the area of the varicose veins, and the isolated damage of venous valves. Besides local complications, CM also causes general effects in 1.5% of all cases. An extreme case of this is allergic shock which demands immediate intubation of the patient with additional oxygen ventilation and measures to stabilize circulation. In addition, application of cortisone preparations (25 mg–1 g) is necessary.

More harmless phenomena are considered to be pruritus, urticaria, edema, and erythema of the whole integument. These can arise within 10 min after application of the CM and are still detectable for up to 12 h (MAY and NISSL 1959). Allergic effects are characterized by release of histamine which has turned out to be a direct, not an indirect, release through an antigen–antibody reaction. A high osmotic pressure of CM is not crucial for the release of histamine.

Hypervolemia is to be expected after application of high CM doses. According to SCHULZE and KAPS (1977), the anticoagulative property of CM corresponds to diffuse intravascular coagulation with the presence of fibrinolytic split products (FSP), hypofibrinogenemia, and a drop in thrombocytes. It can be explained by a direct link of the CM with different factors of coagulation.

Dehydrated patients can suffer from transient kidney damage caused by osmotic nephrosis of the proximal tubulus cells. Identifiable parameters are the albuminuria and hematuria.

To reduce complications, it is necessary to know about the allergic risks of the patient in order to develop from that preoperative protection with H-1 and H-2 blocking agents and establish venous access.

CM application should not exceed 1–1.5 ml/kg of body weight. The maximum volume should lie between 40–90 ml. The CM concentration for phlebography can total 40%–60%; however, in order to reduce damage to the endothelium, the CM can be diluted with distilled water or NaCl solution.

Considering these aspects, the place of injection is of prime importance because of the CM dilution effect, progressing in a centrally oriented flow. The deep veins of the lower leg are therefore examined by injection of the dorsal foot veins under blocking conditions, the superficial veins as far as possible by varicography, and the pelvic veins by puncture of the common femoral vein. Transosseous preoperative phlebography is today no longer justifiable since the alternative of duplex sonography is available.

13.1.7
Postprocedure Care and Premedication

As immediate postprocedure after a phlebographic examination, injection of heparinized physiological NaCl solution (5000 I.E. heparin in 500 ml NaCl) is recommended in order to flush the CM out of the veins. In addition, the patient should move around after the examination. An elastic bandage or a well-adjusted compression stocking are favorable to drainage of the deep leg veins.

13.1.8
Indications Compared to Other Modalities

Phlebography, with its highest diagnostic accuracy and certainty, is the gold standard. It also involves, however, the risk of CM reaction and can trigger off phlebitis itself. Further development of ultrasound diagnostics (US) with the Doppler and color-Doppler procedures, as well as magnet resonance imaging (MRI), have expanded and changed conventional radiological procedures. Sonography offers many uses for diagnostics because it enables significant and accurate evaluation. Moreover, its application is without risk for the patient, frequently repeatable, and not very expensive.

According to HAERTEN (1994), the short picture build-up with US (20–100 ms), as well as almost totally motionless cuts, are also advantageous.

With regard to diagnostics of acute thrombosis, the Doppler and color-coded duplex sonography (also the angiodynography) is considered as equal to phlebography.

The experienced examiner will prefer to use this simpler method in diagnostics, as well as for process controls, because it saves time. Color-coded Doppler sonography (CCDS), according to MÖDDER (1992), is applied mainly in the case of local findings needing to be described. Only in cases where findings are ambiguous, MOSTBECK et al. (1993) and BOMHARD et al. (1993) recommend radiological diagnostic phlebography. (Fig. 13.11a,b).

According to WUPPERMANN (1994) the Doppler and CCDS are indicated in questions of extent of thrombosis, postthrombotic changes of venous walls and valves, vasodilation of insufficiencies, and collaterals recognized by their coloration. CCDS, just like phlebography, allows visualization of the vascular lumen and blood flow. An additional advantage is the depiction of surrounding soft parts.

Fresh vein thromboses can be recognized with a sensitivity of 96% and a specificity of 97%. While diagnostics in the femoral region do not present any special difficulties, the lower leg poses far more problems due to its anatomy with a large number of vessels. With high specificity the sensitivity sinks to 90% (FOBBE et al. 1989) (Table 13.1). FOBBE reports about tele-thermography, which reaches a similarly high sensitivity to phlebography; on the other hand, due to its low specificity it demands additional diagnostics.

Digital luminescent radiography is being increasingly introduced into clinical routine and is basically suitable to substitute film sheets. It is necessary to optimize specific subsequent processing of the picture. A dose reduction of 4% with regard to the reference system led to no decrease in meaningfulness of interpretation because of the high contrasts present in phlebography, but also to no diagnostic improvement. The technical advantages lie in the absence of faulty exposure, in the possibility of subsequent picture processing, and in digital storage (SCHWERMER et al. 1990).

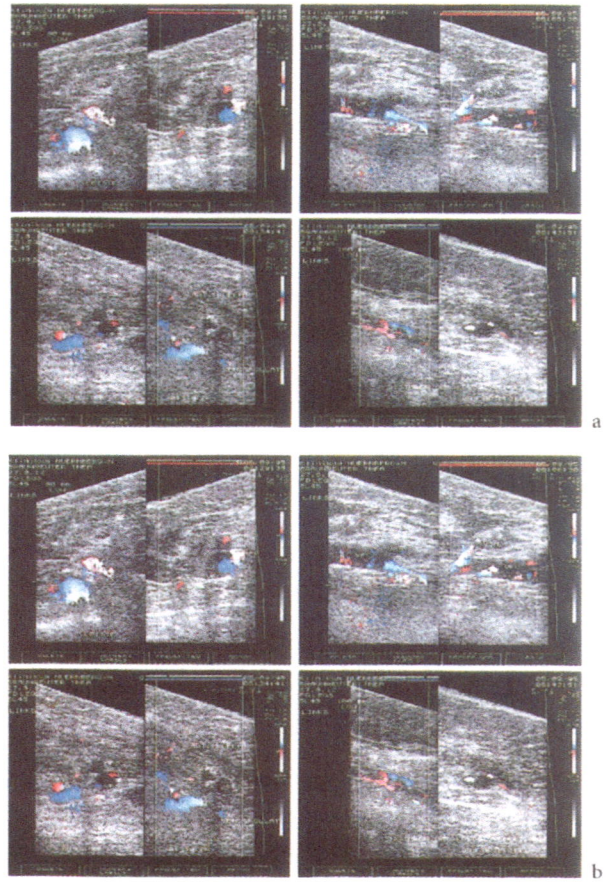

Fig. 13.11. a Venous thrombosis of the lower leg involving the adjacent popliteal segment. **b** Thrombosis of the superficial femoral vein on the left, with formation of collaterals. Also, the transition of the superficial femoral vein into the popliteal vein is thrombosed

Alternative procedures for thrombosis diagnostics include computed tomography angiography (CTA), especially in cases of complete occlusion of the pelvic veins; potentially also MRI. The MR venographic technique, in comparison to phle-bography, does not produce false or negative results. The procedure is well suited to exclude thrombosis proximally to the popliteal vein. A reliable proof of a thrombus in the crural veins cannot successfully be shown. The use of two-dimensional (2D) time-of-flight inflow pictures and secondary three dimensional (3D) maximum intensity projections (MID) reconstructions showed that the sole interpretation of 3D MIP reconstruction does not produce sufficiently reliable results to diagnose deep leg vein thrombosis (SIEWERT et al. 1992; Fig. 13.12).

The MRI technique proved to be superior to duplex sonography and the continuous wave

Table 13.1. Advantages and disadvantages of duplex sonography compared to phlebography (according to DIEHM)

Advantages	Disadvantages
– Reliable visualization of the cross, deep femoral vein muscle veins, and veins of two lumina	– Poor documentation
– Precise diagnostic differentiation (hematoma, arteriovenous fistula, Baker's cyst) and assessment of vascular wall (tumor)	– Poor results in obese patients and in cases of special types of edema
– Assessment of nature of the thrombus	– Long examination time (approximately 20 min/extremity)
– Non-invasive with equally high precision	– Long training
– Repeatable as often as required	– Examiner-dependent
	– Units not installed in sufficient quantity
	– Pulmonary embolism under compression

Doppler in terms of thrombosis of the iliac veins and the vena cava inferior, especially with adipose patients (RICHTER et al. 1993).

In case of progressive changes of chronic venous insufficiency accompanied by subcutaneous fibroses and unspecific infiltration of the remaining extra-fascial zone, CT seems to be slightly more successful than MRI.

One can imagine that it could be used within the framework of posttherapeutic course controls, as well as for medical expertise (GMELIN et al. 1989).

13.1.9
Informed Consent

Before diagnostic procedure, the doctor should explain to the patient why the examination is necessary and how it will be done, including an anatomic briefing. Since an iodine-containing CM is applied, which remains in the body for a short time, possible complications with regard to a thyro-toxicosis risk should be mentioned. In the talk with the patient, the doctor can find out if special preparation for the examination is necessary. The risk of the impending examination is increased by allergic diathesis, thyroid or kidney diseases, or functional impairment of organs. The examination should not be carried out if the presence of phlegmasia cerulea dolens blocks drainage by the obliteration of all veins. Advantages and disadvantages in comparison to other methods should be described; also, possible side effects and subsequent procedures should be mentioned. Judicially, the patient has the right to due consideration of his decision. Therefore, the doctor should have this discussion 1 day prior to the planned procedure or during a normal appointment if there is no presumption of acute thrombosis. Explanations in the radiological room are not tenable in court.

13.1.10
Perspectives

The need for phlebography in cases of varicosis and venous insufficiency is subject to variation. As newer techniques have become available, phlebography is being used less frequently. For the time being, nevertheless, it continues to be indicated preoperatively to every invasive procedure (lysis, cava filter, stent) and in cases of uncertainty following sonographic procedures.

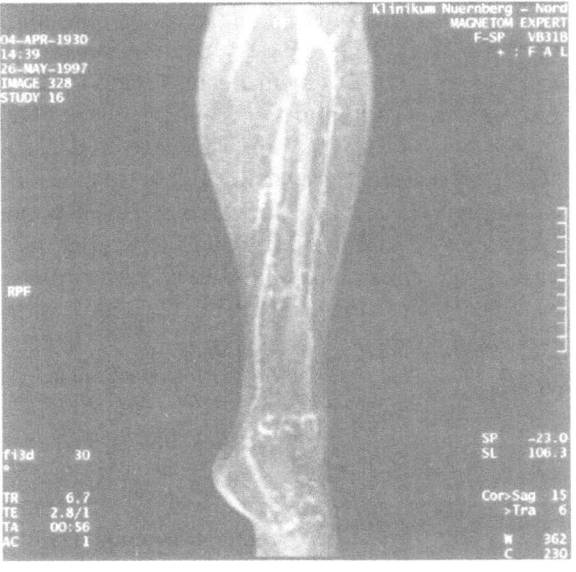

Fig. 13.12. Magnetic resonance phlebography of the lower extremity

References

Bomhard T, Oellinger H, Böttcher H, Flesch U (1993) Stellenwert der farbcodierten Dopplersonographie (FKDS) in der Venendiagnostik der unteren Extremität im Vergleich zur konventionellen Phlebographie. Akthel Radiol 3:279–282

Berberich J, Hirsch S (1923) Die röntgenologische Darstellung an Arterien und Venen am lebenden Menschen. Klin Wochenschr 2:2226

Diehm C, Stammler T, Amendt K (1997) Die tiefe Beinvenenthrombose. Dtsch Aerztebl 94(6):29–39

Fobbe F, Koennecke H-C, El Bediwi M, Heidt P, Boese-Landgraf J, Wolf K-J (1989) Diagnistik der tiefen Beinvenenthrombose mit der farbkodierten Duplexsonographie. ROFO 151(5):569–573

Gmelin E, Rosenthal M, Schmeller W, Tichy P, Busch D (1989) Computertomographie und Kernspintomographie des Unterschenkels bei chronischer Veneninsuffizienz. ROFO 151(1):50–56

Gottlob R (1980) Gefahren und Komplikationen der Phlebographie. In: Hach W (ed) Die Röntgenuntersuchung des Venensystems, vol 22. Schattauer, Stuttgart, pp 161–176

Habscheid W (1992) Diagnostik der tiefen Beinvenen-thrombose Freie Radiol 5/6:26–31

Hach W (1992) Diagnostik der tiefen Beinvenenthrombose. Freie Radiol 5/6:26–31

Hach W, Hach-Wunderle V (1996) Phlebographie der Bein-und Beckengefäße. Schnetztor, Konstanz

Haerten R (1994) Die Rolle der Sonographie in der bildgebenden Diagnostik. Electro Med 2:42–50

Jäger W (1980) Methodik und Technik der Phlebographie. In: Hach W (ed) Die Röntgenuntersuchung des Venensystems, vol 22. Schattauer, Stuttgart, pp 7–18

Maas R, Nicola V, Mügge-Hamann U, Steiner P (1995) Die Phlebographie der oberen Extremität. Teil I. ROFO 162(1):33–38

May R, Nissl R (1959) Die Phlebographie der unteren Extremität. Thieme, Stuttgart

Mödder U (1992) Farbkodierte Duplexsonographie (Angiodynographie). ROFO 157:204–209

Mostbeck GH, Kettenbach J, Henk C (1993) Vergleich der Sonographie mit der Phlebographie in der Diagnose der tiefen Beinvenenthrombose der unteren Extremität. Radiologe 33:498–507

Müller JHA (1994) Phlebographische Thrombosediagnostik unter Benutzung nicht-ionischer Röntgenkontrastmittel. Vasomed 10(6):396–402

Richter CS, Duewell S, Krestin GP, Vesti B, Franzeck UK, Bollinger A (1993) Dreidimensionale Darstellung der Beckenvenen mit Magnetresonanz-Angiographie. ROFO 159(2):161–166

Schubert U, Blank W, Braun B (1992) Realtime-Sonographie zur Diagnostik der Venenthrombose. Krankenhausarzt 65(4):150–156

Schulze B, Kaps HP (1977) Gerinnungshemmende wirkung trijodierter Röntgenkontrastmittel. Arzneimittelforschung 27:972

Schwermer B, Witte G, Nicolas V, Bücheler E (1990) Klinische und technische Erfahrungen mit der digitalen Lumineszenzradiographie bei der Phlebographie des Beines. ROFO 152(2):159–162

Siewert B, Kaiser WA, Layer G, Träber F, Kania U, Hartlapp J (1992) MR-Venographie bei tiefen Bein-und Beckenvenenthrombosen. ROFO 156(6):549–554

Spengel F (1992) Diagnostik der tiefen Beinvenenthrombose. Freie Radiol 5/6:26–31

Strauss AL, Neuerburg-Heusler D (1996) Doppler-und Duplexsonographie bei venösen Abflußstörungen. In: Zeitler E (ed) Klinische Radiologie. Springer, Berlin Heidelbug New York, pp 593–606

Theiss W (1992) Diagnostik der tiefen Beinvenenthrombose. Freie Radiol 5/6:26–31

Wuppermann T (1994) Doppler- und Duplexsonographie der Venen. Internist (Berl) 35:539–545

Zeitler E, Milbert L, Richter E-I, Ringelmann W, Strohm CH (1983) Spezielle Komplikationen der Beinphlebographie. ROFO 138(6):670–677

13.2
Lymphography

13.2.1
Technique

During the 1950s lymphography became a routine procedure as a special, diagnostically relevant method established by KINMONTH (1952). It is a dissective procedure followed by graphic imaging of lymphatic vessels and lymph nodes by means of contrast media (CM) and X-rays. The imaging is on single films. The peripheral puncture of a lymphatic vessel performed in a centripetal flow direction is followed by the slow application of the CM when the intraluminal position of the cannula has been established.

The examination procedure starts with the subcutaneous injection of Patentblau V 2.5% (BYK Gulden, Konstanz, Germany) with a local anesthetic (Xylonest 1% (Astra Yedel)) in a mixed injector between the first and second, as well as the fourth and fifth digit. In rare cases the lymphotropic dye can be applied below the malleolus tibialis (MÜLLER and GÜNTER 1979) and the proximal carpal bones, respectively. As early as 10 min later the dissection of the vessel can start, as distal as possible in the case of repeat lymphography. The blue-greenish colored lymph vessels can be seen through the skin. In the case of lymphography of the upper extremities it may take a little longer until the blue color can be perceived through the skin (Fig. 13.13). A dissective phase follows in which the skin can be incised by longitudinal or crosswise cuts. In the case of a repeat lymphography longitudinal incisions have proved successful.

The uncovered vessel is tied with a stitch proximally (thread 2.5 EP/60 E or Supolene 3 EP/2/0 Ethicon, Norderstadt, Germany) in order to produce resistance for the puncture and the insertion of the cannula (Fig. 13.13).

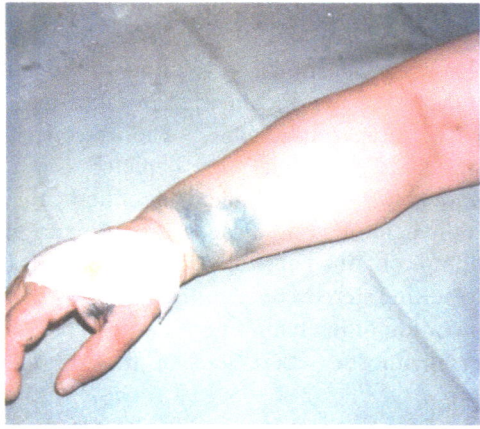

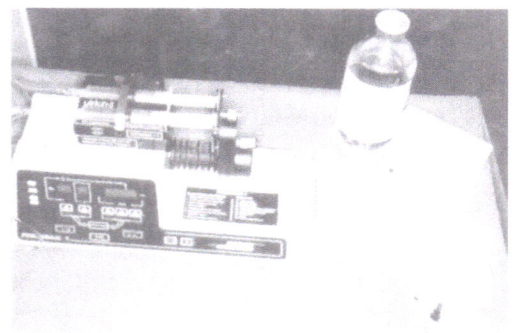

Fig. 13.14. Automatically controlled pressure injection device for lymphography

Fig. 13.13. Diffuse spreading of lymphotrophic color, Patentblau V, above the distal radial region in a woman with breast cancer

Putting the needle as deep as possible into the vessel guarantees that the oily CM (Lipiodol ultrafluid, Byk Gulden, Konstanz) flows freely and undisturbed. The Lipiodol enters the vessel under mechanically constant pressure (0.4 atm). The flow rate is related to the pressure (Fig. 13.14). Correspondingly, the duration of the injection is up to 2 h. To keep the needle safe in the vessel for the time of injection, the needle should be fixed. Losses of CM are avoided compared to newer systems. At the end of the injection phase the skin incision, 0.5–1 cm long, is treated with an adheive plaster. The preparation time until the vessel is connected to the injection system does not last longer than 5–10 min.

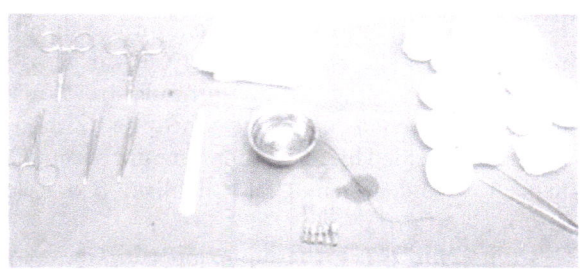

Fig. 13.15. Aseptic table with required instrumentation

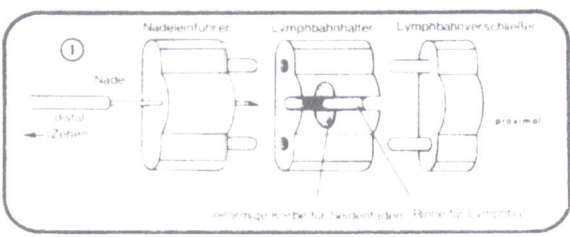

Fig. 13.16. One of the various concepts of lymphography sets

13.2.2
Equipment

Large-scale instruments are not necessary. The sterile table (Fig. 13.15) is equipped with 10-ml one-way syringes for the local anesthetic and the oily CM. Furthermore, there must be a 0.70 × 32-mm injection needle, small flat swabs, sterile stitches made of thread or Pyrolene (approximately two skin clamps 20 cm), and two little anatomic forceps, a scalpel, as well as NaCl 0.9%. Besides the needles with elastic mandrin in different thicknesses designed by RÜTTIMANN and DEL BUONO (1964) according to the Troiquar principle, there are different concepts of lymphography sets available on the market (Angiomed, Ettlingen; Vygon, New Hampshire; biotrol, Melsungen).

They are composed of short, some sharply polished, needles with or without wings and a supply tube made of polyethylene as a one-way system. (Fig. 13.16).

For examiners with poor eyesight a forehead magnifying glass is recommended. Optimal light conditions are essential, e.g., the use of an operating lamp. Engine-operated injectors (Ulrich Ulm-Donau, Braun-Melsungen AG) guarantee constant pressure (0.4 atm) and flow (Fig. 13.17).

Lipiodol ultrafluid (1 ml contains 380 mg iodine), Neo-Hydriol Fluid, and Ethiodol are all oily CM. The amount required is relative to the body weight of the patient. In general, 0.08–0.1 ml/kg body weight

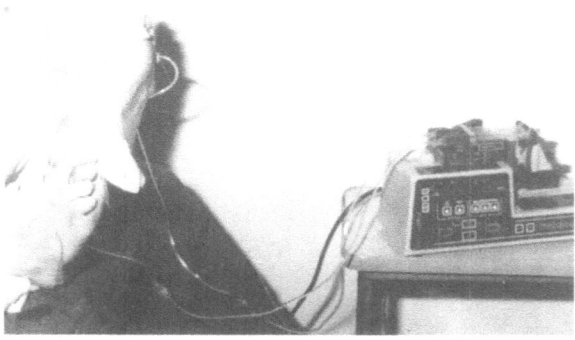

Fig. 13.17. Contrast medium injection phase with elevation of the patient's feet

for adults and 2–5 ml per body side for children. Frequently, 5 ml in total is sufficient for imaging the peripheral vessels. The amount of CM can also be calculated according to the formula by BUHTZ (1974): body length of the person to be examined minus 100 divided by 10. The low amount of oily CM helps to avoid systemic fat embolism (COLLARD 1973).

Urographin 76% (Schering AG, Berlin, Germany) or non-ionic CM (for example Solutrast, (BYK Gulden, Konstanz, Germany) Omnipaque, Schering AG, Berlin, Germany and others) are recommended as non-watersoluble CM with low viscosity. They diffuse through the vessel wall so that blurred outlines, especially of the vessels on the level of the thigh and in the area of the groin, can be seen (SCHMIDT et al. 1978). New CM which can be applied subcutaneously (e.g., Isovist, Schering) with the active substance Iotrolan have a low chemotoxicity. Isovist is non-ionic, lymphotropic and has a very good tissue tolerance. Originally, this CM was used only in the peritoneal, thoracic, and neck areas (TAENZER 1982).

13.2.3
Imaging

13.2.3.1
Conventional

Following mechanical injection of the CM, the imaging of the lymph system is performed on single films with the patient in an a.p. position. The X-ray unit is equipped with a X-ray tube located above the X-ray table and a tube focus of 1.3 mm or smaller (0.6 mm). The focus-film distance is 115 cm. The necessary cassette size is 35 × 43 cm with a class 400 film-foil combination.

At first only the lymphatic vessels are recognizable on the X-ray film. Since the lymph nodes fill themselves proportional to the flow of the CM, the second part of the documentation takes place 24 h after the preparative phase. The retroperitoneal lymph nodes can also be depicted via stereo technique instead of single and oblique imaging. With the help of a binocular it is possible to project the photos obtained optically one on top of the other. The resulting stereoscopic impression allows a better demarcation of the lymph nodes and – above all – a better diagnostic assessment of the lymph node pattern.

VON RAUTENFELD (1993, 1994) reported on lymphography in a new dimension. With the help of a microfocus X-ray technique which enlarges directly (Direct Magnification (DIMA) R-image-intensifier-cinematography) it was possible for the first time to image the initial skin and organ lymph vessels after the application of a CM in permanent infusion and to watch the flow behavior of the lymph.

13.2.3.2
Digital Modalities

Complementary to the endolymphatic method, echography is a valuable diagnostic tool for the pre- and post-therapeutic diagnosis of malignant diseases in lymph nodes. The benefit lies in the outpatient after-care in order to assess lymph node status.

The ultrasound method is indicated in the cranial para-aortic region if, for example, the thoracic duct already starts on the level of L4–5 so that the upper para-aortic lymph nodes cannot be imaged. Or, if the primary lymph node stations of the urogenital organs are only incompletely imaged through the ascending lymphography.

Ultrasound examination is also appropriate for the secondarily blastomatous involvement of lymph nodes in order to assess the full extent of the destruction. In the same way the lymph node stations above a blockade of lymph vessels can be defined by ultrasound. A negative ultrasound diagnosis on the level of a lymphatic blockade requires a search for other reasons. Each echo-free zone of a lymph node in the ultrasound tomogram is related to malignantly changed tissues.

In order to guarantee that it is in fact a lymphocyst, an ultrasound examination alone is enough. However, the distinction between a lymphocyst and a cystically decomposing tumor by ultrasound is not definite. Nevertheless, ultrasound is filling a diagnostic gap. The limitation of the method is the size of the lymph nodes. The minimum diameter required for imaging a lymph node by ultrasound is 2–3 cm (KRATOCHWIL et al. 1975).

Subtly differentiated ways of scanning are possible with differently configured transducers available on the market, whereby width and quality of imaging, and finally also the handling vary (GEBEL 1995).

In the case of the color-coded duplex sonography (angiodynography) the B-mode sonogram is over-laid by colored flow information. Changes in perfusion show the pathology of a lymph node without giving additional CM. Although a definite distinction between a benign and a malignant lymph node has not been possible up to now, improvements in the diagnosis of lymph node metastases from 60% to 73% should be reached via determination of the peripheral flow resistance (TSCHAMMLER et al. 1991).

13.2.3.3
Computed Tomography and Magnetic Resonance Tomography

Due to their normal size of 0.5–1.0 cm in diameter the lymph nodes lie at the lower limit of computed tomographic resolution. Surrounding fat tissue is crucial for recognizing the lymph nodes. In the course of the big vessels of the neck, the thorax, and the abdomen better diagnostic conditions are present, especially when the density of vessels is increased by additional CM.

There are no diagnostic difficulties in lymph node conglomerates in general, even if the liver and spleen hili are considered. The advantage of a lymphography compared to a CT examination is in the recognition of the internal structures of the lymph nodes and lower exposure to radiation, although CT is less invasive and less time-consuming.

If the histology is already known and the CT findings are clear, one can abstain from a dissective ascending lymphography (WEGENER 1992).

As in CT, retroperitoneal lymph nodes are considered normal also in magnetic resonance to-mography (MRT) up to a size of 1.5 cm. They can be seen more rarely in the MRT because of inferior spatial resolution.

The diagnosis of a lymph node metastasis is based on lymph node enlargement and not on signal intensity (SI) behavior. Inhomogeneous SI changes of the lymph node indicate necrolysis or calcifications. On T2 weighted images the devitalized tissue shows a lower SI than vital lymphatic tissue. The nuclear spin technique is preferred for differentiation of scar tissue (weak MR signal) and also for lymph node metastases. Assessing the role of CT and MRT, examination by CT after peroral and i.v. CM has priority in the diagnosis of retroperitoneal and crural lymph node processes (REISER and SEMMLER 1992). With his outlook for the further development of MR CM, LANIADO (1997) hints at the possibility of lymph node imaging in nuclear spin by using rapid sequences.

13.2.3.4
Indirect Methods

In the 1960s lymphology with radionuclides was developed as an alternative procedure to dissective lymphography. Besides its special practicability, the need for this method, performed with [198]Au colloidals, became apparent in patients with malignant tumors necessarily undergoing numerous control examinations over several years in order to recognize lymphatic changes post radiation and to outline the irradiation field. If an ascending lymphography is primarily impossible, this pro-cedure with its partly limited diagnostic value is frequently used (ZUM WINKEL 1972). But isotope lymphography has not died out yet, even if it has lost its original character. The formerly used [198]Au colloid with a half-life of 2.7 days (420 keV, β-radiation) was replaced by [99m]technetium-marked colloids (half-life 6 h, 140 keV, without β-radiation) (ZUM WINKEL 1990). The exposure to radiation after application of 1 mCi (37 MBq) maximum could be reduced drastically and was about 70 rd (700 mGy) at the point of injection and 2.7 rd (27 mGy) at the lymph nodes (MOSTBECK 1986).

Isotope lymphography is preferred for the clarification of functional questions concerning lymphatic transport (THÄMMIG et al. 1993). This includes not only defects in lymphatic drainage in the arms and legs (see Fig. 13.18), but also the selective imaging of the mammaria interna draining areas in the case of breast cancer [e.g., ^{99m}Tc-tincolloid (Nanocoll, Amersham Buchler, Braunschweig, Germany), 2 × 1 MBq s.c.].

In the case of malignant melanoma before surgery, the regional lymphatic drainage vessels are marked s.c. or i.c. scintigraphically (SCHICHA 1991).

In addition, more rare indications for a lymphoscintigraphy are the proof of lymphatic fistula, lymphocysts after kidney transplantation, lympho-drainage due to esophageal carcinoma, examinations concerning lymphokinetics with lymphovenous anastomoses, differentiation of the primary and secondary lymphoedema (Fig. 13.18).

Although until now it was not possible to develop substances for use in clinical routine which deposit preferably at the lymphatic system after i.v. injection, the elegant procedure of indirect lymphography has been revived through the development of the water-soluble, iso-osmolar, nephrotropic CM Isovist (Jotrolan/Schering AG, Berlin, Germany). This technique has been developed by WENZEL-HORA et al. (1985) and clinically proven by PARTSCH et al. (1985). The CM is injected exactly subepidermally into the interdigits or into the swollen areas of the extremity. In this way the initial lymphatics, the precollectors, and the collectors are imaged non-invasively (GMEINWIESER 1988). Isovist is excellently tolerated and can therefore be applied basically in every region of the body. The subepidermal infusion leads to an increase in local tissue pressure, by which a crossing of this CM into the initial lymphatics takes place (WEISSLEDER 1991). Compared with the previously performed conventional lymphography with Lipiodol, it is now possible, according to PARTSCH et al. (1985) to differentiate four forms of the primary lymphedema, the secondary lymphedema, the lipedema, and an edema due to chronic venous insufficiency.

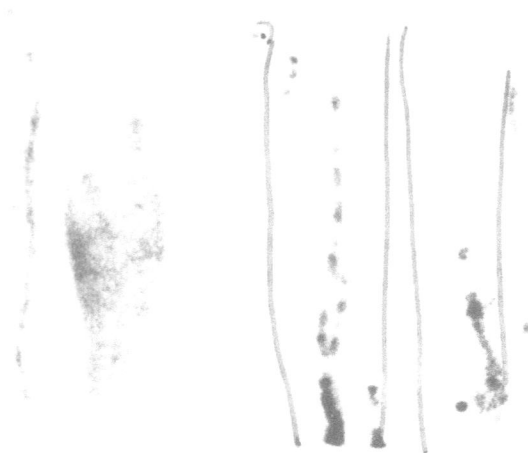

Fig. 13.18. Lymphscintigraphy using 99mTc-Nanocolloid. In the right section of the image the left extremity shows an extremely delayed lymphatic drainage. 2 h later a concentration of nuclide in the soft tissue due to impaired drainage was observed

13.2.4
Indications

With the latest methods such as for example US, CT, and MRT, the number of dissective lymphographies has been minimized. Its use is indicated in the case of localized and generalized soft-tissue swellings of the extremities. Primary and secondary, as well as traumatically caused abnormalities of the lymph vessels which have lead to a lymphedema, can be diagnosed. For the diagnosis of chronic extremity swellings the direct lymphography is obsolete. It is sometimes necessary to prove or to exclude lymphatic damage when artificial lymphedema exists.

13.2.5
Complications

Under normal conditions complications rarely happen. The lymphotropic dye "Patentblau" (2,4-disulfo-5-hydroxy-4′, 4≤bis-diethylamino-triphenylcarbinol monosodium salt) has a high sensitization rate. The dye contains three nuclei with para-amino groups, which are supposed to cause allergic reactions.

This is an immediate reaction which starts locally in most cases and which can very quickly affect the total integument. Life-threatening situations can occur through shock. The assumption is that dyes with triphenyl combinations (food, textiles, agriculture) increase the chance of allergy towards "Patentblau". In such situations it is advantageous to have a venous access in order to infuse 500 ml NaCl almost as bolus to have the circulation diluted quickly. In most cases this is sufficient together with intensive monitoring.

Additional medication is necessary when the state of the patient does not improve. Lipiodol can also cause allergic reactions. In the case of limited lung function and reduced heart function fat emboli of the lung (COLLARD 1973) caused by the CM are life-threatening. The CM given remains in the lung filter 50% longer under these circumstances. The increase in temperature (resorption fever; RICHTER and ZEITLER 1986) during the course of the evening of the examination day is less important. Local lymphangitis, lymph fistula, or pseudo-lymphocysts are detected in 0.1%–1%. Wound infections or wound healing problems should not occur if asepticism is ensured. But this kind of complication is described by FUCHS (1965) and KÖHLER (1968) in connection with disturbances of the arterial circulation and distinct lymphedema. Cerebral incidents are possible because of a right-left shunt of the heart. Paravascular CM is sometimes to be seen in the X-ray picture after the injection phase, pointing to excessive application pressures. The pressure should therefore not go beyond 0.5 (atmospheric excess pressure).

13.2.6
Informed Consent

Before the procedure a conversation between doctor and patient should take place to give the patient the necessary information. The patient is given the reason for the examination, as well as a short outline of the course including an anatomic sketch.

Since an iodine-containing CM will be applied, which remains in the body over a longer period before its metabolism, it is necessary to talk about possible complications. Analyzing the dialogue, the doctor decides whether a special preparation for the lymphography is required (e.g., risk-increasing variants in the case of allergic diathesis, thyroid and kidney diseases) or whether the examination cannot be performed because there is, for example, a right-left shunt of the heart.

The advantages and disadvantages with regard to other methods should be considered, as well as possible subsequent interventions. The patient is legally entitled to think about it and it is therefore sensible to have this conversation 1–2 days prior to the planned procedure. Information in tabula is not legally acceptable.

13.2.7
Pre- and Postprocedure Care

On the evening before the directly ascending lymphography and on the days of examination the patients have to keep a non-fatty diet. The chest X-ray performed 24h following application of the CM determines subsequent diet. On the day of examination the patient need not abstain from food and liquid intake. Potentially existing edemas should be relieved as well as possible in order to make discovering and preparation of the lymphatic vessels easier. If necessary the back of the hand or foot should be shaved; in all cases feet and toes should be cleaned. A short time before the examination feet and hands are cleaned with alcohol and then sprayed with colorless disinfectant. The patient's medical

history and current treatment can be taken from the medical report. A relevant chest X-ray and an ECG should also be presented before the lymphography. Nervous patients receive a sedative with night-time medication and small children up to 6 years of age receive general anesthesia during the procedure. In the case of the latter, the time of examination including the X-ray documentation does not exceed approximately 30 min in total.

There is no special premedication required for lymphography. In the case of existing allergies including hay fever, asthma, or food allergies to citrus fruit, strawberries, milk and mushrooms, and in the case of a plaster, as well as iodine-intolerance, a 3-day preparation with 40 mg corticosteroids every day is indicated. In extreme cases, on the day of examination H_1- and H_2-antagonists are applied i.v. additionally. Venous transbrachial access via angiocath then remains 24 and 48h, respectively.

Since on the day of examination a high resorption fever (39–42°C) can appear, the patient should stay in bed for up to 24h post injection. If generalized distress occurs, it is sufficient to give antipyretics and apply cold compresses to the leg. Constant fever points to complications. A non-fatty diet will be continued until the X-ray series on the second day is completed. The adhesive plaster over the skin incision can be changed after 4 days. Until final healing the small wound area must be kept dry (Hansaplast, Beiersdorf AG, Hamburg, Germany; possibly waterproof), but not treated with powder.

References

Buhtz C, Lüning M, Mach S, Melzer B, Röder K (1974) Standardisierungsempfeh-lungen für die Fußlymphographie. Radiol Diagn 15:503

Collard M (1973) Fettembolie. Witzstrock, Baden-Baden

Fuchs WA (1965) Lymphographie und Tumordiagnostik. Springer, Berlin Heidelberg New York

Gebel M (1995) Sonographie. In: Heuck F, Müller K-HG, Kaiserling E (eds) Klinische Radiologie – Lymphgefäßsystem, Lymphatisches Gewebe Diagnostik mit bildgebenden Verfahren. Springer, Berlin Heidelberg New York, pp 23–29

Gmeinwieser J, Lehner K, Golder W (1988) Indirekte Lymphographie: Indikationen, Technik, klinische Ergebnisse. ROFO 149(6):642–647

Kinmonth JB (1952) Lymphangiography in man. Clin Sci 11:13

Koehler PR (1968) Complications of lymphography. Lymphology 1:116

Kratochwil A, Kärcher K-H, Jentzsch K, Wolf G (1975) Die Wertigkeit und Grenzen der Echographie für die Diagnostik abdomineller Lymphome bei malignen Erkrankungen. ROFO 122(5):410–417

Laniado M (1997) Magnetresonanztomographie-Symposium "Schnelle MR-Bildgebung", February 15, Mannheim

Mostbeck A (1986) Isotopenmethoden. In: Simon HJ, Schoop W (eds) Diagnostik in der Kardiologie und Angiologie. Thieme, Stuttgart, pp 567–571

Müller K-HG, Günter H (1979) Lymphographie. Anatomie-Technik-Diagnostik. Springer, Berlin Heidelberg New York

Partsch H, Wenzel-Hora BJ, Urbanek A (1983) Differential diagnosis of lymphedema after indirect lymphography with Iotasul. Lymphology 16:12–18

Partsch H, Urbanek A, Wenzel-Hora BJ (1985) Indirect lymphography in various forms of primary lymphoedema. In: Bollinger A, Partsch H, Wolfe JHN (eds) The inital lymphatics. Thieme, Stuttgart, pp 147–157

Reiser M, Semmler W (eds) (1992) Magnetresonanztomographie. Springer, Berlin Heidelberg New York

Richter E-I (1995) Voraussetzungen und Methoden zur Darstellung des Lymphsystems. In: Heuck F, Müller K-HG, Kaiserling E (eds) Klinische Radiologie – Lymphsystem, Lymphatisches Gewebe. Springer, Berlin Heidelberg New York, pp 18–23

Richter E-I, Zeitler E (1986) Lymphographie. In: Simon HJ, Schoop W (eds) Diagnostik in der Kardiologie und Angiologie. Thieme, Stuttgart, pp 572–581

Rüttimann A, del Buono MS (1964) In: Ergebnisse der medizinischen Strahlenforschung. vol 1 Schinz HR, Glanner R, Rüttermann A (eds) Thieme Stuttgart, pp 413–434

Schicha H (1991) Kompendium der Nuklearmedizin. Schattauer, Stuttgart, pp 285–287

Schmidt KR, Welter H, Pfeifer KJ, Becker HM (1978) Lymphographische Untersuchungen zum Extremitätenödem nach rekonstruktiven Gefäßeingriffen im Femoropoplitealbereich. ROFO 128(2):194–202

Taenzer V (1982) Lymphography with the water-soluble contrast medium Jotasul. Radiology today II. June 22–27, Salzburg

Thämmig R, Godehardt E, Friedrich M, Herrmann H (1993) Aussagewert der parasternalen Lymphoszintigraphie mit Mikrokolloiden bei der Stadienbe-stimmung und Nachsorge des Mammakarzinoms. ROFO 158(1):62–66

Tschammler A, Gunzer G, Rinhart E, Höhmann D, Feller AC, Müller W, Lackner (1991) Dignitätsbeurteilung vergrößerter Lymphknoten durch qualitative und semiquantitative Auswertung der Lymphknotenperfusion mit der farbkodierten Duplexsonographie. ROFO 154:414–418

Tschammler A, Knitter J, Wittenberg G, Krahe T, Hahn D (1995) Quantifizierung der Lymphknotenperfusion mittels farbkodierter Duplexsonographie ROFO 163(3):203–209

von Rautenfeld, D Berens (1993, 1994) Lymphographie in einer neuen Dimension. Vasomed 5:664–668; vasomed 6:38–43

Wegener OH (1992) Ganzkörpercomputertomographie. Blackwell Wissenschaft, Berlin, pp 459–461

Weissleder H (1991) Indirekte Lymphographie. In: Peters PE, Zeitler E (eds) Röntgenkontrastmittel. Springer, Berlin Heidelberg New York, pp 175–180

Wenzel-Hora BJ, Partsch H, Urbanek A (1985) Indirect lymphography with Iotasul. In: Bollinger A, Partsch H, Wolfe JHN (eds) The initial lymphatics. Thieme, Stuttgart, pp 117–122

Zum Winkel K (1963) Zur Technik der indirekten abdominellen Lypmhkno-tenszintigraphie mit 198 – Au colloidale. Nucl Med 3:148

Zum Winkel K (1972) Lymphologie mit Radionukliden. Hoffmann, Berlin

Zum Winkel K (1990) Nuklearmedizin. Springer, Berlin Heidelberg New York, pp 278–286

14 Out-Patient Angioplasty Management: Organizational Concepts

W. LÖSCH, B. HOLIK and E. ZEITLER

CONTENTS

14.1 Introduction

The evolution in vascular radiology involving the use of ultra-thin catheters and improved techniques has led to a minimization of risks without compromising the quality of percutaneous interventional procedures (GROSS-FENGELS et al. 1998; GÜNTHER 1993; LEMARBRE et al. 1987; MANASHIL et al. 1983; RIESER and RÜCKNER 1995; ROGERS and KRAFT 1990; SOULIER-PARMEGGIAN 1992; STRUK et al. 1993;). These newer developments now enable us to perform such procedures in our private imaging center on an out-patient basis, for which there is growing demand (ZEITLER 1998).

14.2 Diagnostic Work-Up

The diagnostic work-up to percutaneous transluminal angioplasty usually includes Doppler sonography with peripheral pressure gradient measurements and, most importantly of all, a recent angiography, as well as relevant anamnesis and physical and functional examinations. Standard laboratory testing including blood count, thromboplastin time (Quick), partial thromboplastin time, and creatinine and thyroid function tests are obligatory.

Recent vessel occlusions requiring local lysis, carotic, aortic, or renal stenoses, occlusions extending over a distance of more than 10 cm or involving the whole common femoral artery, as well as vessel lesions in uncooperative patients or in the case of adipositas per magna are not considered suitable for out-patient interventions. Severe anemia, bleeding disorders, significant renal failure, or hyperthyroidism should be excluded. Arterial hypertension, as long as it is adequately controlled, should not be considered a contraindication to out-patient intervention.

In general, vascular interventions are indicated in patients showing a clinical Fontaine stage IIb or higher. Patients classified as stage IIa may be considered suitable for intervention should their age, profession, or physical consideration favor such measures. Incidentally, outpatients are selected according to the recommendations set out by the Society of Cardiovascular and Interventional Radiology (see Chap. 5, Sect. 5.1) or the regulations of the German radiological society regarding radiological interventions (LIBICHER et al. 1997).

The patient should be informed of the technicalities of the procedure and possible complications at least 48h prior to the intervention. Follow-up management and required patient compliance should be given special consideration. At least 2 days before the intervention, platelet aggregation blockers, e.g., acetylsalicylic acid 300–500 mg/day, should be prescribed orally and should be continued at a maintained dose of 100 mg/day for at least 6 months. Since older patients with multiple pathology require regular medication, they are given appointments for their intervention between 10 and 12 o'clock so that they can be allowed a light breakfast between 6 and 7 o'clock together with their usual medication.

W. LÖSCH, MD, B. HOLIK, MD, Praxis Drs. Holik–Frank–Meusel–Lösch, Wetterkreuz 21, 91058 Erlangen-Tennenlohe, Germany
E. ZEITLER, Professor, MD, Virchowstraße 13, 90409 Nürnburg, Germany

14.3
Procedure

Balloon angioplasty is performed using modern flat-profile catheters and guidewires introduced through sheaths of 4–7F. At the beginning of the intervention, 5000IU heparin is administered intraarterially; if a stent implant is required, however, 8000IU heparin is infused. Should complications arise, for example, an acute embolus (Fig. 14.1), the intervention must be extended using the appropriate equipment.

14.4
Follow-Up Management

Following a successful intervention, the catheter and sheath are removed and the puncture site is compressed for approximately 15–25min. A compression bandage is then applied for 48h and bed rest is prescribed for 24h. In the case of interventions in the vicinity of the puncture site, a percutaneous hemostatic closure device [for example, Angio-Seal, Kensey Nash Corp., hemostatic puncture closure de-

vice (7–8F), or Perclose, the Prostav system (9–11F)] should be introduced instead. Follow-up management within the practice (out-patient clinic) includes an observation period of 4–6h, with hourly pulse and blood pressure measurements. Following this period, the patient is transported home lying down in an ambulance. The patient is prescribed further bed rest for 24h and should get up only to visit the bathroom.

During the following night, the doctor responsible should remain on call. On the following day, the patient should report back to the clinic on his/her condition during the previous night. Due to the possibility of serious complications occurring, such interventions should be performed in cooperation with a vascular surgical clinic or center for further clinical management. After 4–6 weeks, an out-patient visit to check pulse, peripheral Doppler values and Doppler gradients, together with a duplex sonography of the treated vessel segment is mandatory. Findings should be compared to the pre-intervention status.

To summarize, out-patient angioplasty in itself does not carry a higher risk than a similar intervention performed under in-patient conditions as long

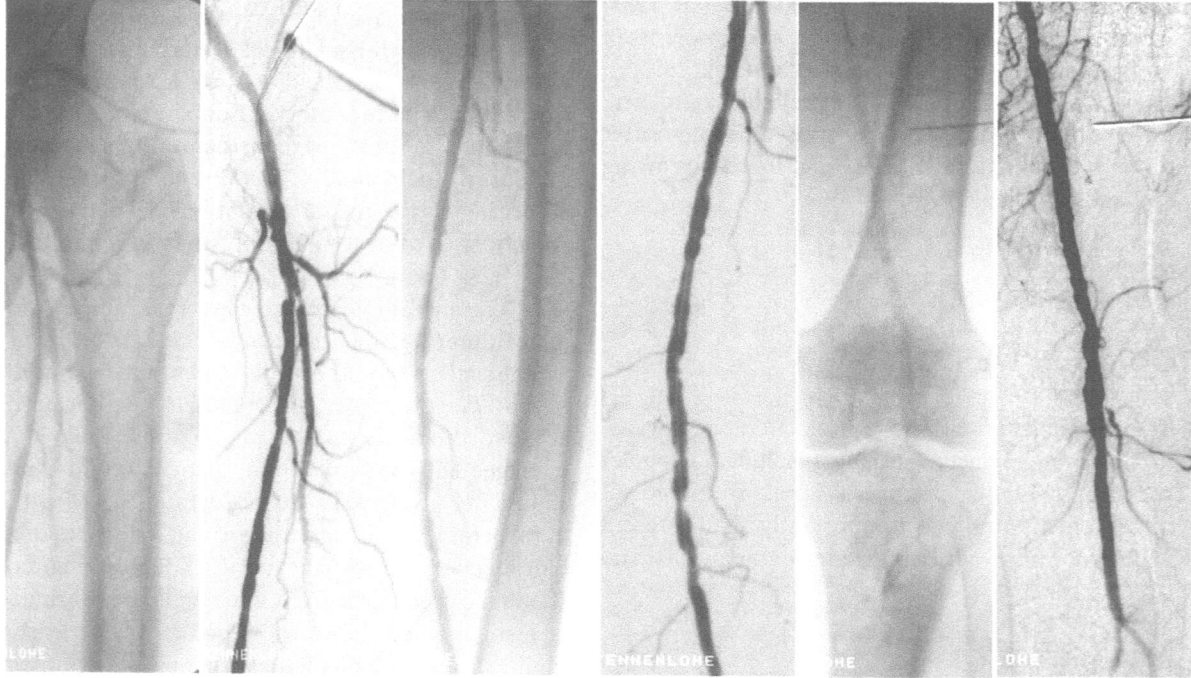

Fig. 14.1 a–c. A 78-year-old overweight patient who has smoked for more than 40 years. Condition following CABG (coronary artery bypass graft) 2 years previously. Walking distance over previous 6 months, less than 150m, Doppler ratio, 0.6. **a** Initial findings. **b** Following percutaneous transluminal angioplasty of superficial femoral artery stenosis, acute embolization to the crural arteries. **c** Following local lysis using 100000IU urokinase and percutaneous aspiration thrombectomy. Follow-up after 4 weeks: Doppler ratio 0.9, subjectively asymptomatic

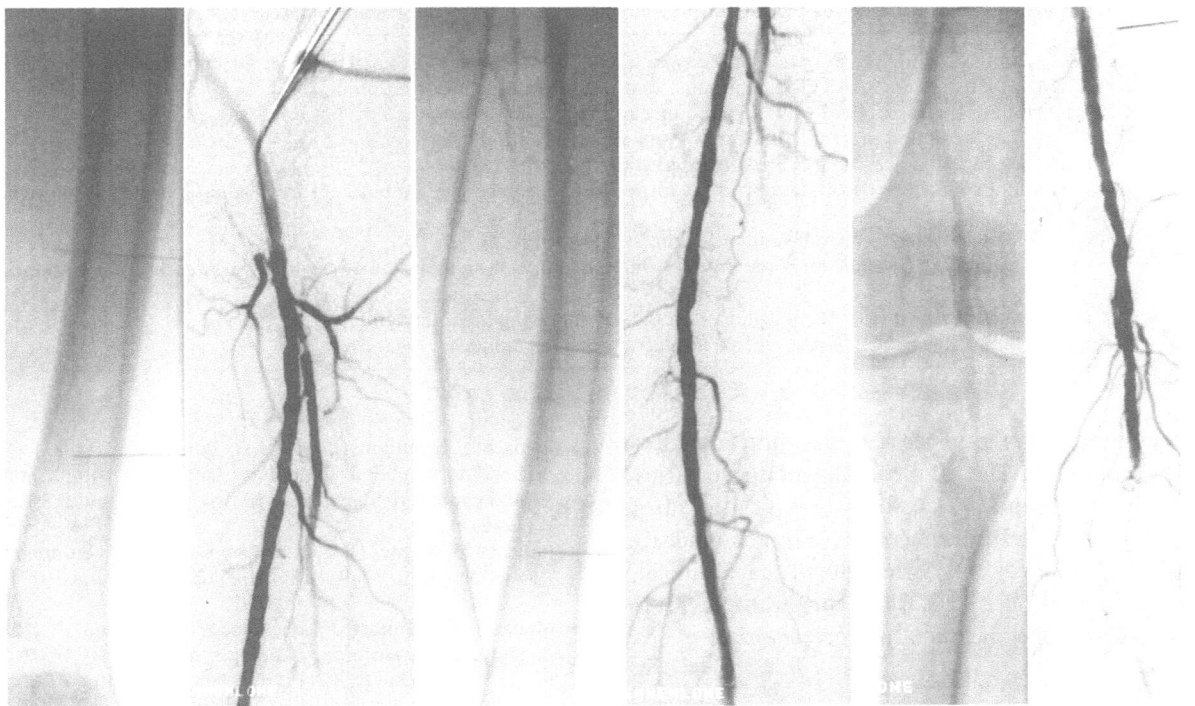

b

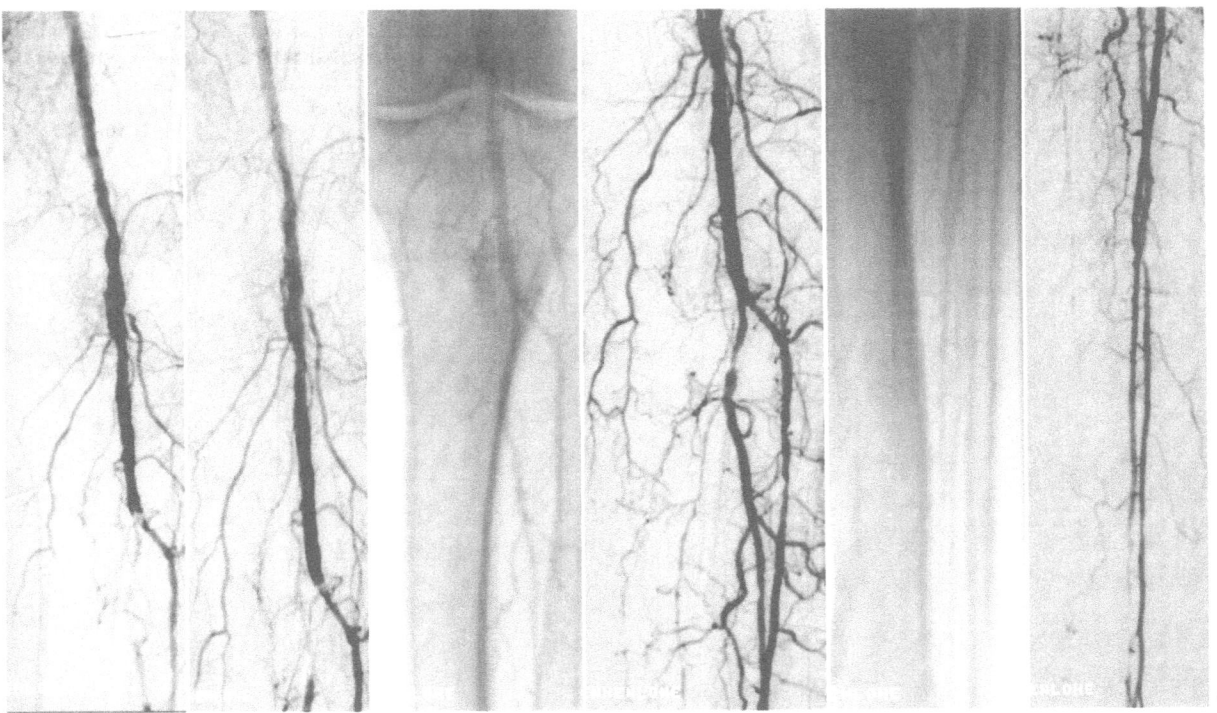

c

Table 14.1. Prerequisites of carrying out an out-patient percutaneous transluminal angioplasty

- Relevant anamnesis with determination of the vascular status, including pulses and peripheral Doppler pressure values
- Availability of a recent angiographic examination in order to plan the intervention
- Determination of the basic blood values, including clotting factors
- Interdisciplinary planning regarding indications and the intervention itself
- Informing the patient at least 48 h before the intervention
- Introduction of adjuvant medical therapy in the form of a platelet aggregation blocker (acetylsalicylic acid 300–500 mg/day)
- Application of a compression bandage for 48 h with strict bed rest for 24 h
- The patient should not be alone on the night following the intervention and should be within easy reach of the responsible doctor/clinic
- The patient should report back (by telephone) on the day following the intervention
- Required technical/medical experience of such interventional techniques

as certain prerequisites are taken into consideration (Table 14.1). The local complication rate varies between 1% and 3% (Gross-Fengels et al. 1998; Rieser and Rückner 1995; Rogers and Kraft 1990; Zeitler 1998), while the primary clinical success rate is over 90%. Close cooperation with a vascular surgical dartment is a prerequisite.

References

Gross-Fengels W, Mückner K, Imig H, Schröder A, Wagenhofer KU, Siemens P (1998) Möglichkeiten und Risiken der ambulanten PTA bei Patienten mit peripherer arterieller Verschlußkrankheit. Fortschr Rontgenstr 168[2]:175–179

Günther RW (1993) Ambulante periphere Angioplastie: Sicherheit und Grenzen. Fortschr Rontgenstr 158:391–392

Lemarbre L, Hudon G, Coche G, Bourassa M (1987) Outpatient peripheral angioplasty: survey of complications and patients' perceptions. AJR Am J Roentgenol 148:1239–1240

Libicher M, Richter GM, Kaufmann GW (1997) Leitlinien für Radiologische Interventionen. Fortschr Rontgenstr 167: L1–L46

Manashil GB, Thunstrom BS, Thorpe CD, Lipson SR (1983) Outpatient transluminal angioplasty. Radiology 147:7–8

Rieser R, Rückner R (1995) Die ambulante PTA zur Behandlung der arteriellen Verschlußkrankheit. Fortschr Rontgenstr 162[4]:330–334

Rogers WF, Kraft MA (1990) Outpatient angioplasty. Radiology 174:753–755

Soulier-Parmeggiani L, Schneider PA, Bounameaux H (1992) Outpatient percutaneous transluminal angioplasty for peripheral arterial disease. Eur J Med 1:13–15

Struk DW, Rankin RN, Eliasziw M, Vellet AD (1993) Safety of outpatient peripheral angioplasty. Radiology 189:193–196

Zeitler E (1998) PTA is an outpatient procedure. J Invas cardiology 10

15 The Vascular Center

B.T. KATZEN and G. J. BECKER

CONTENTS

15.1 Introduction

The 1990s have ushered in new technologies for the treatment of vascular disease at an unsurpassed pace. At the same time, in the United States, changes in the regulatory and economic aspects of medical practice have created unprecedented competitive pressures in the field of vascular care. In other environments, other factors such as ego and political "turf" have contributed to underlying competitive pressures. These pressures have added fuel to an ever-smoldering turf struggle between specialists interested in this field, most notably vascular surgeons, interventional radiologists, and cardiologists, although a few vascular medicine specialists have also participated in conflict. Recently, a considerable amount of rhetoric and commentary regarding perceived roles, responsibilities, and privileges of the various disciplines has been expressed in journals and at meetings of professional societies and postgraduate courses. In hospitals heated credentialing battles have occurred. Pressures to create change undoubtedly create conflicts between affected

parties, but they also create opportunity for innovative solutions to manage change.

The author's observation over many years of practice in university and community hospital settings is that "turf wars" are generally conducted at great cost to all parties. The usual outcome is a hostile environment and the lack of a clear winner. More often than not, everyone involved loses in the end, including the patients. It became clear in my early years of practice that great benefit could be derived from high levels of physician cooperation, benefiting not only the physicians involved, but the systems in which we work, and more importantly the patients whom we serve.

The model of a vascular institute that integrates the knowledge, skills, and practices of the various physicians involved in the care of cardiovascular patients is one that has worked for us at the Miami Cardiac and Vascular Institute (MCVI) (BECKER & KATZEN 1996). The mission of the insitute is to provide the best in the diagnosis, treatment, and prevention of cardiovascular diseases. Pursuit of the goals directed toward this mission has required and continues to require physician leadership, a visionary hospital board and administration, a hospital medical staff whose trust has been earned, and major commitments, primarily to patient care, but also to teaching and research. In the 8 years since the MCVI was founded, all of our plans, policies, procedures, and accomplishments in patient care and research have been outgrowths of our mission and of the commitment of physicians from all cardiovascular disciplines to work together in solving problems of mutual interest. Our patients have been the principal beneficiaries.

15.2 Factors Favoring the Development of Vascular Centers

Vascular surgeons and interventional radiologists are particularly well suited and positioned to com-

BARRY T. KATZEN, MD; G. J. BECKER, MD, Miami Cardiac and Vascular Institute, 8900 North Kendall Drive, Miami, FL 33176, USA

bine efforts and create solutions to suit both their needs and those of their patients with vascular disease. Prominent among the factors making this true are: (a) A common patient base that reflects a common commitment to vascular disorders; (b) complementary skills; (c) a common interest in emerging technologies (this is particularly true in the field of endovascular therapies); (d) a common set of reporting standards in peripheral arterial disease; (e) an increasing tendency in the United States for large purchasers of health care services to purchase these services as a package (i.e., cardiovascular or vascular care services) (SCHWARTZ 1995); (f) an increase in mergers between practices which, although basically defensive in origin, has great potential for spawning creative and productive partnerships (although most mergers represent horizontal integration, i.e., combined practices within the same specialty, vertical integration across specialities is likely to increase in the future); and (g) a current movement afoot within the American Board of Medical Specialties to do away with certificates of added qualifications and special qualifications and replace them with a subcertification process that would enable holders of primary certification under one board to receive subcertification under another.

A review of these factors and their future impact, as well as the solutions of the MCVI follows below. At the Insitute, interventional radiologists practice this specialty full time and in addition accept clinical responsibility for the patients undergoing diagnostic evaluation or therapy. The interventionalist is an activist in the patient care environment, not simply performing procedures. This philosophy has been described previously and has resulted in the equal partnership of interventionalists in patient care.

15.2.1
Common Patient Base

In most hospitals, interventional radiologists and vascular surgeons cooperate and collaborate in the management of patients with vascular disease. In general, patients who are referred to radiology for endovascular therapy are referred by vascular surgeons. However, in many institutions, direct referrals to radiology by primary care specialists, subspecialty internists and others comprise a significant proportion of the interventional practice, making referrals *to* vascular surgeons increasingly common. While some of the latter referrals entail diagnosis and management of peripheral arterial

disease of the lower extremities, a significant proportion are for treatment of renovascular hypertension, vena cava syndromes, and an assortment of other problems for which interventional therapy offers less invasive solutions.

Vascular surgeons are not the only subspecialists to whom peripheral arterial disease (PAD) patients are referred. In many institutions, the cardiologist is the first subspecialist to evaluate the patient with symptoms or signs of PAD, in part because of the coincidence of peripheral and coronary arterial disease. In a few institutions, vascular medicine specialists have assumed this role and in Europe angiologists have a well established history of involvement in management of vascular disease, including the performance of invasive procedures. Interventional radiologists may also be responsible for bringing new peripheral vascular disease patients into the health care system. It is imperative that all interventionalists accepting direct referrals for peripheral vascular disease be knowledgeable and skilled in the diagnostic workup, epidemiology, natural history, and management of these patients and in the detection and management of comorbid conditions, including coronary heart disease and cerebrovascular disease. Only in recent years have subspecialty training programs in vascular and interventional radiology begun to address these concerns. However, now that accreditation of training programs by the Accreditation Council for Graduate Medical Education in the United States is a reality (to date there are 62 in North America and more awaiting accreditation) and now that the American Board of Radiology is offering certifying examinations for added qualifications in vascular and interventional radiology, these educational issues will remain in the foreground. In any event, it is important for interventionalists in all institutions to maintain a close working relationship with vascular surgeons. In this way, patients benefit from the knowledge and expertise of both subspecialists. At the MCVI both a surgeon and an interventionalist are involved in the management of nearly every patient with peripheral arterial disease, even when the patient is referred from elsewhere directly to interventional radiology.

15.2.2
Complementary Skills

Given the generally well-educated population that the MCVI serves, patients often present at a relatively early symptomatic stage of their disease. This is not to say that the disease is in an early stage. On the contrary, the disease is usually moderate to extensive, and *something* can be offered to almost every patient. The treatment philosophy at the MCVI is rather simple: Risk factor reduction receives top priority and monitored exercise is offered through our combined peripheral vascular and cardiac rehabilitation program to all patients with less than category 4 ischemic disease. However, symptom thresholds for percutaneous intervention are lower than those for surgery. When patients are candidates for invasive treatment and endovascular therapy is a reasonable option, patients almost always undergo endovascular therapy as the first line of treatment. MCVI surgeons agree with this philosophy and the collegial atmosphere has served our patients well. Surgical practices have also benefited by this approach. The increased number of patients in the system has led to a more than two-fold increase in the annual number of major vascular reconstructions performed by MCVI surgeons over the past 8 years.

This common treatment philosophy and collegial atmosphere have spawned other benefits that are realized on a daily basis. For example, dealing with such issues as limb salvage, difficult access for transluminal intervention, elective surgical closure after percutaneous intervention, and the moment-to-moment decisions on patients undergoing thrombolytic therapy followed by definitive therapy, has been rendered much simpler by virtue of our close working relationships.

15.2.3
Common Interest in Emerging Technologies

The emerging endovascular treatment of aortic aneurysms, various pseudoaneurysms, and arteriovenous (AV) fistulae has created intense interest by surgeons in endovascular techniques and resulting turf battles in many institutions. At the Institute we have viewed this as an opportunity for further cooperation. To interventional radiologists, these procedures represent an extension of skills long applied to angioplasty, stent deployment, embolization, infusion, intravascular ultrasonography, and other endovascular treatments. However, the patient population is new. Never before has transcatheter therapy been available for these patients. Aside from their role in the diagnostic imaging workup, never before have radiologists been

involved with aortic aneurysm patients. Therefore, interventionalist investigators now involved in clinical endograft protocols have had to learn quickly about the epidemiology, natural history, and conventional surgical management of aortic aneurysms. Without this basic knowledge, investigators would be ill-equipped to counsel patients on the likelihood of complications both with and without treatment. Conversely, surgeons have always been involved in the treatment of aneurysm patients, but with a conventional epidemiologic and surgical approach. Now they are confronted with an entirely new method of therapy that in general requires surgical skills for access, but a different set of skills for safe and proper deployment of an endograft. These essential facts legitimize the roles of both subspecialists in the management of patients with aneurysm.

At the MCVI we have managed to develop a unique routine for handling endograft cases. We perform all of these procedures in a special endovascular suite (KATZEN et al. 1996) in the Institute that has been configured to serve as an operating room. The decision to perform all endograft procedures in the endovascular suite at the MCVI rather than in the operating room was based on the recognition that all of these procedures are extremely imaging-intensive and imaging-dependent. This decision has been universally accepted as an excellent one. The suite meets all of the requirements, including lighting, air exchanges, washable ceiling, seamless floor, traffic handling, infection control, etc. Cases are scheduled not only on the MCVI interventional radiology schedule, but also on the operating room and anesthesia schedules. For each case, all of the necessary equipment and personnel are assembled, and so far this has worked flawlessly, even for the four patients who required abdominal incisions to complete the procedure. As more and more work is done cooperatively in this fashion, creative professional relationships and billing arrangements will certainly evolve.

The functionality of the endovascular suite has led to a realization that various forms of combined treatment (in addition to endograft deployment) can and indeed should be performed in such an optimal imaging environment. As an interventionalist, having surgical access and cooperation has opened many new avenues of combining therapies, without being limited to only percutaneous access. Interventionalists and surgeons have teamed up in the treatment of various types of patients, for example those requiring both iliac artery stent placement and bilateral common femoral endarterectomy and patch angioplasty, and combining carotid endarterectomy with *retrograde* performance of percutaneous transluminal angioplasty (PTA), stenting of a tandem proximal carotid artery lesion.

15.2.4
Common Set of Reporting Standards

In 1986, an ad hoc Committee of the Joint Councils of the International Society for Cardiovascular Surgery (ISCVS) and the Society for Vascular Surgery (SVS) identified a serious lack of uniformity in reporting in the vascular surgery literature that rendered interpretion across studies almost impossible. The committee formulated and published a suggested set of standards for reporting the results of studies concerning the treatment of peripheral arterial disease (RUTHERFORD et al. 1986). By 1991, it was clear that reports on endovascular therapy and those on conventional vascular surgical therapy for peripheral arterial disease should be held to the same standards, since the patient populations and therapeutic goals overlap extensively. A set of standards addressing this concern was published in a special supplement to *Circulation* in 1991 (RUTHERFORD 1991). A modified version was subsequently published the same year in both the *Journal of Vascular and Interventional Radiology* and *Radiology* (RUTHERFORD and BECKER 1991).

15.2.5
Changing Patterns of Health Care Delivery

In the United States it has become obvious that although patients may be the consumers of health care services, they are certainly not the purchasers. Purchasing is done in small part by patients, in larger part by employers, the government, and increasingly by health care corporations, some of whom have their origins and foundations in the insurance industry. The most competitive companies control very substantial market shares and therefore have a great deal of bargaining power, a power which is exerted over hospitals and physicians. Large corporations are currently positioning themselves in the European market and similar changes may take place there in the near future. Purchasing of healthcare services is actually being done in large contracts for tens of thousands and hundreds of thousands of patients at a time. More recently, the

pharmaceutical industry has entered the field as a dominant force. Two large corporations, Merck and Eli Lilly, have purchased health care companies, and now have influence over at least prescriptions and potentially much more for nearly 100 million insured lives (ANONYMOUS 1995). The practical significance of these shifts in health care purchasing is best depicted in those markets that are most affected. In some geographic areas, managed care contracts account for more than half of the health care services rendered. In extremely competitive markets such as California, a handful of companies control so much of the patient population that physicians *must deal with them*. Unfortunately, some of the capitated plans being offered under these conditions have trimmed physician reimbursement so close to the bone that, even though they must, physicians *cannot afford to deal with them*. Viewed from the standpoint of the physician provider, it seems that little can be done to combat such adversity. However, vertical integration of vascular surgical, vascular and interventional radiologic, and other cardiovascular services into a single package with its own outcome and cost statistics renders the vascular center a well positioned bargaining unit in a very competitive environment. This has been the philosophy and the experience of the MCVI.

15.2.6
Increase in Practice Mergers and Establishment of Networks

To combat the loss of bargaining power and the downward spiral in reimbursement, physicians have begun to merge practices and to form networks. In the simplest terms, these maneuvers increase the ability of physicians to bargain with large health care purchasers within a geographic region. However, anti-trust issues have resurfaced. Frustrated by their inability to bargain effectively with large healthcare companies, some physicians have already attempted to unionize. In doing so, they have emphasized their firm belief that current anti-trust law prohibiting physicians as independent contractors from collective bargaining is archaic, because for quite some time physicians have not been in a position to fix prices. Although the outcome is uncertain, it appears that groups will continue to coalesce in some form or another. As they do, those with common interests, such as vascular surgeons and interventional radiologists, may take advantage of the opportunity by creating unique bargaining entities or by merging practices. The concept of the vascular center allows for merging of at least the peripheral vascular surgical and interventional portions of the respective surgical and radiological practices. At the MCVI, substantial progress has been made in this direction in the area of aneurysm treatment. Other segments of practice may follow in the future. This concept is discussed further below. For now, suffice it to say that never before have there been such great technological and economic pressures for vascular surgeons and interventionalists to combine. The institute environment creates an ideal opportunity for these dreams to be realized and for such groups to flourish.

15.2.7
Upcoming Changes in the Process for Subcertification in the United States

In a recent issue of *The ABMS Record*, it was stated that many American Board of Medical Specialties (ABMS) members and many members of ABMS' Committee on Certification, Subcertification, and Recertification (COCERT) feel that the Certificate of Added Qualifications (CAQ), originally designed to curtail fragmentation of primary specialties, has failed to accomplish that goal. Therefore, in June of 1994, COCERT met in a special session. Its preliminary report was presented to the ABMS in September of 1994. The report, which is divided into principles and recommendations, is quoted here directly from *The ABMS Record* (ANONYMOUS 1994).

Principles:
- The certification process should permit movement of qualified individuals across specialties and subspecialties.
- Boards should continue to establish standards and educational and/or practice requirements for admission to their examinations.
- Physicians with knowledge, training, and/or experience in a given area deserve access to certification. The area of knowledge, training and/or experience may be within the purview of a board from which the physician has not received a certificate.

Recommendations:
- Certification other than general certification by an ABMS Member Board can be achieved through two pathways: (a) A member board may establish core requirements for the issuance of a certificate to holders of its general certificate. (b) Two or more Member Boards may jointly establish core requirements for the issuance of an identical certificate.
- ABMS Member Boards should define the primary components of their specialities. Certification in a specialty or subspecialty should indicate mastery of the body of knowledge and skills in the defined components of the specialty or subspecialty.

- Each board should establish criteria by which physicians certified by other ABMS Member Boards may be awarded a certificate issued by that board. In such cases the board should use equivalent training, education, experience and knowledge as criteria for admission to their examination.
- With the institution of the new system, Certificate of Added Qualifications (CAQ) and Certificate of Special Qualifications (CSQ) will no longer be awarded.

The implications of the COCERT principles and recommendations are many and far-reaching. It is easy to imagine subspecialists from several disciplines (such as vascular surgery and vascular and interventional radiology) all engaging in the same type of dedicated practices, all sharing a common subspecialty certificate. How would the new system be handled at the training program level? Would it follow that individuals certified in vascular surgery will be qualified to take a fellowship in vascular and interventional radiology? And vice versa? Only time will tell, but clearly there is opportunity to look at new methods of training and credentialling to accomodate changing technology and physician relationships.

15.3
Leadership of Vascular Centers

The leadership and driving force in the MCVI is and has been provided by vascular and interventional radiologists. Other specialists, including vascular surgeons, cardiovascular surgeons, cardiologists, and neurologists have willingly joined in and profited from this multidisciplinary effort. The result has been an improvement in patient care. Other organizational and leadership patterns for vascular centers may be equally effective and yet better suited to the local situation and personalities. For example, in other circumstances and locations, vascular centers have flourished under the leadership and driving force of a vascular surgeon, and a few vascular centers have been spearheaded by individuals with expertise in vascular medicine or cardiology. Finally, in some circumstances, the dominance and leadership functions may be shared equally between two or more of these specialties. All of these leadership paradigms for a multidisiciplinary vascular center can be equally effective in providing cost-efficient, state-of-the-art quality patient care, when the various specialists work well together and recognize each other's knowledge, skills, opinions, and needs. The essence of an effective vascular center depends more on interspecialty mutual respect and a sharing of responsibilities and resources than it does on which specialty is dominant in a leadership role.

15.4
The Future

What is the appropriate forum for discussion of the future of vascular and interventional radiology and vascular surgery and the future of training in vascular therapeutics? What action can be taken now to move forward? To address these topics, a summit meeting comprising vascular and interventional radiologists and vascular surgeons in the United States was recently held, and follow-up meetings have been ongoing. A six-member task force representing the Society of Cardiovascular and Interventional Radiology met with a six-member task force of the International Society for Cardiovascular Surgery–North American Chapter. Although a resolution of training issues for current trainees could not be achieved, a framework for further discussion was formulated and several areas for mutual cooperation were delineated:

- Joint sponsorship of NIH research initiative meetings
- Evaluation of opportunities to cooperate jointly in educational endeavors
- Begin planning for joint or overlapping annual meetings at a common venue
- Form standing committee to provide liaison
- **Support the concept of the vascular center as a practice model of the future.**

This concept involves encouraging the development of between five and ten pilot centers around the country, in which a unique practice environment will exist (for vascular and interventional radiologists and vascular surgeons already in practice, not those in training). As envisioned, leading physicians from each of these centers would submit their plans for a joint service, to include sharing of inpatient and outpatient care responsibilities, joint clinical decision making, performance of combined procedures, collection of data in a registry, and sharing of revenues.

Our experience at the MCVI supports the notion that today's problems represent the unique opportunities described herein. Because of our experience at the MCVI, we firmly believe that solutions will begin to emerge in vascular centers, rather than in institutions whose leaders hold steadfastly to traditional specialty boundaries. Additionally, all physicians should realize that turf battles are destructive to all parties involved and vehicles for cooperation will result in synergistic increase in qualtiy, numbers of patients, and overall excellence. In vascular centers, the sharing of knowledge and skills will benefit patients and spur the evolution of the hybrid vascular specialist of the future.

References

Anonymous (1994) CAQ/CSQ slated for revision. ABMS Rec 3(4):1, 5

Anonymous (1995) Drug industry takeovers mean more cost-cutting, less research spending. Wall Street Journal, 1 February

Becker GJ, Katzen BT (1996) The vascular center: a model for multidisciplinary delivery of vascular care for the future. J Vasc Surg 23:907–912

Katzen BT, Becker GJ, Mascioli CA, et al. (1996) Creation of a modified angiography (endovascular) suite for tran-sluminal endograft placement and combined interventional surgical procedures. J Vasc Intervent Radiol 7:161–167

Rutherford RB (1991) Standards for evaluating results of interventional therapy for peripheral vascular disease. Circulation 83 Suppl 1: I6–I11

Rutherford RB, Becker GJ (1991) Standards for evaluating and reporting the results of surgical and percutaneous therapy for peripheral arterial disease. J Vasc Intervent Radiol 2:169–174; Radiology 181:277–281

Rutherford RB, Flanigan DP, Gupta SK, et al. (1986) Suggested standards for reports dealing with lower extremity ischemia. J Vasc Surg 4:80–94

Schwartz HW (1995) A contemporary perspective on capitated reimbursement for imaging services. Radiol Manage Winter 36–47

Congenital Vascular Diseases

16 Arteriovenous Malformations

E. Zeitler

CONTENTS

16.1
Definition and Pathogenesis

Since the report published by Klippel and Trenaunay (1900) on a syndrome named *naevus variqueux ostéo-hypertrophique*, which can clearly be described as a combination of local gigantism, nevus flammeus, and varices, but without arteriovenous (av)-shunting blood volume, and the publications by Weber (1907, 1918) on a special syndrome presenting a combination of local gigantism and av-shunt, many discussions regarding the definition and classification of congenital vascular malformations can be found in the literature (Flynn and Mulder 1959; Malan and Puglionisi 1964; Vollmar 1974; Belov et al. 1989, among others). Vollmar (1974) put together some published classifications (Malan 1974; Schobinger 1977; Flynn and Mulder 1959), site by site, and clearly demonstrated that it is most important in the interests of patients to distinguish between congenital vascular malformations *with* and *without av-shunts, single direct shunts, and multiple shunts with several feeding arteries* (Fig. 16.1). For the radiologist, it is of the utmost importance to detect the existence of

av-fistulas and to define the influence of organs, bones, and tissue located far from the diseased skin, a process which can only be carried out by imaging methods.

The elimination of av-fistulas with increasing shunt volume as early as in childhood influences the growth of the skeleton. Thus, the elimination or reduction of the shunt volume is also important for the prevention or limitation of local gigantism and varying longitudinal growth in the arms or legs (Gomes et al. 1982; Schobinger 1989). Table 16.1 represents the modified classification according to Vollmar (1974), which includes clinical aspects and experience gained from advances in diagnostics and treatment over the years.

Another view was to differentiate between primary vascular malformations in terms of truncular or extra-truncular malformations (Belov et al. 1989). Some definitions state that unidentified initial phenomena lead to truncular anomalies in arteries, veins, and lymphatic vessels. In contrast, diagnostic errors lead to the persistence of the av-communication by lack of involution of the reticulum, or by lack of its organization, with the reticulum remaining immature and preserving its plastic potential. These inter-truncular malformations are active or inactive av-fistulas, capillary or phlebectatic malformations (Kaufman et al. 1980; Malan 1974; Schobinger 1995). During lifetime, secondary disorders can develop in the venous system, bones, skin, and subcutaneous tissues (Leu 1990; Vollmar 1996).

At a symposium held in 1988 (Belov et al. 1989), an attempt was made to establish a new standardized classification of vascular defects according to their type and anatomical form (Table 16.2). Diagnosis and treatment of congenital vascular defects (angiodysplasia) requires specific knowledge to prevent poor outcome (Loose 1993).

E. Zeitler, Professor, MD; Virchowstraße 13, D-90409 Nürnberg, Germany

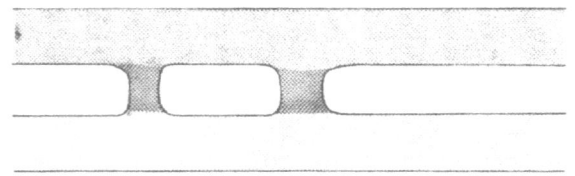

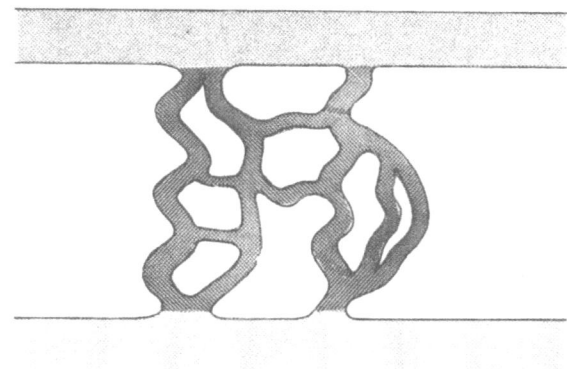

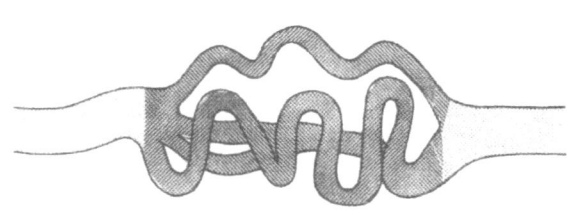

Fig. 16.1 a–c. Types of congenital arteriovenous shunts according to Vollmar (1963). **a** Type I: treatment, surgery; **b** type II: treatment, embolization; **c** type III: treatment, surgery and laser therapy

In contrast to congenital av-malformations (AVMs) with shunt, there are also acquired av-fistulas resulting from traumatic injury, iatrogenic activity (dialysis shunt; av-fistulas after venous thrombectomy), or complications after surgery or interventions (VOLLMAR 1996). They all need clear angiographic documentation for the smallest and best intervention, if intervention is deemed necessary.

16.2
Classification of Congenital Arteriovenous Malformations with Shunt

Type 1. This is an isolated, direct av side-to-side communication (Fig. 16.2), which nearly always presents an important shunt volume exerting a negative long-distance effect on the heart. Typical examples include patent ductus arteriosus (Botallo's duct) and the aortopulmonary window close to the heart. In addition, it also comprises almost all acquired av-fistulas, irrespective of whether these are caused by trauma, shot wounds, surgical measures, angiographies, or vascular interventions (VOLLMAR and NOBBE 1976).

The *patent ductus arteriosus (Botallo)* (PDAB) occurs in 12%–14% of congenital heart defects and is one of the most common central anomalies of the cardiac vascular system, the ratio of affected women compared to men being 2:1. There is a typical systolo-diastolic murmur, and a chest X-ray can clearly demonstrate the condition. There is a shunt between the pulmonary bifurcation and the thoracic aorta, behind the branching of the subclavian artery. At the age of one year, the ductus is only open in about 1% of babies, its dimensions varying between 0.5–1.0 cm in diameter and 0.7–1.0 cm in length in

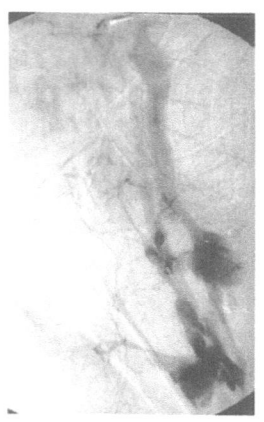
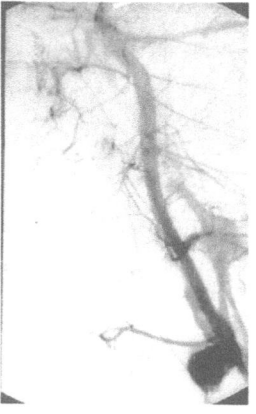
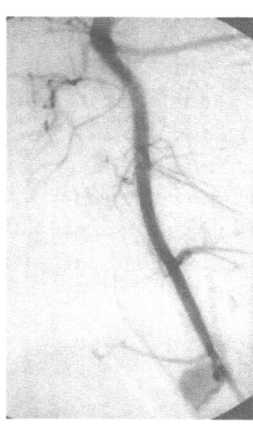

Fig. 16.2. Arteriovenous shunt type I (duct of Botallo-type). A 30-year-old woman with direct shunt between the brachial artery and the brachial vein, resulting in an enormously varicose vein on the upper arm. Shunt volume, 25%. Systolic–diastolic murmur on the upper arm. *Treatment: Vascular surgery, ligation with partial resection of the varicose veins. (Operation performed by Professor Dr. D. Raithel, Nuremberg)*

Table 16.1. Classification of congenital angiodysplasias according to clinical symptoms and findings in medical history

A	**Arterial dysplasias**	B	**Venous dysplasias**	
	1. Abnormalities at the origin, e.g., ischiatic artery		1. Hamartomas Cavitary hemangiomas Systematized hemangiomatosis	*(Possibly gigantism type Klippel-Trenaunay)*
	2. Aplasia or hypoplasia of single arteries e.g., nonexistence of the dorsal pedal artery		2. Hypo- or aplasia of deep veins 3. Avalvular veins 4. Duplication, abnormalities of the course and openings of veins	
C	**Arteriovenous fistulas**	D	**Lymphatic**	
	Type I: Direct transverse axis shunt		1. Aplasia or hypoplasia = primary lymph edemas 2. Ectasia of the lymph vessels	
	Typ II: Indirect multiple transverse axis shunts (mainly one extremity) *(Frequently localized gigantism (60%–90%) type F.P. Weber)*			
	Typ III: Longitudinal axis shunts (angioma racemosum), mainly at the head			
E	**Combined forms** B und D particularly common		*(Frequently gigantism, type F.P. Weber)*	

Table 16.2. New classification of vascular defects according to their type and anatomic form [BELOV et al. (1989) Hamburg/Germany]

Predominant defects	Anatomic form	
Arterial	Truncular:	Aplasia/obstruction Dilatation
	Angiomatous form[a]	
Venous	Truncular:	Aplasia/obstruction Dilatation
	Infiltrating form[a]	
	Angiomatous form[a]	
AV shunting	Truncular:	Deep av-fistulae Superficial av-fistulae
	Infiltrating form[a]	
	Angiomatous form[a]	
Combined vascular	Truncular:	Arterial and venous Hemolymphatic, with or without shunt
	Hemolymphatic angiomatous forms[a]	

[a] Extra-truncular forms.

babies. If it remains patent, both the diameter and length can double. As pressure and resistance in the major circulation are higher than in the minor circulation, arterial blood flows from the aorta via the ductus arteriosus into the pulmonary artery, where it mixes with venous blood from the right ventricle. The shunt volume leads to an enlargement of the aortic arch down to the branching of the duct, the pulmonary vessels, and the left heart chambers. PDAB can be classified into three stages (SCHAD 1968):

- Stage 1: In about 75% of affected patients, the pressure in the pulmonary circulation is not dramatically elevated. Shunt volume is about 40% of the left ventricle volume.

- Stage 2: Elevated systolic pressure in the right ventricle, up to 75% of the systemic pressure.

- Stage 3: There is an adjustment in pressure between the two circulations, with the risk of a right-to-left shunt.

Aortopulmonary window. The defect is located at between a few millimeters and 2 cm above the coronary ostia at the left anterior wall of the aorta or the right wall of the main pulmonary trunk in front of the ostium of the right pulmonary artery, with diameters ranging between 0.5 and 3.0 cm.

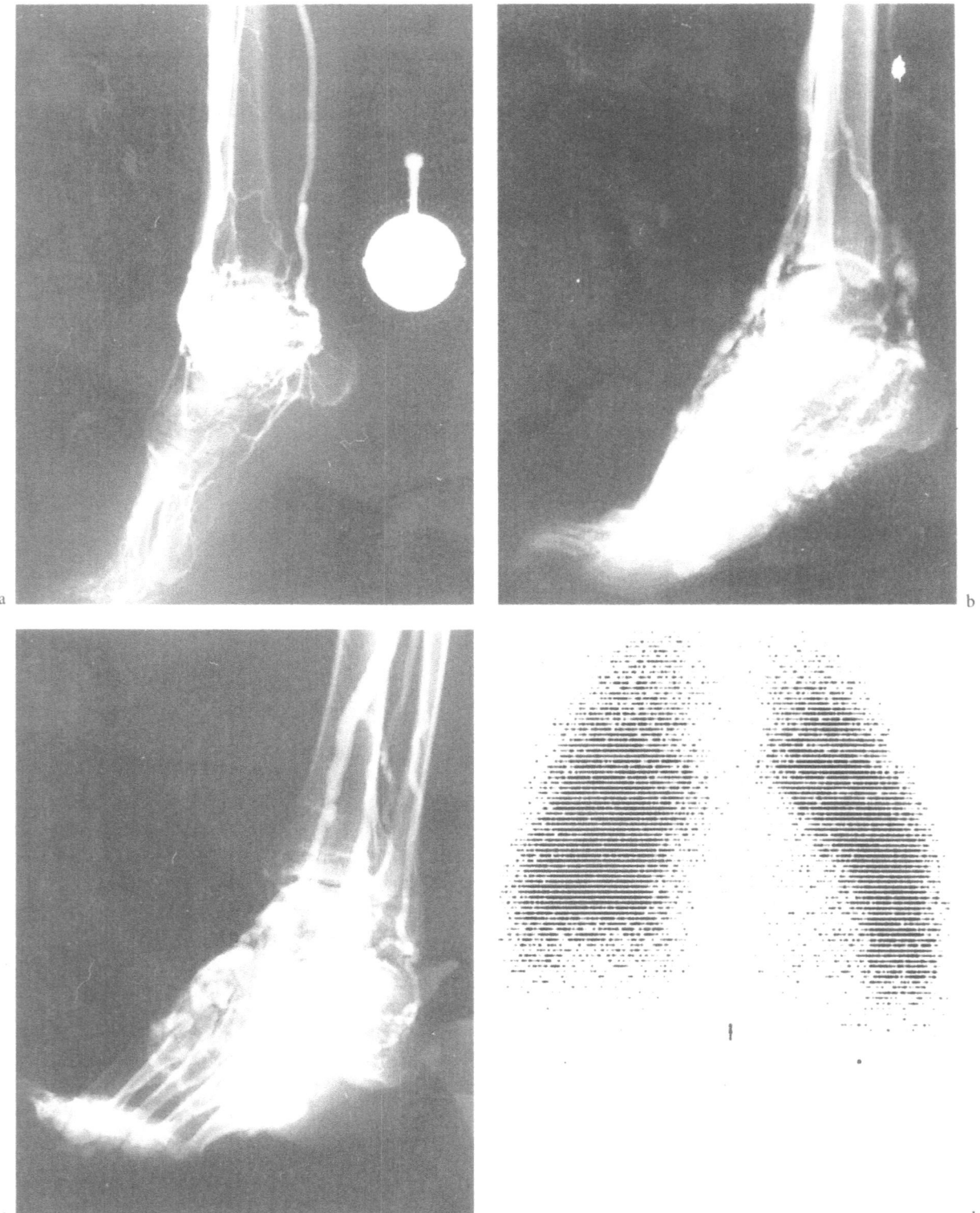

Fig. 16.3 a–d. Congenital vascular malformation with shunt, type II (F.P. WEBER-type). A 36-year-old woman, femoral arteriography. **a** Arterial phase with extensive arteriovenous shunts with reduced flow to the plantar arteries, and good flow to the dorsal arteries of the foot. **b** Extensive contrast filling of the ectatic veins on the foot. **c** Dilatation of the deep venous system of the calf, in addition to superficial varicose veins. **d** Total lung scan after i.a. injection of 200 µCi J[131]-MAA into the superficial femoral artery, demonstrating a shunt volume of 30% in contrast to the radioactivity accumulation after i.v. injection

Type II. Type II is the most common congenital type of vascular malformation showing av-fistulas with multiple av or arteriolo-venous shunts, (see, for example, Figs. 16.3, 16.9, 16.10), mainly affecting an extensive vascular area of the extremities (foot, knee, thigh, or pelvis), an entire extremity, or one side, including the lower and upper extremities (F.P. WEBER 1907, 1918). In such situations, an infiltration of soft-tissue or skeletal segments with the pathologically hemangiomatous vascular convolution can be identified. Increased blood volume may impair the growth of the epiphysis during the growth phase and result in local gigantism of an extremity or toe.

Type III. This is a congenital, local shunt along the longitudinal axis, which mostly develops into the clinical picture of a pulsating vascular tumor (angioma racemosum) in individuals of middle or advanced age. Due to progressive dilatation of the supplying arteries draining directly into the veins, the result is a tumor-like impression. This type more often manifests itself intracranially, in the face and on the neck (Fig. 16.4).

16.3
Diagnostics

Without question, the patient's personal history and physical examination are the most common diagnostic methods. The urgency of intervention is mainly determined by the clinical stage of an AVM. Schobinger (1995) has defined four stages:

- Stage I: Cutaneous blush/warmth
  No or minimal radiographic evidence may give the impression of a venous malformation
  Diagnosis with 20 mHz Doppler

- Stage II: Warmth, bruit, pulsations
  Active shunting detected on color Doppler image (see Fig. 16.5a)
  Imaging diagnostics by magnetic resonance imaging (MRI) or digital angiography (see Fig. 16.5b)

- Stage III: Trophic changes, ulceration, infection, bleeding, pain (Fig. 16.6b)
  Locally invasive, destructive to bones and soft tissues
  Diagnosis with color Doppler or MRI provides highly reliable information (Fig. 16.7b)
  Objective diagnosis with selective arterial angiography (Fig. 16.6c)

- Stage IV: Stage III plus systemic manifestation
  Non-healing ulcers or necrosis Frequent daily bleeding
  Cardiac decompensation with heart insufficiency and cardiomegaly (Fig. 16.8).

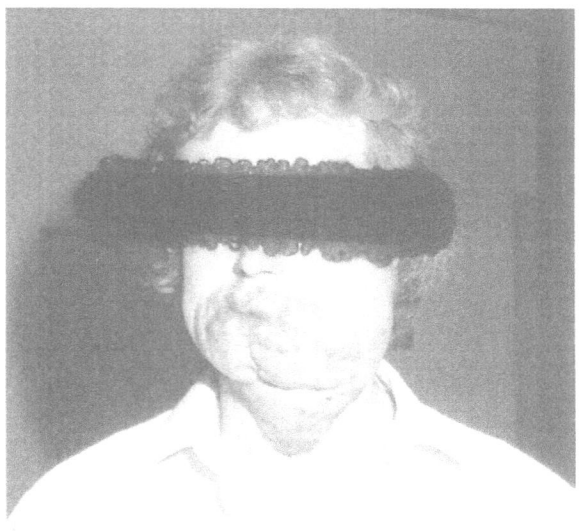

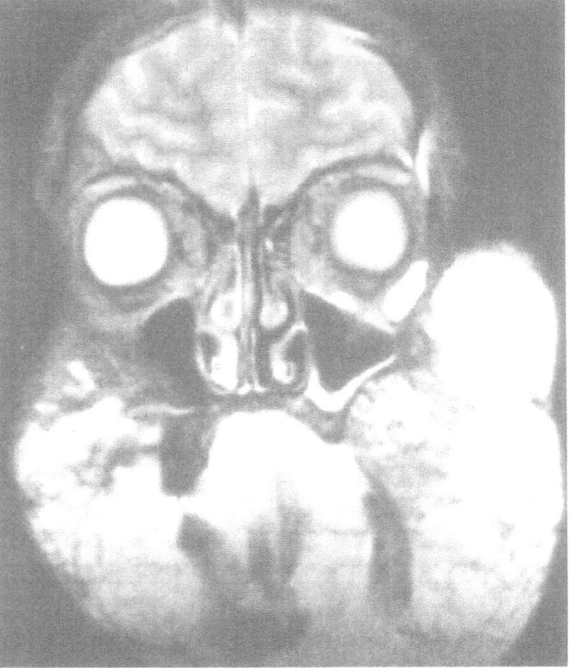

Fig. 16.4. a,b. Arteriovenous malformation type III, tumor formation. **a** Situation after combined surgery, followed by embolization. **b** MR-Image

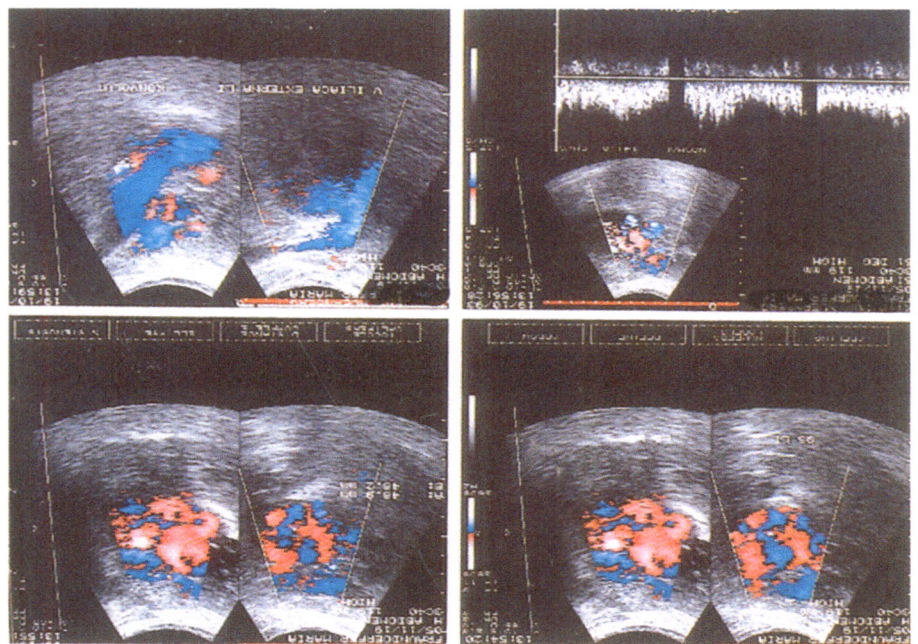

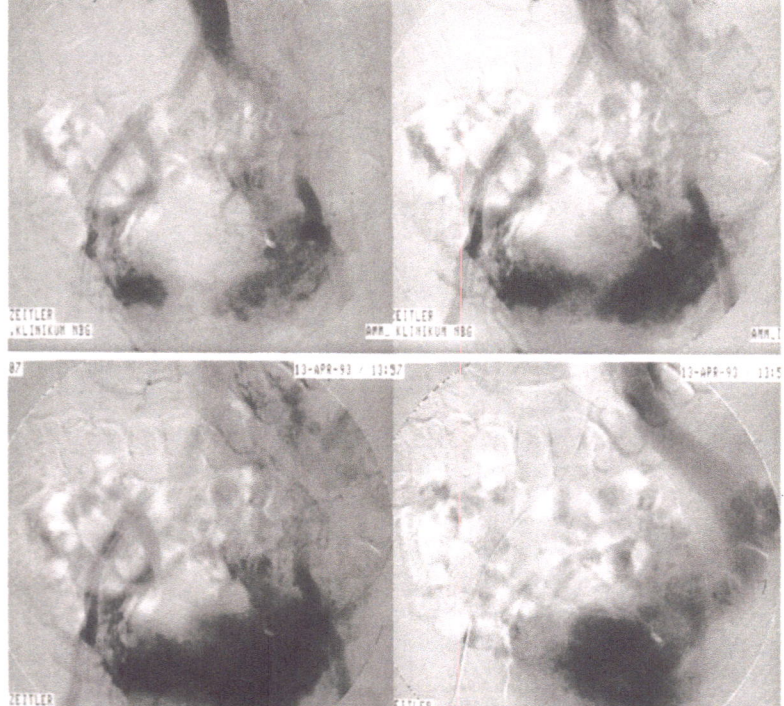

Fig. 16.5 a,b. Extensive arteriovenous malformation in the pelvis. **a** Different images with color-coded duplex sonography, showing the extensive shunt volume. **b** Arteriography with contrast medium injection into the infrarenal aorta, demonstrating an extensive av-shunt from the left internal iliac artery to left- and right-side veins in the pelvis (situation before embolotherapy). (Same patient as in Fig. 16.8)

Large av-fistulas can be suspected from the presence of systolic–diastolic murmurs and palpable thrill with intensified venous filling. If these exist over a long period of time, the formation of excessive varices results. Trophic disorders, such as necroses on the fingers or toes, may develop as a result of ischemia distal of the av-shunt. Typical complications of AVMs, divided into local and systemic, can be seen in Table 16.3. The most common incidence of congenital av-fistulas is on the head and in the brain, followed by the extremities and intestinal organs.

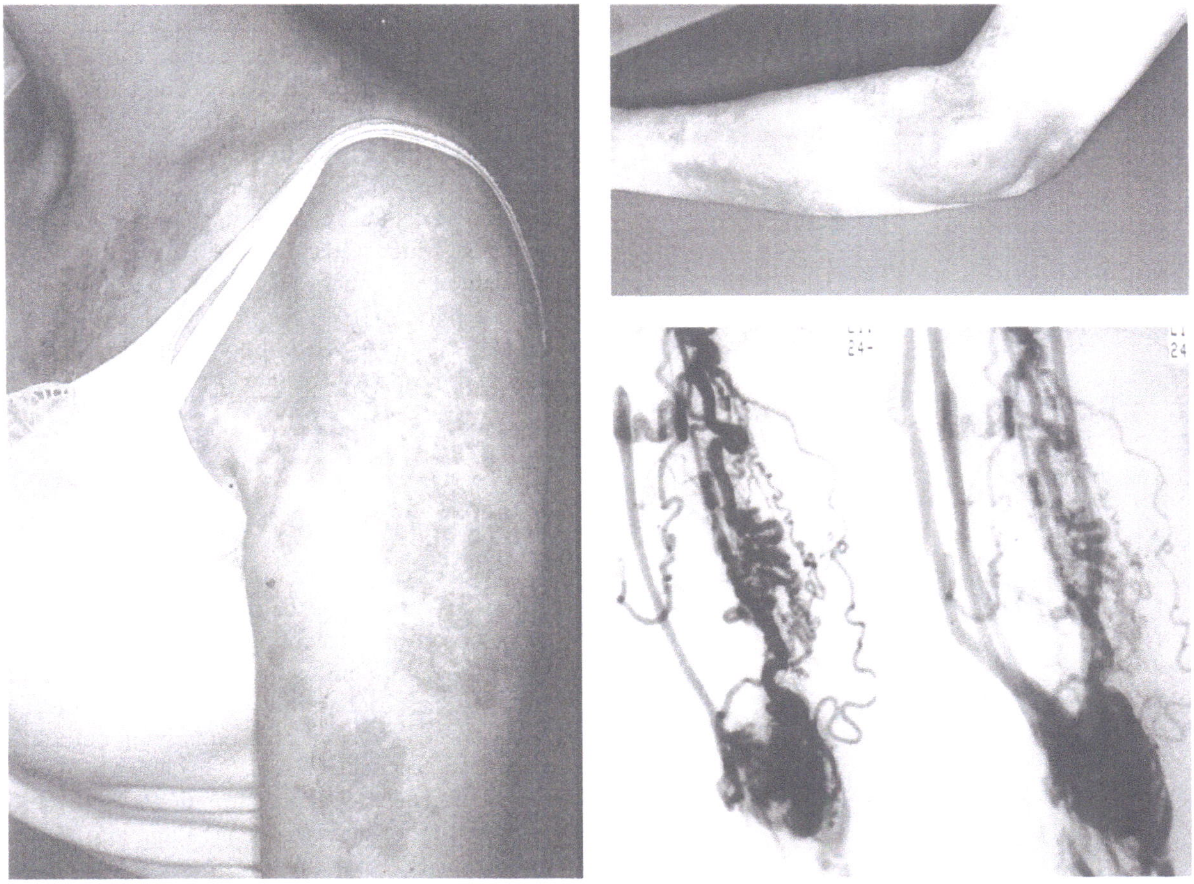

Fig. 16.6 a–c. A 46-year-old woman with extensive nevus flammeus on the left arm, and repeated surgery for varices with arterial ligation on the upper arm and in the shoulder region since childhood. **a** Nevus flammeus. **b** Local hematoma after trauma, with extensive bleeding from the arteriovenous malformation and destroyed head of the radius. **c** Av-shunt type II (F.P. WEBER type) prior to stepwise embolization with Ethibloc. On control 10 years later, no further destruction of the radius head, no new varices, and no shunts were demonstrated using color-coded duplex scanning

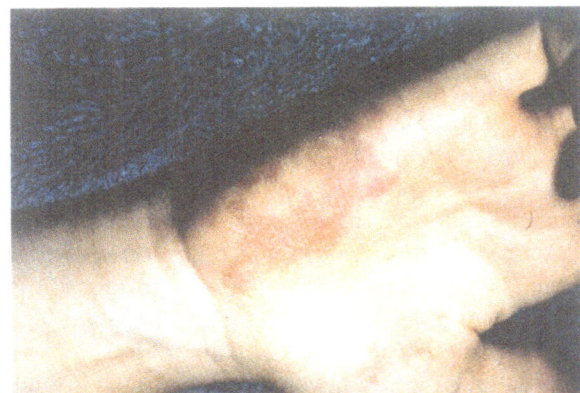

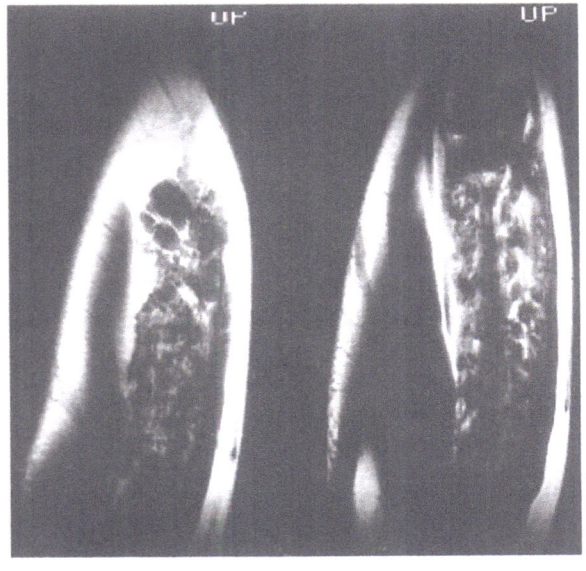

Fig. 16.7. a A 19-year-old woman with varices on the left lower and upper arm, and nevus flammeus on the hand. **b** Extensive arteriovenous malformation demonstrated on T_1-weighted spin-echo magnetic resonance images

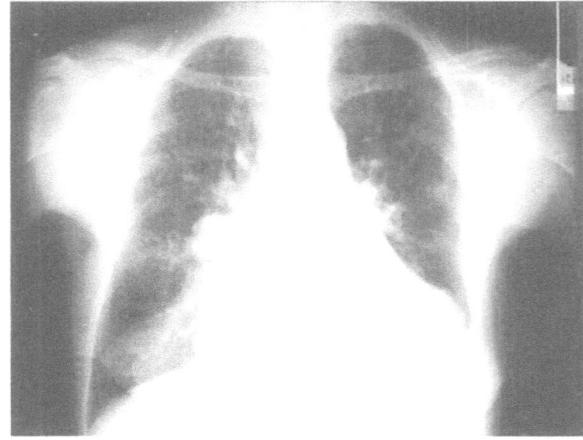

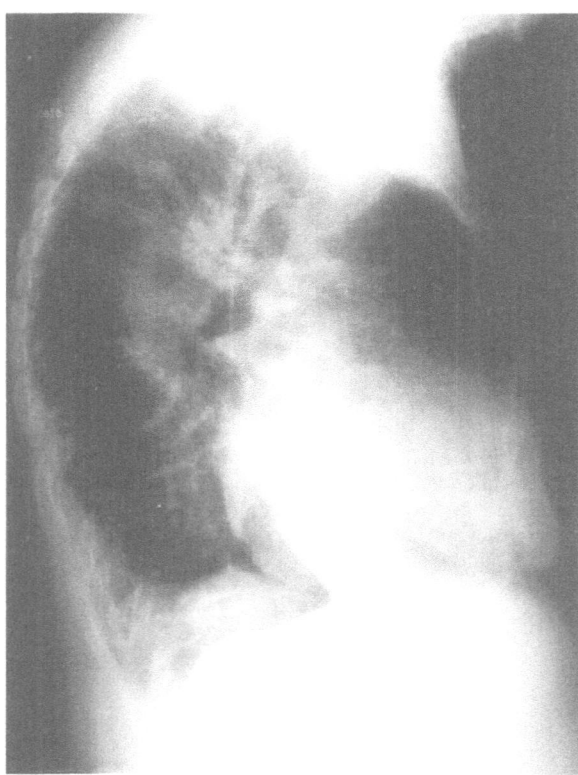

Fig. 16.8 a,b. Cardiomegaly and cardiac insufficiency in a 74-year-old woman with extensive arteriovenous malformation in the pelvis. **a** Sagittal chest image; **b** lateral chest image

Table 16.3. Typical complications of arteriovenous malformations

Local	Systemic
Reduced peripheral circulation with ischemia, necrosis	Cardiomegaly
Hemorrhage, hematoma	Cardiac insufficiency
Bone destruction	Anemia
Local gigantism	

In the case of AVMs with a large shunt volume exceeding 25% of the cardiac output, cardiovascular complications may occur as a reaction to the chronic volume load to the heart. The clinical signs of this are left-sided heart insufficiency with dyspnea after exercise. The hemodynamic effect of palpable av-fistulas can be demonstrated by manual compression of the fistula, which leads to a decrease in the heart rate (Nicoladoni's Branham's sign). As a result of cardiac insufficiency, chest X-rays (Fig. 16.8) show enlargement of the heart and pulmonary stasis, including signs of intrapulmonary interstitial fluid.

16.3.1
Imaging Methods

Diagnostics using imaging systems is capable of confirming a diagnosis, defining the extent of intertruncular changes, defining feeding arteries, and characterizing the nidus in complex type II shunts. In many cases, sonography and Doppler ultrasound enable an assessment of the underlying pathomorphology of the vascular anomaly in benign hemangiomas, venous or arterial malformations, as well as in rare cases of malignant degeneration into hemangiosarcoma. However, they are not capable of demonstrating the entire extent and hemodynamic situation. In the case of clinically suspected vascular malformations, the interstitial extension can be best determined using MRI (see Fig. 16.4). In all cases involving any type of complication or clinical symptoms, their cause and existence must be confirmed or ruled out.

To enable the classification of an AVM, angiography is indispensable. Up to now, a combination of arterial and selective angiography has mainly been used to differentiate between av-, arteriolo-venous, and arteriolo-venolous shunts (ATHANASOULIS 1982; ALLISON and KENNEDY 1989; LOOSE 1989; ROCHE 1990). This differentiation is important for planning "tailored treatment" (WHITE et al. 1980; STÖSSLEIN et al. 1985; WIDLUS et al. 1988). *Combined treatment of selective embolization with total or partial exclusion of the shunt, followed by surgical resection*, if possible, is of the utmost importance in the treatment of all congenital AVMs with shunt.

If total exclusion is not possible, at least a partial reduction of the shunt volume is important, in adults to prevent general complications such as cardiac insufficiency or distal necrosis, and in children to arrest the effects of abnormal growth and reduce the risk of partial gigantism (Fig. 16.9) (VAN DONGEN et al. 1985; WIDLUS et al. 1988; ROCHE 1990; WEBER 1990; VOLLMAR 1996).

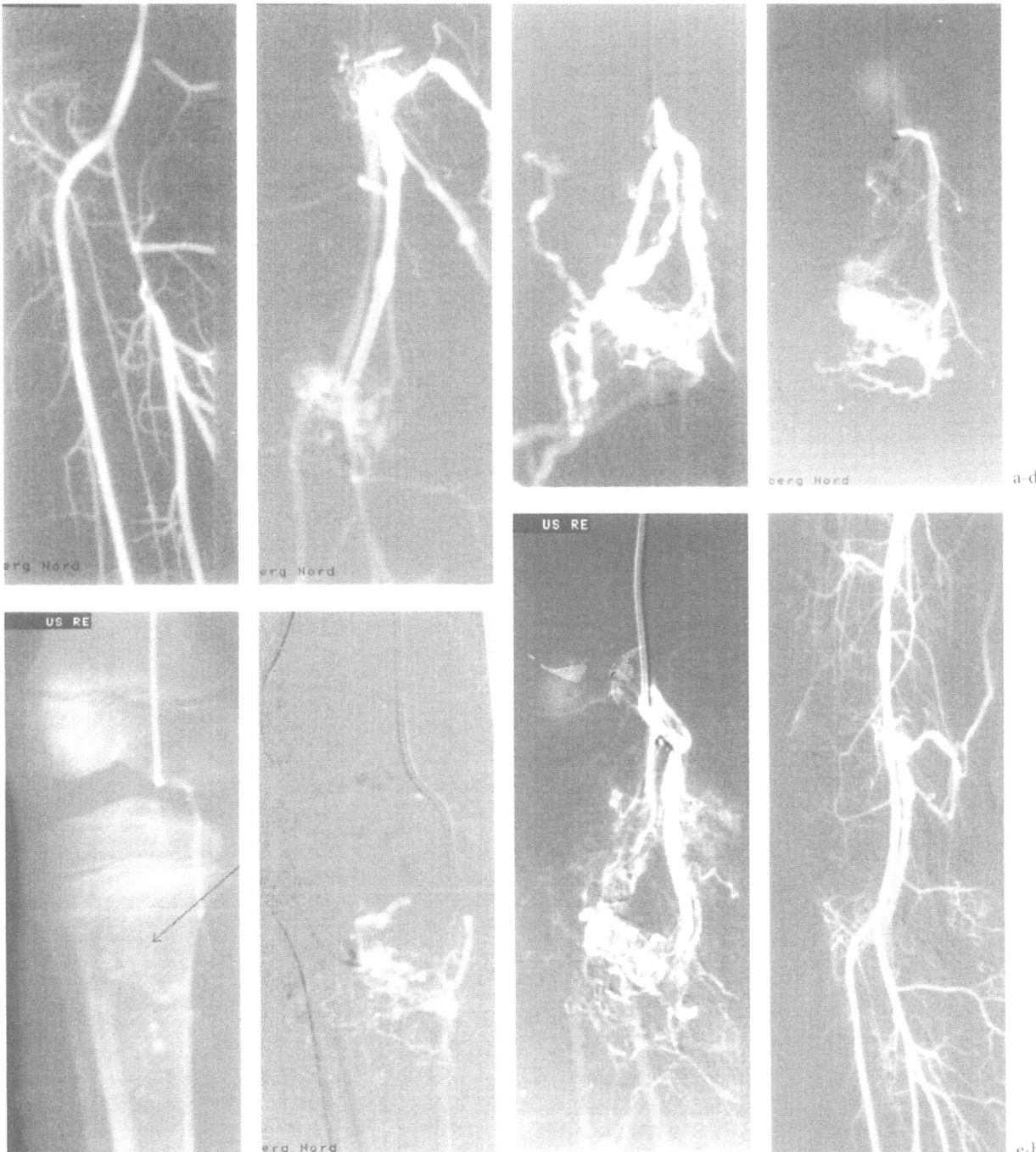

Fig. 16.9 a–h. Arteriovenous malformation (AVM) type II, 5-year-old girl with big toes one and two on the right foot, and AVM in the proximal calf. **a** Selective lower-leg arteriography demonstrating normal peripheral arteries. **b,c** Arteriography with contrast medium injection directly at the height of the av-shunt in the knee region, demonstrating several collateral vessels around the ostium, because of ligation performed prior to embolization treatment, with (**c**) demonstrating several shunting vessels of a localized malformation distal of the proximal tibia epiphysis. **d,e** Superselective catheterization of the important feeding artery, and embolization with Histoacryl. **f,g** Images after several step-by-step injections of Histoacryl. **h** Final control angiogram after central occlusion of the AVM shunts

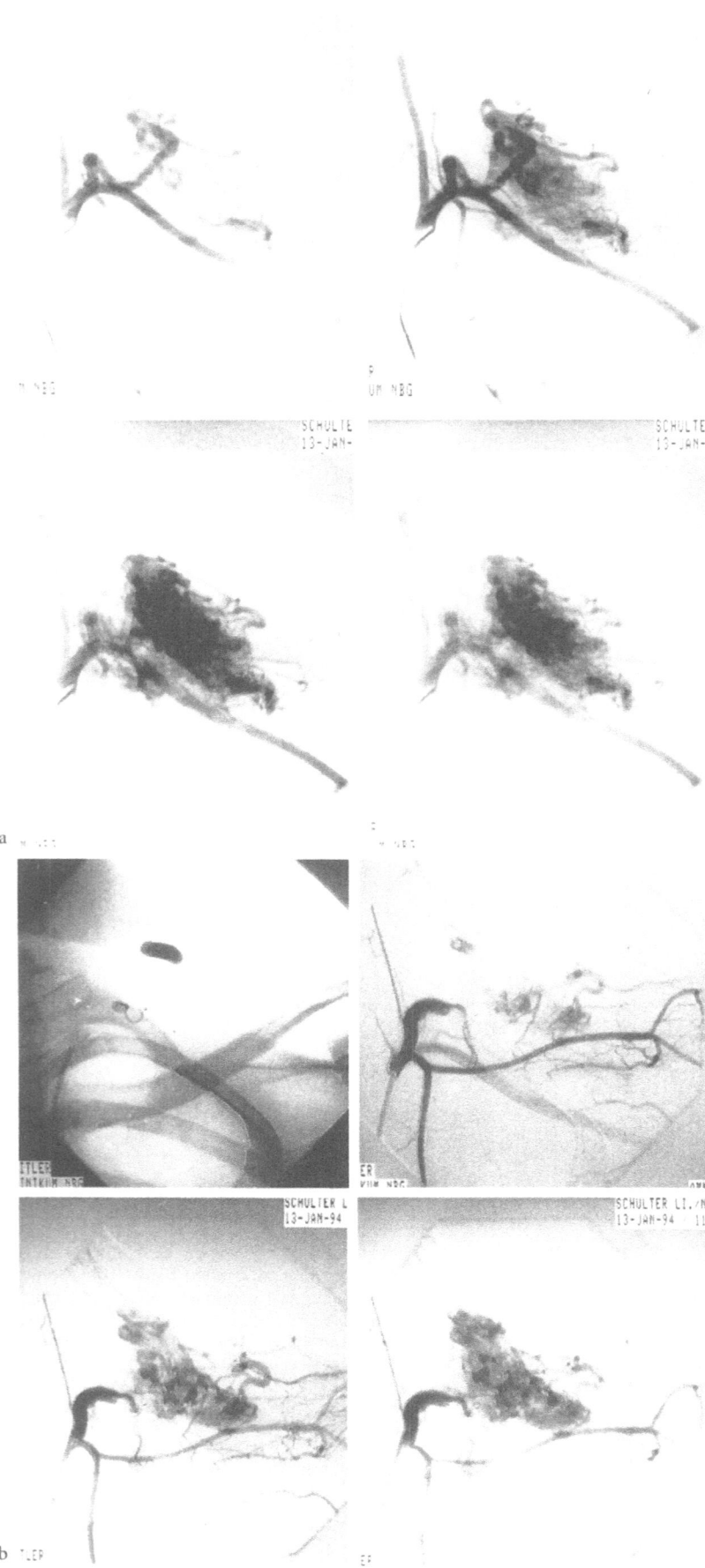

Fig. 16.10 a,b. An 18-year-old man with arteriovenous malformation type II (F.P. WEBER-type). **a** Selective subclavian arteriography, left side. Early and late filling, demonstrating the multiple arterio-capillary and capillary-venous shunting system. **b** Selective angiographic control after embolotherapy, combined with detachable balloon "Stösslein-Münster" (Cook company), in combination with contrast-enhanced Ethibloc. Spasm in the subclavian artery. Free flow in the internal thoracic artery. Last clinical control 26 months later, revealing neither murmur nor shunt, but residual palpable varices on the upper chest

In the interests of clear indications for an angiographic work-up in questionable situations involving AVMs, ALLISON (1989) differentiates between three groups: (1) Situations with pulsatile swelling and bruit; (2) patients with a cosmetic problem, but severe symptoms, e.g., bleeding, necrosis; (3) non-pulsatile swelling, which can be easily emptied by compression. In addition, the exclusion of varices is important prior to or after reduction or exclusion of the av-shunts. This can be done surgically, as well as by using sclerosing therapy in some situations (ALLISON and KENNEDY 1989; LOOSE 1989; WEBER 1990). Surgeons recommend surgery, if possible, and a percutaneous intervention only as a complementary therapy (VAN DONGEN et al. 1985; VOLLMAR 1996).

In the different diagnostic examinations for av-malformations with shunt, Osler-Rendu-Weber disease (OSLER 1915) should be considered as one underlying cause. This term comprises hereditary telangiectasias with formation of multiple angiomatous telangiectasias as autosomal dominant hereditary disease (WHITE 1992). Its pathologic changes are reddish-brown nodules of 1–3 mm in diameter which manifest themselves mainly in the face and under the fingernails, in the nasal or oral mucosa, and on the lips and inner organs. Very often, they occur in combination with av-fistulas in about 50% of cases (RÖMER et al. 1992), particularly in the region of the lung. They become symptomatic with hemoptysis, epistaxis, and also gastrointestinal bleeding. To occlude pulmonary and cerebral AVMs, WHITE et al. (1980; WHITE 1983), STÖSSLEIN et al. (1984) and WEBER (1990) have recommended the use of special types of detachable balloons (Fig. 16.10).

The presence of vascular malformations, therefore, requires a thorough check of all regions that may be affected and, in the case of suspected av-malformation, a chest image (see Fig. 16.8) and ultrasound examination (see Fig. 16.5) or MRI must follow for clarification.

While the clinical symptoms in arms (see Fig. 16.6) and legs (Fig. 16.11) are the same, they cause different clinical effects and symptoms according to their location. As the majority of hemangiomas can be checked visually, they belong to the area of responsability of dermatologists and pediatricians. In clinical and angiological diagnostics, the following questions need to be answered:

- Etiology: acquired or congenital shunt (fistula)?

- Morphology: is the lesion single, multiple, localized on one extremity or one side (arm, body, and leg)?

- Is there a concomitant difference in length of one or two extremities, or limited gigantism (toes or fingers)?

- Location: peripheral (knee, lower leg, foot, and/or elbow, lower arm, hand), or central (shoulder girdle, upper arm, pelvis, or proximal thigh)?

- Is the lesion hemodynamically effective, e.g., with major or minor shunt volume, or without av-shunt?

If an av-shunt has been identified, its extent must be determined.

16.3.2
Noninvasive Tests

Prior to any angiographic diagnosis, the following noninvasive examinations can be helpful (SCHOBINGER 1995) (a) Measurement of segmental limb systolic pressure, (b) segmental plethysmography, (c) arterial velocity wave-form analysis. In cases of large av-fistulas, segmental limb pressures and segmental plethysmographic tracings will be increased proximal to and at the level of the fistula. Similarly, depending on its hemodynamic significance, the values of these studies will be normal or decreased distal of the fistula.

In over 90% of patients with AVMs, the extremities are elongated by 2–4 cm. Extreme elongations requiring surgical orthopedic repair, however, are rare. Early elimination of av-fistulas, as early as in childhood, also leads to a retardation of abnormal skeletal growth, thus emphasizing its therapeutic priority. Av-fistulas – both congenital ones or acquired pathological changes with shunt – can cause local and systemic complications (see Table 16.3). Local complications comprise necrosis on the toes or feet, as well as on fingers, as the effects of ischemia or pressure lesions. Pulsating av-shunts and marked varicosis can result in the localized destruction of bones (radius, tibula, skeleton of the hand and foot). Additional traumata can lead to severe bleeding of an arterial or venous nature (see Fig. 16.6b).

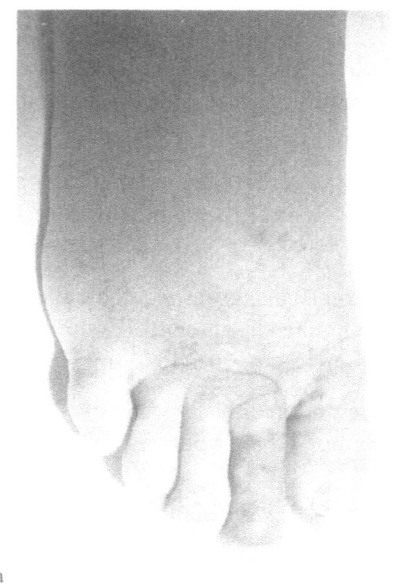

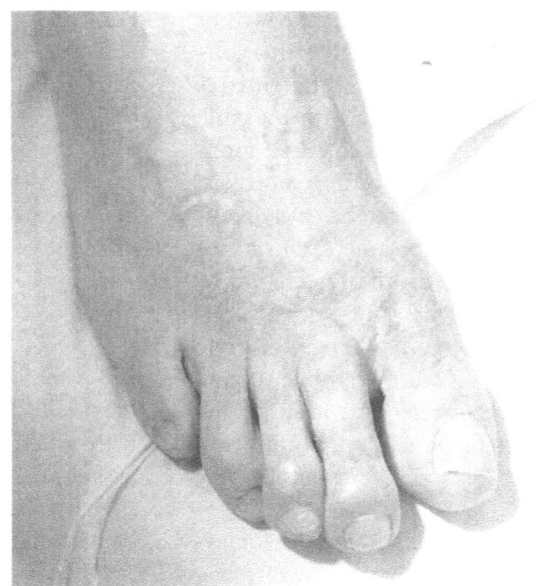

a

b

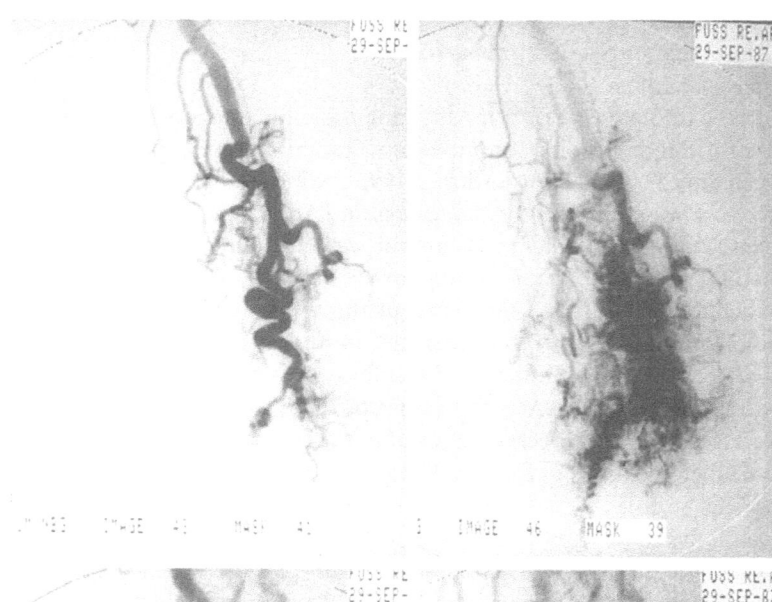

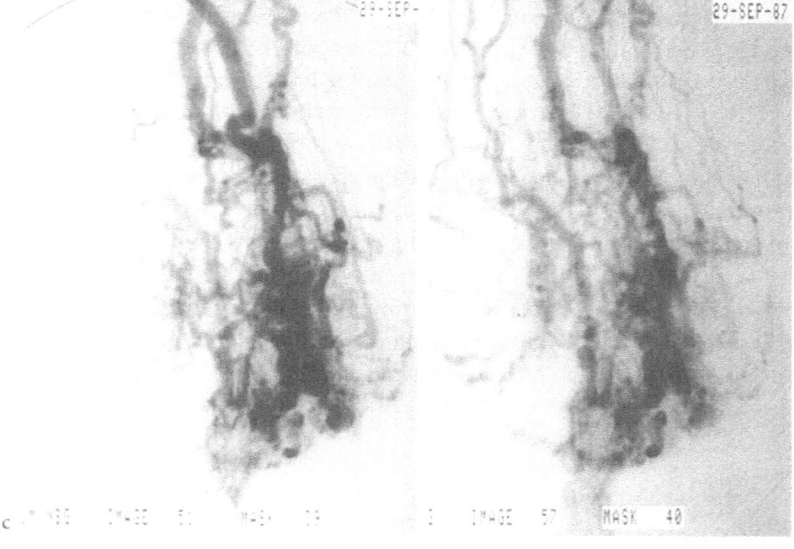

c

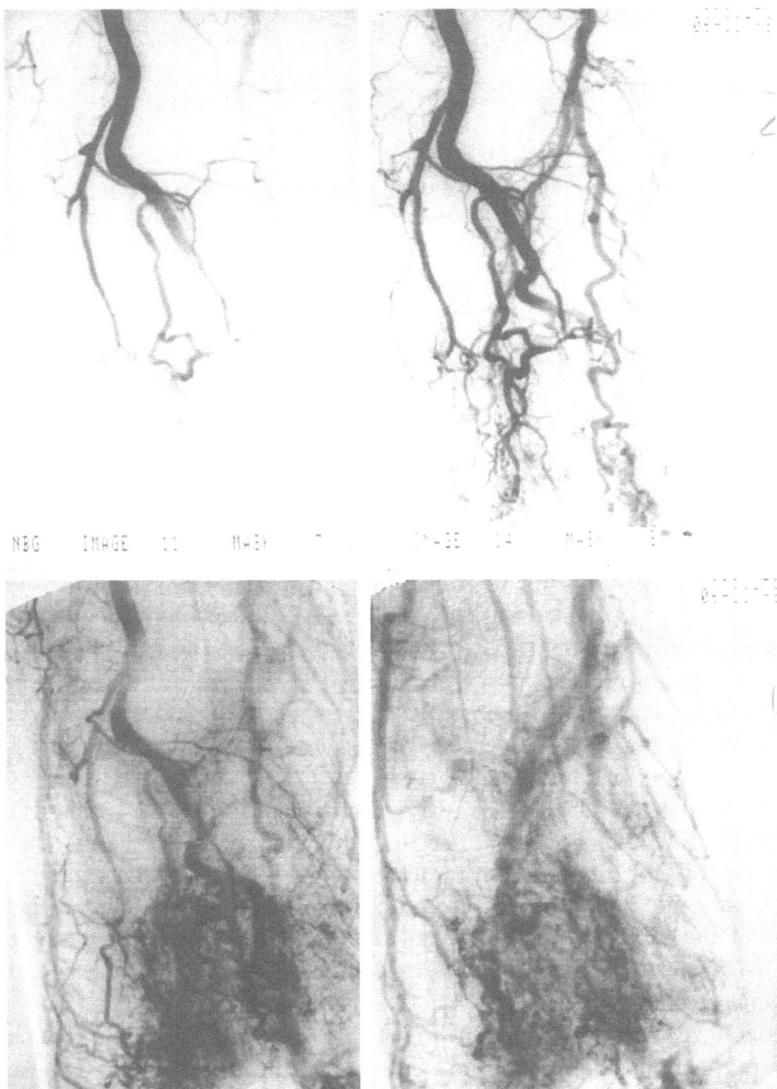

Fig. 16.11 a–d. A 69-year-old woman with extensive varicose veins on the right foot and calf. Situation after resection of varices and repeated sclerosing therapy. **a** Situation before embolotherapy. **b** Situation after embolization, with local ischemia in toes three to five, which persisted for only 24 h. **c** Selective foot arteriography demonstrating the arteriovenous malformation with early venous filling. **d** Angiography after superselective embolization using Ethibloc. Enormous reduction of the varicose veins. The transient ischemia could be controlled within days

16.4
Quantification of Arteriovenous Shunting in the Extremities

Following intraarterial injection of radioactive labeled macroaggregated albumin (MAA) particles (in earlier years ^{133}J, nowadays ^{99m}Tc) into the feeding artery of av-shunts, the particles go through the av-shunts by venous flow into the pulmonary artery bed, resulting in an increase in radioactivity, whereby shunts become identifiable (LOFFERER et al. 1971; PARTSCH et al. 1975; HÖFER et al. 1979; RUTHERFORD 1977). The increase in activity above the lung following an arterial injection in front of the AVM (within the framework of quantifying activity above the lung) enables a proportional determination of the shunt volume, compared to the increase in radioactive counts above the lung after previous intravenous injection. The quantification is calculated according to HANDA et al. (1968).

The following formula should be used to quantify the av-shunt using radionuclide macroaggregates:

$$\text{Shunt (\%)} = \frac{(\text{Pa} - \text{Bg})}{\text{Pv} - \text{Pa}} \times \frac{I_{v1} - I_{v2}}{I_{a1} - I_{a2}} \times 100$$

where Bg is background pulmonary counts per unit time; Pa, pulmonary counts per unit time after arterial injection; Pv, pulmonary counts per unit time after venous injection; I_{v1}, counts per unit time of

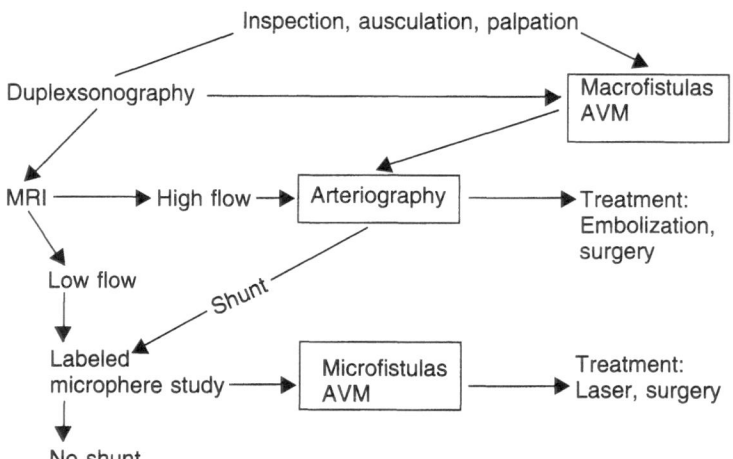

Fig. 16.12. Diagnostic approach to peripheral arteriovenous malformations (*AVM*). *MRI*, magnetic resonance imaging

venous syringe before injection; I_{v2}, residual counts per unit time of venous syringe after injection; I_a, counts per unit time of arterial syringe before injection; I_{a2}, residual counts per unit time of arterial syringe after injection.

Under normal conditions, physiologic shunting in an extremity is almost negligible, in the range of up to 3%. It can be increased by heat application, inflammation, or after sympathectomy. This test can be used in combination with angiography, if the technical equipment can be used in the angiographic room. If not, the catheter or needle can be placed in the supplying artery before or after angiography and the radionuclide study can be carried out in the nuclear medicine department. The albumin microspheres are relatively small in number compared to the dimensions of the vascular tree. They are metabolized and contain a radionuclide with a very short half-life (^{99m}Tc). Thus, there is negligible radiation exposure. To overcome problems arising in the diagnosis of patients with congenital AVMs or angiodysplastic defects, I, as a radiologist, recommend diagnostic and therapeutic management in steps (Fig. 16.12).

16.5
Management of AVMs

16.5.1
Peripheral AVMs

Many congenital vascular defects are treated conservatively. Vascular surgery is the treatment of choice in patients with direct or inter-truncular av-shunts (VAN DONGEN et al. 1985; LOOSE 1989; VOLLMAR 1963). In the case of type I lesions (see Fig. 16.2), surgical ligation is the most common treatment,

while interventional procedures can also be used in special cases. Interventional techniques include percutaneous occlusion with the help of covered stents or detachable balloons (see also Chaps. 17 and 24), in combination with permanent embolization using coils, Histoacryl, or Ethibloc (WHITE 1983; STÖSSLEIN et al. 1984; ALLISON and KENNEDY 1989; WEBER 1989).

Case 1 (see Fig. 16.13). A 19-year-old woman with extensive varicosis of the left upper and lower arm. Distinct swelling of the lower arm and hand, with clear asymmetry to the opposite side. Nevus flammeus on the upper and lower arm. X-rays of the lower arm and hands clearly demonstrate soft-tissue swelling, as well as multiple phleboliths.

Selective arteriography of the brachial artery: The upper arm shows a *direct av type I shunt*, with early venous filling. Additional aneurysmatic dilatations of the brachial artery and brachial vein. Angiography of the hand did not reveal an av short circuit. Normal arteries. Multiple phleboliths in the venous dilatations.

Therapy: Operative ligation of the direct shunt. Complementary sclerotherapy, and compression treatment of the varicosis.

In *type II av-shunt malformations*, in which surgical management is very difficult, the most common type of treatment is the combination of embolization and sclerotherapy (ALLISON and KENNEDY 1989; HEMMINGWAY et al. 1989; HUNTER and AMPLATZ 1989; WIDLUS et al. 1988; ROCHE 1990). Materials for embolization mainly include particles of gelfoam, fibrospum, Gianturco-Wallace coils, detachable balloons, Histoacryl, or Ethibloc (see also Chap. 5, table listing embolization materials). Materials for sclerotherapy with good results are Ethanol, Aethoxysclerol and Sotradecol.

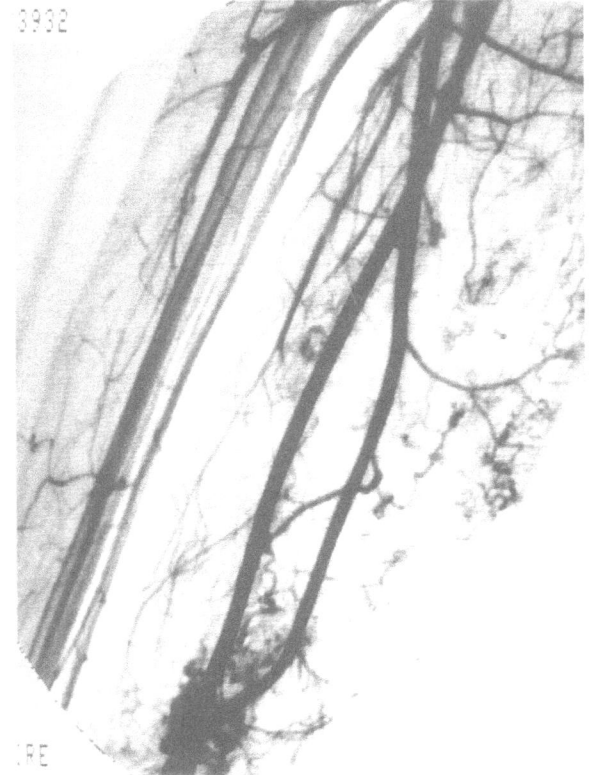

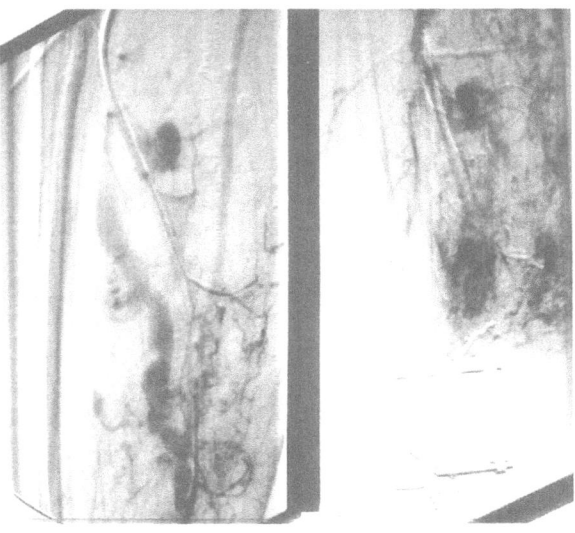

Fig. 16.13 a,b. Selective arm arteriography demonstrating arteriolo-venolous and arteriovenous shunts at several levels of the lower arm and wrist, with extensive varicose filling

Case 2 (see Fig. 16.6a–c). A 44-year-old woman, 7 months after the birth of her second child. As the result of a fall, severe swelling of the left elbow occurred (see Fig. 16.6b). Clinical examination revealed distinct nevi flammei on the left upper and lower arm. Mild varicosis. On sonography, the swelling corresponded to a hematoma. Additional signs of an AVM with dilated veins, also of the deep veins, could be seen on the MR image. An X-ray of the elbow demonstrated clear destruction at the head of the radius, in the form of a pressure defect. No fracture. The angiogram (see Fig. 16.6c) shows a type II av-malformation (F.P. WEBER type). The patient's history included several types of resection and sclerosing therapy of superficial varices in the past.

Therapy: Firstly, puncture of the hematoma and application of a compression bandage. Then, after the disappearance of local symptoms, step-by-step embolization of the av-shunts, first with Gianturco-Wallace coils and gelfoam. Three months later, a second embolization, this time using Ethibloc with glucose close to the coils, as recommended by KAUFFMANN et al. (1977). Finally, after 1 year, repeated embolization of shunts in the proximal upper arm. Circulation in the hand and wrist was at that time normal, and the shunts in the upper arm had been considerably reduced.

After 10 years, only the nevus flammeus persisted, while bone destruction stagnated. No cardiac hypertrophy or heart insufficiency. Duplex sonography demonstrated no major av-fistula (Fig. 16.14).

Case 3 (see Fig. 16.11). A 69-year-old woman with extensive varicosis of the forefoot (Fig. 16.11) and calf (the healthy foot took a smaller shoe size). A history of surgery twice for varices and one ligation of av short-circuit communications on the distal foot. Selective angiography of the femoral artery still showed an AVM of type II (F.P. WEBER) (Fig. 16.11c). Despite the previous ligation, the patient's condition remained symptomatic, with pulsating arteries on the second toe.

Therapy: Selective embolization using Ethibloc plus glucose into the nidus, superselectively. Embolization succeeded in sealing the av-shunts. Localized ischemia in the third to fifth toes and a hematoma on the second toe. Additional pharmacotherapy with analgesics for 3 days. Pain was eased and the ischemia regressed. Sonography did not reveal any av-shunt. The shunt, identified by ^{99cm}Tc MAA decreased from 18% to 5%.

In type III av-malformations with shunt, vascular surgery, sometimes total resection, or in combination with laser-therapy, is principally indicated. In

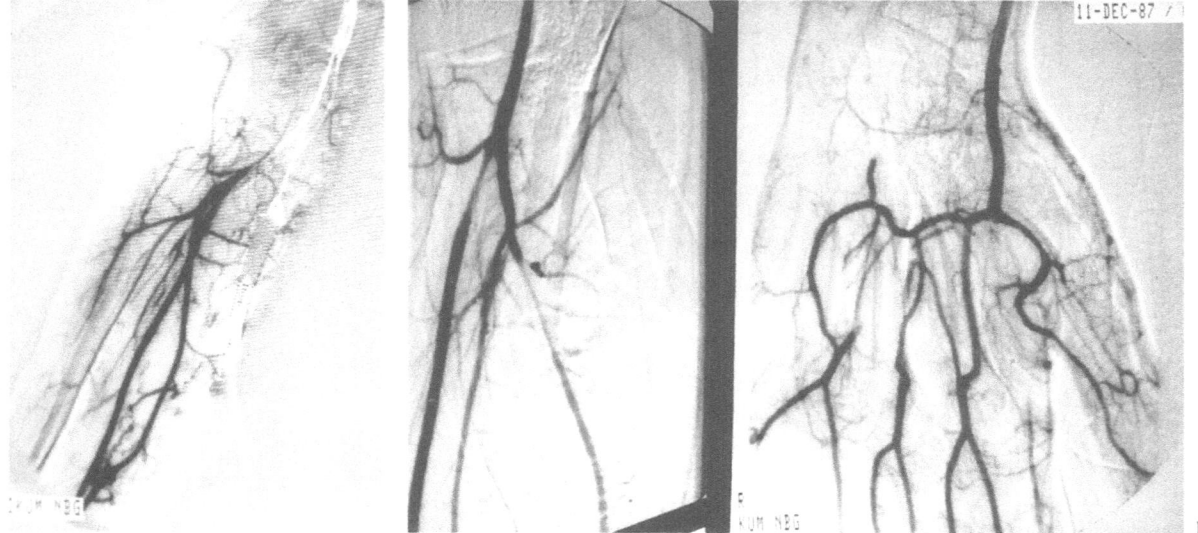

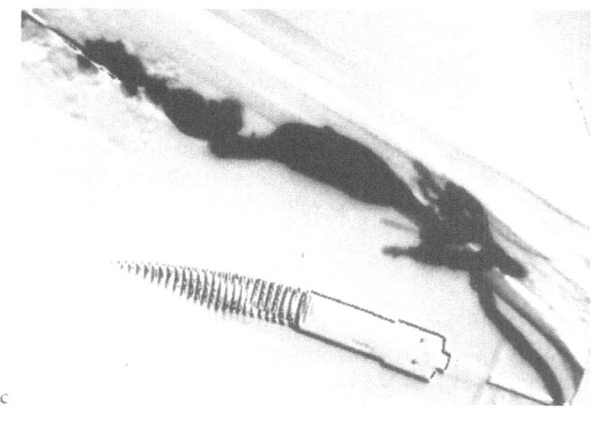

Fig. 16.14 a–c. Same patient as in Figs. 16.7 and 16.13. Control angiograms after superselective embolization with IBC and sclerosing of varices under X-ray and ultrasound control. **a,b** No av-shunts demonstrated, but small residual shunts on the arteriolo-venous level. **c** Selective phlebography at the time of sclerosing of the veins after shunt occlusion

several cases, partial embolization is capable of reducing mass formation prior to laser treatment or surgery.

Embolization of AVMs is not without risk (Novak 1990). Possible complications are summarized in Table 16.4.

16.5.2
Pelvic AVMs

Av-shunts in the pelvic region can be divided into inner and outer shunts. The clinical situation may become obvious by the asymmetrically developed buttock, auscultable systolic–diastolic murmur, and a flow rate curve on Doppler ultrasound. Mean flow on the symptomatic side is increased, depending on the size of the cirsoid aneurysm. On the other hand, the diagnosis may be established during gynecological examinations, possibly during pregnancy, or rectosigmoidoscopy due to increased vascular marking.

The diagnosis in any of these cases is backed up either by arterial angiography, MR angiography, or spiral computed tomography angiography (Fakhri et al. 1987; Weber 1990; Zeitler 1996).

Case 4 (see Fig. 16.15). 33-year-old woman, wishing to have a child. Several gynecological examinations due to internal bleeding. Sonography revealed an increase in vessels in the small pelvis, close to the uterus. The clinical inspection showed asymmetric buttocks. On auscultation, a systolic–diastolic murmur was heard, both above the buttocks and above the symphysis. The patient had been on strict contraception, due to the risk of bleeding during pregnancy and delivery. During previous vascular surgery, attempts had been made to stop progression of the malformation by ligation of the internal iliac artery on the right side.

Despite ligation of the internal iliac artery, the angiogram (Fig. 16.15a) shows an AVM affecting both the uterine and superior and inferior cluteal

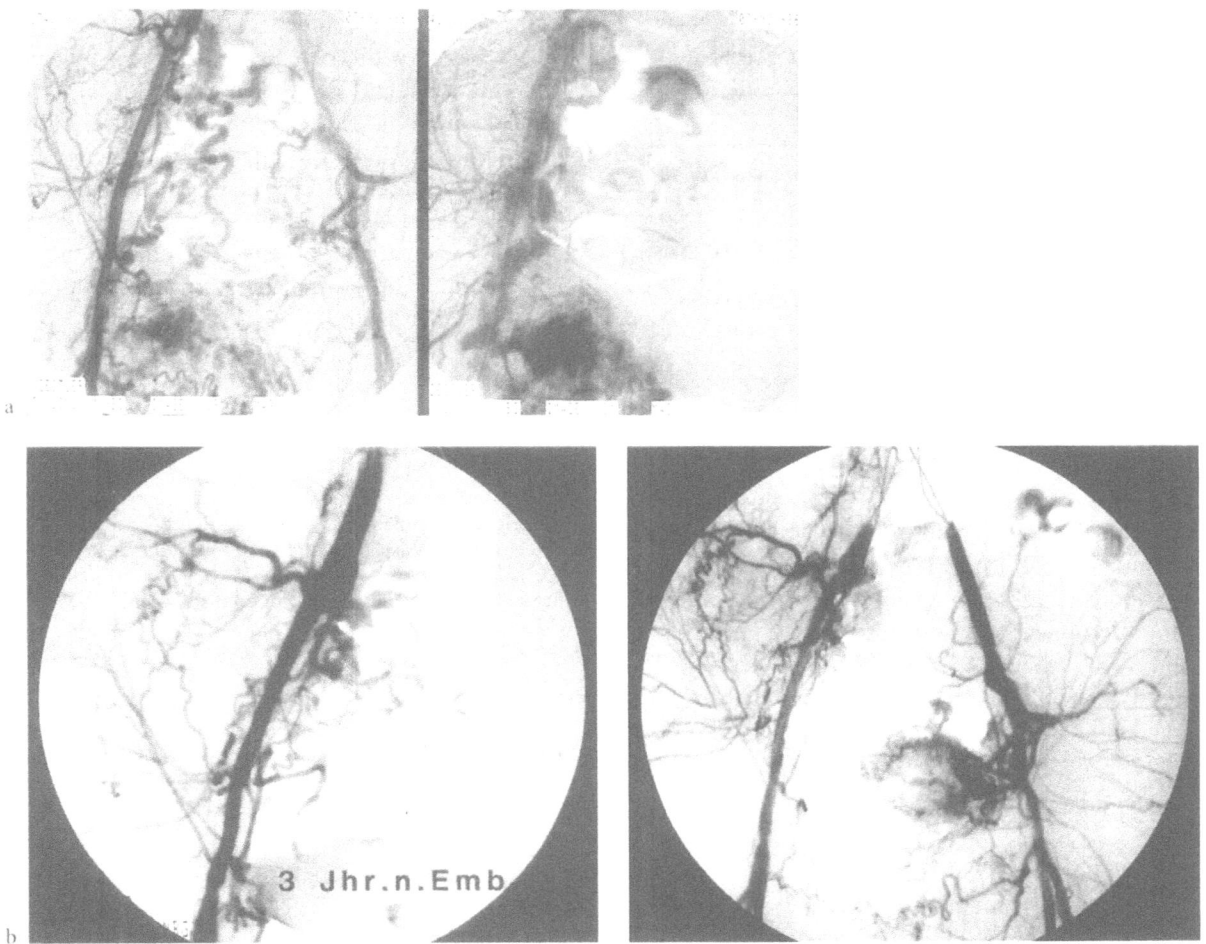

Fig. 16.15. a A 33-year-old woman with av-malformation type II with shunt. Angiography following ligation of the internal iliac artery prior to embolotherapy. **b,c** Control study 3 years following initial embolization and sclerosing of extensive pelvic varices

arteries, fed mainly from the right side. After selective injection of ^{99cm}Tc MAA particles into the common iliac artery on the right, a shunt volume of 77% was clearly identified.

Therapy: Superselective embolization with gelfoam particles into the uterine artery, and Ethibloc plus glucose into the gluteal artery. In total, three superselective embolizations performed over 18 months. Contraception was stopped 3 years after the last embolization (Fig. 16.16b). Within 2 years, the woman became pregnant and a healthy girl was born via cesarean section. A follow-up control 8 years after the first embolization still revealed small av-shunts from the superior gluteal artery on the right. The gynecological examamination was without pathological findings. The lady occasionally senses dragging pain in the pelvis. No cardiac hypertrophy or heart insufficiency.

Due to the foreseeable stress to the heart, which in turn depends on the shunt size, urgent therapy is necessary. On the other hand, therapy may be indicated due to impairment to neighboring organs, rectum, urinary bladder, and uterus, especially when pregnancy is planned, and due to bleeding in the intestinal or urogenital region. Only a limited number of reports dealing with embolotherapy of pelvic AVMS with major shunt volume have been published (WIDLUS et al. 1988; HEMMINGWAY et al. 1989). To the previously published 15 patients over the years, we were glad to add five similar cases in which a good outcome was achieved.

The chances of success with the various therapies are very difficult to define. In too many cases in the past, simple ligation of the internal iliac artery made subsequent types of therapy using embolization very difficult. The best results – based on the scant literature published and own experiences – can be achieved with a combination of interventional radiological and surgical treatment, i.e., superselective embolization and occlusion of the feeding artery

Table 16.4. Complications following embolization of arterio-venous malformations. (According to Allison and Kennedy 1989 and Novak 1990)

Immediate	Delayed
Pain	Post-embolization syndrome (PES)
Nausea	Infection
Embolization of normal structures	Necrosis of normal tissue
Pulmonary embolization	Extension of thrombus into nearly normal vessels
Reaction to embolic materials	

to the shunt vessel, followed by surgical resection, if feasible. If this should be excluded, sclerotherapy Aethoxysklerol, 4%; Kreussler, Wiesbaden) of the venous part of the av-malformation, or percutaneous sclerotherapy under ultrasonographic control, can also be helpful. The combined possibilites of interdisciplinary treatment can be best characterized by the term "tailored embolotherapy" (Widlus et al. 1988; Loose 1989; Weber 1990; Zeitler 1996).

16.6
Conclusion

Without question, the advice of experienced vascular surgeons, like Rutherford and Vollmar, can be followed:

The management of congenital vascular malformations is indeed difficult, and is particularly frustrating in that in most cases complete cure is not possible by surgery or therapeutic embolism. However, the majority of patients with peripheral congenital vascular malformations can be well managed by conservative measures, and this provides some consolation in those cases. Nevertheless, it is important to be able to make a reasonable prognosis, and set forth a therapeutic plan to the patient or the patient's parents, when the patient first presents.

Undoubtedly, congenital vascular malformations require interdisciplinary team work with good collaboration between all specialists contributing to this difficult and important field of diagnostics and therapy. To date, the specialists involved have been represented mainly by pediatricians, dermatologists and, more recently, colleagues in angiology, vascular surgery, and interventional radiology (Belov et al. 1989).

Superficial vascular malformations are a rare entity, associated with great psychological problems. Their management is ideally carried out by multidisciplinary working groups. For special information and questions, the International Society for the Study of Vascular Anomalies (ISSVA) can be contacted at the following address: Centre de Malformations Vasculaires, Clinique Universitaire Saint Luc, 10 avenue Hippocrate, 1200 Bruxelles/Belgium, Fax: 00 32 27626284.

References

Allison DJ, Kennedy A (1989) Embolization techniques in arteriovenous malformations. In: Belov S, Loose DA, Weber J (eds) Vascular malformations. Einhorn, Reinbeck, pp 261–269

Athanasoulis CH (1982) Interventional radiology. Saunders, Philadelphia

Belov S, Loose DA, Weber J (eds) (1989) Vascular malformations. Einhorn, Reinbeck

Fakhri A, Fishman EK, Mitchell SE, Siegelman SS, White RJ (1987) The role of the CT in the management of pelvic arteriovenous malformations. Cardiovasc Intervent Radiol 10:96–98

Flynn PJ, Mulder DG (1959) Congenital arteriovenous fistula. Western J Surg 67:31

Gomes A, Malli WP, Oppenheim WL (1982) Embolization therapy in the management of congenital arteriovenous malformations. Radiology 144:41–49

Handa J, Owayma K, Yonekava Y, Yoshida Y, Handa H (1968) The use of MAA J-131 in cerebral arteriovenous fistulas. Am J Roentgenol 104:18–22

Hemmingway AP, Smith EJ, Allison DJ (1989) Cardiac failure secondary to giant systemic arteriovenous malformations: treatment by embolization. In: Belov S, Loose DA, Weber J (eds) Vascular malformations. Einhorn, Reinbeck, pp 275–278

Höfer R, Willvonseder R, Bergmann H (1979) Nuklearmedizinische Möglichkeiten zur qualitativen Beurteilung arteriovenöser Shunts im Körperkreislauf. In: Zeitler E (ed) Diagnostik mit Isotopen bei arteriellen und venösen Durchblutungsstörungen der Extremitäten. Huber, Bern, pp 138–144

Hunter DW, Amplatz K (1989) Sclerotherapy of peripheral AVMs and hemangiomas through a retrograde transvenous approach. In: Belov S, Loose DA, Weber J (eds) Vascular malformations. Einhorn, Reinbeck, pp 279–280

Kaufman SL, Kumar AA, Roland JMA, et al. (1980) Transcatheter embolization in the management of congenital arteriovenous malformations. Radiology 137:21–29

Kauffmann GW, Hoffmann V (1997) Arteriovenöse Dysplasie. In: Zeitler E (ed) Arterien und Venen. Springer, Berlin Heidelberg New York, pp 313–341

Kauffmann GW, Wimmer B, Bischoff W, et al. (1977) Experimentelle Grundlagen für therapeutische Gefäßverschlüsse mit Angiographie-Kathetern. Radiologe 17:489

Klippel M, Trenaunay P (1990) Du naevus variqueux ostéohypertrophique. Arch Gen Med. Paris 3:641–672

Leu HJ (1990) Pathomorphology of vascular malformations. Analysis of 310 cases. Int Angiol 9:147–154

Lofferer O, Mostbeck A, Partsch H (1971) Die quantitative Shuntvolumenbestimmung bei a.v.-Anastomosen und Fisteln. In: Bollinger A, Brunner U (eds) Meßmethoden bei arteriellen Durchblutungsstörungen. Huber, Bern, p 114

Loose DA (1989) Surgical strategy in congenital venous malformations. In: Belov S, Loose DA, Weber J (eds) Vascular malformations periodica angiologica, vol 16. Einhorn, Reinbeck

Loose DA (1993) Angiodysplasien. In: Alexander K (ed) Gefäßkrankheiten. Urban and Schwarzenberg, Munich, pp 599-610

Malan E (1974) Vascular malformations. Carlo Erba Foundation, Milano

Malan E, Puglionisi A (1964) Congenital angiodysplasias of the extremities. J Cardiovasc Surg 5:87-130

Novak D (1990) Complications of arterial embolization. In: Dondelinger R, Rossi P, Kurdziel S, Wallace S (eds) Interventional radiology. Thieme, Stuttgart, pp 314-324

Osler W (1915) Arterio-venous aneurysm. Lancet I:949-953

Partsch H (1975) Venenverschlußplethysmographie und Doppler-Sondenuntersuchung als Suchmethoden zum Nachweis von a.v.-Fisteln bei gemischten Angiographien der Extremitäten. VASA 3:310-319

Partsch H, Lofferer O, Mostbeck A (1975) Zur Diagnostik von arteriovenösen Fisteln bei Angiodysplasien der Extremitäten. Kriterien für eine Operationsindikation. VASA 4:288-291

Roche A (1990) Peripheral arteriovenous malformations. In: Dondelinger R, Rossi P, Kurdziel JC, Wallace S (eds) Interventional radiology. Thieme, Stuttgart, pp 518-528

Römer W, Bürk M, Schneider W (1992) Hereditäre hämorrhagische Teleangiektasie (Morbus Osler). Dtsch Med Wotherschr 117:669-675

Rutherford RB (1977) Clinical applications of a method of quantitating arteriovenous shunting in extremities. In: Rutherford RB (ed) Vascular surgery. Saunders, Philadelphia

Schad N (1968) Die angeborenen Anomalien des Herzens und der großen Gefäße. In: Schinz HR, Baensch WE, Frommhold W et al. (eds) Lehrbuch der Röntgendiagnostik, vol IV/1: Herz und große Gefäße. Thieme, Stuttgart, pp 27-33

Schobinger RA (1977) Periphere Angiodysplasien. Huber, Bern

Schobinger RA (1989) Arterial malformations. In: Belov S, Loose DA, Weber J (eds) Vascular malformations. Einhorn, Reinbeck, pp 110-111

Schobinger RA (1995) Clinical staging of arterio-venous malformations. Lecture held at CIRSE 1995, Lyon/France, journée consacrée aux malformations vasculaires superficielles

Stösslein F, Speder J, Neugebauer K (1984) Neuer ablösbarer Ballon zur therapeutischen Gefäßembolisation - experimentelle Untersuchungen. Radiol Diagn 25:517-523

Stösslein F, Münster W, Schildhaus I (1985) A new system for safe and simple filling and detaching of intravascular latex balloon. Ann Radiol 28:153

Van Dongen RJAM, Earwegen MGMH, Kromhout JG, et al. (1985) Angeborene arteriovenöse Dysplasie: Behandlungsindikation, angiographische Dokumentation, kombinierte percutane und operative Behandlung. Chirurg 56:65-72

Vollmar JF (1963) Arteriovenöse Fisteln: ihre Pathophysiologie, Klinik und Behandlung. Med Welt 15:793-802

Vollmar JF (1974) Zur Geschichte und Terminologie der Syndrome nach F.P. Weber und Klippel-Trenaunay. VASA 3:231-237

Vollmar JF (1996) Rekonstruktive Chirurgie der Arterien. Thieme, Stuttgart, pp 154-176

Vollmar JF, Nobbe FP (eds) (1976) Arteriovenöse Fisteln - dilatierende Arteriopathien (Aneurysmen). Thieme, Stuttgart, pp 38-49, 56-76

Van der Stricht J (1990) The sclerosing therapy in congenital vascular defects. Int Angiol 9:224-227

Weber FP (1907) Angioma formation in connection with hypertrophy. Br J Dermatol 19:231-235

Weber FP (1918) Hemangiectatic hypertrophy of limbs - congenital phlebarteriectasis and so-called congenital varicose veins. Br J Child Dis 15:13-16

Weber J (1989) Embolizing materials and catheter techniques for angiotherapeutic management of the AVM. In: Belov S, Loose DA, Weber J (eds) Vascular malformations. Einhorn, Reinbeck, pp 252-260

Weber J (1990) Techniques and results of therapeutic catheter embolization of congenital vascular defects. Int Angiol 9:214-223

White RJ Jr (1983) Embolotherapy with detachable balloons. In: Abrams H (ed) Angiography, 3rd edn, vol III: angiography. Little Brown, Boston, pp 2211-2222

White RJ Jr (1992) Pulmonary arteriovenous malformations: how do we diagnose them and why is it important to do so? Radiology 182:633-638

White RJ Jr, Barth KH, Kaufman SL, De Caprio V, Strandberg JD (1980) Therapeutic embolization with detachable balloons. Cardiovasc Intervent Radiol 3:229-236

Widlus DM, Murray RR, White RI, et al. (1988) Congenital arteriovenous malformations: tailored embolotherapy. Radiology 193:583-586

Zeitler E (1996) Pelvic shunts. In: Sigwart U, Bertrand M, Serruys PW (eds) Handbook of cardiovascular interventions. Churchill Livingstone, New York, pp 925-931

Aortic and Paraaortic Diseases

17 Aortic Diseases

E. Zeitler, D. Raithel, P. Heilberger, C. Schunn, and D.M. Williams

CONTENTS

E. Zeitler, Professor, MD, Virchowstraße 13, D-90409 Nürnberg, Germany
D. Raithel, Professor, MD, Klinik für Gefäßchirurgie, Städtisches Klinikum Süd, Breslauer Straße 201, D-90471 Nürnberg, Germany
P. Heilberger, MD, Klinik für Gefäßchirurgie, Städtisches Klinikum Süd, Breslauer Straße 201, D-90471 Nürnberg, Germany
C. Shunn, MD, Klinik für Gefäßchirurgie, Städtisches Klinikum Süd, Breslauer Straße 201, D-90471 Nürnberg, Germany
D.M. Williams, Associate Professor, MD, University Hospitals B1-D530, 1500 East Medical Center Drive, Ann Arbor, MI 48109-0030, USA

Introduction

E. Zeitler

The aorta is the major artery transporting blood from the heart to the peripheral arteries. Thanks to its elasticity and windkessel function, it is capable of stabilizing the systolic–diastolic pressure variations between the aortic valve and the aortoiliac bifurcation, mainly in the ascending aorta and the aortic arch, thereby ensuring a more balanced blood flow in the peripheral arteries. To a certain degree, the arterial system, mainly in the region of the major arteries, can be simply interpreted according to hemodynamic principals, whereas in the distal territories of the arterial vascular system, temperature and biochemical aspects have more influence on perfusion. The aorta constitutes an elastic resistance to intraarterial pressure, whereby its elasticity increases during the growth period, by enlargement of the aortic volume, reaching its peak at the end of adolescence. With the beginning of the aging process, the aorta enlarges further and loses its elasticity. Laminar flow is more often transformed into turbulent flow in the area of branching points and due to the formation of arteriosclerotic changes.

In the aorta and the major arteries, the mean pressure remains nearly stable, whereas it decreases dramatically in the region of the arterioles. The highest flow resistance can be found here, in the resistance vessels. Due to the intermittent activity of the left ventricle, temporal fluctuations (systolic–diastolic) of the flow velocity, pressure, and arterial volume take place. These spread from the aorta into the arterial system (HENSEL 1955). From the aorta to the peripheral vessels, the amplitude of the flow pulse continually decreases, whereby the flow velocity and duration of the backflow in the aorta and vessels close to the aorta increase, which can be observed as pendulum flow in the cineangiogram, and also in magnetic resonance MR measurements. Only flow in a peripheral direction is identifiable in the peripheral arteries, and flow variations are reduced. Changes in the vessel wall developing with age cause a loss in elasticity of the aorta and arteries. Further effects of these changes include elongation and kink formation which, in the chest image, may render the interpretation of and clear distinction from abnormalities and pathologic processes (coarctation, aortic dissection) difficult (EDWARDS et al. 1965; SCHOOP 1974).

Congenital variations in the aorta are mainly found in the region of the aortic arch (see Chap. 35, Sect. 35.1). Along the course of the aorta, only the persistence of the right aortic arch – high right position of the aortic arch with varying branching of the aortic arch arteries – and the double aortic arch are clinically important. In its further course under normal conditions, a gradual transition from the descending aorta into the abdominal aorta, mainly left of the midline in the thoracic region, and left before or beside the lumbar spine in the abdominal region, are the rule.

While the area near the ostia of arteries branching off from the aorta are typically predisposed sites of age-related degenerative changes, this area is also of great importance to the peripheral circulation, both supraaortic to cerebral and arm arteries and aortoiliac to the pelvic and leg vessels. The course of the thoracic aorta, from Valsalva's sinus on wards, presents extensive identifiable pathologico-anatomic arteriosclerotic changes which, however, seldom result in clinical pathologic conditions with hemodynamically effective stenoses. The influence of arteriosclerosis, including increased hardening of the aorta with age, is not dealt with here.

The radiologically and clinically important pathologic changes along the aorta include:
- Non-valvular congenital and acquired aortic stenoses
- Aortic occlusions
- Aortic aneurysms
- Aortic dissection and ruptures
- Postoperative complications of the aorta, including arteriovenous and aortocaval fistulas.

17.1
Aortic Obliterations

17.1.1
Coarctation of the Aorta and other Congenital Defects

The most common congenital stenosis of the thoracic aorta is localized *coarctation* (AMPLATZ 1986; VOLLMAR 1996b); very rare ones include generalized hypoplasia (BACHMANN et al. 1964; BLECKAT and STRUBE 1967), tubular hypoplasia of the aortic isthmus, and aortic-arch interruption (VOLLMAR 1996c).

In its classical form, aortic coarctation occurs only at the junction of the distal aortic arch behind the ostium of the subclavian artery, at the beginning of the descending thoracic aorta. Its incidence is between 5% and 9% of all congenital heart defects (SCHAD 1968; AMPLATZ 1986). The male-to-female ratio is between 2 (–4):1; in patients with isolated coarctation and/or other cardiac anomalies, there is no difference between the sexes (SCHAD 1968; AMPLATZ 1986). The greatest morphologic difference exists between the localized coarctation (Fig. 17.1a) and the diffuse form of coarctation of the aorta (Fig. 17.1b), which is similar to the term "tubular hypoplasia of the aortic isthmus". Aortic coarctation may be either a localized stenosis located opposite the ductus arteriosus Botalli, or a hypoplastic stenotic segment involving the entire aortic isthmus.

Histologically, the primary lesion is a thickened media, composed of fibromuscular tissue combined with an intimal component (CLAGETT et al. 1954). With increasing age, the intima gradually thickens and the stenosis becomes more hemodynamically evident. With all imaging methods, the stenosis demonstrates a notch in the lateral, ventral, and/or dorsal aortic wall, and a medial bulge jutting out into the lumen. The extent of stenosis, therefore, can not be concluded from the outer contour of the aorta with chest images alone. Thus, contrast-enhanced angiography with clear information about the lumen and aortic arch arteries is required (Fig. 17.2), spiral computed tomography (CT) imaging, MR angiography (MRA), or two-dimensional (2D) echocardiography. Due to the arterial ligament, the stenosis is often displaced in a medial direction. The location of the stenosis in relation to the ostium of the left subclavian artery and to the patent ductus arteriosus Botalli is important. The coarctation can be located preductally, juxtaductally, or postductally. In 80% of patients, coarctation is located distal to the ductus, whereas it is located preductally in only 20%.

The tubular type of coarctation can include not only the postsubclavian part of the aorta, but also the part of the aortic arch between the ostium of the left common carotid and the ostium of the left subclavian artery. Physical examination demonstrates a reduced bilateral femoral pulse, increased blood pressure in both arms in contrast to the legs, and auscultation can demonstrate a systolic–diastolic murmur on the back. Chest images may show an

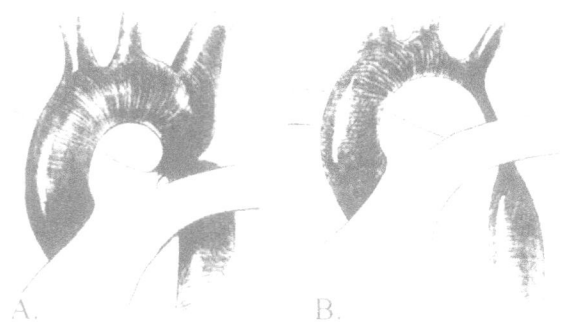

Fig. 17.1 a,b. Coarctatio aortae. **a** Typical segmental type distal of the subclavian artery. **b** Diffuse or dysplastic type, distally located, or including the subclavian artery ostium

ectatic ascending thoracic aorta, and sometimes elongation of the aortic arch. On the left edge, the aorta may present an incision, and "notching" as a typical sign of collaterals can be found on the rips as a result of craniocaudal collateral circulation (EDWARDS et al. 1965; HEBERER et al. 1966b; AMPLATZ 1986).

In the case of coarctation in combination with a patent ductus arteriosus, the hemodynamic situation is that the blood flows from the aorta through the ductus arteriosus proximal to the coarctation into the pulmonary artery, where it mixes with venous blood if there is a postductal isthmic stenosis in the case of a patent ductus arteriosus. The hemodynamic situation is determined by the degree of obstruction, the position of the coarctation in relation to the site of the patent or occluded ductus arteriosus, and the presence of collateral pathways.

Before birth, no pressure gradient exists between the ascending and descending aorta. After birth, the

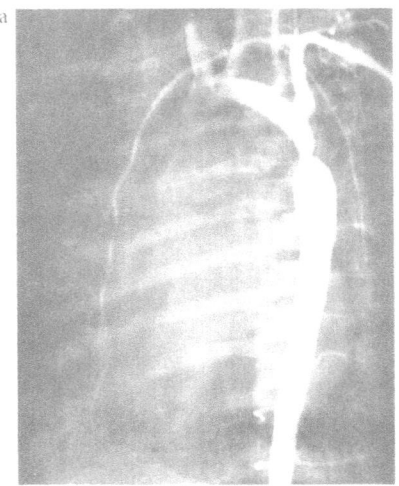
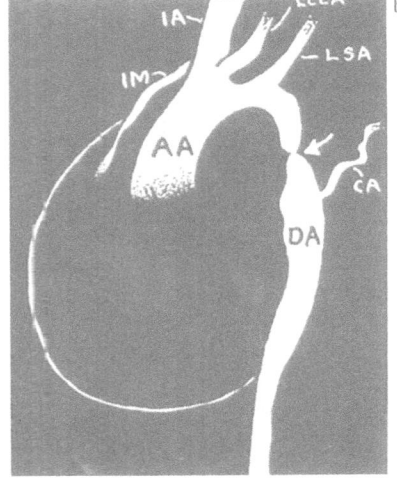

Fig. 17.2 a,b. Coarctatio aortae, segmental type. **a** Cineangiography, transfemoral catheterization. **b** Schematic drawing

collateral circulation develops because of the pressure gradient across the area of the coarctation. The collateral channels enlarge with age. The important collateral pathways include:

- The internal thoracic arteries, which communicate with the epigastric arteries (WINSLOW's collateral pathway)
- The intercostal arteries, between the first two intercostal arteries and the lower intercostal arteries develop bridging branches, and all together drain into the internal thoracic arteries
- The mediastinal collateral arteries (KIRKS et al. 1986).

The high-pressure arteries coming from the ascending aorta via the subclavian arteries give collaterals to the low-pressure arteries, which are located distal of the coarctation. Also, alongside the vertebral column and the spinal cord, a collateral circulation develops between vertebral arteries from the cranial to the anterior spinal artery, as well as from the cervical arteries, periscapular artery collaterals go to intercostal and lateral thoracic arteries (Fig. 17.3), bypassing the coarctation.

This pressure- and flow-dependent collateral circulation from the upper to the lower of the body can also occur from the lower to the upper part in patients with aortic-arch syndrome (upper pulseless disease) and was first described by WINSLOW in 1753. The collateral vessels can be best demonstrated by thoracoabdominal aortography with contrast medium (CM) injection into the ascending thoracic aorta, or bilaterally into the subclavian arteries. Without question, the total collateral circulation can also be imaged using contrast-enhanced MRA after intravenous CM injection (e.g. Magnevist, gadolinium-diethylenetriaminopentoacetic acid).

The preferred standard imaging modality for

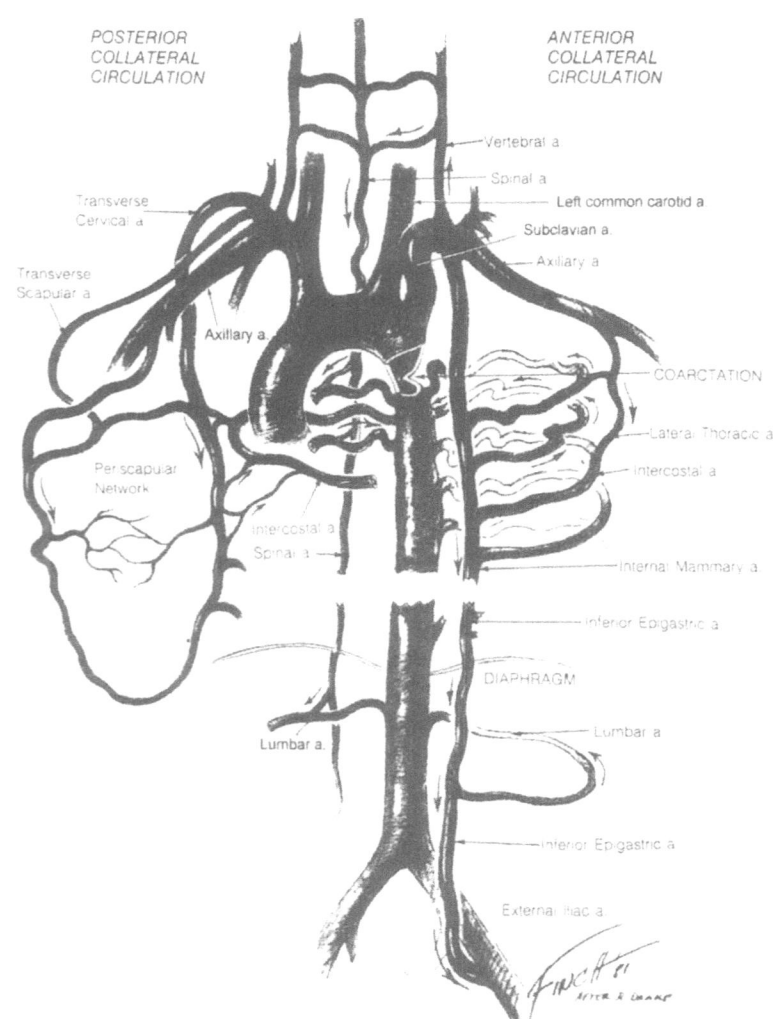

Fig. 17.3. Collateral circulation from the aortic arch arteries to the descending aortal arteries. (According to AMPLATZ 1986)

several decades was thoracic aortography (ABRAMS and JÖNSSON 1983) after arterial catheterization, or via angiocardiography with CM administration into the right or left ventricle. Today, biplane echocardiography, transesophageal echocardiography, and MRA can precisely demonstrate abnormalities in the thoracic artery without radiation exposure. This is particularly advantageous in newborns and infants.

Very rarely, aortic coarctation is present in a family as a result of a genetic defect (KUHN et al. 1963). Therefore, a family history and physical examination of the patient's sisters and brothers is recommended. Each second child with aortic coarctation presents additional defects, such as a ventricular septal defect, aortic valvular stenosis, or patent ductus arteriosus Botalli. Proximal to the coarctation, the diameter of the aorta is larger, and smaller behind the stenotic area. In contrast to this pressure-related lumen reduction, there is generalized hypoplasia of the aorta (BACHMANN et al. 1964). *Generalized hypoplasia of the aorta without a ventriculo-aortal pressure gradient* is a very rare, isolated congenital specialty. In some cases, the normal arterial wall has been documented without degenerative or inflammatory changes (BLACK and CARTER 1963). The aorta had a very small diameter, and the heart a left-ventricle hypertrophy. Diagnosis did not result in an active type of treatment, and co-existent peripheral vascular disease was not observed. So, in combination with aortic stenoses, localized pressure-dependent smaller diameters behind stenoses will assume a normal diameter if the stenosis is successfully treated.

Aortic-arch stenosis, which is very rare, is located between the left common carotid and left subclavian artery. It is present mainly in combination with the patent ductus arteriosus Botalli. Also, combinations with various other heart defects, such as ventricular septal defect (VSD), aplastic left common carotid artery, or aberrant right subclavian artery (SUNDER-PLASSMANN et al. 1963), were found. Therefore, all patients with aortic coarctation or other aortic-arch defects need a complete angiographic study, including aorta, heart, and supraaortic arteries.

One of the anomalies combined with aortic coarctation can be the aberrant right subclavian artery (arteria lusoria), which can impair swallowing, but not the peripheral circulation, if no additional failures are present. If coarcation is combined with the origin of the right subclavian artery behind it, reduced blood pressure in the right arm can be found (SOKOL et al. 1967). The existence of an arteria lusoria may also be suspected on esophageal contrast studies (KLINKHAMER 1965), which also give information about impression into the esophagus ventrally or dorsally. Angiographic documentation is only necessary, therefore, in the case of clinical symptoms or when there are particular problems in differential diagnosis.

Clinical symptoms in early childhood include: (a) Dyspnea, (b) upper respiratory infections, and (c) poor weight gain. In adults, common symptoms include headaches, nose bleeds, sensation of coldness, and leg pain. The *treatment* of aortic coarctation in symptomatic patients is surgery (VOLLMAR 1996b). In localized coarctation without cardiac anomalies, percutaneous balloon dilatation (PTA) has been increasingly used (SINGER et al. 1982; BUSSMANN et al. 1985; SIEVERT et al. 1987; ROCCHINI and BEEKMANN 1986; REDINGTON et al. 1993; FAWZY et al. 1993; BANK et al. 1987). Before its clinical use, percutaneous transluminal dilatation of coarcations of the thoracic aorta was studied post mortem (SOS et al. 1979), which demonstrated its technical possibilities.

The indication for balloon angioplasty in cases of aortic coarctation is still under discussion, since long-term results are available in only a limited number of studies (RAO 1996; ANJOS et al. 1992). Further studies for comparison with surgical treatment need to follow, and thorough selection of patients is a prerequisite (SHADDY et al. 1993; VOLLMAR 1997). However, in highly symptomatic small children, balloon dilatation can be performed as an initial treatment, to be followed after several years, medical condition permitting, by surgical reconstruction at the age of 5 to 6 years, if clinical symptoms exist or recoarctation has been documented.

In the interests of clear decision-making prior to the various surgical techniques or endovascular transfemoral treatment with balloon dilatation or stent application, ABRAMS and JÖNSSON (1983) defined four types of localized coarctatio aortae based on the distance between the subclavian artery and the stenosed area:

- Type I: The distal part of the aortic arch is relatively long and wide
- Type II: The distal part of the aortic arch is relatively long, but narrowed
- Type III: The distal part of the aortic arch is short, or the ostium of the subclavian artery is directly located in the stenotic area
- Type IV: The distal part of the aortic arch is atretic.

While in types I and II aortic resection or balloon dilatation can be discussed, in types III or IV surgical treatment should be preferred. For types I and III demonstrating a short stenosis between two wide aortic segments, resection and end-to-end anastomosis is recommended (HEBERER et al. 1966; ABRAMS and JÖNSSON 1983; VOLLMAR 1996). For types II and IV, mainly implantation of a prosthetic graft is recommended (VOLLMAR 1996). There are various techniques of operative repair, which have been discussed in detail in the surgical literature (VOLLMAR 1996). Operative mortality in the latest literature varies between 1% and 4%. Late local complications following surgery and balloon angioplasty include aortic aneurysm, dissection, or recurrent coarctation, which can be observed after surgery in 6%–10% of patients (CLARK et al. 1979).

Restenosis following surgical treatment of coarctation can be managed successfully using balloon dilatation (ANJOS et al. 1992; RAO et al. 1988; ROCCHINI and BEEKMAN 1986). In recent years, a general consensus has been emerging that balloon dilatation in neonates and small infants offers a relatively safe and effective alternative to surgical repair. With angioplasty, operative interventions may be avoided entirely, or at least be postponed until the children are older and taller, when surgical results are generally much betten. Should recurrence occur following angioplasty, or should an aneurysm develop at the site of dilatation, the infant may undergo surgical resection at a later date. After several papers on early results (Table 17.1) and a small number of long-term follow-up controls (ANJOS et al. 1992; RAO 1996), more studies are important. The incidence of post-dilatation aneurysms following balloon dilatation of native coarctation (14%) or recoarctation (15%) is not statistically significant (RAO 1996).

Recoarctation is defined as a pressure gradient in excess of 30 mmHg and was observed in three of 20 recoarctation PTAs, and in 18 of 90 PTAs of native

coarctation. The event-free survival curves (Fig. 17.4) following initial balloon angioplasty suggest that the event-free rates are better ($p = < 0.001$) for children (1–15 years old) than for infants (1–12 months old) and neonates (1–30 days old). In the majority of children, the blood pressure gradient between arms and legs remained low. Control angiograms following balloon angioplasty demonstrated, both directly after dilatation and later, a marked decrease in collateral vessels. The recurrence of collateral circulation, therefore, indicates new intraaortal pressure measurements and an interdisciplinary discussion about further therapy.

Complications both after balloon dilatation and surgery, such as aneurysm formation (CHENG 1991), or recoarctation (VON SCHULTHEISS et al. 1986),

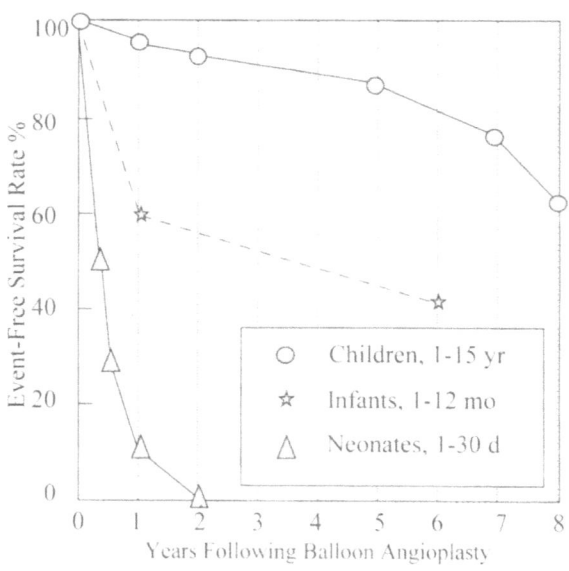

Fig. 17.4. Long-term results after balloon angioplasty for treatment of aortic coarctation (according to RAO 1996). Event-free survival curves of neonates, infants, and children

Table 17.1. Aortic coarctation: results in adult patients with pressure gradient pre- and post-percutaneous transluminal angioplasty. (According to RAO 1996)

Patients (n)	Age (years)	Pressure gradient (mmHg)		Follow-up (months)	Reference
		Pre	Post		
7	28 ± 14	59 ± 22	6 ± 9	6	ERBEL et al. 1990
35	23 ± 7	81 ± 23	15 ± 13	13	TYAGIE et al. 1992
23	23 ± 9	66 ± 19	8 ± 9	15	FAWZY et al. 1992
Complications (n = 60):		1 Aortic perforation	(1.6%)		
		5 Aneurysms	(8.3%)		
		1 Intimal dissection	(1.6%)		

as well as a good outcome, can be documented first with MR imaging (MRI) or 2D echocardiography in combination with duplex flow measurements. The mortality rate following balloon angioplasty of recoarctation was, according to a registry, 2.5% (5 of 200 patients), and 0.7% (1 of 141 patients) after angioplasties of native coarctations. Femoral artery complications were observed in 8.5% and neurologic events in 1.5% (RAO 1996). Meanwhile, coarctatio aortae in children and adults has also been treated by the transfemoral route using balloon-expandable stents (Palmaz stent) (REDINGTON et al. 1993; SUAREZ DE LENZO et al. 1995; O'LAUGHLIN et al. 1991).

In addition, with much less experience and fewer results of PTA of coarctation available than in surgery, angioplasty has proven so far to have the following advantages: intubation, repeated thoracotomy, the risk of spinal-cord injury, and the stay in an intensive-care unit can all be avoided. Moreover, the hospitalization time after balloon angioplasty is shorter and impairment of the peripheral circulation can be treated as effectively as with surgery. The future of stent-assisted balloon angioplasty of coarctation is still open, and prospective studies are required. Atypical coarctation will be discussed in the following chapter.

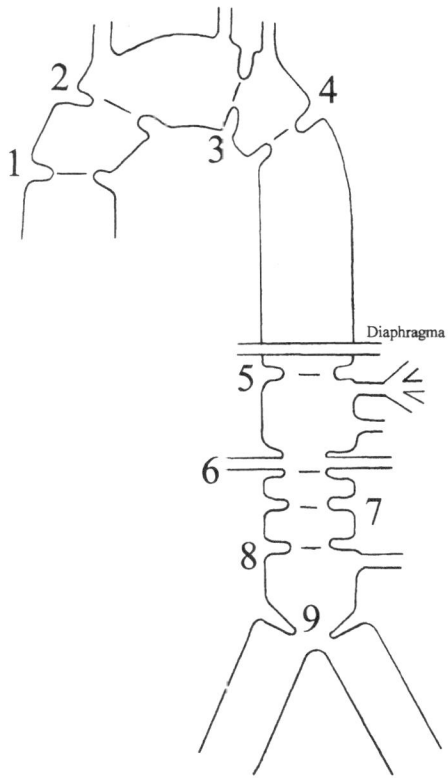

Fig. 17.5. 1–9 Different locations of stenoses in the thoracic and abdominal aorta

17.1.2
Aortic Stenoses

Standard monographies (SCHAD 1968; ABRAMS and JÖNSSON 1983; AMPLATZ 1986) describe exclusively those stenoses close to the aortic valve as "aortic stenoses", in addition to coarctatio aortae:
- Valvular aortic stenoses
- Membranous subaortic stenoses
- Muscular subaortic stenoses
- Supravalvular aortic stenoses.

In view of the peripheral circulation, some additional aortic stenoses exist between the ostia of the coronary arteries and the aortoiliac bifurcation (Fig. 17.5). All of these can result in peripheral occlusive vascular disease with reduced blood pressure in the lower extremities, sensation of coldness, claudication, or symptoms that are typical of all peripheral vascular diseases. Several of these require active treatment, such as vascular surgery or, if possible, percutaneous treatment with balloon angioplasty, or the minimally invasive application of stent grafts.

Regardless of history and etiology, i.e., congenital or acquired stenoses, stenoses as a result of degenertive arteriosclerotic disease, inflammatory disease (endangiitis, aortitis), or previous surgery, the most important clinical symptoms include absent or lowered pulse in the arteries of the groin and feet, and reduced bilateral blood pressure measured on the thigh or ankle in contrast to the brachial blood pressure. We need to differentiate here between aortic stenoses of different location and etiology. These include:
1. Supravalvular aortic stenoses, directly above Valsalva's sinus
2. Supravalvular aortic congenital stenoses in the ascending aorta
3. Aortic arch stenoses
4. Coarctation of classic location
5. Suprarenal thoracoabdominal aortic stenoses
6. Interrenal abdominal aortic stenosis
7. Infrarenal abdominal aortic coarctation and abdominal Takayasu's disease
8. Infrarenal abdominal aortic stenoses – mainly of arteriosclerotic or thrombotic origin

9. Aortoiliac bifurcational stenoses – mainly arteriosclerotic disease in Europe (in southeast Europe and Asia more commonly known as arteriitis).

17.1.2.1
Supravalvular Aortic Stenoses (1 and 2)

Supravalvular aortic stenosis is the least frequent form of aortic stenosis (PETERSSON et al. 1965; HEBERER et al. 1966). Three anatomic types of this anomaly have been described: (1) Narrow membrane directly above Valsalva's sinus, (2) hour-glass deformity of the ascending aorta, and (3) diffuse hypoplasia of the ascending aorta. The last is the same congenital defect as that described as "aorta agusta". The first two forms reflect different degrees of the same condition, causing generalized involvement of the aortic wall (AMPLATZ 1986). AMPLATZ described histologic appearances of the ascending aorta and other involved arteries. The histologic changes show disorganization of the media and a mosaic pattern representing irregular medial fibres. Also, fatal endocarditis has been discussed, and idiopathic hypercalcemia (BLACK and CARTER 1963), combination with Marfan's syndrome, coarctatio aortae, stenoses of brachiocephalic arteries, and peripheral pulmonary artery stenosis.

Moreover, a positive family history has also been discussed (UNDERHILL et al. 1971). The children have signs and symptoms resembling idiopathic hypercalcemia in infancy with slow growth and mild mental retardation. The facies have been described as "elf-like" or "elfin". AMPLATZ saw several such patients and demonstrated excellent angiographies. The results of surgery were published by WEISZ et al. in 1976.

If the stenosis is located in the ascending aorta, arm and leg blood pressures are similar and the elevated systolic pressure can only be measured by heart catheterization. The best imaging method to define the lesion and its extension is thoracic aortography, combined with direct pressure control in front of and behind the stenosis. The indication for treatment exists whenever the pressure gradient is above 40 mmHg.

17.1.2.2
Aortic Arch Stenoses (3)

Arch stenoses are of segmental nature, varying from mild incision, over a strongly segmental, high-grade stenosis to the complete interruption of the aortic arch, typically located between the left common carotid and left subclavian arteries. Another location is betweeen the brachiocephalic trunk and the left common carotid artery. There are three types of complete interruption of the aortic arch (CELORIA and PATTON 1959): In 50% of cases, it is located between the left carotid and left subclavian artery, in 46% of cases between the left subclavian artery and the patent ductus arteriosus, while in only 4% it was seen between the brachiocephalic trunk and the left carotid artery (VOLLMAR 1996b). This type of congenital defect is regularly combined with a patent ductus arteriosus, and mostly with a VSD. Life-expectancy is short, and babies often die during the first months after birth. The diagnosis has to be complete, including the heart chambers and supra-aortic arteries. Treatment, if feasible, can be very complex and requires pediatric cardiac surgery.

17.1.2.3
Abdominal Coarctation

Atypical locations of coarctation include the descending thoracic aorta, and the suprarenal and infrarenal abdominal aorta. SEN et al. (1962) published their study of 81 patients, of which 25 presented the condition in the descending thoracic aorta, 14 in the suprarenal, and 42 in the infrarenal abdominal aorta (n, 73). Meanwhile, this condition has been reported on in many more affected patients (CLAGETT et al. 1954; PIERACH and KATKOW 1972; HEJHAL et al. 1973; MÜLLER-WIEFEL et al. 1973; KREMER et al. 1975; VOLLMAR et al. 1976; CASALINI and SFONDRINI 1994). In several cases, the stenosis cannot be clearly defined as congenital, degenerative, or inflammatory (Fig. 17.6); therefore, the clinical situation was also described as "mid-aortic syndrome" (SEN et al. 1959; LEVIS et al. 1988). Several papers have favored the congenital, others the inflammatory etiology of such atypically localized or hypoplastic stenoses of the abdominal aorta (DEBAKEY et al. 1967; HEBERER et al. 1971; PIERACH and KATKOW 1972; HEJHAL et al. 1973).

In more than 70% of patients, there is a short-segmental stenosis, and in 22% a long hypoplastic aorta, including ostial stenoses in the renal and mesenteric arteries (VOLLMAR 1996). The different types and locations of abdominal coarctation (Fig. 17.8) were compiled in a schematic drawing by VOLLMAR in 1976. The clinical picture of suprarenal and infrarenal locations varies. Therefore, in view of the clinical symptomatology, the appropriate type of treatment, and also the diagnostic imaging methods, we have to distinguish between:

- A Suprarenal aortic stenoses (Fig. 17.5; 5)
- B Interrenal aortic stenoses (Fig. 17.5; 6) (Figs. 17.6 and 17.7)
- C Infrarenal abdominal aortic stenoses (Fig. 17.5; 7).

The suprarenal type of abdominal coarctation was mostly diagnosed in individuals aged between 20 and 51 years. In the literature review (HEBERER et al. 1975), the outcome in nearly 400 patients was discussed. The mean age of this operated patient population was 28.5 years.

The clinical symptoms in patients with suprarenal and interrenal coarctation include:

- Arterial hypertension (in nearly all patients)
- Headache (in 33%)
- Cardiac symptoms with palpitation, dyspnea, or others
- Symptoms of reduced lower-leg circulation, such as pulse- and blood-pressure reduction, and intermittent claudication.

Physical examination can detect a systolic–diastolic murmur above the aorta. A narrowing of the aorta can be identified with duplex sonography, MRA, as well as with CT angiography. The blood pressure controlled in the thigh or ankle is reduced compared to the blood pressure in the arms. In such cases, if no abnormality can be found in classical lower-leg angiographies, thoracic aortography, including demonstration of the thoracic and abdominal aorta, becomes necessary.

As in most patients with unclear arterial hypertension, particularly with elevated diastolic blood pressure, aortography is indicated in addition to non-invasive imaging methods (KIRKS et al. 1986; KREMER et al. 1975; KULGATZ 1964; PIERACH and KATKOW 1972; WENZ 1972; MÜLLER-WIEFEL et al. 1973; LIPCHIK et al. 1964; VOLLMAR et al. 1976). Aortography is indicated prior surgery in the following situations:

1. Suspected atypical location of aortic stenoses, because of the different types which include stenoses on side branches and the existence of hypoplastic or aplastic segments

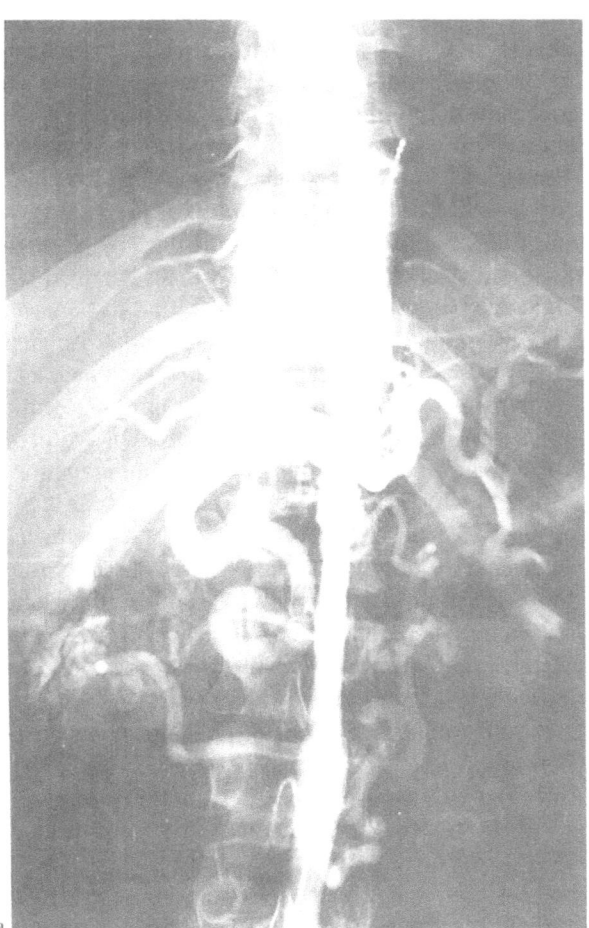
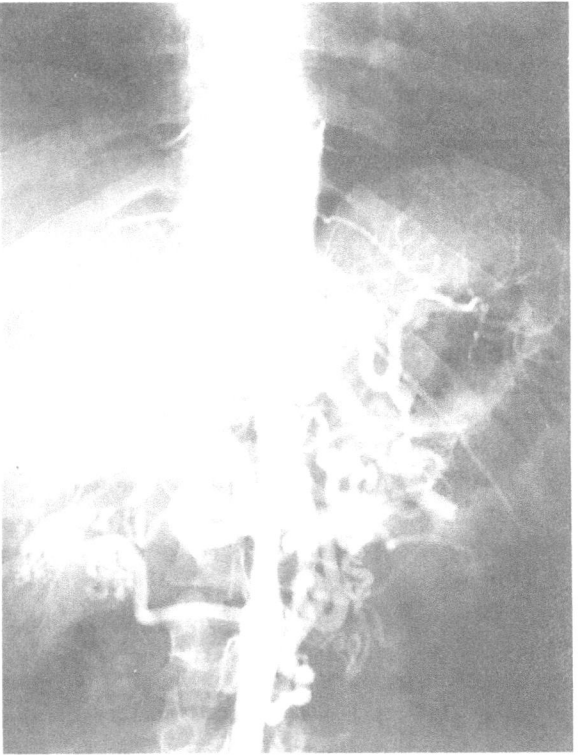

Fig. 17.6 a,b. Abdominal coarctation including the renal arteries. Collateral circulation from the celiac and cranial mesenteric arteries, and intercostal arteries to the infrastenotic aorta and inferior mesenteric artery. Early (**a**) and late (**b**) phase (as observed by Professor Löhr, Essen)

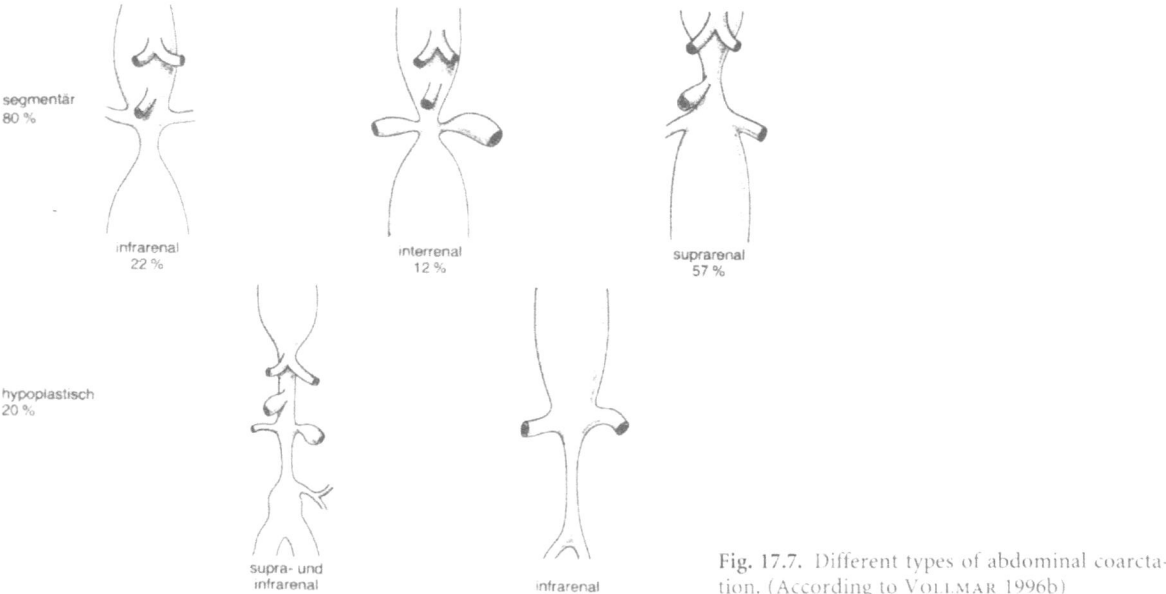

segmentär
80 %

infrarenal
22 %

interrenal
12 %

suprarenal
57 %

hypoplastisch
20 %

supra- und
infrarenal

infrarenal

Fig. 17.7. Different types of abdominal coarctation. (According to VOLLMAR 1996b)

2. To exclude pre- and poststenotic aneurysms
3. In the case of restenoses, complications, and unclear symptoms after surgery or interventional treatment.

In the 20% of hypoplastic aortic stenoses above and below the renal artery, all side branches are usually included (Fig. 17.7). Collateral channels come from the intercostal, celiac, and mesenteric arteries. As similar angiographies have been published in patients with inflammatory disease, all laboratory parameters must be controlled. In any inflammatory etiology, medical treatment using antibiotics and corticosteroids is recommended prior to surgery or interventional treatment. The extraanatomic bypass from the descending thoracic aorta to the lower abdominal aorta (Fig. 17.8) is mostly successful in these situations, with the lowest complication rate.

The possibility of obliterations above or below renal arteries indicates, additional angiographic documentation of the aortic arch, as well as of the pelvic and femoropopliteal arteries. The treatment of all patients with suprarenal or interrenal aortic stenoses is mainly surgery. The recommended techniques include: (a) Localized patch-plasty, or (b) resection of the stenosed segment with interposition of a Dacron graft, in situ bypass, or free extraanatomic bypass (turn-down and turn-up principle, respectively) (VOLLMAR 1996). In some situations, stenosis of the renal, mesenteric, or celiac artery needs to be treated simultaneously by thromboendarterectomy (TEA) or bypass.

17.1.2.4
Infrarenal Aortic Stenoses

Infrarenal aortic coarctation has been defined in the literature in one third of all atypical cases of coarctation (HEBERER et al. 1975). Arterial hypertension exists only if the renal arteries are simultaneously involved. Without the influence of renal arteries, the clinical symptomatology imitates aortoiliac vascular disease, also known as Lériche's syndrome. Intermittent claudication typically produces pain in the back and thigh, before pain in the calf is sensed. Pulses in the groin are lowered and blood pressure in the thigh and ankle is reduced in contrast to that in the arm. The differential diagnosis must rule out an isolated or simultaneous claudication with low-back pain and neurologic deficiency. Of particular importance is the exclusion of a disk prolapse, a congenital or acquired narrowing of the lumbar channel, and inflammatory or degenerative changes in the lumbar vertebrae in the form of marked deforming spon-dylarthritis. Infrarenal aortic stenoses need to be classified into short segmental stenoses (Figs. 17.9 and 17.10) or long severe, irregular arterioscler-otic stenoses (Fig. 17.11). Moreover, there are excentric stenoses of the infrarenal abdominal aorta (Fig. 17.12).

While isolated stenoses of the infrarenal aorta were considered a rare exception in earlier years, since the first descriptions of balloon angioplasty of isolated infrarenal aortic stenoses (VELASQUEZ et al. 1980; ZORN-BOPP et al. 1981), such stenoses have been more frequently diagnosed, resulting in percutaneous treatment of the narrowed vessel. Interestingly, in most cases, women aged between 30 and 60 years are affected. In addition to cigarette-smoking, long-term use of oral contraceptives was found to be a risk factor. However, also within the framework of multilocular arteriosclerosis, infrarenal aortic stenoses exist in combination with arteriosclerotic obliterations in iliac and leg arteries, and these are more common in men.

In the case of extensive obliterations, or a very wide diameter of the infrarenal aorta, a surgical approach by means of TEA, or the application of an endograft, can be performed if the symptoms are clear. The clinical symptoms of an isolated aortic stenosis largely correspond to those of POVD of the pelvis, with bilateral symptoms in the form of intermittent claudication, lowered pulse in the groin, and reduction of pressure in foot and thigh arteries, determined by means of Doppler measurements.

17.1.2.5
Interventional Radiology of Infrarenal Aortic Stenoses

After the publication of initial results with balloon dilatation of infrarenal aortic stenoses by VELASQUEZ et al. (1980) and ZORN-BOPP et al. (1981; INGRISCH et al. 1984), angioplasty was primarily performed using the "kissing-balloon technique" (see Fig. 17.10). On both sides of the groin, one Grüntzig-balloon catheter, each with balloons of the largest diameter as used in earlier years (8–10 mm), were advanced under angiographic control to the level of the stenosis. Simultaneously, the balloons were flushed with a mixture of contrast agent and saline, which resulted in a widening of the inner aortic lumen. If the aorta had a large diameter, or if the outcome of balloon dilatation – controlled by means of the pressure gradient and the angiographic result – was not satisfactory, a further, third balloon catheter could be advanced either via the transbrachial or transaxillary route (see Chap. 8, Sect. 8.2.4) into the aortic stenoses. Three balloons were then dilated simultaneously (triple-balloon dilatation). Optimum control of balloon dilatation in the aorta and the iliac arteries requires direct control of the pressure gradient (see Fig. 17.10).

Reports published on more than 100 patients and 112 balloon angioplasties in the registry of the Working Group on Interventional Radiology (AGIR; ZEITLER 1993) demonstrated a mean pressure gradient of 44 ± 12 mmHg before PTA and 7 ± 5 mmHg after successful dilatation. The infrarenal

aortic stenoses have so far been successfully dilated mainly with the kissing-balloon technique using two or three balloon catheters (MORAG et al. 1987; ODURNY et al. 1989; GROSS-FENGELS et al. 1990; EL ASHMAOUI et al. 1991; CASALIN and SFONDRINI 1994; RAVIMANDALAM et al. 1991; HALLISEY et al. 1994). If the size of the aorta permits, and if balloon catheters as used for valvuloplasty (diameter, 12–15 mm) are available, dilatation with one single balloon can be effected via a sheath of 10 F in diameter (ROTH et al. 1988).

Between 1979 und 1981, INGRISCH et al. (1983) treated seven single aortic stenoses using the kissing-balloon technique. Still, follow-up controls up to 30 months have shown that, unless restenosis had developed within the first year, long-lasting patency was the result of the treatment. Between 1980 and 1994, we treated 23 patients at the General Hospital of Nuremberg using transfemoral angioplasty. The mean age among women was 53 and among men 58 years. In all, 19 were treated with

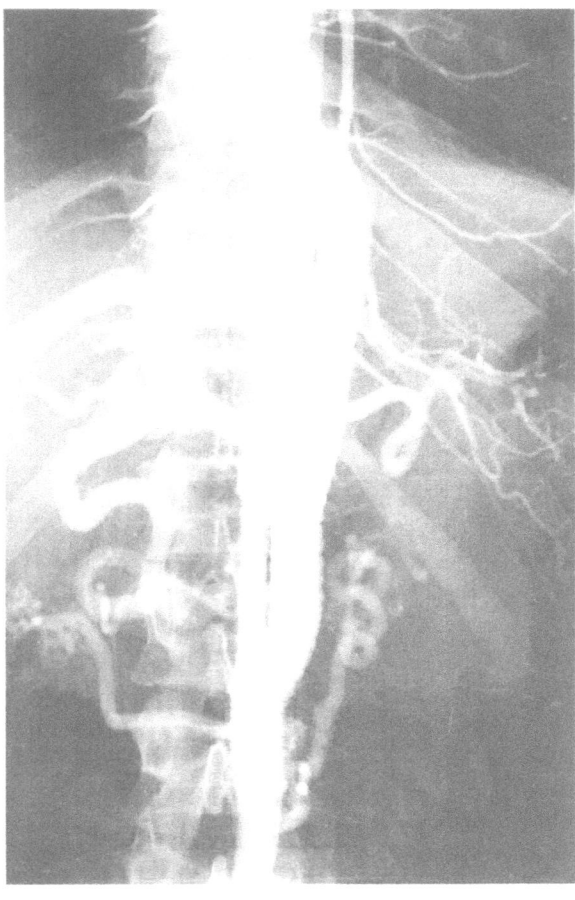

Fig. 17.8. Postoperative angiography demonstrating the aorto-aortal bypass with reduced collateral circulation (same patient as in Fig. 17.6)

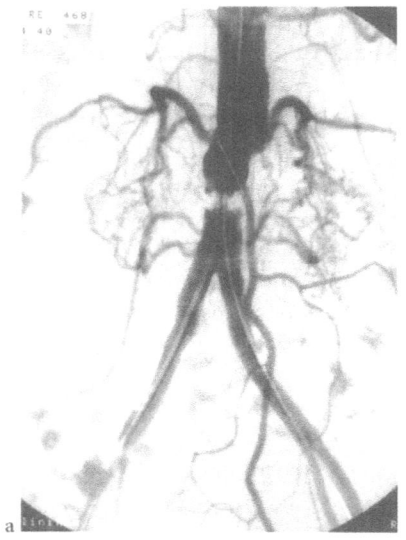
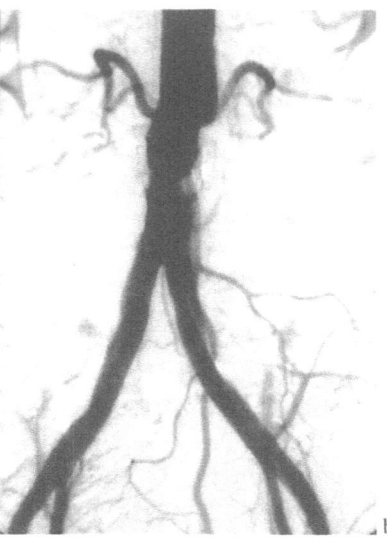

Fig. 17.9 a,b. Segmental infrarenal aortic stenosis. a Segmental type with collateral circulation from the upper lumbar arteries to the lower lumbar arteries, and to the internal iliac artery. b Control angiography after kissing-balloon angioplasty with three balloons

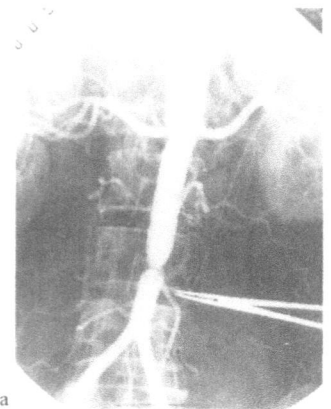
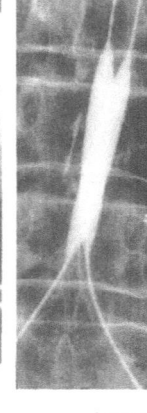
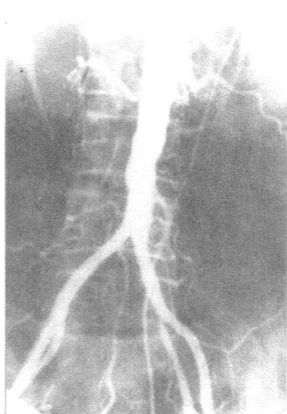

Fig. 17.10 a–c. Kissing-balloon angioplasty of an infrarenal aortic stenosis. a Before treatment, b kissing balloons, c after successful percutaneous transluminal angioplasty (*PTA*), d blood pressure in the right and left groin before PTA, e blood pressure in the aorta and left iliac artery after PTA

Right   Left   Aorta 160 mmHg   External iliac 150 mmHg
100 mmHg   98 mm Hg

d   e

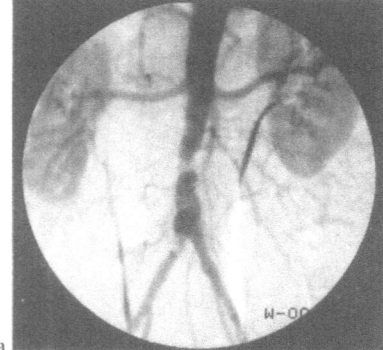
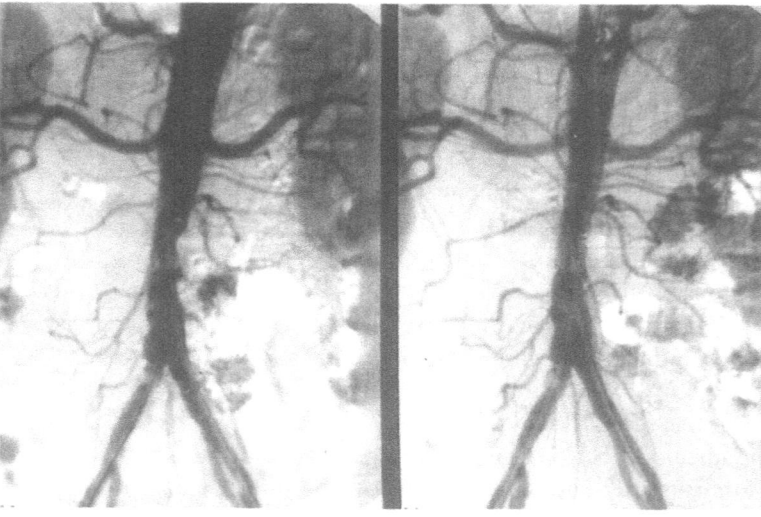

Fig. 17.11 a–c. Irregular infrarenal abdominal aortic stenosis. a Pre-treatment angiography. b,c Control angiographies after successful balloon angioplasty

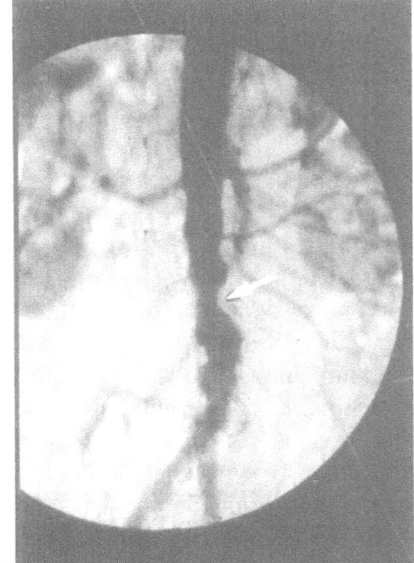

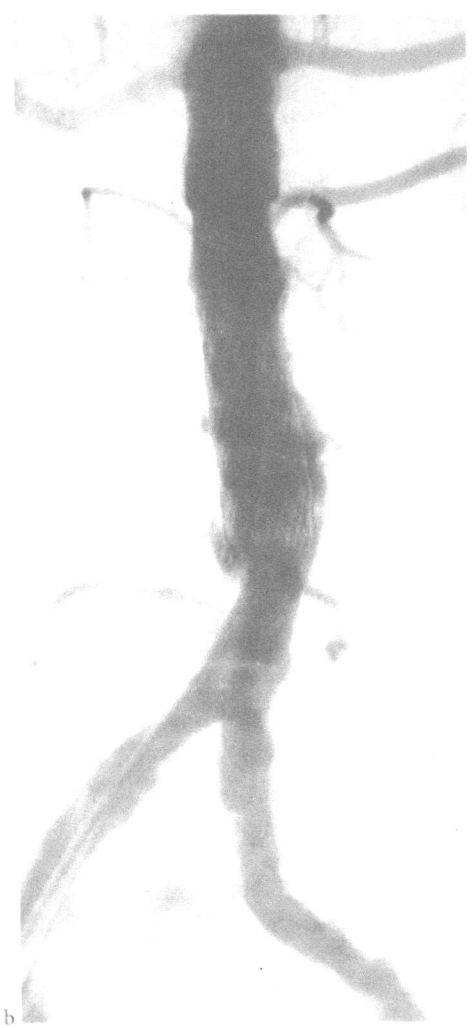

Fig. 17.12. a Infrarenal irregular abdominal arteriosclerotic stenosis. b Control angiography after application of a Palmaz stent in combination with balloon dilatation using the valvuloplasty balloon

the kissing-balloon technique, two with the triple-balloon technique (Fig. 17.9), and two with the single-balloon technique. In three patients with failed dilatation or long-segmental stenoses, we implanted a balloon-expandable Palmaz stent as a second intervention with excellent long-term results (Fig. 17.12). Only one patient received a covered Cragg stent directly after an unsuccessful kissing-balloon technique.

Complications included: hematomas in the groin (2), and in one patient, thrombotic occlusion of the abdominal aorta after 3 months, which was managed surgically. The primary patency rate controlled by ankle blood pressure, Doppler index, and imaging control using digital subtraction angiography (DSA) or spiral CT was 82.6%. The mean follow-up period was 8.7 years (3–16), and the patency rate was 70% after 5 years according to the life-table method. Two patients died of coronary heart disease after seven and 12 years. In addition, the published case reports and literature reviews demonstrated a primary success rate after 3 years of about 89%, and a complication rate of 4%–7%.

Since the establishment of endovascular treatment of abdominal aortic aneurysms (AAA) with tube grafts, all patients with infrarenal-aorta diameters exceeding 20 mm should be treated rather with one of the endovascular grafts (see Sect. 17.4).

The demonstration of the technical principles of "kissing-" or "triple-balloon dilatation" showed that several areas of stenotic material are not treated accurately, which may cause peripheral embolization or acute thrombosis. Also, blue-toe syndrome can be the result of aortic stenosis.

After the successful treatment of a high-grade infrarenal aortic stenosis (see Fig. 17.11), control angiography demonstrated lateral irregularities and intimal flaps, but a pressure gradient of only 12 mmHg. Up to now (4 years after triple-balloon dilatation), this patient is patent and the ankle–arm pressure gradient is 0.85. However, in principle, the application of an endograft should be the preferred alternative in the future. To define the normal diameter of the infrarenal abdominal aorta above and below the stenotic area, cross-sectional measurements with CT angiography are very important. They provide the possibility of choosing the exact diameter of the balloon, stent, or endograft. Also, follow-up controls with spiral CT and color-coded duplex sonography are capable of demonstrating both early and later results, including possible dissection or restenosis. Where stent implantation after balloon dilatation in AAA was indicated, TRILLER et al. (1993) successfully used self-expanding stents. In one of our patients, in Nuremberg, we implanted a self-expanding Wallstent in an aorta of 18 mm in diameter, where the diameter inside the stenosis had narrowed to 6 mm. It was not possible to anchor the stent since it was very soft and easily compressed by the blood pressure, whereupon it had to be removed like a foreign body since thrombotic occlusion occurred. Therefore, in my opinion, the accurate determination of the diameter of the aortic lumen in front of and behind the stenosis is mandatory in order to select the appropriate stent or tube graft.

17.1.2.5
Aortoarteriitis (Takayasu-Type Angiitis)

This inflammatory disease with arterial obliteration, primarily occuring in the area of the aortic arch arteries, is found more often than the purely degenerative arteriosclerotic aortic and arterial obliterations in Japan, China, and India. Histology shows a diffuse thickening and proliferation of the endothelium. The inflammatory process affects all vascular wall layers. On angiogram, there is a smooth rim to the arterial lumen in nearly all cases. This form of obliterating vascular disease has also been observed – albeit in significantly lower numbers – outside Asia (HIRSCH et al. 1964). The variety of publications in Asian countries (Japan, China, India, Korea, Vietnam, Thailand, and the Philippines) (RAU 1970) report that mainly women are affected. The onset of the disease in Asian countries occurs significantly earlier than observed in the US and Europe. The clinical picture of "middle-aortic syndrome" (SEN et al. 1959) does not differentiate between congenital atypical coarctation and stenosis caused by arteriitis of the aorta. Only to a limited degree, the patient's age or, possibly, simultaneous involvement of the abdominal and thoracic aorta, and laboratory data indicate the inflammatory situation.

Histology shows a chronic productive inflammation stretching into the adventitia. Alongside the vasa vasorum, there are focal diffuse round-cell infiltrations. If the condition develops over a long period of time, the signs of inflammation regress, and calcifications appear (ITO 1966). Angiogram demonstrates plaque-shaped, long-segmental lumen narrowings (GROLLMANN and HANAFEE 1964), which reach as far as into the ostia of the branching-off mesenteric and renal arteries. Experience gained in balloon angioplasty for aortoarteriitis in iliac and renal arteries (FAVA et al. 1993) has shown that the removal of the stenosis with balloon catheters is con-

siderably more complicated than in arteriosclerotic isolated stenoses. Therefore, stent implantation seems to be the better approach.

17.1.3
Aortic Occlusions

Aortoiliac obliterations occur in three types (Fig. 17.13), for which the clinical situation is similar: (a) Type I was observed in 37%, (b) type II, the classical Lériche's syndrome, in 55%, and (c) type III in 8%–12% (ROB and VOLLMAR 1959). While the majority of patients with aortoiliac obliterations start with a distal arteriosclerotic stenosis followed by an ascending thrombosis, symptoms can increase slowly, in contrast to the aortoiliac embolic occlusion. Also, "high aortic occlusion" (Fig. 17.14) often occurs as a sudden dramatic event. When no pulse at all is palpable in the groin and auscultatory examination reveals no stenotic murmur above the pelvic arteries, aortic occlusion is the clear diagnosis. What remains to be clarified, then, is the extension of the aortic occlusion, both in a cranial direction, including the renal arteries, and in a caudal direction, to determine the involvement of the pelvic arteries in the occlusive process. The male-to-female ratio varies between 11–19:1 (VOLLMAR 1996).

Angiography is the most effective diagnostic method to define the location and extension of aortic and aortoiliac occlusions (WENZ 1972; ABRAMS and JÖNSSON 1983). As there is no pulse in the groin, the only route for contrast agent administration is the high translumbar aortic puncture (Fig. 17.14a) or, as with more up-to-date methods, retrograde transbrachial catheterization with 3–5-F catheters, and intravenous DSA with pre-atrial contrast medium administration (SEYFERTH et al. 1982; GMELIN and ARLART 1987; DARCY 1991; FINK 1991; ZEITLER and HEUCK 1997).

A diagnosis of aortic occlusion with an approximate determination of the proximal end of the occlusion can also be achieved using duplex sonography, spiral CT, or MRA. For meticulous operation planning and monitoring, however, DSA with a catheter inserted brachially and advanced into the descending thoracic aorta is the preferred technique. Important postoperative information can also be obtained by intravenous DSA or spiral CT. Prior to surgical therapy, either in the form of TEA of the aorta or implantation of an aortofemoral or aortoiliac Dacron bypass graft, it is crucial to assess to what extent the mesenteric or renal arteries are involved in the thrombotic process.

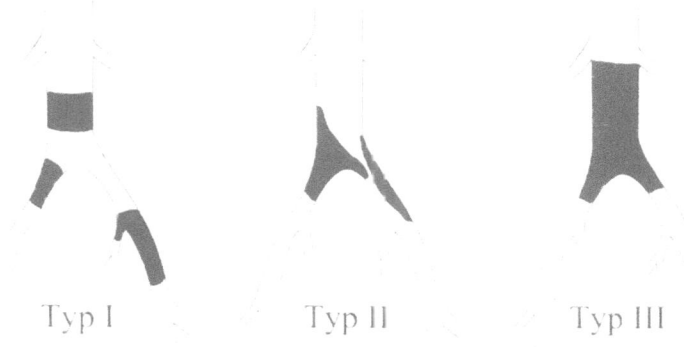

Fig. 17.13. Typ I-III. Typical anatomical situations in aortoiliac obliterations. (According to VOLLMAR 1996)

Typ I   Typ II   Typ III

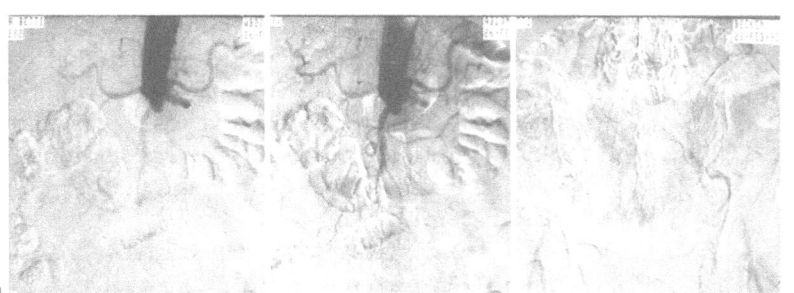

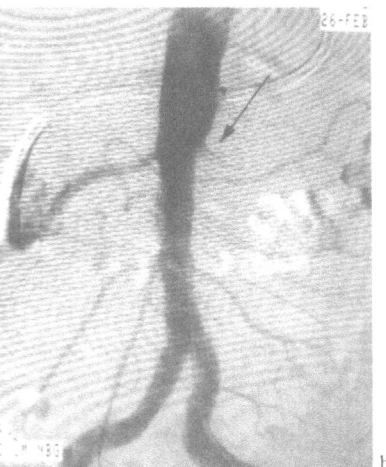

Fig. 17.14 a,b. High aortic occlusion. **a** Angiography before treatment. **b** Control angiography after vascular surgery (operator, Professor D. Raithel, Nuremberg)

The existence of a horseshoe kidney should be excluded in the same way, by means of an X-ray of the abdomen after angiography, as this anatomic anomaly requires specific preparation on the surgeon's part (SCHWILDEN 1978). To obtain optimum information, abdominal aortography should therefore be carried out by a second (oblique or lateral) projection. Three dimensional (3D) scanning methods (spiral CT and MRA) provide the optimum opportunity to analyze anomalies and atypical obliterations at branching points, due to the feasibility of analysis in as many projections as required, without the use of arterial catheterization and X-rays.

In chronic aortic occlusions, there is still a collateral circulation via Winslow's collateral pathways, and from the first and second lumbar arteries to the superior gluteal branches of the internal iliac artery. In these cases, a tiny femoral pulse is palpable, if there is good collateral circulation.

Morphologic studies had already shown in earlier years (MITTELMEIER 1959) that chronic aortic occlusions also contain non-organized thrombi, even after

several months. The results of systemic thrombolysis (SCHOOP et al. 1968) and ultra-high systemic lysis therapy with streptokinase (MARTIN and FIEBACH 1985; SPENGLER et al. 1991; HEIMIG and MARTIN 1997) have demonstrated that aortic occlusions in preselected collectives with occlusions of a clinically assumed existence of 1–6 months could also be dissolved in 57% and 86%, respectively (SCHOOP et al. 1968; SPENGEL et al. 1991). Angiograms following successful thrombolysis (Fig. 17.15a,b) of high aortic occlusions (ZEITLER et al. 1969) demonstrate the extent of the thrombosis amenable to lysis in the vascular lumen, and to what extent the organization of thrombotic material has progressed from the aortic wall. On the other hand, such angiograms also explain the high risk of embolism associated with intraluminal mechanical manipulations in the aorta for the management of aortic occlusions.

Calcifications are observed in many, but not all, patients with aortic occlusion. On the other hand, aortic calcification is part of general arteriosclerosis. There is a certain likelihood that both the calcifica-

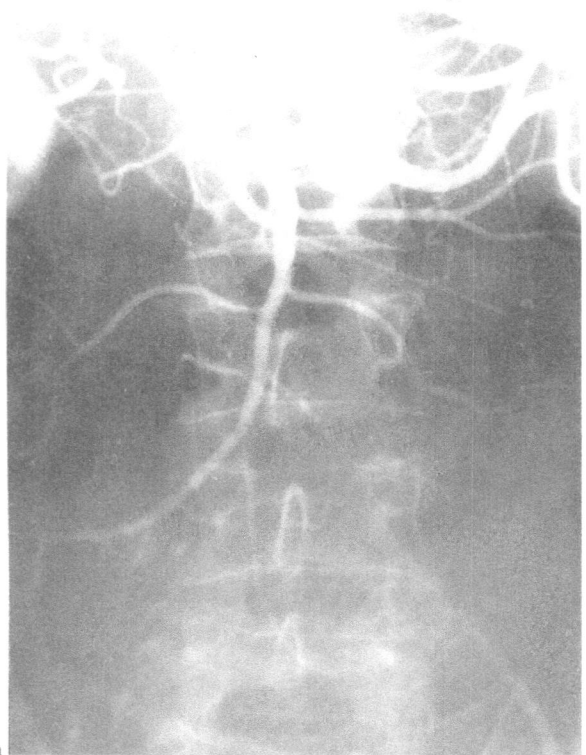

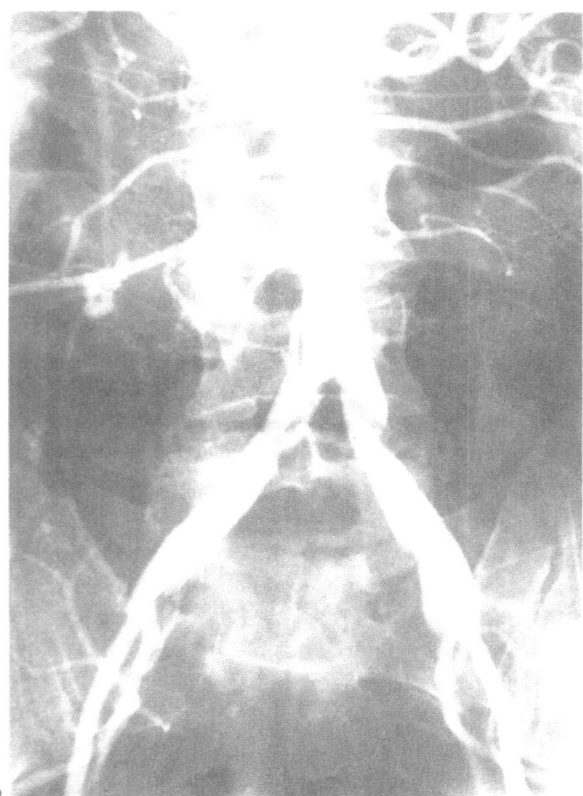

Fig. 17.15. a High aortic occlusion. Translumbar aortography and sacciform aneurysm on the right renal artery. **b** Control angiography after successful systemic thrombolytic treatment with streptokinase. (MARTIN and FIEBACH 1985, Aggertal Clinic, Engelskirchen)

tion of the aortic wall and large vascular diameters might prevent speedy connective-tissue organization of the thrombus.

Peripheral arterial vascular occlusion is a single-level disease only in persons of less than 50 years of age. With increasing age, obliterations on two or three levels (in pelvic, thigh, and lower-leg arteries) are more common. Therefore, detailed angiographic documentation of the inflow and outflow arteries, i.e., of the abdominal aorta including the renal arteries and the leg arteries down to the lower leg and foot, is always necessary.

Therapy should be chosen according to the urgency of intervention as determined by clinical symptoms. While an acute aortic occlusion requires immediate action, a slowly developing pathologic condition leaves sufficient time for appropriate diagnostic measures. Irrespective of the possibilities offered by systemic thrombolysis, acute aortic occlusion is primarily a disease requiring a surgical reconstructive operation.

Only in patients with high operative risk, or other unfavorable conditions for surgery, can thrombolytic treatment under in-patient conditions, including the control of coagulation parameters, be recommended as an alternative (see Chap. 22). Since mechanical recanalization of iliac occlusions has already been associated with a risk of embolization in about 10% of cases, attempts at mechanical recanalization of the aorta, or local thrombolysis of the same, should not be used as a primary treatment.

17.1.3.1
Collateral Circulation in Aortoiliac Occlusions

Typical collateral pathways (Fig. 17.16) for bypassing aortic obliterations at different levels include:
- Thoracic-epigastric circulation (Winslow's collateral pathway)
- Mesenteric circulation (Riolan's collateral pathway)
- Lumbar-iliac collateral vessels
- Mesenteric-iliac collateral circulation
- Obdurator profunda collateral circulation.

Other collateral vessels at different levels, particularly in the area of the pelvic arteries, crossing the two sides, but also between the iliac, spinal, and epigastric system, have been observed.

Angiography should always depict the existent collateral circulation, including its origin and direc-

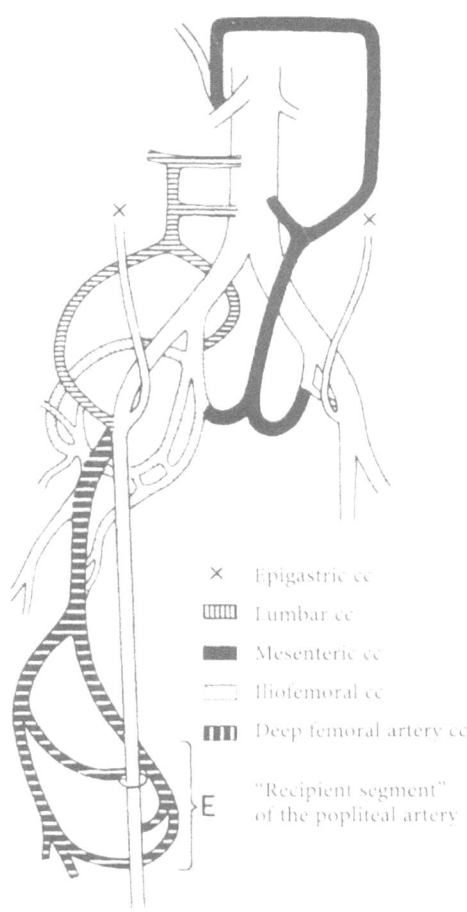

× Epigastric cc

▥ Lumbar cc

▬ Mesenteric cc

▭ Iliofemoral cc

▥ Deep femoral artery cc

"Recipient segment"
of the popliteal artery

Fig. 17.16. Typical collateral pathways in aortoiliac oliterations. *cc*, collateral circulation (According to VOLLMAR 1997)

tion. Consequently, this may necessitate the injection of (CM) at an atypical site. For example, in order to visualize Winslow's collaterals, the contrast agent must be injected in the ascending thoracic artery, or into the two subclavian arteries. The documentation of Riolan's collateral circulation requires the injection of CM into the abdominal aorta above the celiac and mesenteric arteries.

MRA has proven superior to classical angiography with X-rays in demonstrating the total extension of collateral arteries, since it does not document the immediate flow of the injected contrast agent, but the distribution of the intravenously applied CM throughout the whole collateral system, thus later enabling a general overview.

17.2
Surgical Treatment of Aortoiliac Disease

D. RAITHEL and E. ZEITLER

17.2.1
Introduction

The indication for peripheral reconstruction has changed substantially over the past years. Nowadays, reconstructions are mostly undertaken for limb-salvaging, at stages III and IV of POVD. This applies particularly to infrainguinal vascular occlusions. In the area of the pelvic vessels, the indication is now made in a greater number of patients and alternative treatments, such as extraanatomic bypasses (Fig. 17.17) and PTA, are increasingly performed. These techniques take into account the fact that 43%–66% of patients with POVD are suffering from multiple occlusions; in our own population, the rate was 63%.

Reconstruction of an occluded arterial vessel in the sense of a "complete correction" is no longer necessary today. A fact that deserves attention in the reconstruction of pelvic vessels, however, is that severe stenoses at branching points of the deep femoral artery have to be included in the reconstruction. Several criteria need to be considered prior to the indication for surgical therapy. These include: (1) multiple occlusions, (2) singular or multilocular lesions of the pelvic vascular level, (3) the patient's age and operative risk, and (4) the stage of POVD, i.e., urgent or elective reconstruction. Thus, thorough documentation of the peripheral vessels is a prerequisite for any reconstruction. In patients with obliterations of the pelvic vessels, intraarterial DSA after transbrachial catheterization with 4-F catheters is sufficient nowadays. In patients with crural obliterations, arterial fine-needle angiography, including documentation of the plantar arch, is often necessary. Also, duplex sonography can provide additional information In all other cases, however, we are autious in the use of transfemoral arteriography, if reconstruction is planned for a later time, because of the elevated risk of infection. This, of course, is also true for patients with previous interventional treatment.

If possible, whenever a vascular reconstruction is taken into consideration or planned, the vascular system should be assessed by means of arterial DSA performed from the contralateral side, or, if this should be excluded, transbrachially.

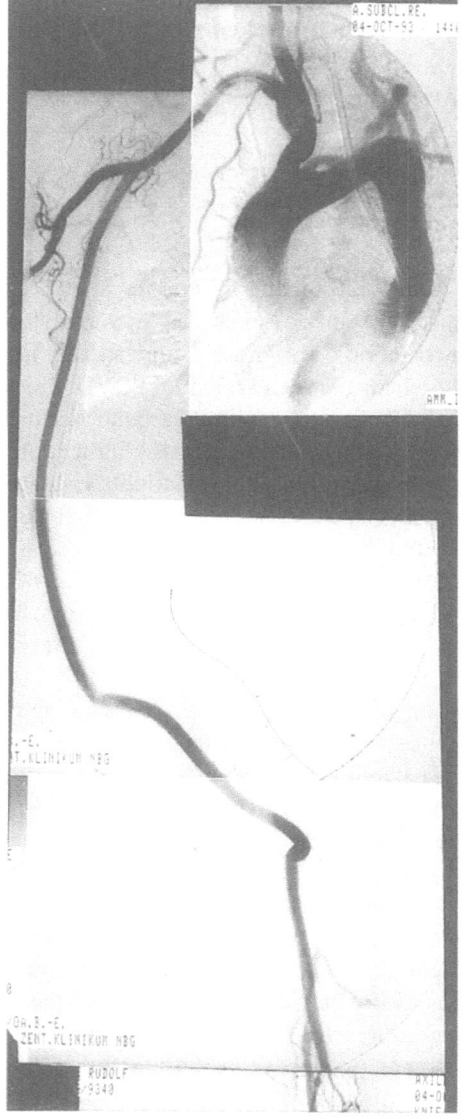

Fig. 17.17 Extraanatomotic subclaviafemoral Bypass right

17.2.2
Pelvic Vessels

Selection of the therapeutic measure depends mainly on the severity and location of the occlusion in the aortoiliac segment and, of course, on the patient's individual operative risk. In the case of isolated short-segmental occlusions and moderately severe stenoses, a transluminal angioplasty, including stent implantation if necessary, is recommended, particularly in the region of the common iliac artery. Longer occlusions, however, require surgical management, either in the form of direct vascular reconstruction

or one of the so-called alternative treatments (see Sect. 17.2.2.3).

17.2.2.1
Indication for Surgery

The indication for a surgical approach in the sense of a direct correction of the aorta or/and the pelvic vessels in elderly patients is only established in stages III or IV of POVD, i.e., in limb-threatening situations. Even stage IIb involving reduced quality of life, with a walking distance of about 50–100 m, should not be corrected in the elderly or high-risk patient (RAITHEL 1990). In isolated iliac occlusions, all of the conservative therapeutic measures should be applied first. Moreover, the indication for PTA is made less restrictively in such cases.

Following assessment of the cardiopulmonary risk, it can be decided whether the pelvic level can be reconstructed by direct, i.e., aortobifemoral or aortofemoral, reconstruction, or whether an extra-anatomic bypass should be preferred over a direct correction in high-risk patients.

17.2.2.2
Operative Techniques: Uni- and Bilateral Reconstruction

In general, unilateral occlusions are corrected via the retroperitoneal and bilateral occlusions via transperitoneal access. In high-risk patients, bilateral correction of the pelvic vascular level can also be effected via retroperitoneal access.

I and my team prefer bilateral over unilateral reconstruction since we have observed a high percentage of occlusions in the contralateral side after unilateral reconstruction during the follow-up period. Therefore, whenever the patient's general condition permits, both pelvic levels should be reconstructed by means of a plastic bifurcated endoprosthesis.

For unilateral reconstructions, we are currently using 8-mm polytetrafluoroethylene (PTFE) prostheses, but Dacron prostheses of the same diameter can also be applied. The implantation is performed beginning with the proximal anastomosis at the aorta and the bifurcation of the common iliac artery from the aorta. The distal connection is located in the segment of the common femoral artery, provided the superficial femoral artery is patent. If the latter is occluded, the deep femoral artery needs to be included in the central reconstruction, in the form of a profundaplasty.

For bilateral occlusions, we prefer Dacron prostheses with diameters of 16×9 or 14×8 mm. This bifurcated prosthesis is anastomosed end-to-end with the infrarenal aorta. Both legs of the prosthesis are pulled through in a retroperitoneal direction, and anastomosed end-to-side on the femoral bifurcation opposite the branching point of the deep femoral artery. Also in this situation, central reconstruction must be combined with profundaplasty. This leads to improved run-in into the deep fermoral artery and an increase in the collateral run-in into the distal popliteal artery in the case of a femoral occlusion located in Hunter's channel.

Obliterations of the renomesenteric vascular level are corrected in the same setting by transaortic endarterectomy or bypass. When Y-shaped prostheses are used, high-positioned end-to-end anastomosis in an infrarenal position has proven to be a reliable technique. It provides several advantages: The re-occlusion rate is lower than that of end-to-side anastomoses and local complications, such as aortoduodenal fistuals, occur less frequently.

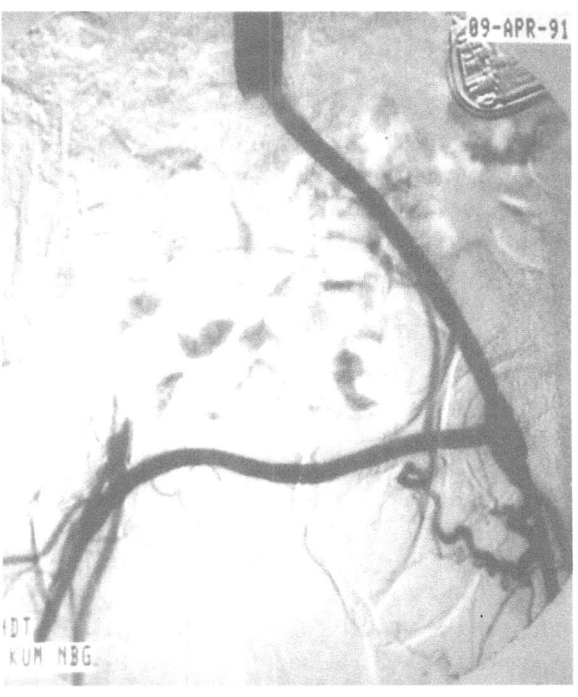

Fig. 17.18. Femorofemoral cross-over bypass (operator, D. Raithel, Nuremberg)

17.2.2.3
Extraanatomic Bypasses: Alternative Techniques

Alternative techniques have gained in importance in reconstructive vascular surgery over recent years, particularly femorofemoral bypasses for the correction of unilateral iliac artery occlusions (Fig. 17.18). This operation is feasible whenever a good pulse is palpable on the contralateral side. Should, however, a marked stenosis be present on the donor side, the latter can be dilated by means of PTA either pre- or intraoperatively. This enables the indication for femorofemoral bypassing to be made less restrictively. The procedure is performed using either Dacron or PTFE prostheses of 8 mm in diameter.

The prosthesis is attached at the highest possible point on the patent iliac artery of the donor side, then subcutaneously led to the contralateral side above the pubis, and finally anastomosed on the recipient segment, much in the sense of a profundaplasty. The intervention can be performed without problems under regional or local anesthesia (in high-risk patients).

The indication for axillofemoral and axillobifemoral bypasses was handled very carefully in earlier years since these transplants involved the disadvantage of higher reocclusion rates. By implanting

ringed PTFE prostheses, the outcome, however, could be considerably improved, which has led to some widening of the indication for axillofemoral bypasses. However, we are still highly autious when establishing the indication for axillofemoral bypassing. The donor artery is then the axillary artery and the prosthesis is conducted laterally alongside the thoracic and abdominal wall to the femoral bifurcation, where it is anastomosed with elongation into the deep femoral artery (see Chap. 8).

17.2.2.4
Results of Surgical Therapy

In our own population, we had a mortality rate of 0.8% following implantation of a Y-shaped prosthesis (RAITHEL 1987). Patency rates after 5 and 10 years were 86% and 81%, respectively. The cumulative survival rate of these patients was 76% after 5, and 57% after 10 years. The crucial aspect determining late results both of uni- and bilateral reconstructions is the optimum correction of the run-in in the connection segment of the profunda. If this is performed successfully, many patients can be spared further peripheral infrainguinal reconstruction. Currently, only some 8% of patients with multiple occlusions require peripheral reconstruction after central reconstruction. Between 1976 and 1979, this rate was only 21%, compared to 69% between 1966 and 1972 (RAITHEL 1987).

Should the control examination following central reconstruction reveal a persistant significant stenosis of the profunda in the presence of a superficial femoral occlusion, we recommend PTA of the profunda stenosis, prior to additional peripheral infrainguinal reconstruction.

The results of alternative techniques have shown that femorofemoral bypassing is associated with a minimal mortality rate of less than 1%. Patency after femorofemoral bypass creation in our population was 92% after 1 year, and 87% after 6 years (SCHWEIGER et al. 1984; SCHWEIGER and RAITHEL 1984; RAITHEL 1990). The correction of unilateral occlusions by means of aortofemoral prostheses resulted in 1.6% of lethal cases, at a patency of 73.4% after 5, and 69.8% after 10 years (RAITHEL 1987; RAITHEL 1990). The femorofemoral bypass even produced better long-term results than unilateral correction of the pelvic vessels (SCHWEIGER and RAITHEL 1984). The results of axillofemoral bypass are less satisfying: Even though death occurs in no more than 1.6% of patients, the patency rates bear no comparison whatsoever with those of femorofemoral bypassing. After 3 years, only 68% of these reconstructions are still patent (TAYLOR et al. 1991).

17.2.25
Renal Vessels

Many of our patients are hypertensive and have renal artery stenoses. In those patients with isolated renal artery stenoses without other significant pathologic changes of the pelvic vessels requiring correction, we try to dilate the stenoses first. Should the dilatation fail, or not be indicated due to vascular findings, reconstruction of the renal vessels is indicated in the interests of salvaging the kidney and achieving reduce pressure.

The procedure is different in patients with renal artery stenoses and concomitant occlusions of the pelvic vessels and aortic aneurysms requiring correction. In such combined occlusions, we always recommend the correction of the renal artery stenosis in the course of reconstruction of the pelvic arteries or resection of the aneurysm. This simultaneous reconstruction of the renal kidneys is, to our mind, only justified when elevated creatinine levels suggest disturbed perfusion of the kidneys, or if the patient has

renal hypertension which is difficult to stabilize (DEAN and KIMBERLEY 1991). The preferred reconstruction principle in such cases is the correction of the renal vessels by means of transaortic endarterectomy of the renal kidneys.

17.2.3
Peripheral Vessels

Prior to any correction of the peripheral vessels, it must be borne in mind that unconsidered stenoses of the pelvic vessels can jeopardize, or at least negatively influence, the operative outcome. Thus, reconstruction of the pelvic vessels has priority over the correction of the peripheral vessels. As a rule, only a sufficient run-in will guarantee a good long-term result after infrainguinal vascular reconstruction. The indication for preoperative dilatation of the pelvic vessels should therefore be made generously, even in cases with a groin pulse that is no more than acceptable. Treatment via a contralateral or transbrachial approach is possible to dilate inflow pelvic artery stenoses.

17.2.3.1
Indication for Surgery

Today, we almost exclusively consider patients with occlusive vascular disease stages III–IV, i.e., in limb-threatening situations, as candidates for infrainguinal vascular reconstruction. Only in exceptional cases, we consider the indication for peripheral vascular reconstruction in stage-IIb patients, provided there is satisfactory run-in and -off. Therefore, in such cases, at least two patent run-off arteries in the lower leg should have been documented before hand.

Since, in general, these are long segmental obliterations of the femoral and popliteal arteries, partially including the lower leg vessels, a thorough evaluation of the operative and interventional procedure is necessary. Undoubtedly, it is not always appropriate to burden the patient with extensive, strenuous crural reconstructions for stenoses of the popliteocrural segment, which, in addition, bear the risk of high reocclusion rates should the transplant material used be inappropriate. In many cases, it is more useful to choose the least strenuous intervention, e.g., correction of the upper thigh vessels by means of a bypass, which, in many cases, is feasible despite the long-segmental obliterations stretching down into the lower leg arteries. Should such a femoropopliteal reconstruction fail to dramatically improve the vascular condition, including an improvement in the Doppler index to above 0.5, a control angiography can facilitate the decision of whether a further peripheral reconstruction is useful, or whether PTA would be a better approach to eliminating stenoses located further down. This applies, in particular, to bypass stenoses in the vicinity of the anastomosis and obliterations located behind.

When establishing the indication for surgery, one must not neglect the assessment of the deep femoral artery which, in many cases even at a patent pelvic-vessel situation, is narrowed by arteriosclerotic plaque at its branching point. An attempt should then be made to dilate this profunda stenosis. Should this fail, a profunda plasty (patch plasty) is then indicated. Every occlusion of the superficial femoral artery involves a relative bifurcational stenosis of about 50%, while minor plaque formation of the profunda ostium increases this effect by another 14%–20% (BERGUER et al. 1975). Therefore, the prerequisite of optimizing the profunda circulation in the event of an occluded superficial femoral artery is a long segmental dilatation of the deep femoral artery or, if this is excluded on technical grounds, dilatation of the profunda. HEYDEN et al. (1979) highlighted the importance of the deep femoral artery and emphasized that the profunda must always be included in the central correction of the pelvic level.

17.2.3.2
Surgical Technique

Endarterectomies of femoral or popliteal occlusions have largely been given up. Currently, the correction of such occlusions is mainly performed with the autologous great saphenous vein, or with alloplastic materials (Dacron, PTFE) (Fig. 17.19). The prerequisite of bypassing a femoropopliteal/crural occlusion by means of the autologous vein is a functioning great saphenous vein. According to our experience, it should have a minimum diameter of 4 mm; if the diameter is smaller, immediate reocclusion is the result in a high percentage of cases.

As regards alloplastic materials, PTFE prostheses of 6 mm in diameter have proven to be reliable, even though 8-mm Dacron prostheses are still implanted in a few cases. Biological materials (umbilical veins, collagen prostheses) can also be implanted. These transplants, however, have the disadvantage of bio-degeneration in the long run, with formation of anastomotic or bypass aneurysms, which may result in occlusion.

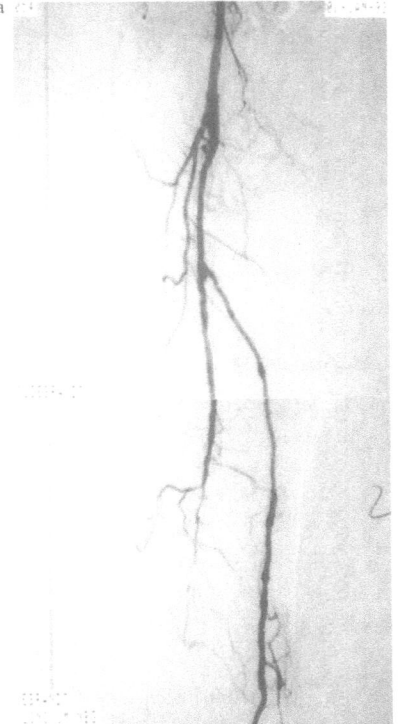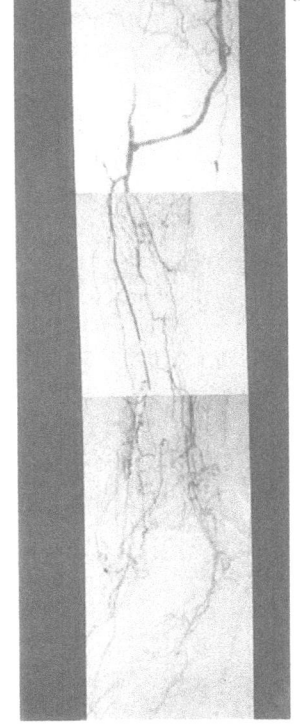

Fig. 17.19 a,b. Angiography demonstrating a femoropopliteal bypass bridging a distal femoropopliteal obliteration

Since alloplastic prostheses involve a higher reocclusion rate when used across joints, primary implantation of plastic prostheses is only performed above the knee joint. For reconstructions onto popliteal segment III and the lower leg artery, either a ringed PTFE prosthesis or biological materials (umbilical vein or collagen prosthesis) should be implanted in the event of non-availability of the great saphenous vein. Moreover, so-called composite grafts have proven helpful whenever reconstructions need to cross the knee joint. For the central segment up to popliteal segment 1, a plastic prosthesis is implanted which is anastomosed using an end-to-end technique with a segment of the great saphenous vein. This saphenous segment is used for reconstruction bridging the joint.

In the case of a bad run-off (e.g., partial occlusion of the plantar arch), the additional creation of an arteriovenous fistula at the level of, or peripheral to, the distal anastomosis has often been recommended. This has been done with a view to improving the rate of flow and consequently the patency of long transplants.

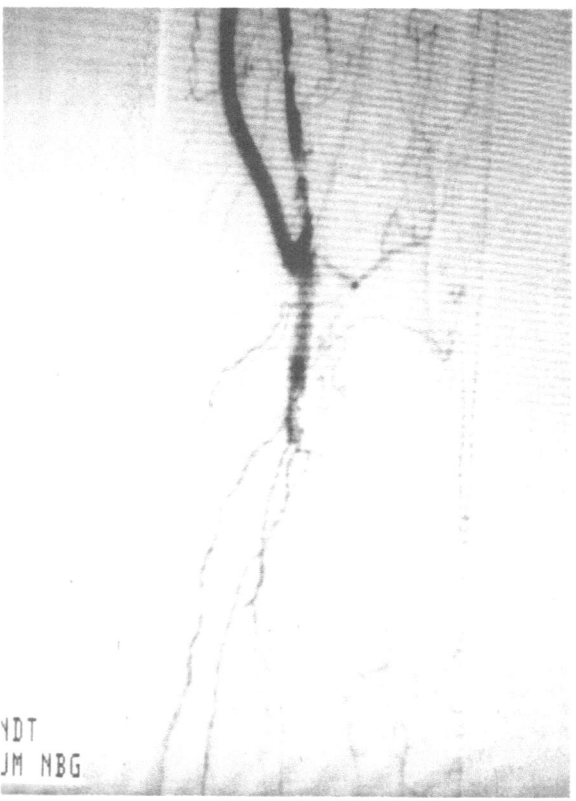

Fig. 17.20. Angiography demonstrating the result of bypass surgery with an isolated popliteal segment after a third reoperation (operator, D. Raithel, Nuremberg)

Long segmental reconstructions from the groin down to the ankle or dorsal pedal artery are technically feasible, but limited because of inadequate autologous transplant material. In many patients, the saphenous vein is not available in its complete length, with the result that ringed PTFE prostheses or biological materials need to be used. In some cases. however, this crural reconstruction is not necessary if angiography demonstrates an "isolated popliteal segment" in the case of a femoral occlusion and an obliteration of the popliteocrural segment (Fig. 17.20). Such isolated popliteal segments drain very effectively into the lower leg level via their collaterals and yield better long-term results as regards their patency rates than direct reconstructions at the level of the mid or distal lower leg in the form of crural reconstruction. The preferred material for the reconstruction of isolated popliteal segments is a 6-mm PTFE prosthesis.

17.2.3.3
Results of Surgical Therapy

The results of reconstruction in the peripheral vascular system depend on the stage of arterial occlusive disease, the run-off situation into the lower leg, and the transplant material used. Among the risk factors, only diabetes has an influence on the later outcome (RAITHEL et al. 1983). Mortality following infrainguinal reconstruction is minimal – below 1% – particularly if the operation is performed under spinal or epidural anesthesia.

The autologous great-saphenous-vein bypass has a patency rate of 72% after 3 years, and 65% after 5 years, according to a collective study by MEHTA (1980). In our own population, we saw patency rates of 66% after 3 years, and 50% after 5 years following reconstruction above the knee joint using the autologous great saphenous vein. Patency rates for reconstructions above the knee joint using PTFE prostheses was 64% after 3, 52% after 5, and 37% after 10 years. Below the knee joint, patency was 40% after 3 years, 32% after 5 years, and 27% after 8 years (RAITHEL 1992). Results after the use of PTFE prostheses for solely crural reconstructions were essentially poorer, with patency rates of 37% after 3 years, and only 28% after 5 years.

The composite graft (PTFE–saphenous vein) achieved a patency of 57% even after 3 years, and of 53% after 5 years following reconstruction onto popliteal segment III. An analysis of our PTFE reconstructions revealed that late results are highly dependent on the preoperative stage of the patients and the run-off situation (RAITHEL 1991).

In patients with intermittent claudication (stage II), patency after reconstruction above the knee joint was 63%, 53%, and 42% after 5, 8, and 10 years, respectively. After reconstruction for limb-salvage, patency rates were no more than 49% after 5 years, and 34% after 8 years (RAITHEL 1992). Related to the run-off situation, the patency after 5 and 8 years was 59% and 49%, respectively, in patients with a run-off over two to three patent lower leg vessels, but only 51% and 48%, respectively, in patients with a run-off over only one patent lower leg vessel. Extremities could be salvaged by reconstructions using PTFE prostheses above the knee joint in 82% after 5 years, in 78% after 8 years, and 74% after 10 years.

The results in our patients who underwent reconstruction using PTFE prostheses clearly demonstrate that the amputation rate was dependent on the preoperative stage and on the run-off situation into the lower leg. Patients who were operated for intermittent claudication had an amputation rate of 10% after 5 years, whereas patients in stage IV had an amputation rate of 31% after 5 years (RAITHEL 1991).

The most impressive results were achieved in reconstruction onto an isolated popliteal segment, compared to the results of the purely crural reconstruction: After crural reconstruction, a primary occlusion rate of 16% was found, in contrast to only 6% after reconstruction of an isolated popliteal segment. After 5 years, 53% of our reconstructions onto an isolated popliteal segment still functioned (RAITHEL 1992).

Biological materials, such as the umbilical vein or collagen prostheses, have a limited long-term prognosis as they tend to produce aneurysms followed by thombotic occlusion. Nevertheless, in our own patient collective, we achieved good long-term results with the umbilical vein: After 6 years, 46.7% still worked, whereas the collagen prostheses only worked in 42.4% of patients after 4 years.

17.3
Aortic and Other Aneurysms

E. ZEITLER

17.3.1
Definition

Aneurysms are localized permanent dilatations of the aorta or other artery due to disease in the vascular wall. Aneurysms can be classified as true or false. A true aneurysm results from a weakening of the vascular wall caused by congenital atrophy or acquired destruction of the elastic fibers in the media. Aneurysms are localized, often thrombosed, and bag-shaped dilatations of the aorta and arteries. We further distinguish between true, false, and dissecting aneurysms (see Fig. 17.21b+c). The true aneurysm (Fig. 17.21a) can be ball-shaped, spindle-shaped, sacciform, or of fusiform formation, while the generalized ectasia, especially of the aorta, is related to physiological sclerosis in old age, developing more predominantly in patients with arterial hypertension.

While in the abdominal aorta, the most common site of aneurysms (Fig. 17.22), the shape identifiable in the angiogam is mainly determined by the extent of thrombosis, aneurysms of the peripheral and cerebral arteries typically show a local out-pocketing (Fig. 17.23). Diffuse aneurysms in the peripheral arteries, spindle- or ball-shaped (Fig. 17.24), can be found close to the aorta, or in the framework of a global and multilocular dilating arteriopathy, respectively, also defined as "arteriomegaly" (CARLSSON et al. 1975).

The more dilating forms of arteriopathy (HEBERER et al. 1974; VOLLMAR and NOBBE 1976; ZEITLER 1976), which LERICHE (1943, 1947) described as *dystrophie polyanévrysmale*, are likely to be caused by extensive degenerative changes to the arterial wall (STAPLE et al. 1966; WALZ and DEININGER 1974). The patient's age and an analysis of risk factors involved suggest, unlike excentric aneurysms which are found mostly in subjects aged

Fig. 17.21. a Various types of true aneurysm: (*left* to *right*) globular, sacciform, spindle-like. b aneurysma spurium c aneurysma dissecans (From ZEITLER 1997)

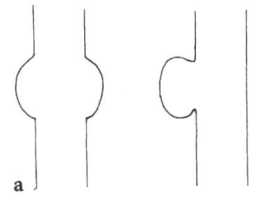
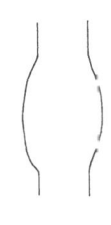
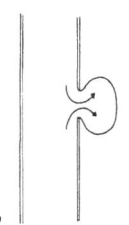
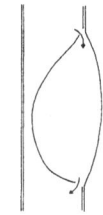

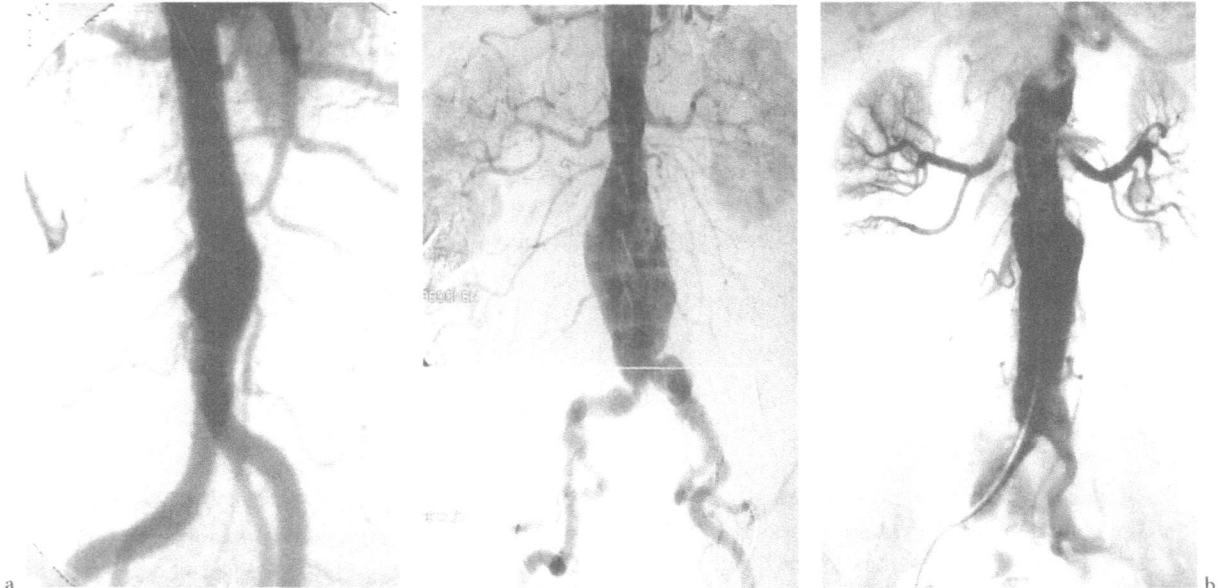

Fig. 17.22 a–c. Various abdominal aortic aneurysms. **a** Ball-shaped (63-year-old man), **b** spindle-shaped (80-year-old man), c fusiform (73-year-old man)

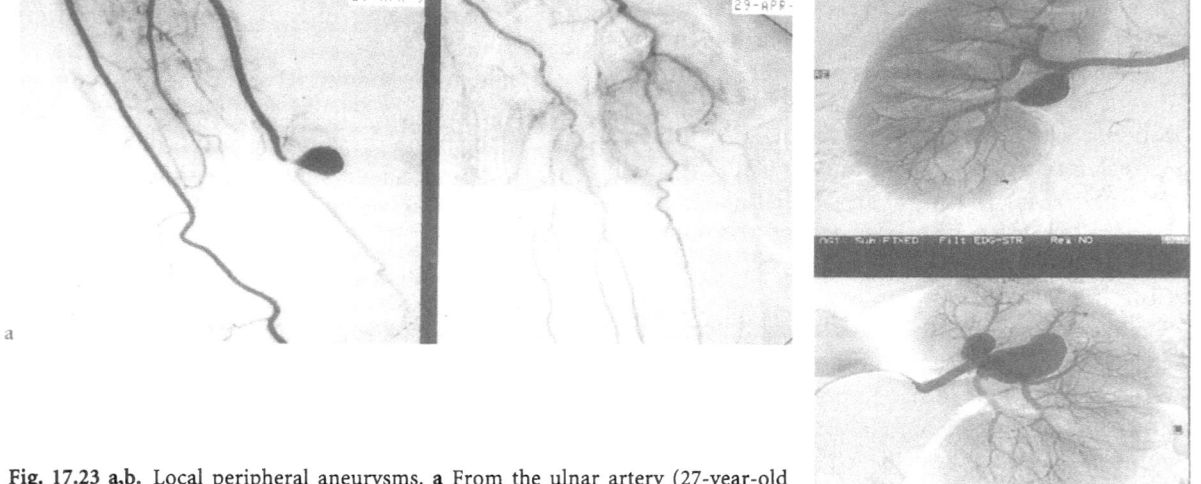

Fig. 17.23 a,b. Local peripheral aneurysms. **a** From the ulnar artery (27-year-old woman). **b** Right and left renal arteries (36-year-old woman)

between 50 and 70 years of age, that this disease is a special type of arteriosclerosis occurring from the age of 70. An apparent fact is that the triglyceride values of patients with extensive polyaneurysmal arteriopathy are often elevated, apart from the presence of other risk factors, such as nicotine abuse or hypertension. Angiograms show either an obliterating, a dilating, but also a combined form of arteriosclerosis (Fig. 17.25).

According to WHITE (1992), the primary effect of aneurysm formation is more the elastolysis of the adventitia and less the degeneration of the media. The elastolysis proportion of the media in patients with aneurysms is said to be reduced by over 80%, in contrast to non-aneurysmatic arteries.

The etiology of aneurysms of the aorta and peripheral arteries is therefore a special type of arteriosclerosis, the result of different kinds of congenital defects (YOUNG and OSTERTAG 1987), or, rarely, infection. In addition, there are posttraumatic, postoperative, and true or false aneurysms after interventional procedures (ANDERSON et al. 1974;

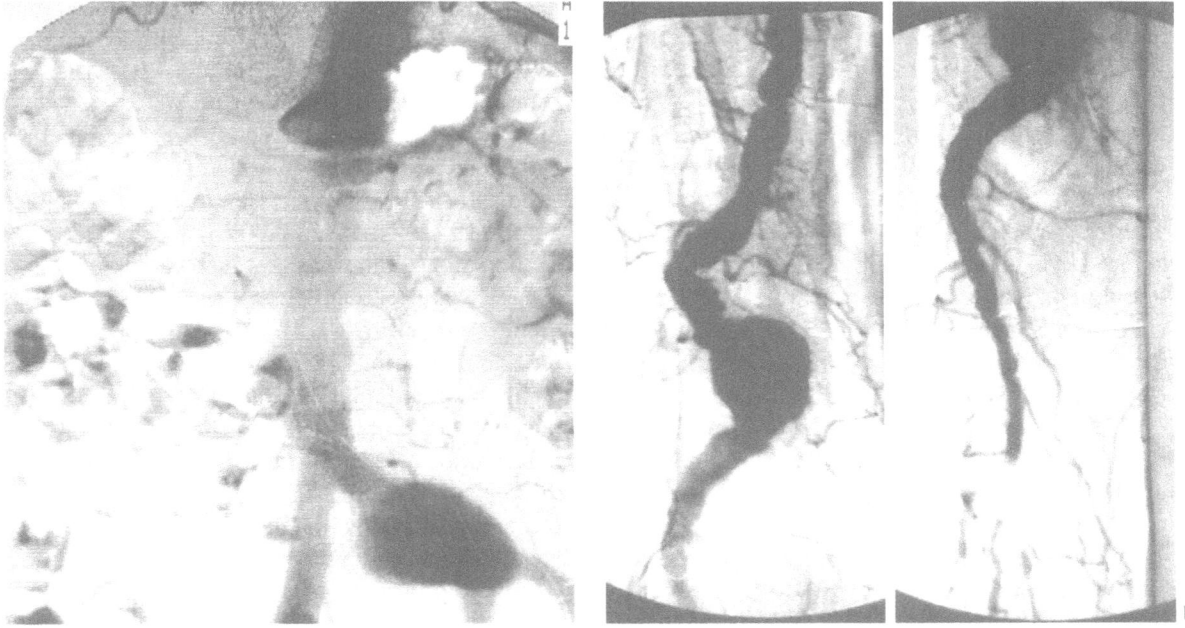

Fig. 17.24. a Spindle-shaped aneurysm of the common iliac artery in an 80-year-old man. **b** Ball-shaped aneurysm as part of dystrophic polyaneurysmal disease (Leriche syndrome) in a 75-year-old man with embolic occlusion

CRAWFORD et al. 1985; REDDY 1986; BECKER et al. 1991).

Idiopathic medionecrosis, Erdheim-Gsell's necrosis, manifests itself as a destruction of all components of the media (collagen, musculature, and elastica), and conversion into large cysts with mucoid contents and intact elastic structure of the surrounding tissue. Marfan's syndrome produces smaller mucoid cysts in the media, with fragmented elastic structures, but is basically no aneurysm. Marfan's syndrome was detected by LEU (1976) in 3.4% of patients in postmortem studies. In radiological examinations (CT or angiography), it appears as ectasia and can induce dissection of the ascending aorta.

Irrespective of the histologic characteristics, including etiology, aneurysms can be classified according to their type and location. Common *locations* of arterial aneurysms impairing the peripheral circulation in the extremities include:

- Abdominal, thoracic, and thoracoabdominal aortic aneurysms
- Iliac and common femoral aneurysms
- Femoral and popliteal aneurysms
- Subclavian and arm artery aneurysms
- Aneurysms in intestinal (renal, splenic, and other) arteries
- Postoperative aneurysms.

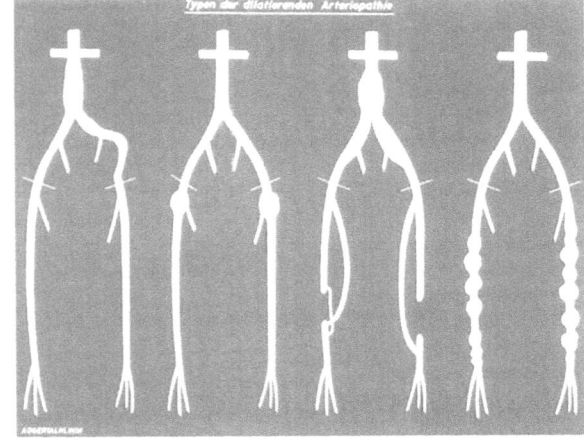

Fig. 17.25 a–d. Types of dilating arteriopathy (according to ZEITLER 1976). **a** Aortoiliac dilatation (pre-aneurysmac). **b** Iliac or common femoral dilatation, or still aneurysm. **c** Combined occlusive and dilating arteriopathy: aortoiliac aneurysm plus femoropopliteal occlusions? **d** Bilateral dystrophic polyaneurysmal disease (Leriche)

17.3.2
Incidence and Location of Aneurysms

Statistical data from postmortem studies report aneurysms to be present in 3%–5% of patients (LEU 1976; KUNZ 1980; OSTERTAG and YOUNG 1987). In the course of analysis carried out over 25 years

(KUNZ 1980), 1344 aneurysms of the aorta and other arteries, including 362 inferior cerebral arteries, were evaluated. Arteriosclerosis was identified as the cause of the aneurysms in 80%. Idiopathic medial necrosis (Erdheim-Gsell) with dissecting aneurysm was identified in 9.7% of aneurysms by KUNZ (1980), and in 4.8% by LEU (1976). Men were typically affected before the age of 70, women in contrast before the age of 60. Syphilitic aneurysms were still found in 3.7% at that time. However, these have decreased considerably over the past 20 years. Infectious aneurysms (in earlier years known as mycotic aneurysms) were found in 1% (LEU 1976; KUNZ 1980).

The increase in *arteriosclerotic* aortic aneurysms, which account for 90%-95% of aneurysms in the area of the abdominal aorta, has been attributed to the recent higher life expectancy (DEBAKEY et al. 1958; CRAWFORD and CRAWFORD 1988; SANDMANN and KNIEMEYER 1991; VOLLMAR 1996). In Switzerland, for example, this rose from 50 years of age in 1900 to 70 years of age in 1980. True aneurysms (A. verum) were observed in 83.6%, dissecting aneurysms (aortic dissection) in 15%, and false aneurysms (A. spurium) in 1.4%.

False aneurysms result from an acute perforation of the aorta or artery, and are contained only by perivascular connective tissues and organized blood clots. Thus, the wall of a false aneurysm does not contain the usual three arterial layers. The most commonly occurring false aneurysm is localized in the groin, following arterial catheterization. In its early stage, it is a "pulsating hematoma".

Aortic aneurysms were seen in 4.8% (217 of 7262 autopsies), and multiple aneurysms in 11% of all aneurysms. A comparison of men versus women revealed a ratio of 2:1 (LEU 1976) in Zürich and 9:1 (YOUNG and OSTERTAG 1987) in Hannover. A comparison of locations of aortic aneurysms (Table 17.2) highlights the dominance of AAAs. It demonstrates the location of the 241 aortic aneurysms in 217 patients out of 7262 autopsies. Of these, 31% were ruptured, and one in four were ruptured from the ascending aorta into the pericardium.

Aneurysms of the extremities are underrepresented in autopsy studies, and are more commonly seen in pathologic institutes after surgical resection (LEU 1976). Of 52, the majority were located in the iliac or femoropopliteal arteries.

The situation is different in vascular surgical departments (DENCK 1976) (Table 17.3). Clinical studies demonstrate that 70% of all non-aortic operations were performed in the popliteal artery

Table 17.2. Localization and incidence of aortic aneurysms (AA): 217 patients with 241 aneurysms in 7262 autopsies. (According to LEU 1975)

Type	Incidence (%)
Abdominal AA	65
Ascending thoracic AA	13
Thoracoabdominal AA	7.5
Descending thoracic AA	7.0
Arcus aortae aneurysm	6.5
Sinus Valsalva aneurysm	1.0

Table 17.4. Complications of aortic and peripheral arterial aneurysms

Complication	Incidence (%)
Rupture of the abdominal aorta or arterial aneurysm	≈15
Thrombosed (occluded) aneurysm	≈24
Peripheral embolization	≈13

Table 17.3. Localization and incidence of 57 aortic and 55 peripheral arterial aneurysms operated in a vascular surgery clinic. (According to DENCK 1976)

Localization	n (%)	Rupture	Thrombosed	Embolization
Abdominal aortic aneurysm	45 (79)	14	–	3
Aortic arch aneurysm	8 (14)	2	1	–
Descending thoracic aneurysm	4 (7)	–	–	1
Femoral artery	16 (29)	1	9	3
Subclavian artery	14 (25)	–	9	5
Popliteal artery	11 (20)	–	5	2
Iliac artery	7	–	1	–
Axillary artery	2	–	1	–
Brachiocephalic artery	2	–	1	–
Radial artery	1	–	–	–
Ulnar artery	1	–	–	–
Dorsal interosseous forearm artery	1	–	–	–

(SANDMANN and KNIEMEYER 1991; VOLLMAR 1996a; BRUNNER and HUWYLER 1975). We have seen 30 patients with popliteal aneurysms out of 4480 vascular patients. Between 50% and 60% of popliteal aneurysms are found bilaterally (BRUNNER and HUWYLER 1975; VOLLMAR and NOBBE 1976; VOLLMAR 1996).

The fate of patients with aneurysms, or poly-aneurysmatic disease (LÉRICHE's *méga-artère dolicho*) mainly depends on their complications (Table 17.4). While LEU (1976) found ruptured aortic aneurysms in 31% at autopsy, KUNZ (1980) diagnosed ruptured aneurysms in only 17% of aneurysms in all locations.

Since angiography has become standard in the clinical management of patients with suspected aortoiliac disease (ABRAMS and JÖNSSON 1983; WENZ and BEDUHN 1976; HEBERER et al. 1966), more patients with aneurysms have been diagnosed and received elective surgical treatment before aneurysmal rupture. In a clinical summary of 154 aneurysms (DENCK 1976), 14% of all aneurysms, but 31% of AAAs, were ruptured. Therefore, in aortic aneurysms, the risk of dying from one of the complications can be reduced if diagnosis by means of imaging methods begins in an asymptomatic stage (HEBERER et al. 1996; VOLLMAR 1997). It could be shown that an AAA screening program for all males over the age of 50 (MORRIS et al. 1994; HOLDSWORTH 1994; ZEITLER 1991) can reduce the high complication rate of AAAs, such as rupture, with subsequent high operative mortality (NOPPENEY and RAITHEL 1990). In screening programs with abdominal sonography in males over the age of 60, asymptomatic AAAs could be detected in up to 8%.

17.3.3
Imaging of Aneurysms

Diagnosis with imaging techniques has contributed considerably to the impressive success of modern vascular and cardiac surgery for aortic aneurysms (DEBAKEY et al. 1958; HEBERER and REIDEMEISTER 1974; CRAWFORD et al. 1985, 1988; SZILAGYI et al. 1966; MORRIS et al. 1994; SANDMANN and KNIEMEYER 1991; VOLLMAR 1996c), and similarly to the application of endovascular stent grafts (see Sect. 17.4). The various imaging systems (Table 17.5) have gained greatly in importance in the early diagnosis of aneurysms. These techniques are described and their results demonstrated in various chapters of this book.

Table 17.5. Imaging Systems in the Diagnosis of aneurysms

- Duplex and color-coded sonography (CCDS)
- Echocardiography and transesophageal echocardiography (TEEC)
- Contrast-enhanced computed tomography (CT) and spiral CT
- Thoracic and abdominal aorto arteriography
- Digital subtraction angiography (DSA)
- Magnetic resonance imaging (MRI)
- Magnetic resonance angiography (MRA)

To establish a precise differential diagnosis of pathologic vascular findings, their operability, and in order to plan an operation or interventional therapy, non-invasive screening methods, (such as US, MRI, or MRA) are not necessarily superior to invasive radiological vascular examinations using catheters and contrast-enhanced angiography (conventional angiography, DSA). Clinical symptoms, and the spectrum of therapies and their prognosis, is determined to a great extent by the location of the aneurysm.

An aneurysm of the aorta is primarily an indication for vascular surgery. New endovascular techniques have gained in importance in the treatment of high-risk patients and small aneurysms, but require more precise diagnostic quantitative measurements in order to reduce complications.

17.3.4
Abdominal Aortic Aneurysms

The infrarenal AAA in 90%–95% of patients is an arteriosclerotic aneurysm which remains asymptomatic in most cases until rupture occurs (DARLING 1970; FAGGIOLOI et al. 1994). Modern vascular surgery, however, is capable of managing such ruptures, provided the patients come directly to the clinic and the diagnosis is established quickly (DEBAKEY et al. 1958; SZILAGYI et al. 1966; HEBERER et al. 1966; CRAWFORD and CRAWFORD 1988; VOLLMAR 1996; BECKER et al. 1991; DARLING 1970; EGLOFF et al. 1983; GIESSLER and HEBERER 1968; SANDMANN and KNIEMEYER 1991; SZILAGYI et al. 1972). In such critical situations with shock, a pulsating abdominal mass, or sudden heavy abdominal pain, possibly with a systolic murmur, the chest image, plain abdominal X-ray image, abdominal sonography, or emergency CT deliver all the required information. If necessary, any type of angiography can be ignored to spare time.

If the limits of the pulsating tumor can be fixed below the costal arch, it can be assumed that it is an infrarenal aortic aneurysm (HEBERER et al. 1966). If not, a differential diagnosis to exclude a thoraco-AAA needs to be made. Depending on the equipment available, spiral CT, MRA, and digital thoraco-abdominal aortography are capable of answering all important questions. The right-sided transbrachial arterial access to the ascending thoracic aorta, but also intravenous DSA, should be preferred over high translumbar aortography, which was preferably used in earlier years. Thanks to modern soft-tip catheters of 3–5 F, inserted via a flexible-tip guidewire, there are no contraindications to transfemoral catheterization, if this is the best access. Embolization initiated by catheter angiography – formerly a feared risk – belongs nowadays in the past (ZEITLER 1991; ZEITLER and HEUCK 1997).

The selection of the appropriate diagnostic imaging modality is determined by the clinical symptoms, the urgency of the case, and the equipment immediately available until an operating theatre is free (Table 17.5). In all patients with stable circulation, the situation should be clarified as quickly as possible. The best-suited technique for preoperative or preinterventional diagnosis of symptomatic AAA, dissection, or similar disease, including acute aortic occlusion, or in the case of threatening rupture, is either axial CT using intravenous power contrast injection in spiral-CT technique (Fig. 17.26), or arterial DSA (Fig. 17.27), in biplane mode if possible. The radiologic signs of a partially thrombosed AAA can be summarized as follows:

- The diameter of the free lumen of the infrarenal aorta is equal to, or larger than, that of the suprarenal aorta.
- Presence of a uni- or bilateral dilatation.
- The border of the aortic lumen shows an alternation of dilatations and constrictions (step-like).
- There is kinking of the aorta with large distances between the front edge of the vertebra and the contrast column in the aorta in lateral projection.
- The lumbar arteries and inferior mesenteric artery are not identifiable.
- Complete absence of collateral vessels in the aorta's environment.
- A collateral circulation to the pelvic arteries via the internal iliac artery, from the suprarenal mesenteric arteries or the lumbar arteries, is identifiable.

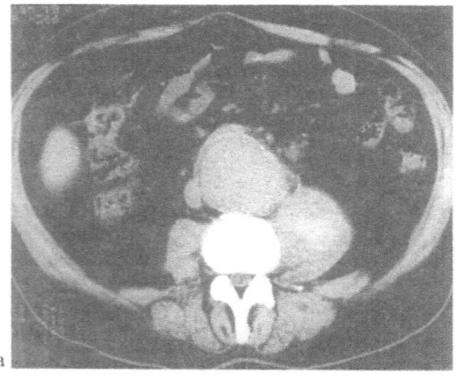
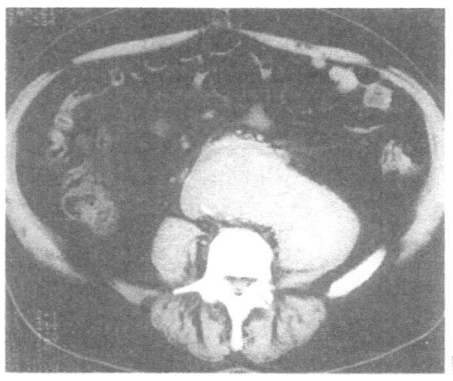
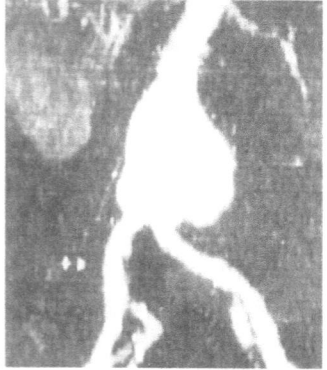
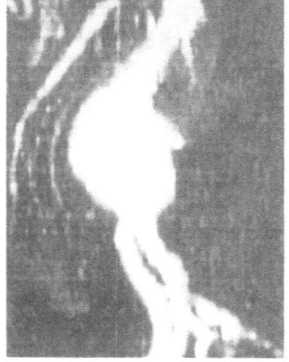

Fig. 17.26 a–d. Infrarenal abdominal aortic aneurysm (AAA) with penetration into left retroperitoneal direction. a,b Axial computed tomography (CT) scans. c,d Angio-spiral CT demonstrating the fusi-sacciform AAA in anteroposterior and oblique projections, including the iliac arteries and the occluded lumbar arteries, but patent renal and mesenteric arteries. (From ZEITLER 1997)

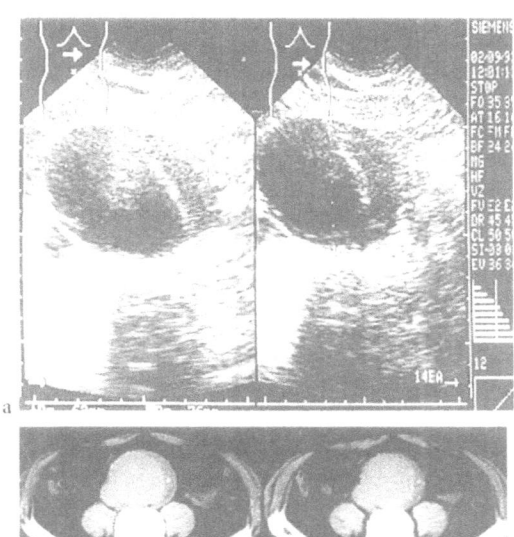
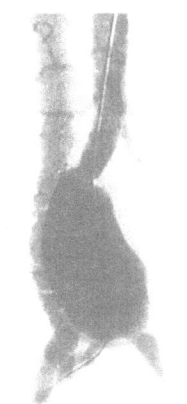
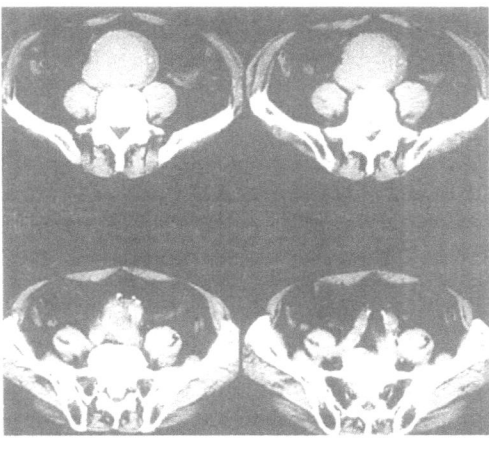

Fig. 17.27 a–c. Infrarenal abdominal aortic aneurysm with perforation into the inferior vena cava. **a** Sonography. **b** four computed tomography images; same contrast in the free aortic lumen and the vena cava. Calcifications in the iliac arteries, with patent lumen. **c** Transfemoral digital subtraction angiography of the iliac arteries, demonstrating the extension of the aneurysm and aortocaval perforation. (From ZEITLER 1997)

Selection of the appropriate imaging technique will always be determined by the urgency of intervention and interdisciplinary cooperation with the surgeon, as the latter can choose from varying operative techniques. CT images provide the advantage of clear assessment of the aneurysm, including extent of the thrombus, wall thickness, calcification, perforation, and its direction (Figs. 17.26, 17.28). 2D sonography can also demonstrate the free lumen, the thrombosed part of the aneurysm (Fig. 17.27a), and flow-related changes. Because of different open surgical techniques and minimally-invasive interventional types of treatment, it is necessary to define the aneurysm in its diameter and extent (Fig. 17.29) with a scanning system (spiral CT or MRA), and additional abdominal aortography with the use of an AAA vessel-sizing catheter.

An existing shunt after aortocaval perforation (Fig. 17.27c) can be best demonstrated and localized using DSA. In several patients, only a combination of angiography plus CT or MRA can give optimum information. Since angiography may overlook the thrombosed part and is not capable of demonstrating the post-perforation hematoma, direction of perforation or penetration, the dissecting membrane,

or a leak following endovascular repair, US and CT provide clear information about contact zones between different vascular structures (Fig. 17.28), or contact to parts of the intestine or neighboring organs.

The non-perforated AAA has no specific symptoms. Lumbago, unclear abdominal pain, gastrointestinal or nephrourologic symptoms can mimic the situation, and still neurologic symptoms can result from direct nerve compression or vertebral destruction. Therefore, imaging methods are of great importance for early and precise diagnosis.

As a result of stenoses or kinking of the aorta or peripheral embolization, intermittent claudication can also be the first symptom of an AAA (HEBERER and REIDEMEISTER 1974). Therefore, in patients with a pulsating abdominal mass, unclear lumbar pain with erosion of the spine, peripheral embolisms in the leg arteries, or POVD, angiography provides additional detailed information to US, CT, or MRA alone.

Besides clinically- or US-detected arterial obliterations, or popliteal aneurysms, aortic aneurysms have been frequently and unexpectedly identified. This resulted over recent decades in an increase in AAAs being operated in their asymptomatic stages,

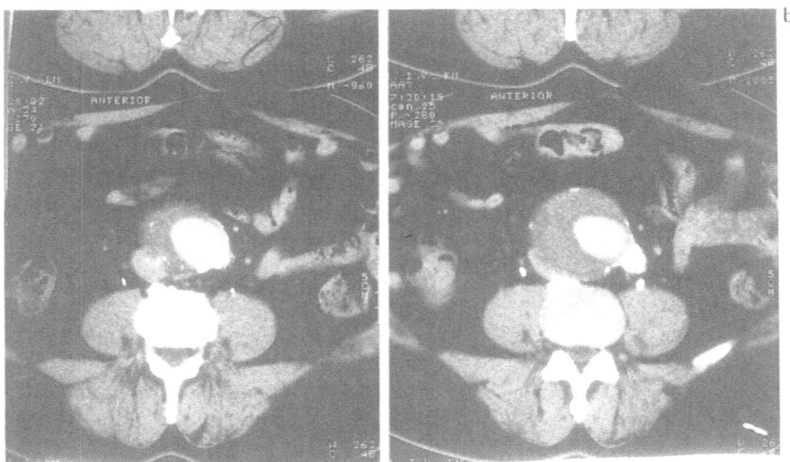

Fig. 17.28. Abdominal aortic aneurysm with extensive thrombus formation and secondary occluded aortocaval fistula as a result of thrombus formation

for example, in Nuremberg from 63% before 1959 to 83% in the 1985 (NOPPENEY and RAITHEL 1990). Nevertheless, the number of operations of ruptured aortic aneurysms only decreased from 19% to 12%. During the same period of time, the perioperative 30-day mortality rate dropped from 20.2% to 4.5% in asymptomatic AAAs, and from 45.1% to 9.1% in symptomatic aneurysms. In contrast, the mortality rate among the smaller number of ruptured aortic aneurysms has not changed, remaining at 60%.

The indication for active therapy is recommended in AAAs with a diameter exceeding 4 cm. Small aneurysms require regular US controls at 6-month intervals. Important information which angiography, in contrast to other methods, provides with great precision includes:

· Existent renal artery stenosis
· Mesenteric artery occlusion
· Existent horseshoe kidney
· Accessory existent renal arteries and renal infarction
· Occluded lumbar arteries
· Kinked or stenosed abdominal aorta
· Precise extension of the infrarenal aorta and the aneurysm in comparison to the lumbar spine
· Demonstration of the collateral circulation (from lumbar, mesenteric, and other arteries)
· Demonstration of the thoracic aorta during the same procedure
· Demonstration of the iliofemoral arteries during the same procedure.

While the future of imaging lies in US and MRI, angiography will still be indicated and of help in numerous patients in the coming years. It is also a method for controlling new types of treatment.

17.3.5
Inflammatory Aneurysms

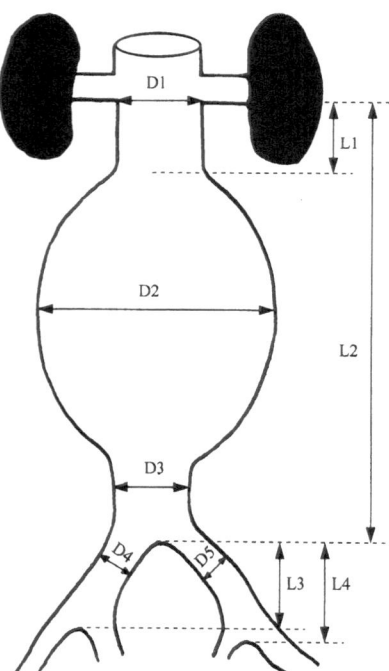

Fig. 17.29. Diameters and extensions necessary for a quantitive assessment prior to endovascular grafting via the transfemoral route (Parodi's technique described in Sect. 17.4). *D*, diameters; *L*, length

The *inflammatory* AAA is more often seen in men than in women. Ureteral obstruction or compression can be the first signs of an inflammatory AAA, occasionally causing hydronephrosis (Fig. 17.31). According to WALKER et al., ureteral obstruction is an important sign of inflammatory AAA, occurring in 10% of cases. This type of AAA has a higher risk of complications and mortality, and therefore necessitates a special therapeutic concept. The number of ruptures is relatively low compared to the collective figures. In Düsseldorf (SANDMANN and KNIEMEYER 1991), for example, ruptures were observed in 35% of AAA patients, compared to 17% in patients with inflammatory AAA. However, the average age of the patients with inflammatory AAA, 65 ± 8 years of age, corresponds to that of all other AAAs. Endocarditis and intestinal infection are predominantly discussed as causes of inflammatory aneurysms (ANDERSON et al. 1974; PATEL and JOHNSTON 1977; GOLDSTONE et al. 1978; CRAWFORD et al. 1985).

As a rule, inflammatory AAAs are symptomatic. The patients present with pain in the abdomen and back, and recurrent abdominal complaints of unknown origin. Often, there is an excessive weight loss of about 10 kg within a few weeks. The blood sedimentation rate (BSR) in the first hour is mostly above 40 mm. Penetration occurs against the spine, but is more commonly a covered perforation. Intraoperatively, a hard fibrous aortic wall with a reddish or grey-whitish surface is found. Accordingly, CT and MRI depict a very thick wall with contrast absorption. In a serial CT, the contrast absorption in the inflammatory, thickened aortic wall can also be identified on histogram (Fig. 17.30). Angiography and sonography do not provide any indication of inflammatory nature. According to VALESKY et al., CT using CM is the only preoperative imaging technique enabling the detection of an inflammatory aneurysm.

The causes of inflammatory reactions are as yet unknown. Partial aspects include: chronic aortic leakage, blockage of lymphatic channels, and adhesion of aneurysms and portions of the intestine. There are also distinct indications suggesting involvement of the immunological system. The inflammatory aortic aneurysm has been observed in the abdominal infrarenal, suprarenal, and thoracic arteries, and inguinal false aneurysms.

With axial CT (Fig. 17.30) or MRI scans, for example, the very thick aortic walls of inflammatory AAAs, sometimes including gas bubbles, and compression and distention of the kidney and ureter, become visible. The causes of inflammation can include penetration into parts of the intestine or immunological situations. The same situation has also been defined as "endoluminally infected aneurysmal abscess", but the former definition, mycotic aneurysm, is no longer recommended (VOLLMAR 1997).

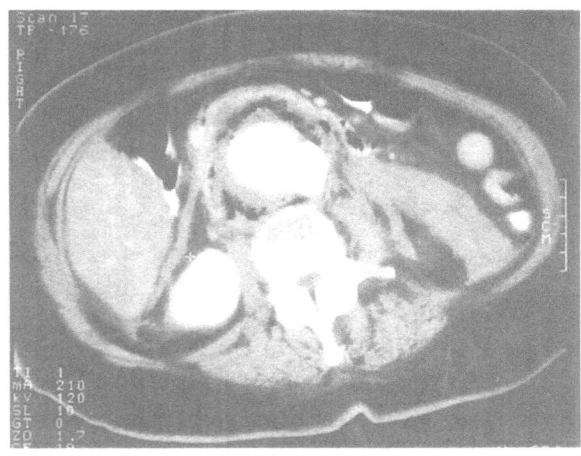

Fig. 17.30. Inflammatory abdominal aortic aneurysm after penetration and intestinal perforation, with a thickened aortic wall and gas accumulation in the wall, and retroperitoneal and intraperitoneal hematoma

As resection or direct graft implantation are not feasible in such situations, an external thoracoaortal or axillofemoral bypass must be created for the long period of antibiotic therapy aimed at eliminating the source of infection (Fig. 17.31b).

The *mycotic aneurysm*, with its controversial definition, was defined by OSLER in 1885 as an "endoluminal, infected aneurysmatic abscess"; he used this description because of the appearance of the disease, which resembles a spore fungus. Endocarditis has been considered the main source of infection, and the risk of hemorrhage or sepsis is relatively high. Atypical locations (e.g., suprarenal, or iliofemoral and intracerebral) underline the highly embolic nature of the disease. As surgery foresees neither resection, nor an endovascular prosthesis, a careful diagnosis is necessary in the patient's interest. In particular, the possible existence of a mycotic or inflammatory AAA should, provided there is sufficient time, result in the performance of an angiography *and* an axial scanning method. Only this combination enables protective measures to be taken against septic spreading of germs, to choose the best-suited vascular prosthesis, or to decide for a bypass operation.

Today, in the age of antibiotics and modern microbiology, the inflammatory aortic aneurysm occurs far more seldom. The definition "mycotic aneurysm" – used only for a short time – has been broadened to include its occurrence in the aorta and peripheral arteries (ANDERSON et al. 1974; PATEL and JOHNSTON 1977). Before the introduction of antibiotics, of 217 mycotic aneurysms, 25% each

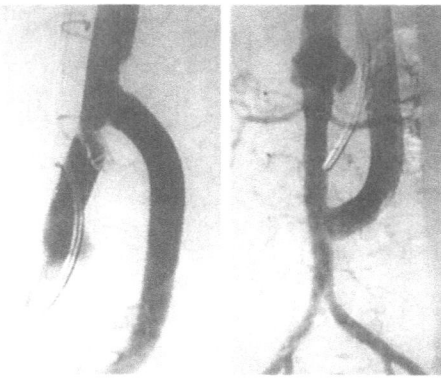

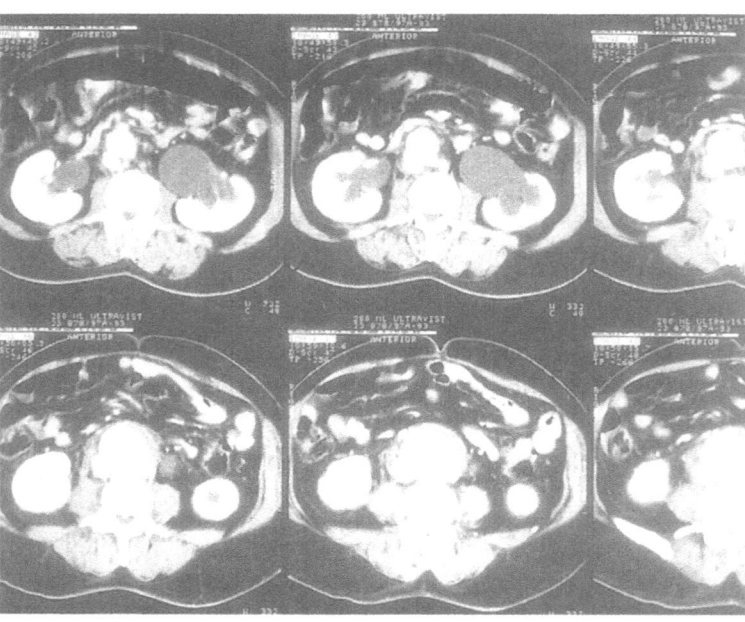

Fig. 17.31 a,b. a Inflammatory abdominal aortic aneurysm (AAA) with compression of both ureters, resulting in bilateral ectasia of the renal pelvis, with right-sided hydronephrosis. b Inflammatory AAA located close to the superior mesenteric artery. Digital subtraction angiography for control of the exclusion with the aortoaortal extraanatomic bypass without resection of the aneurysm. (From ZEITLER 1997)

were found in the aorta, visceral arteries, and intracranial and extremity arteries. In the 1980s (REDDY 1986), in contrast, the femoral artery in the groin was the most common site in the US, with 72%, of which 92% were identified as having long-term drug abuse as an etiologic factor. As the disease is also amenable to conservative therapies, CT, in addition to angiography, will gain in importance also in this medical field.

17.3.6
Ruptured Abdominal Aortic Aneurysm

The rupture of an aneurysm is a severe life-threatening situation to the patient which, without immediate treatment for shock and surgical intervention, usually leads to death (DARLING 1970; HEBERER and REIDEMEISTER 1974; CRAWFORD and CRAWFORD 1988). The situation requires immediate and determined action by an experienced team. The fact that 30%–35% of all symptomatic aortic aneurysms show signs of rupture emphasizes the necessity to be prepared for the situation. From the onset of symptoms to the time of operation, the mean time interval was 10h for those who survived, but 50h for those who died. One cause of interventions coming too late is a step-by-step diagnostic concept in many cases. Another is the pathoanatomical development from a penetration of the aneurysm over a covered perforation to the secondary, or final, free retroperitoneal bleeding (VOLLMAR 1996). Clinical symptoms include: (a) Acute abdominal pain, (b) palpable tumor

in the abdomen, and (c) hypovolemic depression of the circulatory system. *The suspected rupture of an AAA should lead to the patient's immediate referral to a vascular surgical centre.*

Typical false diagnoses include lumbago, ureteral colic, perforation of the intestine, ileus, or pancreatitis. In cases of unclear abdominal symptoms, imaging of the abdomen in left-side and flat position and abdominal sonography are necessary. A CT with CM, however, can be carried out immediately, simultaneous to shock treatment.

In patients with unstable circulation, CT or angiography cannot be performed, and the patient can be operated without prior imaging examination. If there is sufficient time, however, these technique enable the detection of abnormalities in neighboring organs and appropriate surgical planning. Among the abnormalities of special importance are the horseshoe kidney and other kidney abnormalities, but any inflammatory situation also needs to be identified.

SCHWILDEN et al. (1978) gave the following classification of kidney abnormalities in the case of aortic aneurysms:

- Type A: Accessory renal arteries at the proximal end of the AAA
- Type B: Accessory renal artery in the distal area of the AAA
- Type C: One kidney is supplied by a renal artery branching in the AAA
- Type D: Both kidneys are supplied by several renal arteries arising from the aneurysm.

Effective surgical planning, quick action, and the best therapeutic results can only be achieved by optimum cooperation between the physician who treats the patient first, the ambulance service which has the addresses of clinics spezialized in vascular surgery, and a cooperative radiological institute with all necessary diagnostic imaging modalities. A simple sonography or angiography alone is not sufficient for a differentiated diagnosis in these patients. The radiological department must provide a 24-h service.

Spiral CT and ultrafast CT, already feasible during the administration of shock treatment, have essentially contributed to a further improvement in good vascular surgical results. To what extent additional techniques, such as the semiinvasive application of endoprostheses or percutaneous inner fenestration, are capable of improving the initial and late outcome, remains to be investigated.

17.3.7
Aortocaval Perforation

Not only can the AAA compress and displace, it can also perforate the vena cava caudalis (BURKE and JAMIESON 1983; CRAWFORD and CRAWFORD 1988) (Fig. 17.27) and, in the case of a covered perforation, initiate the formation of aortointestinal fistulas. Aortocaval fistulas are observed in up to 2% of patients with AAAs (STIRNEMANN et al. 1986; VOLLMAR 1997). Their prognosis is better than that of patients with free rupture. However, the result is venous insufficiency due to blood accumulation, and the large shunt volume results in cardiac insufficiency.

17.3.8
Aortointestinal Fistula

The literature has reported on approximately 400 aortointestinal fistulas, 100 of which occurred primarily, the majority, however, following the implantation of endoprostheses in the aorta. They are mainly located in the horizontal and ascending parts of the duodenum – in primary aortointestinal fistulas in 81.6%, in secondary in 94% (WEIMANN and FLORA 1991) – and escape primary endoscopic examination. Only in cases of suspected aortoduodenal fistulas, an endoscopy reaching beyond the duodenal papilla and the flexura caudalis is performed, making it the most important diagnostic technique. Perforation into the

stomach and intestine is also possible. The incidence is 0.04%–1.7% since elective AAA resection has been the method of choice (VOLLMAR 1996), and 0.6% after vascular surgery. A secondary formation of fistulas can occur in about 1.7% of patients after an AAA operation, whereby an exploratory laparotomy should be avoided. The clinical picture is mostly a case history of often repeated bleeding over several days, the cause of which is frequently recognized too late. CT and angiography are helpful in these cases, and an endoscopy is necessary. In some cases, only a scintigraphy using gallium helps to detect an aortoenteral fistula. For precise localization, further, and if necessary selective, angiographic techniques are required, unless the fistula is located in the aortal region or close to the anastomosis.

Aortointestinal fistulas can also be the result of perforation of a duodenal ulcer into the aorta. As a rule, it should be remembered that: *Gastrointestinal bleeding in a patient with aortic prosthesis is likely to be an aortointestinal fistula, unless another underlying cause is identified.*

17.3.9
Postoperative Anastomotic Aneurysms

Immediate problems following aortoiliac surgery are generally related to technical errors which may result in thrombosis or hemorrhage. Doppler US or arteriography can be indicated to minimize the risks of reoperation (CRUMMY 1983; ZEITLER and HEUCK 1997). Typical complications following operation of an AAA, but also after implantation of an endoprosthesis due to POVD, are aneurysms at the proximal or distal anastomosis of the implanted prosthesis. After AAA operations, such anastomotic aneurysms were found in 2.9% of patients after 5 years, and in 11.1% after 10 years (PLATE et al. 1985). The formation of an anastomotic aneurysm is influenced by the material of the prosthesis and of the suture. In most patients (68%) with aneurysms at the end of the implanted graft, the material was Dacron (SANDMANN and KNIEMEYER 1991).

Patients with hypertension have a three- to four-fold higher risk of developing an anastomotic aneurysm than healthy persons (WEIMANN and FLORA 1991). According to WEIMANN and FLORA's findings, aneurysms at the suture occur more frequently in end-to-side anastomoses (7.3%) than in end-to-end anastomoses (WEIMANN, FLORA 1991).

Etiologic factors under discussion include dilatation due to prostheses, infections, and limited collateral vessels in the case of an AAA. More than half of the patients present an anastomotic aneurysm on both sides of the groin. Anastomotic aneurysms at the proximal anastomosis do occur more seldom, but involve the elevated risk of developing an aortointestinal fistula with gastrointestinal bleeding.

Anastomotic aneurysms can be diagnosed by palpation and auscultation during regular sonography in the course of follow-up controls. In the case of a suspected anastomotic aneurysm in one side of the groin, DSA needs to clarify whether there is also a proximal anastomotic aneurysm. The differential diagnosis has to consider the possibility of a false aneurysm after diagnostic angiography, the existence of enlarged lymphatic nodes, or an inguinal hernia. The differential diagnosis alone emphasizes the important role of sonography, mainly for long-term controls. Moreover, sonography provides the feasibility of functional tests and, with color-coded duplex sonography, of detecting changes in the flow profile.

17.3.10
Thoracic Aortic Aneurysms

The different forms of this type of aneurysm require varying radiological approaches: (a) The true aneurysm of the thoracic ascending aorta, (b) the traumatic aneurysm and the aortic rupture, and (c) the dissecting aneurysm, or acute aortic dissection. Their incidence varies considerably in the operation statistics (Table 17.6), demonstrating the need for close cooperation between all medical specialities and first aid personnel.

The varying distribution of the different types of aneurysm in the mainly cardiac surgical centers underlines the various criteria of selection of patients for surgery. This can be, for example, an involvement of the aortic valve, or an existing perforation with or without involvement of the pericardium. In a collective of 85 patients with aneurysms in the ascending aorta and aortic arch, BORST (1991) demonstrated the effectiveness of endoluminal endoprostheses as a therapy concept; he was able to reduce the primary mortality rate to 8.2%, and the late mortality rate to 7.7%. In every aneurysm and dissection close to the heart, the protective measures employed are decisive for the prognosis. Particularly in these cases, diagnostics is an essential tool for therapy planning.

17.3.11
Imaging Diagnostics of the Thoracic Aortic Aneurysm

The basic diagnostic tool (HEBERER et al. 1974; KAPPERT 1976) in the case of symptomatic (post-traumatic or dissecting) or asymptomatic thoracic AAAs is the chest X-ray (Fig. 17.32). It plays an important role in the differential diagnosis between mediastinal tumors, esophagogastral hernias, and postoperative conditions of varying nature. In old age, ectasia and elongation of the aorta with kinking also have to be considered, as the vertebral fractures due to osteoporosis can lead to compression of the aorta. Due to the lack of elasticity of the aorta in old age, a thoracic or thoracoabdominal aneurysm can often only be excluded by a technique using CM (STEINBERG and STEIN 1966; BERGAN and YAO

Table 17.6. Incidence, operative mortality, and risk of ischemic myelitis (paraplegia). (According to CRAWFORD et al. 1990; SEGESSER and TURINA 1990; VOLLMAR 1997)

Type of aortic aneurysm		Incidence (%)	Operative mortality (%)	Ischemic myelitis (%)
DeBakey dissecting aneurysm	Stanford			
I	A	55	7–30	<1
II		10		
III	B	35	10–14	5–15
Non-dissecting thoracoabdominal aortic aneurysm, or two aneurysms		5–10		
	Elective surgery		<10	<5
	Emergency surgery		30–50	<20
Traumatic aortic rupture (TAR) → False aneurysm of the descending thoracic aorta (TAR)	20% of patients survive. TAR accounts for 5% of all vascular traumatic patients in vascular surgery clinics		10–30	5–8

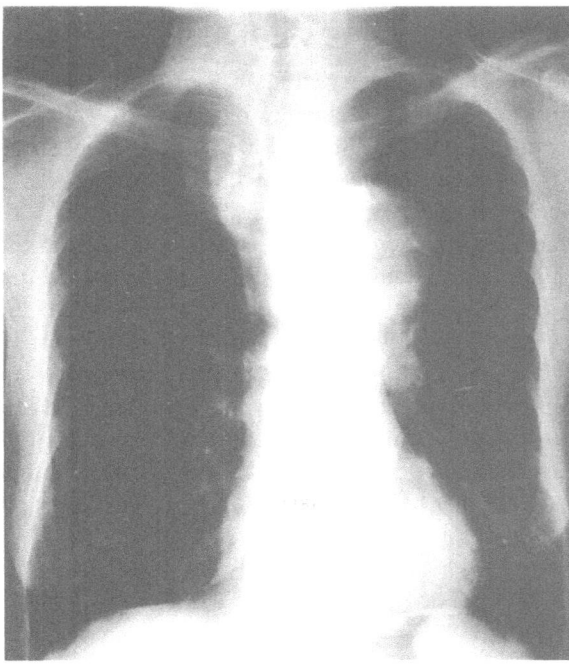

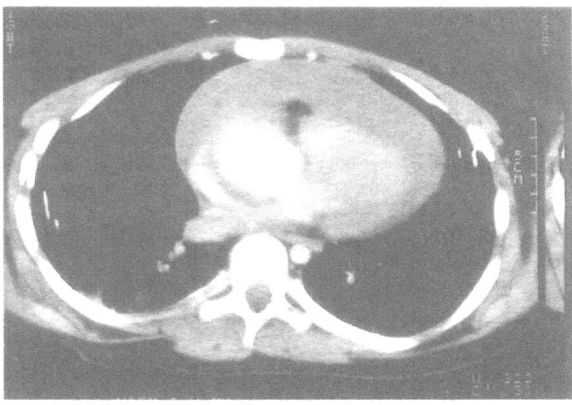

Fig. 17.33. One axial computed tomography scan in a patient with perforation of an ascending aortic aneurysm into the pericardium

Fig. 17.32. Chest image of a 66-year-old male 4 months after a car accident. Widening of the mediastinum with a posttraumatic false thoracic aortic aneurysm after conservative treatment

1982; ZEITLER and HEUCK 1997), unless MRI is used. Patients with Marfan's syndrome are mainly younger, while arteriosclerotic patients are older, which has to be considered when selecting the imaging technique to be used. The most common diagnostic methods are echocardiography, axial scanning techniques, CT, and MRI. CT, preferably performed as spiral CT, is best suited for a simultaneous shock treatment of patients suspected of having an acute dissection. In the intensive care unit or at the time of primary shock treatment, transthoracic echocardiography (TTE) can be utilized for detection of dissections or aneurysms in the region of the ascending aorta, and transesophageal sonography (TES) is helpful in cases of suspected aortic rupture or dissection of the descending aorta. The sophistication of equipment has enabled 3D reconstruction in spiral- or ultrafast-CT diagnostics, which may sometime replace angiography. Angiography is, however, the appropriate method of diagnosis in the aortic valve, with simultaneously performed coronarography.

In the case of aneurysms of the ascending aorta, it should be clarified whether a perforation into the pericardium in the environment of the valve ring (Fig. 17.33) has occurred, and whether there is an aortic vitium, an aneurysm of Valsalva's sinus, or a rupture.

In the event of aneurysms in the aortic arch, it should be clarified whether the branching vessels of the aortic arch are involved, and whether the dissections reach as far as into the major branches of the aortic bow or are limited to the ascending aorta.

X-ray fluoroscopy helps to determine whether a shadow is pulsating or not. The absence of pulsation can indicate a tumor, but also a thrombosed thoracic aortic aneurysm. Using contrast-enhanced CT or angiography, a thoracic aortic aneurysm can be differentiated from a tumor, and its location, extension, and type can be demonstrated (see Chap. 9). Angiography is inevitable prior to surgery, (BRODÉN et al. 1949), as the elongation of the aorta with kinking, especially behind the branching of the left subclavian artery, can mimic an aneurysm. We use various angiographic techniques, which are applied according to the clinical findings. Vascular imaging with the lowest risk is intravenous DSA, with CM injection into the cranial vena cava. But also the transfemoral retrograde or transbrachial arterial access, mainly from the right side, is then possible. In cases where heart catheterization is indicated, CM injection can also be performed intracardially. For an assessment of the branches of the aortic arch, an aortography of the left anterior oblique projection is always required. To assess the plane of the aortic valve,

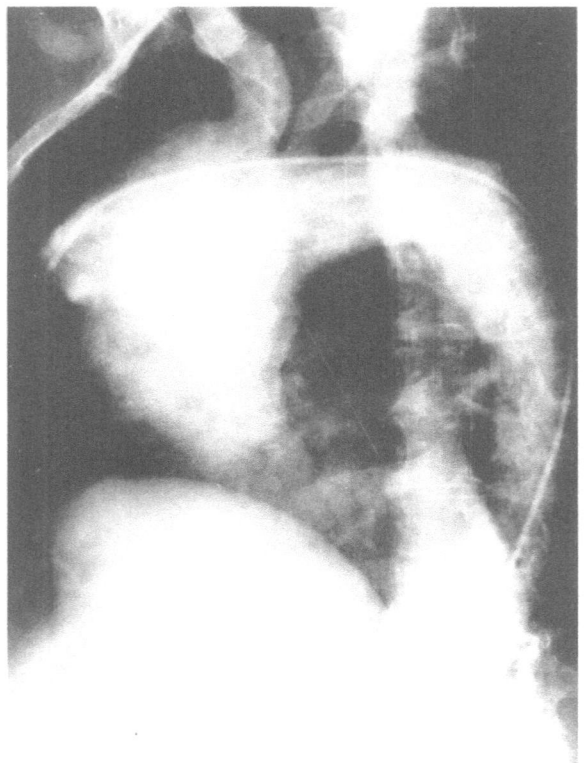

Fig. 17.34. Ascending luetic thoracic aortic aneurysm. Trans–fermoral thoracic aortography from 1973

in contrast, the right anterior oblique projection has to be documented for an analysis of insufficiency and to demonstrate Valsalva's sinuses. The indications for angiography of the thoracic aorta, still today, include: unclear situations in patients with aortic coarctation, thoracic aneurysm, unclear congenital conditions, and aortic arch syndrome (Abrams and Jönsson 1983; Heberer et al. 1974; Rau 1970).

True Aneurysm of the Thoracic Ascending Aorta

The isolated aneurysm of the ascending aorta is found relatively seldom to day; the most common cause is lues (Fig. 17.34), and in rare cases also a fuisform aneurysm of the ascending aorta of arteriosclerotic genesis. Sometimes, it reaches into the aortic arch, and can be present also in patients with idiopathic medionecrosis. It was only after the introduction of the inlay-technique by (Rawford and Crawford (1988), that surgery became possible also in asymptomatic stages, with relatively low surgical mortality. In diagnosis, it is sometimes difficult to clearly distinguish a fusiform aneurysm from an isolated aortic ectasia. The severity of symptoms should then guide the decision regarding appropriate therapy.

17.3.13
Dissecting Aneurysms or Acute Aortic Dissection

According to the DeBakey (1958) classification (Fig. 17.35), there are three types:
- The type I dissection has its source in the ascending aorta, close to the aortic valve ring. It stretches in varying lengths in a distal direction, up to the abdominal, suprarenal, or infrarenal aorta. In many cases, it reaches also into the iliac artery and ends at the iliac bifurcation (Fig. 17.36).
- The type II dissecting aneurysm is restricted to the ascending aorta and can stretch into the aortic arch, up to one of the vessels branching there. The dissection can reach either into the brachiocephalic trunk or into the left carotid common artery. This type is very rarely clearly identified preoperatively.

17.3.12

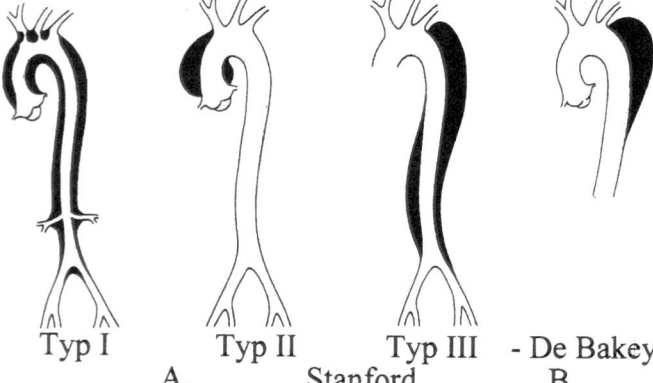

Fig. 17.35. Modified types of dissecting aneurysms. (According to DeBakey et al. 1958)

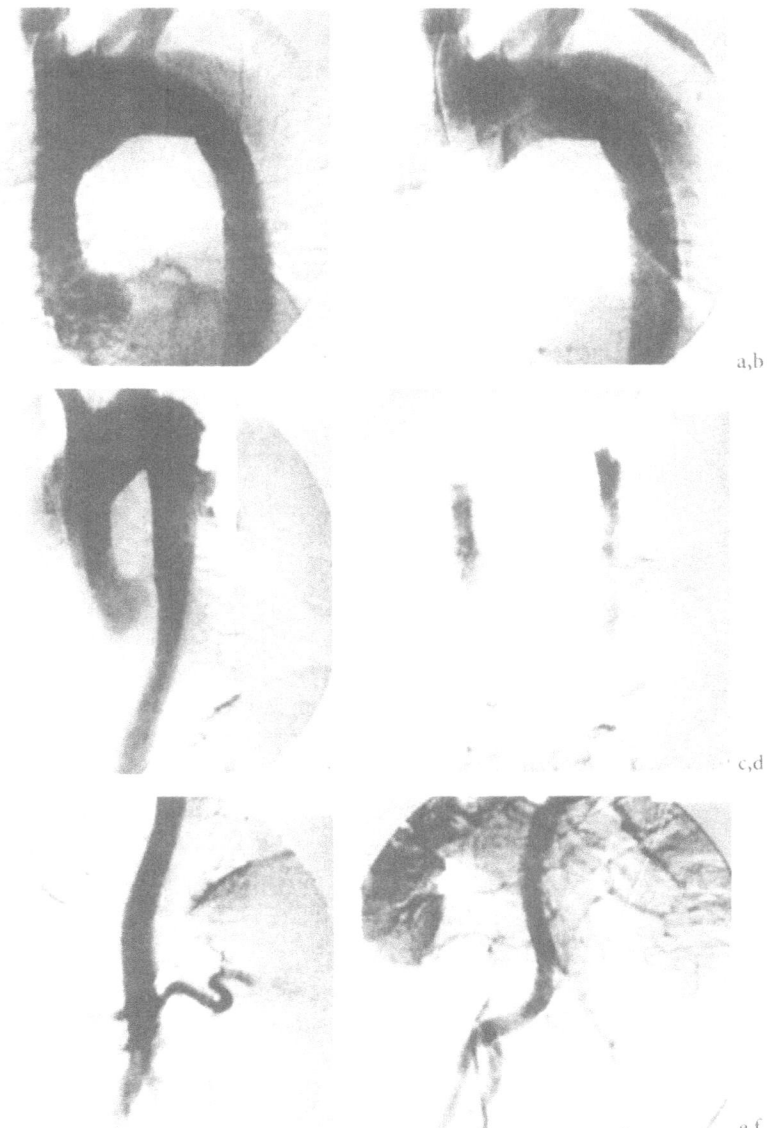

Fig. 17.36 a–d. Thoracoabdominal dissecting aneurysm. DeBakey type 1. Thoracic aortography (digital subtraction angiography with catheterization from the right brachial artery. **a,b** Two parts of the ascending aorta and aortic arch with different contrast intensity; Stanford type A dissection. **c,d** Descending thoracic aorta. **e** Abdominal aorta. **f** Left iliac artery occlusion from the dissection (From ZEITLER 1997)

– In type III, the dissection begins in the distal aortic arch, very close to the left subclavian artery (Fig. 17.37), and stretches down to the abdominal aorta at varying levels. Both spontaneous perforation into the free aortic lumen or displacement of arterial branches (celiac artery, renal artery) can occur. In many cases, the dissection changes from a lateral beginning in a cranial direction to a more medially placed dissecting membrane (BEDUHN et al. 1973).

All dissections in the region of the aorta follow the direction of the blood flow; *a retrograde dissection is an extremely rare exception.* However, the latter was observed after operations at the aortic arch (e.g., after aortocoronary venous bypass) or other operations in the area of the aortic arch, and after

intraluminal seminvasive diagnostic or thrapeutic interventions, as a iatrogenic consequence. The clinical symptoms can be characterized by four different situations: (1) The thoracic syndrome, (2) the abdominorenal syndrome, (3) the peripheral occlusive syndrome, and (4) the neurologic syndrome. This recommendation can serve as guideline when considering to what extent CT or angiography should be performed (HEINZ and LINDHEIMER 1965).

Aortic dissections have increasingly been classified according to Stanford's type A or B, which has facilitated the indication for either heart or vascular surgery. The classification distinguishes between dissections beginning in the ascending aorta (type A) (Fig. 17.38), and others beginning at or behind the

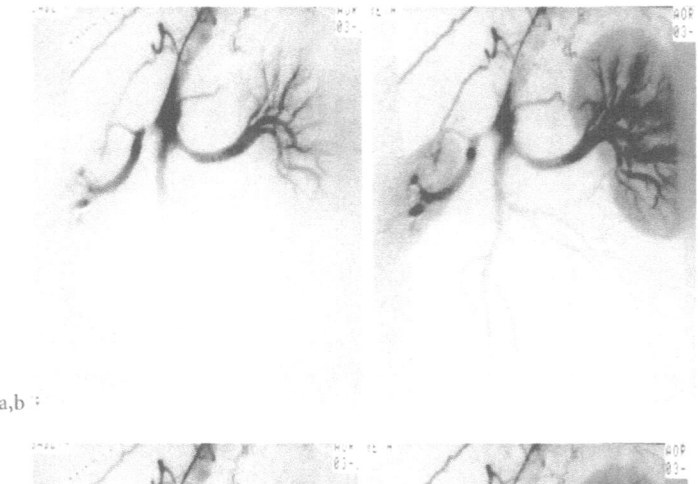

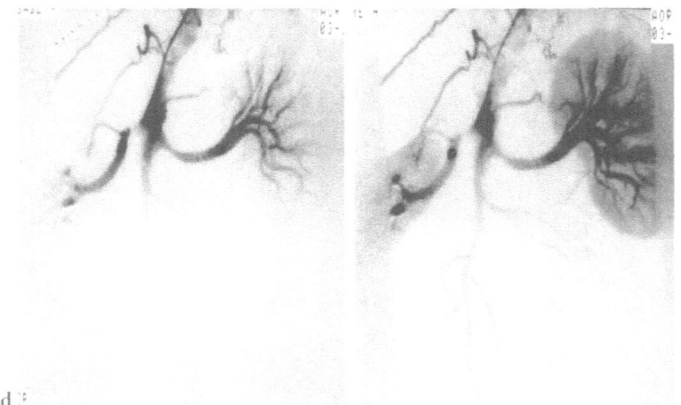

Fig. 17.37 a–f. Thoracoabdominal dissecting aneurysm, DeBakey type III. Thoracic aortography with right transbrachial catheterization. a–d Aortic arch in left anterior oblique projection demonstrating the dissecting membrane which begins directly at the ostium of the left subclavian artery (*arrow*). e,f Upper abdominal angiography depicting contrast enhancement in the true lumen and no contrast in the dissecting parts, with the result of aortic occlusion at the height of the renal arteries (Stanford type B dissection)

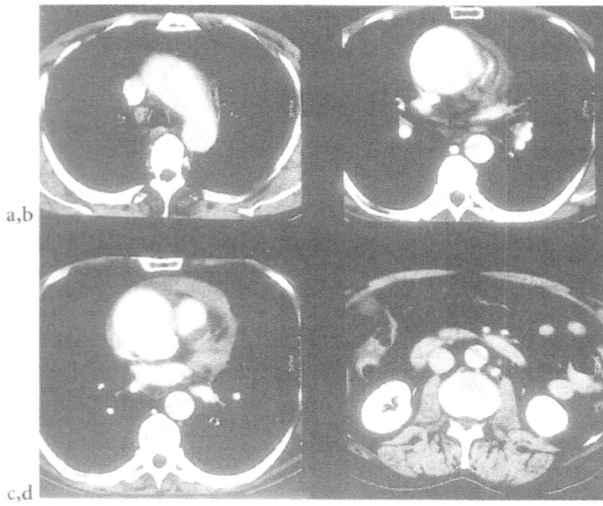

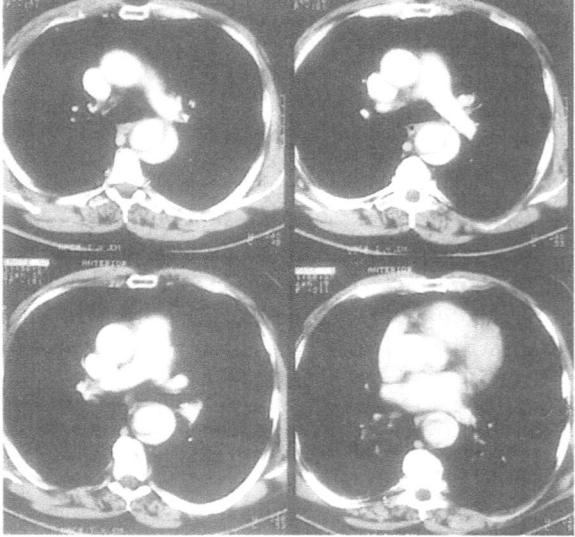

Fig. 17.38 a–d. An 81-year-old female patient with a Stanford type A dissection. In the computed tomography scans, the dissecting membrane can be seen in (a) the aortic arch, (b,c) ascending aorta, (c,d) in the descending and abdominal aorta

Fig. 17.39. A 63-year-old man. Computed tomography scans demonstrate the dissecting membrane and two lumina only in the descending thoracic aorta. The ascending aorta is normal

left subclavian artery (type B) (Fig. 17.39), both of which can also be diagnosed with CT (Figs. 17.38, 17.39) and MRA. The angiographic and spiral CT criteria of dissecting aneurysms include: (a) Double lumen; (b) intimal flap; (c) compression and spiral-shaped picture of the dissection; (d) intimal step at the entry; (e) the time needed for contrast filling in the true and false lumens varies; (f) absence of contrast filling of vesssels branching from the aorta in the area of the dissection.

The major complications of thoracic aortic aneurysms include perforation into the mediastinum, perforation into the pericardium, and free perforation into the pleural space with pleural effusion. The aneurysm can also rupture Valsalva's sinus, with the creation of an aortic insufficiency. In the case of acute clinical symptoms, the chest X-ray can be followed by the quickest diagnosis with spiral CT under intravenous CM administration while the patient is receiving treatment for shock (Figs. 17.38, 17.39). Figure 17.40 shows CT scans of a DeBakey type-II aneurysm, or aortic dissection of Stanford type A with perforation into the pericardium.

Acute dissections of the Stanford type B seem to be well amenable to semiinvasive interventions using percutaneously or surgically implanted endoprostheses through the groin or abdominal aorta (see Sect. 17.4). An important problem in the diagnosis of thoracic aneurysms and dissections is the difficulty in localizing the supply to the spinal cord in order to reduce the risk of paraplegia (CRAWFORD et al. 1990; SEGESSER and TURINA 1990), which can also be caused by an inlay-technique with displacement of the branching arteries to the spinal cord, with severe complications.

In contrast to acute dissections, the luetic forms of thoracic aortic aneurysm of the ascending aorta often show effects of compression and the beginnings of calcification in the marginal area. For the purposes of differential diagnosis of non-dissecting thoracic aortic aneurysms (Marfan's syndrome with diffuse ectasia, or luetic aortic aneurysm), in the case of Marfan's syndrome with a type A dissection, the aorta is not calcified, but an ectasia in the anuloaortic ring is identifiable. The typical patient is relatively young and female.

The location of luetic aneurysms, which are rare nowadays, was mainly the ascending aorta. Calcifications are present, the aortic wall is enlarged and hard, and only in exceptional cases is an extension beyond the aortic arch found, whereas the dilated aorta in patients with Marfan's syndrome extends to the descending thoracic aorta.

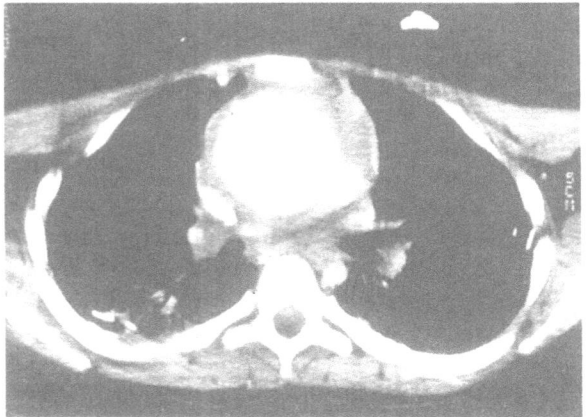

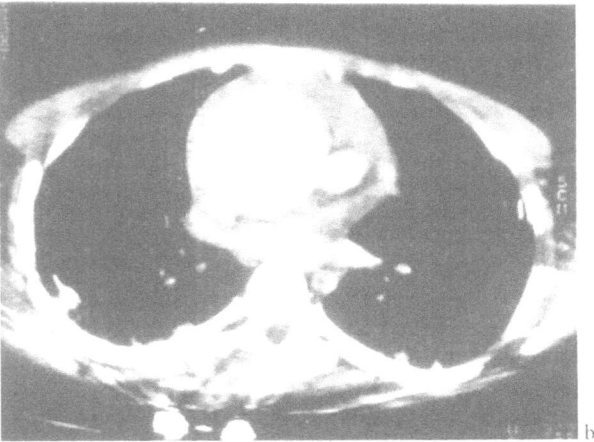

Fig. 17.40 a,b. Dissecting aneurysm DeBakey type II, or Stanford type A. Computed tomography scans show extra-aortic contrast enhancement and hemopericardium. (From ZEITLER 1997)

Irrespective of the type of dissection and the form of the aneurysm, the aim of CT examinations with CM, preferably using the bolus technique, is to demonstrate the extension of the aneurysm, the entry of the dissection, and its re-entry (PINET et al. 1972; GUILLAT et al. 1979; DeSANCTIS et al. 1987; HEBERER et al. 1966; KAPPERT 1976; ZEITLER and HEUCK 1997). Such examinations also need to determine the vessels branching from the aorta as regards their patency, or involvement by dissection. Angiography, therefore, should be performed in two planes, if possible, unless CT or MRI have already povided the necessary information. Also, the scanning methods have to depict the two lumina in case of a dissection, to clearly outline the intimal border, and to demonstrate the extent of a thrombosis. Indications of threatening perforation include isolated contrast accumulations within the thrombus or a thinning of the aortic wall in non-calcified areas.

Diagnostic accuracy in the detection of an acute dissection is over 80%, both with angiography and CT. The combination of transthoracic and transesophageal echocardiography gives approximately the same result (80%–90%) in experienced hands. Again, the advantages of CT, i.e., speed and operator-independent use during simultaneous shock treatment, need to be emphasized. In principle, however, each of the three scanning modalities (US, CT, MRI) can serve for the initial examination and, depending on their findings, the decision should be made as to whether to perform an additional angiography or to operate without delay. This applies, in particular, to hospitals where Stanford type A dissections cannot be treated. In this case, the patient should be transferred immediately after the scanning examination to a hospital with a cardiac surgery department.

17.3.14
Traumatic Aortic Perforation (Posttraumatic Thoracic Aortic Aneurysm)

Given the frequency of road accidents today, the traumatic thoracic aortic aneurysm occurs relatively often (see Table 17.6). The patients have mostly suffered a contusion trauma or a whiplash injury to the chest, and consequently the first examination has to be a chest X-ray and echocardiography to detect a possible aortic rupture, the signs of which include: (a) Enlargement of the mediastinum, (b) displacement of the trachea and esophagus, (c) narrowing of the retrosternal space, and (d) a suspect enlargement of the prominent thoracic aortic segment.

If these signs are not detected at the first examination, and if the patient is observed in an intensive care unit, without the need for immediate clarification with axial scanning methods or angiography, a control X-ray examination has to follow within 2–3 h to detect possible enlargement of the mediastinum, which is the case in mediastinal bleeding. If such an enlargement is identified within 2 h (after the first examination), a contrast study of the thoracic aorta with CT and/or angiography is urgently required. Thoracic posttraumatic aortic aneurysms are located mainly in the area of the left subclavian artery (SCHLOSSER and FAEDRICH 1990; BECKER et al. 1991), but they have also been seen in children in the ascending aorta (GRAJO et al. 1979). Rupture at multiple sites in the thoracic aorta (LIVONI et al. 1982) have also been seen. Modern imaging methods provide good chances of a quick diagnosis if the patient arrives at the clinic in time (BOONJE 1977). In non-acute traumatic lesions, the differential diagnosis

(versus an extreme ectasia of the thoracic aorta with partial thrombosis) presents only minor problems. Without a definite anamnesis, and particularly when the aortic arch is involved, conservative treatment is often considered as an alternative as soon as the acute stage is over, whereby the permanent risk of perforation is neglected.

As for the diagnosis of thoracic aortic aneurysms, dissections, and dilatative angiopathies, diverse imaging modalities are available and it is useful to attempt a clarification using thoracic aortography (Fig. 17.41) as soon as the suspicion arises. But this

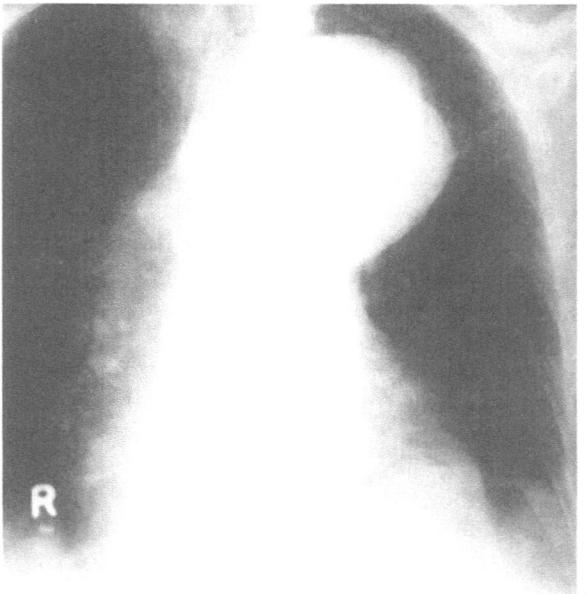

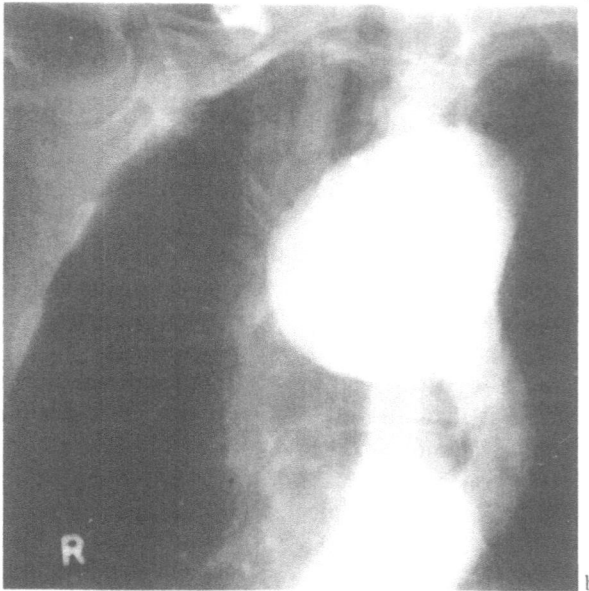

Fig. 17.41 a,b. Posttraumatic aneurysm of the thoracic aorta 2 years after a car accident and conservative treatment. (From ZEITLER 1997)

can also be done primarily under non-invasive conditions using MRI, MR angiography, or CT with the bolus or spiral technique. If findings permit operative treatment or interventional therapy, angiography needs to determine the extension of the lesion and any involvment of neighboring organs. The possibility of a coronary angiography during the first angiography with imaging of the level of the aortic valves should be taken into consideration.

If the patient has already undergone an operation on the thorax, particularly vascular or cardiac surgery, the environment of the anastomosis (e.g.,

after aortocoronary bypasses) has to be closely controlled, as dissections can emerge from these anastomoses.

Posttraumatic aneurysms in the sense of false aneurysms can occur not only in the area of the aorta, but also in other thoracic and abdominal arteries and veins (VOLLMAR 1996). In several chronic arterial aneurysms, a distinction between spontaneous true or posttraumatic aneurysm is impossible with angiography alone. Color-coded duplex sonography can sometimes precisely demonstrate the rupture and wall defect.

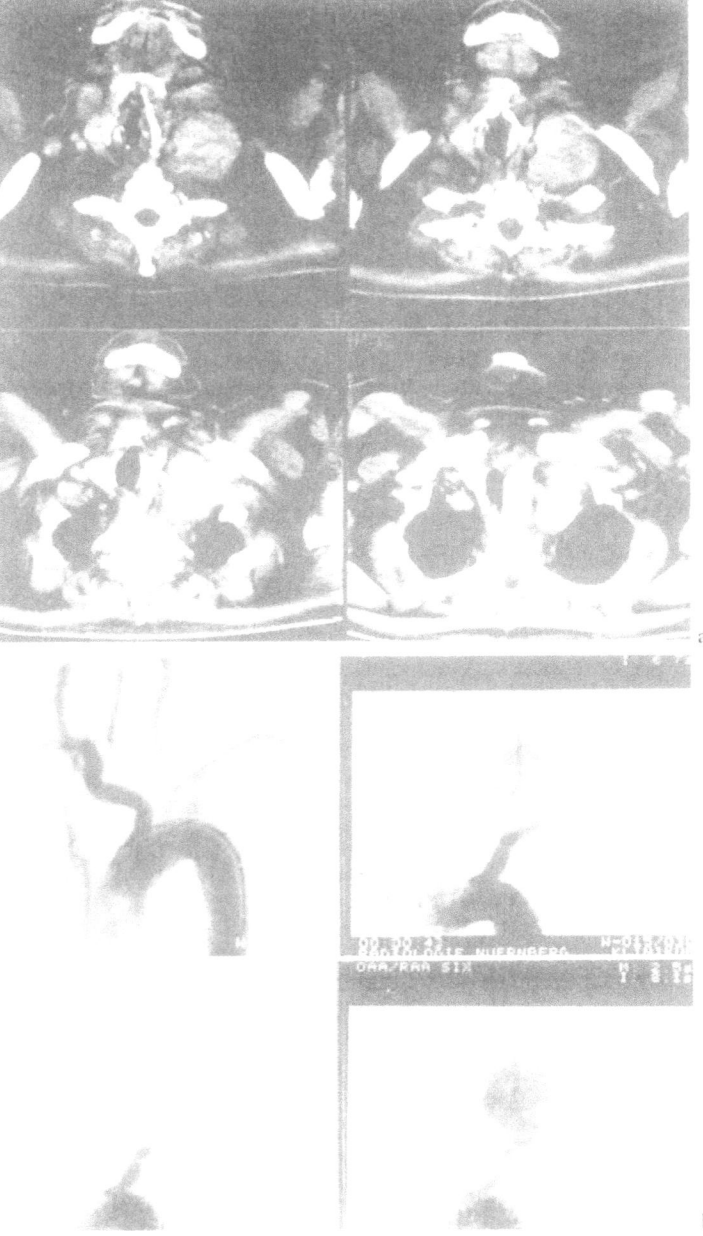

Fig. 17.42 a,b. Posttraumatic aneurysm of the left subclavian artery 3 months after a motorcycle accident. **a** Axial computed tomography scans before and after contrast medium enhancement. **b** Digital subtraction angiography of the thoracic aorta and left shoulder in early and late images. (From ZEITLER 1997)

Figure 17.42 shows a posttraumatic aneurysm of the left subclavian artery in very close proximity to the branching vertebral artery. A contusion trauma has caused the laceration of all layers of the aortic wall, which initiated the formation of an extensive ball-shaped false aneurysm within 3 months. Clinically, it was palpable as a pulsating tumor in the supraclavicular fossa, and could easily be identified with CT and angiography. Nevertheless, DSA with long imaging series proved to be superior to conventional angiography. Such aneurysms, however, are also easily detectable with color-coded duplex sonography (see Chap. 10).

17.3.15
Peripheral Aneurysms

While aneurysms and dissections of the aorta are life-threatening situations and require urgent medical or surgical intervention, aneurysms in other arteries often also present radiologists and surgeons with problems. Autopsy findings have revealed the pelvic, upper-leg, and knee arteries to be the most common locations of peripheral aneurysms. Aneurysms in the extremities, however, often escape detection at autopsy, as autopsies in the extremities are not routinely performed. While aortic aneurysms are found in 3% (1.8%–6.6%) of autopsies, the rate of peripheral aneurysms is about 1%–15% of that of adominal aneurysms. It should be remembered, in this context, that 20% of patients with aortic aneurysms have additional aneurysms in other arteries.

As a consequence of the above, the detection of a peripheral aneurysm will always lead to an angiographic examination of the abdominal aorta. Whereas rupturing is the most common complication of AAAs, peripheral aneurysms bear the risk of thrombosis and embolism. The existence of an aneurysm has to be assumed whenever clinical examination reveals a pulsating tumor, a palpable thrill, or a systolic murmur at auscultation. In earlier days, these were often misinterpreted as a benign or malignant tumor, an abscess, effects of an injury, or a Baker's cyst, and the aneurysm was only recognized when complications occurred. The widespread use of sonography has facilitated the diagnosis. Nevertheless, CT and angiography can provide very helpful information for therapy planning in the differential diagnosis. Non-aortic aneurysms, except those in cerebral arteries, can be differentiated on the basis of their etiology, in those in the lower and upper extremities arteries and those of organ arteries.

17.3.16
Aneurysms of the Lower Extremities

Contrary to autopsy findings, experience in vascular surgical departments has shown that aneurysms of the pelvic and femoropopliteal arteries account for about 40% of all aneurysms treated. With a share of 70%, aneurysms at the femoropopliteal origin and in the poplitea itself are the most common peripheral dilating arteriopathies (VOLLMAR and NOBBE 1976). The age of these patients varies between 40 and 90 years of age (mean age 67), and 90% are men (DENCK 1976).

The femoral artery, which is dilated over long distances and has local excessive dilatations (polyaneurysmatic dystrophy) (LÉRICHE 1943; RANDALL et al. 1979), can be distinguished from small, ballshaped aneurysms at the back of the knee. A total of 40%–60% of patients have similar aneurysms in both legs (ECOIFFIER et al. 1968; BRUNNER and HUWYLER 1975). Patients mostly present acute symptoms because of an embolism in the lower leg (Fig. 17.44), or an acute thrombotic occlusion of the popliteal artery in one leg. Therefore, systematic angiography of both legs is essential to establish a precise diagnosis. The thrombotic occlusion is often preceded by a long asymptomatic period of time during which, in addition to dilatation, longitudinal growth of the artery with kinking takes place (Fig. 17.43). These kink stenoses can lead to claudication and changes in blood flow. Long-segmental stenoses change into arteriomegalies (LÉRICHE 1943; LEA THOMAS 1971; STAPLE et al. 1966; WALZ and DEININGER 1974; ZEITLER and HEUCK 1997).

Changes in circulatory dynamics can be analyzed both qualitatively and quantitatively with pulsed Doppler US, cineradiography within the framework of angiographies, and MRI. Inside fusiform aneurysms, slowing of the blood flow compared to the run-in and run-off can be observed. Inside ballshaped aneurysms, there is circular blood flow with turbulence due to varying flux. The varying flow properties within aneurysms complicate the exact determination of the portion which is already thrombosed; this applies to day to MRI, as formerly to cineangiography, and emphasizes the essential improvement in the accurate assessment of aortic and peripheral aneurysms afforded by DSA.

As regards the analysis of complications of aneurysms and their effects on neighboring organs, CT

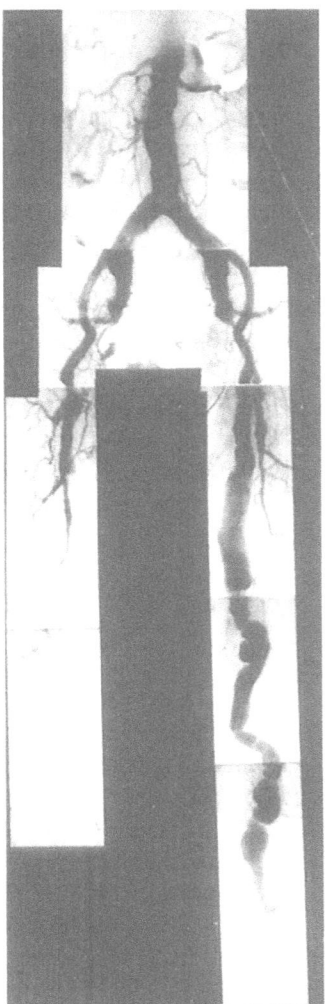

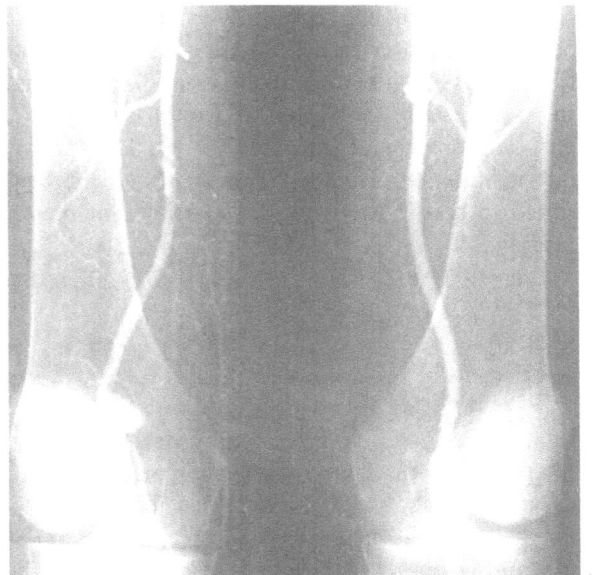

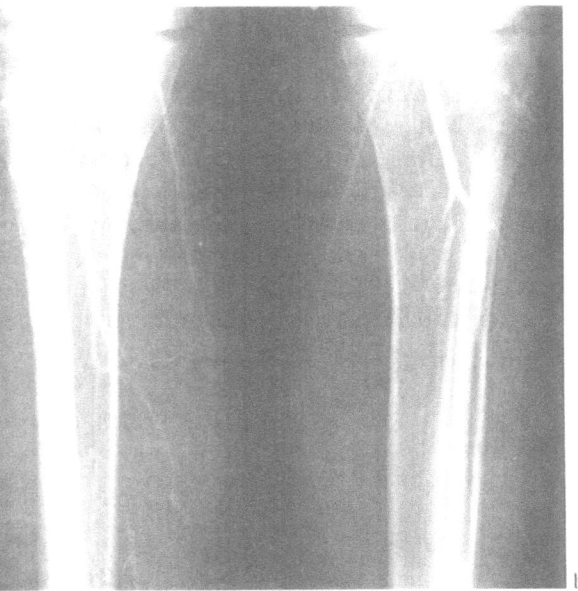

Fig. 17.43. Polyaneurysmatic dysplasia or diffuse femoropopliteal aneurysms in the left leg, with several stenoses, elongation, kink stenoses, and emboli into the tibioperoneal arteries of the right leg due to a totally thrombosed femoropopliteal artery aneurysm

Fig. 17.44 a,b. Bilateral poplitea aneurysm with peripheral embolization. **a** Aortoarteriography with catheter demonstrating partially thrombosed aneurysms on both legs. **b** Angiography of lower-leg arteries with embolus on the popliteal bifurcation on the right leg

and MRI have contributed to a better preoperative diagnosis and detection of postoperative complications. This has been the case in aneurysms of the body trunk and in the region of the knee. US, CT, and MRI have contributed to popliteal and other aneurysms being increasingly detected at asymptomatic stages. As therapy, which is performed only after thrombotic occlusion with acute ischemia, is associated with a relatively high rate of amputations of the lower leg (20% compared to 2%), the elimination of aneurysms in their asymptomatic stage is recommended. This can be done with an endograft, a stent, or a bypass. The latest designs of polyester-coated endoprostheses have opened up the possibility of a useful percutaneous or minimally-invasive therapy. These "EndoPro" stents, like other modifications, can be inserted via a 10-F sheath into the groin under local anesthesia. In Nuremberg, seven popliteal aneurysms have been eliminated to date using this intervention, which has also been increasingly accepted in other clinics (e.g., Munich and Nancy). Studies on long-term results, however, are not yet available.

Aneurysms of the lower leg arteries, such as the posterior tibial or foot arteries, are only reported in case studies, whereby they are mainly of posttraumatic or postoperative origin. Their development can be controlled with sonography at short intervals. For surgical planning, the identification of additional complications, such as arteriovenous fistulas or stenoses (which are clinically symptomatic), can be valuable. An arterial DSA using a simple needle technique as angiography is sufficient in most cases. In these cases, MRI or spiral CT with 3D reconstruction can also provide clear information. Prior to any intervention, the vascular surgeon should be consulted to take precautions for possible emergency cases.

17.3.17
Aneurysms of the Upper Extremities

Dilating degenerative arteriopathy develops in old age, mainly in patients over the age of 70, particularly if these suffer from hypertension, are overweight and/or have high triglyceride values, without the risk factor of cigarette-smoking. Not only the aorta, but also the supraaortal arteries, the anonyma artery, and the carotid and subclavian arteries are affected. Significant dilatations of the subclavian arteries can mainly be observed as poststenotic processes in the case of subclavian stenoses or thoracic outlet syndrome. A few cases of aneurysms of the radial or ulnar arteries have been reported (see Fig. 17.23a). More common are the diffuse and limited dilatations of the arm arteries following surgery, especially after the creation of arteriovenous shunts for dialysis purposes, or posttraumatic aneurysms (see Fig. 17.42).

17.3.18
Aneurysms of the Renal Arteries

Due to the widespread use of renal angiography, the incidence of renal artery aneurysms is well known. It has been reported at a rate of 0.5%–0.8%, depending on whether the fibromuscular forms are included or not. The following forms are distinguished:
- The *sacculated aneurysm*, which is mostly located close to the hilus, in the region of the bifurcation of the renal arteries (see Fig. 17.23b).
- The *fusiform aneurysm*, which is often only a poststenotic dilatation in the case of renal artery stenosis. To distinguish it from fibromuscular dysplasia is often impossible.
- The *intrarenal microaneurysm*, which is mainly detected in examinations for a systemic disease, such as panarteritis nodosa or lupus erythematosus.

The age of the patients with aneurysms of the renal arteries varies between 20 and 90 years of age (mean age: 61). Often, a concomitant hypertension is detected. The correlation between sacculated renal artery aneurysms and hypertension, contrary to that of fibromuscular dysplasia, has not as yet been proven. Clinical symptoms are observed in about 20% of patients with renal artery aneurysms: pain in the abdomen, hematuria, or disturbed renal function. In patients with hypertension, a medicamentous treatment prior to operative resection on the opened kidney (microsurgery) is recommended. Renal artery aneurysms have diameters of 0.3–4 cm. During 19 years of practice, I myself have detected seven sacculated aneurysms of between 0.5 and 3 cm in diameter, and five microaneurysms smaller than 0.5 cm.

17.3.19
Isolated Iliac Aneurysms

This type of aneurysm (see Fig. 17.24) was already identified in 1966 with the Steinberg angiography (STEINBERG and STEIN 1966). While in the autopsy statistics its frequency is only 1%, clinical collectives have reported on 40 isolated iliac aneurysms out of 476 aortoiliac aneurysms (8%), while other clinics found it in only 1.5% of all aneurysms. A total of 95% of persons affected are men. The age of patients varies widely from 7 to 88 years (mean age, 67), suggesting, apart from arteriosclerosis, also a congenital, local, or traumatic origin as regards etiology (HEBERER and REIDEMEISTER 1974; WENZ and BEDUHN 1976; ZEITLER 1976; VOLLMAR 1996).

Often, diagnosis is an incidental finding in angiographic, CT, or US examinations. Clinically observed symptoms include lumboinguinal pain, which can be misinterpreted as ureteral colic. Other patients complain of gastrointestinal tenesmus and obstipation. Symptoms caused by ureteral compression or pressure on the sciatic nerve are described. On rectal palpation, pulse-synchronous resistance may be felt. I myself found the latter quite often in pelvic arteriovenous malformations. The variety of symptoms often leads to diagnostic misinterpretations, until an angiography is performed.

BÄR and NACHBUR (1991) reported that in Bern, 14 of 40 patients with isolated iliac aneurysms required surgery due to rupturing. Of these patients, eight had received incorrect treatment due to diagnoses such as inguinal hernia, renal colic, or diverticulitis over a period of between 1 and 14 years. The use of sonography and CT should contribute to a faster detection of the causes of pelvic compression syndromes before perforation occurs. Iliac aneurysms can also occur in the common, external, and internal arteries. These regions are suited to implantation of polyester-coated stents, so-called endoprostheses, via percutaneous access within the framework of interventional radiology or endovascular surgery (see Sect. 17.4).

17.3.20
Postoperative and Other Iatrogenic Aneurysms

Anastomotic aneurysms are considered to be a tribute to the progress of vascular surgery (RAITHEL 1973; CRUMMY 1983; CRAWFORD and CRAWFORD 1988), and mostly occur after the application of synthetic materials (GIESSLER et al. 1968). They develop within 5–12 years after the primary operative intervention, in most cases after implantation of a Y-shaped prosthesis. A total of 60% of patients have aneurysms in both inguinal arteries, and a proximal anastomotic aneurysm in the aorta. Following surgery for abdominal aortic aneurysms, 2.9% of patients developed a suture aneurysm in the groin after 5 years, and 11.1% of patients after 10 years (WEIMANN and FLORA 1991). Other studies have reported on a frequency of 4.5%–15%. Besides the material of the prosthesis and the suture, arterial hypertension is mentioned as one of the underlying causes of such postoperative aneurysms. In hypertensive patients, anastomotic aneurysms occur about four times as often within 10 years (VOLLMAR 1996).

For the evaluation of anastomotic aneurysms, follow-up controls over several years with sonography or angiography have proven the effects of the material and determined the time of surgical resection. The future will show whether new graft materials or endovascular therapies are capable of preventing or reducing the incidence of anastomotic aneurysms.

Every radiologist should be familiar with the symtoms, diagnostic procedure, and treatment of iatrogenic aneurysms. For diagnostic catheter angiographies using Seldinger's technique, the diameter of the catheters could mostly be reduced to 5F or less, which has led to a reduction in typical complications after puncture, such as false aneurysm or arteriovenous fistula in the groin (<0.1%). Other

diagnostic examinations, such as ECG in combination with levocardiography, mostly require a 7-F introducer-sheath system. While hematomas after puncture almost exclusively develop in patients under anticoagulation, or in the event of disturbances in coagulation after catheterization for diagnostic or interventional purposes (e.g., percutaneous transluminal coronary angioplasty or cerebral embolization), the potential of complications due to prophylactic heparinization has to be taken into account (Fig. 17.45). VOLLMAR (1996) reported on vascular complications in the groin or axilla after catheter techniques, requiring surgical treatment in 1% of all procedures, the majority of these after cardiac catheterization.

For radiological interventions, the use of sheaths of up to 14F will become increasingly common in indications such as the treatment of aneurysms or arterial obliterations, or the treatment of intracranial aneurysms with coaxial catheter systems. Given this, the following precautions need to be observed:

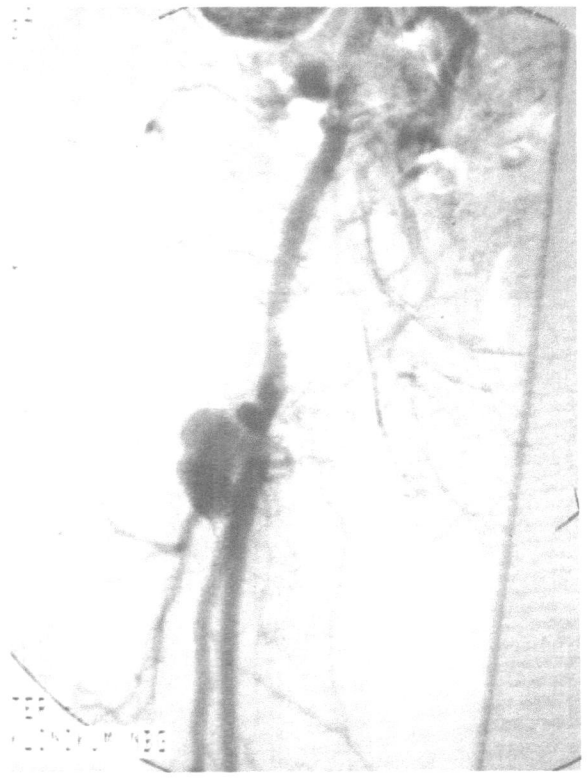

Fig. 17.45. False aneurysm in the right groin, or pulstating hematoma. After transfemoral left heart and coronary angiography in a 77-year-old woman with severe angina pectoris. Transbrachial arterial digital subtraction angiography also demonstrating a femoropopliteal bypass on the right leg

1. *Prophylaxis of complications at the puncture site:* A properly performed puncture should seek to avoid any injury to the arterial back wall. This can be achieved by determining the location of the artery using the Doppler technique, and by the use of puncture needles without stylet.
2. *Postinterventional bleeding control:* After diagnostic catheterizations or therapeutic percutaneous interventions, an experienced physician should seal the puncture hole either by manual compression or with a pressure-controlled pneumatic compressor until bleeding stops, despite anticoagulation.

In the case of puncture holes of over 7F, a mechanical puncture-hole closure device (Angioseal, Perclose, Vasoseal ES) should be used. These devices function either on the basis of a collagenous plug (Fig. 17.46a-c), or a percutaneous vascular suture (Fig. 17.46a-c). Also, after the use of this type of bleeding control, the patient should remain under the physician's control for at least 2h, otherwise a control over 4h is recommended. Complications after the use of percutaneous closure devices with local stenoses in the femoral artery and acute leg ischemia, were observed after the use of Vasoseal in 0.3%-2.0%, with major complications requiring surgical repair in 0.1% (Schräder et al. 1993; Sanborn et al. 1994). After the use of the Angioseal device, an incidence of five local stenoses in the femoral artery – out of 1500 applications – has been published (Steinkamp et al. 1999). In these patients representing 0.3%, the local obliteration was treated with laser-assisted balloon PTA. If erroneous application leads to a total occlusion of the femoral artery because the occluded system lies completely intraarterially (Silber et al. 1998), surgical resection with patch-plasty becomes necessary.

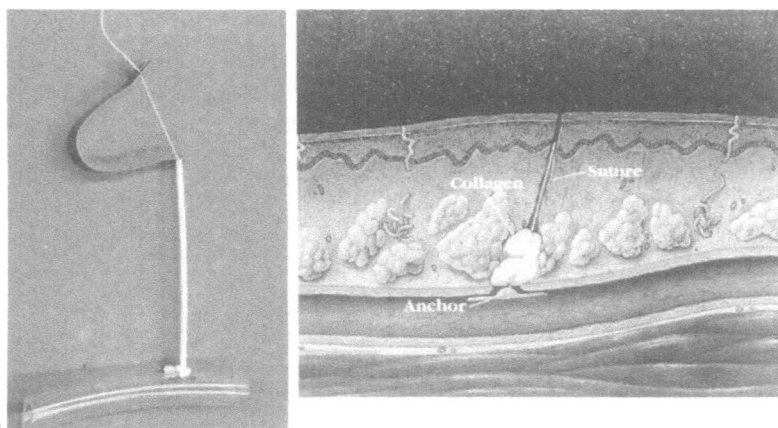

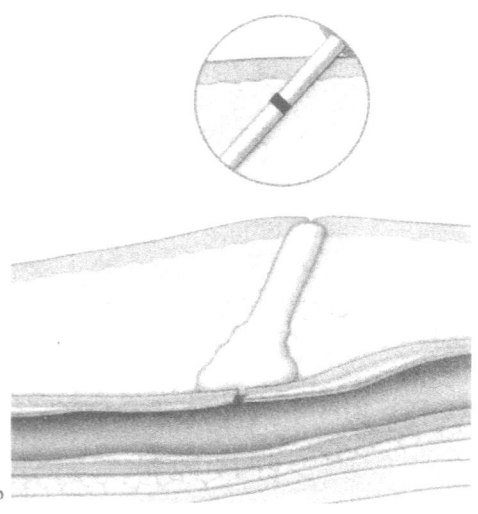

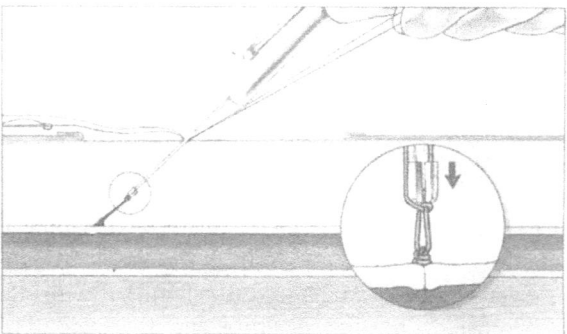

Fig. 17.46 a–c. Puncture-hole closure devices. **a** AngioSeal, **b** Vasoseal ES (Datascope), **c** Prostar (Perclose)

3. *When the bleeding stops:* a solid bandage should be applied around the hip and groin, unless the patient is still under the physician's control.

If, despite these precautionary measures, a false aneurysm develops, the puncture site can be compressed under US monitoring. Several studies have shown that in this way an operation can become superfluous. In the case of extensive bleeding that cannot be controlled, however, the vascular suture and removal of the hematoma with subsequent drainage for at least 48 h to prevent infection become necessary. Every radiologist should be capable of managing such interventional situations and, if necessary, the vascular surgeon should be consulted.

References

Abrams HL, Jönsson G (1983) Coarcation of the Aorta. In: Abrams HL (ed) Angiography, 3rd edn., vol I. Little Brown, Boston, pp 382–412

Aker TU, Kensey R, Heuser R, et al. (1994) Immediate arterial hemostasis after cardiac catheterization. Cardiovasc Diagn 31:228–232

Alevizacos P, Hegenscheid M, Hepp W (1964) Autogene Rekonstruktion bei mykotischem imaginalem Aneurysma – Langzeitergebnisse. VASA 23:164

Amplatz K (1986) Coarctation of the aorta. In: Amplatz K (ed) Radiology of congenital heart disease, vol I. Thieme Medical, New York, pp 461–490

Anderson CB, Butcher HR, Ballinger WF (1974) Mycotic aneurysms. Arch Surg 109:712–717

Anjos R, Oureshi SA, Rosenthal E, et al. (1992) Determinants of hemodynamic results of balloon dilatation of aortic recoarctation. Am J Cardiol 69:665–671

Bachmann D, Dressler F, Schmutzler H (1964) Supravalvuläre Aortenstenose mit primärer Aortenhypoplasie und Koronararterienanomalie. Fortschr Rontgenstr 100:460–468

Bank EZ, Aisen AM, Rocchini AP, Hernandez RJ (1987) Coarctation of the aorta in children undergoing angioplasty: pretreatment and posttreatment MR imaging. Radiology 162:235

Bär W, Nachbur B (1991) Beckenarterienaneurysmen. In: Sandmann W, Kniemeyer HW (eds) Aneurysmen der großen Arterien. Huber, Berlin, pp 286–293

Bariéty M, Paulet J, Terris G (1961) Les dolicho-méga-artéries. Buell Mem Soc Med Hop Paris 77:394–412

Bean WJ, Rodan BA, Thebant AL (1985) Leriche syndrome: treatment with streptokinase and angioplasty. AJR 144:1285

Becker HM, Ramirez VE, Heberer G (1991) Traumatic aneurysms of the descending aorta. Ann Vasc Surg Marker ••

Beduhn D, Büsing CM, Roth E (1973) Angiographie einer akuten ausgedehnten Aortendissektion. Munch Med Wochenschr 115:193–196

Benson LN, Freedom RM, Wilson GJ, et al. (1986) Cerebral complications following balloon angioplasty of coarctation of the aorta. Cardiovasc Intervent Radiol 9:184

Bergan JJ, Trippel OH (1963) Management of juxtarenal aortic occlusions. Arch Surg 87:230–238

Bergan JJ, Yao JSt (1982) Aneurysms – diagnosis and treatment. Grune and Stratton, New York

Berger T, Sorensen R, Konrad J (1986) Aortic rupture: complication of transluminal angioplasty. AJR 146:373

Berguer R, Higgins RF, Cotton LT (1975) Geometry blood flow and reconstruction of the deep femoral artery. Am J Surg 130:68–71

Black JA, Carter REB (1963) Associations between aortic stenosis and facies of severe infantile hypercalcaemia. Lancet II:745–748

Bleckat G, Strube G (1967) Die generalisierte Hypoplasie der Aorta. Munch Med Wochenschr 109:1851–1854

Boonje AH (1977) Traumatic aneurysm. VASA 6 (4):372

Borst HG (1991) Chirurgische Therapie chronischer Aneurysmen der Aorta ascendens und des Aortenbogens. In: Sandmann W, Kniemeyer HW (eds) Aneurysmen der großen Arterien. Huber, Bern, pp 185–187

Brecht G, Brecht T, Lackner K, Thurn P (1979) Die Computertomographie in der Untersuchung großer Arterien. In: Hild R, Spaan G (eds) Therapiekontrolle in der Angiologie. Witzstrock, Baden-Baden, pp 272–276

Brodén B, Jönsson G, Karnell J (1949) Thoracic aortography. Acta Radiol 32:498–508

Brunner U, Huwyler R (1975) Das arteriosklerotische femoropopliteale Aneurysma in chirurgischer Sicht. In: Brunner U (ed) Die Kniekehle. Huber, Bern, pp 51–56

Burke AM, Jamieson GG (1983) Aortocaval fistula associated with ruptured aortic aneurysm. Br J Surg 70:431

Bussmann WD, Reifart N, Sievert H, Kaltenbach M (1985) Transfemorale Angioplastik der Aortenisthmusstenose. Dtsch Med Wochenschr 110:1839–1841

Carlson DH, Gryska P, Sebetz J, Armstrong S (1975) Arteriomegaly. Am J Roentgenol Rad Ther Nucl Med 125:553–558

Casalini E, Sfondrini MS (1994) Abdominal aortic coarctation treated with percutaneous transluminal angioplasty: case report. Eur Radiol 4:382–384

Celoria GC, Patton RB (1959) Congenital absence of aortic arch. Am Heart J 58:407

Cheng TO (1991) Aneurysm formation after repair of coarctation of the aorta. Radiology 181:905

Clagett OT, Kirklin JW, Edwards JE (1954) Anatomic variations and pathologic changes in coarctation of the aorta. Surg Gynecol ••:98

Clark RA, Colley DP, Siedlecki E (1979) Later complications at repair site of operated coarctation of aorta. AJR 133:1071

Crawford ES, Crawford JL (1988) Diseases of the aorta. Williams and Wilkins, Baltimore

Crawford ES, Coselli JS, Svensson LG, et al. (1990) Diffuse aneurysmal disease (chronic aortic dissection, MARFAN and MEGA aorta syndromes) and multiple aneurysm. Treatment by subtotal and total aortic replacement. Ann Surg 211:521–537

Crawford JL, Stowe CL, Safi HJ, Hallmann CH, Crawford ES (1985) Inflammatory aneurysms of the aorta. J Vasc Surg 2:113

Crummy AB (1983) Arteriography of the patient with previus aortoiliac surgery. In: Abrams HL (ed) Angiography, 3rd edn, vol III. Little Brown, Boston, pp 1819–1833

Cullenward MJ, Scanlan KA, Pozniav MA, Acher CA (1986) Inflammatory aortic aneurysm (perioaortic fibrosis): radiologic imaging. Radiology 159:75

Darcy MD (1991) Lower-extremity arteriography: current approaches and techniques. Radiology 178:615–619

Darling RC (1970) Ruptured arteriosclerotic abdominal aortic aneurysm. A pathologic and clinical study. Am J Surg 119:397–401

Dean RH, Kimberley JH (1991) Prophylactic renal revascularization: has it a role? In: Veith FJ (ed) Current critical problems in vascular surgery, vol 3. Quality Medical Publ, St. Louis

DeBakey M, Cooley DA, Crawford ES, Morris G (1958) Aneurysms of the thoracic aorta. J Thorac Cardiovasc Surg 30:393–420

DeBakey ME, Garrett HE, Howell JE, Morris GG Jr (1967) Coarcatio of the abdominal aorta with renal arterial stenosis: Surgical considerations. Ann Surg 165:830

Denck H (1976) Chirurgie der peripheren Arterien. In: Vollmar JF, Nobbe FP (eds) Arteriovenöse Fisteln – Dilatierende Arteriopathien (Aneurysmen). Thieme, Stuttgart, pp 133–138

DeSanctis R, Doroghazi RM, Austen GW, Buckley MJ (1987) Aortic dissection. N Engl J Med 317:1060–1067

DeSwart H, Dijkman L, Hofstra L, et al. (1993) A new hemostatic puncture closure device for immediate sealing of arterial puncture sites. Am J Cardiol 72:445–449

Deutsch V, Wexler L, Deutsch H (1974) Takayasu's arteriitis, an angiographic study with remarks on ethnic distribution in Israel. AJR 122:13

Drexler ChJ, Stewart JR, Kincard OW (1964) Diagnostic implications of rib notching. Am Journal Roentgenol 91:1064–1074

Ecoiffier J, Laval-Jeantet M, Kauffmann E (1968) Cinéartériographie fémorale dans les artheromatoses avec dolicho-méga-artère. J Radiol 49:294–296

Edwards JF, Carey LS, Neufeld HN, Lester RG (1965) Congenital heart disease. Correlation of pathologic anatomy and angiocardiography. Saunders, Philadelphia, pp 677–698

Egloff L, Dimai W, Schneider E, Kugelmeier J, Turina M, Senning A (1983) Das Bauchaortenaneurysma beim über 70jährigen Patienten – soll es in jedem Fall operiert werden? Schweiz Med Wochenschr 113:208–211

El Ashmaoui A, Do DD, Triller J, et al. (1991) Angioplasty of the terminal aorta: follow-up of 20 patients treated by PTA or PTA with stents. Eur J Radiol 13:113–117

Faggioloi GL, Stella A, et al. (1994) Morphology of small aneurysms: definition and impact on risk of rupture. Am J Surg 168:131–135

Fava MP, Foradori GB, Garcia CB, et al. (1993) Percutaneous transluminal angioplasty in patients with Takayasu arteritis: five-year experience. JVIR 4:649–653

Fawzy ME, Dunn B, Galal O, et al. (1993) Balloon coarctation angioplasty in adolescents and adults: early and intermediate results (abstract). JVIR 4:158

Fink U (1991) Peripheral DSA with automatic stepping. Eur Radiol 13:50–55

Fontaine R, Fruehling L, Grey J (1944) La dystrophie polyanévrysmale ou variqueuse des artères à évolution thrombosante. Chir Lyon 39:575

Giessler R, Heberer G (1967) Diagnose und Therapie des rupturierten Aneurysmas der Bauchaorta. Chirurg 38:514–520

Giessler R, Gehl H, Heberer G (1968) Das Nahtaneurysma nach alloplastischem Gefäßersatz. Arch Klin Chir 322:992–996

Gmelin E, Arlart JP (1987) Digitale subtraktionsangiographie. Thieme, Stuttgart

Goldstone J, Malone JM, Moore WS (1978) Inflammatory aneurysms of the abdominal aorta. Surgery 83:425

Grajo GA, Kook Sang LW, Young OH (1979) Traumatic aneurysm of the ascending aorta in a child. Pediatr Radiol 8:263–265

Grollmann JH, Hanafee W (1964) The roentgen diagnosis of Takayasu's arteriitis. Radiology 83:387–392

Gross-Fengels W, Steinbrich W, Pichlmaier H, Erasmi H (1990) Die perkutane transluminale Angioplastie (PTA) der infrarenalen Aorta abdominalis. Radiologe 30:235–241

Guillot M, Froment JC, Touboul P, Delahaye JP, Pinet F (1979) Dissections aortiques aigues. Facteurs prognostiques, indications thérapeutiques, 137 observations. L Nouv Presse Med 8:2603–2607

Hallisey MJ, Meranze SG, Parker BC, et al. (1994) Percutaneous transluminal angioplasty of the abdominal aorta. JVIR 5:679–••

Heberer G, Reidemeister JC (1974) Aneurysmen und Elongationen der Arterien. In: Heberer G, Rau G, Schoop W (eds) Angiologie, 2nd edn. Thieme, Stuttgart, pp 555–571

Heberer G, Rau G, Löhr HH (1966a) Aorta und große Arterien. Springer, Berlin Heidelberg New York

Heberer G, Rau G, Löhr HH (1966b) Typische Coarctatio aortae ("Aortenisthmusstenose"). In: Heberer G (ed) Aorta und große Arterien. Springer, Berlin Heidelberg New York, pp 716–764

Heberer G, Zumtobel V, Eigler FW, Rau G (1971) Behandlung atypischer suprarenaler Stenosen der Aorta bei Hypertonikern. Dtsch Med Wochenschr 96:615

Heberer G, Rau G, Schoop W (1974) Angiologie, 2nd edn. Thieme, Stuttgart

Heberer G, Schildberg FW, Becker HM, Stelter WJ, Zumtobel V (1975) Die atypische suprarenale Aortenstenose als Ursache eines juvenilen Hypertonus. Dtsch Med Wochenschr 100 (13):649–660

Heimig T, Martin M (1997) Thrombolyse. In: Zeitler E (ed) Klinische Radiologie: Arterien und Venen. Springer, Berlin Heidelberg New York, pp 193–198

Heinz N, Lindheimer W (1965) Zur Klinik der dissezierenden Aortenruptur. Dtsch Med Wochenschr 90:1349

Hejhal L, Hejhal J, Firt P (1973) Coarctio of the abdominal aorta. J Cardiovasc Surg 14:168

Hensel H (1955) Über die Steuerung der peripheren Durchblutung. Arch Phys Ther (Lzg) 7:60–68

Heyden B, Vollmar J, Voss FU (1979) Therapiekontrolle bei Zweietagenverschlüssen (aorto-iliakal und femoropopliteal). Zentralbl Chir 104:519–528

Hirsch MS, Aikat BK, BASU AK (1964) Takayasu's arteriitis: report of 5 cases with immunologic studies. Bull Johns Hopkins Hosp 115:29••

Holdsworth JD (1994) Screening for abdominal aortic aneurysm in Northumberland. J Surg 81:10–12

Inada K (1965) Atypical coarctation of the aorta with special reference to its genesis. Angiology 16:608

Ingrisch H, Seyferth W, Kufter G (1984) Percutaneous transluminal angioplasty in cases of stenosis in the region of the infrarenal abdominal aorta and the aortoiliac bifurcation. In: Dotter CT, Grüntzig AR, Schoop W, Zeitler E (eds) Percutaneous transluminal angioplasty. Springer-Verlag, Berlin Heidelberg New York

Ito J (1966) Aortitis syndrome with reference to detection of anti-aorta antibody from patients sera. Jpn Circulat J 30:75

Jones KL, Smith DW (1975) The Williams elfin facies syndrome: a new perspective. J Pediatr 86:718

Kappert A (1976) Lehrbuch und Atlas der Angiologie, 7th edn. Huber, Bern

Kappestein AP, Zwinderman AH, Bogers AJJC, et al. (1995) More than thirty-five years of coarctation repair: unexpected high relapse rate. Radiology 194:591

Kirks DR, Currating G, Chen JTT (1986) Mediastinal collateral arteries: important vessels in coarctation of the aorta. AJR 146:757

Klinkhamer AC (1965) Diagnose von abweichenden Arterien im oberen Mediastinum mit Hilfe des Esophagogramms. Rontgen Agfa Gevaert 3:9–12

Kremer K, Loose DA, Moschinski D, Kleinschmidt F, Kovacicek S, Benesch L (1975) Coarctatio aortae abdominalis. VASA 4:125–131

Kuhlgatz G (1964) Die Isthmusstenose der Aorta – Irrwege der Diagnostik. Padiatr Pry 3:363–370

Kuhn E, Kohn R, Schönthal H, Schaaf J (1963) Familiäre Coarctatio aortae (Aortenisthmusstenose). Z Kreislaufforsch 52:1120–1124

Kunz R (1980) Aneurysmata bei 35.380 Autopsien. Schweiz Med Wochenschr 110:142–148

Lea Thomas M (1971) Arteriomegaly. Br J Surg 58:690–694

Lériche R (1943) Dolicho et méga-artère dolicho et méga-veine. Presse Med 51:554–555

Lériche R (1947) Les symptômes douloureux des dolicho-artéries. Presse Med 55:641

Leu HJ (1976) Pathomorphologie und Ätiologie der dilatierenden Arteriopathien. In: Vollmar JF, Nobbe FP (eds) Arteriovenöse Fisteln – Dilatierende Arteriopathien (Aneurysmen). Thieme, Stuttgart, pp 93–97

Lewis VD III, Meranze SG, McLean GK, O'Neill JA Jr, Berkowitz HD, Burke DR (1988) Midaortic syndrome: diagnosis and treatment. Radiology 167:111

Lipchik EO, Rogoff StM (1983) The abnormal abdominal aorta: arteriosclerosis and other diseases. In: Abrams HL (ed) Angiography, 3rd edn, vol II. Little Brown, Boston, pp 1057–1078

Lipchik EO, Rogoff SM (1983) Aneurysms of the abdominal aorta. In: Abrams H (ed) Angiography, vascular and interventional radiology. Little Brown, Boston, pp 1079–1089

Lipchik EO, Rob CG, Schwartzberg S (1964) Obstruction of the abdominal aorta above the level of the renal arteries. Radiology 82:443–446

Livoni JP, Bogren HG (1982) Multiloculated chronic post-traumatic aneurysm of the thoracic aorta with late acute rupture. Cardiovasc Intervent Radiol 5:227–229

Maekawa M, Ishikawa K (1966) Occlusive thromboaortopathy. Jpn Circ J 30:79

Martin M, Fiebach BJO (1985) Die Streptokinase-Behandlung peripherer Arterien- und Venenverschlüsse unter besonderer Berücksichtigung der ultrahohen Dosierung. Huber, Bern

Mehta S (1980) A statistical summary of the results of femoropopliteal bypass surgery. Gore, Newark

Mendelsohn AM, Lloyd TR, Crowly DC, et al. (1995) Late follow-up of balloon angioplasty in children with a native coarctation of the aorta. Radiology 195:591

Miani S, Giorgetti PL, et al. (1994) Spontaneous aortocaval fistulas from ruptured abdominal aortic aneurysms. Eur J Vasc Surg 8:36–40

Mittelmeier H (1959) Pathologische Anatomie der obliterierenden Gefäßerkrankungen. In: Hess H (ed) Die obliterierenden Gefäßerkrankungen. Urban and Schwarzenberg, Munich

Morag B, Rubinstein Z, Kessler A, et al. (1987) Percutaneous transluminal angioplasty of the distal abdominal aorta and its bifurcation. Cardiovasc Intervent Radiol 10:129–133

Morris GE, Hubbard CS, Quick CR (1994) An abdominal aortic aneurysm screening programme for all males over the age of 50 years. Eur J Vasc Surg 8:56–60

Müller-Wiefel H, Brieler HS, Müller W (1973) Coarctatio aortae abdominalis mit Beteiligung der Nierenarterien. Thoraxchir Vasc Chir 21:81–86

Nakao K, Ikeda M, Kimata SJ, et al. (1967) Takayasu's arteriitis. Clinical report of eighty-four cases and immunological studies in seven cases. Circulation 35:1141

Noppeney T, Raithel D (1990) Age as high risk factor in the treatment of abdominal aortic aneurysm. Vasc Surg 24:2741–2276

Odurny A, Colapinto RF, Sniderman KW, Johnston KW (1989) Percutaneous transluminal angioplasty of abdominal aortic stenoses. Cardiovasc Intervent Radiol 12:1–6

Noppeney T, Kasprzak P, Raithel D (1991) Die Bedeutung der Risikofaktoren bei Operationen eines abdominalen Aortenaneurysmas. In: Sandmann W, Kniemeyer HW (eds) Aneurysmen der großen Arterien. Huber, Bern

O'Laughlin MP, Perry SB, Lock JE, et al. (1991) Use of endovascular stents in congenital heart disease. Circulation 83:1923–1939

Orend KH, Becker HM (1991) Dissektion und dissezierendes Aortenaneurysma. In: Sandmann W, Kniemeyer HW (eds) Aneurysen der großen Arterien. Huber, Bern, pp 213–215

Ostertag H, Young R (1987) Ätiologie und Rupturrisiko des Aortenaneurysmas. DMW 112 33:1253–1256

Patel S, Johnston KW (1977) Classification and management of mycotic aneurysms. Surg Gynecol Obstet 144:691–694

Peterson TA, Todd DB, Edwards JE (1965) Supravalvular aortic stenosis. J Thorac Cardiovasc Surg 50:735

Pierach CA, Katkow F (1972) Coarctation of the abdominal aorta. Vasc Surg 6:159–166

Pinet F, Amiel M, Clermont A, Rubet A, Karim A, Froment JC (1972) L'aortographie des anévrysmes disséquants de l'aorte. Ann Radiol 5–6:381–391

Plate G, Hollier LA, O'Brien R, Pairolero PC, Cherry KJ, Kazmier FJ (1985) Recurrent aneurysms and late vascular complications following repair of abdominal aortic aneurysms. Arch Surg 120:590

Raithel D (1973) Das Anastomosenaneurysma als Früh- und Spätkomplikation nach Gefäßrekonstruktion im aorto-poplitealen Abschnitt. Chirurg 44:235–238

Raithel D (1984) Die Belastbarkeit des Patienten in der Gefäßchirurgie. Langenbecks Arch Chir 364:177–180

Raithel D (1988) Operative Therapie der Bein- und Becken-arterienverschlüsse. In: Trübestein G (ed) Therapie der arteriellen Verschlußkrankheit. Zuckschwerdt, Munich pp 197–203

Raithel D (1990) Gefäßchirurgie im Alter. In: Platt D, Voßschulte K, Fahlbusch R (eds) Handbuch der Gerontologie, vol 4.1. Fischer, Stuttgart, pp 344ff

Raithel D (1991) Role of PTFE grafts in infrainguinal arterial reconstructions: a 10-year experience. In: Veith FJ (ed) Current critical problems in vascular surgery, vol 3. Quality Medical Publ, St. Louis, pp 66ff

Raithel D (1992) Das isolierte Popliteasegment-eine Alternative zum Kruralen Bypass. In: Hepp W, Palenker J (eds) Femorokrurale Arterienverschlüsse. Steinkopff, Darmstadt

Raithel D, Franke F, Gall FP (1983) Spezielle Probleme der Revascularisation bei Diabetikern im Bereich des Unterschenkels. Therapiewoche 33:2269

Randall PA, Omar MM, Rohner R, Hedgcock M, Brenner RJ (1979) Arteria magna revisited. Radiology 132:295–300

Rao PS (1995) Coarctation of the aorta. Semin Nephrol 15:87–105

Rao PS (1996) Aortic coarctation. In: Sigwart U, Bertrand M, Serruys PW (eds) Cardiovascular Interventions. Churchill Livingstone, New York, pp 757–781

Rao PS, Najjar HN, Mardini MK, et al. (1988) Balloon angioplasty for coarctatio of the aorta; immediate and longterm results. Am Heart J 115:657–665

Rau G (1970) Verschluß-Syndrom der Aortenbogenäste oder Aortenbogen-Syndrom. Ergeb Inn Med. Springer, Berlin Heidelberg New York, pp 116–126

Ravimandalam K, Rao VRK, Kumar S, et al. (1991) Obstruction of the infrarenal portion of the abdominal aorta: results of treatment with balloon angioplasty. AJR 156:1257

Reddy DJ (1986) Infected femoral artery aneurysm. In: Ernst CB, Stanley JC (eds) Current therapy in vascular surgery. Decker, Philadelphia

Redington AN, Hayes AM, Ho SY (1993) Transcatheter stent implantation to treat aortic coarctation in infancy. Br Heart J 69:80–82

Rob CG, Vollmar JF (1959) Die Chirurgie der Bauchaorta. Ergeb Chir Orthop 42:569

Rocchini AP, Beekman RH (1986) Balloon angioplasty in the treatment of pulmonary valve stenosis and coarctation of the aorta. Texas Heart Inst J 13:377–385

Roth FJ, Heimig Th, Berliner P, Grün B, Koppers B, Krings W (1988) Perkutane Rekanalisation peripherer Gefäße. In: Günther RW, Thelen M (eds) Interventionelle Radiologie. Thieme, Stuttgart, pp 20–44

Sanborn TA, Gibbs HH, Brinker JA, et al. (1994) Multicenter randomized trial comparing a percutaneous collagen hemostasis device with conventional manual compression after diagnostic angiography and angioplasty. JVIR 5:395–399

Sandmann W, Kniemeyer HW (eds) (1991) Aneurysmen der großen Arterien. Huber, Bern

Schad N (1968) Die angeborenen Anomalien des Herzens und der großen Gefäße. In: Schinz HR, Baensch WE, Frommhold W, et al. (eds) Lehrbuch der Röntgendiagnostik, vol IV, 6th edn, ••

Schlosser V, Faedrich G (eds) (1990) Aneurysmen der thorakalen Aorta. Steinkopff, Darmstadt

Schoop W (1974) Pathophysiologie der arteriellen Durchblutung. In: Heberer G, Rau G, Schoop W (eds) Angiologie, Grundlagen, Klinik, Praxis, 2nd edn. Thieme, Stuttgart

Schoop W, Martin M, Zeitler E (1968) Beseitigung alter Arterienverschlüsse durch intravenöse Streptokinase-Infusion. Dtsch Med Wochenschr 48:2321–2324

Schweiger H, Raithel D (1984) Der femoro-femorale Bypass beim einseitigen Beckenarterien-verschluß: Alternative oder Verfahren der Wahl? VASA 13:147

Schweiger H, Raithel D, Franke F (1984) Die quere femoro-femorale Umleitung beim unilateralen Beckenarterienverschluß. Angio 6:55

Schräder R, Steinbacher S, Burger W, et al. (1993) Collagen application for sealing of arterial puncture sites in comparison to pressure dressings: randomized trial. JVIR 4:590–593

Schwilden ED, Barwegen M, von Dongen R (1978) Aortenaneurysma und Hufeisenniere – Kasuistik und Literaturübersicht. Langenbecks Arch Chir 346:135–148

Segesser LV, Turina M (1990) Die Vermeidung von Rückenmarksschäden bei chirurgischer Rekonstruktion von thorako-abdominalen Aortenaneurysmen. In: Schlosser LV, Faedrich G (eds) Aneurysmen der thorakalen Aorta. Steinkopff, Darmstadt, pp 133–140

Selby JB, Tegtmeyer CJ (1991) Angioplasty of abdominal aortic stenoses. In: Kadir S (ed) Current practice of interventional radiology. Decker, Philadelphia, pp 389–394

Sen PK, Egineer SD, Paruckar GB (1959) The middle aortic syndrome. Br Heart J 25:610

Sen PK, Kinare SG, Kulkarni TP, Parulkar GB (1962) Stenosing aortitis of unknown etiology. Surgery 51:317

Seyferth W, Marhoff P, Zeitler E (1982) Transvenöse und arterielle digitale Videosubtraktionsangiographie (DVSA). Fortschr Rontgenstr 136:301–309

Shaddy RE, Boncek MM, Sturtevant JE, et al. (1993) Comparison of angioplasty and surgery for unoperated coarctation of the aorta. JVIR 4:584

Sievert H, Bussmann WD, Pfrommer W, Reuhl J, Kaltenbach M (1987) Transluminale Angioplastik der Aortenisthmusstenose bei Jugendlichen und Erwachsenen. Dtsch Med Wochenschr 112:1371–1373

Silber S, Schön N, Seidel N, Heiß-Bogner J (1998) Akzidenteller Verschluß einer A. femoralis communis nach Angio-Seal Applikation. Z Kardiol 87:51–55

Singer MJ, Rowen M, Dorsey TJ (1982) Transluminal aortic balloon angioplasty for coarctation of the aorta in the newborn. Am Heart J 103:131–132

Sokol S, Narkiewicz M, Malecka-Dymnicka S, Mierzejewski T (1967) Arteria lusoria mit Aortenisthmusstenose bei einem 12jährigen Knaben. Zentralbl Chir 92(47):2884–2888

Sos T, Sniderman K, Rettek-Sos B, et al. (1979) Percutaneous transluminal dilatation of coarctation of thoracic aorta post mortem. Lancet 2:970–971

Spengel FA, Anton B, Küffer G (1991) Ultrahohe systemische Lyse bei Strombahnhindernissen der Aorta und der A. iliaca bei 14 Patienten. VASA [Suppl] 33:128 (abstract)

Sperling DR, Dorsey TD, Rowen M, et al. (1982) Percutaneous transluminal angioplasty of congenital coarctation of the aorta. Clin Res 30:1121

Staple WT, Friedenberg MJ, Anderson MS, Butcher HR Jr (1966) Artérie magna et dolicho of Lériche. Acta Radiol 193–305

Steinberg JH, Stein HL (1966) Aorteriosclerotic abdominal aneurysms. Report of 200 consecutive cases diagnosed by intravenous arteriography. J Amer Med Assoc 195:1025

Steinkamp HJ, Scheiert D, Hettwer H, et al. (1999) PTLA – Rekanalisation von Femoralarterienstenosen/-okklusionen nach Angio-Seal™ Applikation. Fortschr Rontgenstr 170:105–108

Stirnemann P, Ritz S, Senna A (1986) Die aorto-kavale Fistel als Komplikation des Aortenaneurysmas. VASA 15:245–250

Suarez de Lezo J, Pan M, Romero M, et al. (1995) Balloon-expandable stent repair of severe coarctation of the aorta. Am Heart J 129:1002–1008

Sunder-Plassmann P, Menges G, Ruland L (1963) Aorten-Arkusstenose mit abnormem Abgang aller Hals- und Armgefäße, •• der A. carotis sinistra und offenem Ductus arteriosus Botalli. Med Klinik 56 (13):574–579

Szilagyi DE, Smith RF, DeRusso FJ, Elliott JP, Sherrin FW (1966) Contribution of abdominal aortic aneurysmectomy to prolongation of life. Ann Surg 164:678–699

Szilagyi DE, Elliot JP, Smith RF (1972) Clinical fate of the patient with asymptomatic abdominal aortic aneurysm and unfit for surgical treatment. Arch Surg 104:600–606

Taylor DB, Blaser SI, Burrows PE, et al. (1991) Arteriopathy and coarctation of the abdominal aorta in children with mucopolysaccharidosis: imaging findings. AJR 157:819

Taylor LM Jr, Hamre D, Moneta GL, Yeager RA, Porter JM (1991) Axillobifemoral bypass. In: Veith FJ (ed) Current critical problems in vascular surgery, vol 3. Quality Medical Publishing, St. Louis, pp 261–269

Tegtmeyer CJ, Moore TS, Chandler JG, et al. (1979) Percutaneous transluminal dilatation of a complete block in the right iliac artery. AJR 133:532–535

Triller J, Do-Dai DD, Stirnemann P, et al. (1993) Balloon-resistant stenosis of the distal abdominal aorta: treatment with self-expandable stents. Eur Radiol 3–5:463

Underhill WL, Tredway JB, D'Angelo GJ, Baay JEW (1971) Familial supravalvular aortic stenosis. Am J Cardiol 27:560

Van Heuvn LWE, Wong CM, Siegelhalter DJ (1995) Surgical treatment of aortic coarctation in infants younger than three months: 1985 to 1990 success of extended end-to-end arch aortoplasty. Radiology 194:591

Velasquez G, Castaneda-Zuniga AW, Formanek A, et al. (1980) Nonsurgical aortoplasty in Leriche Syndrome. Radiology 134:359–363

Vollmar JF (1996a) Aorto-iliacale Verschlüsse. In: Vollmar J: Rekonstruktive Chirurgie der Arterien, 4th edn. Thieme, Stuttgart, pp 207–241

Vollmar JF (1996b) Neonatale Mißbildungen der Arterien: coarctatio aortae. In: Vollmar J (ed) Rekonstruktive Chirurgie der Arterien, 4th edn. Thieme, Stuttgart, pp 50–69

Vollmar JF (1996c) Aneurysmen. In: Vollmar JF (ed) Rekonstruktive Chirurgie der Arterien, 4th edn. Thieme, Suttgart, pp 96–153

Vollmar JF, Nobbe FP (1976) Arteriovenöse Fisteln – Dilatierende Arteriopathien (Aneurysmen). Thieme, Stuttgart

Vollmar J, Voss EU, Nadjafi AS, Heymer B (1976) Die atypische Coarctatio aortae. Atypical Aortic Coarction. Thoraxchirurgie 24:107–118

Vollmar JF, Paes E, Pauschinger P, Heze E, Friesch A (1989) Aortic aneurysms as late sequela of above-knee amputation. Lancet 2 (8667):834–835

von Schulthess GK, Higashino SM, Higgins SS, et al. (1986) Coarctation of the aorta: MR imaging. Radiology 158:469

Walz H, Deininger HK (1974) Das Krankheitsbild der polyaneurysmalen Dystrophie. Fortsch Geb Rontgenstr Neuen Bildgeb Verfahr 121:394–398

Weimann S, Flora G (1991) Anastomosenkomplikationen nach abdominalem Aortenaneurysma: Anastomostenaneurysma, aortoduodenale Fistel. In: Sandmann W, Kniemeyer HW (eds) Aneurysmen der großen Arterien. Huber, Bern, pp 116–122

Weisz D, Hartmann AF Jr, Weldon CS (1976) Results of surgery for congenital supravalvular aortic stenosis. Am J Cardiol 37:73–76

Wenz W (1972) Abdominale Angiographie. Springer, Berlin Heidelberg New York

Wenz W, Beduhn D (1976) Extremitätenarteriographie. Springer, Berlin Heidelberg New York

White JV (1992) The role of adventitial defects in the pathogenesis of aortic aneurysms. In: Veith FJ (ed) New techniques in vascular surgery (19th annual symposium). Quality Medical Publishing, St. Louis

Winslow JB (1753) Expositio anatomica structurae corporis humani, vol 3. Paris, paragraphs 89, 90

Witsenburg M, The SHK, Bogers AJC, et al. (1994) Balloon angioplasty for aortic recoarcation in children: initial and follow-up results and midterm effect on blood pressure. JVIR 5:180

Young R, Ostertag H (1987) Häufigkeit, Ätiologie und Rupturrisiko des Aortenaneurysmas. Eine Autopsiestudie. Dtsch Med Wochenschr 112:1253–1256

Zeitler E (1974) Aortaarteriographie. In: Heberer G, Rau G, Schoop W (eds) Angiologie, 2nd edn. Thieme, Stuttgart, pp 283–285

Zeitler E (1976) Röntgenologische Diagnostik der dilatierenden Arteriopathien – Aneurysmen der Aorta und der Gliedmaßenarterien. In: Vollmar JF, Nobbe FP (eds) Arteriovenöse Fisteln – Dilateriende Arteriopathien (Aneurysmen). Thieme, Stuttgart, pp 107–124

Zeitler E (1991) Diagnostik von Aneurysmen der großen Arterien mit bildgebenden Verfahren. In: Sandmann W, Kniemeyer HW (eds) Aneurysmen der großen Arterien. Huber, Bern, pp 41–49

Zeitler E (1993) Cardiovascular and interventional radiology – the German perspective. Cardiovasc Intervent Radiol 16:1–2

Zeitler E (1995) Peripheral vessels. In: Rosenbusch G, Oudkerk M, Ammann E (eds) Radiology in medical diagnostics – evolution of x-ray applications 1895–1995. Blackwell Science, Oxford, pp 236–247

Zeitler E (1997) Klinische Radiologie: Arterien und Venen. Springer, Berlin Heidelberg New York

Zeitler E, Heuck FHW (1997) Aneurysmen und Dilatative Angiopathie. In: Zeitler E (ed) Klinische Radiologie: Arterien und Venen. Springer, Berlin Heidelberg, New York, pp 277–312

Zeitler E, Martin M, Schoop W (1969) Angiographische Befunde bei chronischer arterieller Verschlußkrankheit vor und nach Streptokinasebehandlung. Fortschr Rontgenstr 111:498–510

Zorn-Bopp E, Ingrisch H, Mietaschk A, Frey KW (1981) Transluminale Gefäßdilatation der distalen Bauchaorta der Arterie iliaca communis und externa. Fortschr Rontgenstr 134:471–475

17.4
Conventional and Endovascular Therapy of Infrarenal Abdominal Aortic Aneurysms

P. HEILBERGER, C. SCHUNN, and D. RAITHEL

17.4.1
Epidemiology

According to recent publications the incidence of infrarenal aortic aneurysms in the industrialized world varies between 12 and 36 cases per 100000 inhabitants. In the population over 60 years of age the incidence ranges between 2% and 5% (ERNST 1993; GOLDSTONE 1993). Improved screening methods using ultrasound technology have raised the number of aortic aneurysms diagnosed in a population of over 55-year-old patients in Scotland from 25.8 per 100000 inhabitants in 1971 to 63.6 in 1984 (NAYLOR et al. 1988).

Department of Vascular Surgery, Nuremberg Southern Hospital (Chief of Service: Prof.Dr.med.D.Raithel)

17.4.1.1
Risk of Rupture

The risk of rupture of aneurysms greater than 5 cm reaches 25%–41% within 5 years after diagnosis (ERNST 1993; KNIEMEYER and SANDMANN 1992). Currently about 15 000 aneurysm ruptures with lethal outcome are documented in the US per year. The spontaneous mortality of patients with aneurysms greater than 6 cm in diameter has been noted to be 72% for the first 2 years after diagnosis (SZILAGYL et al. 1972). However, also smaller aneurysms (<5 cm) may rupture. In a large autopsy study 18% of ruptured aneurysms measured less than 5 cm (DARLING 1970).

17.4.2
Treatment Modalities of Aortic Aneurysms

After standardization and simplification of the conventional operative approach to aortic aneurysmal disease by DeBAKEY and others in the 1950s and 1960s, the introduction of endovascular therapy using endoluminal stent grafts in the 1990s may be considered the next milestone in the therapeutic evolution for this disease (Tables 17.7 and 17.8).

Despite improved screening methods approximately 20%–30% of all aortic aneurysm repairs

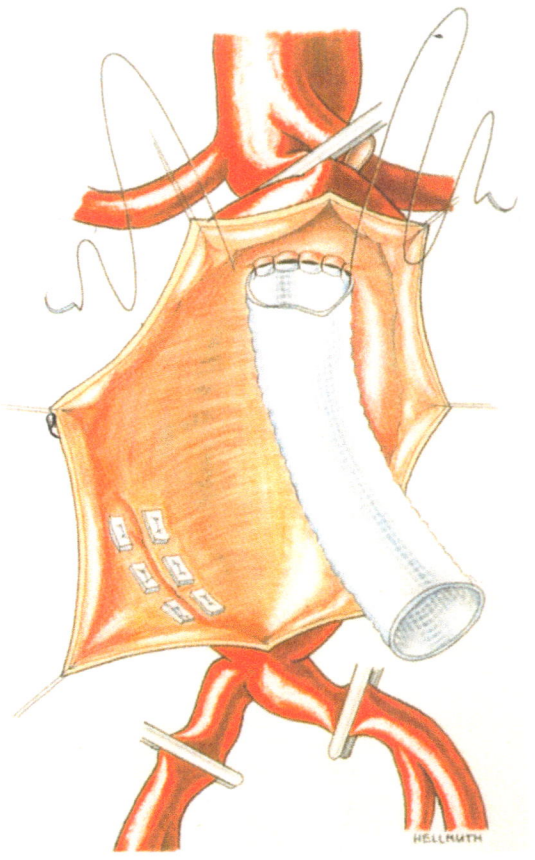

Fig. 17.47. Conventional aortic reconstruction (inlay technique)

Table 17.7. History of conventional operative therapy of abdominal aortic aneurysms

Treatment	Ref.
– Aneurysm ligation	(MATS 1925)
– Thrombosing of the aneurysm by wiring	(POWER 1921)
– Resection and reconstruction of the aneurysm	(DUBOST 1952)
– Aortic graft inlay technique	(CREECH 1960; DeBAKEY et al. 1964) (Fig. 17.47)
– Aneurysm exclusion and reconstruction with axillo-bifemoral bypass	(BLAISDELL et al. 1965)
– Rigid prosthesis with proximal and distal ligature	(LEMOLE et al. 1984)

Table 17.8. Endovascular therapy of abdominal aortic aneurysms (AAA)

Treatment	Ref.
– Endoluminal placement of vascular prostheses into an aneurysm in a canine model	(DOTTER 1969)
– Endoluminal use of a stented graft	(CRAGG et al. 1983)
– Transfemoral implantation of a stented polyurethane graft	(BALKO et al. 1986)
– Use of a stented nylon prosthesis in a canine model	(MIRICH et al. 1991)
– Endoluminal implantation of a vascular prosthesis into an AAA	(VOLODOS et al. 1991)
– Exclusion of aortic aneurysms in humans using endovascular stent grafts	(PARODI et al. 1991)
– US Patent EVT device	(LAZARUS 1992)

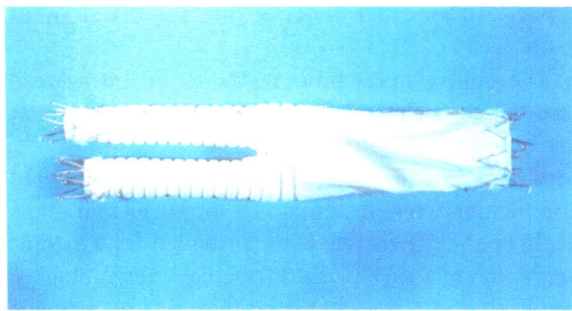

Fig. 17.48. Single unit stent graft (EGS, Endovascular Technologies, Menlo Park, Calif., USA)

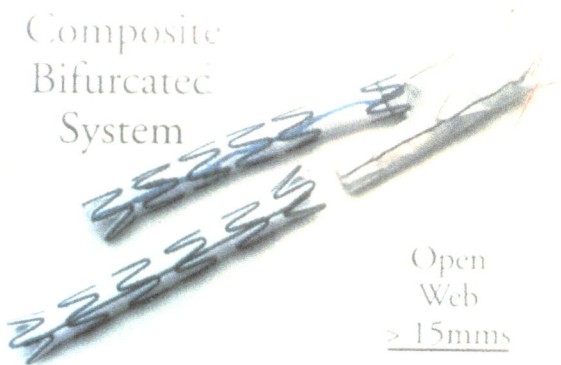

Fig. 17.49. Modular stent graft (Talent, World Medical, Sunrise, Fla., USA)

still occur under emergency conditions. Despite improvements in intensive care and operative methods the mortality of patients presenting with free rupture who undergo surgical repair remains basically unchanged at between 35% and 50%, according to the literature and in our own patient population (CAPPEUER et al. 1996; HEPP et al. 1980; NAYLOR et al. 1988).

In large contemporary series the hospital mortality after conventional elective aneurysm repair ranges between 2.8% and 6.2%, with coronary artery disease being the major risk factor for postoperative death (CAPPELLER et al. 1996).

Length of hospitalization is the most important determinant of overall cost for patients undergoing elective aneurysm repair. It has been reported as a mean of 17.4 days by CAPPELLER and is 12.9 days in our hospital (CAPPELLER et al. 1996).

17.4.3
Stent Graft Systems and Technique of Aortic Stent Graft Implantation

The main objective of endovascular therapy for abdominal aortic aneurysm disease is to lower perioperative mortality, particularly in high risk cardiac patients. By lowering the length of hospitalization a marked overall cost reduction should be achievable.

Minimally invasive aortic surgery involves the implantation of a balloon-expandable or self-expanding stent which is covered with ultra-thin prosthetic material. This is implanted trans-

femorally. These stent grafts may be assembled by the surgeon or are industrially manufactured from individual components (Tables 17.9 and 17.10).

Notable differences exist between the implantation of modular systems and endografts made of one piece.

17.4.3.1
Implantation of Modular Stent Grafts

Completely stented tube grafts are transfemorally implanted and need to have an exact fit at the proximal and distal aneurysm neck (see Fig. 17.58). Variation in length is only possible using a second stent graft which is placed in the proximal endograft using the stent-in-stent modular technique. This "trombone" system is a primary feature of the Baxter straight endograft system (Baxter Vascular Systems, Irvine, Calif., USA).

Modular tubes as well as modular bifurcated stent grafts are assembled endoluminally. By docking several iliac limbs in series the total length of stented aneurysm becomes variable. Graft systems with inner lamination are available in order to reduce intimal hyperplasia in the iliac limbs (Talent).

Tapered grafts may be custom-made for special indications (i.e., exclusion of internal iliac aneurysms, aorto-monoiliac stenting) (Fig. 17.50).

Advantages of modular systems:
- Much less prosthetic material needs to be in stock as prosthetic length may be varied using modular components.
- Deployment of tube grafts is technically simple.

Table 17.9. Components of stent grafts

Stents	Materials	Function
Gianturco	Steal	Self-expanding
Palmaz	Steal	Balloon-expandable
Strecker	Tantalum	Balloon-expandable
Wallstent (Schneider)	Steal	Self-expanding
Cragg	Nitinol	Self-expanding
Graft Materials:		
Dacron		
PTFE		
Polyurethane		

PTFE, polytetrafluoroethylene.

Table 17.10. Endovascular abdominal aortic aneurysm repair: commercially available devices

AneuRx 1997
Cook 1998
EVT 1995
Gore 1998
Talent 1996
Vanguard 1996

Disadvantages of modular systems:
- Risk of secondary leaks or thrombosis at the docking zone.
- Docking maneuver for bifurcated modular stent graft systems is technically demanding.
- Rigidity of the stented system in a milieu of continuous pulsatile wall stress may cause fractures of stent struts.
- Exact distal fit to the millimeter is necessary for tube grafts as intra-operative correction of length is impossible.

17.4.3.2
Implantation of Single Unit Stent Grafts

Single unit stent graft systems (e.g., EVT, Endovascular Technologies, Menlo Park, Calif., USA; Chuter device, Chuter et al. 1997) are straight and bifurcated stent grafts made out of one piece and armed with stents and anchoring systems only at the proximal and distal end of the prosthesis. Due to the crimping of the prosthetic graft material of these devices they allow for some variability in length (1–1.5 cm). This greatly enhances the

chances of an exact distal fit into the distal aneurysm neck.

The contralateral limb needs to be introduced into the contralateral iliac artery using a crossover maneuver (Fig. 17.51).

This endograft concept has now been expanded to also include tapered stent grafts for aorto-monoiliac deployment. These may be provided as custom-made models (EVT, Endovascular Technologies, Menlo Park, Calif., USA). However, currently only a 50% taper between proximal aortic and distal iliac diameter of the device is available.

Advantages of single unit stent grafts. Variability in length of the crimped prosthetic material helps to avoid docking problems and enhances a precise distal fit.

Disadvantages of single unit stent grafts. The implantation of this device is technically demanding. Iliac prosthetic limbs may be narrowed at the distal aortic neck or aortic bifurcation. There is a significant risk of torsion of the iliac limbs causing stenosis or limb occlusion. Custom-made prosthetic devices need to be manufactured individually for each patient according to preoperative measurements.

Currently endovascular stent grafting is limited to controlled clinical human and animal trials. A few standardized grafts (Vanguard, Boston Scientific, Oakland, N.J., USA; Talent, World Medical, Sunrise, Fla., USA) have already become commercially available on the European market.

Therefore, it is imperative to follow strict guidelines for patient selection according to the aneurysm type and diameter, and to adhere to a strict follow-up

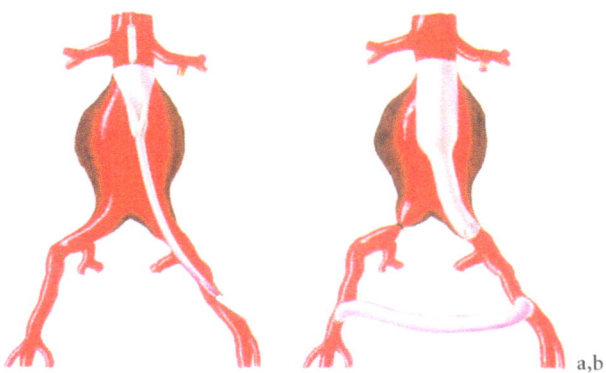

Fig. 17.50 a,b. Aorto-monoiliac reconstruction with femorofemoral crossover bypass. **a** Introduction of stent graft. **b** Released stent graft, femoro–femoral bypass

protocol to identify treatment failures and typical complications of this method. This will assure that further interventions, such as overstenting or conversion to conventional open reconstruction, may be performed in a timely fashion.

17.4.4
Classification of Infrarenal Aortic Aneurysms for Endovascular Reconstruction

Suitability of infrarenal aortic aneurysms for endovascular exclusion is determined using the morphologic classification established by ALLENBERG and SCHUMACHER et al. (Fig. 17.52) (ALLENBERG and SCHUMACHER 1995; SCHUMACHER et al. 1997).

Aneurysms of type I (straight graft) and IIa and IIb (bifurcated graft) can be treated by endovascular reconstruction. Unsuitable for endovascular recon-

struction are aneurysms of type IIc (due to necessary occlusion of the internal iliac artery) and type III (due to inadequate proximal anchoring site).

We have added type Ib, an infrarenal aortic aneurysm with adequate proximal and distal necks and an additional iliac artery aneurysm. In our opinion this anatomical constellation may also be treated with the straight stent graft. The isolated iliac artery aneurysm is thus left untreated. Only when there is an increase in size documented during follow-up may this be excluded using a covered iliac stent.

Similar classifications have been published by BLUM and DÜBER (types A–D), HARRIS (types A–E) and AHN (types I–IV) (AHN et al. 1997; BLUM et al. 1997; DÜBER et al. 1996; HARRIS et al. 1997). The preoperative classification by AHN also involves the clinical stage, aneurysm diameter, the angulation of the proximal neck, as well as the quality of the iliac arteries (AHN et al. 1997).

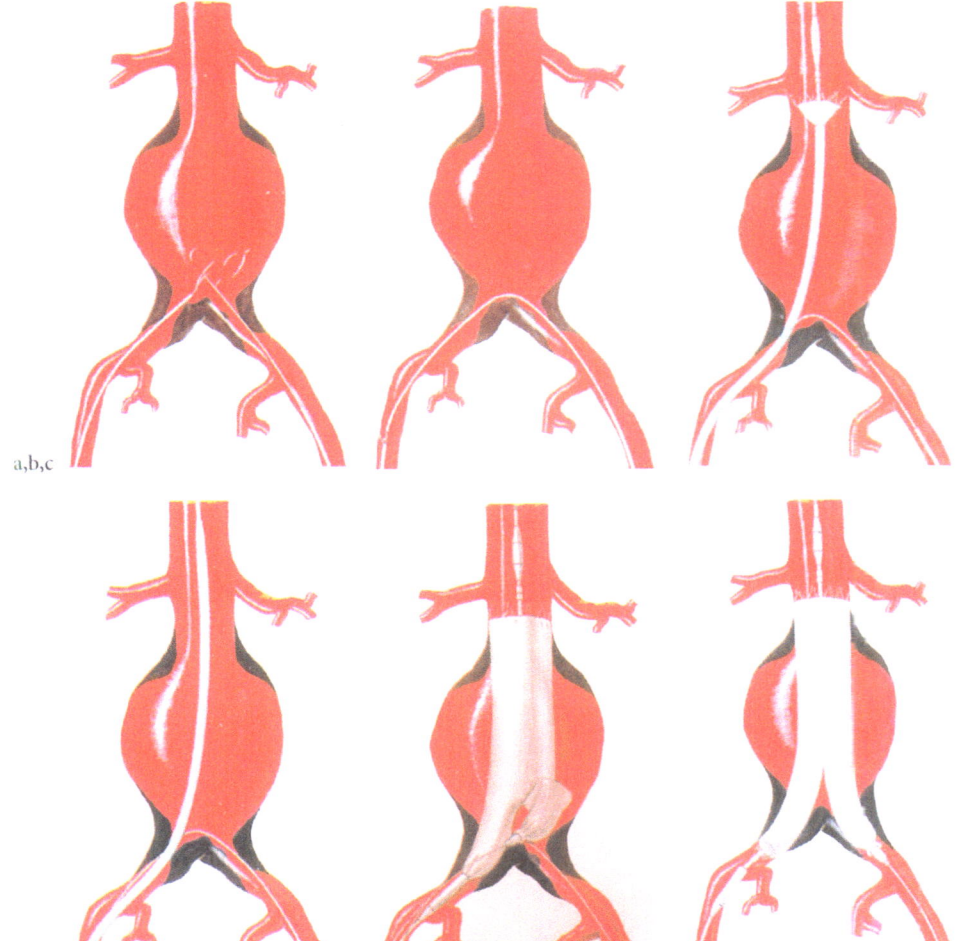

a,b,c

d,e,f

Fig. 17.51 a–f. Implantation of a bifurcated stent graft (single unit). Endovascular cross-over maneuver step-by-step. a Crossover manoeuver I; b crossover manoeuver II; c introduction of prosthesis; d releasing of the graft; e cross-over placement of the contralateral limb; f modeling the distal right limb

17.4.5
Preoperative Diagnosis and Differential Diagnosis

After clinical or ultrasound diagnosis of an aortic aneurysm the vascular surgeon and radiologist will have to answer the following questions:

(1) Is there an aneurysm that needs to be treated?
(2) Which therapeutic option is best suited to treat this aneurysm?
(3) What is the operative risk of this patient?

To answer these questions the following diagnostic approach is suggested:

1. Clinical assessment
   - History
     Pain, symptoms of congestive heart failure or coronary insufficiency, aneurysm enlargement or penetration, cerebrovascular insufficiency, claudication, clinical stages (AADAHL et al. 1997)
   - Physical examination
     Pulse status, ankle brachial index, abdominal findings of palpation and auscultation, signs of congestive heart failure.
2. Ultrasound examination
   - Carotid duplex
   - Aortic duplex
   - Duplex of ilio-femoral vessels
   - Cardiac echo with determination of ejection fraction.
3. Radiological evaluation
   - Spiral computed tomography (CT) of the abdomen with i.v. contrast (3–5-mm slices with multiplanar reconstructions (MPR)
   - Transarterial digital subtraction angiography (DSA) with graded measuring catheter (15 cm marked at 1-cm intervals)
   - Standard measurements (AHN et al. 1997; YUSUF et al. 1997):
   - Diameter and length of proximal and distal aortic neck

   - Length between lowest renal artery and aortic bifurcation or iliac bifurcation
   - Common iliac artery and/or external artery diameters
   - Angulation at the proximal aortic neck
   - Angulation of the iliac arteries.
4. Evaluation of operative risk
   - Electrocardiography (ECG)
   - Coronary stress tests
   - Pulmonary function
   - Routine laboratory values including creatinine.

According to the recommendations of the Society of Vascular Surgery (SVS) abdominal aortic aneurysms of greater than 4 cm diameter should be electively corrected (HOLLIER et al. 1992). This recommendation should also be followed for endovascular aneurysm therapy. However, with an increasing level of expertise and lower complication rates this treatment modality may surely be used safely for aneurysms of less than 4 cm in diameter. It should be kept in mind that even aneurysms of less than 4 cm may have an up to 10% risk of rupture (JOHANSSON et al. 1990). Furthermore, small and particularly sacciform aneurysms often have a longer proximal and distal neck well suited to anchoring an endovascular stent graft (ALLENBERG and SCHUMACHER 1995).

Patients with significant cardiac risk factors or multiple previous abdominal procedures may benefit most from endovascular stent graft therapy. However, indication for endovascular repair, as well as preoperative patient preparation, should generally follow the guidelines for conventional therapy as conversion to open surgical repair may become necessary any time during endovascular aortic stent grafting. Inadvertent occlusion of renal arteries, distal misplacement of the prosthetic device with acute outflow obstruction, aortic dissection, or a large proximal leak which could not be managed by further endovascular manipulations were all causes for emergent conversion to conventional therapy in 11

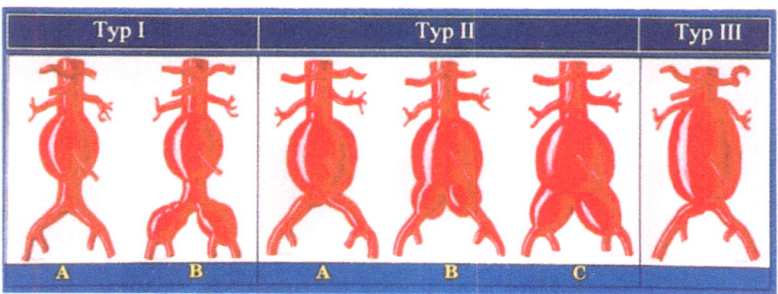

Fig. 17.52. Classification of infrarenal aortic aneurysms according to ALLENBERG as modified by RAITHEL (ALLENBERG and SCHUMACHER 1995)

of our 131 patients treated with aortic stent grafts (HEILBERGER et al. 1997b).

High grade internal carotid stenoses (>80%), as well as coronary artery stenoses, should be corrected before elective aortic surgery. Pulmonary obstructive disease should be pre-treated for 3–5 days with medication as well as physiotherapy.

A thorough physical examination of the patient and documentation of peripheral pulses, as well as ankle brachial index, are important to help determine the appropriate vascular access and to assess postoperative embolic complications in the vessels of the lower limbs. Endovascular access via a femoral artery with absent or diminished pulses will most likely result in failure, or will at least require an intraoperative iliac percutaneous transluminal angioplasty (PTA) to assure adequate access.

Raised levels of blood urea nitrogen (BUN) and creatinine require careful angiographic evaluation of renal artery anatomy; of course, they also call for conservative intraoperative contrast dosage. In the presence of surgically correctable renal artery stenoses endovascular aortic aneurysm therapy should be avoided. Conventional reconstruction of the infrarenal aorta in conjunction with surgical correction of the ostial renal artery stenosis is preferable. Occasionally PTA (with or without stent) of a non-ostial renal artery stenosis may be performed in conjunction with endovascular exclusion of an aortic aneurysm.

Conventional aneurysm therapy may be based on preoperative duplex scan and abdominal contrast CT alone. Only occasionally angiography will have to be added to elucidate renal and mesenteric artery anomalies or stenoses, as well as peripheral vascular occlusive disease.

Preoperative planning for endovascular therapy on the other hand requires more sophisticated technology, including thin slice spiral CT (3 mm slices) to evaluate the proximal and distal anchoring sites. Arterial DSA using a calibrated intraluminal catheter is mandatory to measure intraluminal vessel diameters at the proximal and distal neck and to determine the required prosthetic length (Fig. 17.53). If duplex sonography documents a type III aortic aneurysm (no adequate proximal neck) further diagnostic work-up and preparation for endovascular therapy are unnecessary and conventional therapy should be planned for (Fig. 17.54).

Anatomic details are transferred from X-ray to a graphic outline and submitted to the manufacturer (see Fig. 17.71). According to these data and drawings either a prefabricated stent graft is chosen or a custom-made model is produced for the individual patient.

Angiography is particularly important to delineate pelvic vascular anatomy, including patency of internal iliac arteries and patent aortic side branches (i.e., lumbar arteries, presacral artery, inferior mesenteric artery), which will be sacrificed by endovascular therapy (Tables 17.11 and 17.12).

Aortic aneurysms limited to the infrarenal aorta with a proximal neck of at least 15 mm in length with a maximum diameter of 26 mm are ideal for endovascular therapy. Aneurysms without suitable distal cuff above the aortic bifurcation with continuation of the aneurysm onto the iliac arteries (type II) require implantation of a bifurcated stent graft. The iliac limbs must find adequate anchoring sites in the common iliac or external iliac arteries. If one iliac artery is too large to anchor the graft but the other side features a suitable anchoring site, implantation of a tapered aorto-monoiliac stent graft with endovascular occlusion or surgical ligation of the contralateral common iliac artery, in conjunction with a femoro-femoral crossover bypass, is another therapeutic option (Tables 17.12 and 17.13) (see Fig. 17.50). When anchoring the iliac limbs care should be taken not to occlude the internal iliac arteries bilaterally to avoid the dreaded complication of intestinal or pelvic ischemia. In isolated case reports, however, this has been well tolerated (BLUM et al. 1996).

Considering all clinical, as well as morphological, prerequisites only about 20%–30% of patients with infrarenal aortic aneurysms will qualify for endovascular therapy (BLUM et al. 1996; SCHUMACHER et al. 1997). Between August 1994 and May 1997 we found 150 (24%) patients with aortic aneurysms suitable for endovascular aortic grafting at our institution. A total of 480 patients (76%) were treated conventionally during this time period.

17.4.5.1
Approach to the Patient with Ruptured Aneurysm

Hemodynamic instability is a contraindication to endovascular aortic therapy. Even under optimal conditions the necessary spiral CT with i.v. contrast, as well as graded catheter DSA, will lead to significant delays in therapy and also involve considerable loads of contrast medium in a patient who is already vitally threatened by prerenal azotemia due to hemorrhagic shock.

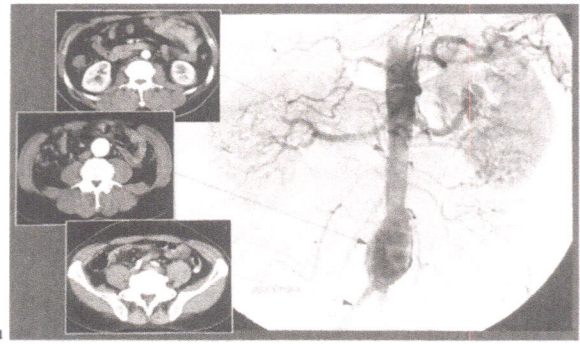

a

b

Fig. 17.53 a,b. Endovascular aortic reconstruction, preoperative planning. **a** Spiral computed tomography (CT)/digital subtraction angiography; **b** spiral CT/3D reconstruction

17.4.5.2
Approach to the Patient with Contained Ruptured or Symptomatic Aortic Aneurysm

Hemodynamically stable patients with contained ruptured or symptomatic aortic aneurysms may be considered for endovascular therapy provided that a suitable prosthesis is readily available. Tapered aorto-iliac stent grafts have been found particularly valuable in this clinical scenario (YUSUF et al. 1997).

17.4.6
Intraoperative Diagnostic Tools

Intraoperative proceedings vary greatly between patients and may be dependent on the prosthetic device that is being used. Therefore only general principles shall be outlined in the following section (Tables 8–14).

The implantation of aortic stent grafts should be performed only in an operating room environment where emergent conversion to conventional transabdominal therapy is feasible. A mobile C-arm with DSA and road-mapping capabilities needs to be available (Fig. 17.56).

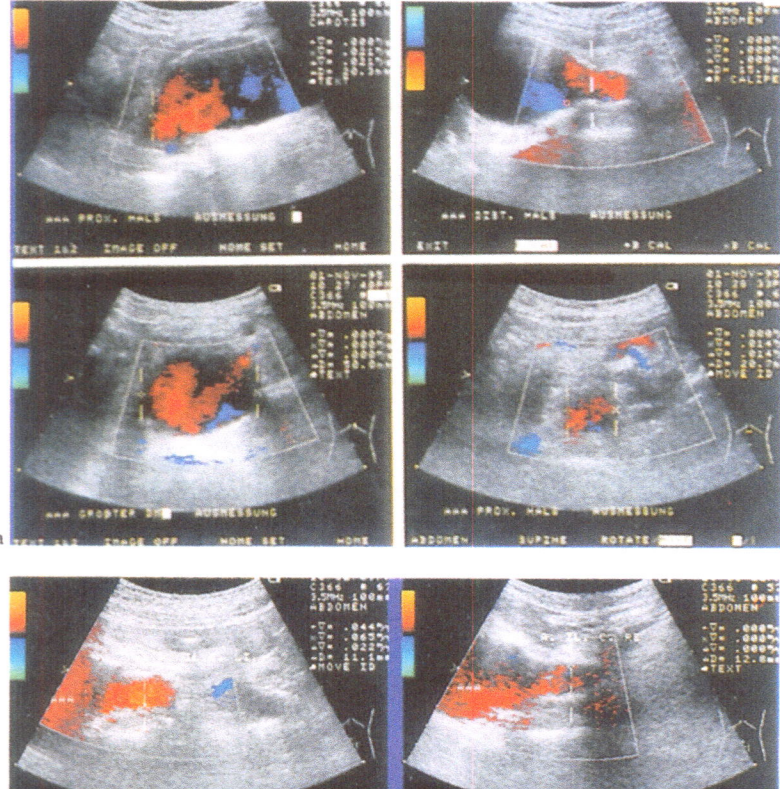

a

b

Fig. 17.54 a,b. Endovascular aortic reconstruction, preoperative duplex scanning. **a** Assessment of infrarenal aorta; **b** assessment of iliac arteries

After placement of the angiography catheter the exact localization of the renal arteries, as well as the aortic bifurcation, is determined using DSA. We use 18-G intradermal needles as skin markers.

After implantation of the endograft a completion angiogram documents patency of the renal arteries as well as the pelvic run-off. The protrusion of the soft latex aortic balloon into both iliac orifices during the final dilation of the distal stent after tube graft placement serves as an indirect sign of correct distal positioning (the so-called double-bubble sign). In case a straight endograft is placed too low at the aortic bifurcation acute occlusion of pelvic outflow may occur. This can frequently be corrected by repositioning the stent graft using a balloon introduced from the contralateral groin. Should this prove to be impossible a femoro–femoral crossover bypass or urgent conversion to conventional surgery will be required.

Finally the intraoperative DSA serves to document complete exclusion of the aneurysm. Discrete contrast leakage into the aneurysm sack may be tolerated as this frequently represents transient seepage through the unclotted Dacron graft which may be expected to disappear spontaneously within several hours.

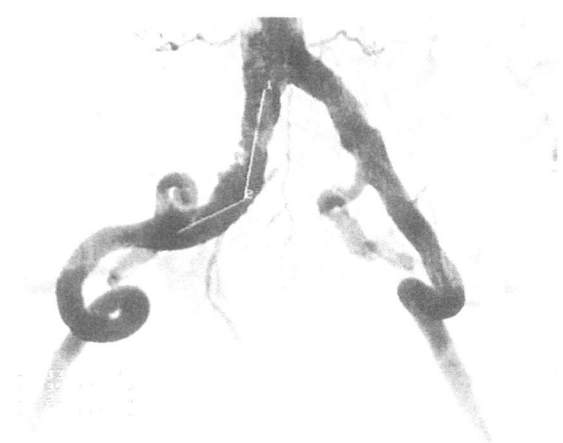

Fig. 17.55. Endovascular aortic reconstruction, preoperative aortogram. Contraincication to endovascular aortic grafting: severe bilateral iliac artery tortuosity

Table 17.11. Contraindications for endovascular aortic reconstruction: inadequate vascular access

- Extreme kinking or coiling of the iliac arteries (Fig. 17.55)
- Small caliber iliac arteries (<8 mm)
- Long, high grade iliac artery stenoses or occlusions

Table 17.12. Contraindications for endovascular aortic reconstruction: aneurysm morphology

- Unsuitable proximal aortic neck (length <15 mm, diameter >26 mm, wall adherent thrombus or major wall calcifications in the proximal neck), aortic angulation
- Unsuitable iliac anchoring sites
  Bifurcated stent grafts: common or external iliac artery >12 mm
  Tapered aorto-iliac grafts: common or external iliac artery >20 mm
- Aortic aneurysm side branches
  - Prominent patent IMA after sigmoid colon resections
  - Patent IMA with prominent arc of Riolan in the presence of SMA occlusion
  - Large accessory renal arteries originating from aneurysm
  - High-grade renal artery stenosis unsuitable for PTA with or without stent

IMA, inferior mesenteric artery; SMA, superior mesenteric artery; PTA, percutaneous transluminal angioplasty.

Table 17.13. Anatomic requirements for aortic stent grafts

	Tube	Bifurcated	Tapered aortoiliac
Proximal infrarenal neck (length)	>15 mm	>15 mm	>15 mm
Proximal infrarenal neck (diameter)	<26 mm	<26 mm	<30 mm
Distal aortic anchoring site (length)	>15 mm	–	–
Distal aortic anchoring site (diameter)	<26 mm	–	–
Iliac anchoring site	–	<12 mm	<15 mm

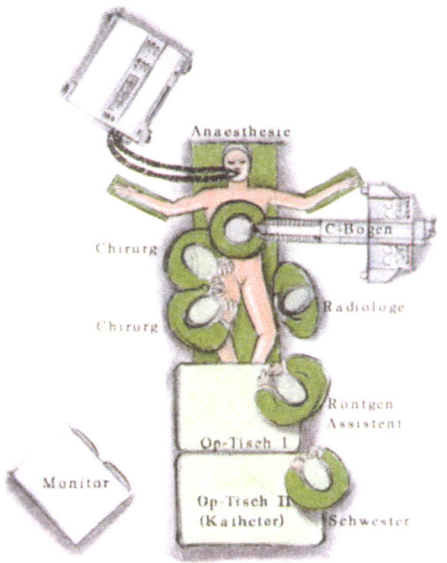

Fig. 17.56. Endovascular aortic reconstruction; operating room set-up

Particularly proximal endoleaks with significant contrast flow into the aneurysm sack, however, should be corrected at the time of the primary procedure, if possible. Otherwise surgical conversion is called for.

Most aortic stent grafts have a proximal portion of uncovered stent protruding from the actual graft to enhance anchoring properties. When this uncovered part of the stent comes to overlie the renal artery ostium this may theoretically result in thrombosis of the renal artery. In these patients postoperative angiography should be performed within 1–2h after the procedure to assure renal artery patency, or else the opportunity for renal salvage may be missed.

Table 17.14. Vascular access for aortic stent grafts

- 5-cm Femoral incision approximately 1–2 cm lateral to the common femoral artery
- Dissection of the femoral bifurcation for separate clamping
- Tourniquet control of the common femoral artery at its most proximal portion (depending on the prosthetic device a uni- or bifemoral approach will be required)
- Full anticoagulation with heparin sodium (125 IU per kg body weight)
- Separate clamping of superficial and deep femoral arteries allows for appropriate flushing maneuvers (in order to avoid peripheral embolization)
- Puncture of the common femoral artery using Seldinger's technique

Some authors describe the intentional placement of the uncovered part of the stent across the renal artery orifices to enhance anchoring at the proximal neck (STELTER et al. 1996).

17.4.7
Postoperative Diagnostics

On the first postoperative day we perform an abdominal CT of the infrarenal aorta using i.v. contrast (Fig. 17.59; Table 17.21).

On the same day a duplex ultrasound examination of the aorta is performed before the patient receives food. The patient's aorta is examined according to the criteria outlined in Table 17.22 (Fig. 17.60).

Angiography is only performed in selected patients to assess renal perfusion, stenosis of the pelvic outflow tract, or to clarify suspected intestinal ischemia (Fig. 17.61).

When an endoleak is detected by CT or duplex (Fig. 17.62), angiography is performed to localize the origin of the leak and to plan for further treatment (Figs. 17.63, 17.64).

The following features should be assessed during postoperative duplex scanning:
- Adequate intraprosthetic flow
- Investigate aneurysm sack for flow phenomena, inhomogeneous thrombus, and high pulsatility
- Document adequate apposition of the proximal and distal anchoring stents to the aortic wall
- Assess renal artery and iliac artery take-off
- Compare Doppler curves of iliac and femoral vessels with preoperative tracings

A postoperative baseline of infrarenal and mid-aneurysmal diameter needs to be established by duplex and CT to assure recognition of progressive aneurysm dilatation during follow-up.

Any problems detected during the first follow-up check, for example, graft dislodgment, large endoleaks (Fig. 17.64), in particularly proximal endoleaks, iliac limb stenosis (Fig. 17.65) or occlusion (Fig. 17.66) should be corrected immediately by interventional or surgical treatment.

17.4.8
Follow-up Examinations

Implantation of aortic stentgrafts at the current time should only be performed as part of a clinical trial. It is mandatory to adhere to a strict follow-

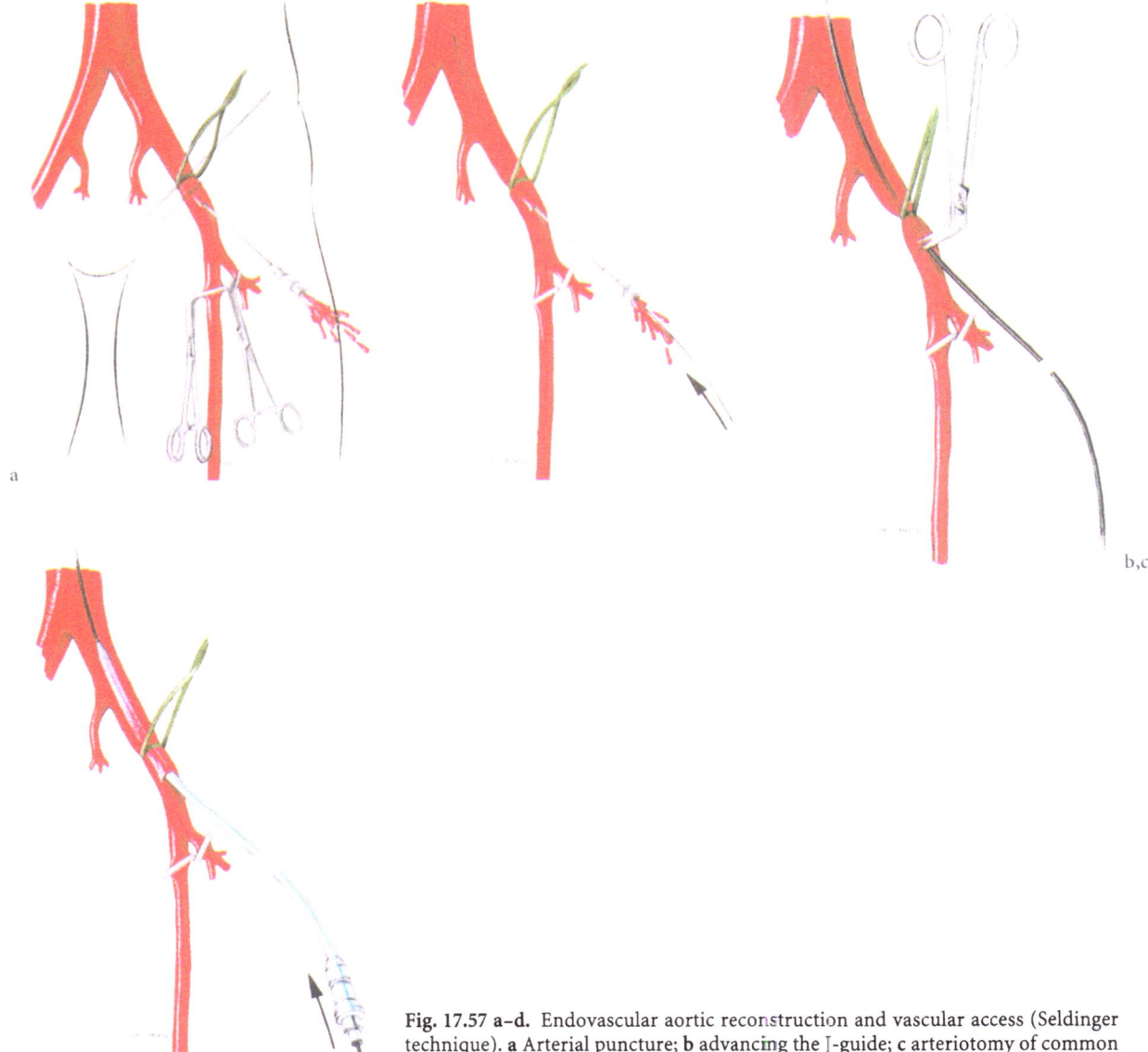

Fig. 17.57 a–d. Endovascular aortic reconstruction and vascular access (Seldinger technique). **a** Arterial puncture; **b** advancing the J-guide; **c** arteriotomy of common femoral artery; **d** introduction of the delivery system

up protocol. Our current follow-up schedule for patients not included in clinical trials is outlined in Fig. 17.67.

Abdominal plain X-rays (auteroposterior and lateral) should be obtained every 12 months to check for stent migration and changes of stent configuration. We have observed structural changes (fracture of stent struts, breakage of sutures aligning stent components) in 24% of first generation Mihaile stentor devices (MinTec, Freeport, Bahamas) (Fig. 17.68).

Plain films of EVT (Endovascular Technologies, Menlo Park, Calif., USA) bifurcated systems demonstrate parallel markers at both sides of the iliac limbs

and thus serve to determine adequate alignment of the endograft and to detect torsion of a limb.

17.4.9
Discussion and Review of Current Results of Endovascular Aortic Grafting

Current controversy centers on the relevance of small endoleaks, therapy of thrombotic complications, indications for conversion to conven-tional therapy, advantages of different prosthetic devices, and indication for repair of small aneu-rysms using endovascular aortic grafting (EAG) (see Table 17.23).

Table 17.15. Implantation of aortic stent grafts: interventional maneuvers

- Puncture of the common femoral artery using Seldinger's technique (Fig. 17.57a)
- Advancement of the J-guide to a level above the renal arteries (Fig. 17.57b)
- Placement of a graded angiography catheter (pigtail or cobra catheter)
- Diagnostic aortography using the graded catheter to define the lowest renal artery orifice and the aortic bifurcation using DSA road map technique, on-table marker board (Endovascular Technologies) or intradermal needles serve to set landmarks
- Transverse arteriotomy at the common femoral puncture site (Fig. 17.57c)
- Implantation of the delivery sheath with its hemostatic valve (Fig. 17.57d)
- PTA of preexisting iliac stenoses as necessary

DSA, digital subtraction angiography; PTA, percutaneous transluminal angioplasty.

Table 17.16. Implantation of a straight endograft (EGS, Endovascular Technologies)

- After unpacking, check the original prosthetic device for manufacturing defects
- Introduce the EGS delivery sheath including obturator and dilator (this may require enlargement of the arteriotomy)
- Attach pressurized heparinized saline i.v. lines to the flushing channel of the gate
- Introduce the prosthetic device through the gate, positioning it exactly under the lowest renal artery orifice
- Release the proximal anchoring system
- Mold the proximal stent to the aortic wall using the aortic balloon of the stent system (rotating the balloon three times)
- Precise placement of the distal stent in the most distal protion of the aneurysm neck above the bifurcation and release of the distal anchoring system
- Molding of the distal stent using the aortic balloon at three different levels rotating the balloon three times
- Remove application system and replace over guidewire with angiography catheter
- Final DSA to check for renal artery patency, effective exclusion of the aneurysm and to identify outflow problems

DSA, digital subtraction angiography.

Table 17.17. Implantation of a straight endograft (EGS, Endovascular Technologies)

- Bilateral introduction of the femoral sheaths
- Introduction of the crossover wire which is caught using a snare from the contralateral groin
- Introduction of the stent graft to a level above the renal arteries
- Withdrawal of the outer sheath releasing the contralateral limb, which is pulled down into the iliac artery, controlling for rotational problems
- Lowering of the endograft to below the renal artery orifice and release of the proximal attachment system
- Balloon modeling of the proximal attachment system (three positions)
- Release of the iliac attachment systems
- Balloon dilatation of the iliac limbs
- Control DSA to assess renal artery patency and leak-proof repair

DSA, digital subtraction angiography.

Table 17.18. Implantation of a straight aortic stent graft (type Vanguard)

- Unpack original prosthesis and check for manufacturing problems
- Flush applicator system with ice saline (nitinol stent needs cooling before insertion)
- Introduce prosthesis through arteriotomy (Fig. 17.58a) and position exactly below most inferior renal artery orifice. *Note:* Proximal marker 1 corresponds to uncovered upper end of the proximal stent, marker 2 corresponds to upper end of covered portion of the proximal stent
- Advance balloon into suprarenal aorta
- Fractionated release of the prosthetic device by stabilizing the internal pusher with one hand and withdrawing the outer sheath with the other (Fig. 17.58b)
- Molding of the released proximal and distal stent with the aortic balloon (Fig. 17.58c,d)
- Completion of DSA and removal of the applicator system

DSA, digital subtraction angiography.

Table 17.19. Implantation of a bifurcated aortic stent graft (type Vanguard)

The main body of the stent graft is implanted following the steps for a tube graft:
- Advancing the main body of the stent graft. Any rotation needs to be avoided. The docking zone of the contralateral limb faces the orifice of the contralateral common iliac artery
- Introduction of the main body of the stent graft
- Markers at the distal end of the contralateral docking site should come to lie in a frontal plane appearing as parallel lines on the flow image
- Release of the main body of the stent graft. A guidewire is advanced from the contralateral groin to pass through this docking site into the main body of the stent
- The iliac limb is advanced over this guide wire and released by withdrawing the outer sheath over a pusher. A balloon is used to "mold" the docking zone for a tight fit
- Completion of DSA and removal of the applicator system

DSA, digital subtraction angiography.

Table 17.20. Endovascular aortic stent graft: surgical completion

- Removal of all applicator systems
- Separate flushing maneuvers of superficial, deep, and common femoral arteries
- Vascular closure
- Complete hemostasis after heparin reversal with protamine
- Insertion of closed circuit suction drains
- Surgical closure of the wound

Table 17.21. Postoperative computed tomography scanning after aortic stent graft implantation

- Always use i.v. contrast
- Maximum slice thickness should be no greater than 4–5 mm
- Note adequate bilateral enhancement of renal parenchyma
- Stent graft should be completely filled with contrast
- Check for appearance of contrast in the aneurysm sack (endoleak)
- Check for signs of incomplete thrombosis of the aneurysm sack
- Use fractionated contrast injections and delayed cuts to identify opacification of inferior mesenteric and lumbar arteries

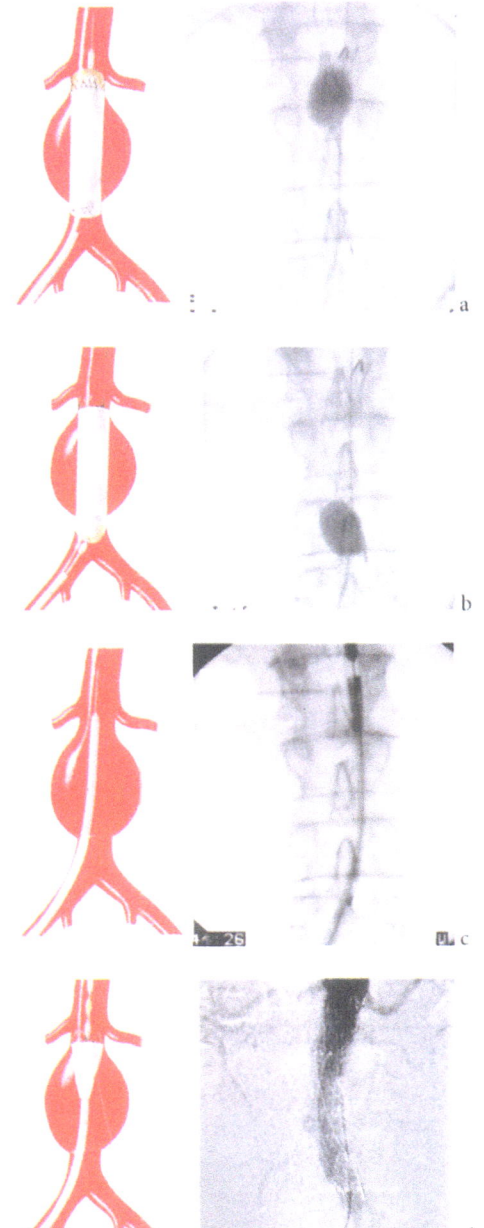

Fig. 17.58 a–d. Implantation of a Vanguard straight endograft (intraoperative digital subtraction angiography; Boston Scientific, Oakland, N.J., USA) **a** Introduction of the delivery system; **b** releasing the proximal stent graft; **c** modeling the proximal stent with balloon dilatation; **d** modeling the distal stent graft with balloon dilatation

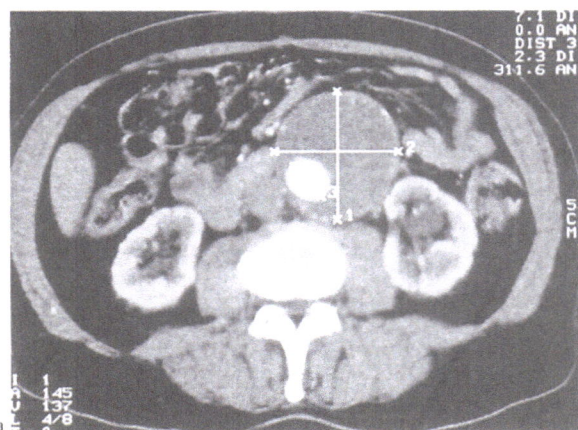
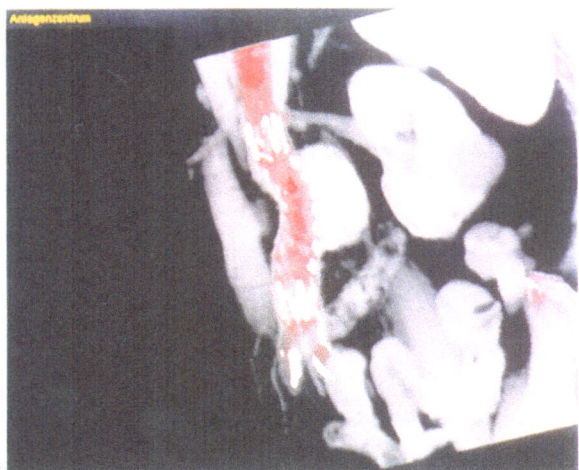

Fig. 17.59 a,b. Endovascular aortic reconstruction and postoperative contrast computed tomography (CT). **a** Spiral CT. **b** Two-dimensional reconstructions (EGS, Endovascular Technologies, Menlo Park, Calif., USA)

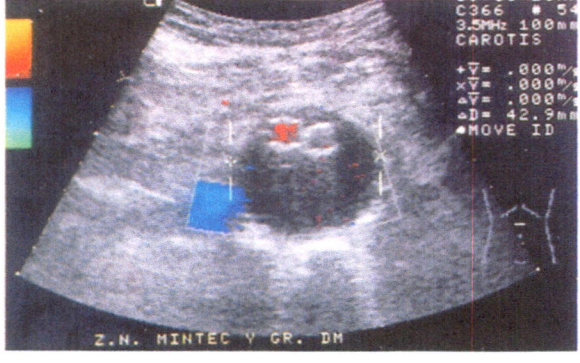

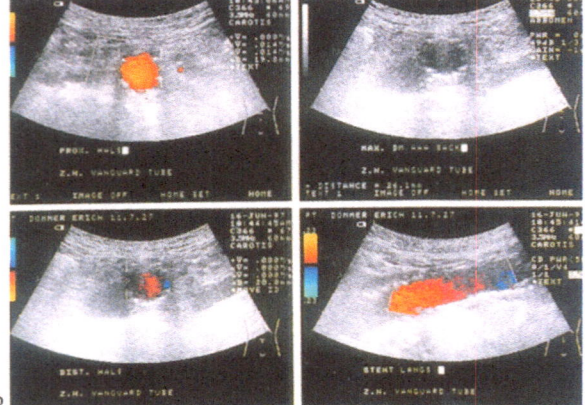

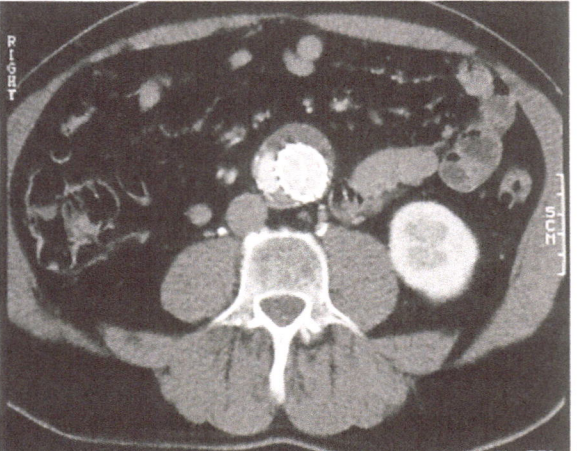

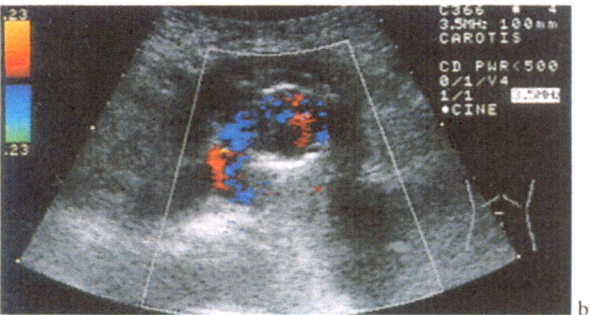

Fig. 17.60 a,b. Endovascular aortic reconstruction, postoperative duplex scanning, standard views. **a** Largest aneurysm diameter (MinTec bifurcated endograft, Freeport, Bahamas); **b** standard views (MinTec tube endograft, Freeport, Bahamas)

Fig. 17.62 a,b. Proximal and distal anchoring endoleak (MinTec straight endograft) **a** Contrast computed tomography (proximal endoleak); **b** duplex scan (transverse), proximal endoleak

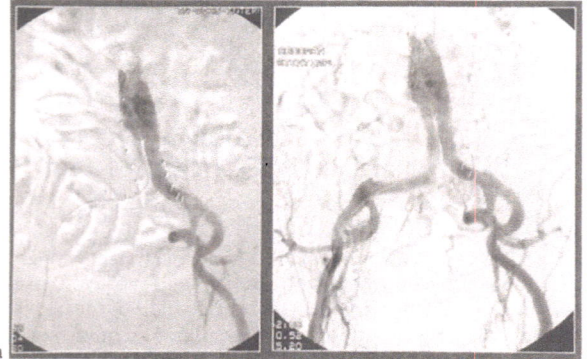

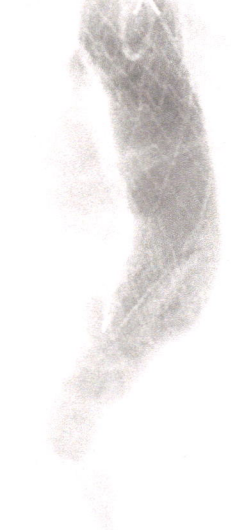

Fig. 17.61 a,b. Endovascular aortic reconstruction and postoperative digital subtraction angiography. **a** EVT bifurcated endograft, occlusion of right iliac limb. **b** Right iliac limb, status post suction thrombectomy and percutaneous transluminal angioplasty

Fig. 17.63. Digital subtraction angiography (MinTec straight endograft), proximal and distal anchoring leak

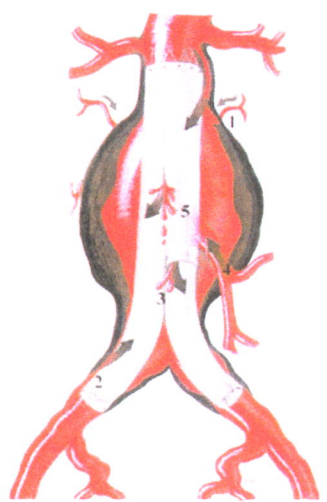

Fig. 17.64. Classification of endoleaks. *1* Proximal anchoring leak; *2* distal anchoring leak; *3* intraprosthetic leak; *4* side branch endoleak; *5* leak at docking site

Table 17.22. Postoperative duplex scanning of aortic stent grafts

Standard views include:
- Infrarenal aorta longitudinal
- Aorta transverse (greatest diameter of the aneurysm)
- Transverse cut of the aorta at the level of the proximal neck (infrarenal)
- Transverse aortic cut at the distal neck (at the bifurcation)

Additional views after implantation of bifurcated stent grafts:
- Right iliac axis longitudinal with Doppler interrogation
- Left iliac axis longitudinal with Doppler interrogation

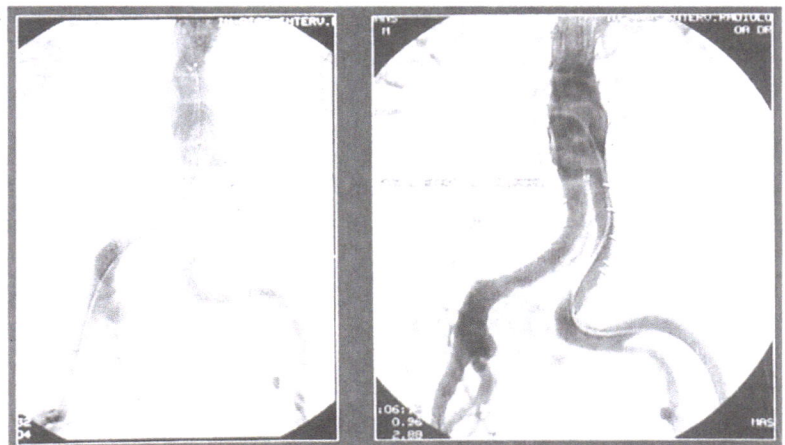

Fig. 17.65. Postoperative digital subtraction angiography (status post EVT bifurcated stent graft). **a** Bilateral iliac limb stenosis. **b** Status post bilateral percutaneous transluminal angioplasty and implantation of wall stents

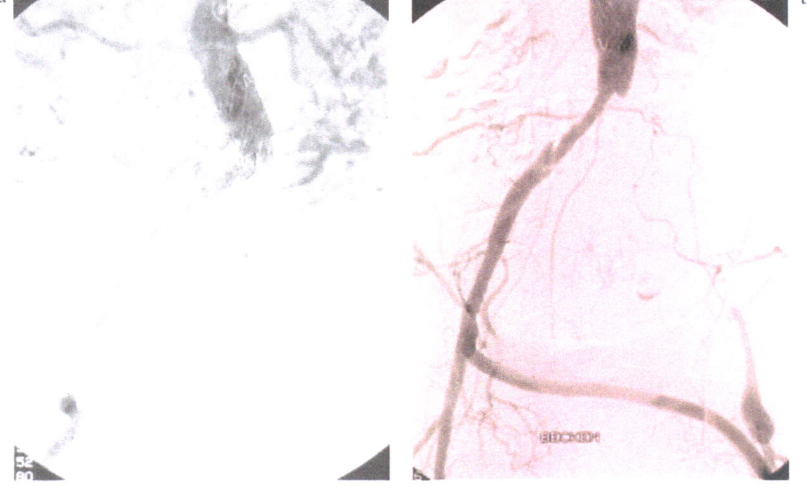

Fig. 17.66 a,b. Postoperative digital subtraction angiography (status post MinTec bifurcated endograft). **a** Left iliac limb occlusion. **b** Status post reconstruction with femoro-femoral crossover bypass

17.4.9.1
Aneurysm Size and Endovascular Aortic Grafting

Smaller aneurysms are technically easier to reconstruct. This is reflected in current literature where the treatment of patients with minor (<4cm) and small (<5cm) aortic aneurysms is reported with increasing frequency. We found the mean aortic diameter of patients undergoing repair of infrarenal aneurysms ranging between 45.2 and 60mm (BLUM et al. 1996; CHUTER et al. 1997; DÜBER et al. 1996; HEILBERGER et al. 1997a,b; MALINA et al. 1997; MARIN et al. 1995; MAY et al. 1996; MOORE and RUTHERFORD 1996; PARODI 1996; STELTER et al. 1996; YUSUF et al. 1997).

Lower perioperative mortality rates after endovascular reconstruction compared to conventional aortic repair seem to justify aggressive therapy of small aneurysms.

Furthermore, up to 18% of ruptured aortic aneurysms have been observed to be smaller than 5cm in diameter (DARLING 1970). At our institution we repair fusiform aortic aneurysms greater than 40mm. Patients with sacciform aneurysms or local signs of impending rupture on contrast CT are selected on an individual basis according to aneurysm morphology.

17.4.9.2
Prosthetic Devices

A number of different devices are currently available for endovascular aortic reconstructions (Table 17.23). After initial self-made devices various industrially manufactured products (MinTec, Freeport, Bahamas, Vanguard, Boston Scientific, Oakland, N.J., USA; EGS, Endovascular Technologies, Menlo Park, Calif., USA, Talent, World Medical, Sunrise, Fla., USA) are now commercially available combining a variety of graft materials and stent models.

We may distinguish between *modular systems*, which are usually completely stented (i.e., the stent stabilizes the vascular graft along its entire length) and *single unit devices*, which consist of a tube or bifurcated graft made out of one piece which is only stented at its proximal and distal ends.

Aortic vascular anatomy and investigator preference dictate the use of either tube grafts, bifurcated grafts, or aorto-monoiliac tapered grafts in conjunction with occlusion of the contralateral iliac limb and a femoro–femoral crossover bypass. Particularly during our earlier experience we limited endovascular aortic therapy to selected patients with type I infrarenal aortic aneurysms which could be reconstructed using a straight endograft (HEILBERGER et al. 1997b).

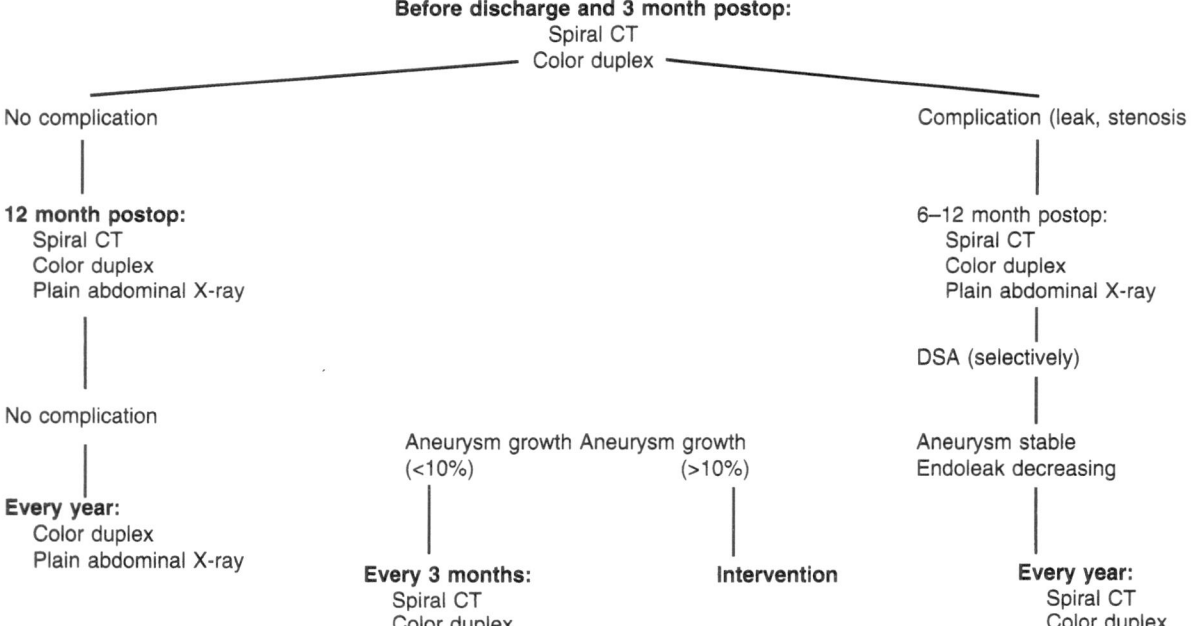

Fig. 17.67. Follow-up protocol for patients with aortic endograft. *CT*, computed tomography; *DSA*, digital subtraction angiography

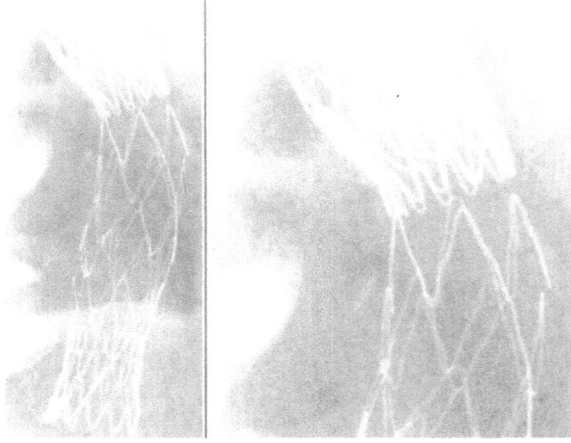

Fig. 17.68. Status post-MinTec straight endograft implantation, stent fracture (X-ray)

17.4.9.3
Conversion to Conventional Reconstruction

Conversion to conventional surgical therapy, according to current experience (Table 17.23), has been required in 0%–16% of patients undergoing endovascular aortic reconstruction. In our own experience this was necessary in 10% (HEILBERGER et al. 1997a,b).

The indication for conversion to conventional therapy may occur at any point in time during endovascular reconstruction (occlusion of renal arteries, stent dislodgment, outflow obstruction, vascular disruption or dissection, etc.). Thus the implantation of aortic endografts should only be performed in a well-equipped vascular operating theater.

Late conversion to open surgery may become necessary for:
- Patients with persistent endoleaks not treatable by endovascular means
- Patients with >10% increase in aneurysm diameter
- Patients with secondary distal aneurysms
- Patients with endoleaks due to prosthetic defects or defects of the stent
- Patients with thrombotic occlusion of the aortic portion of the stent.

17.4.9.4
Perioperative Mortality After Endovascular Therapy

Reported mortality after endovascular aortic reconstruction varies between 0% and 28% (Table 17.23). High-end mortalities reported by some investigators (MARIN et al. 1995) are based on their patient selection, offering endovascular therapy on a compassionate basis to high risk patients who would normally not be candidates for conventional aortic repair. Perioperative mortality after conventional aortic reconstructions in the literature ranges from 2.8% to 6.2%. According to average mortality rates, perioperative mortality after conventional aortic reconstructions is thus higher than average mortality after endovascular reconstruction (BLUM et al. 1996; CAPPELER et al. 1996; DÜBER et al. 1996; HEILBERGER et al. 1997a,b; MALINA et al. 1997; MAY et al. 1996; YUSUF et al. 1997).

17.4.9.5
Primary and Secondary Endoleaks

The main risk after EAG relates to endoleaks. Incomplete exclusion of the aneurysm, i.e., the occurrence or persistence of a primary or secondary endoleak, may result in aneurysm growth and ultimately in rupture. LUMSDEN et al. reported two fatal ruptures after endovascular aortic reconstructions which had persistent endoleaks (LUMSDEN et al. 1995).

Therefore, peri – and postoperative diagnostic tools need to detect primary and secondary endoleaks with adequate sensitivity and specificity. Comparing contrast spiral CT (Fig. 17.69) to duplex scan with adjunctive ultrasound contrast (Levovist Schering A.G., Berlin, Germany), we found comparable sensitivity and specificity of >90% for both diagnostic tools to detect and quantify postoperative endoleaks (HEILBERGER et al. 1997a) (Fig. 17.70).

Once an endoleak has been identified its origin needs to be defined by duplex, CT, and angiography to plan for appropriate endovascular or surgical therapy according to our classification (Fig. 17.71). We distinguish proximal and distal anchoring leaks, docking leaks (modular systems with stent-in-stent arrangement), leaks due to prosthetic defects (tear of the graft fabric, unraveling of suture lines, etc.), and

Table 17.23. Results after endovascular aortic reconstruction

	Blum et al. (1997)	Düber et al. (1996)	Marin et al. (1995)	Malina et al. (1997)	May et al. (1996)
Number of patients	154	19	18	35	85[a]
AAA diameter (mm)	54	53	>50	52	~58
Type of endograft	MinTec/Vanguard	MinTec	Homemade/Endovascular Technologies	Homemade	EVT/Chuter/Sydney
Straight/bifurcated/tapered (%)	22/132/0 14%/86%/0	3/16/0 16%/84%/0	12/0/6 67%/0/33%	Bifurcated + tapered = 35	33/3/11 70%/6%/24%
Conversions	3 (2%)	0	0	1	14 (16%)
Mortality	1 (0.7%)	0	5 (28%)	0	5 (6%)
Primary endoleaks	17 (11%)	4 (21%)	6 (33%)	7	5/47 (11%)
Secondary endoleaks	7 (4.5%)	0	–	6	(including secondary leaks)
Primary success	87%	15 (79%)	16 (88%)	28/35 (80%)	n.r.

	Chuter et al. (1997)	Stelter et al. (1996)	Moor and Rutherford (1996)	Parodi (1996)	Yusuf et al. (1997)
Number of patients	52	69	46	87	30[b]
AAA diameter (mm)	n.r.	n.r.	52	38–120?	60
Type of endograft	Dacron + Gianturco homemade	MinTec	Endovascular Technologies	Palmaz + Dacron	Dacron + Gianturco
Straight/bifurcated/tapered (%)		10/59/0 14%/86%/0	46/0/0 100%/0/0	45/0/42 52%/0/48%	0/0/30 0/0/100%
Conversions	13 (25%)	3 (4%)	9 (20%)	3 (3%)	2 (7%)
Mortality	1 (2%)	5 (7%)	0 (<30T)	9% (<30 d)[c]	2 (7%)
Primary endoleaks	5 (10%)	7 (13%)	17 (13%)	6 (7%)	2 (7%)
Secondary endoleaks	7 (13%)	7 (13%)	n.r.	8 (9%)	3 (10%)
Primary success	94%	86%	85%	65/87/3Konv. (75%)	25 (83%)

[a] Only 47 patients analyzed.
[b] Two emergencies, two inflammatory aneurysms.
AAA, abdominal aortic aneurysm.
[c] Four patients died secondary to embolization.

side-branch leaks due to retrograde perfusion of the aneurysm sack via side branches (inferior mesenteric artery, lumbar arteries) (see Fig. 17.64).

During the first 12 months after endovascular aortic reconstruction change of aneurysm morphology may be slow to occur and is difficult to detect by duplex and CT scan. However, the detection of endoleaks may serve as a marker for future aneurysm growth. MAY et al. have documented decreasing aneurysm size in 39 patients without endoleaks. In eight patients with increases in aneurysm diameter MAY found five endoleaks (MAY et al. 1996).

Endoleaks occurring in the immediate perioperative period (primary endoleaks) have been described in 7%–33% of patients after endovascular aortic reconstruction. The occurrence of an endoleak after initially successful exclusion of the aneurysm (secondary endoleak) has been observed in 0%–13% of patients (Table 17.23).

In our own experience a relatively high number of secondary endoleaks have occurred predominantly after aortic reconstructions using straight endovascular devices (HEILBERGER et al. 1997b).

These were usually secondary distal anchoring leaks which occurred after implantation of completely stented rigid endografts anchored in a relatively short distal neck. During implantation this rigid system offers no variability in length. A second mechanism is the secondary dislodgment of a limb extension graft out of its proximal anchoring site (HEILBERGER et al. 1997b).

17.4.9.6
Early Results of Endovascular Aortic Reconstruction

Successful aneurysm therapy using endovascular aortic stent grafts may be achieved in 74%–94% of patients (Table 17.23).

The results of different investigators, however, are difficult to compare since criteria for successful endovascular therapy vary considerably.

In our opinion successful endovascular aortic reconstruction requires: (a) Complete exclusion of the aneurysm; (b) absence of thrombotic or obstructive complications; (c) anchoring of the stent graft in healthy, non-aneurysmal arterial anatomy; and (d) absence of any endoleaks.

17.4.9.7
Thrombotic Complications

Thrombosis of a straight aortic endograft is a rare occurrence, usually involving major technical mishaps. The occlusion of an iliac limb of a bifurcated endograft, however, is a complication that may be seen in up to 25% of patients independent of the type of prosthetic device used (HEILBERGER et al. 1997a,b). In modular systems the critical point for thrombosis of the outflow tract is usually the docking site between the main body of the aortic endograft and the iliac limb. This was corrected by the implantation of a femoro–femoral crossover bypass in four patients (HEILBERGER et al. 1997b).

Bifurcated endografts manufactured as a single unit (e.g., the EGS system by EVT or the Chuter device) run a high risk of limb occlusion due to ex-

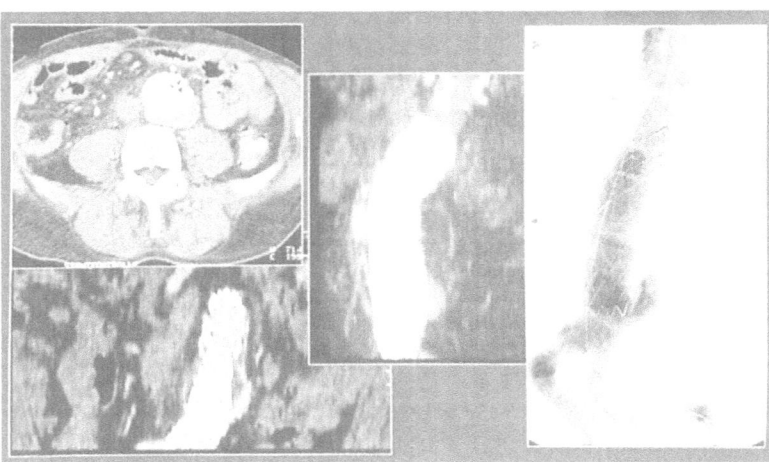

Fig. 17.69. Distal prosthetic endoleak (MinTec, Tube), spiral computed tomography, two-dimensional reconstruction, digital subtraction angiography

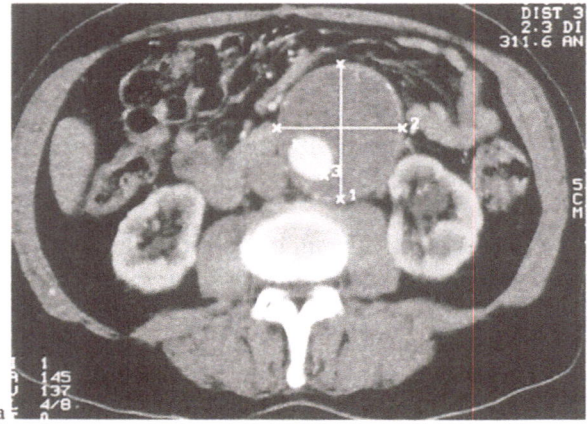

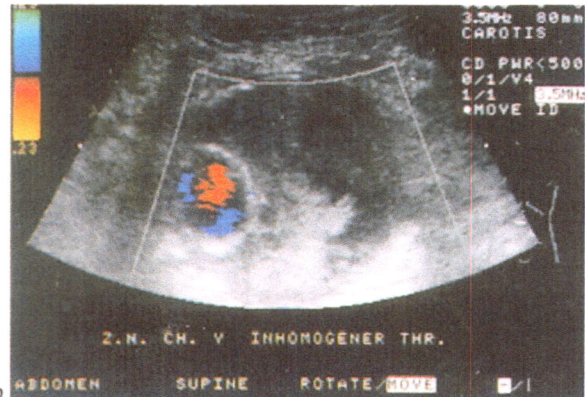

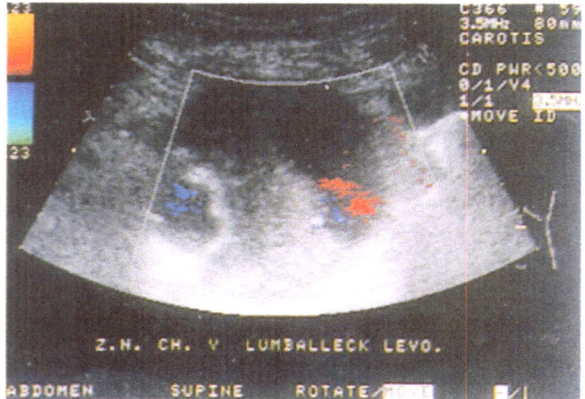

trinsic compression of the unstented iliac limb in its course through a narrowed atherosclerotic native iliac artery. Any torsion of these unstented limbs may also lead to stenosis and subsequent thrombosis. Kinking of the graft resulted in thrombosis of an iliac limb in five of CHUTER's patients who subsequently underwent conversion to conventional repair (CHUTER et al. 1997). The routine implantation of wall stents in the iliac limbs in their course through the three narrowings at the distal aneurysm neck, aortic bifurcation, and proximal iliac arteries may solve this problem (CHUTER et al. 1997) (Fig. 17.65).

Iliac limb occlusions after implantation of a bifurcated EVT device were successfully recanalized using transfemoral percutaneous implantation of a wall stent in three of our patients (HEILBERGER et al. 1997).

17.4.9.8
Expanding Indications for Endovascular Aortic Reconstructions

With increasing experience endovascular aortic exclusion has also been performed in patients with inflammatory aneurysms, as well as hemodynamically stable patients with contained aortic ruptures (BOYLE et al. 1997; YUSUF et al. 1997). Urgent as well as emergent endovascular therapy is limited by the necessity to stock a large array of prosthetic devices of varying lengths and diameters. With increasing

Fig. 17.70 a–c. Endovascular aortic reconstruction, status post-CHUTER bifurcated endograft, follow-up examinations. **a** Contrast computed tomography. **b** Duplex ultrasound without i.v. ultrasound contrast. **c** Duplex ultrasound with i.v. ultrasound contrast (Levovist, Schering A.G., Berlin, Germany)

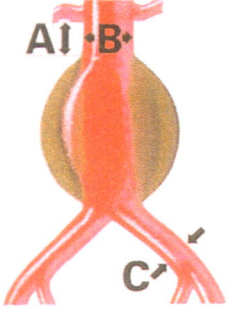

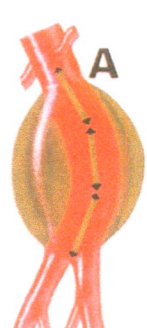

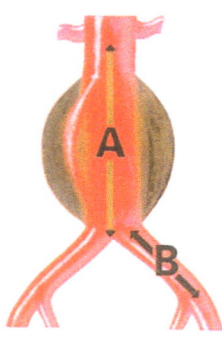

Fig. 17.71. Endovascular aortic reconstruction, preoperative evaluation

usage, however, a decrease in prosthetic prices may be anticipated and stocking of a sufficient number and variety of devices may become financially feasible.

Mycotic aneurysms are not suitable for endovascular therapy as we have observed early prosthetic infections using this therapeutic modality. Conventional surgical therapy remains the mainstay to treat these difficult patients. After endovascular therapy of mycotic aneurysm of one iliac artery and one thoracic aorta in two of our patients, septic rupture of the vessel wall occurred in both patients.

17.4.10
Summary

In the hands of experienced vascular surgeons and interventional radiologists, endovascular aortic therapy is an attractive minimally-invasive alternative therapy for infrarenal aorto-iliac aneurysms.

Although this therapeutic option may be performed with a very low mortality rate, it is still fraught with high complication rates involving the occurrence of endoleaks and thrombotic outflow obstruction.

High primary success rates may be achieved using standardized implantation techniques. The long-term goal must now be to improve secondary success rates by diligent follow-up and an aggressive approach to interventional therapy of endoleaks and thrombotic complications.

Industry must strive to improve stent design and durability of materials used. Stent application systems need to become thinner and easier to handle. Stent attachment systems need improvements to minimize risks of dislocation and secondary endoleak.

Endoleaks following endovascular repair of aortic aneurysms can be optimally diagnosed by angio-CT or contrast-enhanced duplex sonography. CT examinations revealed endoleaks according to our current knowledge (1999) in 20%–30% of patients. On CT, leaks located in a ventral direction from the prosthesis are fed almost exclusively by the inferior mesenteric artery. The endoleak has to be embolized via the superior mesenteric artery in the direction of Riolan's anastomotic collateral circulation. If the leak goes to dorsolateral, it is supplied by either the lumbar or median sacral artery, via the hypogastric artery. In this case, embolization of the feeding lumbar or median sacral arteries has been recommended (GÖRICH et al. 1999). All patients with endoleaks need short-term follow-up controls with contrast-enhanced ultrasound or spiral CT with 3D reconstruction.

References

Aadahl P, Lundbom J, Hatlinghus S, Myhre HO (1997) Regional anesthesia for endovascular treatment of abdominal aortic aneurysms. J Endovasc Surg 4:56–61

Ahn SS, Rutherford RB, Johnston KW, May J, Veith FJ, Baker JD, Ernst CB, Moore W (1997) Reporting standards for infrarenal endovascular abdominal aortic aneurysm repair. J Vasc Surg 25:405–410

Allenberg JR, Schumacher H (1995) Endovaskuläre Rekonstruktion des infrarenalen abdominellen Aortenaneurysmas (AAA). Chirurg 66:870–877

Balko A, Piasecki GJ, Shah DM, Carney WI, Hopkins RW, Jackson BT (1986) Transfemoral placement on intraluminal polyurethane prosthesis for abdominal aortic aneurysm. J Surg Res 40:305–309

Blaisdell FW, Hall AD, Thomas AN (1965) Ligation treatment of abdominal aortic aneurysms. Am J Surg 109:560–565

Blum U, Langer M, Spillner G, Mialhe C, Beyersdorf F, Buitrago-Tellez C, Voshage G, Düber C, Schlosser V, Cragg AH (1996) Abdominal aortic aneurysms: preliminary technical and clinical results with transfemoral placement of endovascular self-expanding stent-grafts. Radiology 198:25–31

Blum U, Voshage G, Lammer J, Beyersdorf F, Töllner D, Kretschmer D, Spillner G, Polterauer P, Nagel G, Hölzenbein T, Thurnher S, Langer M (1997) Endoluminal stent-grafts for infrarenal abdominal aortic aneurysms. N Engl J Med 336:13–20

Cappeler WA, Hinz MH, Lauterjung L (1996) Das infrarenale Aortenaneurysma – 10-Jahres-Verlauf nach Ausschaltungsoperation mit Kostenanalyse. Chirurg 67:697–702

Chuter TA, Wendt G, Hopkinson BR, Scott RA, Risberg B, Kieffer E, Raithel D, van Bockel JH (1997) European experience with a system for bifurcated stent-graft insertion. J Endovasc Surg 4:13–22

Cragg A, Lund G, Rysavy J (1983) Nonsurgical placement arterial endoprothesis: a new technique using nitinol wire. Radiology 147:261–263

Creech O (1960) Endoaneurysmorrhaphy and treatment of aortic aneurysm. Ann Surg 164:935–946

Darling RC (1970) Ruptured arteriosclerotic abdominal aortic aneurysms: a pathological and clinical study. Am J Surg 119:397–401

DeBakey ME, Crawford ES, Cooley DA (1964) Aneurysm of abdominal aorta: analysis of results of graft replacement therapy one to eleven years after operation. Ann Surg 160:622–631

Dotter CT (1969) Transluminally-placed coil spring endarterial tube grafts: long term patency in canine popliteal artery. Invest Radiol 4:329–332

Düber VC, Schmiedt W, Pitton M, Neufang A, Eberle B, Wollmann JC, Oelert H, Thelen M (1996) Endovaskuläre Therapie aortaler Aneurysmen: erste klinische Ergebnisse. Rofo Fortschr Geb Rontgenstr Neuen Bildgeb Uerfehr 164(1):1–94

Dubost C, Allary M, Oeconomos N (1952) Resection of an aneurysm of the abdominal aorta: reestablishment of the continuity by a preserved arterial graft, with the result after five months. Arch Surg 64:405–408

Ernst CB (1993) Abdominal aortic aneurysms. N Engl J Med 328:1167–1172

Goldstone J (1993) Aneurysms of the aorta and iliac arteries. In: Moore WS (ed) Vascular surgery: a comrehensive review, 4th ed. Saunders, Philadelphia, p 401–423

Görich J, Rillinger N, Sokiranski R, et al. (1999) Classification of endoleaks after endovascular repair of aortic aneurysms, based on findings at computed tomography, angiography and radiography (in press)

Harris PL, Buth J, Mialhe C, Myhre HO, Norgren L (1997) The need for clinical trials of endovascular abdominal aortic aneurysm stent-graft repair: the Eurostar Project. J Endovasc Surg 4:72–77

Heilberger P, Schunn C, Ritter W, Weber S, Raithel D (1997a) Postoperative color flow duplex scanning in aortic endografting. J Endovasc Surg 4:262–271

Heilberger P, Ritter W, Schunn C, Gabriel P, Raithel D (1997b) Ergebnisse und Komplikationen nach endovaskulärer Rekonstruktion von Aortenaneurysmen. Zentralbl Chir 122:762–769

Hepp W, Vollmar J, Krier S (1980) Das Aneurysma der infrarenalen Aorta abdominalis. Chirurg 51:330–335

Hollier LH, Taylor LM, Ochsner J (1992) Recommended indications for operative treatment of abdominal aortic aneurysms. J Vasc Surg 15:1046–1056

Johansson G, Nydahl S, Olofsson P, Swedenborg J (1990) Survival in patients with abdominal aortic aneurysms. Comparison between operative and nonoperative management. Eur J Vasc Surg 4:497–502

Kniemeyer HW, Sandmann W (1992) Operationsindikation beim abdominellen Aortenaneurysma. Dtsch Med Wochenschr 117:583–587

Lazarus HM (1992) Endovascular grafting for the treatment of abdominal aortic aneurysms. Surg Clin North Am 72:959–968

Lemole GM, Spagna BM, Strong MD (1984) Rigid intraluminal prothesis for replacement of the thoracic and abdominal aorta. J Vasc Surg 1:22–26

Lumsden AB, Allen RC, Chaikof EL, Resnikoff M, Moritz MW, Gerhard H, Castronuovo JJ Jr (1995) Delayed rupture of aortic aneurysms following endovascular stent grafting. Am J Surg 170:174–178

Malina M, Ivancev K, Chuter TA, Lindh M, Länne T, Lindbald B, Brunkwall J, Risberg B (1997) Changing aneurysmal morphology after endovascular grafting: relation to leakage or persistent perfusion. J Endovasc Surg 4:23–30

Marin ML, Veith FJ, Jacob Cynamon, Sanches LA, Lyon RT, Levine BY, Bakal CW, Suggs WD, Wengerter KR, Rivers SP, Parsons RE, Yuan JG, Wain RA, Ohki T, Rozenblit A, Parodi JC (1995) Initial experience with transluminally placed endovascular grafts for the treatment of complex vascular lesions. Ann Surg 222:449–469

Mats R (1925) Ligation of the abdominal aorta: report of the ultimate result, one year, five months and nine days after the ligation of the abdominal aorta for aneurysm of the bifurcation. Ann Surg 81:457

May J, White G, Yu W, Waugh R, Stephen M, Harris J (1996) A prospective study of anatomico-pathological changes in the abdominal aortic aneurysms following endoluminal repair: is the aneurysmal process reversed? Eur J Vasc Endovasc Surg 12:11–17

Mirich D, Wright KC, Wallace S (1991) Percutaneously placed endovascular grafts for aortic aneurysms: feasiblity study. Radiology 170:1033

Moore WS, Rutherford RB (1996) Transfemoral endovascular repair of abdominal aortic aneurysm: results of the North American EVT phase 1 trial. J Vasc Surg 23:543–553

Naylor AR, Webb J, Fowkes GR, Ruckley CV (1988) Trends in abdominal aortic aneurysm surgery in Scotland (1971–1984). Eur J Vasc Surg 2:217–221

Parodi JC (1996) Endovascular repair of aortic aneurysms, arteriovenous fistulas, and false aneurysms. World J Surg 20:655–633

Parodi JC, Palmaz JC, Barone HD (1991) Transfemoral intraluminal graft implantation for abdominal aortic aneurysm. Ann Vasc Surg 5:491–499

Power DA (1921) The palliative treatment of aneurysms by "wiring" with Colt's apparatus. Br J Surg 9:27

Schumacher H, Eckstein HH, Kallinowski F, Allenberg JR (1997) Morphometry and classification in abdominal aortic aneurysms: patient selection for endovascular and open surgery. J Endovasc Surg 4:39–44

Stelter WJ, Umscheid T, Ziegler P (1996) Schwierigkeiten und Komplikationen der transfemoralen Implantation von Stent-Prothesen beim infrarenalen Bauchaortenaneurysma (BAA). Zentralbl Chir 121:734–743

Szilagyi DE, Elliott JP, Smith RF (1972) Clinical fate of the patient with asymptomatic abdominal aortic aneurysm and unfit for surgical treatment. Arch Surg 104:600–606

Volodos NL, Karpovich IP, Troyan VI (1991) Clinical experience of the use of self-fixing synthetic prosthesis for remote endoprosthetics of the thoracic and the abdominal aorta and iliac arteries through the femoral artery and as intraoperative endoprothesis for aorta reconstruction. Vasa Suppl 33:93–95

Yusuf SW, Witaker SC, Chuter TAM, Ivancev K, Baker DM, Gregson RHS, Tennant WG, Wenham PW, Hopkinson BR (1997) Early results of endovascular aortic aneurysm surgery with aortouniiliac graft, contralateral iliac occlusion, and femorofemoral bypass. J Vasc Surg 25:165–172

17.5
Diagnosis and Management of Branch-Vessel Compromise in Aortic Dissection

D.M. WILLIAMS

17.5.1
Introduction

Aortic dissection is a disease process with overlapping clinical and pathological definitions. Strictly speaking, aortic dissection is a blood-filled cleavage plane in the aortic media, and this process is associated with diseases of diverse etiology. The clinical presentation of classic aortic dissection, in one patient stereotypical and catastrophic-like tearing chest pain, in another patient bizarre and indolent-like intermittent gastrointestinal bleeding, evokes powerful clinical reflexes based on nearly 50 years' experience of treating the disease with the latest medical and surgical advances.

Aortic dissection with branch vessel compromise has an ominous natural history and presents a formidable challenge to the clinician. By wide consensus, dissection involving the ascending aorta (Stanford A, DeBakey I and II) requires emergent surgical aortic reconstruction. However, paraplegia, renal, or mesenteric ischemia complicating aortic dissection is associated with an operative mortality of approximately 50% (CAMBRIA et al. 1988; FANN et al. 1990) and is a relative contraindication to immediate aortic reconstruction. Dissection sparing the ascending aorta (Stanford B, DeBakey III) may be managed medically. Generally accepted exceptions to medical management are evidence for extension of the dissection (such as unrelenting pain or documented growth of the false lumen) or aortic branch vessel obstruction involving a limb or critical organ. Thus, in the setting of both type I and type III aortic dissection, branch vessel compromise is an important determinant of patient treatment and prognosis. Radiology has an important role in both establishing a firm diagnosis and providing safe and efficacious treatment of this devastating complication of aortic dissection.

17.5.2
Anatomy of Branch Vessel Obstruction

Aortic dissection leads to branch vessel obstruction by two principal mechanisms, both of them depen-dent on the haphazard spiraling course of the dissection as it propagates past the level of branch arteries (Fig. 17.72) (WILLIAMS et al. 1997b). Based on the anatomic relation of the dissection flap to the ostia of branch arteries, obstruction is classified as static (when the flap intersects a vessel origin) or dynamic (when the flap spares a vessel origin but prolapses across the origin like a curtain or narrows the true lumen above the origin). This distinction has not been recognized in the surgical or pathological literature because the dynamic type of obstruction disappears once the aorta is directly inspected, either at surgery after clamping and aortotomy or at autopsy, and is evident only at cross-sectional imaging studies such as transesophageal echocardiography (TEE), computed tomography (CT), and magnetic resonance aortography (MRA). Moreover, the distintion is important since it determines how the branch vessel obstruction is relieved.

Other causes of branch vessel obstruction can be observed in the setting of aortic dissection. An embolism from the true or false lumen may lodge peripherally. A chronic asymptomatic atherosclerotic narrowing may become critical after proximal compromise of the true lumen acutely lowers perfusion pressure and flow below a physiologically tolerated threshold. We have also observed a patient in whom foot pulses disappeared and reappeared during closely monitored observation in an intensive care unit. Examination in this case established no fixed anatomic cause of obstruction, suggesting either intermittent dynamic obstruction of the distal aorta or intermittent peripheral vasospasm. Finally, patients with ischemic syndromes may actually have no ongoing anatomic obstruction, and the clinician and angiographer may be observing a post-ischemic sequella such as acute tubular necrosis or spinal cord stunning following temporary ischemia and reperfusion.

17.5.3
Diagnosis of Branch Vessel Obstruction

The goal of cross-sectional imaging such as CT or MRA is to rule out ischemic anatomy, either by demonstrating that the flap spares major vessel origins (no static obstruction present) or by demonstrating an adequate aortic lumen from the heart to the level of the critical vessel origin (no dynamic obstruction present). When either static or dynamic obstruction is suspected, angiographic evaluation is indicated (Table 17.24).

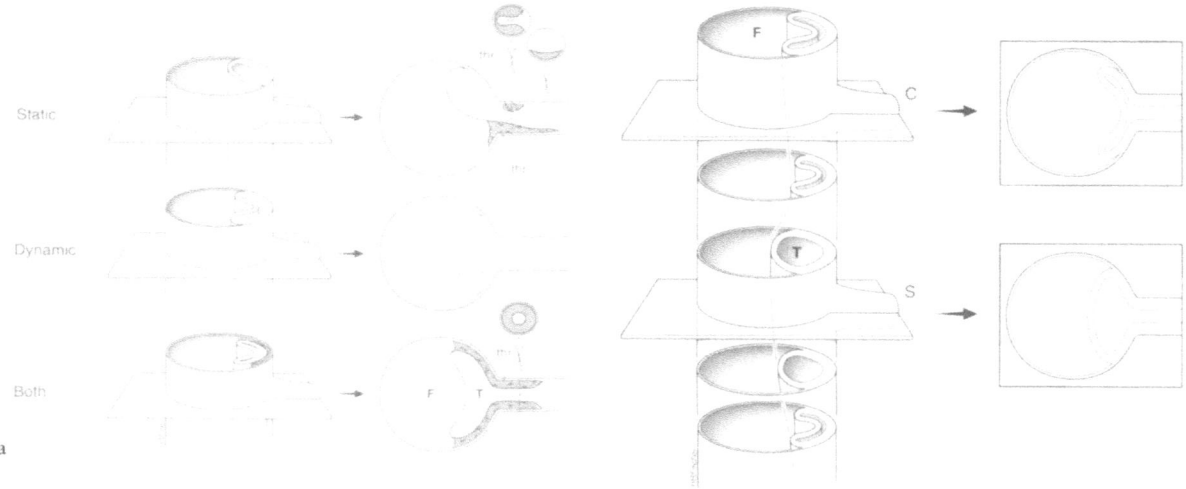

Fig. 17.72 a. Two types of branch vessel obstruction by aortic dissection. In static obstruction, the dissection flap intersects the branch vessel origin. In dynamic obstruction, the flap does not intersect the origin, but prolapses across the origin, covering it like a curtain. **b** Dynamic obstruction of the aorta above a branch-vessel origin will also compromise that vessel, such as *S* in, even though the flap appears to spare the vessel origin itself. (Reprinted with permission from WILLIAMS et al. 1997b)

Table 17.24. Static and dynamic obstruction of aortic branch vessels: angiographic features and treatment

	Static	Dynamic
Dissection flap	Intersects vessel origin	Does not intersect vessel origin, is concave toward false lumen, covers vessel origin like a curtain
Manometry	Pressure gradient between organ hilum or limb and the parent aortic lumen	Pressure deficit between aortic true and false lumens
Treatment	Stent in branch vessel origin	Balloon fenestration, possible stent in aortic true lumen

Angiographic work-up includes true and false lumen aortography and manometry, intravascular ultrasound (US), and selective renal, mesenteric, or lower extremity arteriography and manometry. Intravascular US within the aortic true and false lumens identifies the true and false lumens, demonstrates the relations of the dissection flap with the aortic branch artery origins, depicts the size of the aortic lumens from the aortic valve to the bifurcation, and documents the spatial relation of the true and false lumens to guide balloon fenestration (LEE et al. 1997). Aortography within the aortic true and false lumens and selective arteriography demonstrate patency and flow dynamics of lumens and branch arteries. Manometry in the aortic true and false lumens and in branch arteries is useful to document perfusion pressure deficits which need to be addressed by interventional means. Equipment capable of dual pressure measurements allows rapid assessment of pressure gradients.

The exact features of the angiographic work-up depend on the availability of intravascular US, the acuity of the dissection, and the suspected malperfusion syndrome (renal, mesenteric, lower extremity, or clinically indeterminate combination). A negative work-up ends with the demonstration of normal flow and perfusion pressures from the aortic valve to the limb(s) or organ(s) at risk. For example, in the setting of abdominal pain and suspected mesenteric ischemia, a negative work-up might consist of intravascular US to examine the superior mesenteric and celiac origins (flap does not intersect origins and the aortic true lumen appears of adequate caliber from the aortic valve to the visceral origins); pressure measurements in the ascending aorta and in the aortic true and false lumens at the level of the superior mesenteric artery (all pressures equal, confirming the intravascular US findings); and selective superior mesenteric arteriography (patent superior mesenteric artery and vein, patent portal vein).

17.5.4
Percutaneous Balloon Fenestration

The technical skills required for this procedure are in the repertoire of most interventional radiologists. The absolute prerequisites are to know the spatial relationships of the aortic true and false lumens from the diaphragm to the aortic bifurcation and to know which lumen supplies each of the major branch arteries. In addition, it is helpful to be able to catheterize the aortic true and false lumens at will, and so it is helpful to know the location of naturally occurring reentry tears. The technique is illustrated in (Fig. 17.73) (WILLIAMS et al. 1997a).

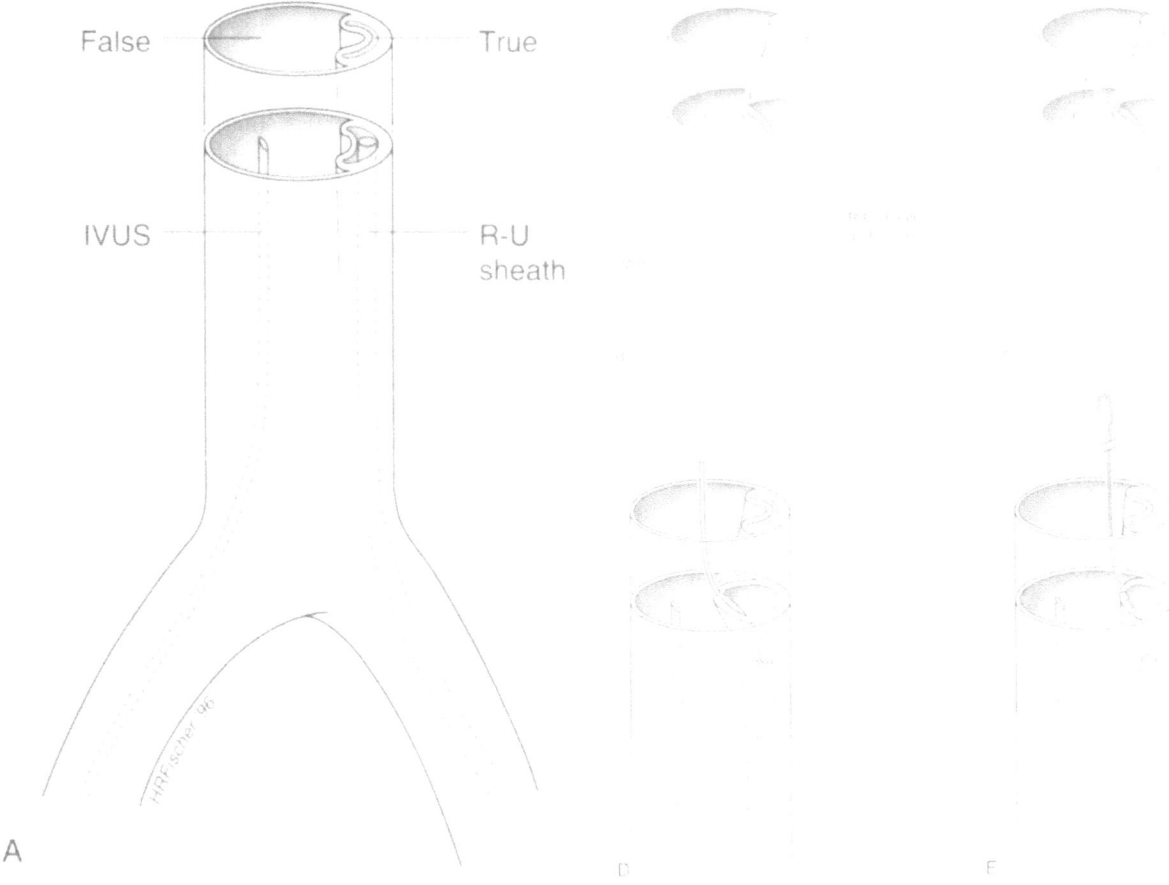

Fig. 17.23 a–g. Technique of percutaneous balloon fenestration using intravascular ultrasound (IVUS) guidance. In the absence of IVUS monitoring of the procedure, an angioplasty balloon or wire basket may be placed in the target lumen to guide needle-perforation of the dissection flap. In (**a**), the IVUS probe is in the false lumen, the Rosch-Uchida (R-U) sheath (Cook Inc, Bloomington, IN, USA) in the true lumen. The R-U needle assembly is aimed toward the false lumen approximately perpendicular to the flap (**b**), whereupon the trocar is advanced across the flap in a short quick thrust (**c**). The inner 5-F catheter is advanced over the trocar, and the trocar is removed (**d**). Contrast or saline is injected to verify (by fluoroscopy or IVUS, respectively) that the catheter has crossed to the opposite lumen. A guidewire is then placed across the flap (**e**), and the perforation is extended with a 14-mm angioplasty balloon (**f**) to create the gaping fenestration or reentry tear (**g**). (Reprinted with permission from WILLIAMS et al. 1997a

17.5.5
Treatment of Branch Vessel Obstruction

Approximately 90% of branch vessel obstructions due to acute type I aortic dissection respond to aortic reconstructive surgery. However, advanced mesenteric or lower extremity ischemia is a relative contraindication to emergent surgical repair because of the attendant high mortality. When aortic reconstructive surgery is not indicated, conventional treatment of branch vessel obstructions is surgical bypass of the threatened organ or limb, the complication-specific approach (ELEFTERIADES et al. 1992). Recent reports indicate that these branch vessel obstructions can be managed effectively by percutaneous means (SLONIM et al. 1996; WALKER et al. 1993; WILLIAMS et al. 1997a).

17.5.5.1
Dynamic Obstruction

In dynamic obstruction, aortic branch arteries are sequestered from the hemodynamically competent lumen by the dissection flap, which prolapses across branch origins like a washcloth over a bathtub drain. In the classic dissection with an entry tear in the proximal third of the thoracic aorta, compromised branches almost always originate from the true lumen, and true lumen pressure is less than or equal to false lumen pressure. Treatment of dynamic obstruction requires establishing interluminal flow between the hemodynamically competent (usually the false) lumen and the compromised (usually the true) lumen. Percutaneous balloon fenestration creates a transverse tear in the dissection flap, resulting in interluminal pressure equilibration and blood flow. At times, the true lumen remains collapsed despite restoration of flow at one level, and in these cases it is necessary to supplement fenestration by deployment of an uncovered stent in the segment of aortic true lumen between the fenestration tear and the critical artery. When possible, we avoid deploying a stent across the superior mesenteric and renal artery origins.

17.5.5.2
Static Obstruction

In static obstruction, the dissection enters a branch artery and narrows the lumen. In our experience, these lesions are highly elastic, are unresponsive to unassisted balloon angioplasty, and are best treated

by primary stenting. As noted above, branch arteries thus compromised are usually served by the true lumen, and the stent is deployed from the branch lumen, across the origin, into the aortic true lumen. In certain circumstances it may be necessary to stent from the branch artery into the aortic false lumen.

One caveat should be kept in mind: Restoration of aortic true lumen flow into newly opened large branch arteries can initiate or exacerbate dynamic obstruction of the true lumen. Consequently, following treatment of static obstruction, the aortic lumens should be resurveyed by intravascular US and manometry (Fig. 17.74) (WILLIAMS et al. 1997a).

When obstruction has both dynamic and static components, we favor correcting the dynamic component first for two reasons. Firstly, as noted above, treatment of significant static obstruction can initiate or exacerbate dynamic obstruction. Secondly, the overall pressure deficit is the sum of a central (aortic) deficit due to dynamic obstruction and a peripheral (branch artery) deficit due to the oroficial stenosis by the dissection flap. Attempting to correct the peripheral deficit first may be misleading in that flow across the stenosis may not be optimal (and consequently a hemodynamically significant stenosis may be masked) until the central perfusion deficit is corrected. Fenestration equalizes pressures between the true and false lumens, and the branch artery stent equalizes pressure between the organ/limb and its parent lumen.

17.5.5.3
Other Obstructions

As noted above, branch vessel obstructions can be due to distal emboli as well as transformation of a sub-critical stenosis to a critical lesion by the dissecting flap. These obstructions are treated using conventional interventional techniques, with the exception of the relative contraindication to urokinase or other pharmocologic lytic therapy in this clinical setting.

17.5.6
Clinical Results

17.5.6.1
Technical Success and 30-Day Mortality

In our recently reported series of 24 patients with infradiaphragmatic branch vessel compromise due to aortic dissection (summarized in Table 17.25), obstruction was present in 77 out of 144 branch arteries (including celiac, superior mesenteric, right and left main renal, and right and left common iliac arteries). Obstruction was static in 12 arteries, dynamic in 45, both static and dynamic in 17, and indeterminate in three. Percutaneous techniques resulted in restoring flow to 71 (92%) of the obstructed branch arteries. Six patients died within 1 month (25% 30-day mortality): two due to systemic inflammatory response syndrome 1 day and 3 days, respectively, after successful restoration of flow to the superior mesenteric artery; one due to renal failure 1 day after restoration of flow to one kidney in a patient whose family refused dialysis; one due to tamponade 7 days after fenestration and stenting of the aortic true lumen; one due to rupture of the false lumen 10 days after fenestration while awaiting aortic reconstructive surgery; and one during aortic reconstructive surgery 17 days after fenestration.

17.5.6.2
Technical Complications

In two patients, potentially major technical complications occurred after restoration of flow to branch arteries compromised by static obstruction. In both patients, restoration of flow to statically obstructed branches resulted in collapse of the aortic true lumen and in the development of dynamic obstruction of several branch arteries, some of which were previously well perfused. Fortunately, both complications were recognized immediately and successfully managed percutaneously. In this respect, intravascular US allows rapid re-survey of the aorta during the procedure, whereas a pre-procedural MR or CT aortogram might be misleading due to intraprocedural changes in the aortic lumens.

17.5.6.3
Fate of the False Lumen

In 46 patients with classic aortic dissection who underwent angiography and manometry, pressure in the false lumen exceeded pressure in the true lumen in 16 and equalled it in 30. Percutaneous treatment did not alter false lumen pressure, but, by increasing true lumen pressure, reduced the peak systolic interluminal pressure gradient from a mean of 28 mmHg to 2 mmHg. The question arises whether thus decompressing the false lumen affects the long-term tendency of the false lumen to dilate. In our series, three

patients died due to complications of the false lumen, despite successful correction of flow abnormalities and equalization of pressures between the true and false lumens: one 10 days after fenestration, before proximal aortic reconstruction could be undertaken, and two with enlarging false lumens 3 months and 7 months, respectively, after fenestration. Thus, following aortic intervention for ischemic complications, the false lumen remains at risk of aneurysmal degeneration, and patients with a patent false lumen must be followed for life at intervals appropriate for the diameter of their aorta, blood pressure, symptoms, and clinical risk factors (WILLIAMS et al. 1997a).

17.5.7
Future Developments

There may also be a role for fenestration to create a reentry tear in the treatment of the dead-end false lumen, which can be associated with thrombotic and embolic complications and false lumen rupture. The role of stent-grafts in excluding the false lumen must be defined once devices of a suitable diameter are generally available. Although percutaneous methods are highly successful in restoring blood flow to compromised aortic branches, technical success does not always lead to clinical success. Improvements in clinical success of reperfusion techniques requires advances in preventing or treating systemic inflammatory response syndrome.

17.5.8
Conclusion

Contemporary cross-sectional imaging and manometry clarify the mechanisms of branch vessel obstruction in aortic dissection and modify earlier notions based on cross-clamped or post-mortem aortas. Intravascular US greatly facilitates evaluation of the aorta and its branch arteries and guides percutaneous treatment. Fenestration and stent deployment are safe and effective means of restoring blood flow in branch arteries compromised by aortic dissection. Despite the high technical success of these reperfusion techniques, the 30-day mortality is high, although favorable compared to surgical approaches to the same patient population. In our experience, mortality is due primarily to development of systemic inflammatory response syndrome and, in unoperated patients with type I dissection, to the fate of the false lumen.

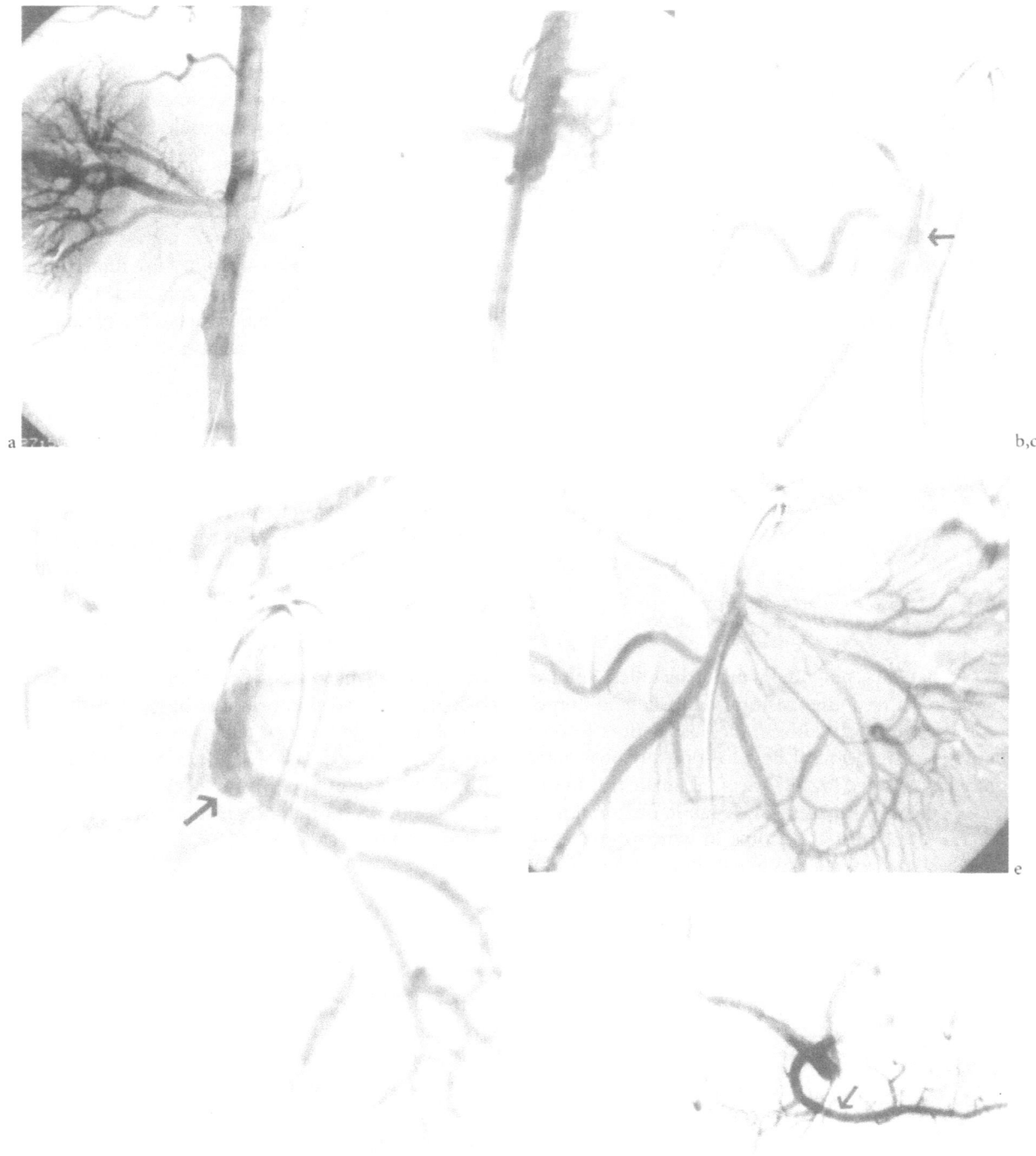

Fig. 17.24 a–j. Images from a 48-year-old male with acute type III dissection and heme-positive nasogastric aspirate. Aortic false lumen pressure was 15 mm higher than aortic true lumen pressure, indicating mild dynamic obstruction. Contrast injection into the aortic true lumen in anteroposterior (**a**) and lateral (**b**) projections filled the main and accessory right renal arteries and showed proximal occlusion of the celiac and superior mesenteric arteries (SMAs). The left renal artery filled from the false lumen (not shown). Selective injection of the true (**c**) and false (**d**) lumens of the SMA showed extensive dissection, which was associated with a 60-mm systolic gradient between the level of the right colic artery (*arrow* in **c**) and the aortic true lumen. The patent portion of the false lumen extended to the mid-jejunal level (*arrow* in **d**). Injection into the celiac trunk filled inferior phrenic arteries (not shown). Static obstruction of the superior mesenteric and celiac arteries was treated with deployment of 10-mm × 42-mm and 8-mm × 40-mm Wallstents (Schneider, Minneapolis, MN, USA), respectively. Selective injection of the superior mesenteric (**e**) and celiac (**f**) arteries after stent deployment showed filling of distal mesenteric branches, the dorsal pancreatic (*arrow* in **f**), and left gastric artery, from which the left hepatic artery originated. The right hepatic and splenic arteries did not fill. Repeat contrast injection of the aortic true lumen in anteroposterior (**g**) and lateral (**h**) projections showed improved filling and washout compared to baseline aortography, indicating relief of static (Continued on next page)

Fig. 17.24 a–j. (Continued) . . . obstruction (**i**, *top left*), which was confirmed by manometry. Following restoration of celiac and SMA flow, the aortic true lumen at the level of the SMA was unchanged (**i**, *bottom left*; *arrowhead* points to Wallstent). However, at the level of the main right renal artery (*arrow* in **i**, *bottom middle*) and accessory right renal artery (*curved arrow* in **i**, *bottom right*), the aortic true lumen had collapsed, consistent with the development of dynamic obstruction, which was confirmed by manometry. Following fenestration and stenting of the aortic true lumen just above the level of the SMA, the aortic true lumen at the level of the main right renal artery (RR) returned to its baseline size (**j**). (Figures 17.24**b**,**i** and **j** are reprinted with permission from WILLIAMS et al. 1997a)

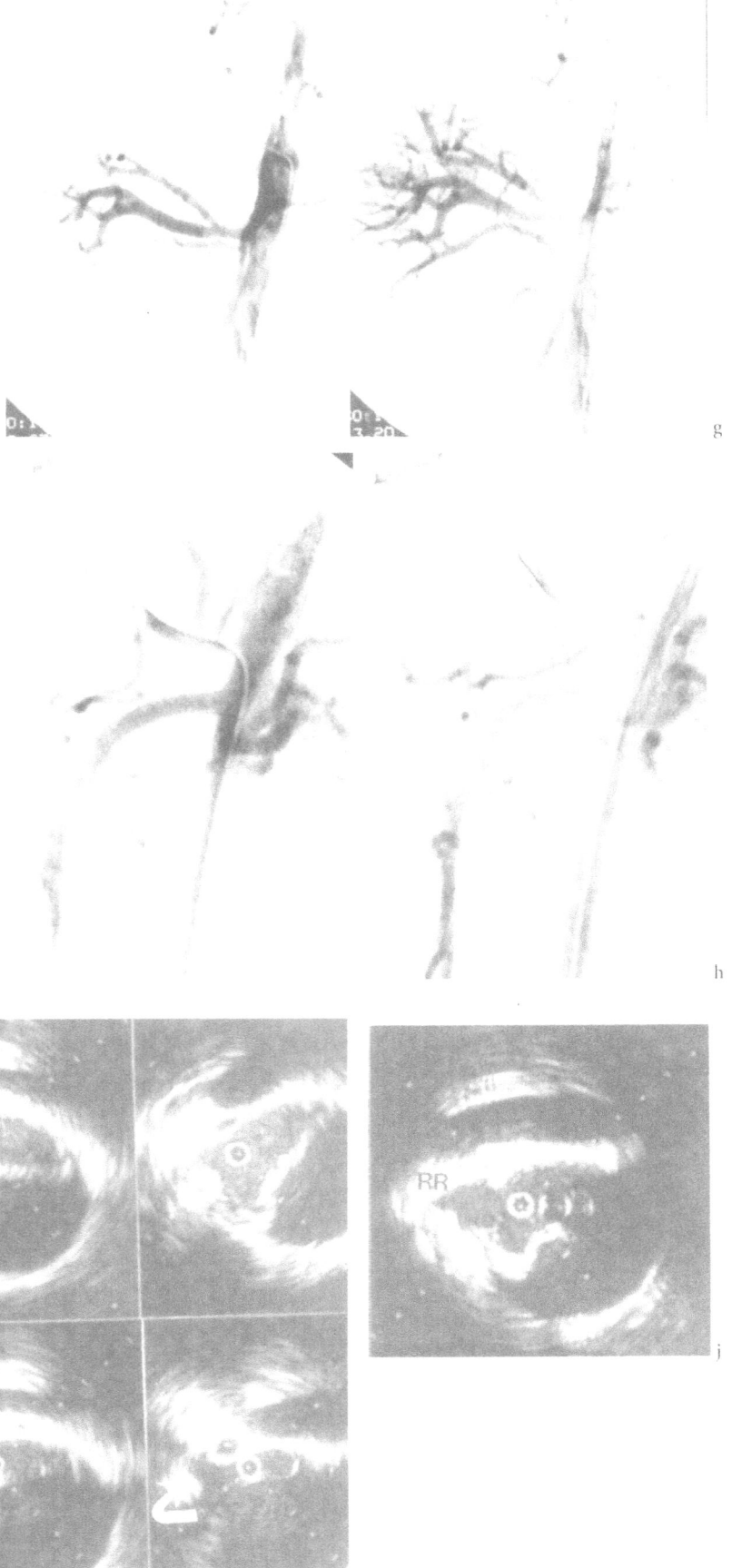

Table 17.25. Summary of treatment results

Patients (*n*)	24	
Arteries (*n*)	144	
Obstructed arteries (*n*)	77	
Type of obstruction		
Static	12	(16%)
Dynamic	45	(58%)
Static and dynamic	17	(22%)
Indeterminate	3	(4%)
Success in flow restoration	71/77	(92%)
30-Day mortality	6	(25%)
Systemic inflammatory response syndrome	2	
Renal failure	1	
Cardiac tamponade (post-operative)	1	
False lumen rupture (pre-operative)	1	
Intraoperative hemorrhage	1	

References

Cambria RP, Brewster DC, Gertler J, et al. (1988) Vascular complications associated with spontaneous aortic dissection. J Vasc Surg 7:199–209

Elefteriades JA, Hartleroad J, Gusberg RJ, Salazar AM, Black HR, Kopf GS, Baldwin JC, Hammond GL (1992) Long-term experience with descending aortic dissection: the complication-specific approach. Ann Thorac Surg 53:11–21

Fann JI, Sarris GE, Mitchell RS, Shumway NE, Stinson EB, Oyer PE, Miller DC (1990) Treatment of patients with aortic dissection presenting with peripheral vascular complications. Ann Surg 212:705–713

Lee DY, Williams DM, Abrams GD (1997) The dissected aorta. II. Differentiation of the true from the false lumen with intravascular US. Radiology 203:32–36

Slonim SM, Nyman UR, Semba CP, Miller DC, Mitchell RS, Dake MD (1996) True lumen obliteration in complicated aortic dissection: endovascular treatment. Radiology 201:161–166

Walker PJ, Dake MD, Mitchell RS, Miller DC (1993) The use of endovascular techniques for the treatment of complications of aortic dissection. J Vasc Surg 18:1042–1051

Williams DM, Lee DY, Hamilton B, Marx MV, Narasimham DI, Kazanjian SN, Prince MR, Cho KJ, Andrews JC, Deeb GM (1997a) The dissected aorta. Percutaneous treatment of ischemic complications – principles and results. J Vasc Intervent Radiol (in press)

Williams DM, Lee DY, Hamilton B, Marx MV, Narasimham DI, Kazanjian SN, Prince MR, Cho KJ, Andrews JC, Deeb GM (1997b) The dissected aorta. III. Anatomy and radiologic diagnosis of branch-vessel compromise. Radiology 203:37–44

18 Paraaortic Diseases

E. ZEITLER

CONTENTS

Disorders of the mesenteric and renal arteries occur either in isolation, or in the framework of generalized arteriosclerosis and a number of systemic diseases [arterial embolisms, diabetes mellitus, fibromuscular dysplasia (FMD), Recklinghausen's disease, among others]. The radiologist should always consider, in the form of a general overview, the possibility of other pathologic conditions, or of a dominating clinical condition of the renal and unpaired arteries (Table 18.1) (MORRIS et al. 1966; RÖSCH and STECKEL 1972; WENZ et al. 1972). Abdominal aortography provides excellent information on all intestinal, renal, and pelvic arteries (Fig. 18.1).

18.1
Celiac and Mesenteric Arteries

Via its branches, the celiac trunk supplies the digestive system from the stomach to the duodenum, the liver, the pancreas, and the spleen. The superior mesenteric artery feeds the small bowel and the colon, down to the flexura lienalis. The inferior mesenteric artery is the vessel supplying the descending colon, sigmoid colon, and rectum. Both the celiac trunk and the superior and inferior mesenteric artery arise from the front of the aorta. (RÖSCH and STECKEL 1972; ABRAMS 1983; BOIJSEN 1983). The celiac trunk is an arterial segment of 1–4 cm in length, which

Table 18.1. Paraaortic arterial diseases

Acute mesenteric ischemia
Angina abdominalis
Renovascular hypertension

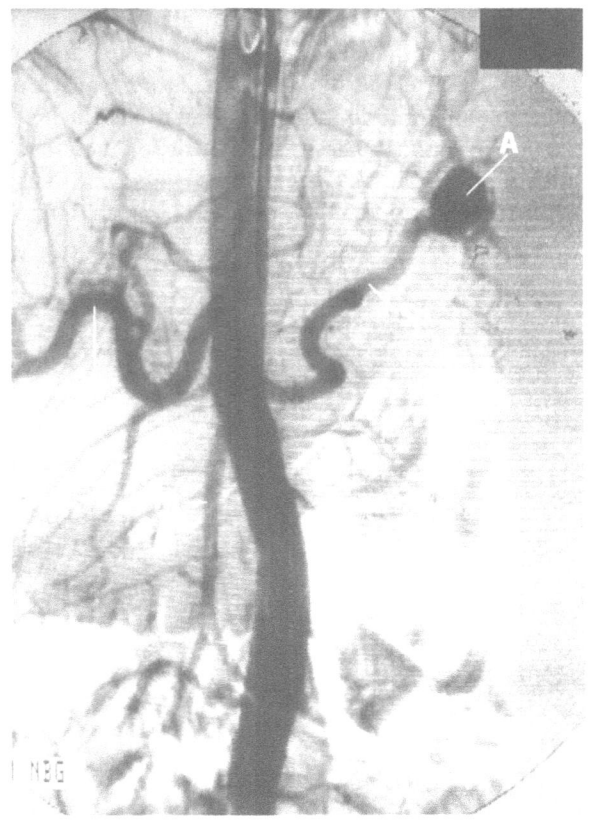

Fig. 18.1. Abdominal aortography in a patient (51-year-old man) with bilateral renal shrinkage, demonstrating the hepatic (H), splenic (Sp), superior mesenteric (m), renal (r), and gastroduodenal (g) arteries, and a splenic artery aneurysm (A)

E. ZEITLER, Professor, MD, Virchowstraße 13, D-90409 Nürnberg, Germany

originates directly below the diaphragm. In exceptional cases (about 0.4%), the celiac trunk and the superior mesenteric artery have a common main trunk. In 65% of cases (KADIR 1991), the celiac trunk splits up into three arteries, the lienal artery, the common hepatic artery, and the left gastric artery (Fig. 18.1). In 18%–20% of instances, the superior mesenteric artery extends one artery to the liver, typically the right hepatic artery, which arises from the superior mesenteric artery. The common hepatic artery arises from the superior mesenteric artery in 2.5% of cases (KADIR 1991). On aortography or selective arteriography, the supplying arteries to the pancreas and adrenals can often provide important information (ATHANASOULIS et al. 1982; BOOKSTEIN 1983; VAN DONGEN 1988).

18.1.1
Acute Mesenteric Ischemia

Acute obstruction of the branching point of the celiac trunk can be caused by an arterial embolism, arterial thrombosis, aortic dissection, abdominal aortic aneurysm, trauma, or external compression. In 90% of cases, acute obliterations of the superior mesenteric artery are embolisms. Other causes of superior mesenteric artery obliterations include: aortic dissection, arterial thrombosis, or the effects of abdominal trauma (ATHANASOULIS 1982; MORRIS et al. 1966; ROB 1966; GIESSLER 1974; VAN DONGEN

are the most common predisposing condition, and the superior mesenteric artery is the most frequently affected, with important clinical consequences (BOIJSEN 1983b).

Embolism of the mesenteric arteries (Fig. 18.2) always results in mesenteric infarction, unless a collateral circulation has developed beforehand, or an aggressive roentgenologic and surgical approach is initiated as early as possible (BOLEY et al. 1973). The formation of the mesenteric infarction depends on the site of occlusion.

The symptoms of mesenteric artery embolism include:
- Diffuse, persistent pain of varying intensity in the abdomen.
- Initially, obstipation occurs, later diarrhea.
- In the acute stage, the first symptom can be cardiovascular shock.
- Clinically, there is a differentiation between the initial stage (1–6 h), and the silent, symptom-free interval (7–12 h), during which phase there is tolerable persistent pain. With the disappearance of bowel peristalsis, the patient's general condition deteriorates.
- The final stage, occurring 12–48 h after onset, involves the manifestation of peronitis, paralytic ileus, and protracted shock. The second stage is that of a deceptive silence, during which an invasive diagnosis should be forced (ATHANASOULIS 1982; BOLEY et al. 1973).

Most of the specific literature only describes the

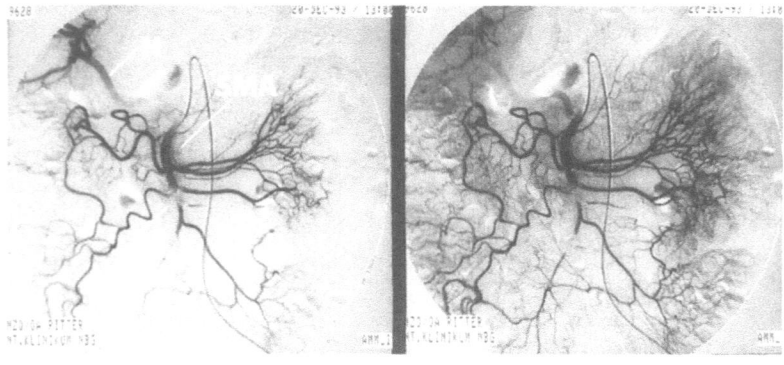

Fig. 18.2 . Selective arteriography of a superior mesenteric artery (*SMA*), demonstrating embolic occlusions. The right hepatic artery arises from the superior mesenteric artery

1988; VAN DONGEN and SCHWILDEN 1976; VOLLMAR 1996).

According to an analysis of all arterial embolisms (see Chap. 19, Sect. 19.1), those of the mesenteric arteries account for about 6% of cases, those of the branches of the celiac trunk and renal arteries for about 5%, whereas the incidence of embolisms of the pelvic and leg arteries is about 50%. Cardiac diseases

roentgenologic situation in general X-rays of the abdomen in standing, side, and supine positions whereby a positive finding is only achieved during the stage of paralytic ileus. Also, sonography provides additional information at this stage, unless the exclusion of other pathologic conditions is the main purpose of the examination. If the anamnesis includes known cardiac diseases, including the risk of embolism, selective mesentericography should be performed without delay (WENZ et al. 1972; BOLEY et al. 1973; ATHANASOULIS 1982; BOIJSEN 1983; VOLLMAR 1996).

While embolisms in the area of the vessels of the celiac trunk mostly have a promising prognosis, that of embolisms of the superior mesenteric artery is poor. In such cases, an interdisciplinary therapeutic concept should be quickly formulated (BOLEY et al. 1973). After selective arteriography and diagnostic confirmation of either an acute thrombosis of the mesenteric artery, or one or several embolic occlusions, arterial pump infusion of papaverin (60 mg/h) can be started immediately (ATHANASOULIS 1982). In addition, local thrombolysis can follow promptly. Apart from the publication of individual cases, however, the result of the latter in a larger patient population with embolism of the mesenteric artery is not yet available. The currently recognized therapeutic concept (VOLLMAR 1996) is orientated by the findings of mesentericography. Only if mesentericography cannot be performed, or results are not available, is a primary laparotomy, as well as a second-look operation, recommended. In the case of occlusion of a major trunk, embolectomy takes priority, which, in the event intestinal necrosis has already developed, additionally requires intestinal resection (BOLEY et al. 1973; VOLLMAR 1996).

Irrespective of the outcome, a repeat angiography and secondary laparotomy (second-look operation), including the vitality test of the intestine, may become necessary. The patient requires close follow-up on an intensive-care unit, with ultrasound or computed tomography (CT) checks, and measures to prevent deep venous thrombosis.

18.1.2
Chronic Intestinal Ischemia (Abdominal Angina, Intestinal Angina, Maladie d'Ortner)

Arteriosclerotic changes at the celiac trunk and the superior and inferior mesenteric artery are considered causes of chronic perfusive disorders (FRY and KRAFT 1963; MORRIS et al. 1966; ROB 1966; VAN DONGEN and SCHWILDEN 1976; VOLLMAR 1976). A clinical picture rarely occurs in the case of isolated obliteration of one of these three unpaired vessels. This is attributable to the existence of preformed collateral arteries between the celiac trunk and the superior mesenteric artery (Fig. 18.3), and to Riolan's collateral between the middle colic artery and the left colic artery, which connects the arterial

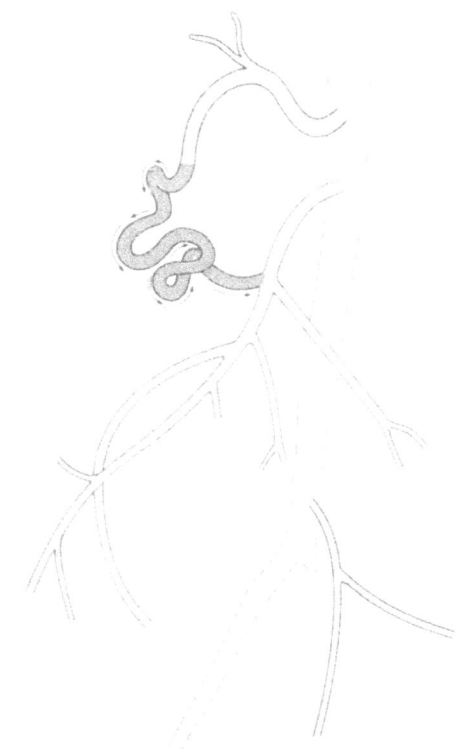

Fig. 18.3. Communication between superior and inferior gastroduodenal artery, the important pre-existing collateral pathway between the celiac and superior mesenteric arteries

area of the superior mesenteric artery and inferior mesenteric artery (Figs. 18.4 and 18.5) (DIEMEL et al. 1964; WENZ et al. 1972; GIESSLER 1974).

In the case of infrarenal aortic occlusion, Riolan's collateral is capable of bridging the aortic occlusion, bypassing the superior mesenteric artery via the inferior mesenteric artery to the hypogastric artery in a craniocaudal direction; or, conversely, caudocranial collateral circulation in the case of occlusion of the superior mesenteric artery and/or obliterations of the celiac trunk (Fig. 18.5). This example of a patient with abdominal angina shows how, from the inferior mesenteric artery, via Riolan's collateral, the last vessel depicted is the celiac trunk, including its branches (Fig. 18.5c and 18.6). Figure 18.5 shows a simultaneous occlusion of the common iliac artery on the left side, which is bypassed by both the mesenteric artery and the lumbar arteries, to the hypogastric artery. The lateral projection of the abdominal aorta (Fig. 18.6) demonstrates stenosis of the celiac artery and superior mesenteric artery occlusion. Combined obliterations of intestinal and extremity arteries demonstrate the general arteriosclerotic diseases.

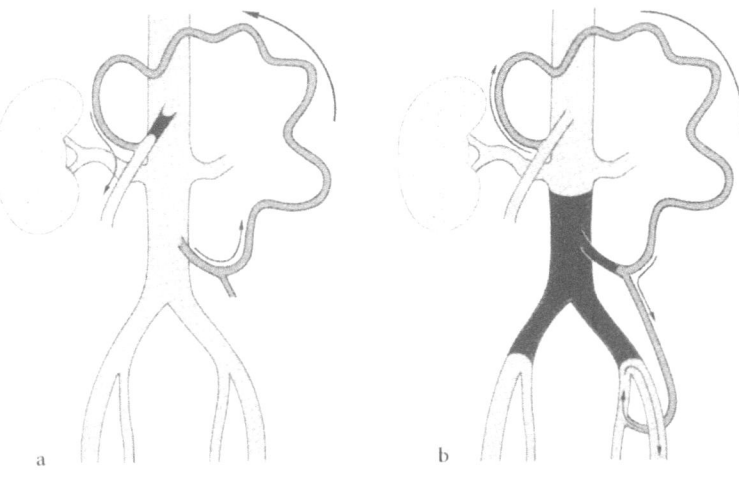

Fig. 18.4 a,b. Riolan's collateral circulation between the middle colic and left colic arteries. **a** Occlusion of the superior mesenteric artery (SMA), blood-flow direction from below (inferior mesenteric arteries) to the SMA. **b** Occlusion of the infrarenal aorta and common iliac arteries. Blood-flow direction from above (SMA) to below (inferior mesenteric artery), bypassing the occlusion, and flow into the left hypogastric artery

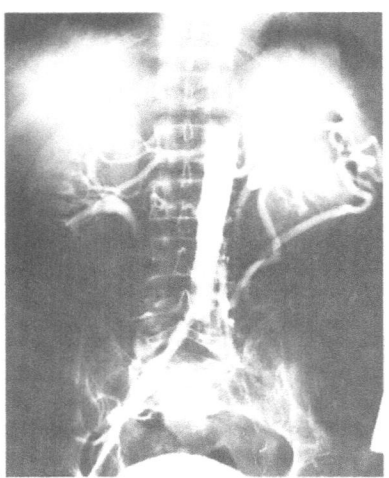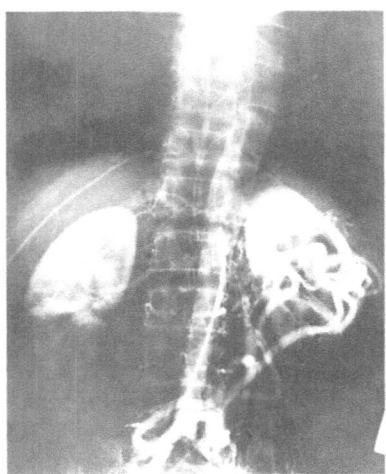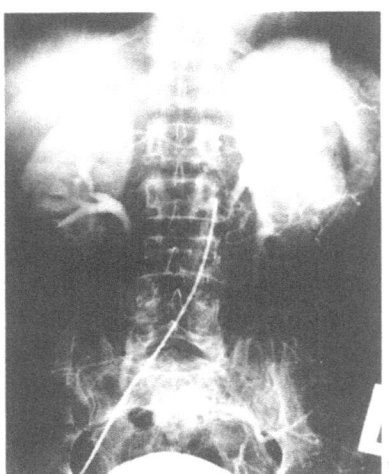

Fig. 18.5 a–c. Aortography of a 55-year-old man with abdominal angina (Ortner's syndrome). **a** Caudocranial contrast enhancement of Riolan's artery; **b** additional occlusion of the left common iliac artery; **c** late contrasted branches of the celiac trunk, behind the stenosis

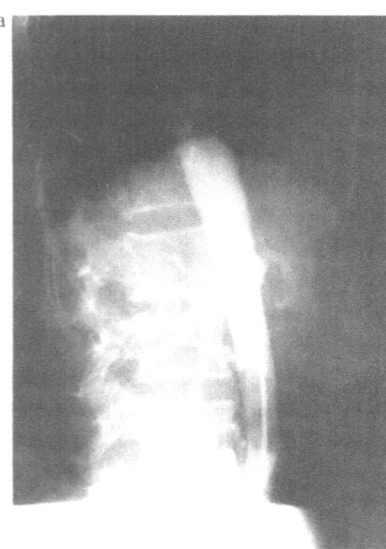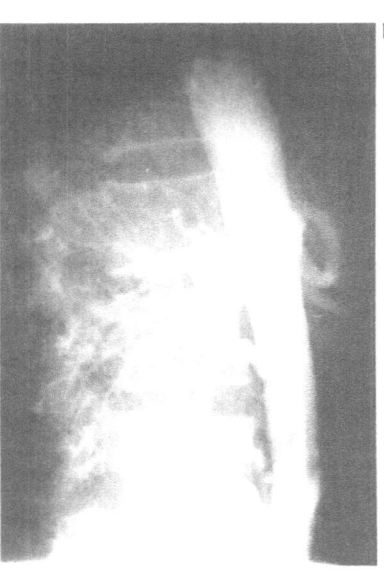

Fig. 18.6 a,b. Same patient as in Fig. 18.5. Aortography, lateral projection. **a** Stenosis of the celiac artery and occlusion of the SMA. **b** Retrogarde filling through Riolan's artery

In Fig. 18.7, this is the case in a patient with arterial hypertension, claudication with pain in the buttock and thigh, as well as in the calf, and abdominal pain which starts on walking exercise. The angiography demonstrates in an anteroposterior projection (Fig. 18.7a,b) extensive arteriosclerotic changes in the left renal artery, with a left shrinking kidney, stenosis of the inferior mesenteric artery, and a left common iliac artery occlusion with collateral circulation from the inferior mesenteric artery to the hypogastric artery and external iliac artery.

The lateral view (Fig. 18.7c) demonstrates a circular stenosis of the celiac trunk. The differential diagnosis between arteriosclerotic stenosis and compression of muscle fibers from the diaphragm is not easy. Therefore, the treatment was thromboendarterectomy of the left common iliac artery, whereupon the steal disappeared. There was no further need for surgery in the area of the celiac trunk and left kidney.

Creatinine levels demonstrated compensated renal function.

This situation has been described several times (MAY and NISSL 1965; BÜCHELER et al. 1967; ABRAMS 1983a). In an important article on the problems of steal syndromes, VOLLMAR (1971) postulated that:

1. Syndromes only exist if clinical symptoms exist, such that the demonstration of a collateral circulation alone does not necessarily indicate a syndrome, but at most an effect (e.g., subclavian steal effect).
2. It is more realistic to name the syndrome according to the artery that steals the blood. Working on this premise, the collateral circulation mentioned here is not a mesenteric steal syndrome, but a "hypogastric steal syndrome".

The symptoms of abdominal angina include colic

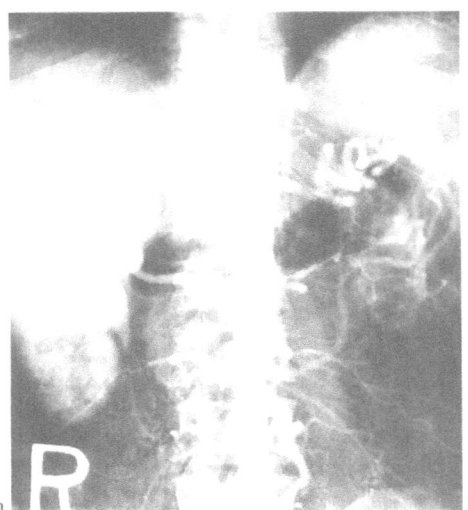
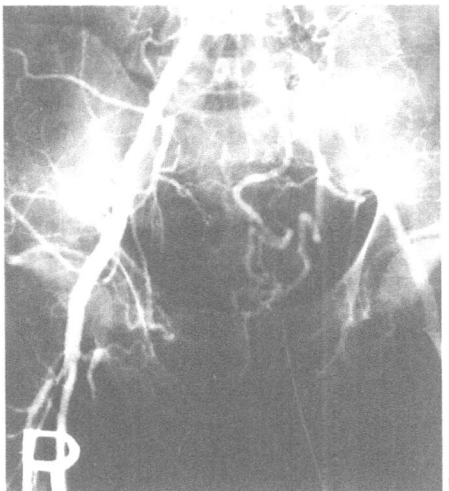
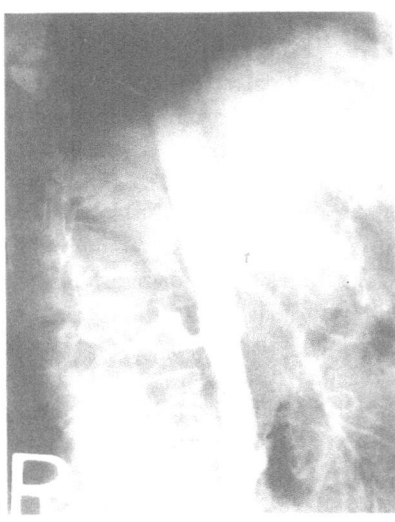

Fig. 18.7 a–c. Aorto-arteriography (59-year-old man), multilocular arteriosclerotic obliterations. Claudication of the left leg: "hypogastric steal syndrome" (mesenteric steal syndrome). Left shrinking kidney with diffuse arteriosclerotic obstructions. a Arteriosclerotic narrowing of the left renal artery, stenosis of the inferior mesenteric artery. b Occlusion, common iliac artery on the left; collateral pathway to the hypogastric artery. c Lateral projection with stenosis of the celiac and inferior mesenteric arteries

pain in the epigastric region and mediate abdominal cavity, occurring as a rule 30–60 min after a meal and eating within 1–2 h. The fear of strong pain following substantial meals leads the patient to consume only small meals ("small meal syndrome") (Rob 1966). The consequence is an increasing loss of appetite, whereby vomiting provides relief. This reinforces the vicious circle of increasing loss of appetite (Giessler 1974).

Abdominal angina can often be found in patients with simultaneous coronary or peripheral comorbidity, but in whom only the abdominal symptoms are dominant. The diagnosis needs to be confirmed if sonography has produced suspicious findings. Although to date a reliable imaging technique has been biplane catheter aortography, angiography with three-dimensional (3D) imaging using new scanning systems, such as spiral CT or magnetic resonance angiography (MRA) (Schoenberg et al. 1999), can also be considered capable of optimum visualization of obliterations and collateral circulations (see Chap. 12). Any abdominal angina not attributable to vascular disorders, but rather tumor compression (Borm and Müller-Wiefel 1970) and hemorrhage, can thus be identified and localized.

On the other hand, the low-toxic, non-ionic contrast agents and atraumatic soft-tip catheter systems currently used have also reduced the risk associated with digital subtraction angiography (DSA) to such an extent that it now offers a fast diagnosis at low risk (Boley et al. 1973; Athanasoulis 1982). The advantage of angiography, therefore, is the possibility of starting an immediate therapeutic approach in the case of acute perfusive disorders of the visceral arteries. In the same way, the therapeutic procedure of balloon dilatation for chronic obliterations can be completed, if necessary, by stent implantation, whereby the patient needs to be informed accordingly beforehand.

The first balloon dilatation performed for upper abdominal pain was the dilatation of a superior mesenteric artery stenosis (Furrer et al. 1980). A summary of about 50 cases of PTA in visceral arteries was provided by Mahler in 1990. Of these cases, 13 were dilatations of celiac artery stenoses, while the majority were stenoses of the superior mesenteric artery. A total of 20% required redilatation, which corresponds to the incidence of restenoses in the coronary arteries. Mahler attributes the rare cases of dilatations of visceral arteries to the fact that abdominal angina is not a common clinical picture, the majority of patients being first referred to visceral surgery, and that the PTA technique in the visceral

arteries is somewhat difficult to perform. A fact worthy of attention is that external compression can also narrow the visceral arteries, such that in all cases, including suspected compression by a tumor, a precise diagnostic examination using a scanning method (CT or MRI) should precede any further therapeutic decisions.

However, several authors (Diemel et al. 1964; Morris et al. 1966; Cen et al. 1972; Van Dongen 1976; Vollmar 1996) have reported on patients who were completely symptom-free, despite existing stenoses or even occlusions.

The decisive aspect that can be derived from questionable abdominal complaints is that, in patients with arterial vascular diseases, the physician should not only concentrate on the feet, coronary arteries, and brain, but also consider other regions, although abdominal angina is a rare diagnosis. The patient suffers considerable loss in weight.

Figure 18.8 shows an example of a concentric stenosis of the celiac and superior mesenteric arteries in a patient before and after balloon dilatation. In the Nuremberg clinics, of five stenoses of visceral arteries which we treated by dilatation, one case included stent implantation, and four cases needed balloon dilatation only. One stenosis was dilated a second time 3 months later, and no operative treatment became necessary.

18.2
Renal Artery Obliterations

The lumbar and renal arteries are regularly documented within the framework of aortography. At this time, the existence of multiple renal arteries can often be clearly identified, which may also pose some problems in the differential diagnosis. In the angiographic literature (Boijsen 1983), multiple renal arteries were reported in 20%–27%. Sometimes, very small additional renal arteries are too small, with the result that they are misinterpreted as capsular arteries. Collateral vessels to the kidneys can indicate a collateral circulation in renal artery obliterations (Abrams 1983a; Boijsen 1983).

In kidneys with multiple arteries, one main stem usually arises from the aorta at a normal level. Most of the supplementary arteries go to the lower renal pole, some to the upper pole (Figure 18.9). Supplementary arteries arising from the aorta are segmental, or subsegmental arteries. Supplementary renal arteries also can arise from the iliac, mesenteric, and lumbar arteries. The wide variations in the origin

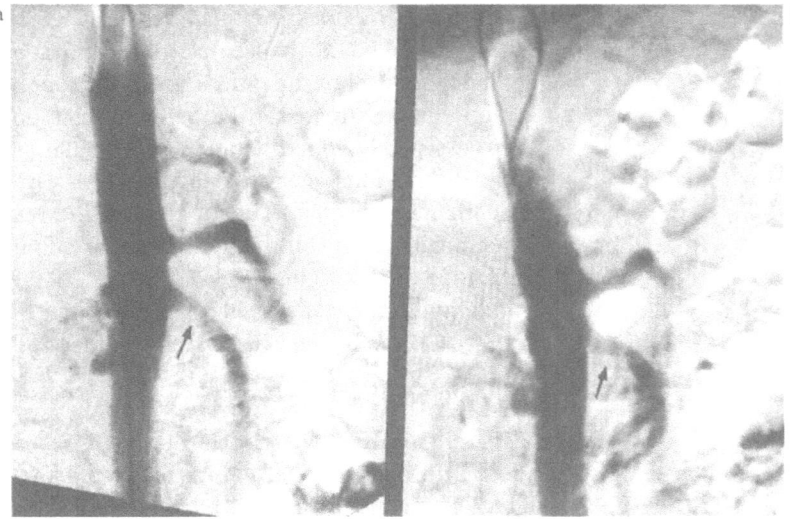

Fig. 18.8 a,b. Aortography (lateral projection) of a patient with angina abdominalis and stenoses in the celiac artery, superior mesenteric artery (SMA), and inferior mesenteric artery (IMA) occlusion: before (**a**), and after balloon dilatation (**b**)

and course of multiple renal arteries was well explained by the development of the mesonephric arteries (FELIX 1911). These arteries develop on each side of the aorta and are distributed from the sixth cervical to the third lumbar segments. The appearance of vascular anomalies is thus the result of unusual parts in the primitive vascular plexuses and the persistence of vessels normally obliterated.

18.2.1
Stenoses and Occlusions

In the diagnosis of renovascular hypertension, it is important to make the diagnosis not only with selective renal angiographies, because of several obliterations at the ostium of renal arteries (Fig. 18.10), and also of supplementary renal and visceral arteries (Fig. 18.7). In addition, midaortic stenoses, which are also summarized under abdominal coarctation, can

also induce arterial hypertension. Therefore, selective and semi-selective renal angiography is only an additional procedure for the diagnosis of intrarenal arterial lesions (Figs. 18.11 and 18.12), and part of the renal artery interventions (ABRAMS 1983a; ARLART 1997).

The most common cause of renal artery stenosis is arteriosclerosis. It is usually observed in patients over 40 years of age, and is more common in men. A distinction is made between three different types of arteriosclerosis in renal arteries:

1. *Ostial stenoses:* These are stenoses close to the inner lumen of the aorta, which are partially the result of arteriosclerotic degeneration of the aorta itself (Fig. 18.10). These types of arteriosclerotic renal artery stenoses have a limited chance of being successfully treated by balloon dilatation alone. Therefore, vascular surgery or stent-assisted balloon angioplasty are indicated as alternative treatments.

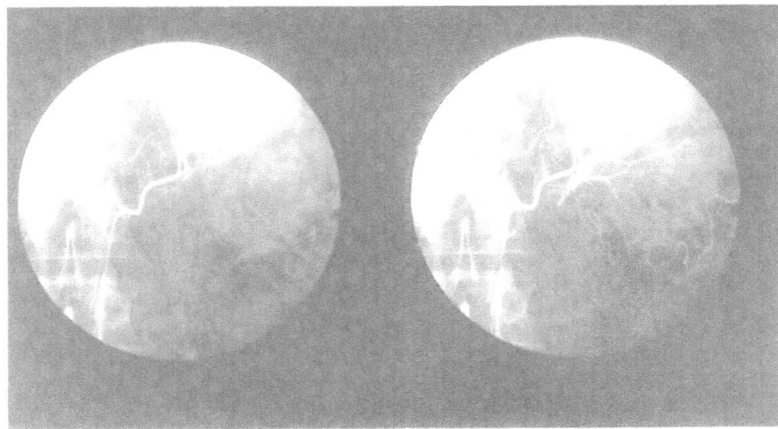

Fig. 18.9. Renal artery occlusion (51-year-old male patient). Selective arteriography of the upper pole artery demonstrates good run-off behind the total obliteration. Vascular surgery was successfully performed with aorto-renal bypass (operator, Prof. Raithel)

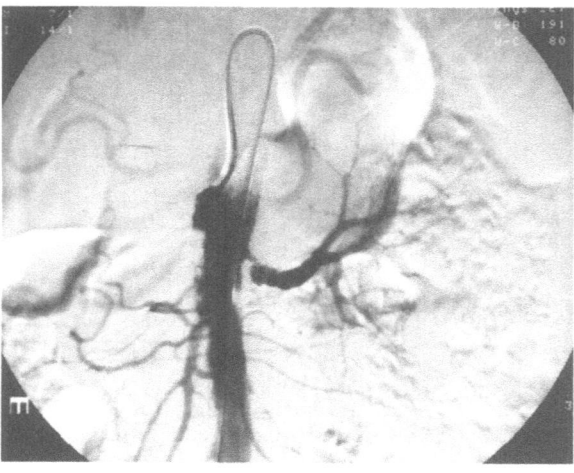

Fig. 18.10. Aorto-arteriography (54-year-old woman with renal insufficiency and arterial hypertension): arteriosclerotic ostial stenosis (left), and extensive atheromatous plaques in the aorta

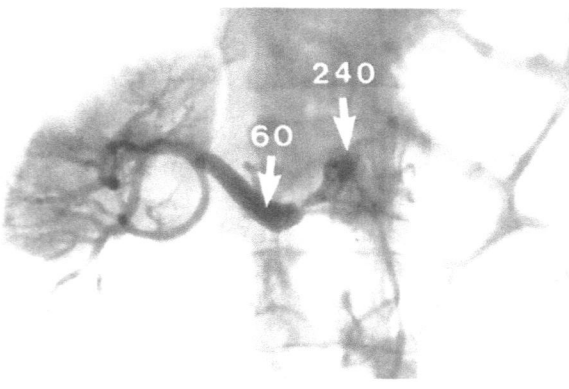

Fig. 18.11. Postostial renal artery stenosis; directly measured peak systolic blood pressure (46-year-old woman)

2. *Postostial arteriosclerotic stenoses (Fig. 18.11):* These are stenoses (concentric or excentric) at least 5 mm distal of the inner lumen of the aorta, which can be treated with balloon dilatation, stent-assisted balloon dilatation, or vascular surgery. Bifurcational stenoses (Fig. 18.12) can exist in patients with a short main stem of the renal artery, with early bifurcation. They are found mainly in the left kidney.

3. *A long-distance arteriosclerotic obliteration* (Fig. 18.7a) can be the cause of a non-functioning kidney.

In general, localized arteriosclerotic stenoses are located in the proximal third of the main stem of the renal artery. In some patients, bilateral renal artery stenoses are present (Figs. 18.14 and 18.15), and the mean age in men is 50–55 years of age, in women 60–65 years of age.

Fibromuscular dysplasia (FMD) (Fig. 18.18) is found even in children and young women, the diagnosis being mostly established between the ages of 25–45. The female-to-male incidence of FMD is 4:1 (ABRAMS 1983a). The disease is not only localized in the renal arteries, but also in the mesenteric, carotid, and external iliac arteries (see also Chap. 27). The classification, according to early histologic studies (HARRISON and McCORMACK 1971) distinguishes between the rarer forms of intimal fibrodysplasia, and adventitial or periarterial fibrosis, as well as the most common fibrodysplasia of the media including multiple aneurysmatic deformations (Fig. 18.19). Even though a histologic evaluation within the framework of interventional therapy – unlike surgical therapy – is not possible, at least a differentiation

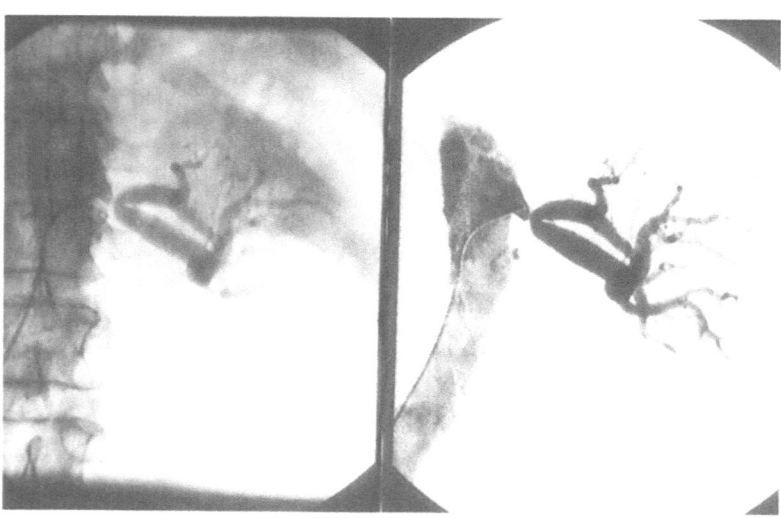

Fig. 18.12. Bifurcational renal artery stenosis; arteriosclerotic or intimal fibromuscular dysplasia is unclear without histology (47-year-old woman, blood pressure 170/105 mmHg)

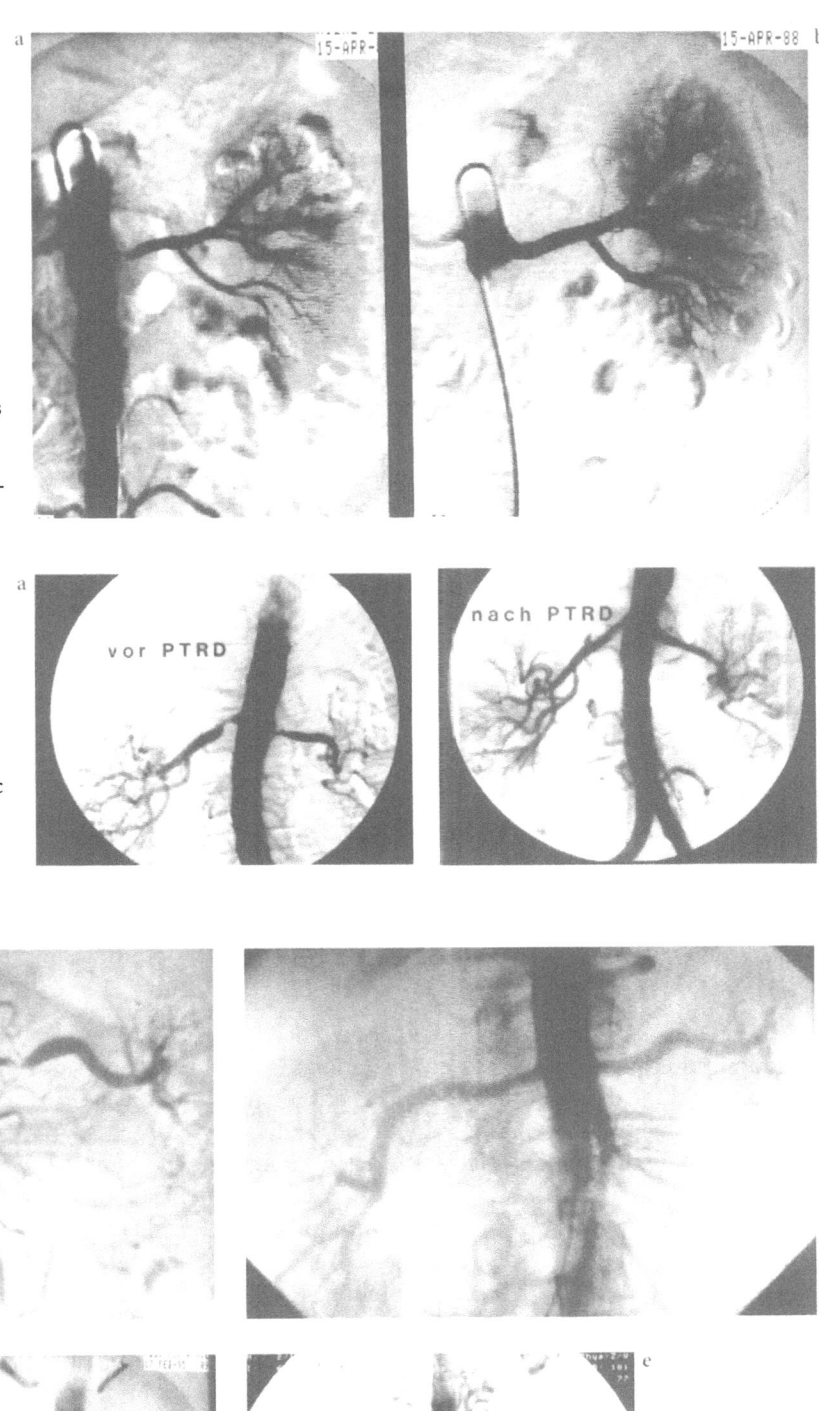

Fig. 18.13 a,b. Postostial atheromatous RAST. Angiography before (**a**) and after (**b**) successful percutaneons transluminal renal dilatation; pressure-gradient dropped from 70 to 8 mmHg

Fig. 18.14 a,b. Bilateral arteriosclerotic renal artery stenosis before (**a**) and after (**b**) successful percutaneous transluminal renal dilatation

Fig. 18.15 a–e. Bilateral renal artery stenosis (RAS), primary treatment with Palmaz stents; in-stent hyperplasia and balloon dilatation. **a** Bilateral RAS postostial (55-year-old woman with RAH). **b** Result after primary balloon dilatation and stent application. **c** 5 Months later, in-stent stenosis. **d** Directly after balloon dilatation. **e** 5 Months after dilatation of the stent stenosis; blood-pressure improvement

a

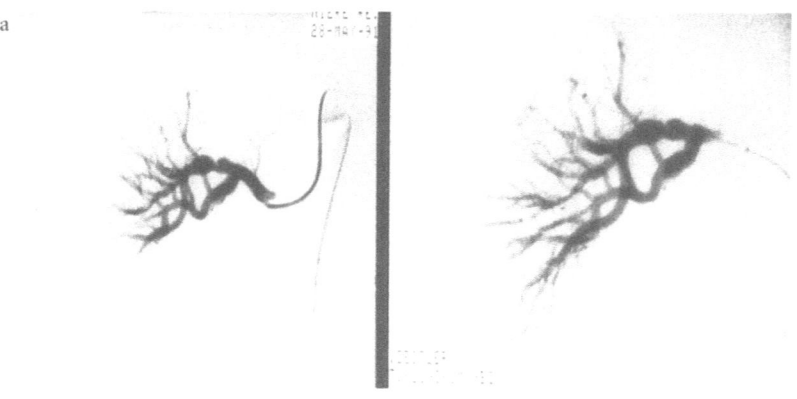

b

Fig. 18.16 a,b. Postbifurcational RAST before (a) and after (b) successful balloon dilatation (41-year-old male patient)

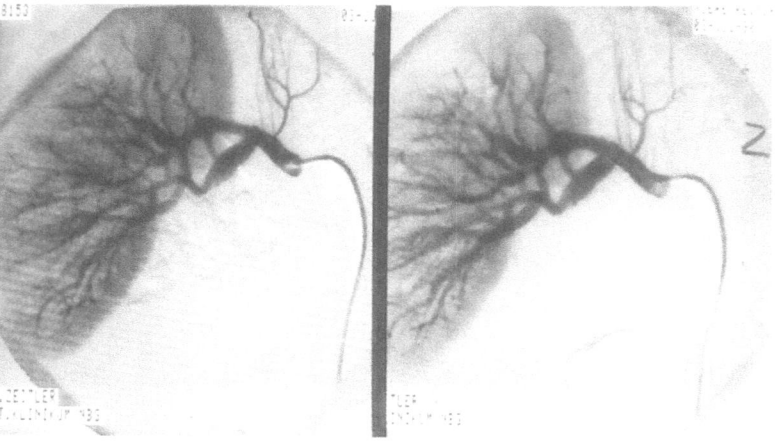

Fig. 18.17. Selective renal arteriography 14 months after percutaneous transluminal renal dilatation (same patient as in Fig. 18.16)

between the aneurysmatic medial occurrence, including multiple narrowings and dilatations in the second and third part of the main trunk of the renal arteries, is helpful in defining FMD of the media on the basis of pathologic correlations to arteriography. Difficulty, however, can arise in the differentiation between arteriosclerotic, intimal fibroplastic, and periarterial stenoses.

The classic picture of FMD resembles a string of beads (see Figs. 18.18 and 18.21), where short segmental aneurysms alternate with ring-shaped constrictions. The initial outcome of percutaneous transluminal renal dilatation (PTRD) for fibromuscular dysplasia is cleary better than that of arteriosclerotic renal artery stenoses, in view of the morphologic removal of the stenosis, and the positive long-term effects on arterial hypertension (Sos et al. 1983; Martin et al. 1986; Baert et al. 1990; Mahler 1990).

18.2.2
Diagnosis of Renovascular Hypertension (RVH) and Renal Artery Stenosis (RAS)

The radiologist, who, as a rule, is not the first physician to examine the patient, needs to establish a therapeutic indication based not only on the angiographic findings, but by also taking into consideration the clinical laboratory parameters documenting the degree of renal insufficiency, the period of time for which the arterial hypertension has been present, and which therapeutic medications have already been administered. Atheromatous obstructions or stenoses of other origins can be diagnosed with several imaging modalities. While conventional or digital angiography was the gold standard for diagnosing renal artery obliterations in the 1970s and 1980s, MRA, spiral CT, or 3D ultrasound will be the primary methods of imaging in the near future. Several factors indicate the existence of RAS (Table 18.2).

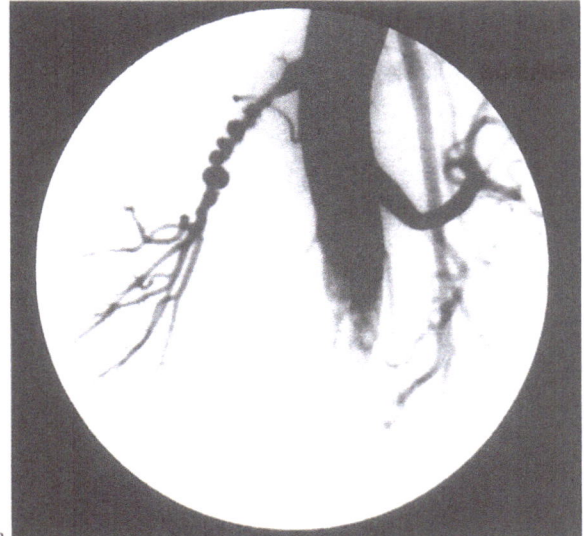

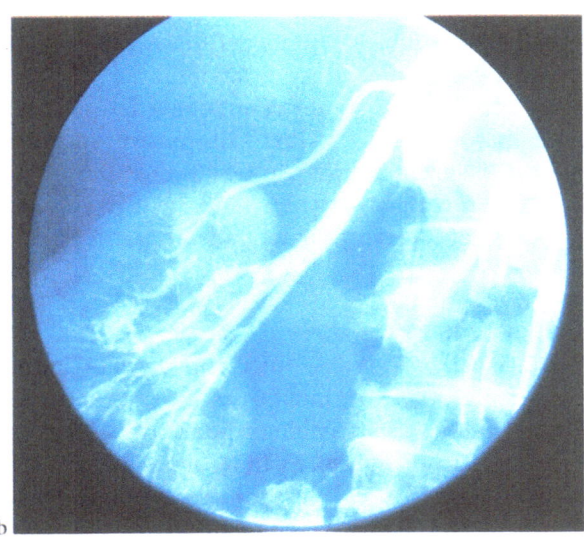

Fig. 18.18 a,b. Fibromuscular dysplasia, medial type, right renal artery and nephroptosis. **a** Diagnostic aortography. **b** Selective arteriography following successful balloon dilatation

The findings of renal angiography with the questionable diagnosis "renovascular hypertension (RVH)" had formerly indicated:

1. *Blood sampling* of venous blood from the right and left renal vein and measurement of the renin levels in each, followed by an evaluation of the effects of the angiotensin-converting enzyme inhibitor, captopril.

   In unilateral RASs, the ratio of renin between the stenotic and the normal side is defined as positive if it is above 1.5:1. In bilateral RAS, the additional blood sample of the infrarenal vena cava can help to define the kidney with the more effective stenosis.

2. *Angiography* needs to be performed in an antero-posterior and two oblique projections to additionally define the ostia of the renal arteries.

3. Each aorto- and renovasography needs to be followed by documentation of the excretory organs, i.e., kidneys, ureter, and urinary bladder.

Whereas non-functioning kidneys also demonstrate diffuse arteriosclerosis, the reduction of the kidney's length by more than 1 cm is very common in patients with unilateral renal artery stenoses. The definition of RAS is given in Table 18.2.

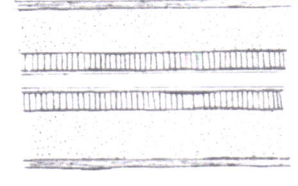 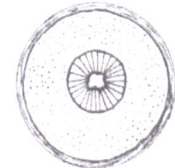

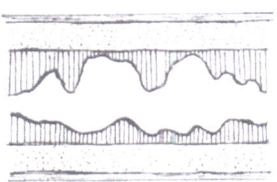 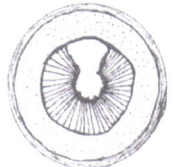

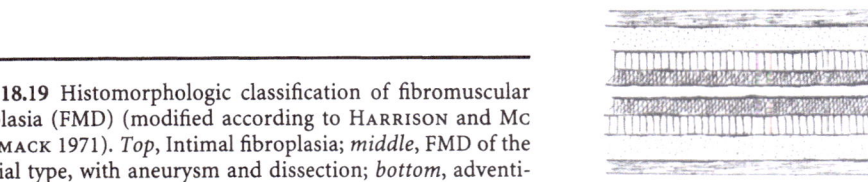 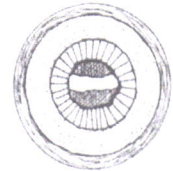

Fig. 18.19 Histomorphologic classification of fibromuscular dysplasia (FMD) (modified according to HARRISON and MC CORMACK 1971). *Top*, Intimal fibroplasia; *middle*, FMD of the medial type, with aneurysm and dissection; *bottom*, adventitial and periadventitial fibrosis

With the new, non-invasive methods of 3D imaging, information on the thickness of the aortic wall can provide a more precise definition of ostial stenoses, and prevent complications or unsuccessful treatment. An oblique view at the time of PTRD is important for precise stent positioning, if required. Indications for PTRD are summarized in Table 18.3.

18.2.3
Important Strategies

There are clear recommendations regarding the diagnosis of renovascular hypertension using laboratory tests and imaging methods. However, successful cure, and improved condition in patients with FMD and postostial arteriosclerotic stenoses (Sos et al. 1982; PUIJLAERT et al. 1983; MARTIN et al. 1986; BAERT et al. 1990; RAMSEY and WALLER 1990; ZEITLER et al. 1993) is also possible with normal laboratory tests following PTRD.

The diagnosis of RVH can be based on physiologic tests: measurement of plasma renin levels with the Captopril-test, and renal vein sampling, with measurement of the renin levels, with or without angiotensin-converting enzyme inhibition. Plasma renin levels in the peripheral veins are not sensitive enough to diagnose RVH. The captopril test, however, has a high sensitivity (71%–100%) and specificity (82%–95%) (MULLER 1986; MANN and PICKERING 1992).

MULLER (1986) recommends the captopril test as follows:

- After 3 weeks without antihypertensives, the test is performed in a seated position, and three baseline renin levels are drawn. A dose of 50 mg of dissolved captopril is then given under blood-pressure monitoring for 60 min. Blood samples are obtained and renin levels determined.
- The test is positive with a stimulated plasma renin level of at least 12 ng/ml/h, and an absolute increase in renin activity of at least 10 ng/ml/h, as well as an at least 150% increase in plasma renin levels, or a 400% increase in baseline renin level of less than 3 ng/ml/h.
- This test should be given to hypertensive patients, whereby RVH should be considered after imaging methods.

The imaging methods need to define which morphologic type of RAS exists:
- The majority are arteriosclerotic stenoses, in the first third of the artery distal of the aorta.
- Ostial stenoses are the result of aortic-wall thickening and can be best diagnosed, including calcified plaques, with spiral CT and 3D images
- FMD of renal arteries is the most common cause of RVH in younger patients, particularly in females.
- Most common is medial fibroplasia (Figs. 18.20 and 18.21).
- Renal artery stenoses of different types include arteriitis, which are multiple and, in most cases, distal of the renal artery bifurcation of the kidney, and are of an inflammatory nature, or FMD (Fig. 18.22).
- Postsurgical and posttransplantation stenoses (Fig. 18.23) are defined by their history and location.

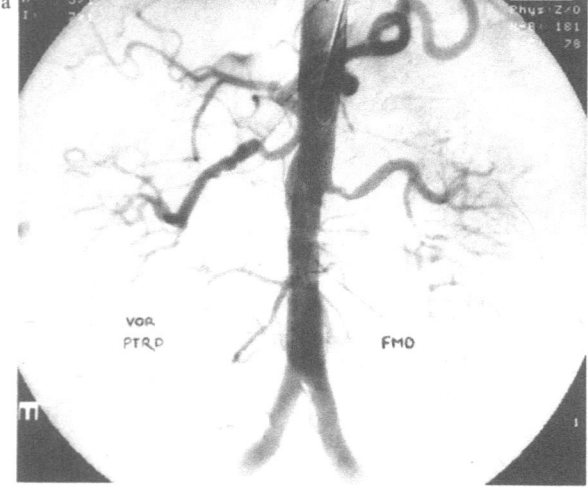

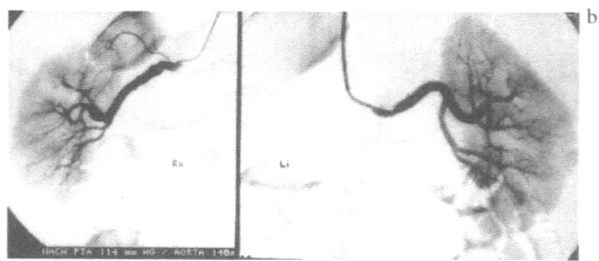

Fig. 18.20 a,b. Transaxillary aortography and percutaneous transluminal renal dilatation (PTRD). Fibromuscular dysplasia, right renal artery; left, postostial arteriosclerotic (?) renal artery stenosis. a Diagnostic arterial digital subtraction angiography before treatment. b Arteriography after successful PTRD (72-year-old woman with renovascular hypertension of 30 years standing). Blood pressure did not improve

Table 18.2. Definition of renal artery stenosis

Lumen reduction
More than 50%
Diameter reduction
More than 30%
Renin ratio: stenosed/not stenosed renal artery
Over 1.5:1.0
Intraarterial pressure gradient in front to behind stenoses
More than 20 mmHg
Successful PTRD
Reduction of pressure gradient to
below 10 mmHg

PTRD, percutaneous transluminal renal dilatation.

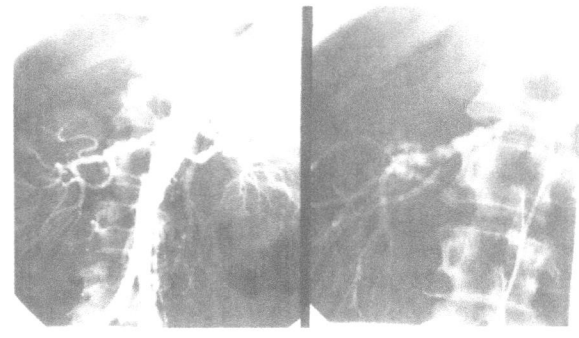

Fig. 18.21 a,b. Bilateral fibromuscular dysplasia (43-year-old woman with renovascular hypertension). **a** Diagnostic arteriography. **b** Small perforation with Terumo straight glide-wire. The patient was transferred directly to an operating theater and successfully operated with aorto-renal bilateral bypasses

18.2.4
Technique of PTRD

The first published cases in which successful balloon dilatation of RAS could be documented with the coaxial catheter system (Fig. 18.24) came from the Zürich team, Dr. MAHLER and Dr. GRÜNTZIG (GRÜNTZIG et al. 1978; MAHLER et al. 1979). As the result of clinical laboratory and imaging tests, the indication for PTRD (Table 18.3) is the result of cooperation between nephrologists, angiologists, vascular surgeons, and the interventional radiologist. Whereas ostial stenosis is still a primary indication for vascular surgery, FMD and nonostial

arteriosclerotic stenoses are good primary indications for PTRD (MAHLER et al. 1979; BUSSMANN et al. 1982; MARTIN et al. 1986, 1988; SLATER 1986; INGRISCH 1988; KLINGE et al. 1989; BAERT et al. 1990; MAHLER 1990; RAMSEY and WALLER 1990; SOS 1991; ZEITLER et al. 1993).

Having provided clear information and obtained informed consent from the patient, inpatient treatment starts following agreement (Table 18.4) on the day and time of the procedure with the vascular surgeon, since, in a small percentage of cases (1%–3%), emergency surgery is required (TEGTMEYER and

Table 18.3. Indications to percutaneous transluminal renal dilatation (PTRD)

1. Clinical	Renovascular hypertension with positive captopril test
	– Elevated diastolic blood pressure 95 <
	– Unsuccessful medicamentous treatment
	– Suspected RAS (US, MRI, or CT)
	– Renal insufficiency
2. Angiography	– FMD
	– Clear RAS
	– Elevated intraarterial pressure gradient
	– Location of RAS:
	Postostial – primary treatment:
	Balloon dilatation
	Ostial – and without aortic problems:
	Stent-assisted PTRD
	Ostial and non-ostial in combination with AAA
	or aortic obliteration:
	Vascular surgery
	– Bifurcational RAS vascular surgery or combined with
	endovascular treatment, kissing balloon-technique

RAS, renal artery stenosis; US, ultrasound; MRI, magnetic resonance imaging; CT, computed tomography; PTRD, percutaneous transluminal renal dilatation; AAA, abdominal aortic aneurysm.

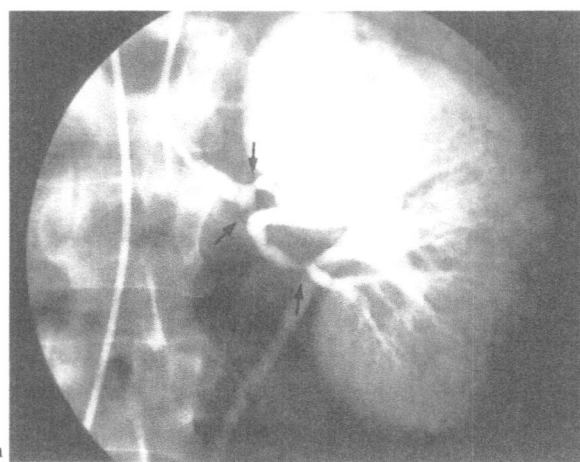
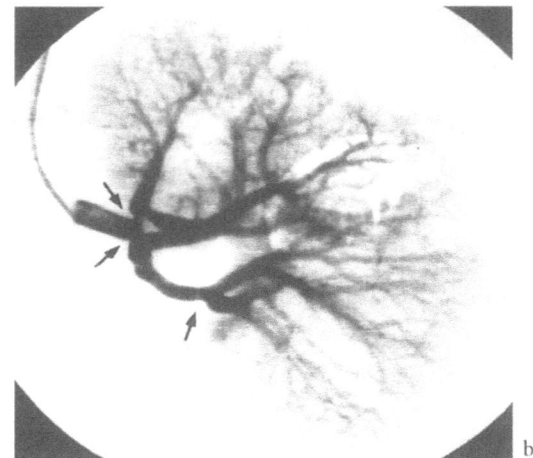

Fig. 18.22 a,b. Multiple congenital renal artery stenosis in segment arteries (35-year-old male patient). Same patient had fibromuscular dysplasia (FMD) (histologically controlled) in the carotid, external iliac, and superior mesenteric arteries, and femoropopliteal aneurysms on both legs. It should be also FMD in the kidneys. After percutaneous transluminal renal balloon dilatation, the antihypertensive medication dropped from 3 to 1 antihypertensives, and could be controlled for 11 years

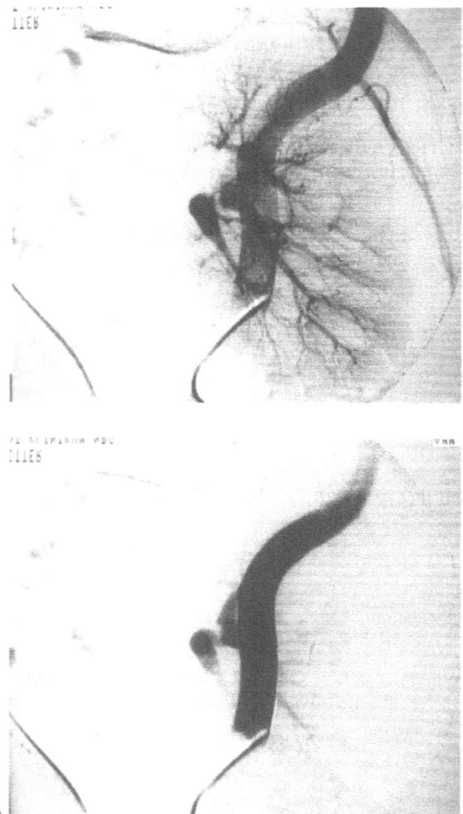
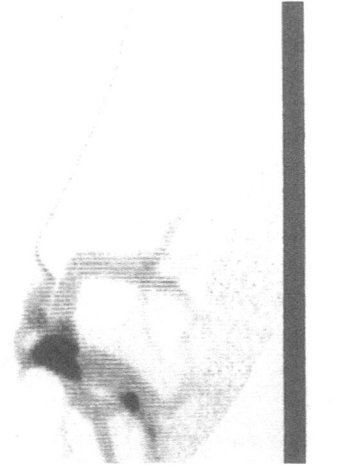
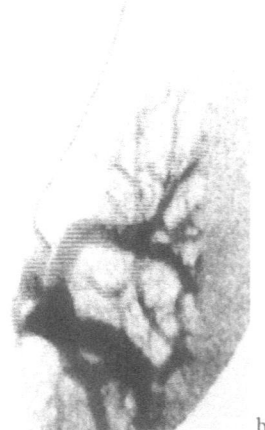

Fig. 18.23 a,b. Renal artery stenosis in a transplanted kidney (31-year-old male patient). **a** Documentation of the stenosis with selective arteriography from the contralateral groin. **b** Control after balloon dilatation. However, 5 months later, surgical treatment of the stenosis became necessary

Table 18.4. Organization of percutaneous transluminal renal dilatation (PTRD)

Pre-PTRD	After interdisciplinary indication
	Chest X-ray
	Duplex sonography of carotid arteries
	Patient information
	Premedication:
	Thrombocyte aggregation inhibitors
	ASS or clopidogrel
	Controlled or reduced antihypertensive medications
	PTRD in clinical treatment with 3-day follow-up control
	Informed vascular surgeon (indication, time of intervention)

Sos 1986; ZEITLER et al. 1982; PUIJLAERT et al. 1983; Sos 1991).

The technique of PTRD (Figs. 18.24 and 18.25) has the following steps after premedication:

1. Arteriographic documentation and definition of the location and size of the RAS.

2. With coaxial guiding and a side-winder catheter in the ostium, injection of contrast medium for safe localization of the catheter tip, followed by 100–300 µg of nitroglycerine, is carried out. Greater safety can be achieved with a second Cobra or pigtail catheter in the aorta (INGRISCH 1988).

3. Atraumatic crossing of the stenotic lesion, first with the guidewire [for optimum safety: (a) a steerable platinum coronary guidewire, 0.018 in., or the 0.035-in. open-ended guidewire for simultaneous blood-pressure measurment], followed by the 5-F guiding catheter.

4. Exchange of the guidewire for: (b) a stiffer, 0.035-in., "heavy duty" guidewire with a short, floppy tip, and a 1.5-mm tight J at its end.

5. In some situations, transbrachial access (see Fig. 18.20) for angioplasty of RAS or stenoses of the splanchnic arteries is also very helpful.

The balloon size is selcted by measuring the renal artery diameter on the arteriogram. FMD stenoses in the distal third of the renal artery are dilated with balloons with a diameter of between 5 and 6 mm, and in some FMD patients, with a balloon length of 4 cm.

In the case of arteriosclerotic stenoses in the proximal third, I prefer to start with a balloon of 5 mm in diameter and 2 cm in length. Pressure control with an open-ended wire or small-diameter catheters distal of the lesion and the guiding catheter in the aorta, demonstrates the pressure gradient, in addition to the control arteriography after successful balloon dilatation with a pressure of 5–6 atm (ZEITLER et al. 1982; INGRISCH 1988).

If the residual stenosis exceeds 30%, a second, larger-diameter (7–8 mm) balloon catheter is chosen. If important dissections occur, or the result is hemodynamically, or on arteriography, insufficient, the implantation of a Palmaz stent is indicated. This requires a stiff guidewire and precise imaging control. If, at the time of balloon dilatation, a small rupture occurs (see Fig. 18.21), the best first step to control this situation is to place the inflated balloon

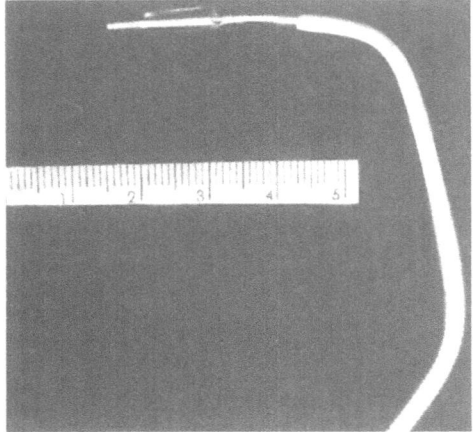

Fig. 18.24. Original coaxial catheter set for treatment of renal artery stenosis, by A. GRÜNTZIG

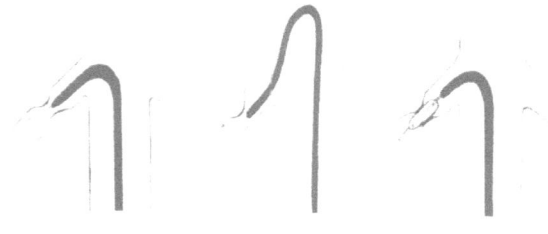

Fig. 18.25 a–c. Techniques of percutaneous transluminal renal dilatation. **a** Femoro-renal catheters or cobra catheters and direct use of a guidewire. **b** Selective catheterization with side-winder catheter without coaxial technique, and exchange of catheters over the wire. **c** Use of coaxial catheters in addition to the guidewire and balloon catheter

E. Zeitler

at the site of the perforation, prepare a covered stent, and change the above guidewire and guiding catheter at the defect. If this is not possible, direct transfer to the operating theater is necessary.

18.2.5
Results of PTRD

Primary technical success of PTRD in postostial arteriosclerotic and FMD stenoses is over 90% (Sos et al. 1983; MARTIN et al. 1986; INGRISCH 1988; MAHLER 1990; ZEITLER et al. 1991). It has been shown (MARTIN et al. 1986) that, with experience, both the technical and the clinical results can improve. In patients with the indication of RVH, a large number of papers have documented their results. Their definition mainly follows the surgeon's guideline

(MAXWELL et al. 1972; Sos et al. 1983) to defining cured and improved renovascular hypertension.

Table 18.5 summarizes some results following PTRD in patients with renovascular hypertension divided into arteriosclerotic postostial stenoses and FMD stenoses. The results in the Nuremberg clinics (Fig. 18.26a,b) include primary patency, control by angiography, and second intervention.

Several papers (BUSSMANN et al. 1982; KLINGE et al. 1989; MARTIN et al. 1986; MAHLER 1990; ZEITLER et al. 1993) have also shown the change in the systolic and diastolic blood pressure over time, as well as the percentage of patients requiring no antihypertensive medication (Fig. 18.27), as did Sos and coworkers in 1983.

Without question, with recurrent blood-pressure elevation, as well as controlled pathologic radionuclide studies, early restenosis can be estimated

Table 18.5. Results of percutaneous transluminal renal dilatation (PTRD). Result definition of renovascular hypertension (MAXWELL et al. 1972; Sos et al. 1983; MAHLER 1990)

Arteriosclerotic stenoses (n)	Cured[a]	(%)	Improved[b]	Fibromuscular stenoses (n)	Cured[a]	(%)	Improved[b]	Reference
94	16	80	64	28	65	87	22	MAHLER (1990)[c]
252	25	80	55	31	52	81	29	Sos et al. (1983); Sos (1991)[d]
?	50	75	25	?	60	90	30	LAMMER (1991)
189	24	66	42	36	62	80	18	ZEITLER (1993)[e]

[a] Blood pressure normalized to below 140/90 mmHg; no medication.
[b] Blood pressure reduction: systolic, below 160 mmHg; diastolic, below 95 mmHg; or diastolic blood pressure 15% reduced and reduction of antihypertensive medications.
[c] Primary success after 36 months.
[d] Primary success after 24 months.
[e] Primary success after 48 months and angiographic control without restenosis of over 50%.

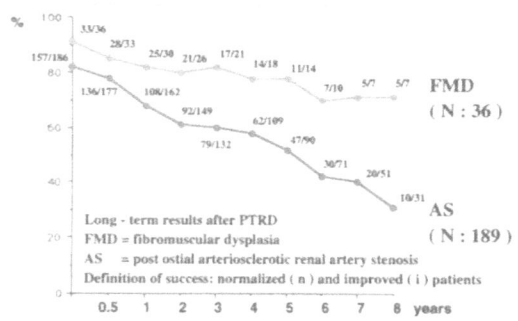

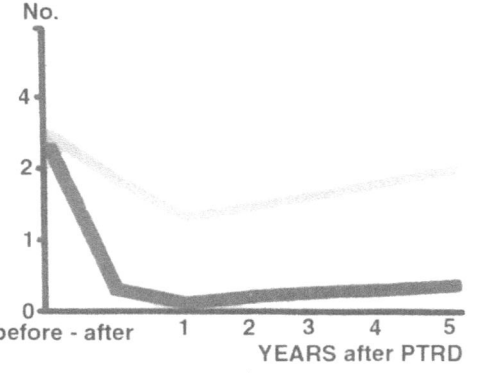

Fig. 18.26. a Long-term results after percutaneous transluminal renal dilatation (Nuremberg Clinic, North). **b** Mean number of antihypertensive medications used in the same patient group

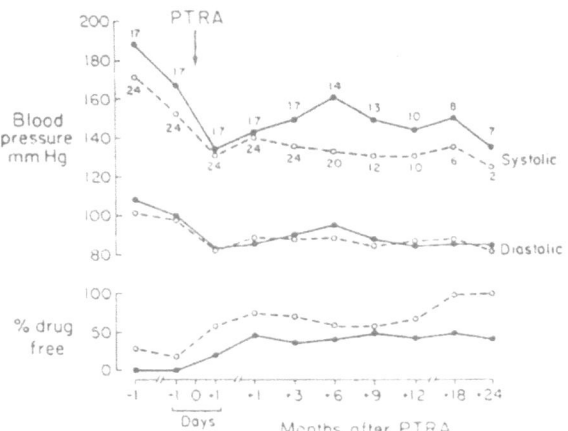

Fig. 18.27. Long-term effects of successful percutaneous transluminal renal angioplasty (*PTRA*) on blood pressure in patients with unilateral atheromatous (*filled circles*) or fibromuscular (*clear circles*) stenoses (*upper portion*). Figures at the points indicating systolic-pressure values denote number of patients. The *lower portion* of the figure shows percentage of patients requiring no antihypertensive medications. [Modified according to Sos (?)]

(ZEITLER et al. 1982) and indicate repeated imaging of the renal arteries. If, again, an important RAS exceeding 50% can be diagnosed, I favor a second PTRD before referring the patient to surgery (Fig. 18.28). In the time between the third and ninth month, a second intervention was performed in 10% of patients with FMD, and in 25% of patients with postostial arteriosclerotic stenoses. Undoubtedly, each patient with ostial stenoses we had dilated twice, and implanted the Palmaz stent during the third intervention. The results following Palmaz stent treatment are shown in Table 18.6.

The treatment of ostial stenoses, in general, has gained practical interest with the advent of the new types of vascular endoprostheses (the new, uncovered Palmaz stent, the covered "Wallgraft" stent, and other types of flexible endoprostheses). After more casuistic and technical publications, BLUM et al. (1997) demonstrated improved results using stents following failed balloon dilatation.

The results summarized in Table 18.5 demonstrate, as with most papers, a superior effect on blood pressure in FMD patients, in contrast to arteriosclerotic cases. The effects of PTRD in patients with renal insufficiency (azotemia) is less well documented, and only followed by an improvement in the form of a decrease in serum creatinine levels over several months up to 1 year (Sos 1991; MAHLER

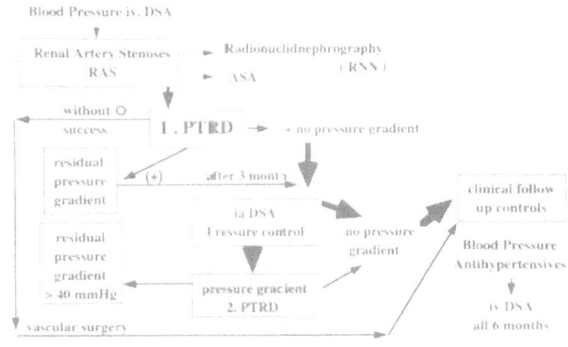

Fig. 18.28. Steps to control and treat patients with renal artery stenosis or renal insufficiency by means of percutaneous transluminal renal dilatation or vascular surgery

Table 18.6. Renal artery stenting. Palmaz stents in 21 renal artery stenoses (RAS)

15 Unilateral RAS
3 Bilateral RAS
  14 Ostial stenoses
   4 Restenoses – postostial
   3 Primary stenting – RAS
11 Male patients, mean age 64 (49–75) years
 7 Female patients, mean age 53 (30–79) years

Results: Mean follow-up 26 months ± 8 months.
Technical success, 89%; secondary patency, 81% [four redilatations, one vascular surgery (VS)]
Clinical success plus improved blood pressure: 13 out of 18 patients (including VS).

Table 18.7. Complications of percutaneous transluminal renal dilatation

Renal artery rupture
Dissection with renal artery occlusion
Dissection with reduced flow
Acute thromboses of the renal artery
Embolization of cholesterol crystals
Worsening of renal function

1990). In general, the best results can be seen in patients with FMD and unilateral postostial arteriosclerotic stenoses and younger than 60 years of age (Fig. 18.29a–c). The method of PTRD is, in experienced hands, a safe procedure, but back-up to manage complications by intervention or vascular surgery is very important. Strong follow-up surveillance is required to establish the need for secondary interventions.

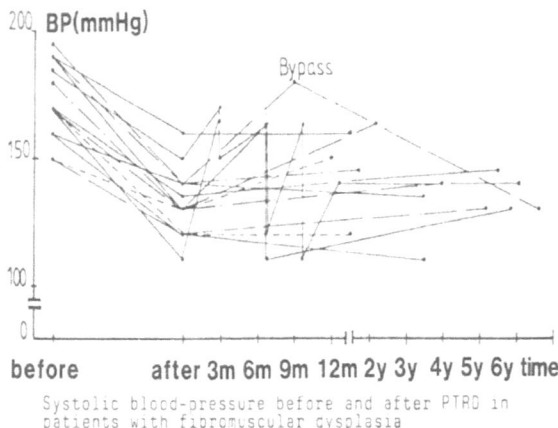

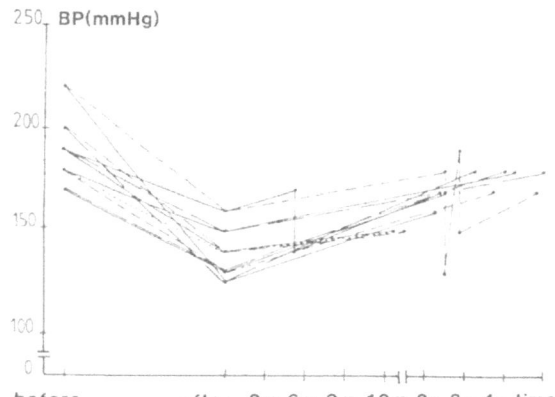

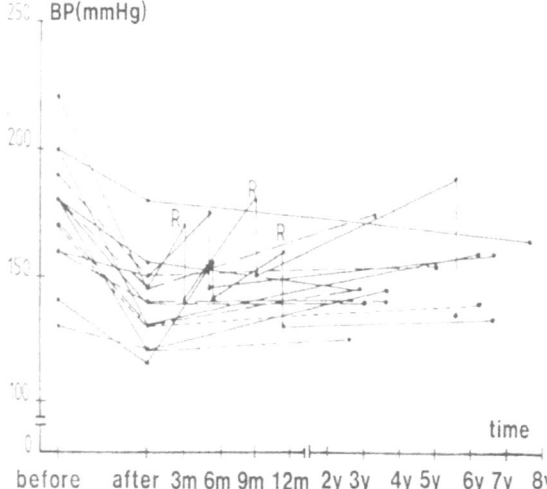

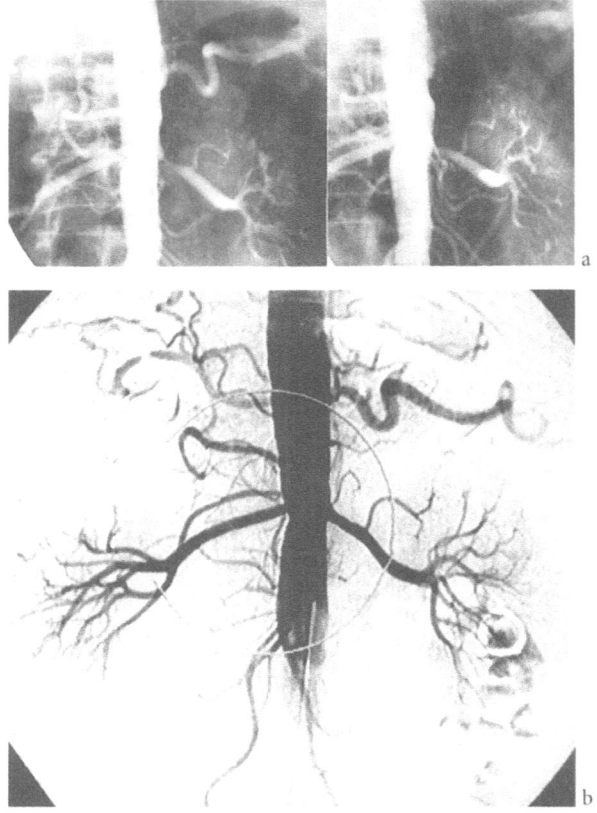

Fig. 18.30 a–c. Postostial unilateral atheromatous renal artery stenosis (60-year-old male patient). **a** Diagnostic angiography with stenoses. **b** Post-percutaneous transluminal renal dilatation angiography with residual stenoses of 20% and a pressure gradient of 10 mmHg. **c** Control digital subtraction angiography 5 years later; patient without antihypertensive medication

Fig. 18.29 a–c. Documentation of blood pressure response to percutaneous transluminal renal dilatation with balloon. Peaks indicate redilatation (second balloon dilatation). **a** Patients with fibromuscular dysplasia (FMD). **b** Female patients younger than 60 years of age; no medial type of FMD. **c** Female patients older than 60 years of age

18.2.6
Complications of PTRD

The primary success rate of PTRD is over 90%, with a complication rate of between 5% and 13% (MAHLER 1990). Among the possible complications (Table 18.7), dissection, perforation, and plaque or cholesterol crystal embolism play a particular role. Perforation and dissection may constitute grounds for immediate surgical intervention, unless they can be managed by stent implantation or a second dilatation. Embolisms due to detached plaque can certainly be avoided to an increasing extent with the help of modern guidewires, soft-tip catheters, and improved coaxial balloon catheters, but also by primary stenting in patients with ostium stenoses. To prevent such embolisms caused by plaque, only small, stiff, highly flexible, soft-tip guidewires are used in catheter angiographies and catheter manouvres performed in extensively arteriosclerotic vessels. These can essentially aid in the prevention of embolisms caused by plaque. Nevertheless, complications can be caused not only by balloon dilatation, but also by a soft-tip guidewire, particularly in vulnerable arteries (see Fig. 18.21).

Between 1978 and 1994, we treated 524 patients with 712 interventional procedures. During this time, we had to operate on three patients: one after guidewire perforation, one after balloon dilatation, and one to explant a thrombosed Wallstent.

In all patients treated with PTRD, it is necessary to carry out angiographic checks not only directly after the intervention (Figs. 18.14–18.18), but also to obtain angiographic results between 3 and 6 months, and even later in some cases (Fig. 18.30). Clinical checks for blood pressure, as well as ultrasound, are basic control techniques, but arterial DSA or the excellent 3D MRA are very important for good long-term results.

References

Abrams H (1983a) Renal arteriography in hypertension. In: Abrams H (ed) Angiography, vol 2, 3rd edn. Little Brown & Co., Boston, pp 1247–1297

Abrams H (1983b) Inferior mesentic arteriography. In: Abrams H (ed) Angiography, vol 2, 3rd edn. Little Brown & Co., Boston, pp 1701–1736

Arlart IP, Gerlach A (1997) Renovaskuläre Hypertonie. In: Zeitler E (ed) Arterien und Venen. Springer, Berlin Heidelberg New York, pp 413–429

Athanasoulis CA, et al. (1982) Interventional radiology. Saunders, Philadelphia

Athanasoulis CA (1982) Bowel ischemia. In: Athanasoulis CA (ed) Interventional radiology. Saunders, Philadelphia, pp 334–342

Baert AL, Wilms G, Amery A, et al. (1990) Percutaneous transluminal renal angioplasty: initial results and long-term follow-up in 202 patients. Cardiovasc Intervent Radiol 13:22–28

Baert AL (1994) Renal artery stent placement. Radiology 191:619–621

Blum U, Krumme B, Flügel P, et al. (1997) Treatment of ostial renal artery stenoses with vascular endoprothesis after unsuccessful ballon angioplasty. N Engl J Med 336:459–465

Boijsen E (1983a) Renal angiography anomalies and malformations. In: Abrams H (ed) Angiography, vol 2, 3rd edn. Little Brown & Co., Boston, pp 12–17

Boijsen E (1983b) Superior mesenteric arteriography. In: Abrams H (ed) Angiography, vol 2, 3rd edn. Little Brown & Co., Boston, pp 1623–1668

Boley SJ, Sprayregen S, Veith FJ, et al. (1973) An aggressive roentgenologic and surgical approach to acute mesenteric ischemia. In: Nyhus LM (ed) Surgery. Annual New York Appleton-Century-Crofts, pp 355–370

Bookstein JJ (1983) The roles of angiography. In: Abrams H (ed) Angiography in adrenal disease, vol 2, 3rd edn. Little Brown & Co., Boston, pp 1395–1424

Borm D, Müller-Wiefel H (1970) Angina abdominalis infolge Tumorkompression der Arteria mesenterica superior. Munch Med Wochenschr 112:1145–1147

Bücheler E, Düx A, Rohr H (1967) Mesenterica-Steal-Syndrom. Fortschr Rontgenstr 106:313

Bussmann WD, Dowinsky S, Rummel D, et al. (1982) Percutaneous transluminal angioplasty in the treatment of renovascular hypertension. In: Kaltenbach M, Grüntzig A, Rentrop K, Bussmann WD (eds) Transluminal coronary angioplasty and intracoronary thrombolysis. Springer, Berlin Heidelberg New York, pp 431–439

Cen M, Kämmerer K, Neef H (1972) Verschluß der drei unpaaren Eingeweide-arterien ohne klinische Symptomatik. Dtsch Med Wochenschr 97:197–200

Diemel H, Rau G, Schmitz-Dräger HG (1964) Die Riolansche Kollaterale. Ihre diagnostische Bedeutung für die Angiographie bei Verschlußkrankheiten der Mesenterialarterien. Fortschr Rontgenstr 101:253–257

Felix W (1922) Die Entwicklung der Harn- und Geschlechtsorgane. In: Keibel F, Mall FP (eds) Handbuch der Entwicklungsgeschichte des Menschen, vol 2. Hirzel, Leipzig, pp 7–32

Fry WI, Kraft RO (1963) Visceral angina. Surg Gyn Obst 117:417–420

Furrer J, Grüntzig A, Kugelmeier J, Goebel N (1980) Treatment of abdominal angina with percutaneous dilatation of an arteria mesenterica superior stenosis. Cardiovasc Radiol 3:43–44

Gellens M, Martin KJ (1999) Renovascular hypertension: a clinical overwiew. In: Kadir S (ed) Teaching atlas of interventional radiology. Thieme, Stuttgart, pp 21–27

Giessler R (1974) Chronische Verschlüsse der Darmarterien. In: Heberer G, Rau G, Schoop W (eds) Angiologie. Thieme, Stuttgart, pp 517–522

Grüntzig A, Kuhlmann U, Vetter W, et al. (1978) Treatment of renovascular hypertension with percutaneous tansluminal dilatation of renal artery stenosis. Lancet 1:801–802

Harrison EG, Mc Cormack LJ (1971) Pathologic classifications of renal arterial disease in renovascular hypertension. Mayo Clin Proc 46:161–167

Ingrisch H (1988) Perkutane Rekanalisation der Nierenarterien. In: Günther RW, Thelen M (eds) Interventionelle Radiologie. Thieme, Stuttgart, pp ••

Kadir S (1991) Atlas of normal and variant angiographic anatomy. Saunders, Philadelphia

Klinge J, Mali WPTM, Puijlaert CBAJ, et al. (1989) Percutaneous renal angioplasty: initial and long-term results. Radiology 171:501–506

Lecky JW (1972) Renal angiography. In: Hanafee W (ed) Selective angiography. William & Wilkins, Baltimore, pp 216–226

Lüscher TF, Kaplan PL (1992) Renovascular and renal parenchymatous hypertension. Springer, Berlin Heidelberg New York

Mahler F, Krneta A, Haertel M (1979) Treatment of renovascular hypertension by transluminal renal artery dilatation. Ann Intern Med 90:56–57

Mahler F (1990) Katheterinterventionen in der Angiologie. Thieme, Stuttgart

Mann SJ, Pickering TG (1992) Detection of renovascular hypertension: state of the art 1992. Ann Intern Med 117:845–853

Martin LG, Casarella WJ, Alspaug H, Chuang VP (1986) Renal artery angioplasty: increased technical success and decreased complications in the second 100 patients. Radiology 159:631–634

Martin LG, Casarella WJ, Gaylord GM (1988) Azotemia caused by renal artery stenoses: treatment by percutaneous angioplasty. AJR Am J Roentgenol 150:839–844

Maxwell MH, Bleifer KH, Franklin SS, Varady PD (1972) Cooperative study of renovascular hypertension. Demographic analysis of the study. JAMA 220:1195–1204

May R, Nissl R (1965) Das "mesenteric-steal-syndrom". Med Welt 18.N.F.:1270

Mc Cormack LJ, Poutasse EF, Meaney TF, et al. (1966) A pathologic-arteriographic correlation of renal arterial disease. Am Heart J 72:188

Morris GC, DeBakey ME, Bernhard V (1966) Abdominal angina. Surg Clin N Am 46:919

Puijlaert CBAJ, Geyskes GG, Ruijs JHJ, et al. (1983) Renal angioplasty in hypertension: technique, radiological and clinical results and complications in 134 dilatations. In: Dotter CT, Grüntzig AR, Schoop W, Zeitler E (eds) Percutaneous transluminal angioplasty. Springer, Berlin Heidelberg New York, pp 279–280

Ramsey LE, Waller PC (1990) Blood pressure response to percutaneous transluminal angioplasty for renovascular hypertension: an overview on published series. Brit Med J 300:569–572

Rob C (1966) Surgical diseases of the coeliac and mesenteric arteries. Arch Surg 93:21–25

Rösch J, Steckel RJ (1972) Selective angiography of the abdominal viscera. In: Hanafee WN (ed) Selective angiography. Williams & Wilkins, Baltimore, pp 17–87

Schoenberg SO, Knopp MV, Bock M, et al. (1999) Bildgebung der Nieren. Radiologe 39:373–385

Slater EE (1980) Renal artery angioplasty versus surgery: a hypertensionologist's dilemma. AJR Am J Roentgenol 135:961–962

Sos TA, Sniderman KW, Pickering T, Vaughan ED Jr, Case D, Laragh JH (1982) Percutaneous transluminal renal angioplasty: experience in over 100 arteries. In: Kaltenbach M, Grüntzig A, Rentrop K, Bussmann WD (eds) Transluminal coronary angioplasty and intracoronary thrombolysis. Springer, Berlin Heidelberg New York, pp 412–425

Sos TA, Pickering TG, Phil K, et al. (1983) Percutaneous transluminal renal angioplasty in renovascular hypertension due to atheroma or fibromuscular dysplasia. N Engl J Med 309:274–279

Sos TA (1991) Angioplasty for the treatment of azotemia and renovascular hypertension in arteriosclerotic renal artery disease. Circulation 83[Suppl 2]:162–166

Tegtmeyer CI, Sos AJ (1986) Techniques of renal angioplasty. Radiology 161:577–586

Van Dongen RJAM, Schwilden ED (1976) Die chronischen intestinalen Durchblutungsstörungen. Chirurg 47:366–379

Van Dongen RJAM (1988) Renal and intestinal artery occlusive disease. World J Surg 12:777–787

Vaughan ED, Bühler FR, Laragh JH, et al. (1973) Renovascular hypertension: renin measurements to indicate hypersecretion and contralateral suppression, estimate renal plasma flow, and score for surgical curability. Am J Med 55:402–409

Vollmar J (1971) Steal-Syndrome. Münch Med Wochenschr 13:501–506

Vollmar J (1996) Verschlußprozesse der Viszeralarterien. In: Vollmar J (ed) Rekonstruktive Chirurgie der Arterien. Thieme, Stuttgart, pp 364–389

Weibull H, Bergquist D, Bergentz SE, et al. (1993) Percutaneous transluminal renal angioplasty versus surgical reconstruction of atherosclerotic renal artery stenoses: a prospective randomized study. J Vasc Surg 18:841–850

Wenz W, van Kaick G, Beduhn D, Roth FJ (1972) Abdominale Angiographie. Springer, Berlin Heidelberg New York

Zeitler E, Grosse-Vorholt R, Gessler U, Krönert E, Lux E (1982) Percutaneous, transluminal dilatation (angioplasty) in renal arteries. In: Kaltenbach M, Grüntzig A, Rentrop K, Bussmann WD (eds) Transluminal coronary angioplasty and intracoronary thrombolysis. Springer, Berlin Heidelberg New York, pp 426–430

Zeitler E, Richter EI, Wachter G (1993) Renovaskuläre Hypertonie: invasive perkutane Diagnose- und Therapiemöglichkeiten. Wien Klin Wochenschr 105:365–370

Acute Arterial Diseases

19 Arterial Embolism

D. Raithel and E. Zeitler

19.1
Introduction and General Remarks

The definition of embolism is the intravascular transmission of formed, non-physiologic material which causes occlusion of one or several vessels (VOLLMAR 1996; HEBERER and VAN DONGEN 1987).

19.1.1
Prevention of Pulmonary Embolism

In the *venous* circulation, both the air or fat embolism can have an immediate lethal outcome, depending on the quantity of embolic material. Venous thromboembolism can result in pulmonary embolisms with clinical symptoms of varying severity. This situation requires, first and foremost, preventive measures to avoid embolisms caused by large thrombi, leading to death. In approximately 2%–15% of all lethal cases, pulmonary embolism is the cause (CREUTZIG 1993). While in earlier years up to 5% of operated patients suffered a lethal pulmonary embolism, this rate has dropped to 0.2%–0.5%, due

D. RAITHEL, Professor, MD, Klinik für Gefäßchirurgie, Städtisches Klinikum Süd, Breslauer Straße 201, D-90471 Nürnberg, Germany
E. ZEITLER, Professor, MD, Virchow Straße 13, D-90409 Nürnberg, Germany

to effective and widely administered thrombosis prophylaxis with anticoagulants.

In cases where this effective anticoagulation is absolutely contraindicated, the embolism of large thrombi, or the risk of recurrent pulmonary embolism, can be reduced by implanting a vena cava filter. However, the efficacy of the different permanent, or temporary, cava filters for the prevention of pulmonary embolism has not been clearly proven to date, particularly when adequate anticoagulation therapy is possible.

19.1.2
Heparin and Heparin-Induced Thrombocytopenia

Heparin is the most important drug for the prophylaxis and therapy of thromboembolic diseases. In rare cases, bleeding complications due to high doses may occur. In addition to this, heparin may cause a severe side effect, the "white clot syndrome": heparin-induced thrombocytopenia type II (HIT type II) – (WARKENTIN et al. 1995; GREINACHER 1996).

Low-molecular weighted heparins (LMWH) represent the most effective prophylaxis of thromboembolisms (KEMKES-MATTHES 1997). Apart from their anticoagulative effect, the inhibition of fibroplastic material and retardation of the growth of smooth muscle cells are also attributed to heparins. The fractional LMWHs have a lower molecular weight of approximately 4000–7000 (in contrast to $12\,000 \pm 10\,000$). The half-life of LMWHs is 3–5 h, at a considerably higher bioavailability than those of the ultra-filtered heparins (30–150 min). In our departments, we have been using the LMWH nadroparine (Fraxiparin, Sanofi-Winthrop, Germany), both for perioperative thrombosis prophylaxis and the therapy of deep venous thrombosis.

A severe side effect is heparin-induced thrombocytopenia. Two types can be differentiated between (KEMKES-MATTHES 1997), as shown in Table 19.1.

Table 19.1. Differentiation between heparin-induced thrombocytopenia (HIT) types I and II. [according to KEMKES-MATTHES (1997)]

	HIT Type I	HIT Type II
Incidence	5%–30% of all patients treated with heparin	Approximately 0.5% of all patients treated with heparin
Heparin	Mostly high doses of UFH, i.v.	Regardless of the type of heparin, mode of administration, and dosage
Cause	Direct interaction: heparin–thrombocyte	Immunologic reaction
Thrombocytes	In rare cases, decrease to 100 000/µl	In most cases, clearly under 100 000/µl
Onset	During initial days of heparin therapy	Typically between the fifth and twentieth day
Complications	Unknown	"White clot syndrome" Venous and/or arterial thromboses
Mortality rate	None	Approximately 20%

UFH=unfractionated heparin

In severe cases, the platelet count can drop below 30 000/µl. The critical period is between the fifth and the twentieth day following re-exposure. At the slightest suspicion of HIT type II, heparin therapy must be stopped immediately. The following clinical symptoms indicate HIT type II:

- Decline in thrombocytes to 50% of initial value
- Occurrence or deterioration of arterial or venous thromboses
- No changes in partial thromboplastin time (PTT) under heparin therapy
- Local reactions at subcutaneous injection site.

Whenever a change in therapy becomes necessary, hirudin or the heparinoid Orgaran (Azko-Organon, The Netherlands) is recommended.

Foreign-body embolisms occur mainly within the framework of medical interventions. They are the result of migration of catheter parts, guidewires, or embolizing materials inserted for therapeutic purposes (coils, microcoils, cava filters), or broken metal or plastic fragments of different catheters, such as cava catheters, pacemaker catheters, or catheters for long-term therapy). Their removal can be achieved percutaneously, with the help of varying adjunctive instrumentation, via the femoral artery or vein. Typical purpose-designed catheters and seizing instrumentation is shown in Chap. 5. A detailed summary has been elaborated by MATHIAS (1988) and ROSSI and PAVONE (1990). This interventional radiological technique is not practically feasible without image-intensifier television fluoroscopy, and an alternative is often only transthoracic surgery involving high risk.

19.2
Arterial Embolism: Incidence and Etiology

In 80%–90% of patients suffering arterial thromboembolism, a cardiac disease is the underlying cause: atrial thrombi and atrial fibrillation, cardiac aneurysm following myocardial infarction, thrombi as a result of myocardial infarction, and valvular defects. While embolisms to the arm and cerebral arteries mainly originate from the heart, aortic aneurysms to the pelvic and leg arteries also represent a source of embolism that always needs to be excluded (BAIRD 1964). Drawing on data from several publications, the localizations of embolic occlusions are distributed over the arterial system, as shown in Fig. 19.1.

Of 143 patients operated for peripheral embolisms (RAITHEL and WALZ 1972), the source of embolism was localized in the left heart in 75%. The range of sources of embolism was as follows:

- Absolute arrhythmia in 26%
- Valvular defects in 22%
- Coronary heart disease in 15%
- Arteriosclerotic changes along the course of the aorta with thrombi in 14%
- Myocardial infarction in 12%.

In 11% of these patients, the source of embolism could not be determined. Emboli patients who reach a clinic alive, already represent a selection (VOLLMAR 1996). The embolism is localized in 75%–83% between the caudal aorto-bifurcation, and the popliteal bifurcation (Fig. 19.2) BREWSTER et al.

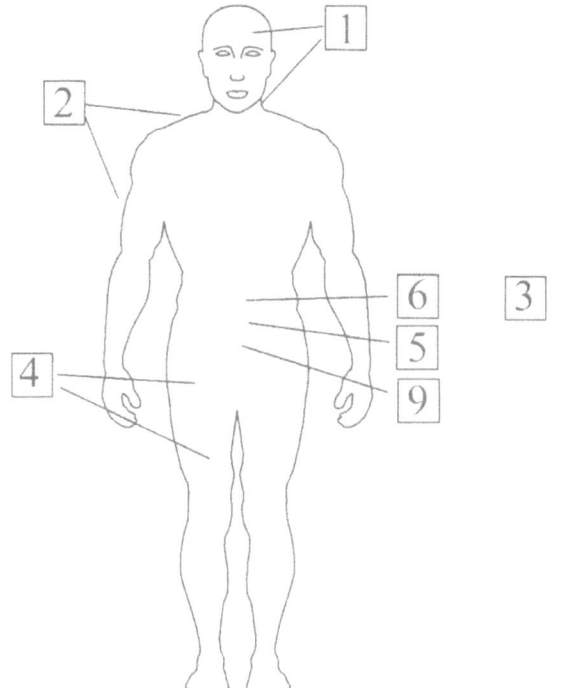

Fig. 19.1. Distribution of arterial emboli throughout the arterial system. *1*, Intracerebral and carotid arteries (15%); *2*, shoulder and arm arteries (15%); *3*, abdominal, *5*, renal, *6*, splanchnicus *9*, aorta arteries (20%); *4*, iliofemoral, lower extremity, femoropopliteal arteries (50%)

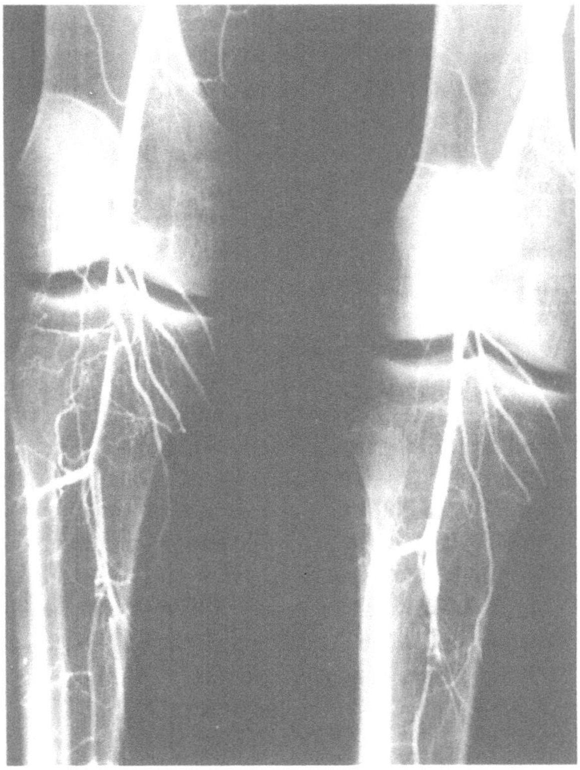

Fig. 19.2. Aorto-arteriography with bilateral extremity embolic occlusions. *Right*, embolus at the popliteal bifurcation and popliteal occlusion; *left*, embolic occlusion at the bifurcation of the tibiofibular trunk

1989). Paradoxical embolisms from the venous system at an existing open foramen ovale are a rare exception, and are identified as such in less than 5%. The mean age of patients with arterial embolism ranges from 65 to 75 years of age, and both sexes are almost equally affected (MÜLLER-WIEFEL and SELLE 1973; RAITHEL 1980; BREWSTER et al. 1989; VOLLMAR 1996). In patients with mitral vitium and sinus rhythm, arterial embolism was observed in 6%–10%, in patients with atrial fibrillation in 34% (DUNANT 1988). TURINA et al. (1988) reported 49% of embolisms from the heart to occur in patients with atrial fibrillation, 10% from abdominal aortic aneurysms, whereby the source of embolism may remain unidentified in up to 40%.

The mortality rate following embolisms in the extremity arteries has been reported at between 4% (TURINA et al. 1988), and 10% (DUNANT 1988), whereas after surgery of aortoiliac bifurcational embolisms, the mortality rate varies between 26% and 34% (DUNANT 1988; MÜLLER-WIEFEL and SELLE 1973; VOLLMAR 1996). The rate of amputations varies between 1% (TURINA et al. 1988) and 7.5% (DUNANT 1988). More than 50% of these patients die within 1 year due to cardiac insufficiency or coronary heart disease. In the past, the femoral bifurcation in the groin and the popliteal bifurcation were commonly considered more important localizations of embolisms requiring surgery than the aortoiliac bifurcation. Re-embolectomy needs to be carried out in about 10% of patients. Up to 40% of patients die within 1 year due to severe underlying basic disease.

The acute event of arterial occlusion in the extremities is thromboembolism in about 70% of cases, acute thrombosis in about 20%, and the result of trauma in less than 10%. Moreover, dissecting aneurysms, particularly in the aorta and the pelvic arteries, can also result in an acute occlusion.

In the area of the lower extremities, peripheral embolisms following local thrombolysis and catheter recanalization have also gained in importance since the use of interventional techniques. As regards the therapy, the advantage lies in the fact that this can be started immediately after the embolism has been detected. Embolisms within the framework of local thrombolysis, angioplasty, and percutaneous aspiration thromboembolectomy are observed in 3%–10% of arterial interventions.

Similarly, embolisms of the cerebral and arm arteries can arise from catheter maneuvers performed in the aortic arch and left heart. Due to the introduction of the so-called floppy guidewires and soft-tip catheters, the risk of thromboembolisms and cholesterol crystal embolisms induced by instrumentation will probably decrease further.

19.3
Clinic of Acute Thromboembolism

The sudden occurrence of ischemia in one or several arteries indicates thromboembolism. The symptoms of acute ischemia in the leg and arm arteries are characterized by the six "P"s (PRATT 1954):

- Pain
- Paleness
- Pulselessness
- Paresthesia
- Paralysis
- Prostration.

On clinical examination, a cold, white extremity is discovered. In the case of complete ischemia

due to arterial embolism, the surgeon calls for embolectomy according to FOGARTY and Coworkers (1971), by means of a catheter, either through the groin or elbow, to be performed immediately following heparinization (HEBERER and VAN DONGEN 1987; FOGARTY et al. 1971; GARCIA-GALLONT and KLEMPNAUER 1991; VOLLMAR 1996; CLASON et al. 1989; VARTY et al. 1992).The clinical findings need to be rapidly distinguished in order to decide either on surgery or the appropriate imaging system, possibly including an intervention (Table 19.2).

By dispensing with further diagnostic techniques and quickly performing embolectomy, the severe consequences of complete ischemia of an extremity (Table 19.3) can be avoided (PISTORIUS and WALTER 1996).

19.4
Indication to the Imaging Methods

In order to plan therapy, a differentiation between embolism and arterial thrombosis is essential since, as a rule, embolectomy is ineffective in patients with the latter (JIVEGARD et al. 1986; SCOTT et al. 1989; MARBET 1988). Whenever the differentiation is successful in case of acute severe ischemia of an extremity, based on the anamnesis and clinical findings, immediate heparinization and catheter embolectomy are recommened, instead of unneccessary diagnostic imaging to avoid prolongation of the ischemia condition. As only 75% of all embolisms present with a dramatic onset (VOLLMAR 1996), and 15% take a rather slow development, a precise diagnosis by means of angiography is often still necessary. An emergency operation without previous angiography is recommended by DUNANT (1988) only in cases of absolute ischemia of the extremity. Arterial digital subtraction angiography (DSA), if performed promptly and provided there is free access via the groin or elbow, can positively assist in quickly determining the suitable therapy (SCHMITT et al. 1988; PISTORIUS and WALTER 1996). In Basel (SCHMITT et al. 1988), for example, of 88

Table 19.2. Categories of acute ischemia

Category	Sensory loss	Muscle weakness	Doppler arterial signal
Viable	None	None	Audible
Threatened (acutely)	None or minimal (toes)	None	Inaudible
Immediate	More than toes, with rest pain	Mild, moderate	Inaudible
Irreversible	Profound, anesthetic	Profound paralysis	Inaudible

Table 19.3. Late sequelae of ischemia and reperfusion to the organism (Tourniquet syndrome)

Acidosis
Hyperkalemia
Hemolysis
Microembolisms
Myoglobulinuria
Kidney failure
Cardiopulmonary disorders
Postischemic syndrome

Table 19.4. Angiographic symptoms of arterial embolic occlusion

Abrupt occlusion
Contrast-agent surrounded, convexly bent filling defect
Intact vascular system proximal and distal of the embolic occlusion
Multiple occlusions
Occlusions at bifurcations

patients with acute occlusion of leg arteries, 73 (83%) were amenable to arteriography. Their mean age varied between 70 years for men, and 77 years for women.

Angiographic signs (Chap. 25, Fig. 25.3) of arterial embolic occlusions are shown in Table 19.4. Angiography provides a more precise differentiation between arterial embolism and local arterial thrombosis. In view of this, vascular surgeons also recommend an angiographic examination in unclear situations, despite the time delay involved. This is based on the fact that embolectomy is useless in falsely interpreted thromboses, and can even be associated with a higher mortality rate (JIVEGARD et al. 1986; SCOTT et al. 1989).

The larger variety of imaging techniques for visualizing arteries and veins has widened the technical spectrum to establish a quick, objective diagnosis. In addition to DSA, which, if possible, should not be performed through the groin or elbow as these are possible access sites for embolectomy, we use spiral computed tomography (CT) preceded by intravenous administration of iodinated contrast agents, magnetic resonance angiography (MRA) without X-rays, and high-resolution color-coded duplex sonography.

19.5
Vascular Surgery and Results

Embolectomy is the most common vascular surgical emergency situation. Whenever an embolism is localized proximal to the knee or elbow joint, this constitutes a severe ischemic syndrome. The preferred therapy is balloon embolectomy according to FOGARTY and Coworkers (1971) (GREEN et al. 1975; HEBERER and VAN DONGEN 1987; VOLLMAR 1996; RUTHERFORD 1986). The aim of every embolectomy performed early is to avoid any unnecessary prolongation of the ischemic condition. At the same time, the formation of a massive apposing thrombosis can thus be prevented. Embolectomy can clear the major vessels. Side branches and peripheral vessels, however, may then still obstruct a free perfusion. To avoid any migration of embolic material into arteries of second order, manual compression of the side branches should be carried out during embolus extraction (PISTORIUS and WALTER 1996). For embolectomies of a riding embolus in the area of the aortic bifurcation, access from both groins is required. A temporary blockade by means of a balloon catheter from the contralateral side is recommended to avoid

Table 19.5. Different therapeutic indications in patients with acute arterial embolism

Localization of embolism	Therapy	Specific techniques
Aortic bifurcation and both iliac arteries	Surgery	Retrograde embolectomy with balloon catheter
Femoral bifurcation (SFA and deep femoral artery)	Surgery	Retro- and prograde balloon catheter embolectomy
Brachial and popliteal bifurcations	PAT or surgery	Balloon catheter embolectomy or PAT plus local thrombolysis
Lower leg and forearm arteries	PAT and/or catheter thrombolysis	In all situations, additional systemic heparinization

SFA, superficial femoral artery; PAT, percutaneous aspiration thromboembolectomy.

the transposition of a white thrombus. To complement embolectomy of the major vessels, it can be performed in combination with local intraarterial thrombolysis within the framework of the operation.

The options relating to the various therapeutic techniques are chosen on the basis of interdisciplinary consultation (Table 19.5) and require that the physician, as well as the radiologist, remain on call for 24 h. In questionable situations without prior angiography, an intraoperative check using angiography or angioscopy is a suitable alternative (RAITHEL and WALZ 1972; VOLLMAR 1996).

Catheter embolectomy according to FOGARTY is feasible under local anesthesia in the majority of patients. Depending on the localization of the embolus and following interdisciplinary agreement, percutaneous thrombus aspiration (SCHNEIDER and LARGADIÈR 1987), and rotational aspiration thrombectomy (RAT)-PAT (STARCK et al. 1985), or local catheter lysis (HESS et al. 1987) can also be employed as alternatives to embolectomy. The differentiated indications are shown in Table 19.5.

The therapeutic aim is the complete removal of the embolus and white thrombus, to obtain a free arterial blood flow, whereby a transposition of thrombotic material into the periphery should be avoided under all circumstances (Chap. 25, Fig. 25.5). Simultaneously, a reliable stabilization of the circulatory system must be achieved. This needs to be followed by effective heparinization, which finally changes into oral anticoagulation using Marcumar. The aim is to eliminate an identified source of embolism, followed by clinical symptoms.

In situations of acute vascular occlusion, the patient's care is unequivocally in the hands of the vascular surgeon, with the radiologist and anaesthesiologist offering the best possible cooperation according to the local situation.

In view of possible late sequelae, such as a reperfusion syndrome, tourniquet syndrome, or postischemic syndrome (see Table 19.3), subsequent follow-up for the prevention of general complications is very important (PAETZ and ALLENBERG 1992).

Incorrect medical practice to be *strictly avoided* (VOLLMAR 1996) includes:

- High positioning of the extremities
- Fixation of the ischemic extremity on a brace
- Local application of cold or heat
- Administering vasodilators.

The outcome of treatment of arterial embolisms has been considerably improved by remote embolectomy using balloon catheters, both in the aortoiliac segment and the extremity arteries. This is attributable, in particular, to the possibility of performing such remote embolectomies, including the possibility of local anesthesia even in patients with severe cardiac and/or circulatory disturbances. The mortality rate on the aortoiliac level could be reduced from 55% to 35%, and from 37% to 23% in embolectomies of the extremities, while the amputation rate among patients who survived dropped from 43% to 3% during the years between 1955 and 1988 (VOLLMAR 1996). More recent publications (PISTORIUS and WALTER 1996), and own results have shown that a further reduction in the mortality rate down to 15% or even 10% is possible by means of modified indications to the various therapeutic methods (DURHAM and RUTHERFORD 1994). The current, and still relatively high, mortality rate is attributable to the changed age structure of patients with embolism (above 70 years of age) and the high proportion of coronary disease and other comorbidities, as well as additional postischemic syndromes. Due to closer cooperation between vascular surgeons, interventional radiologists, and hemostasiologists, the therapy can probably be further optimized (SCHNEIDER and LARGADIER 1987).

19.6
Postoperative Imaging

During the postoperative phase, mainly the recurrence of embolism and complications resulting from muscle ischemia need to be considered. The imaging methods suited to follow-up checks include color-coded duplex sonography and simple arterial needle angiography. In addition, a possible aortic aneurysm at risk of rupturing, or presenting a possible cause of embolism, has to be ruled out. For that purpose, the ultrasound examination can be followed by spiral CT or an immediate DSA, to back up the diagnosis. In the detection of the source of embolism, ECG and echocardiography are very helpful.

References

Baird RJ, Lajos TZ (1964) Emboli to the arm. Ann Surg 160:905
Brewster DC, Chin AK, Fogarty TJ (1989) Arterial thromboembolism. In: Rutherford RB (ed) Vascular surgery, 3rd edn. Saunders, Philadelphia, pp 548–564

Clason AE, Stonebridge PA, Duncan AJ, et al. (1989) Morbidity and mortality in acute lower limb ischaemia. A 5-year review. Eur J Vasc Surg 3:339–343

Creutzig A (1993) Lungenembolie. In: Alexander K (ed) Gefäßkrankheiten. Urban & Schwarzenberg, Munich, pp 688–696

Dunant JH (1988) Der akute Arterienverschluß: chirurgische Therapie. In: Widmer LK, Zemp E (eds) Angiologie 86. Huber, Bern, pp 78–80

Durham JD, Rutherford RB (1994) Standards for reporting lower extremity ischemia. In: LaBerge JM (editor in chief), Darcy MD (ed) Peripheral vascular interventions – SCVIR Syllabus. Congress catalogue number: 94-069675, pp 206–215

Fogarty TJ, Daily PO, Shumway NE, et al. (1971) Experience with balloon catheter technique for arterial embolectomy. Am J Surg 122:231–236

Garcia-Gallont R, Klempnauer J (1991) Akut erforderliche Operationen an peripheren Arterien und an der abdominellen Aorta. In: Pichlmayer R, Lohlein D (eds) Chirurgische Therapie. Springer, Berlin Heidelberg New York, pp 656–674

Green RM, DeWeese JA, Rob CG (1975) Arterial embolectomy before and after the Fogarty catheter. Surgery 77:24–33

Greinacher A (1996) Heparin-induzierte Thrombozytopenien. Internist 37:1172–1178

Heberer G, van Dongen RJAM (1987) Gefäßchirurgie – Kirschnersche allgemeine und spezielle Operationslehre, vol XI. Springer, Berlin Heidelberg New York, pp 373–382

Hess H, Mietaschk A, Rückel R (1987) Peripheral arterial occlusions: a 6-year experience with local low-dose thrombolytic therapy. Radiology 163:753–758

Jivegard L, Holm J, Schersten T (1986) The outcome in arterial thrombosis misdiagnosed as arterial embolism. Acta Chir Scand 152:251–256

Kemkes-Matthes B (1997) Nebenwirkungen der Heparin-Behandlung. Vasomed 9:288–292

Marbet GA (1988) Systemische Lyse beim akuten Arterienverschluß. In: Widmer LK, Zemp E (eds) Angiologie 86. Huber, Bern, pp 81–85

Mathias K (1988) Perkutane transvasale Fremdkörperextraktion. In: Günther R, Thelen N (eds) Interventionelle Radiologie. Thieme, Stuttgart, pp 272–282

Müller-Wiefel H, Selle N (1973) Peripheral arterial embolism – experiences with 174 treated extremities. J Cardiovasc Surg 14:312–316

Paetz B, Allenberg JR (1992) Behandlung des Reperfusionsschadens nach akuter Extremitätenischämie. Chirurg 63: 90–97

Pistorius GA, Walter F (1996) Die chirurgische Therapie der arteriellen Embolie. Vasomed 8:320–327

Pratt GH (1954) Cardiovascular surgery. Kimpton, London

Raithel D, Walz K (1972) Die chirurgische Behandlung der peripheren Embolie. Klinikarzt 1:165–169

Raithel D (1980) Spätergebnisse nach arterieller Embolektomie VASA 9:211–213

Rossi P, Pavone P (1990) Foreign body-retrieval. In: Dondelinger RF, Rossi P, Kurdziel JC, Wallace S (eds) Interventional radiology. Thieme, Stuttgart, pp 717–729

Rutherford RB, Flanigan DP, Gupta S, Johnston KW, et al. (1986) Suggested standards for reports dealing with lower extremity ischemia. J Vasc Surg 4:80–94

Schmitt HE, Biland L, Widmer LK (1988) Der akute Arterienverschluß der unteren Extremität: Thrombose oder Embolie? In: Widmer LK, Zemp E (eds) Angiologie 86. Huber, Bern, pp 74–77

Schneider E, Largadièr J (1987) Therapiekonzept beim akuten Verschluß der Extremitätenarterien. Ther Umsch 44:653–660

Scott DJ, Davies AH, Horrocks M (1989) Risk factors in selected patients undergoing embolectomy. Ann R Coll Surg Engl 71:229–232

Starck EJ, McDermott A, Crummy A, et al. (1985) Percutaneous aspiration thromboembolectomy. Radiology 156: 61–66

Turina M, Siebenmann R, Soterion M (1988) Kardiochirurgische Aspekte beim akuten Arterienverschluß. In: Widmer CK, Zemp E (eds) Angiologie 86. Huber, Bern, pp 86–89

Varty K, St Johnston JA, Beets G, Campbell WB (1992) Arterial embolectomy. A long-term perspective. J Cardiovasc Surg 33:79–84

Vollmar J (1996) Rekonstruktive Chirurgie der Arterien. Thieme, Stuttgart, pp 179–193

Warkentin TE, Levine NW, Hirsch J, et al. (1995) Heparin-induced thrombocytopenia in patients treated with low-molecular weight heparin or unfractionated heparin. New Engl J Med 332:1130–1334

20 Acute Thrombosis in Extremity Arteries

D. Raithel and E. Zeitler

20.1
Definition and Incidence

Acute arterial thrombosis is mostly a complication of pre-existent arterial wall diseases, for the most part, arteriosclerosis. In a smaller number of cases, it is the result of a hemorheologic disorder of the coagulation system (BREWSTER et al. 1989). The latter may occur in pathophysiologic disorders of the circulation, such as shock, cardiac insufficiency, hyperglobulinemia, possibly also without disorders of the arterial wall. Thrombotic arterial occlusions always present a similar, acute symptomatic clinical picture as thromboembolic vascular occlusions. Of acute arterial occlusions in extremities, 30%–40% are thrombotic, while 60%–70% are arterial embolisms.

The acute progression of peripheral occlusive vascular disease (POVD) – from stenoses to complete occlusion – has been observed in the upper thigh arteries five times as often as in the pelvic arteries (VOLLMAR 1996). According to HUMPHRIES et al. (1963), these rates were 33% in the upper thigh, and 6%–8% in the pelvis. Frequent stenoses of the femoral arteries (a typical localization of POVD) change within 2 years, unless treated, into arterial occlusion in about 50% of cases due to local thrombosis. If this process develops slowly, a collateral pathway varying in importance develops, mean while, due to the pressure gradient at the site of the arterial stenosis. The most important collateral artery for the upper thigh is then the deep femoral artery, the efficacy of which depends on the site and extent of the femoral artery occlusion. As a rule, if an isolated, single-level occlusion occurs, there will be sufficient compensation. On the other hand, in the case of pre-existent arterial occlusions, compensation may be impeded proximal to or distal of these (SCHOOP 1988).

20.2
Clinical and Differential Diagnoses

Acute ischemia is categorized as "viable", "threatened", or "irreversible" (DURHAM and RUTHERFORD 1994). "Viable" describes a limb that is not acutely threatened. An acutely "threatened" limb is salvageable, if promptly treated. An "irreversible" limb has major tissue loss or permanent nerve damage.

Since the therapy for acute thromboembolism, in contrast to acute arterial thrombosis within the framework of POVD, varies, a precise diagnosis is essential. Important signs, therefore, can be anamnestic data, as given in Table 20.1. These differential diagnostic considerations must be made prior to any indication to angiography (RAITHEL 1980; RUTHERFORD 1989), in the same way as a clinical angiological examination is performed mainly to determine the exact site of an acute occlusion: aortoiliac or in the lower leg.

The tentative clinical diagnosis of an acute pelvic artery occlusion is based on a non-palpable pulse. Ischemic syndromes may affect the toes, extending up to the mid upper leg. Thus, a differential diagnosis needs to distinguish between a possible thromboembolism, acute arterial thrombosis, and a dissecting aneurysm. Color-coded duplex sonography (NEUERBURG-HEUSLER and HENNERICI 1999), prior to angiography, can sometimes provide the relevant data in such cases. However, obesity, quality of ultrasound equipment, and lack of ex-

D. RAITHEL, Professor, MD, Klinik für Gefäßchirurgie, Städtisches Klinikum Süd, Breslauer Straße 201, D-90471 Nürnberg, Germany
E. ZEITLER, Professor, MD, Virchowstraße 13, D-90409 Nürnberg, Germany

Table 20.1. Clinical differences of acute extremity ischemia (data taken from case histories)

Arterial embolism	Arterial thrombosis
Absolute arrhythmic disorders	Existent POVD, claudication
Postmyocardial infarction syndrome	Diabetic vascular disease
Mitral or aortic-valve disease	Existent coronary heart disease, thus far no myocardial infarction
Aneurysm of left ventricle or aorta	Existent stenosis in carotid arteries, symptomatic or asymptomatic
Previous embolism	

POVD, peripheral occlusive vascular disease.

perience among physicians available in the night may interfere with this. Angiography, promptly performed, therefore provides a risk-free means of reaching a clear decision regarding what to do next.

In the case of acute occlusions in the femoral and popliteal area, there is severe ischemia of the whole leg. The inguinal pulse is palpable or strong, whereas popliteal and foot pulses are absent. In the case of acute lower leg artery occlusions – thrombosis or embolism – local ischemic symptoms occur, which only exceptionally lead to massive complications. On examination, no foot pulses are palpable.

In the differential diagnosis, traumatic injuries and acute venous thrombosis should also be clinically considered. A specific clinical situation is phlegmasia cerulea dolens. This is a combined arterial and venous occlusive symptomatology, characterized by acute onset of pain (RUTHERFORD 1989; SENN and GAENGER 1992). Primarily, it is a massive blockade of the whole venous system of one extremity. Secondarily, within hours or days, an additional blockade of the arteries takes place. The latter is not necessarily a thrombosis, but can also be compression caused by the surrounding edema. The consequence can be complete ischemia of the affected extremity, with distal necroses. The phlebothrombosis can be clearly identified by means of duplex sonography. On arteriography, an extremely narrow position of the arteries, with no contrast in the periphery, can be observed (VOLLMAR 1996). Therapy consists of a combined conservative treatment, including systemic thrombolysis, anticoagulation, and venous thrombectomy with primary fasciotomy. This needs to be decided in interdisciplinary cooperation.

20.3
Angiography

Needle angiography, or catheter angiography with a 3- or 4-F catheter using the digital subtraction angiography (DSA) technique remain the gold stan-

dard in the diagnosis of acute ischemic syndrome (Fig. 20.1), as well as bypass occlusions. These can be performed via a transfemoral or transbrachial access and provide a fast and precise diagnosis.

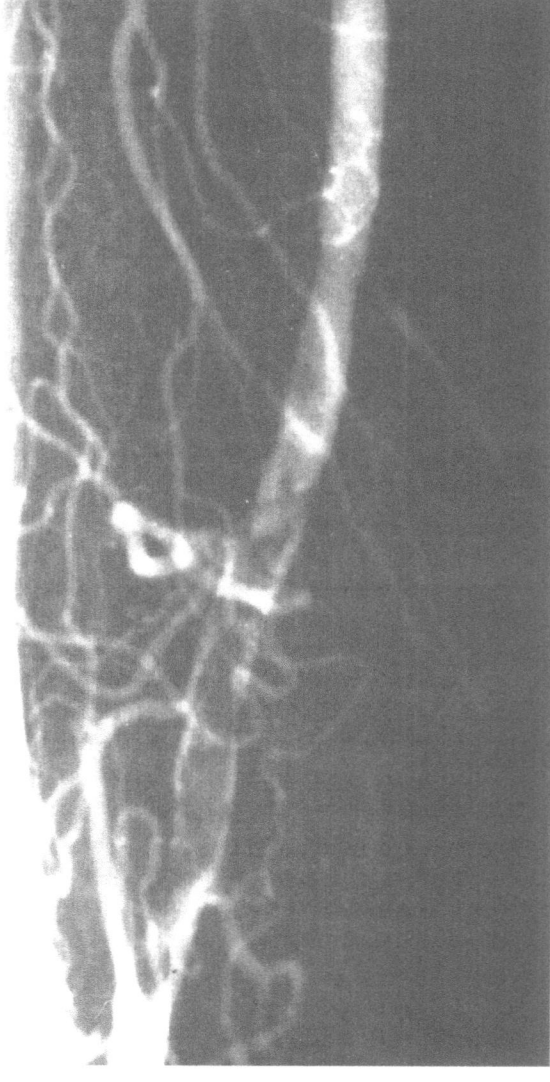

Fig. 20.1. Transfemoral aorto-arteriography from the contralateral femoral artery (*detail*). Local thrombus in the femoral saphena bypass with chronic occlusion of the superficial femoral artery (*left*)

The initial angiologic diagnosis indicates the access site for the needle and catheter. With absent pulses in the groin bilaterally, transbrachial catheterization of the descending aorta, translumbar aortography, or intravenous DSA can be chosen. With good pulse in the groin and unilateral ischemia, orthograde femoral catheterization is indicated, which may be followed by thrombus aspiration or percutaneous aspiration thrombectomy–rotational aspiration thrombectomy (PAT–RAT). In uncertain situations, transfemoral aorto-arteriography with puncture at the less involved site is also possible.

The criteria indicating a thrombotic occlusion on angiogram, in contrast to an embolus, can be seen in Table 20.2. After an early diagnosis, and in addition to anticoagulation, it is necessary to restore a free lumen. Thrombotic occlusions in surgically created bypasses are mainly located distally, close to the anastomosis (Fig. 20.1). This is very quickly followed by the total bypass thrombosis.

Table 20.2. Angiographic criteria of thrombotic occlusion

Blurred, cloudy demarcation
Identified arteriosclerotic calcified changes to the vascular wall
Arterial stenosis
Identified thrombus, in addition to irregularities above and below the thrombus
Pre-existent collateral circulation of varying importance

20.4
Vascular Surgery and Interventional Therapy

The following treatment principles for acute arterial thrombosis have been defined (VOLLMAR 1996):

1. To consider the underlying diseases: coronary heart disease, heart insufficiency, diabetes mellitus, pulmonary dysfunction
2. To always perform a preoperative angiography, to demonstrate not only the occlusion, but also possible co-existent lesions, collateral pathways, and important run-off vessels
3. To choose the least invasive intervention or operation first.

In contrast to clear embolic occlusions in the aorta, down to the femoral arteries, the indication for surgery is limited to patients with arterial thrombosis. It is only immediately indicated in the case of a com-

plete ischemic syndrome (VOLLMAR 1996). Irrespective of this, surgical therapy, to be performed after a certain interval, is recommended (WESOLOWSKI and DENIS 1963; SCHNEIDER and LARGIADÈR 1987). The primary intention is to perform the smallest possible intervention, which may be catheter thrombolysis (HESS et al. 1982; OURIEL 1993), PAT, or RAT-PAT (STARCK and WAGNER 1990). Systemic thrombolysis (MARBET 1988) involves more general complications than local thrombolysis.

Cardiovascular comorbidity and risk factors, such as diabetes and others, often restrict immediate operative therapy, particularly in patients with acute arterial thromboses in the aortoiliac region. Provided a viable category of acute ischemia is present, primarily conservative treatment including the control and therapy of risk factors is essential, bringing the patient into a condition enabling angiography and surgery. If, however, the patient presents with a severe acute ischemic syndrome with sensory loss, in addition to conservative treatment with heparin, infusion, and low positioning of the legs, treatment has to be indicated immediately after angiography within the framework of a cooperation between vascular surgeon and interventionalist (PAETZ and ALLENBERG 1992; VOLLMAR 1996). Surgical or interventional therapy needs to be performed within the ensuing few hours, or the next day at the latest.

The results are mainly determined by the patient's age, clinical condition according to the criteria for acute or chronic ischemia, and localization of the occlusion. Since, during an acute event the extremity is threatened and any delay might additionally jeopardize the patient's general condition, urgent referral to a specialized clinic or vascular center should always be made. The results of treatment of acute thrombosis correspond, provided a suitable therapy has been chosen, to those of chronic arterial vascular disease. Balloon thromboembolectomy is *not* the method of choice.

20.5
Postoperative Imaging

Following acute therapeutic methods for arterial thrombosis, control of the result, not only clinically, but also with imaging methods, is necessary. Depending on the localization and extent, duplex sonography may be sufficient, but possibly needs to be complemented by angiography, depending on the clinical situation, and particularly if the clinical picture deteriorates. Thus, the patient's general condition needs to be observed in order to deploy the most suitable and least invasive imaging technique. Follow-up controls at 1, 3, and 6 months are recommended. In most patients, treatment of the basic disease and risk factors, as well as secondary prevention with anticoagulants and platelet-aggregation inhibitors, are necessary.

References

Brewster DC, Chin AK, Fogarty TJ (1989) Arterial thromboembolism. In: Rutherford RB (ed) Vascular surgery, 3rd edn. Saunders, Philadelphia

Durham JD, Rutherford RB (1994) Standards for reporting lower extremity ischemia. In: La Berge JM (editor in chief), Darcy MD (ed) Peripheral vascular interventions-SCVIR Syllabus. Congress catalogue number: 94-069675, pp 206-215

Hess H, Ingrisch H, Mietaschk A, Rath H (1982) Local low-dose thrombolytic therapy of peripheral arterial occlusions. New Engl J Med 307:1627-1630

Humphries AW, de Wolfe VG, Young JR, Lefevre FA (1963) Evaluation of the natural history and the results of treatment on occlusion arteriosclerosis involving the lower extremities in 1850 patients. In: Wesolowski SA, Denis C (eds) Fundamentals of vascular grafting. McGraw-Hill, New York

Marbet GA (1988) Systemische Lyse beim akuten Arterienverschluß. In: Widmer LK, Zemp E (eds) Angiologie 86. Huber, Bern

Neuerburg-Heusler D, Hennerici M (1999) Gefäßdiagnostik mit Ultraschall. Thieme, Stuttgart

Ouriel K (1993) Thrombolysis versus operation in acute peripheral arterial occlusion. In: Veith F (ed) 20th Annual symposium on current critical problems and new technologies in vascular surgery. New York, November 18-21

Paetz B, Allenberg JR (1992) Behandlung des Reperfusionsschadens nach akuter Extremitätenischämie. Chirurg 63:90-97

Raithel D (1980) Spätergebnisse nach arterieller Embolektomie. VASA 9:211-213

Rutherford RB (1989) Vascular Surgery, 3rd edn. Saunders, Philadelphia

Schneider E, Largiadér J (1987) Therapiekonzept beim akuten Verschluß von Extremitätenarterien. Ther Umsch 44:653-660

Schoop W (1988) Praktische Angiologie. Thieme, Stuttgart

Senn A, Gaenger KH (1992) Phlegmasia coerulea dolens. In: Hornibostel H, Kaufmann W, Siegenthaler (eds) Innere Medizin in Klinik und Praxis, vol I, 4th edn. Thieme, Stuttgart

Starck EE, Wagner HJ (1990) Rotations-Aspirations-Thromboembolektomie. Dtsch Med Wochenschr 116:1-6

Vollmar J (1996) Rekonstruktive Gefäßchirurgie. Thieme, Stuttgart, pp 182-187

Wesolowski SA, Denis C (1963) Fundamentals of vascular grafting. McGraw-Hill, New York

21 Mechanical Thrombolysis

H. Rousseau, P. Perreault, P. Otal, P. Soula, D. Colombier, P. Leger and F. Joffre

CONTENTS

The Fogarty catheter has proven to be an effective tool for the treatment of acute vascular obstructions, particularly when these obstructions are embolic in origin. When utilized for the treatment of thrombosis associated with atherosclerotic disease, there have been many technical problems which have limited the efficiency of this catheter, such as its ability to traverse the obstruction, dissection, arteriospasm, and migration of the thrombus distally in the vascular bed (BLAISDELL et al. 1978; GORDON and FOGARTY 1984). As an alternative treatment method to the Fogarty catheter, intravascular fibrinolysis has been successful in relieving acute obstruction with the added advantage of repermeabilization of distal collaterals (LAMMER et al. 1986; MCNAMARA et al. 1991; MEYEROVITZ et al. 1990). The most recent randomized studies comparing surgical and fibrinolytic therapy reinforce these findings (DIFFIN and KANDARPA 1996; OURIEL et al. 1996). There are, however, several limiting factors associated with intravascular fibrinolytic therapy:

HERVE ROUSSEAU, MD, PIERRE PERREAULT, MD, PHILIPPE OTAL, MD, DANIEL COLOMBIER, MD, FRANCIS JOFFRE, MD, Department of Radiology, C.H.U. Rangueil, 1, Avenue Jean Poulhes, 31054 Toulouse, France
PHILIPPE LEGER, MD, PHILIPPE SOULA, MD, Department of Cardiovascular Surgery, C.H.U. Rangueil 1, Avenue Jean Poulhes, 31054 Toulouse, France

1. The delayed action of these agents (4–48h) eliminates the possibility of treating irreversible acute ischemic episodes (stage III of the Rutherford classification).
2. Side-effects associated with the medication, particularly hemorrhage, which persist despite recent progress in molecular biology and newer methods of administering these products.
3. Elevated cost associated with the technique when the cost of the fibrinolytic agents combined with the necessary intensive care unit monitoring are taken into account.

Because of these limiting factors, other treatment methods such as percutaneous mechanical thrombus disruption techniques have been developed for the treatment of acute vascular obstruction of the lower limbs. These percutaneous mechanical thrombectomy procedures are efficient at relieving the obstruction in a short period of time with little or no use of fibrinolytics and hence increasing the therapeutic efficiency while diminishing the cost of the overall procedure.

Several types of catheters have been developed using three different mechanisms for percutaneous mechanical thrombectomy: (1) Thrombus aspiration type catheters, (2) catheters which function by vortex effect, basically destroying clots without suctioning the subsequent debris, and (3) catheters which function on the basis of the Venturi effect which permit fragmentation and simultaneous aspiration.

This chapter aims to classify the specific clinical indications for each of these methods in the treatment of acute vascular obstructions.

21.1 Thombus Aspiration Devices

21.1.1 Principle

The term thrombus aspiration device embraces all methods which allow aspiration with or without fragmentation of the thrombus responsible for obstruction of a vessel. The principle involved in thrombus aspiration techniques is a simple pressure effect created by aspiration with a syringe which allows evacuation of the obstructing clot. The thrombus is effectively aspirated onto the end of the catheter and can be removed with or without prior fragmentation. The objective of this method is not to have the thrombus aspirated into the catheter, but simply to aspirate and fix the thrombus to the end of the catheter which is eventually retrieved through an introducer of larger diameter with a removable one-way antireflux valve, and hence thrombi of large diameters compared to the diameter of the catheter can be effectively removed.

21.1.2
Materials

Several types of catheters have been utilized for this thrombus aspiration procedure: These catheters all have one feature in common which is a non-traumatic distal end and an internal diameter which is maximized in comparison to the external diameter of the catheter to optimize the aspiration procedure. The diameter of the catheter must relate to the vessel being treated and it has to be sufficiently large to produce an adequate aspiration without, on the other end, traumatizing the arterial walls. Having gained access to the site of arterial obstruction, the aspiration catheter is advanced on a guidewire until it comes into direct contact with the obstructing thrombus. After removing the guidewire, manual aspiration utilizing a 50 cc syringe produces a depression on the thrombus and the material is removed by simply pulling the catheter back through the introducer which is of larger caliber and equipped with a unidirectional valve. The presence of these removable unidirectional valves eliminates the possibility of thrombus obstruction at this site (Fig. 21.1).

When the thrombus does remain obstructed at the distal end of the introducer, a prolonged aspiration technique utilizing the introducer must be undertaken. In these cases, a hydrophilic guidewire is inserted through a Y shaped valve and then the introducer is withdrawn completely while maintaining aspiration pressure with the 50 cc syringe. With this security guidewire in place, the introducer can then be replaced and the whole procedure repeated. Several aspirations may be necessary to complete the thrombus aspiration procedure.

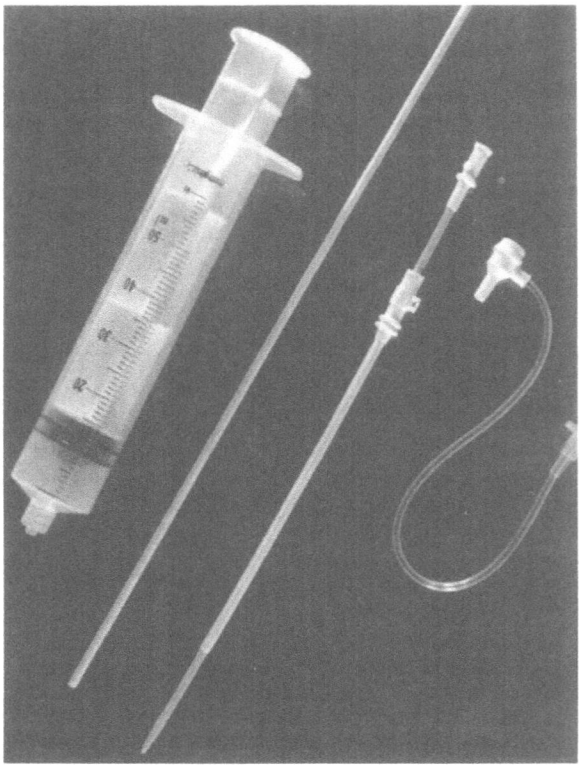

Fig. 21.1. The material required for thrombo-aspiration includes a large syringe, conventional guide wires, and a sheath with a hemostasis valve, removable to facilitate removal of entrapped clot material (BARD MurrayNill, N.J., USA). A large thin-walled, minimally tapered catheter without distal side holes is used. Catheters of 5–9-F are used according to vessel size

In cases of distal obstruction, it is not necessary to put the aspiration catheter in direct contact with the obstructing thrombus as the simple pressure phenomena created by aspirating with the syringe of a catheter which is adjacent to a thrombus results in displacement of the thrombus towards the catheter. To reduce the possibility of arterial spasm vasodilators are systematically utilized for patients with distal obstructions. This thrombus aspiration technique is to be utilized only by ipsilateral puncture to avoid propagation of thrombus material into the contralateral leg.

21.1.3
Indications

Thrombus aspiration techniques are particularly useful in certain clinical settings:

(a) Distal embolic obstructions associated with propagation of cardiac thrombi and/or vegetations or iatrogenic disease secondary to a recent arterial procedure where this thrombo-aspiration technique has several distinct advantages. A percutaneous procedure performed under direct fluoroscopic guidance which enables selective catheterization of the involved vessels and treats all etiologies of obstruction including migration of an atheromatous plaque or acute thrombus, or embolic phenomena with immediate efficient results and an overall low cost associated with the procedure.

(b) For obstruction associated with adjacent atheromatous lesions, this technique can be utilized as the initial treatment method when the thrombotic episode is a recent phenomena. By performing thrombo-aspiration prior to angioplasty, embolic migration of the thrombus can be eliminated (Fig. 21.2).

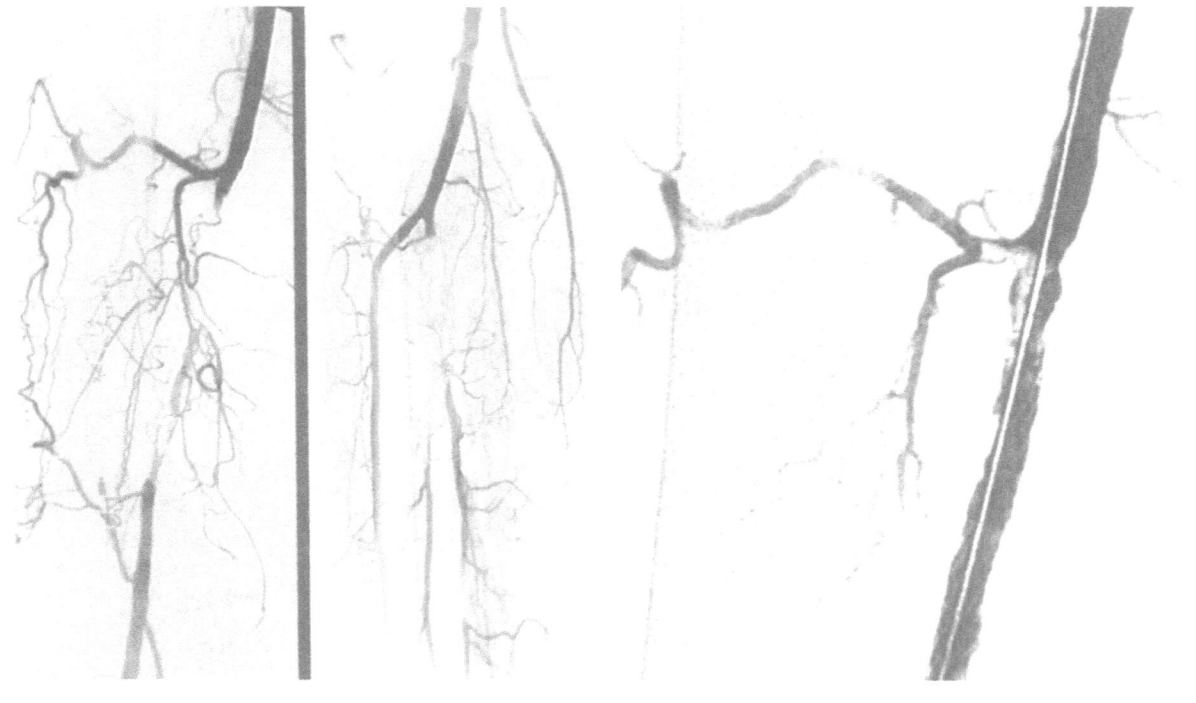

a,b

c

d

Fig. 21.2. a Fresh thombotic occlusion of a femoral stenosis with distal migration. A percutaneous aspiration thrombectomy was performed first and residual stenosis was dilated and then stented. b A residual thrombus in a proximal collateral and at the upper part of the stent was removed by an angulated thrombectomy catheter. c,d Final control arteriogram proximally (c) and distally (d)

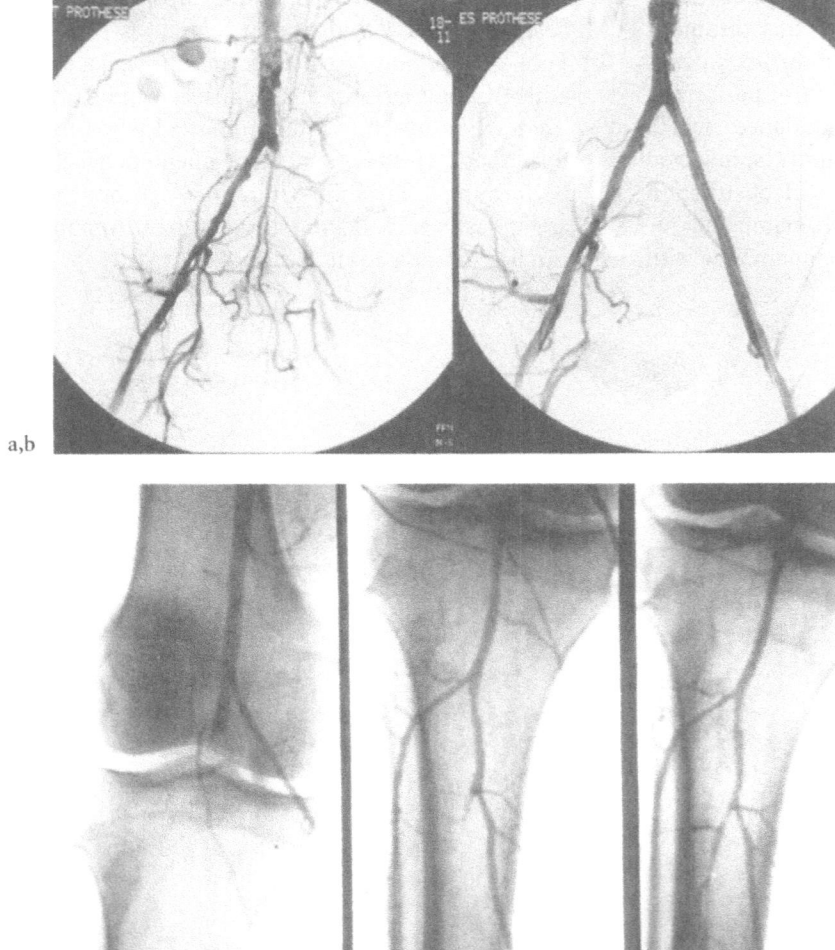

a,b

c,d,e

Fig. 21.3. a,b Occlusion of the left common iliac artery treated by stent and angioplasty with excellent results (**b**). **c** Control angiogram demonstrated an acute embolic controlateral popliteal occlusion. **d** Angiography after first aspiration. **e** After a second aspiration, patency of the three arteries was fully restored

Thrombo-aspiration techniques have also been utilized for treatment of deep venous thrombosis, but due to the volume and size of thrombi and the veins involved, the method is often inefficient and is most often limited to treatment of obstructions of hemodialysis arteriovenous fistulae.

STARCK and MacDERMOTT (1988; WAGNER et al. 1994) noted a 92% success rate in 82 patients treated for arterial obstruction utilizing this thrombo-aspiration technique with only two complications (one case of arterial rupture and one pseudoaneurysm) described in their series. It has been adequately demonstrated, however, that the success of thrombo-aspiration devices depend on the site of obstruction, the length of the thrombus, and the chronicity of the obstruction. It has been shown that for recent obstruction of a small caliber vessel by embolic migration, specifically after endovascular procedures, thrombo-aspiration proved to be a very efficient method (Fig. 21.3). When, however, the thrombotic phenomena is chronic or the artery in question is of larger caliber (common iliac or superficial femoral arteries), and for embolic events from cardiac or aorto-iliac origins, the thrombo-aspiration techniques proved to be less efficient and often need to be replaced with procedures which effectively fragment these larger thrombi.

Thrombo-aspiration procedures have been combined with local fibrinolytic therapy (WAGNER et al. 1994). Thrombo-aspiration performed prior to fibrinolysis increases both the speed and the efficiency of fibrinolytic therapy. Inversely, smaller doses of intravascular fibrinolytics can be a useful adjunct to complete a thrombo-aspiration procedure by effectively causing lysis of distal obstructing thrombi.

Other mechanical methods utilizing the principle of thrombus fragmentation with catheters equipped with either a rotary or metallic drill type apparatus, Dormia catheters or Fogarty catheters, allow simultaneous fragmentation and aspiration of thrombotic material from the involved vessels. These specific apparatus will be addressed later on in this chapter (WAGNER et al. 1994; MATSUMOTO et al. 1992; SCHMITZ-RODE and GÜNTHER 1991; PONOMAR et al. 1991; TEROTOLA et al. 1994; VORWERK et al. 1992; GÜNTHER and VORWERK 1991; HAWKINS et al. 1985; SCHMITZ-RODE et al. 1993).

At the moment, the best indication for thromboaspiration seems to be for an acute short segment obstruction in an artery smaller than 7 mm occurring during a proximal recanalization procedure or spontaneous popliteal emboly for other reasons such as aortic aneurysm or thrombus from the heart.

21.2
Catheters Utilizing the Vortex Phenomenon

21.2.1
Principle

The vortex effect is a mechanical depression created at the end of a catheter (similar to the effect of an object coming into contact with an airplane propeller) which effectively attracts and pulverizes thrombotic material in contact with the distal end of this catheter. There is, however, no mechanism for aspiration of the fragmented particles with this catheter.

21.2.2
Materials

Various catheters, which utilize the vortex effect for fragmentation of thrombotic material, are available:

- The Amplatz catheter (Meditech Boston Scientific, Boston, Mass., USA) has two major components, an 8-F catheter armed with a metallic capsule which has two side holes and which has a drill-like mechanism centrally which rotates at very high speed powered by compressed air (100 000 rev/min). The metallic capsule ensures protection of the vascular walls while the lateral side holes and the rapid rotation mechanism of the central drill are responsible for pulverization and

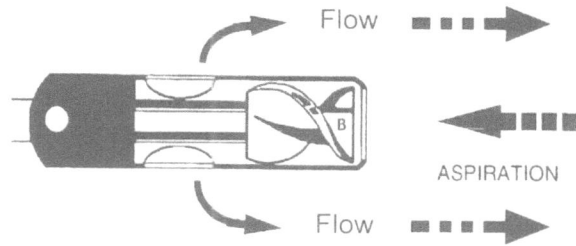

Fig. 21.4. The distal tip of the Amplatz thrombectomy catheter. An impeller covered by a 1-cm metal capsule is driven by a drive shaft at high speed. With the vortex effect the thrombus is aspirated against the impeller, liquefied, and then expelled through side ports (*solid arrows*)

recirculation of these micro-particles fragmented by the vortex effect (Fig. 21.4). The efficiency of this catheter system is directly proportional to the speed and duration of the rotation device (BILDSOE et al. 1989). A study done by YASUI has shown experimentally a 98% efficiency of this apparatus with fragmented particles of the order of 13 μm with no particle larger than 1000 μm ever been liberated (YASUI et al. 1993). Another study done by NAZARIAN demonstrated minimal hemolytic effect associated with this thrombus obliteration but recommended this procedure to be used cautiously in patients who are known to be in chronic renal failure, anemic, or in hypoxic states (NAZARIAN et al. 1996).

- The catheter designed by Kensey utilizing the vortex principle was initially adapted for treatment of atheromatous lesions of the lower limb. It has also shown promise for the treatment of recent thrombotic events but in the absence of a guidewire the risk of perforation of the vessel side walls has caused most investigators to abandon this catheter system.

- The Schmitz-Rode Gunther catheter is essentially a Kensey catheter which has been equipped with a metallic type Dormia cage around the distal end of the catheter to diminish the chance of damage to vessel walls associated with the vortex effect (Fig. 21.5).

- The Thrombolizer (Angiocor – Cordis, Johnson and Johnson Intervention System, Warren, N.J. USA) is essentially made up of two coaxial catheters with one central lumen which allows passage of a guidewire (0.035 in.). The catheter is equipped with clefts in its extremity to allow bending and deformation in this area in response to rotation which is powered by a proximal motor. Although appealing for the obstruction of larger caliber vessels, there is a significant risk of

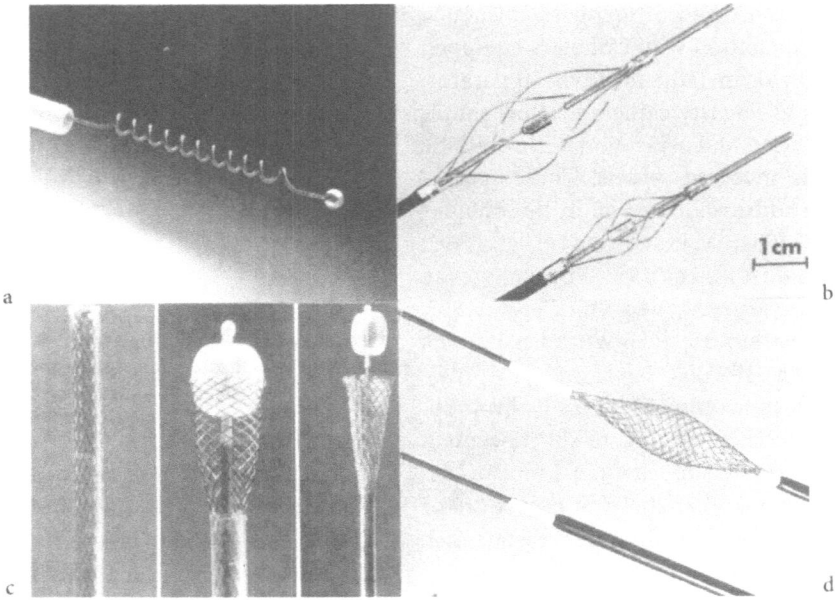

Fig. 21.5. a Rotating aspiration thromboembolectomy (RAT; BARD) is composed of a catheter with a spherical-tipped spiral to facilitate aspiration. **b** Compression thromboem bolectomy catheter using a tulip sheath composed of a covered or non-covered self-expandable stent with a coaxial Fogarty balloon catheter. With the balloon held against the tulip sheath, the thrombus is compressed and then removed through the sheath. **c** The "Mesh Basket" catheter (Schmitz-Rode) constructed by folding both ends of a Wallstent. Self-expansion of the stent is achieved by withdrawing the introducer catheter. The device is turned inside the vessel to remove wall-adherent thrombi. **d** The self-expandable impeller basket catheter (Gunther). An impeller (rotation speed of 100 000 rpm) is protected by a Dormia composed of four spiral-shaped wires to avoid parietal lesion

damage to the side walls of these vessels because of the inability to control the excursion of the drill mechanism during the rotation process. Due to this, modifications have been added (protective cage mechanism) by Schmitz-Rode et al. (1996) which should effectively limit these types of complications.

– Ultrasonic waves (20 kHz) transmitted through a guidewire can also fragment and achieve lysis of thombi utilizing a mixture of cavitation and vortex effect (Schmitz-Rode et al. 1991). To obtain this type of effect, stiff guidewires must be utilized, thus again introducing a risk of vascular perforation. Catheters which are equipped with distal ultrasound transducers at their extremities should alleviate this risk of perforation but necessitate the use of much higher ultrasound frequencies (Shlansky-Goldberg et al. 1994).

21.2.3
Indications and Results

The Amplatz catheter is the only clinically tested system for the moment. Initial studies have demonstrated the system to be efficient in the treatment of

acute thrombosis following graft surgery or for the treatment of thrombosed arteriovenous fistula, but again the absence of a guidewire increases the risk of parietal vascular damage and rules out its use via a contralateral vascular approach (Coleman et al. 1993; Uflacker et al. 1996). In a study done by Uflacker et al. (1996) hemolysis was noted in 63% of patients treated with the Amplatz catheter system; however, no patients demonstrated significant clinical signs associated with this phenomenon.

The major inconvenience of these systems utilizing the vortex effect is the absence of an aspiration-type mechanism, and the significant risk of distal migration of the thrombotic material. Using a compression system concomitantly can diminish the chance of these migrations but does not eliminate them completely. These distal migration phenomena are noted frequently in mechanical recanalization of obstructions of dialysis fistulae but are rarely associated with clinical consequences. Even though clinical consequences are rare, allowing migration distally into the pulmonary bed is an unacceptable complication of thrombectomy, particularly in patients who are dialyzed, of whom up to one third can have elevated arterio-pulmonary pressures and also associated coronary artery disease. In these patients even a minimal embolic phenomenon to the lung bed could possibly cause respiratory decompensation.

On another note, regardless of the method of thrombectomy utilized it is important to prescribe heparin to minimize the bronchospasm which is associated with inhibition of serotonin release in response to an activation of thrombin during the procedure.

In summary, because of the absence of a system of clot aspiration, these catheter systems do not prevent distal embolic migration and necessitate the utilization of fibrinolytics as an adjunct therapy to complete lysis of these distal emboli.

21.3
Catheters Utilizing the Venturi Effect

21.3.1
Principle

Rheolytic catheters are armed with a metallic nozzle at their distal end which allows injection of normal saline under pressure. The retrograde jet of fluid oriented towards the central lumen of the catheter permits destruction of clots by a pressure phenomenon without damaging the vessel walls while permitting aspiration of the fragmented material via the Venturi effect and hence diminishing the chance of distal embolic migration of thrombotic material (Fig. 21.6). The distal metallic nozzle can be simple or complex, armed with one or multiple orifices to increase efficiency of the procedure. The catheter is equipped with a large lumen diameter and hence permits aspiration of fragmented material as well as allowing passage of a guidewire and injection of contrast material to evaluate the progression of recanalization.

21.3.2
Materials

Three types of such catheters are presently available (Fig. 21.7): the Rheolytic Thrombectomy System (Angiojet, Possis Medical Corporation, USA), a 5-F catheter which utilizes a specific injector type (10–15 psi); the Hydrolyser catheter (Cordis) in 7- and 6-F caliber; and a newer catheter of 8-F caliber (OASIS Boston). The last two catheter systems have a major advantage over the Angiojet system in that a standard angiographic injector system (750 psi with a flow rate of 3–5 ml/s) can be utilized.

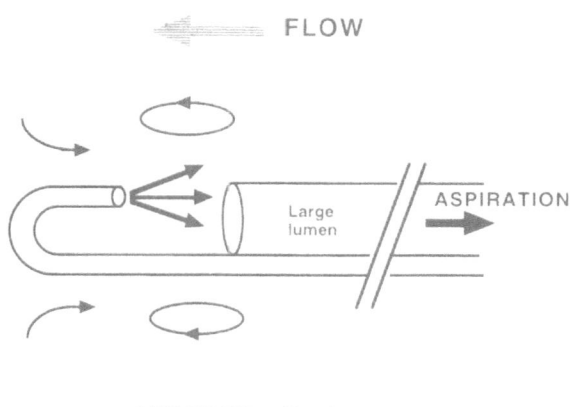

Fig. 21.6. The Venturi effect. The devices using high-pressure water jets allow three functions: (1) The mechanical force of the fluid jet attacks the clot, breaking it up into fragments. (2) The returning jet stream results in a slight negative pressure at the catheter tip (Venturi effect). Therefore, the clot is sucked towards and into the jet. (3) The remaining jet velocity transports the fragmented clot material through the discharging lumen into a collecting bag

21.3.3
Indications and Results

These catheters all have the common feature of being flexible and maneuverable on a guidewire. By utilizing the Venturi effect, thrombus fragmentation and aspiration are achieved while theoretically eliminating distal embolic phenomena. In vitro documentation confirms the efficiency of this system in limiting distal embolic fragment migration, particularly when a distal occluding cuff is utilized which effectively diminishes the flow and increases the recirculation of blood (BALLINI et al. 1995; BUCKER et al. 1996). Histological analysis after use of this system shows remarkably little endothelial damage, that is to say greatly reduced as compared to the changes noted with the Fogarty catheter (VAN OMMEN et al. 1994). Moreover, hemolysis is not significant with these types of catheter.

The first clinical applications of these new catheter systems seem to have generated significant interest and enthusiasm for their abilities (DRASLER et al. 1992; REEKERS et al. 1993) (Fig. 21.8). To our knowledge, only use of the Hydrolyser catheter has been reported many times in the literature (VORWERK et al. 1994; REEKERS et al. 1996; ROUSSEAU et al. 1997).

For hemodialysis fistulae and grafts, the success rate of these catheters is on average around 93%, the main causes of failure being aneurysms, kinks, and organized thrombi. Complications associated

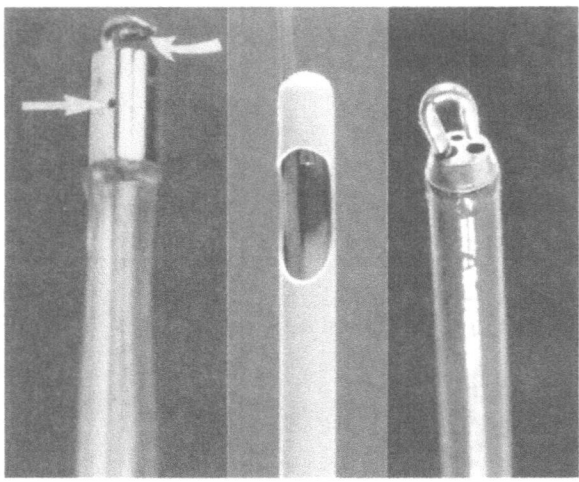

Fig. 21.7. Three catheters using the Venturi effect are available: (1) The rheolytic thrombectomy system (Angiojet Possis Minneapolis, Minn., USA) is a 5-F dual-lumen tubing. The smaller lumen contains a high pressure stainless-steel tubing for high-pressure water jets. A special pump is required to achieve a pressure of 10000 psi. The exhaust lumen is operated by a roller pump. (2) The Hydrolyser (Cordis) is a 65-cm long, straight, 6–7-F double-lumen catheter, with a 6-mm side hole located 4mm from the distal tip. (3) The OASIS Catheter (Boston) is an 8-F, three-lumen catheter. These three catheters are flexible and can follow a guidewire of 0.0018, 0.0025, and 0.0014 in., respectively. The Hydrolyser and OASIS at catheters need a conventional contrast injector to achieve the high-pressure jets

with thrombectomy of hemodialysis shunts are infrequent and are usually due to venous dissections which can be easily treated by installating an endoprosthesis at the dissection site.

For native arteries and bypass grafts thrombotic events in the lower limb, the success rate is lower, 73% and 53%, respectively, and in 58% of these successful cases no adjunct fibrinolytic therapy was necessary (ROUSSEAU et al. 1997). The most notable complication is distal embolic migration which is most often noted in recanalization procedures of infrapopliteal bypass graft thrombosis. The literature documentation has demonstrated, however, that these distal embolic migration phenomena can be avoided if certain basic rules are followed: (a) Begin the injection of normal saline at a thrombusfree area and at a significant distance from the obstructive site to optimize the Venturi effect before beginning the recanalization procedure; (b) never traverse the distal lesion with the catheter; and (c) systematically use a compression system to diminish the distal flow and facilitate the thrombectomy procedure.

21.4
Discussion

Generally speaking, percutaneous thrombectomy provides an efficient mechanism for relieving vascular obstruction and produces results in minutes as opposed to several hours when compared to fibrinolytic therapy, with the added benefit of decreased

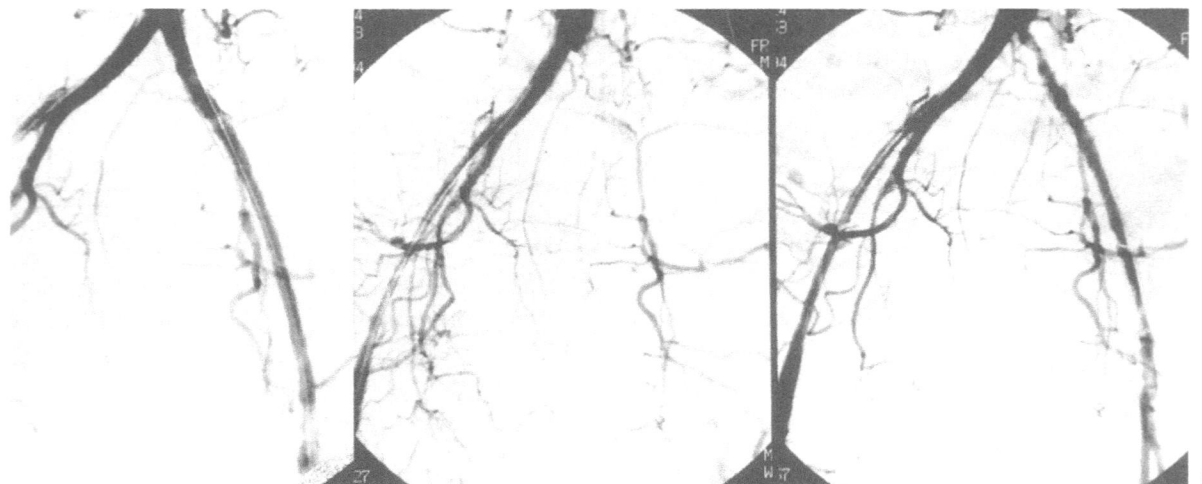

Fig. 21.8 a–c. Woman with 200-m claudication of 6 days' duration. (a) Initial angiogram demonstrates a totally occluded left iliac artery (a Wallstent was implanted 6 months earlier for a chronic external iliac artery occlusion). **b,c** Angiogram, obtained just after Hydrolyser thrombectomy (via a retrograde left femoral approach), shows a widely open lumen with proximal and distal residual stenoses (**b**), successfully treated by balloon dilatation (**c**)

morbidity and diminished overall cost. These procedures, however, are to be viewed as complementary to rather than in direct competition with thrombectomy procedures.

The choice of a particular treatment method must take into account several factors:

The patient: age, clinical setting, degree of ischemia, contraindications to possible fibrinolytic therapy.
The etiology of the obstruction: emboli, thrombosis on a pre-existing atheromatous lesion, iatrogenic complication associated with arterial catheterization, obstruction of bypass graft surgery, etc.
Type of obstruction: proximal or distal, diameter of the artery, length of the obstruction, state of the distal vascular bed.

Classically, embolic phenomena involving the aorta or iliac artery have been treated with the classic Fogarty catheter technique, whereas, in our opinion, distal obstructive phenomena and obstructions which occur on pre-existing pathological arterial beds are better treated with percutaneous endovascular techniques.

Rheolytic over-a-wire catheter systems which permit simultaneous thrombolysis and thromboaspiration of thrombotic debris are the preferred method of treatment of long obstructed segments in the femoropopliteal region with or without short-term adjuvent in situ fibrinolytic therapy. Conversely, distal vascular lesions and embolic migration phenomena secondary to a proximal dilatation are better treated by a simple thromboaspiration technique. Finally, thrombosed popliteal aneurysm which are symptomatic should be primarily treated with in situ fibinolysis to liberate the distal vascular bed of thrombotic material, hence optimizing subsequent bypass graft surgery.

In summary, the ideal catheter system for percutaneous thrombectomy should be of the smallest diameter possible and capable of limiting the distal embolic migration phenomenon and/or damage to the vascular wall while treating all forms of obstruction regardless of the size of the artery or vein in question. Catheters utilizing the Venturi effect seem to be best equipped to fulfill the above-mentioned criteria as a method of percutaneous thrombectomy. In our present socio-economic context, these types of percutaneous procedures should prove to be highly efficient and diminish the need for adjuvent fibrinolytic therapy to justify the increased cost associated with this treatment, which has not been clearly demonstrated in the literature thus far.

References

Reekers JA, Kromhout JG, Van Der Waal K (1993) Catheter for percutaneous thrombectomy: first clinical experience. Radiology 188:871–874

Reekers JA, Kromhout JG, Spithoven HG, Jacobvs MJHM, Mali MPHM, Schultze-Kool LJ (1996) Arterial thrombosis below the inguinal ligament: percutaneous treatment with a thrombosuction catheter. Radiology 198:49–53

Rousseau H, Sapoval M, Ballini P, Dubé M, Joffre F, Gaux JC, Cercueil JP, Krause D, Moulin G, Bartoli JM (1997) Percutaneous recanalization of acutely thrombosed vessels by hydrodynamic thrombectomy (Hydrolyser). Eur Radiol (in press) 1997; 7:935-941

Schmitz-Rode TH, Günther RW (1991) New device for percutaneous fragmentation of pulmonary emboli. Radiology 180:135–137

Schmitz-Rode TH, Günther RW, Muller-Leisse C (1991) US-assisted aspiration thrombectomy: in vitro investigations. Radiology 178:677–679

Schmitz-Rode TH, Bohndorf K, Günther RW (1993) New «mesh basket» for percutaneous removal of wall-adherent thrombi in dialysis shunts. Cardiovasc Intervent Radiol 16:7–10

Schmitz-Rode TH, Adam G, Kilbinger M, Pfeffer J, Biesterfeld S, Günther RW (1996) Fragmentation of pulmonary emboli: in vivo experimental evaluation of two high-speed rotating catheters. Cardiovasc Intervent Radiol 19:165–169

Shlansky-Goldberg RD, Sehgal C, Redd DCB (1994) Use of high-frequency ultrasound for thrombolysis (Abstr). Society of Cardiovascular and Interventional Radiology, 19th Annual Scientific Meeting, San Diego

Hawkins IF, Helms R, Spencer C, Hawkins MC (1985) Mechanical spiral embolectomy catheter. Semin Intervent Radiol 2(4):414–418

Lammer J, Pilger E, Neumayer K, Schreyer H (1986) Intraarterial fibrinolysis: long term results. Radiology 161:159–163

Matsumoto AH, Sarosi MG, Selby JB, Tegtmeyer CJ (1992) Thromboembolectomy with the transluminal extraction catheter (TEC) as an adjunct to thrombolysis. J Vasc Intervent Radiol 3:491–495

McNamara TO, Bomberger RA, Merchant RF (1991) Intraarterial urokinase as the initial therapy for acutely ischemic lower limbs. Circulation 83(Suppl 1):I–106, I–119

Meyerovitz MF, Goldhaber SZ, Reagan K et al. (1990) Recombinant tissue-type plasminogen activator versus urokinase in peripheral arterial and graft occlusions: a randomized trial. Radiology 175:75–78

Nazarian GK, Qian Z, Coleman CC, Rengel G, Castaneda-Zuniga WR, Hunter DW, Amplatz K (1996) Hemolytic effect of the Amplatz thrombectomy device. J Vasc Intervent Radiol 5:155–160

Ouriel K, Veith FJ, Sasahara AA (1996) Thrombolysis or peripheral arterial surgery: phase I results. J Vasc Surg 23:64–75

Ponomar E, Carlson JE, Kindlund A, Rodriguez JP, Castaneda-Zuniga WR, Hunter DW, Yedlicka JW, Amplatz K (1991) Clot-trapper device for transjugular thrombectomy from the inferior vena cava. Radiology 179:279–282

Ballini P, Dubé M, Rousseau H, Otal P, Sentenac B, El Khouri J, Joffre F (1995) The hydrolyser catheter: in vitro testing to evaluate distal embolisation. J Vasc Intervent Radiol 18 Suppl 1

Bildsoe MMC, Moradian GP, Hunter DW, Castaneda-Zuniga WR, Amplatz K (1989) Mechanical clot dissolution: new concept. Radiology 171:231–233

444

Blaisdell FW, Stelle M, Allen RE (1978) Management of acute lower extremity ischemia due to embolism and thrombosis. Surgery 84:822–834

Bucker A, Schmitz-Rode TH, Vorwerk D, Günther RW (1996) Comparative in vitro study of two percutaneous hydrodynamic thrombectomy systems. J Vasc Intervent Radiol 7:451–454

Coleman CC, Krenzel C, Dietz CA, Nazarian GK, Amplatz K (1993) Mechanical thrombectomy: results of early experience. Radiology 189:803–805

Diffin DC, Kandarpa K (1996) Assessment of peripheral intraarterial thrombolysis versus surgical revascu-larization in acute lower-limb ischemia: a review of limb-salvage and mortality statistics. J Vasc Intervent Radiol 7:57–63

Drasler W, Jenson ML, Wilson GJ, Thielen MT, Protonarios EI, Dutcher RG, Possis ZC (1992) Rheolytic catheter for percutaneous removal of thrombus. Radiology 182:263–267

Gordon RD, Fogarty TJ (1984) Peripheral arterial embolism. In: Rutherford RB (ed) Vascular surgery, 2nd edn. Saunders, Philadelphia, p 451

Günther RW, Vorwerk D (1991) Minibasket for percutaneous embolectomy and filter protection against distal embolization: technical note. Cardiovasc Intervent Radiol 14:195–198

Starck EE, MacDermott JC (1988) Rotating aspiration thromboembolectomy. Radiology 169(P):366

Terotola SO, Lund GB, Scheel PJ, Savader SJ, Vembrux AC, Osterman FA (1994) Thrombosed dialysis access grafts: percutaneous mechanical declotting without urokinase. Radiology 191:721–726

Uflacker R, Rajogopalan PR, Vujic I, Stutley JE (1996) Treatment of thrombosed dialysis access grafts: randomized trial of surgical thrombectomy versus mechanical thrombectomy with the Amplatz device. J Vasc Intervent Radiol 7:185–192

Van Ommen GVA, Van Der Veen E, Daemen M, Habets J, Wellens HJ (1994) In vivo evaluation of the safety to the vessel wall of the hydrolyser hydrodynamic thrombectomy catheter (Abstr). Society of Cardiovascular and Interventional Radiology, 19th Annual Scientific Meeting San Diego

Vorwerk D, Günther RW, Clerc C, Schmitz-Rode TH, Imbert C (1992) Percutaneous embolectomy: in vitro investigations of the self-expanding tulip sheath. Radiology 182:415–418

Vorwerk D, Sohn M, Schurmann K, Hoogeveen Y, Gladziwa U, Günther RW (1994) Hydrodynamic thrombectomy of hemodialysis fistulas: first clinical results. J Vasc Intervent Radiol 5:813–821

Wagner HJ, Starck EE, Reuter P (1994) Long-term results of percutaneous aspiration embolectomy. Cardiovasc Intervent Radiol 17:241–246

Yasui K, Oian Z, Nazarian GK, Hunter DW, Castaneda-Zuniga WR, Amplatz K (1993) Recirculation-type Amplatz clot macerator: determination of particle size and distribution. J Vasc Intervent Radiol 4:275–278

22 Pharmacological Thrombolysis - Systematic Therapy

M. MARTIN

22.1
Introduction

The development of chronic arterial occlusion is due to three processes: the first step is an arteriosclerotic lesion of the intima. Causes under discussion are: radiation (NYLANDER et al. 1978; SILVERBERG et al. 1978), carbon monoxide (MARSHALL et al. 1978), high blood pressure (WOOSHMANN and NITSCHKOFF 1966), lipid infiltration (DOERR 1963; KANNEL et al. 1979), and old age (SCHOOP and SCHMIDTKE 1973).

Subsequently, smooth muscle cells from the vessel wall and monocytes from the blood stream invade this area. Some of these clusters of intimal cells become foam cells by the accumulation of lipids. Another feature are caps of fibrocollagenous tissue bulging into the lumen of the artery affected (ROBBINS and ANGELL 1976). Platelets play a role here as they secrete platelet derived growth factor (PDFG) (HARKER et al. 1975) which stimulates the devision and accumulation of fibrocytes.

Platelet accumulation is followed by fibrin deposition leading, over months and sometimes years, to an arteriosclerotic vessel occlusion. If these narrowings meet in the center of the vessel, blood flow stops and a coagulation thrombus builds up extending to the branches of the next collaterals upstream and downstream. By this, the length of the occlusion is given (Fig. 22.1).

M. MARTIN, MD, Professor, Angiologische Praxis, Klinikum Duisburg, Zu den Rehwiesen 3, 47055 Duisburg, Germany

22.2
Fibrinolytic Treatment of Chronic Arterial Occlusions

In 1968 five papers were published independently (ALEXANDER et al. 1968; EHRINGER and FISCHER 1968; KAINDL et al. 1968; SCHOOP et al. 1968a,b) dealing with streptokinase treatment in patients with chronic arterial occlusions and stenoses (Table 22.1). These early clinical trials showed that even long-standing arterial obstructions could be fibrinolytically removed. The occlusion period, however, had its limit and occlusions of many months or years standing had a poorer prognosis than younger obstructions. Therefore, study groups dealing with patients suffering from a very long claudication history (e.g., 3–15 months) did not find favorable clinical results (KAINDL et al. 1968). Others who treated patients with a shorter occlusion history (1 to several weeks) were much more successful in that a considerable number of chronic arterial occlusions could be removed (ALEXANDER et al. 1968; EHRINGER

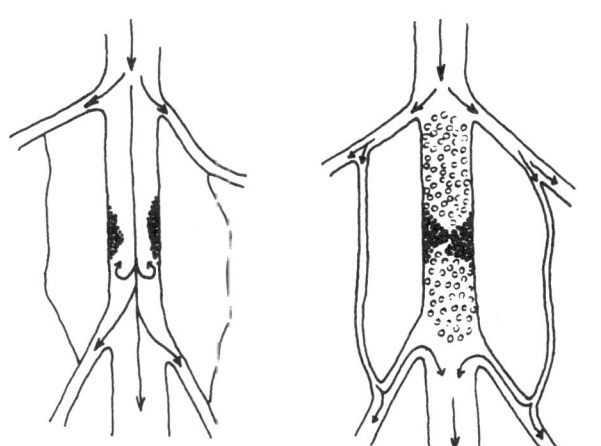

Fig. 22.1 a,b. The development of a chronic arterial occlusion. a Mural thrombi have sedimented at an atherosclerotic part of the inner face of the artery. b A pressure gradient builds up between the lumina proximal and distal to the stenosis which is a stimulus for collaterals to grow

Table 22.1. Accumulation of reports dealing with removal of chronic arterial occlusions and widening of stenoses

Author	Type of obstruction						Therapeutic results and comments
	Femoral		Iliac		Aortic		
	St	Oc	St	Oc	St	Oc	
ALEXANDER et al. (1968)	2	23	5	5	–	–	Removal of four femoral occlusions 5 weeks–9 months old Removal of two iliac occlusions 5 weeks–6 weeks old
EHRINGER and FISCHER (1968)	–	8	–	1	–	–	Removal of five femoral occlusions 5 days–5 weeks old
KAINDL et al. (1968)	–	10	–	1	–	–	No success. Occlusions 5–15 months old
SCHOOP et al. (1968a) old	–	34	–	43	–	7	Removal of one femoral occlusion 10 months old Removal of seven iliac occlusions 5 weeks–4 years Removal of three aortic occlusions 6 months–7 years old
SCHOOP et al. (1968b)	11	–	5	–	1	–	Widening of three femoral stenoses Widening of five iliac stenoses Widening of one aortic stenoses
MARTIN et al. (1970)	25	98	73	97	4	15	Removal of four femoral occlusions Removal of 16 iliac occlusions Removal of four aortic occlusions Widening of five femoral stenoses Widening of 42 iliac stenoses Widening of three aortic stenoses
VERSTRAETE et al. (1971)	5	17	16	11	1	2	Removal of one femoral artery 21 days old Removal of one iliac artery 4 months old Removal of one aortic occlusion 1 year old Removal of one iliac occlusion 14 days old
DEUTSCH and EHRINGER (1972)	–	53	–	13	–	–	Removal of 14 femoral occlusions 6 days–6 weeks old Removal of two femoral occlusions 6 weeks–6 months old Removal of seven iliac occlusions 6 days–6 weeks old Removal of two iliac occlusions 6 weeks–6 months old
HEINRICH and SCHMUTZLER (1972)	6	22	–	31	2	6	Removal of eight femoral occlusions less than 8 weeks old Widening of three femoral stenoses less than 2 years old Removal of three iliac occlusions less than 1 year old Widening of 13 iliac stenoses less than 2 years old Removal of one aortic occlusion
LE VEEN and DIAZ 1972	–	26	–	3	–	1	Removal of ten femoral occlusions 6h–9 months old
DOTTER et al. (1972)	–	2	–	2	–	1	Removal of two fresh iliac occlusions and one 3–4-week-old subclavian occlusion
PERSSON et al. (1973)	–	14	–	4	–	–	Therapeutic failure in eight femoral and one iliac occlusion of several months or years standing. Clearance in six femoral and three iliac occlusions less than 10 days old
MARTIN (1982)	–	22	–	136	–	31	Removal of 20 femoral, 33 iliac and ten aortic occlusions Good results if occlusions younger than 6 weeks old, poorer if occlusions older

St, stenosis; Oc, occlusion.

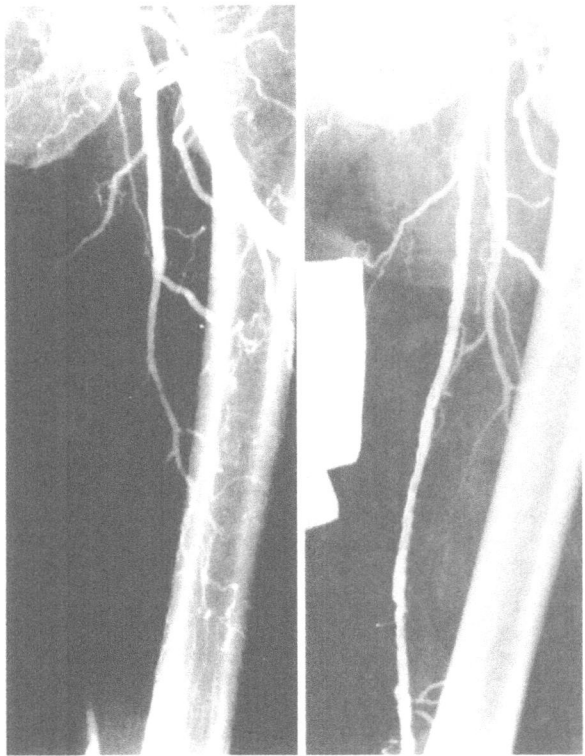

a,b

Fig. 22.2 a,b. Type I lysis. **a** Occlusion of the femoral artery over its entire length. **b** Complete clearance after systemic short-term ultrahigh streptokinase treatment

and FISCHER 1968; SCHOOP et al. 1968a; MARTIN et al. 1970; DEUTSCH and EHRINGER 1972; HEINRICH and SCHMUTZLER 1972; LE VEEN and DIAZ 1972; DOTTER et al. 1972; PERSSON et al. 1973; MARTIN 1982).

It became evident that two basically different situations exist: in one an artery is obstructed by a thrombus which can be cleared completely by fibrinolytic treatment (Fig. 22.2), and in the other, fibrocollagenous organization tissue forms beneath a mural thrombus. In this situation a connective tissue-type stenosis forms which persists after lysis but may be widened by further percutaneous transluminal angioplasty (PTA) (Fig. 22.3).

22.3
Conventional Streptokinase Treatment

In 1970 a first monograph was published on thrombolytic therapy of chronic arterial occlusions (MARTIN et al. 1970). According to this report best results were achieved in the common iliac artery, poorest in the femoral segment. Arterial stenoses were also treated and could be widened if they were located in relatively large vessels (e.g., aorta, iliac arteries) and

displayed special morphologic features such as short extension, of crumbly and asymmetric shape.

Second and third mongraphs on the same subject were published by HEINRICH in 1975 and MARTIN in 1982. In the former, seven angiologic departments reported on their results in 708 patients receiving fibrinolytic treatment for chronic arterial occlusions and stenoses. In the latter monograph the results of the Aggertal Clinic between 1967 and 1977 were summarized. It covered a 1–3-day streptokinase infusion treatment administered to 600 patients with arterial occlusions and stenoses. The results of both studies were quite similar. Clearance rates of around 70% were achieved up to 2 weeks (femoral occlusion) and 6 weeks (iliac occlusion) after onset of symptoms, respectively. Femoral arteries were virtually non lysable after 3 months, and iliac occlusions after 6 months.

One of the most important side effect of streptokinase treatment using the 100 000 IU/h regimen was cerebral bleeding. A total rate of 2.8% bleeds were recorded. Of these 0.83% were reversible (no neurological deficits at hospital discharge), 1.3% led to irreparable neurological deficits, and 0.67% were fatal.

22.4
Short-Term Ultrahigh Streptokinase Treatment

A new era of fibrinolytic treatment of chronic arterial occlusion came with the advent of a newly developed short-term ultrahigh streptokinase dosage regimen (UHSK). To date this treatment form replaces the 100 000 IU/h scheme in most German hospitals. UHSK consists of one or more 6-h series of 9 million IU each. Dependent on the clinical outcome, up to five series can be given on 5 subsequent days.

In the Duisburg trial (MARTIN and FIEBACH 1994) three aortic occlusions, 73 iliac artery occlusions, and 286 femoropopliteal occlusions were treated with UHSK. Two of the three aortic occlusions were dissolved following between one and four UHSK series, respectively. In the other cases where a stenosis remained or where, after fibrinolytic therapy, the arteries still remained occluded, a subsequent PTA was performed. The total patency rate for iliac artery occlusion treated with UHSK-PTA was 46 of 73 (63.0%). Stratification into occlusions of shorter duration improved this last figure in that the clearance rate of occlusions less than 3 months old rose to 33 of 49 (67.3%) and the clearance rate of occlusions less than 3 weeks to 26 of 34 (76.5%).

Femoropopliteal occlusions were another target for UHSK therapy. The global clearance rate for

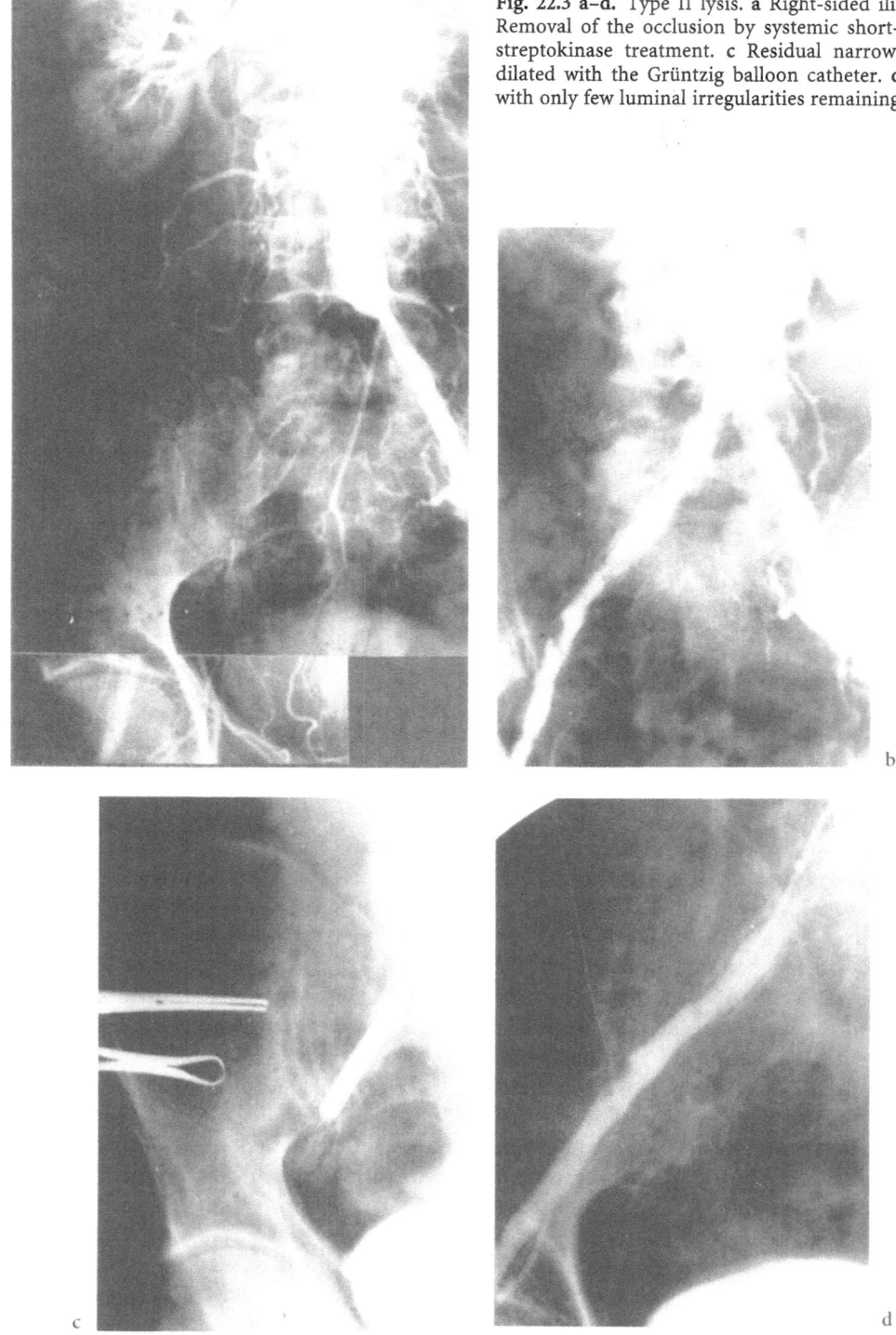

Fig. 22.3 a–d. Type II lysis. **a** Right-sided iliac occlusion. **b** Removal of the occlusion by systemic short-term ultrahigh streptokinase treatment. **c** Residual narrowings are being dilated with the Grüntzig balloon catheter. **d** Vessel patent with only few luminal irregularities remaining

femoral artery occlusions treated with UHSK in combination with PTA was 143 of 268 (53.4%). Of great importance for the removal rate of femoral occlusions was the outflow situation of the calf. A rise of patency from 53.4% to 67.5% was seen if two or

three calf arteries were open. Less important was the occlusion age in the ≤6-week group (rise of patency from 53.4% to 60.5%) and the occlusion length in the ≤15-cm group (rise of patency from 53.4% to 59.2%). A particularly good result was recorded in patients with a short history, a limited occlusion length, and a good outflow tract. Here the opening rate was 55 of 68 (80.9%) with UHSK therapy alone or in combination with PTA.

Six cerebral bleedings (0.836%) were recorded in 718 patients treated with UHSK. Four patients (0.557%) died directly through the impact of bleeding. The cerebral bleeding was correlated with the number of UHSK series (fall to 0.598% if only one or two series were given) and with the patient age (no bleeding in patients under 55 years of age).

22.5
Mechanisms of Lytic Removal of Chronic Arterial Occlusions

On the clinical level, three different mechanisms of lysis exist:

1. Fibrinolytic therapy leads to clot removal (see Fig. 22.2);

$$\text{Occlusion} \xrightarrow{\text{Lysis}} \text{Clearance}$$

2. Only partial clearance can be achieved. Residuals stenoses remain which can be dilated by PTA (see Fig. 22.3):

$$\text{Occlusion} \xrightarrow{\text{Lysis}} \text{Residual stenosis}$$

$$\text{Residual stenosis} \xrightarrow{\text{PTA}} \text{Clearance}$$

3. After fibrinolytic treatment the vessel is still blocked. However, by introducing a wire or a catheter, clearance is restored immediately even in long-extended occlusions which normally do not respond to PTA technique. In this case thrombus material becomes fluid, but vessel patency is not restored because of tiny crumbs of undissolved thrombi or thin flaps of organization material spreading within the vessel's lumen (Fig. 22.4):

$$\text{Occlusion} \xrightarrow{\text{Lysis}} \text{"softening" of the occlusion}$$

$$\text{Softened occlusion} \xrightarrow{\text{PTA}} \text{Clearance}$$

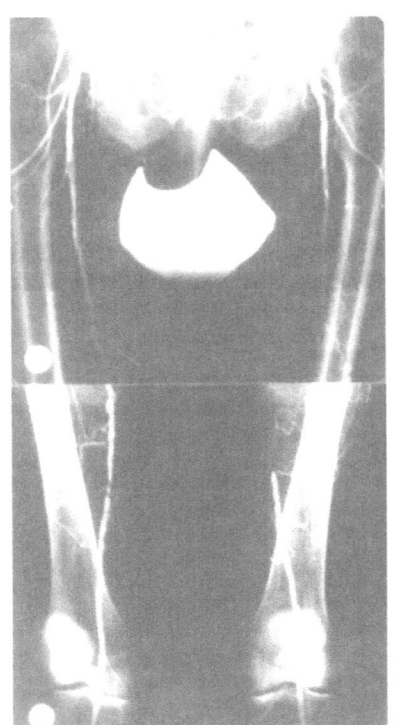
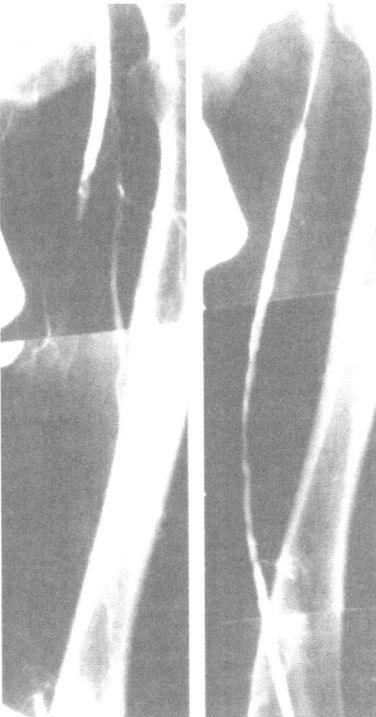

Fig. 22.4 a–c. Type III lysis. a Left-sided femoral occlusion. b After systemic short-term ultrahigh streptokinase treatment partial clearance of the upper part of the vessel. A distal occlusion is still in place. c The femoral artery becomes patent at full length merely by intraarterial introduction of the Grüntzig catheter (without balloon inflation)

22.6
Conclusion

Systemic fibrinolytic therapy in combination with PTA was an effective tool for the removal of arteriosclerotic vessel occlusions and the widening of arterial stenoses. When the claudication history did not exceed 6 weeks, good results were achieved in aortic, iliac, and femoral occlusions. In femoral occlusions the calf run-off situation was of great importance. For satisfying results, two or three calf arteries had to be open. Arterial stenoses responded to lytic treatment if certain morphological features were present and the vessel was not too small.

The cerebral bleeding rate as the most important side effect of lytic treatment was 2.83% in patients treated with a conventional 100 000 IU streptokinase per hour regimen and 0.836% with the newly devised short-term UHSK. This reduction in bleeding accidents speaks in favor of the latter treatment form and was recently confirmed by a controlled multicenter study (conventional streptokinase regimen versus UHSK regimen) (HEINRICH and HEINRICH 1996).

The efficacy of systemic fibrinolytic treatment compared with other forms of treatment (e.g., intraarterial lysis) is difficult to assess. Up to now no systematic study has been conducted to answer this question. Future trials need to compare groups in which essential characteristics for good or poor prognosis, such as occlusion age, occlusiong length, and run-off situation, are evenly distributed.

References

Alexander K, Buhl U, Holsten D, Poliwoda H, Wagner HH (1968) Fibrinolytische Therapie des chronischen Arterienverschlusses. Med Klin 63:2067–2070

Deutsch E, Ehringer H (1972) Thrombolytic therapy in chronic arterial occlusions. J Clin Pathol 25:644–645

Doerr W (1963) Perfusionstherorie der Arteriosklerose. Thieme, Stuttgart

Dotter CHT, Rosch J, Seaman AJ, Dennis D, Massey WH (1972) Streptokinase treatment of thromboembolic disease. Radiology 102:283–290

Ehringer H, Fischer M (1968) Erfolgreiche thrombolytische Therapie bei subakuten arteriellen Thrombosen. Med Welt:1726–1730

Harker LA, Ross R, Slichter SJ (1975) Chronic endothelial cell injury and platelet-factor induced arteriosclerosis (Abstr). Vth Congress of the International Society on Thrombosis and Haemostasis, July 21–26, Paris, p 56

Heinrich F (1975) Streptokinase-Therapie bei chronischer arterieller Verschlußkrankheit. Ergebnisse einer multizentrischen Studie. Medizinische Verlagsgesellschaft Marburg

Heinrich F, Heinrich U (1996) Ergebnis der Nordbadischen Venen-Lyse-NBVL-Studie. Prospektive phlebographisch kontrollierte randomisierte multizentrische Prüfung der Wirkung von ultrahoher versus konventionell dosierter Streptokinase bei frischen Thromben in tiefen Bein-Becken-Venen. Med Klin 91:1–13

Heinrich F, Schmutzler R (1972) Ergebnisse der Thrombolysebehandlung chronischer Gliedmaßenarterienverschlüsse. Dtsch Med J 23:351–358

Kaindl F, Pilgerstorfer HW, Weidinger P, Fischer M (1968) Untersuchungen zur Thrombolyse älterer arterieller Verschlüsse mit Streptokinase. Med Welt:1731–1733

Kannel WB, Castelli WP, Gordon T (1979) Cholesterol in the prediction of atherosclerotic disease. Ann Intern Med 90:85–95

Le Veen HH, Diaz CA (1972) Venous and arterial occlusive disease treated by enzymatic clot lysis. Arch Surg 105:927–936

Marshall M, Hess H, Staubesand J (1978) Experimentelle Untersuchungen über den Risikofaktor Rauchen. VASA 7:389–397

Martin M (1982) Streptokinase in chronic arterial disease. CRC Press, Boca Raton

Martin M, Fiebach BJO (1994) Fibrinolytische Behandlung peripherer Arterien- und Venenverschlüsse. Huber, Bern

Martin M, Schoop W, Zeitler E (1970) Thrombolyse bei chronischer Arteriopathie. Huber, Bern

Nylander G, Pettersson F, Swedenborg J (1978) Localized arterial occlusions in patients treated with pelvic field radiation for cancer. Cancer 41:2158–216

Persson AV, Thomson JE, Patmann D (1973) Streptokinase as an adjunct to arterial surgery. Arch Surg 107:779–784

Robbins SL, Angell M (1976) Basic pathology. Saunders, Philadelphia

Schoop W, Schmidtke I (1973) Spontane Lumenerweiterungen von Arterienstenosen. Herz Kreisl 5:9

Schoop W, Martin M, Zeitler E (1968a) Beseitigung alter Arterienverschlüsse durch intravenöse Streptokinaseinfusion. Dtsch Med Wochenschr 93:2312–2324

Schoop W, Martin M, Zeitler E (1968b) Beseitigung von Stenosen in Extremitätenarterien durch intravenöse Streptokinase -Therapie. Dtsch Med Wochenschr 93:1629–1633

Silverberg GD, Britt RH, Don Goffinet R (1978) Radiation-induced carotid artery disease. Cancer 41:130–137

Verstraete M, Vermylen J, Donati MB (1971) The effect of streptokinase on chronic arterial occlusions and stenoses. Ann Intern Med 74:377–382

Wooshmann H, Nitschkoff ST (1966) Histochemische Untersuchungen an Aortenläsionen nach experimenteller Hypertonie. Acta Biol Med Ger 16:70–78

23 Catheter Interventions in Acute and Subacute Occlusions of Peripheral Arteries

F. Mahler and D.-D. Do

CONTENTS

23.1
Introduction

The catheter-based approach to the problems of acute and subacute occlusion of peripheral arteries, besides vascular surgery, is increasing in importance, particularly when alternative interventional methods to local thrombolysis, such as pharmaco-mechanical dissolution and aspiration of the thrombus material, are included. In this chapter, the experiences of our group, as well as those given in the literature concerning interventional therapy, are summarized. We will present evidence to support the proposition of a complex percutaneous catheter approach in each case by using various appropriate techniques, including catheter thrombus aspiration, percutaneous transluminal angioplasty (PTA), and local thrombolysis.

23.2
Catheter-Guided Methods of Thrombolysis

First attempts at thrombolysis in thromboembolic lesions were published by Dotter et al. (1974), and later by Dembski and Zeitler (1978). It was not before Hess et al. (1982) had published a large series of patients that the method gained some popularity and standardization. Historically, systemic intravenous infusion for thrombolysis was introduced for peripheral arteries prior to intraarterial application, but it has been almost completely abandoned at present. Although this method is the current therapy for coronary artery occlusions, its efficacy in large peripheral arteries and the occurrance of complications make it clearly inferior to the direct intraarterial approach (Working party on thrombolysis in the management of limb ischemia 1996).

In intraarterial catheter-guided thrombolysis, two principal methods can be distinguished: The first, used more in Anglo-Saxon countries, consists of regional intraarterial infusion of thrombolytics, even though the catheter is initially placed close or into the occluding thrombus; the second consists of direct infiltration of the thrombus by the thrombolytic agent by means of different catheter techniques. Infiltration techniques have been applied mainly in Europe and, recently, also in Anglo-Saxon countries in the form of pulsed-spray techniques. The following sections briefly review the methods currently available and outline their advantages and disadvantages.

23.3
Techniques of Local Thrombolysis

23.3.1
Intraarterial Infusion

This method is preferred by most authors from the American continent (Working party on throm-

F. Mahler, Professor, MD, D.-D. Do, MD, Angiologische Abteilung, Inselspital, CH 3010 Bern, Switzerland

BOLYSIS IN THE MANAGEMENT OF LIMB ISCHEMIA 1996). The thrombolytic agent is delivered by an intraarterial catheter placed proximal or within the occluding thrombus with the intention of maximizing the concentration of the drug in the vicinity of the thrombus. Via the catheter the infusion is started according to one of the dosage schemes reported (McNamara and Fischer 1985). The majority of reports and studies have been carried out according to this principle as summarized in the consensus report on thrombolysis in the management of limb arterial occlusion (Working party on thrombolysis in the management of limb ischemia 1996). One of the largest studies, the TOPAS trial (Ouriel et al. 1998), which compared local thrombolysis with one of these techniques, found no clear advantage over the initial surgical approach, but rather a significant complication rate.

23.3.2
Thrombus Infiltration

The Hess Technique (Hess et al. 1996): The principle of this technique is a stepwise infusion through an end-hole catheter, the tip of which is advanced within the thrombus as soon as the material has dissolved. This method requires only small doses of thrombolytic agent, but necessitates that the patient and the operator remain present in the angiography laboratory during the entire treatment session, which used to last up to several hours.

The Microporous Balloon Technique (Schneider and Hoffmann 1996): Thrombolytic agents are applied to the thrombus via a perforated balloon catheter. By thrombus dilatation and simultaneous infiltration, a pharmaco-mechanical mechanism is exerted and the dissolution of the thrombus accelerated, usually lasting less than 1h. This technique requires, as does the Hess technique, the presence of the operator throughout the procedure for manipulation of the catheter. Introduction of the microporous balloon catheter requires initial guidewire passage through the thrombus.

Pulse-Spray Infusion (Kandarpa et al. 1988; Valji et al. 1993): This technique employs intermittent injection of the thrombolytic agent into the thrombus in order to fragment it and to increase the surface area available for enzymatic action by the plasminogen activator. It requires specially designed infusion catheters with distal side holes introduced over a guidewire. There are varying models of such catheters with different infusion lengths and dis-

tances between the orifices with and without the need for tip occlusion, as well as specially designed intermittent pumps.

23.3.3
Comparison of Techniques

We have chosen to illustrate the efficacy of the infiltration techniques according to Hess (end-hole) and Schneider (microporous balloon) by the preliminary results of a prospective randomized multicenter study comparing urokinase and recombinant tissue plasminogen activator (rt-PA), and the two methods (see Table 23.1). Following thrombolysis, between 70% and 80% of all arteries showed reperfusion, and after the application of additional methods, such as PTA and/or aspiration to terminate the intervention, the success rate was up to 90% regardless of the method or thrombolytic agent employed (Steering committee for study on local thrombolysis, submitted).

Table 23.1. Comparison of infusion versus infiltration methods for thombolysis using recombinant tissue plasimogen activator (based on 16 studies involving 785 patients)

	Time to reperfusion (min)	Total dose (mg)
Infusion	928 ± 965	24.7 ± 21.8
Infiltration	106 ± 263	7.8 ± 13.0

We have performed a retrospective comparison of infusion and infiltration techniques based on 16 studies using rt-PA either by the infusion (532 patients) or the infiltration technique (253 patients), or both. As shown in Table 23.2 for the infiltration techniques, the mean time to reperfusion was nine times shorter ($p < 0.00001$), and the mean total dose three times smaller ($p < 0.00001$) than with infusion techniques. Since adverse events, such as bleeding, amputation, and death, were positively related to the total dose (besides patient age, presence of diabetes etc.), there were significantly more adverse events in the studies using infusion methods.

23.4
Choice and Dosage of Thrombolytic Agents

In the early publications on catheter thrombolysis, streptokinase was almost the only agent available. Hess

Table 23.2. Fluoroscopic (TIMI grade) and angiographic results following local thrombolysis using two infiltration techniques

	rt-PA				Urokinase					
	Hess[a]		Schneider[b]		Hess		Schneider		Both	
	EOL	AI	EOL	AI	EOL	AI	EOL	AI	EOL	AI
TIMI grade 2 + 3	83	90	77	88	73	85	79	89	79	89
Open on angiography	80	90	70	90	72	97	71	90	73	91

EOL, end of lysis without further interventions; AI, after all interventions performed (lysis, percutaneous transluminal angioplasty, aspiration).
[a] Infiltration by end-hole catheter.
[b] Infiltration by perforated balloon.

originally performed catheter thrombolysis by repeated intrathrombus injection of small amounts of streptokinase (1000–3000 IU every 5–15 min), with step-by-step advancement of the catheter between injections up to a total dose of 180 000 IU (HESS et al. 1982).

This regimen was soon replaced by low-dose continuous infusion into the thrombus for up 48–76 h (GRAOR and OLIN 1989), not recognizing the difference in efficacy between the advancement of the catheter and the fixed catheter position. Later, urokinase started to be used to replace streptokinase and, more recently, rt-PA has been introduced into local thrombolysis (VERSTRAETE et al. 1988). While initially low doses of either streptokinase or urokinase were infused, a scheme beginning with a high, but tapered, dose was later proposed (McNAMARA and FISCHER 1985), and became popular (e.g., 240 000 IU of urokinase for 2 h until restoration of antegrade flow, reduced to 120 000 IU/h for another 2 h, and 2600 IU until complete lysis has been achieved). The TOPAS phase I trial (OURIEL et al. 1996) compared three initial doses: 120 000, 240 000, and 360 000 per hour for 4 h, and found 240 000 IU/h the most appropriate regimen, maximizing lytic efficacy (71%) against the risk of bleeding (2%). With this scheme, the total dose amounts to 5 000 000 IU. With rt-PA, the dosage schemes vary from 0.05 mg/h to 10 mg/h. In general, studies comparing doses of rt-PA found no benefit at higher doses.

There are only a few studies comparing different thrombolytic agents, initially in open trials (BELKIN et al. 1986; VAN BREDA et al. 1987; Do et al. 1989), and later in open randomized trials where a greater initial success rate with rt-PA than with streptokinase or urokinase was found (MEYEROVITZ et al. 1990). In the STILE trial (1994), however, there was no difference between urokinase and rt-PA. One recent multicenter study (STEERING COMMITTEE FOR STUDY ON LOCAL THROMBOLYSIS, submitted) compared urokinase and rt-PA in an open randomized fashion in 234 patients in whom either the HESS or the microporous balloon technique were applied. It was observed that, with the HESS technique, rt-PA at a dose of 2.5 mg/h achieved a TIMI grade 3 in significantly more patients than urokinase (100 000 IU/h), while there was no difference with the microporous balloon or when both techniques were employed together (see Table 23.1). Apparently, the dose in all of the agents available depends strongly on the administration mode (see Chap. 1).

23.4.1
General Considerations

There are three thrombolytic agents on which data and recommendations are available regarding how and in what dose they need be applied. Generally speaking, the direct thrombus infiltration techniques require smaller concentrations and overall amounts of agents than the infusion techniques, regardless of the agents employed. It seems that there are also fewer complications (BERRIDGE 1989) and contraindications with the infusion techniques. In resistant cases, infiltration may be continued with a low-dose infusion for several hours to increase the chances of success (Do et al. 1987). Definite recommendations of dosages cannot be given, they depend on the individual laboratories and operators. In any case, recent trends are moving away from streptokinase and favoring urokinase and rt-PA due to certain inflammatory and allergic reactions observed with streptokinase.

23.5
Catheter Thrombus Aspiration

A modality gaining increasing importance in the treatment of subacute and acute peripheral artery occlusions is catheter thrombus aspiration. In our laboratory, it is used with ever greater frequency, and is steadily taking the place of catheter thrombolysis. An example of a procedure including thrombolysis and successful aspiration is shown in Fig. 23.1.

This method was originally introduced by SCHNEIDER (SCHNEIDER and HOFFMANN 1996) and STARCK et al. (1985). Despite its great efficacy and short duration, as well as a low complication rate, it has not yet gained general popularity, perhaps since it requires a certain degree of manual skill in the catheter operator. More recent publications (ZEHNDER et al., submitted) report excellent success, especially in combination with other catheter methods, and aspiration merits further study and improvement. Although many automatic devices have been advertised to deal with fresh thrombotic material, such as the Acolysis and Amplatz systems, Angiojet, Hydrolyser, etc., none of them has offered a better solution, nor proven superior in most of the practical situations we have encountered, with the possible exception of the newly developed "Rotarex" system from Switzerland.

23.5.1
Technique

With catheter thrombus aspiration, a sheath of 6–9 F has to be introduced with detachable hemostatic valves. This is an important feature since the aspirated thrombus may barely fit in the catheter and be pulled through the sheath, but not through the orifice of the valve. There are wide-bore aspiration catheters available in 5 F–8 F. The aspiration catheter is introduced with its tip in the thrombus, and when suction is established using a syringe of at least 50 ml, it is pulled back upstream as long as the vacuum is maintained. In this case, a thrombus may be extracted through the sheath. When blood is aspirated, thrombotic material may be in the syringe or may be lost on the way up. The syringe needs to be rinsed and emptied, and the procedure repeated. The movements should be performed slowly to give the material time to deform and adapt to the instruments. Larger volumes of thromboembolic material need to be sucked out in several steps. Sometimes, large thrombi need thrombolytic pretreatment and/or mechanical detachment from the arterial wall and/or fragmentation by a wire loop or basket.

As an illustrative example, we present results from our laboratory on more than 100 patients treated by aspiration and/or other catheter methods as shown in Table 23.3.

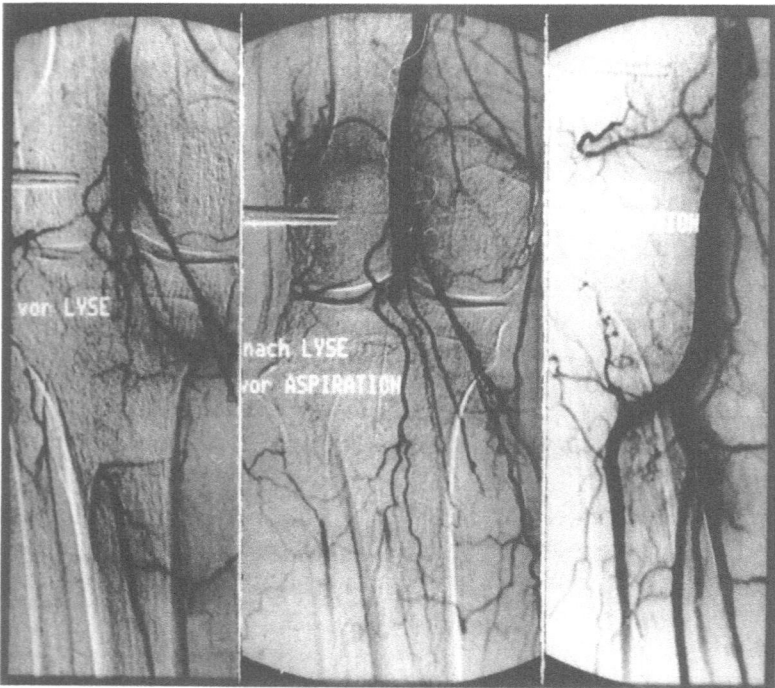

Fig. 23.1. Angiograms of a patient with an embolic occlusion of the popliteal artery before (*left panel*), after thrombolysis by perforated balloon technique (*center*), and after catheter thrombus aspiration (*right panel*)

Table 23.3. Percutaneous catheter thrombus aspiration in 112 patients with acute and subacute occlusions of leg arteries (experience from Inselspital Bern)

Male (*n*)	54
Female (*n*)	58
Age	*71 ± 14 years*
Inital stage III/IV	77%
Additional lyses	19%
Additional PTA	69%
Amputation rate (1 year)	8%
Reintervention (1 year)	30%
Endovascular	17%
Mortality (1 year)	18%

PTA, percutaneous transluminal angioplasty.

23.6
Indications to the Catheter Approach

23.6.1
Acute or Subacute Thromboembolic Occlusions of Arteries and Bypass Grafts

The catheter-based approach is indicated in both of the above situations (GARDINER et al. 1989) as long they are located below the inguinal ligament. It is considered a technical advantage when an access segment of the vessel is free to introduce the sheath, although in special situations thrombolysis (e.g., by pulse-spray infusion) is possible by a cross-over approach.

23.6.2
Embolism and Local Thrombosis

Both conditions may be treated by catheter methods. While embolism may often be treated sufficiently by thrombus aspiration, local thrombosis requires adjunctive thrombolysis and PTA more frequently. It is sometimes difficult to distinguish between the two, and the procedure should be started by probing the thrombus with the wire for its consistency or by the aspiration catheter for its mobility. The methods may be tried in occlusions of up to 12 weeks old, even though the age of the occlusion is sometimes difficult to determine. Catheter methods may also be tried in situations where no run-off vessels are visualized, especially in acute situations.

In general, we do not recommend this procedure for thromboembolic occlusions *above the inguinal ligament*, although some operators perform it. There is a great danger of distal embolization, creating situations which cannot be dealt with in the same session by catheter methods.

Following successful intervention, we recommend initiating anticoagulation, the duration of which should be determined according to the underlying disease.

23.6.3
Contraindications

There are almost no medical contraindications to catheter thrombus aspiration. In local thrombolysis, however, even though low-dose regimens are used, the risk of serious complications, such as cerebral embolism particularly in cases with atrial fibrillation and/or hemorrhage, needs to be considered. For the infusion methods, classic medical contraindications have to be followed: hemorrhagic disorders, previous operations, hypertension, etc.

23.7
General Conclusions

Based on our experience, we recommend a therapeutic catheter approach to acute and subacute thromboembolic occlusions of the leg arteries or bypass grafts by using a variety of methods combining thrombus aspiration, low-dose thrombus infiltration thrombolysis, and PTA if necessary. Success rates in excess of 90% may be achieved by this triple approach, with minimal complications and good long-term results. It should be borne in mind that the patient population in question has very high morbidity and mortality rates (up to 20% per year), and it is precisely for this reason that a minimally invasive catheter procedure may be appropriate as an initial approach.

Acknowledgements. I wish to thank the following coworkers who have contributed over the years to our ever growing experience in dealing with the problem of acute and subacute ischemia: Dr. Iris Baumgartner, Dr. Thomas Zehnder, Dr. Manuela Birrer from the Angiology Division, and Prof. Jürgen Triller from the Institute of Diagnostic Radiology, Inselspital.

References

Belkin M, Belkin B, Buchnam CA, Straub JJ, Lowe R (1986) Intra-arterial fibrinolytic therapy. Efficacy of streptokinase vs urokinase. Arch Surg 121:769–773

Berridge DC, Niakin CS, Hopkinson BR (1989) Local low-dose intra-arterial thrombolytic therapy, the risk of major stroke and haemorrhage. Br J Surg 76:1230–1233

Dembski JB, Zeitler E (1978) Selective arterial clot lysis with angiography catheters. In: Zeitler E, Grüntzig A, Schoop W (eds) Percutaneous vascular recanalization. Springer, Berlin Heidelberg New York, pp 157–159

Do DD, Mahler F, Triller J, Nachbur B (1987) Combination of short- and long-term catheter thrombolysis for peripheral arterial occlusion. Eur J Radiol 7:235–238

Do DD, Mahler F, Triller J (1989) Catheter thrombolysis with streptokinase, urokinase, and rt-PA for peripheral arterial occlusion. In: Zeitler E, Seyferth W (eds) Pros and cons in PTA and auxiliary methods. Springer, Berlin Heidelberg New York, pp 248–253

Dotter CT, Rösch J, Seaman AJ (1974) Selective clot lysis with low dose streptokinase. Radiology 111:31–37

Gardiner GA, Harrington DP, Koltun W, Whittemore A, Mannick JA, Levin DC (1989) Salvage of occluded bypass grafts by means of thrombolysis. J Vasc Surg 9:426–431

Graor RA, Olin JW (1989) Regional thrombolysis in peripheral arterial occlusions. In: Julian DG, Kübler W, Norris RM, Swan HJ, Collen D, Verstraete M (eds) Thrombolysis in cardiovascular disease. Dekker, New York, pp 381–395

Hess H, Ingrisch H, Mietaschk A, Rath H (1982) Local low-dose thrombolytic therapy of peripheral arterial occlusions. N Engl J Med 307:1627–1630

Hess H, Mietaschk A, von Bilderling P, Neller P (1996) Peripheral arterial occlusions: local low-dose thrombolytic therapy with recombinant tissue-type plasminogen-activator (rt-PA). Eur J Vasc Endovasc Surg 12:97–104

Kandarpa K, Drinker PA, Singer SJ, Caramore D (1988) Forceful pulsatile local infusion of enzyme accelerates thrombolysis: in vivo evaluation of a new delivery system. Radiology 168:739–744

McNamara TO, Fischer JR (1985) Thrombolysis of peripheral arterial and graft occlusions: improved results using high-dose urokinase. AJR 144:769–775

Meyerovitz MF, Goldhaber SZ, Reagan K, Polak JF, Krishna K, Grassi CJ, Donovan BC, Bettmann MA, Harrington DP (1990) Recombinant tissue-type plasminogen activator versus urokinase in peripheral arterial and graft occlusions: a randomised trial. Radiology 175:75–78

Ouriel K, Veith FJ, Sasahara AA for the TOPAS investigators (1996) Thrombolysis or peripheral artery surgery (TOPAS) phase I results. J Vasc Surg 23:64–75

Ouriel K, Veith FJ, Sasahara AA for the TOPAS investigators (1998) A comparison of recombinant urokinase with vascular surgery as initial treatment for acute arterial occlusion of the legs. N Engl J Med 338:1105–1111

Schneider E, Hoffmann U (1996) Perkutane lokale Lysetherapie und Thrombenextraktion bei Verschlüssen der Extremitätenarterien. Internist 37:607–612

Steering committee for study on local thrombolysis (submitted) Recombinant tissue plasminogen activator versus urokinase for local thrombolysis of femoro-popliteal artery occlusions: a prospective, randomized multicenter trial

STILE Investigators (1994) Results of a prospective randomised trial evaluating surgery versus thrombolysis for ischemia of the lower extremity. The STILE trial. Ann Surg 220:251–268

Starck EE, McDermott JC, Crummy AB, Turnipseed WD, Archer CW, Burgess JH (1985) Percutaneous aspiration thromboembolectomy. Radiology 156:61–66

Valji K, Bookstein JJ, Roberts AC, Sanchez RB (1993) Occluded peripheral arteries and bypass grafts: lytic stagnation as an end point for pulse-spray pharmacomechanical thrombolysis. Radiology 188:389–394

van Breda A, Katzen B, Deutsch AS (1987) Urokinase versus streptokinase in local thrombolysis. Radiology 165:109–111

Verstraete M, Hess H, Mahler F, Mietaschk A, Roth FJ, Schneider E, Baert AL, Verhaeghe R (1988) Femoro-popliteal artery thrombolysis with intra-arterial infusion of recombinant tissue plasminogen activator – report of a pilot trial. Eur J Vasc Surg 2:155–159

Working party on thrombolysis in the management of limb ischemia (1996) Thrombolysis in the management of limb arterial occlusion. Towards a consensus interim report. J Intern Med 240:343–355

Zehnder T, Birrer M, Do DD, Baumgartner I, Triller J, Nachbur B, Mahler F (submitted) Percutaneous catheter thrombus aspiration for acute or subacute arterial occlusion of the legs: how much thrombolysis necessary?

24 Diagnostic and Therapeutic Strategies for Vascular Injuries (Surgical and Endovascular)

T. Ohki and F.J. Veith

CONTENTS

24.1
Introduction

Vascular injuries due to blunt or penetrating trauma can be challenging to diagnose and treat, particularly when they involve central vessels or occur in patients with other major injuries or comorbidities. Over the past 30 years, the optimal management of these vascular lesions has been refined by both military and civilian trauma experiences (JAHNKE and SEELEY 1953; PERRY et al. 1971; DRAPANAS et al. 1970; BURNETT et al. 1976; FELICIANO et al. 1984; RICH and SPENCER 1978). This chapter describes several general principles which apply to the diag-nosis and traditional surgical treatment of major arterial and venous injuries. In addition, it reviews the indications for various endovascular treatment techniques, the literature on the use of endovascular stented grafts for vascular trauma, and our experience with these grafts for traumatic vascular lesions at the Montefiore Medical Center in New York.

24.2
Principles in the Diagnosis of Major Vascular Injuries

24.2.1
Diagnosis 1: Unstable Patients

The diagnosis of penetrating arterial trauma is obvious in patients who present with life-endangering external bleeding. Such patients should be taken directly to the operating room for exploration without delay. Angiography can be done prior to or during exploration in the operating room if necessary and if appropriate equipment is available.

24.2.2
Diagnosis 2: Stable Patients

Preoperative arteriography is indicated in stable patients with a suspected arterial injury on the basis of a pulsatile or expanding mass, ischemia, or decreased pulses distal to the site of injury. Penetrating wounds in proximity to a major artery and in certain specific locations such as the mediasternum or base of the neck also dictate the need for arteriography. Other conditions that mandate diagnostic angiography include violent decelerating injury, dislocation of the knee, and fracture of the first rib. Since most abdominal injuries are accompanied by other organ injury which will usually require operative treatment, arteriography prior to abdominal exploration is rarely indicated.

Spiral contrast computed tomography (CT) or duplex may obviate the need for arteriography. Intravascular ultrasound which may be performed at the time of angiogram will provide certain details such as the exact location and size of the fistula that are otherwise difficult to obtain, especially when coexisting arteriovenous fistula make the angiographic interpretation difficult (Fig. 24.1). These details may be important for performing an endovascular repair.

TAKAO OHKI, M.D., FRANK J. VEITH, M.D., M.D. Division of Vascular Surgery, Department of Surgery, Montefiore Medical Center, 111 East 210th Street, New York, NY 10467 USA

24.3
Principles for the Treatment of Major Vascular Injuries

It is not necessary to treat all vascular injuries. Occluded minor vessels, including a distal forearm artery or a single tibial artery, can be safely observed. In addition, minor intimal defects, intimal flaps that are adherent downstream, and a pseudoaneurysm less than 5 mm in diameter can be managed conservatively, provided the distal circulation is maintained and no active hemorrhage is present (WEAVER et al. 1989). However, care must be taken not to underestimate the degree of arterial injury based solely on angiogram, since pseudoaneurysms filled with thrombus are incompletely visualized on contrast studies.

If operative treatment for internal or external bleeding is indicated, the patient should be volume resuscitated with crystalloid and blood before the operation. Exposure and dissection of the injured area usually results in significant blood loss due to distorted anatomy, and this is poorly tolerated by the patient in a hypovolemic state. In addition, prevention of hypothermia by using a heating blanket and warming intravenous fluids, the anesthetic gases, and the room are important aspects of intraoperative care.

Hemorrhage from venous injury is best controlled by pressure applied around the injured venous structure and then suture repair of the damaged vein. Ligation is reserved for instances of loss of vein substance or injured small extremity veins.

Inflow arterial control is best obtained in a location proximal and distal to and separate from the area of injury. If remote control cannot be obtained rapidly in the face of active hemorrhage, manual compression should be applied to the area of injury. Alternatively, a Fogarty balloon catheter or an occlusion balloon can be inserted through the injury site into the proximal artery and the balloon inflated.

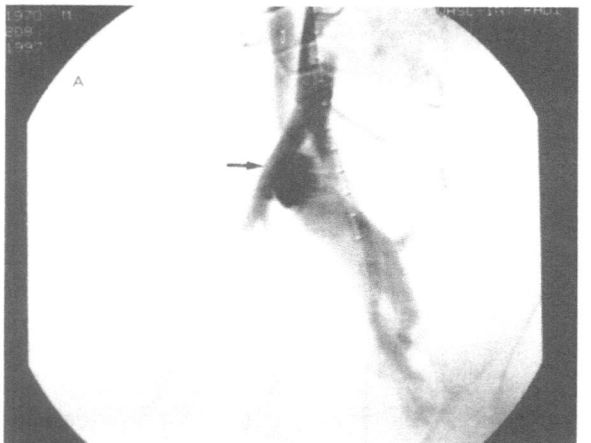

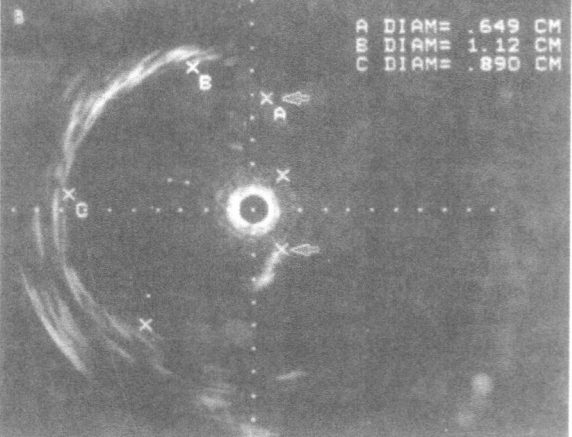

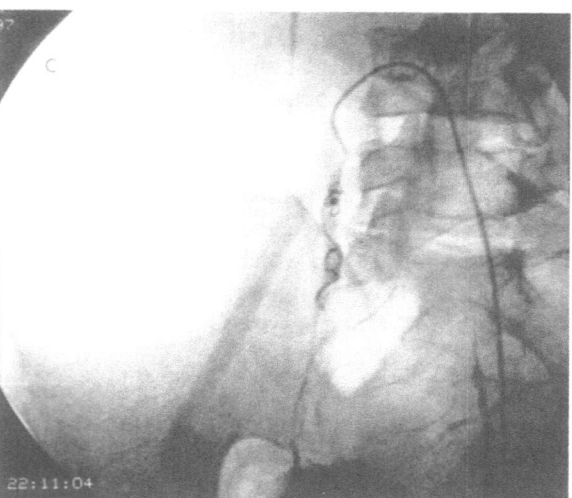

Fig. 24.1. **A** Pre-interventional angiogram of an iatrogenic arteriovenous fistula (AVF) involving the right common iliac artery due to lumbar disc surgery. The left common iliac vein and the inferior vena cava (*i*) is visualized by the contrast flowing through the AVF (*arrow*). However, the exact location of the AVF relative to the internal iliac artery and the precise size of the fistula is not clearly shown. **B** Intravascular ultrasound (IVUS) image taken at the time of angiography. The amount of substance loss and the location (by identifying the location of the probe of the IVUS under fluoroscopy) is well demonstrated (*arrows* denote the extent of the fistula). **C** Coil embolization of the right internal iliac artery. Since the location of the fistula was only 0.5 cm proximal to the origin of the internal iliac artery measured by the technique described above, the internal iliac artery was embolized with multiple coils at the time of angiogram. **D** Completion angiogram. A Corvita graft (10 mm × 6 cm) was used to repair the AVF. Note the preservation of iliac flow and the obliteration of the AVF

Arterial injuries without loss of artery substance are repaired directly or with a patch (vein or prosthetic material). Extremity arterial injuries with loss of substance or extensive damage to an arterial segment are repaired with a saphenous vein graft from the contralateral extremity. Excision of the area of injury with end-to-end anastomosis may be performed for short segment injury. Larger vessels are best treated with Dacron grafts or polytetrafluoroethylene (PTFE) grafts. If the operative field is deemed contaminated from the injury, PTFE grafting may be a better material since it is thought to be more resistant to infection.

24.4
Endovascular Treatment

As described above, surgical repair of vascular injuries may be complicated by the inaccessibility of the vascular lesion when trauma occurs to a vessel within a central body cavity, by distorted anatomy due to large hematoma and false aneurysm, and by venous hypertension when arteriovenous fistulas

are present. These conditions make the use of endovascular techniques appealing, since repair can be performed from a remote access site obviating the need for direct surgical exposure of the hostile injury site, thus reducing the morbidity and mortality rates of the repair.

Endovascular techniques for the treatment of vascular trauma include the use of coil embolization, intravascular stents, and more recently the use of stented grafts. Coil embolization has been used to treat relatively small traumatic arteriovenous fistulas and pseudoaneurysms involving non-essential vessels, such as a lumbar artery, the internal mammary artery or the branches of the hypogastric or deep femoral arteries (ROSCH et al. 1972; PANETTA et al. 1985) (Fig. 24.2). Long-term follow-up of these coil-treated lesions has proven to be favorable. Placement of intravascular stents are useful for the repair of intimal flaps. However, due to their porous nature, it is not indicated for the treat-ment of arteriovenous fistulas or pseudoaneurysms. Although these endovascular techniques proved to be effective in selected cases, the majority of the patients with vascular trauma were not amenable to such therapy.

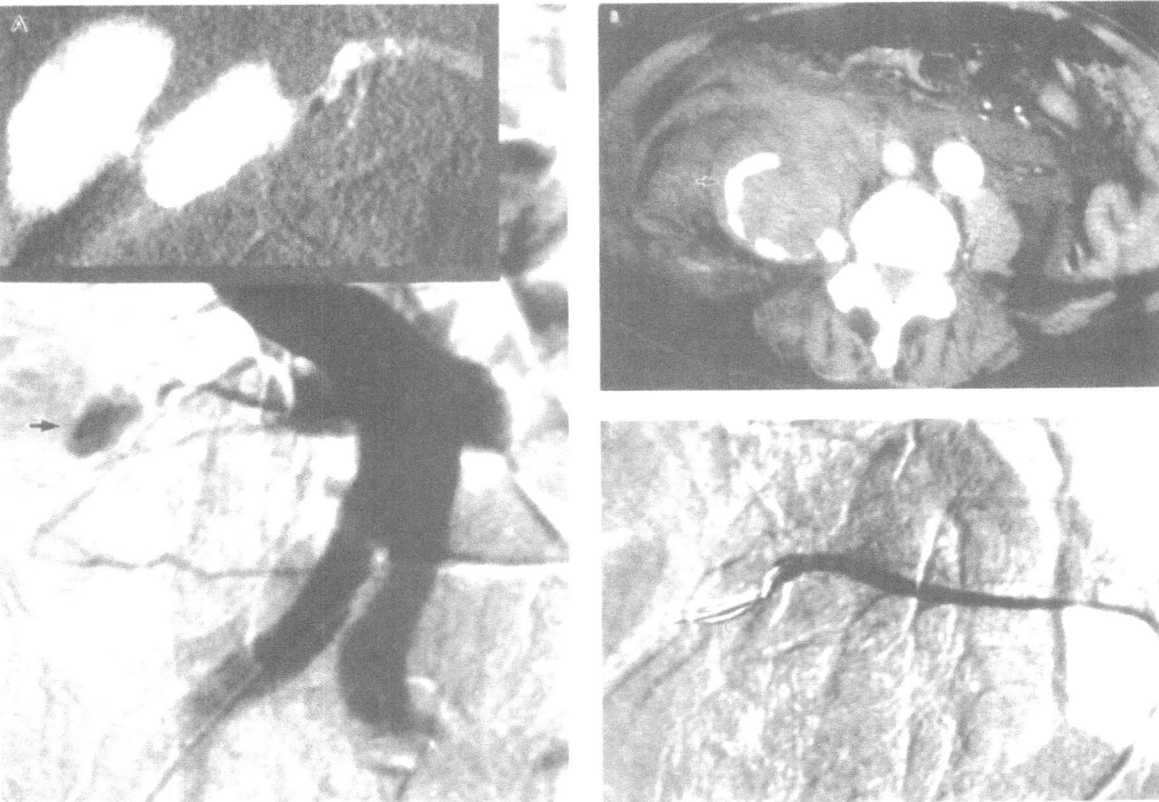

Fig. 24.2. **A** Pre-interventional angiogram of a ruptured spontaneous lumbar artery aneurysm (*arrow*). *Inset* shows magnification of the aneurysm. **B** Enhanced computed tomography image. Contrast extravasation is detected within the retroperitoneal hematoma (*arrow*). **C** Coil embolization. The aneurysm is no longer visualized following placement of multiple embolization coils (*c*)

24.5
Endovascular Stented Grafts

Endovascular grafts were first used to treat human abdominal aortic aneurysms by PARODI et al. (1991). Following this report, the use of endovascular grafts were expanded to include virtually all types of arterial pathology, including occlusive disease and vascular trauma. Endovascular grafts have greatly extended the potential of endovascular therapy for vascular trauma. These grafts have been used to treat almost every kind of injury at various locations in the body. Most of these grafts were used in circumstances in which coil embolization or stent placement were deemed inappropriate (MARIN et al. 1955, 1994, 1996;

PARODI 1995; BECKER et al. 1991, 1995; SCHMITTER et al. 1995; MARSTON et al. 1995; ZAJIKO et al. 1995; DORROS and JOSEPH 1995; ALLGAUER et al. 1996; GOMEZ-JORGE et al. 1996; TERRY et al. 1995; CRIADO et al. 1997; OHKI et al. 1997). In some instances, endovascular grafts have been used to treat life-threatening acute hemorrhage (Fig. 24.3). The types of devices that have been reported are predominantly a combination of a Palmaz stent and an ePTFE graft. Since the traumatized field is often contaminated, the use of a vein graft in combination with a Palmaz stent has also been reported (PARODI 1995; DORROS and JOSEPH 1995) (Fig. 24.4b). Different types of stented grafts that have been reported are summarized in Table 24.1 and shown in Fig. 24.4.

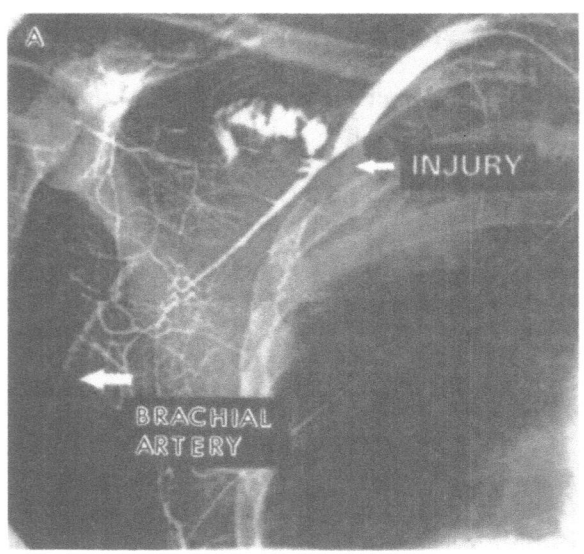

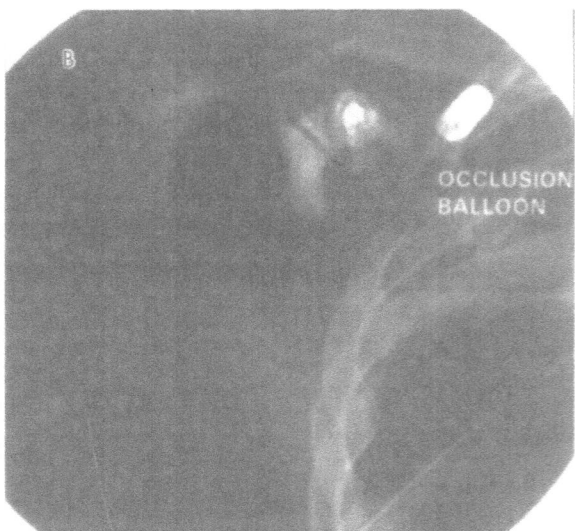

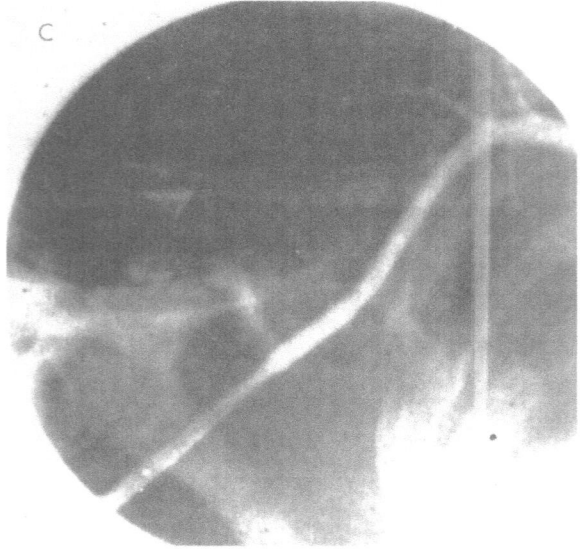

Fig. 24.3 A–C. Angiographic images of a patient who sustained a gunshot wound to the right chest. A Prograde angiogram (femoral artery puncture) shows occlusion of subclavian artery and active bleeding. B An occlusion balloon was placed to achieve hemostasis. C Following hemostasis, the patient was taken to the operating room. A guidewire was successfully passed across the injured artery and was repaired by the insertion of a stented graft of polytetrafluoroethylene (ePTFE and Palmaz stent). (From PATEL et al. 1996)

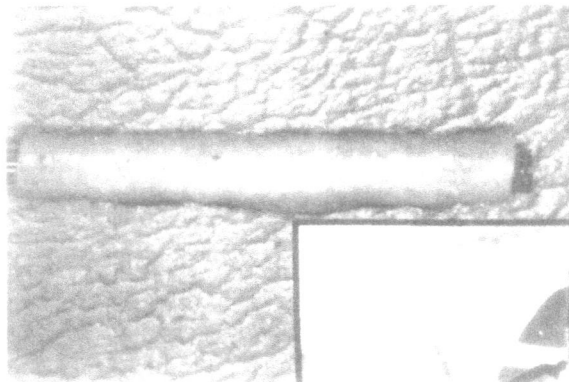

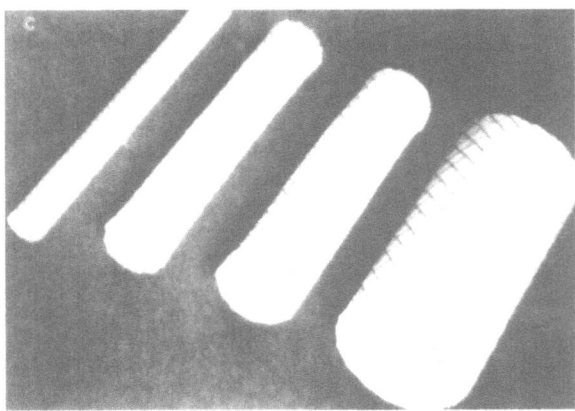

Fig. 24.4 A–C. Endovascular stented grafts. **A** Dacron graft material may be used to cover the balloon expandable stents. **B** Autologous vein can be used to cover stents, creating biological stented grafts. The collapsed stent graft assumes a small profile which effectively covers the struts (*s*) of the stent following deployment (*inset*). **C** Corvita endovascular graft for arterial trauma. This polyurethane covered stent structurally resembles the Wallstent

Lesion characteristics, technical success rate, and outcome of stented grafts in the treatment of vascular trauma has been summarized in Table 24.2. These results have so far been encouraging as shown by the high technical success rate and the low complication rate (Table 24.2), especially when one considers the difficulties in treating these lesions by direct surgical repair as discussed previously. In addition, the minimal invasiveness and cost effectiveness of such endovascular techniques are apparent and the shorter length of stay in patients so treated also represents an advantage (Table 24.2).

24.6
Montefiore Experience with Stented Grafts

24.6.1
Technique and Devices

We have predominantly used the Palmaz stent in combination with a thin-walled PTFE graft covering to perform arterial repairs of pseudoaneurysms and arteriovenous fistulas. The stents varied between 2 and 3 cm in length and were fixed inside 6-mm

Gore-Tex grafts (W.L. Gore, Flagstaff, Ariz., USA) by two "U" stitches (Fig. 24.5a). The stented graft was then mounted on a balloon angioplasty catheter which then had a tapered dilator tip firmly attached to its end (Fig. 24.5b). The entire device was contained within a 12-F delivery system for over-the-wire insertion either percutaneously or through an arterial cut-down.

Alternative devices include the Corvita stent graft (Corvita, Miami, Fla., USA), which is fabricated from a self-expanding stent of braided wire. The stent is covered with polyurethane fibers (see Fig. 24.4c). The stent graft may be cut to the desired length in the operating room using wire cutting scissors and then loaded into a specially designed delivery sheath. This sheath has a central "pusher" catheter which is used for discharging the graft at the desired location.

24.6.2
Results

A total of 16 patients received 16 stented grafts to treat traumatic arterial lesions (Table 24.3). Seven injuries occurred as a result of gunshot wounds (Figs. 24.3, 24.6), one as a result of a knife wound,

Table 24.1. Description of devices for arterial trauma

Type	Combination of Palmaz stent and various grafts				Cragg Endopro	Corvita graft
Stent	Palmaz stent				Nitinol	Self-expanding
Graft material	PTFE	Dacron	Vein	Silicone	Ultrathin woven polyester fabric	braided stent Polycarbonate urethane
Arterial access	1[a] or 2[b]	2	2	1 or 2	2	2
Study	Marin et al. (1994, 1995, 1996); Parodi (1995); Becker et al. (1995) Schmitter et al. (1995); Marston et al. (1995); Zajiko et al. (1995); Criado et al. (1997)	Marin et al. (1996)	Parodi (1995); Dorros and Joseph (1995)	Becker et al. (1991, 1995)	Allgayer et al. (1996)	Marin et al. (1996); Gomez-Jorge et al. (1996)

[a] 1, Open arteriotomy.
[b] 2, Percutaneous.

Table 24.2. Characteristics of lesion and outcome by location of injury

Location of trauma	Axillary-subclavian artery	Aorta or iliac artery	Femoral artery
Cases (n)	18	15	5
Cause of injury	Bullet, 55%; catheterization, 28%; others, 17%	Surgical, 36%, catheterization, 18%; bullet, 9%; others, 36%	Bullet: 60%; catheterization: 40%
Presence of pseudoaneurysm	61%	67%	80%
Presence of AV fistula	44%	73%	40%
Arterial access	Brachial arteriotomy, 39%		
	Brachial percutaneous, 39%	Femoral arteriotomy, 64%	Femoral arteriotomy, 80%
	Femoral percutaneous, 22%	Femoral percutaneous, 36%	Femoral percutaneous, 20%
Technical success rate	94% (17/18)[a]	100%	100%
Complication: Minor	0%	7%	0%
Major	6%[b]	7%[d]	0%
Mean length of stay	3.3 days	4 days	5.3 days
Mean follow-up	18 months	10.5 months	17.4 months
Primary patency	85%[c]	100%	100%
Study	Marin et al. (1955, 1996); Parodi (1995); Schmitter et al. (1995); Marston et al. (1995); Becker et al. (1991); Patel et al. (1996); Criado et al. (1997)	Marin et al. (1955, 1996); Parodi (1995); Becker et al. (1995); Zajiko et al. (1995); Allgayer et al. (1996); Terry et al. (1995)	Marin et al. (1955, 1996); Parodi (1995); Dorros and Joseph (1995)

AV, arteriovenous.
[a] One failure due to mis-diagnosis.
[b] Brachial artery injury during device insertion.
[c] Two failures due to stent deformity.
[d] Distal embolization requiring thrombectomy.

three iatrogenic needle catheterization injuries, two iatrogenic arterial trauma (gynecological surgery, and lumbar disk surgery) (see Fig. 24.1), and three occurred as a result of arterial graft disruptions. All injuries were associated with an adjacent pseudo-aneurysm. In five instances the arterial injury formed a fistula to an injured adjacent vein. Associated injuries were present in seven patients with arterial trauma and in one with an iatrogenic arterial injury (see Table 24.1). One patient who had an axillary pseudoaneurysm repaired with a stented graft required a vein patch of a small brachial artery at the catheter insertion site at the conclusion of the procedure. Stented graft patency was 100% with no early or late graft occlusions. One patient with a left axillary-subclavian stent graft developed compression of the stent at 12 months (Fig. 24.7a). This was treated with balloon angioplasty (Fig. 24.7b). This problem recurred 3 months later and no intervention was required. The device has not thrombosed with follow-up over 3 years. Mean follow-up for all stent grafts was 30 months with a range of 6–46 months.

Table 24.3. Stented grafts for traumatic arterial lesions: Montefiore experience

Sex/age	Mechanism of injury	Vessel(s) involved	PA	AVF	Anesthesia	Associated injuries	Injury to repair time interval	Stent graft length (cm)	Access	Hospital stay (days)	Patency (months)	Complications
M/21	Surgical trauma	RCIA LCIV	Yes	Yes	Local	None	4 weeks	6[b]	RCFA percutaneous	4	5	–
M/22	Bullet	LSFA	Yes	No	Local	Soft tissue injury; left DVT	12 h	3	LSFA arteriotomy	6	8[a]	–
F/85	Surgical trauma	RCIA	Yes	Yes	Local	None	8 years	5[b]	LCFA percutaneous	4	11	Distal emboli[c]
M/49	Catheterization	RCIA	Yes	Yes	Epidural	None	18 months	5	RCFA arteriotomy	5	11	Wound hematoma
M/68	Iliac graft disruption	LCIA	Yes	No	Epidural	None	1 month	9	LCFA arteriotomy	5	8	–
M/66	Aortic graft disruption	Aorta	Yes	No	Epidural	None	1 week	10	LCFA arteriotomy	5	17	–
M/76	Aortic disruption	Aorta	Yes	No	Epidural	None	3 days	7	LCFA arteriotomy	7	19	–
M/18	Bullet	RASA	Yes	No	Local	None	6 h	3	Right brachial artery	3	20	–
M/22	Bullet	RASA	Yes	No	Local	Hemothorax	3 h	3	Right brachial artery	6	20	–
M/18	Bullet	RSA	Yes	Yes	Local	Hemothorax	48 h	3	Right brachial artery	4	29	–
F/78	Catheterization	RSA	Yes	No	Local	Hemothorax	24 h	3	Right brachial arteriotomy	8 weeks	36	–
M/78	Catheterization	LCIA	Yes	No	Epidural	None	4 months	2	LCFA arteriotomy	2	36	–
M/35	Bullet	RASA	Yes	No	Local	Brachial plexus	3 weeks	3	Right brachial arteriotomy	4	37	–
M/24	Knife	LASA	Yes	No	General	Pneumothorax; hemothorax	4 h	3	Left brachial arteriotomy	7	41	Stent compression
M/28	Bullet	RSFA	Yes	No	Local	Left open femur fracture	12 h	3	RSFA arteriotomy	9	44	–
M/20	Bullet	LSFA LSFV	Yes	Yes	General	Soft tissue buttock	36 h	3	LSFA percutaneous	5	46	–

PA, Pseudoaneurysm; AVF, arteriovenous fistula; LSFV, left superficial femoral vein; LSFA, left superficial femoral artery; RSFA, right superficial femoral artery; RSA, right subclavian artery; LCIA, left common iliac artery; RCIA, right common iliac artery; RASA, right axillary subclavian artery; LASA, left axillary subclavian artery; LCFA, left common femoral artery; DVT, deep venous thrombosis.
[a] Died 2 months post-procedure (homicide).
[b] Corvita stent graft.
[c] Treated with catheter suction thrombectomy.
[d] Hospitalized for multiple medical problems.

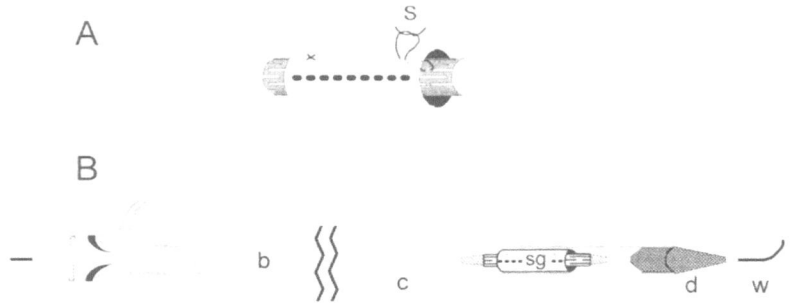

Fig. 24.5 A. An endovascular stented graft or covered stent. A segment of ePTFE is attached to a Palmaz stent using two 5-0 prolene "U" stitches (*s*). **B** The stent graft (*sg*) is mounted on an angioplasty balloon (*b*) and placed into a sheath (*c*) prior to insertion. Note the presence of a dilator tip (*d*) at the end of the balloon catheter which provides a smooth taper within the catheter (*w*, guidewire)

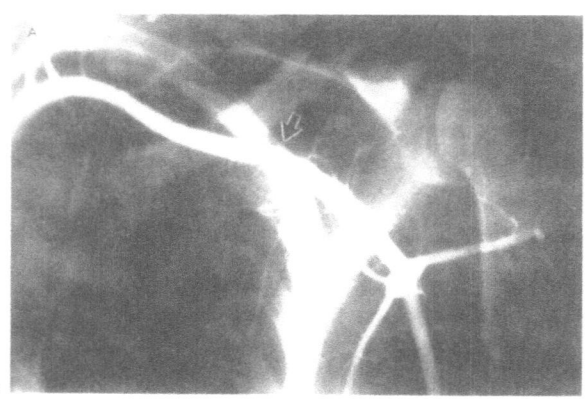
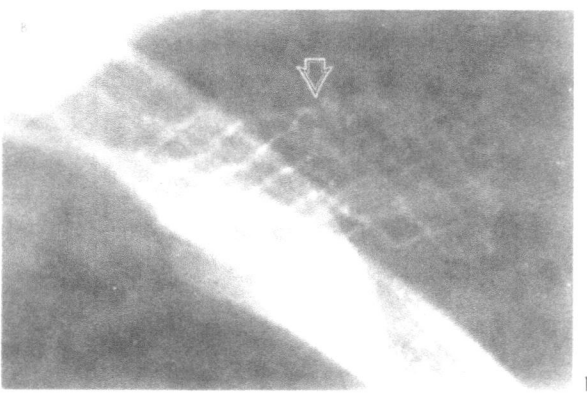

Fig. 24.7 A,B. Eight months following stent graft repair of a left subclavian injury, a patient was found to have external compression of the Palmaz stent. **A** The angiography revealed a proximal stenosis (*arrow*) within the stent. **B** Plain roentgenogram revealed a stent fracture (*arrow*). Balloon dilatation resulted in protracted patency. (From PATEL et al. 1996)

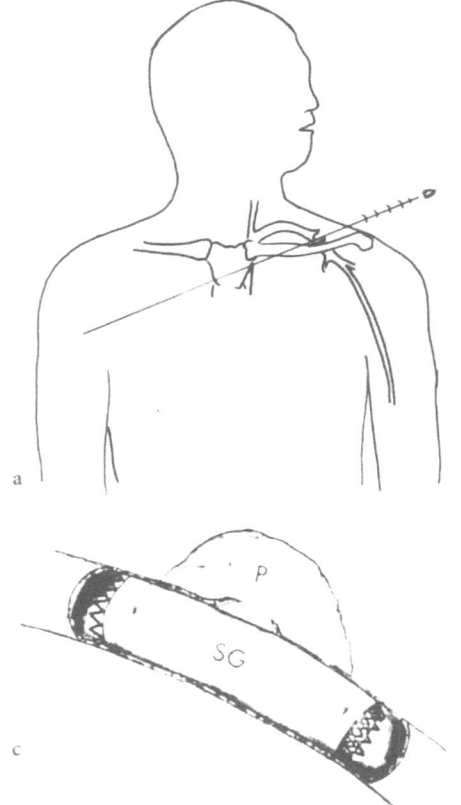
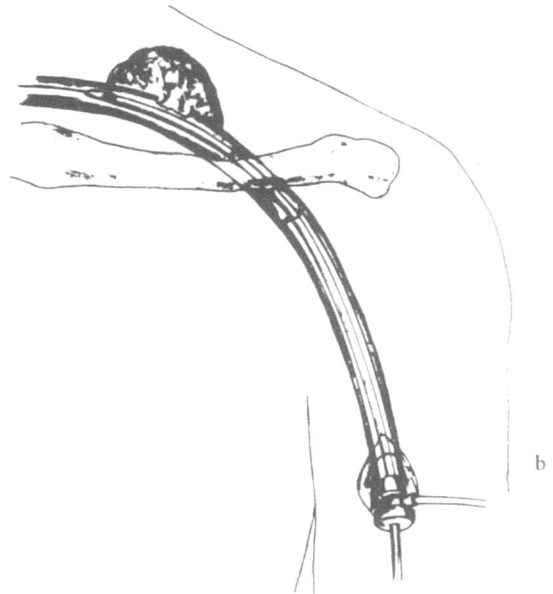

Fig. 24.6 A–C. Stented graft repair of an arterial injury. **A** A bullet wound partially disrupts the wall of the vessel. **B** The stent graft device is delivered to the site of injury via a remote arteriotomy. **C** Once deployed, the stented graft covers the hole in the vessel. (From MARIN et al. 1994)

24.7
Summary

Vascular injuries due to blunt or penetrating trauma can be challenging to diagnose and treat surgically, particularly when they involve central vessels. The use of stented grafts appears to be associated with decreased blood loss, a less invasive insertion procedure, reduced requirements for anesthesia and a limited need for an extensive dissection in the traumatized field. These advantages are especially important in patients with central arteriovenous fistulas or false aneurysms, particularly those who are critically ill from other coexisting injuries or medical comorbidities. In these circumstances, the use of stented grafts already appears justified to treat traumatic central arterial lesions.

Acknowledgments. Supported by grants from the James Hilton Manning and Emma Austin Manning Foundation, the Anna S. Brown Trust, and the New York Institute for Vascular Studies.

References

Allgayer B, Theiss W, Naundorf M (1996) Percutaneous closure of an arteriovenous fistula with a Cragg endoluminal graft. AJR AM J Roentgenol 166:673–674

Becker GJ, Benenatl JF, Zemel G, et al. (1991) Percutaneous placement of a balloon-expandable intraluminal graft for life-threatening subclavian arterial hemorrhage. J Vasc Intervent Rodiol 2:225–229

Becker GJ, Katzen BT, Benenati JF, et al. (1995) Endografts for the treatment of aneurysm and traumatic vascular lesions: MVI experience (Abstr). J Endovasc Surg 2:380–382

Burnett HF, Parnell CL, Williams GD, et al. (1976) Peripheral arterial injuries: a reassessment. Ann Surg 183:701–709

Criado E, Marston WA, Ligush J, Mauro MA, Keagy BA (1997) Endovascular repair of peripheral aneurysms, pseudoaneurysms, and arteriovenous fistulas. Ann Vasc Surg 11:256–263

Dorros G, Joseph G (1995) Closure of a popliteal arteriovenous fistula using an autologous vein-covered Palmaz stent. J Endovasc Surg 2:177–181

Drapanas T, Hewitt RL, Weichert RF, et al. (1970) Civilian vascular injuries: a critical appraisal of three decades of management. Ann Surg 172:351–360

Feliciano DV, Bitondo CG, Mattox KL, et al. (1984) Civilian trauma in the 1980s. A 1-year experience with 456 vascular and cardiac injuries. Ann Surg 199:717–724

Gomez-Jorge JT, Guerra JJ, Scagnelli T, et al. (1996) Endovascular management of a traumatic subclavian arteriovenous fistula. J Vasc Intervent Radiol 7:599–602

Jahnke EJ Jr, Seeley SF (1953) Acute vascular injuries in the Korean war: an analysis of 77 consecutive cases. Ann Surg 138:158–177

Marin ML, Veith FJ, Cynamon J, et al. (1995) Initial experience with transluminally placed endovascular grafts for the treatment of complex vascular lesions. Ann Surg 222:449–469

Marin ML, Veith FJ, Panetta TF, et al. (1994) Transluminally placed endovascular stented graft repair for arterial trauma. J Vasc Surg 20:466–473

Marin ML, Veith FJ, Cikki T (1996) Endovascular stent-grafts for treatment of traumatic pseudoaneurysms and arteriovenous fistulas. In: Yao JST, Pearce WH (eds) Vascular surgery: 20 years of progress, 1st edn. Appleton and Lange, Norwalk, pp 315–327

Marston WA, Criado E, Mauro M, et al. (1995) Transbrachial endovascular exclusion of an axillary artery pseudoaneurysm with PTFE-covered stents (case report). J Endovasc Surg 2:172–176

Ohki T, Marin ML, Veith FJ (1997) Use of endovascular grafts to treat non-aneurysmal arterial disease. Ann Vasc Surg 11:200–205

Panetta TF, Sclafani SJA, Goldstein AS, et al. (1985) Percutaneous transcatheter embolization for arterial trauma. J Vasc Surg 2:54–64

Parodi JC (1995) Endovascular repair of abdominal aortic aneurysms and other arterial lesions. J Vasc Surg 21:549–557

Parodi JC, Palmaz JC, Barone HD (1991) Transfemoral intraluminal graft implantation for abdominal aortic aneurysms. Ann Vasc Surg 5:491–499

Patel AV, Marin ML, Veith FJ, et al. (1996) Endovascular graft repair of penetrating subclavian artery injuries. J Endovasc Surg 3:382–388

Perry MO, Thal ER, Shires GT (1971) Management of arterial injuries. Ann Surg 173:403–408

Rich NM, Spencer FC (1978) Vascular trauma. Saunders, Philadelphia

Rosch J, Dotter CT, Brown MJ (1972) Selective arterial embolization. A new method for control of acute gastrointestinal bleeding. Radiology 102:303–306

Schmitter SP, Marx M Bernstein R, et al. (1995) Angioplasty-induced subclavian artery dissection in a patient with internal mammary artery graft: treatment with endovascular stent and stent-graft. AJR Am J Roentgenol 165:449–451

Terry PJ, Houser EE, Rivera FJ, et al. (1995) Percutaneous aortic stent placement for life threatening aortic rupture due to metastatic germ cell tumor. J Urol 153:1631–1634

Weaver FA, et al. (1989) Injuries to the ascending aorta, aortic arch and great vessels. Surg Gynecol Obstet 169:27–37

Zajiko AB, Little AF, Steed DL, et al. (1995) Endovascular stent-graft repair of common iliac artery-to-inferior vena cava fistula. J Vasc Intervent Radiol 6:803–806

Chronic Arterial Diseases (POVD)

25 Arterosclerotic Diseases

E. Zeitler

25
Arterosclerotic Diseases

In radiologic examinations, only macroscopic arteriosclerotic changes are demonstrable. Luminal narrowings less than 50% are defined as plaques and narrowings exceeding 50% as stenoses, while further partial differentiation is possible based on the structure of the artery's inner surface (Fig. 25.1). Plaques are more easily identified in small arteries than in major arteries due to the lower concentration of contrast medium. In the aorta, plaques appear as irregularities of the intima, but a high concentration of contrast agent can obscure small changes of the vascular wall. Smaller amounts of contrast agent, as are used in the 'transparent technique' using Medichrome film, have demonstrated better detection of plaques (Zeitler and Hüring 1972). Irregularities and arteriosclerotic plaques may become a source of emboli. Prior to establishing therapy and in order to prevent emboli, ulcerating atherosclerotic plaques and associated small thrombi need to be identified (Schmitt et al. 1971). Ulcerations may constitute a source of emboli of cholesterol crystals. A verrucous surface, with different irregularities of the vascular wall, and different types of stenosis lined with

thrombotic material can, in part, be diminished by thrombolysis (Fig. 25.2):

The presence of post-stenotic dilatation and collateral circulation are indicators of the hemodynamic severity of a stenosis. However, they may also be present distal to high-grade stenoses and long-segment arterial narrowings lacking hemodynamic effects, and resolve immediately after removal of the stenosis.

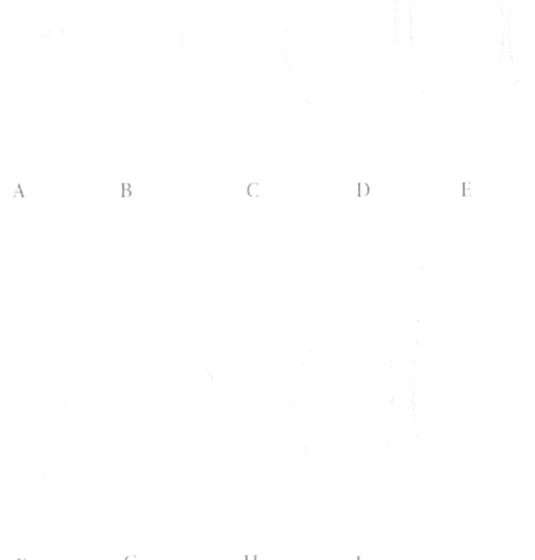

Fig 25.1. Different types of stenosis as seen on angiography. *Upper row:* Stenoses with smooth surfaces. **A** Ring-like; **B** symmetric, central stenosis with poststenotic dilatation; **C** eccentric stenosis, which could be an eccentric plaque or compression from outside; **D** cylindrical stenosis, very common close to an operative anastomoses, after stent implantation, or in intimal hyperplasia; **E** hour-glass stenosis, mainly organized thrombus or intimal hyperplasia; *Lower row:* Stenoses with irregular surfaces and risk of emboli. Possibility of pharmacological thrombolysis. **F** Short central stenosis; **G** Atheromatous ulcer; **H** Eccentric stenosis, with an irregular surface, demonstrating parts of unorganized thrombus; **I** long-irregular stenosis

EBERHARD ZEITLER, MD, Professor, University Erlangen-Nürnberg; Germany
address for correspondence:
Virchowstrasse 13, 90409 Nürnberg, Germany

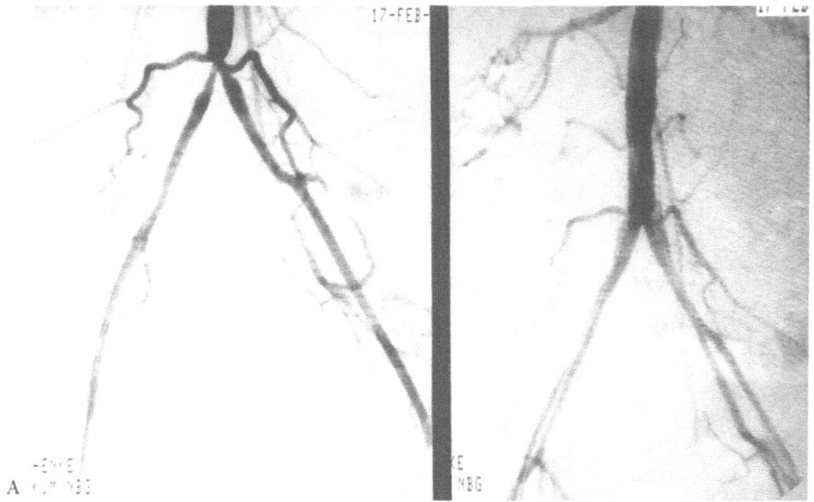

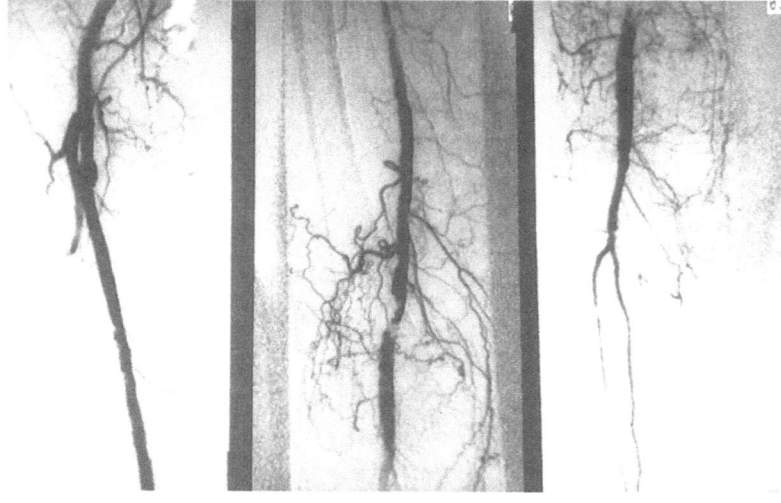

Fig. 25.2. Angiography of various stenoses. A Smooth bi-furcational stenosis before and after safe balloon dilatation – kissing-balloon technique. B Eccentric atheromatous stenosis with irregular surface (type H). C Oblique angiography of pelvic arteries, left: atheromatous ulcer (type G), right: central stenosis with poststenotic dilatation(type B). D Diffusse multiple long arteriosclerotic stenosis (type I).

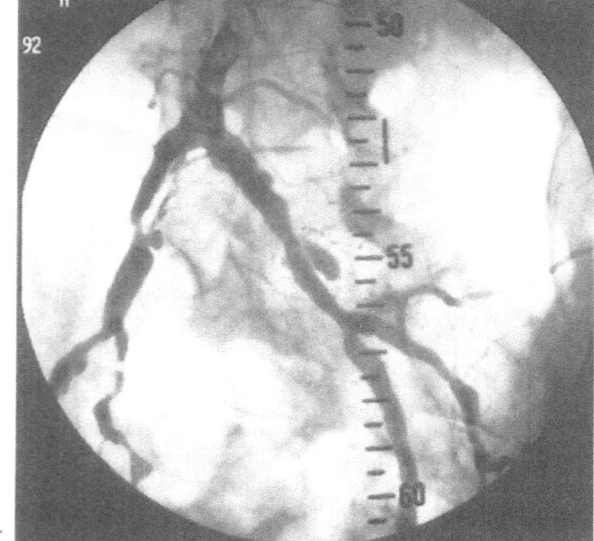

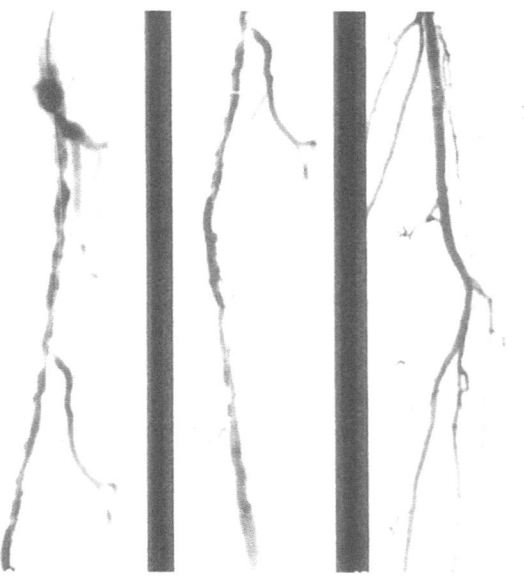

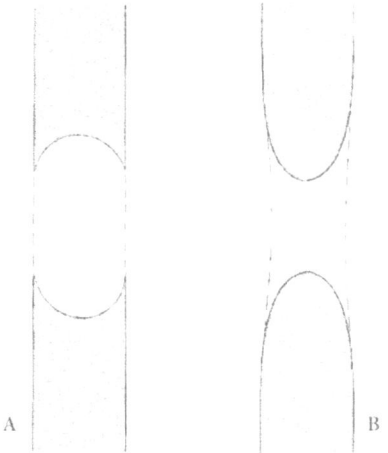

Fig. 25.3. Schematic demonstration of **A** acute thrombotic arterial occlusion; **B** chronic arterial occlusion

The clinically relevant complications of arteriosclerosis are hemodynamically effective stenosis and thrombotic occlusion. The diagnosis of an acute thrombotic occlusion is usually possible clinically (HEBERER et al. 1974; KAPPERT 1985; SCHOOP 1988; PEATT 1954; ALEXANDER 1993; VOLLMAR 1996). Because the differential diagnosis of acute thrombotic occlusion is acute arterial embolism, there may be diagnostic difficulties and angiographic assessment of the contrast agent column at the proximal and distal end of the occlusion merits special attention (Fig. 25.3). Typically, fresh thrombus containing sufficient liquid has a convex outline at its interface with contrast medium, both proximally and distally (Fig. 25.5). The older the thrombotic occlusion, the more the proximal and distal limitation of the contrast column is concave (Fig. 25.5).

Arteriosclerotic changes can either reduce, and ultimately obliterate, the arterial lumen, or have an ectatic / dilative effect resulting in diffuse dilatation or localized dilatation to produce an arteriosclerotic aneurysm (VOLLMAR and NOBBE 1976). Thus, the combination of proximal arteriosclerosis, aneurysm formation and distal obliterative changes (Fig. 25.6) is not an uncommon finding on aorto/arteriography. This underlines the importance of documenting the entire vascular course, from the origin of the renal arteries to the periphery at the ankle joints, possibly including the foot arteries, in patients with peripheral arterial disease (POVD) prior to operation or intervention (ZEITLER 1974; WENZ and BEDUHN 1975; VOLLMAR 1996).

Due to the wider lumen of the aorta and its branches, including the pelvic arteries, stenoses and plaques may be overlooked on angiography undertaken in the AP projection. Therefore, because of the incomplete information obtainable from auscultation, stress tests and AP angiography it is important to depict the vessels in the pelvis in two planes (CRUMMY et al 1978). This is best done, particularly for documentation of the iliac and femoral bifurcations, in an oblique 35° projection (Fig. 25.2c). Color-coded duplex sonography (CCDS) and CT angiography have proven to be superior to angiography in such cases, due to the possibility of multidirectional documentation and 3-D reconstruction (See Chap. 9).

The age of a femoral occlusion can not only be estimated from the appearance of its margins, but also from the type and extent of the collateral circulation (WENZ and BEDUHN 1976). In the collateral arteries, the flow rate increases considerably as a consequence of the pressure gradient between the artery before and after the occlusion. In the distal segment of the

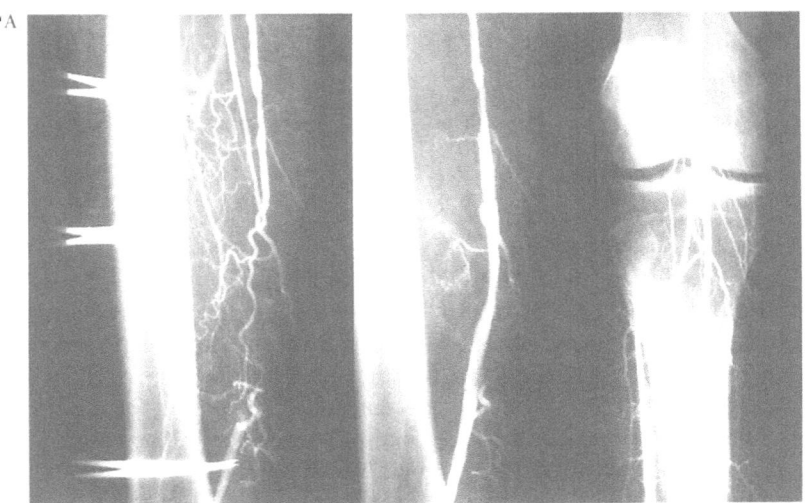

Fig. 25.4. A Chronic occlusion of the superficial femoral artery in Hunter's canal with proximal atherosclerosis. **B** Situation after recanalization and balloon angioplasty, with residual smooth lumen narrowings

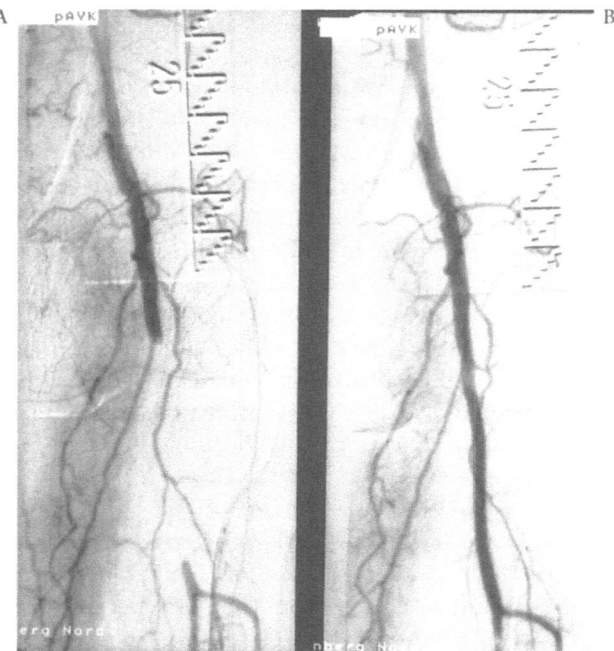

Fig. 25.5. A Acute popliteal artery occlusion. **B** Angiography after mechanical treatment with hydrolyzer

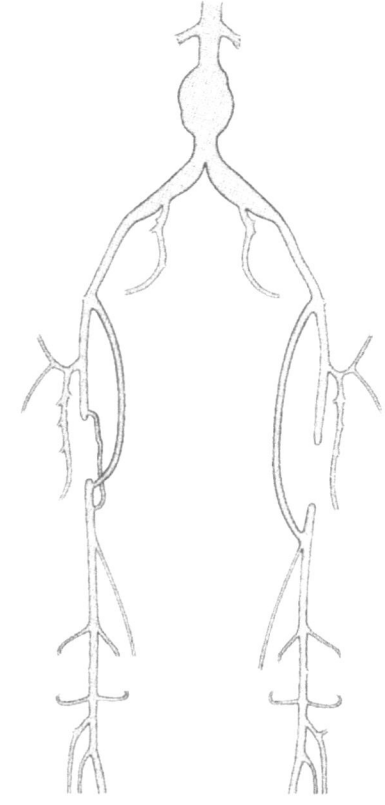

Fig. 25.6 Combined occlusive and dilated arteriopathy. Aorto-iliac aneurysm and SFA occlusion with collateral circulation from the deep femoral artery and direct collaterals to bypass a long SFA occlusion.

collateral system, reverse flow can occur. Chronic arterial occlusions can be distinguished from acute ones by the presence of a developed collateral circulation, dilatation of the distal collateral arteries (Fig. 25.7) and secondary vascular changes, such as a stenosis at the distal supply to the main artery with local dilatation behind it - the so-called 'sinus phenomenon'. Whenever diastolic and mean pressures are decreased distal to a stenoses, the result will be a collateral circulation and peripheral vasodilatation. Typical signs of the collateral arterial system are:
1) Elongation of arteries
2) Meandering
3) Reduced distal diameter
4) Stenosis of the ostium of the collateral artery
5) Distal sinus phenomenon.

Hemodynamically effective stenoses or occlusions can be identified by Doppler demonstration of reduced blood pressure in the foot arteries after application of a blood pressure cuff at the ankle joint, provided there is no significant mediasclerosis (BOLLINGER 1979; SCHOOP 1988). The possibility of other causes of arterial stenoses or occlusions in the pelvic and leg arteries, as well as the shoulder and arm arteries, should always be considered, even though arteriosclerosis is the predominant cause. This is particularly important in young patients. An important clinical aspect is the differentiation of

POVD into iliac, femoro-popliteal, tibio-peroneal, and foot arterial diseases, because of prognosis and complications differ with site.

25.1
Aorto-iliac Localizations

At this site there is a higher likelihood of aneurysms, and stenoses and occlusions caused by the distal end of an aortic dissection should also be considered. Moreover, rare vascular pathologic processes, such as cystic adventitial degeneration (Fig. 27.8; Chap. 27.3) and fibromuscular dysplasia of the external iliac artery (Chapter 27.5) are also found in this vascular territory (RAITHEL and HACKER 1975; KREMER et al. 1977; RÖDL 1980; Arlart 1997).

Narrowing of the external iliac artery can also be the result of external compression by a tumor or scarring after radiation therapy (WENZ 1972; KAPPERT 1985; VOLLMAR 1996). The constrictions of the

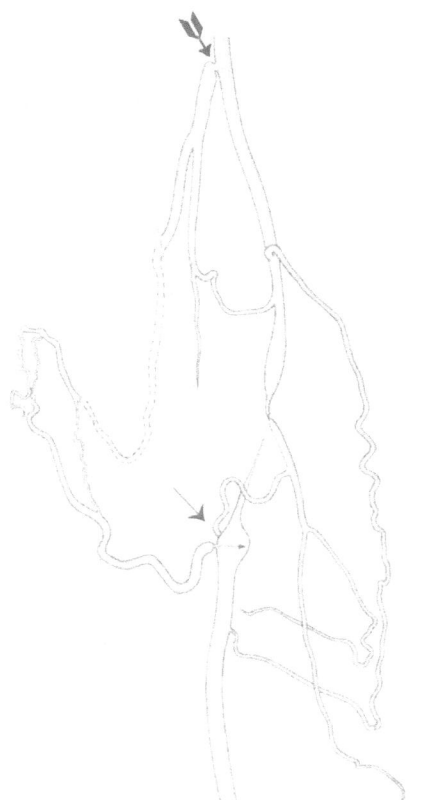

Fig. 25.7. Signs of collateral pathways crossing a long-segment SFA stenosis: elongation of collateral arteries, stenosis at the beginning of the collateral artery (>→) and at the end with sinus phenomenon (→)

pelvic arteries in such cases are mostly long or show smooth distortions without irregularity of the inner vascular surface on arteriography. This differential diagnosis can be achieved most impressively by computed tomography (CT) or magnetic resonance imaging (MRI) especially when the cause is tumor or retroperitoneal hematoma.

25.2
Femoropopliteal Localization

Within the spectrum of femoropopliteal occlusive disease, three segments need to be clearly distinguished. Most common are occlusions of the superficial femoral artery at the level of the adductor canal (Fig. 25.4). This is the arteriosclerotic disease which is most significantly correlated with cigarette smoking as a risk factor (HASSE 1974; WIDMER et al 1981). The proximal superficial femoral artery less often presents isolated arteriosclerotic changes, but is severely involved

in the pathologic process as POVD is progressing (Fig. 25.2d) in heavy smokers, by age, or as thrombus behind short arteriosclerotic occlusions. Complete occlusion of the superficial femoral artery is often bypassed by the deep femoral artery. Surgeons have defined the deep femoral artery as the most important collateral vessel. Under these conditions, a hemodynamically effective stenosis at the branching point of the deep femoral artery deserves special attention (Fig. 25.7).

In the assessment of the femoral bifurcation, profunda stenoses may be overlooked at angiography if the proximal superficial femoral artery is still patent. Proximal occlusions of the superficial femoral artery and common femoral artery are partially bypassed by collaterals from the internal iliac artery. This collateral circulation via the obturator artery develops slower than that via the deep femoral artery. Occlusions in the SFA are primarily fresh thrombus superimposed on arteriosclerotic changes. Within weeks, the thrombus becomes organized and shrinks (Schmitt et al 1971; KUTHAN et al 1971; TILLGREN et al. 1963), followed by a white thrombus which reaches to the next arterial bifurcation.

An important part of radiologic examination of the upper thigh is documentation of the different bypasses, for which either the long saphenous vein or plastic prostheses are used (VOLLMAR 1996). They are undertaken to demonstrate the diameter of the bypass vein or prosthesis and detect possible changes of the wall. The beginning and end of the bypass can become stenosed, either as a result of clamping, intimal hyperplasia or arteriosclerotic progression.

25.3
Popliteal Obliterations

Thrombotic and embolic occlusions of different underlying causes are found in the popliteal fossa. In addition to chronic occlusion (Fig. 25.5), arteriosclerotic popliteal aneurysms (Fig. 25.10), thrombotic occlusions as a result of popliteal compression syndrome (due to a variation of the proximal muscle insertion), and cystic adventitial degenerations (RAITHEL and HACKER 1975; KREMER et al. 1977; RÖDL 1980; ARLART 1997) have to be considered in the differential diagnosis (Fig. 25.8). Several imaging modalities are applicable to the popliteal fossa. Angiography, sonography (Fig. 25.10a), CT (Fig. 25.10b), and MRI provide different information regarding the lumen, the arterial wall, and the surrounding tissues (Fig. 25.10). Con-

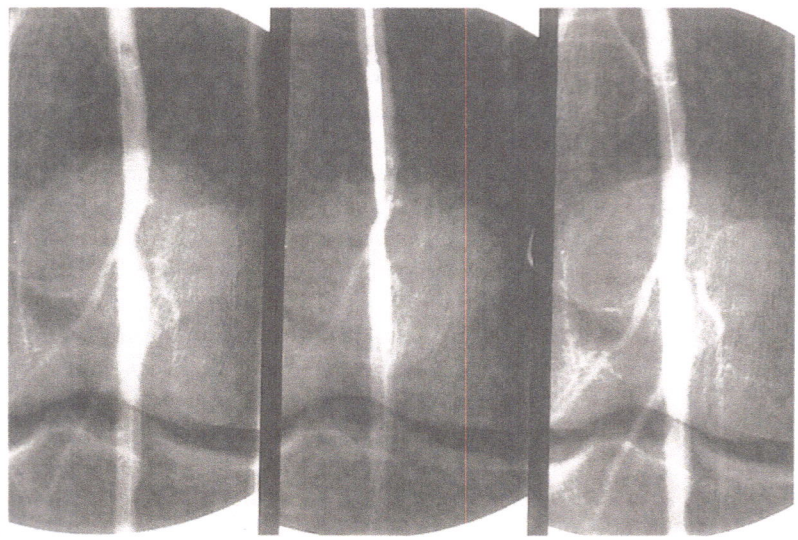

A   C

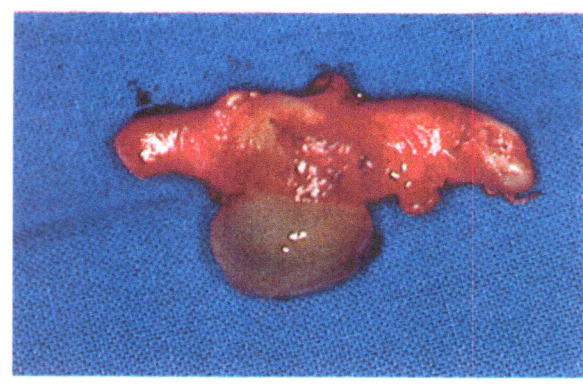

B

Fig. 25.8. Eccentric popliteal stenosis with smooth surface in a patient with cystic adventitial degeneration. **A** Angiography before treatment. **B** Specimen after surgical resection (surgeon: Professor Steckmeier, Munich) **C** Angiography after succesful operation

ventional angiography only provides intra-arterial information on the location, luminal narrowing or dilatation, e.g. aneurysmal sacs, but does not provide information about possible peri-arterial changes.

In contrast, all other modalities enable analysis of the arterial wall, of possible thromboses, and inspection of the extravascular anatomy. Special attention should be paid to changes in the joint, such as a Baker's cyst, and also abnormalities of the run-off arteries and the compressed veins, which can result in a deep venous thrombosis (Fig. 27.9). Particularly in the popliteal fossa, the inclusion of non-invasive imaging modalities is of special importance to establish a clear diagnosis before vascular surgery, intervention or other therapies are discussed.

The prognosis of popliteal artery occlusion depends on:
1) The extension of the occlusion into the tibio-fibular arteries (Fig. 25.11)
2) Patent or occluded sural arteries
3) Occlusion or patency of proximal knee arteries (Fig. 25.9)

25.4
Peripheral Localization

In the lower leg arteries, obliterative changes mainly occur in patients with Buerger's disease (Fig. 25.12) and diabetes mellitus (ALEXANDER 1993 b), but also in the form of embolic occlusions. Arteriosclerosis appears either in the form of isolated segmental occlusions, or in the form of multiple plaques, one behind the other, resulting in hemodynamically effective stenoses. The collateral vessel of importance to bypass occlusions in the lower leg arteries is the peroneal artery, which is rarely occluded (Fig. 25.13). The arteries arising from it to supply the posterior tibial and anterior tibial arteries (the perforating and communicating branches) are then the important collaterals. Their visualization is important prior to any vascular surgical bypass operation or amputation (VOLLMAR 1996). They often provide good arterial perfusion of the plantar and dorsal pedal arteries, respectively, which are essential for a distal anastomosis in the framework of femorocrural or femoropedal bypass operations.

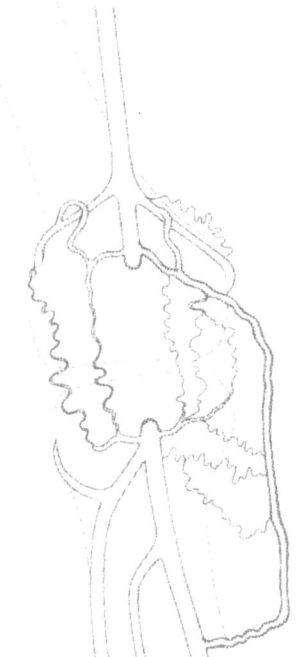

Fig. 25.9. Popliteal artery occlusion and collateral circulation via sural, upper- and lower-knee arteries.

The decisive task of the radiologist is not only to document the existence of occlusions or stenoses, including their precise location, but to determine the etiology of the disease, and to derive possible optimum therapies on the basis of the different morphologies of the stenoses and collateral circulation.

25.5
Age-dependent Arteriosclerosis and Restenosis

As early as the first year of life, lipoid inclusions have been observed in the iliac arteries. At 30 years of age most individuals show lipid incrustation in the aorta, and ten years later also in the SFA (MEYER 1974). With age, arteriosclerotic changes and medial calcification increase. This applies mainly to the arteries in the adductor canal. The definition 'obliterating arteriosclerosis' only applies to some of the individuals with POVD. The arterial lumen is, in most cases, only obliterated by additional thrombosis. In the lower leg, the most common site of arterial occlusions is the posterior tibial artery (RODDA 1960; TILLGREN et al. 1963).

One of the most important problems in the treatment of arterial obliterations after the introduction of percutaneous transluminal angioplasty (PTA) is the high incidence of restenoses after PTA, stent application and other mechanical types of recanalization. Since the first experiences with PTA, we have learned that 70% of patients with treated SFA disease retain patency for 6–12 months, or more (ZEITLER 1974, GRÜNTZIG 1977; SCHOOP 1978). In the common iliac artery and the subclavian artery, this figure reaches about 80% because these arteries have a wider lumen.

After the introduction of percutaneous transluminal coronary angioplasty (PTCA) (GRÜNTZIG et al. 1987), significant restenoses 3–6 months after balloon angioplasty could be diagnosed by coronary arteriography in approximately 30–35% of patients. Coronary arteries have a smaller diameter than iliac and proximal SFA in men. The coronary arteries are also on the surface of a heart beating round the clock. Even though arteriosclerosis is the basic problem in arterial occlusive disease, the pathophysiology of coronary arteries is different from that of extremity arteries. One point is the difference in arterial diameter, the second is that flow in peripheral arteries is less pulsatile, and the third is that pressure and flow in extremity arteries can be non-invasively controlled, in contrast to the coronary arteries. Restenosis can therefore be diagnosed more easily.

Restenoses are defined as late luminal narrowings greater than 50% (LEIMGRUBER et al. 1986). Restenosis appears due to local neointimal hyperplasia, which occurs especially in coronary arteries after balloon angioplasty and in femoral or iliac arteries after treatment with uncovered stents. So, in the long-term treatment of patients with arterial occlusive diseases we have arteriosclerosis with different types of plaque formation, but later there is the problem of neointimal hyperplasia and neointimal hypertrophy. In contrast to the original atherosclerosis, restenosis in extremity arteries in most cases is the result of exuberant healing. However, the change in the clinical situation can also be the result of arteriosclerotic progression close to the site of the primary intervention, or at different locations proximal and distal of the first treated lesion. Therefore, to learn more about the disease and its evaluation, atherectomy, followed by histological studies of the specimen is important. Also, if the long-term results of atherectomy are not better than balloon angioplasty, this technique is necessary for new information in general (HÖFLING et al. 1997), and in each individual patient. Despite important new developments, such as atherectomy, lasers and stenting, balloon angioplasty remains the most appropriate interventional device for most lesions suitable for percutaneous angioplasty (SERRUYS et al. 1992).

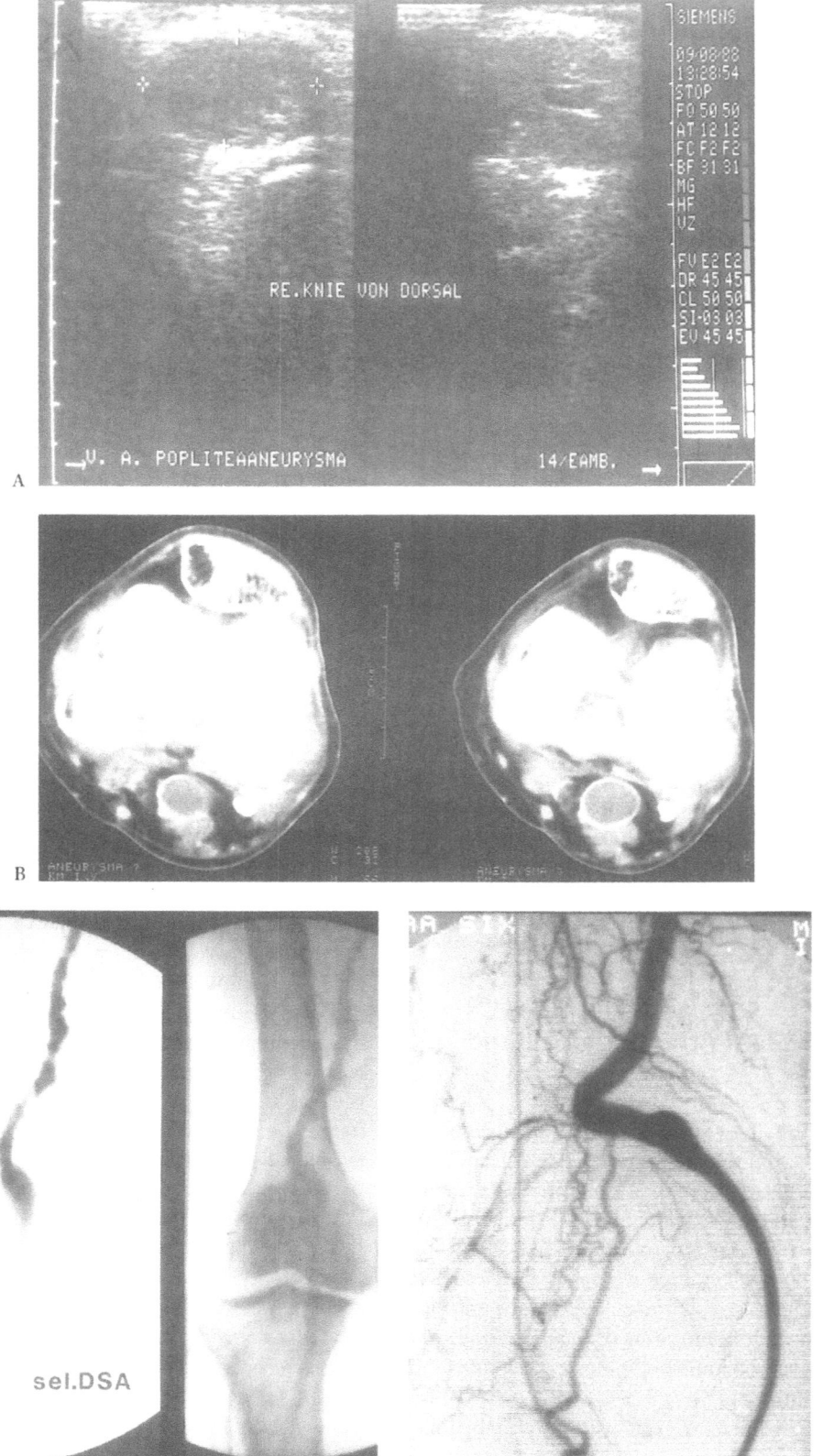

Fig. 25.10. Popliteal artery changes. **A** Popliteal artery aneurysm documented by ultrasound. **B** CT after contrast medium injection, demonstrating a thrombosed popliteal artery aneurysm. **C** Partially thrombosed femoropopliteal aneurysm and diffuse arteriosclerosis. **D** Arteriography demonstrating a thrombosed giant popliteal artery aneurysm with a small residual lumen

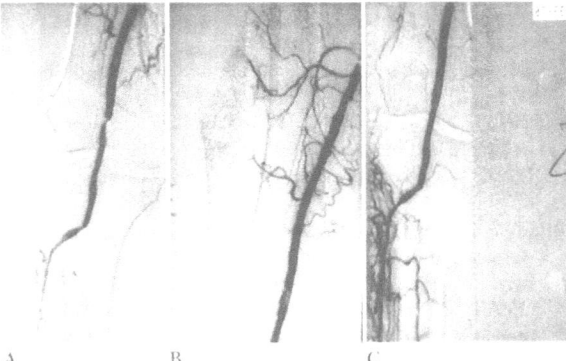

A   B   C

Fig. 25.11. Ring-like atherosclerotic stenosis at the popliteal and anterior tibial artery: also existing occlusion of the tibioperoneal trunk and occlusion of the posterior tibial artery. A Before treatment. B After balloon dilatation with 4-F catheters, 3 and 5 mm balloon diameter, of the proximal obliteratiosn (81-year-old male with forefoot gangrene: risk factors diabetes mellitus and cigarette smoking). C improved tibio-peroneal run-off

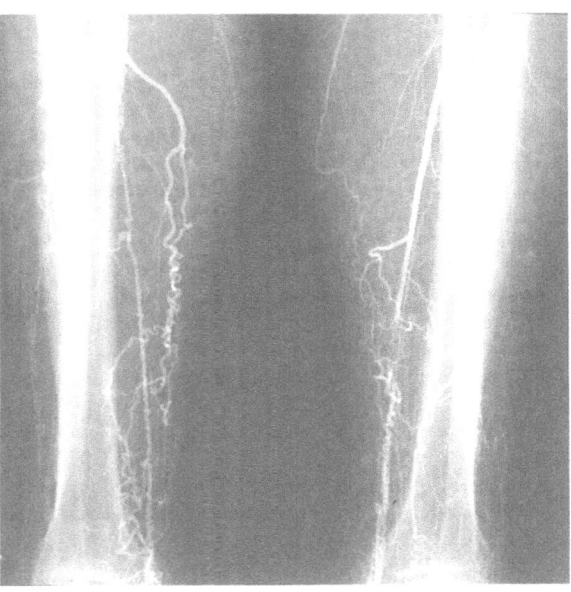

Fig. 25.12. Peripheral type of bilateral POVD with occlusion of all tibioperoneal arteries: cork-screw collateral vessels demonstrating Buerger's disease (43-year-old Male, heavy cigarette smoker)

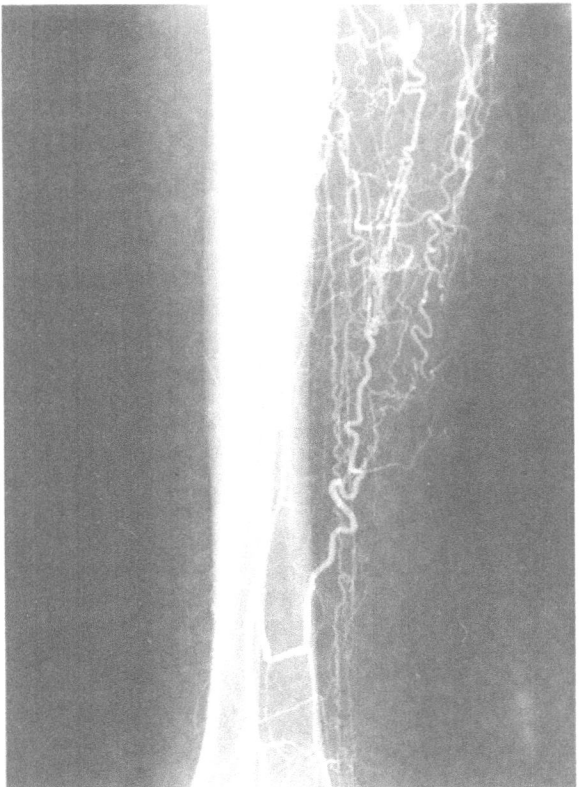

A

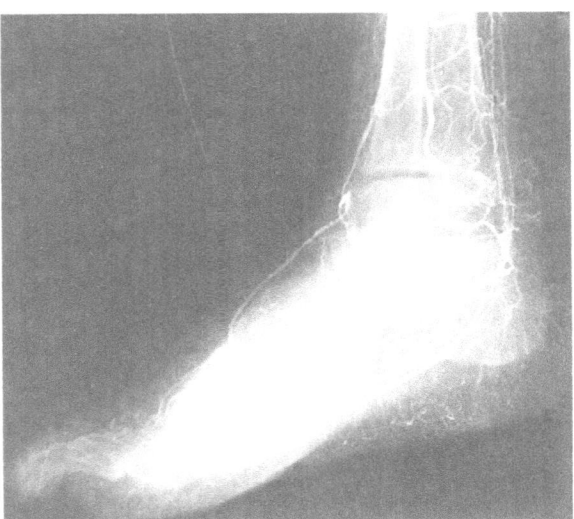

B

Fig. 25.13. POVD, Fontaine stage IV (59-yaer-old male, heavy cigarette smoker). Occlusion of the SFA, popliteal and tibio-peroneal arteries. Tibioperoneal and foot arteries with collateral circulation to the foot from the peroneal artery, through the perforating and communicating arteries to the posterior tibial, plantar and dorsal pedal arteries – prograde catheter arteriography.

References

Alexander K (1993a) Typische Symptome bei arteriellen und venösen Durchblutungsstörungen. In: Alexander K (ed) Gefäßkrankheiten. Urban & Schwarzenberg, Munich, pp 111–124

Alexander K (1993b) Diabetische Angiopathien. In: Alexander K (ed) Gefäßkrankheiten. Urban & Schwarzenberg, Munich, pp 515–531

Arlart IP (1997) Fibromuskuläre Dysplasie – Zystische Adventitiadegeneration – Gefäßwandtumoren. In: Zeitler E (ed) Arterien und Venen. Springer, Berlin Heidelberg New York, pp 355-368

Bollinger A (1979) Funktionelle Angiologie. Thieme, Stuttgart

Bollinger A (1979) Angiitiden. In: Bollinger A (ed) Funktionelle Angiologie, Lehrbuch und Atlas. Thieme, Stuttgart, pp 88-101

Crummy AB, Rankin RS, Turnipseed WD, Berkoff HA (1978): Biplane arteriography in ischemia of the lower extremity. Radiology 126:111–115

Grüntzig A (1977) Die perkutane transluminale Rekanalisation chronischer Arterienverschlüsse mit einer neuen Dilatationstechnik. Verlag G.Witzstrock, Baden-Baden

Hasse HM (1974) Chronische arterielle Verschlußkrankheit. In: Heberer G, Rau G, Schoop W (eds) Angiologie. Thieme, Stutgart, pp 397-431

Heberer G, Rau G, Schoop W (1974) Angiologie. Thieme, Stuttgart

Kappert A (1985) Lehrbuch und Atlas der Angiologie. Huber, Bern

Kremer H, Sprandel U, Marshall M, Baumann G, Hess H (1977) Zystische Gefäßwanddegeneration. Münch Med Wochenschr 119:435–438

Kuthan H, Burkhalter R, Ludin H, et al (1971) Development of occlusive arterial disease in lower limbs: angiographic follow-up of 705 medical patients. Arch Surg 103:545–547

Meyer WW (1974) Atherosklerose. In: Heberer G, Rau G, Schoop W (eds) Angiologie. Thieme, Stuttgart, pp 68–76

Pratt Ch (1954) Cardiovascular surgery. Kimpton, London

Raithel D, Hacker RW (1975) Die zystische Adventitiadegeneration der A. poplitea. VASA 4:353–356

Rodda T (1960) Arteriosclerosis in lower limbs. J Pathol Bacteriol 65:315–322

Rödl W (1980) Die zystische Adventitia-Degeneration der Arteria poplitea. RöntgenBl 33:187–192

Schmitt W, Wack HO, Beneke G (1971) Das Substrat chronischer arterialler Stenosen und Okklusionen. Dtsch med Wochenschr 96:1522–1531

Shoop W (1987) Praktische Angiologie, 4th edn. Thieme, Suttart

Tillgren C, Stenson S, Lund F (1963) Olerative arterial disease of the lower limbs studied by means of repeated femoral arteriography. Acta Radiol (Diagn) 1:161–178

Vollmar J, Nobbe FP (1976) Arteriovenöse Fisteln – Dilartierende Arteriopathien (Aneurysmen). Thieme, Stuttgart

Vollmar J (1996) Rekonstruktive Chirurgie der Arterien, 4th edn. Thieme, Stuttgart

Wenz W (1972) Abdominale Angiographie. Springer Berlin, Heidelberg New York

Wenz W, Beduhn D (1975) Extremitätenarteriographie. Springer Berlin, Heidelberg New York

Widmer LK, Stähelin HB, Nissen C, da Silva A (1981) Venen-, Arterien-Krankheiten, koronare Herzkrankheit bei Berufstätigen. – Prospektiv-epidemiologische Untersuchung Basler Studie I-III 1959-1978. Huber, Bern Stuttgart Wien

Zeïtler E (1974) Aortoarteriographie. In: Heberer G, Rau G, Schoop W (eds) Angiologie. Thieme, Stuttgart, pp 243–302

Zeitler E, Hüring HG (1972) Das Medichrome-Verfahren in der Röntgen-Aufnahmetechnik. Fortschr Röntgenstr 116:402–415

26 Diabetic Vascular Disease

E. ZEITLER

CONTENTS

The clinical picture of diabetic macroangiopathy is determined by the localization and extent of the arterial obliterations. Moreover, additional diabetic microangiopathy and polyneuropathy have a critical influence on the clinical picture, in the form of disorders of the microcirculation, and marked analgesia. According to ALEXANDER (1993), micro- and macroangiopathies are integral components of the diabetic foot changes, and not simply complications of diabetes mellitus. The benefits of insulin and antibiotic therapies have had the effect that patients not only survive, but also suffer from their angiopathy.

26.1
Classification of Diabetes Mellitus

Classification of diabetes mellitus by the American Diabetes Association (ADA) and the WHO (KERNER 1998):
I   Diabetes mellitus type I (beta cell destruction, resulting in complete hypoinsulinemia)
II Diabetes mellitus type II (ranging from predominant insulin resistance with relative hypoinsulinemia to predominant hyposecretion with insulin resistance)

III Other types of diabetes of known causes:
    a) Genetic defects of beta cells
    b) Genetic defects of insulin function
    c) Diseases of the exocrine pancreas
    d) Endocrinopathies
    e) Toxic and drug induced
    f) Infection
    g) Rare immunologic forms
    h) Other syndromes associated with diabetes

26.2
Diagnostic Criteria for Diabetes Mellitus

26.2.1
Symptoms

- Elevated plasma glucose ≥200 mg/dl or ≥11.1 mmol/l (glucose in the capillary whole blood ≥200 mg/dl or ≥11.1 mmol/l) at any time of day
- Polyuria, and unclear weight loss, or
- Fasting glucose ≥126 mg/dl or ≥7.0 mmol/l (glucose in the capillary whole blood ≥110/mg/dl or ≥6.1 mmol/l)
- 'Fasting' means no intake of calories for at least 8h, or 2-h plasma glucose ≥200 mg/dl or ≥11.1 mmol/l (glucose in the capillary whole blood ≥200 mg/dl or 11.1 mmol/l) during an oral glucose tolerance test (OGTT).
  (Glucose tolerance test according to WHO guidelines)

26.3
Histology

From the histological standpoint, diabetic macroangiopathy is a highly severe form of arteriosclerosis (BELL 1956; LINDNER 1977), which occurs prematurely (EGNER et al. 1997) and is mostly of centripetal-progredient type. The muscular arteries tend to

EBERHARD ZEITLER MD, Professor, University Erlangen-Nürnberg, Germany
address for correspondence:
Virchowstraße 13, D-90409 Nürnberg, Germany

produce Mönckeberg's sclerosis, including calcifications which are identifiable on plain radiographs. Arteriolar hyalinosis, rich in arteriosclerosis and lipids, is found in diabetic patients mainly in the kidneys, in the afferent and efferent glomerular arterioles. Diabetic microangiopathy affects the capillaries, whose basal membrane shows defective collagenous reticulum, at a simultaneously elevated glucose level and non-enzymatic carbohydrate bond onto proteins. During that process, they considerably thicken. The major sites of manifestation are kidney and retina.

The characteristics of diabetic macroangiopathy of the extremities (LUNDBAEK 1954, 1973; LEVIN and O'NEAL 1973; HAUPT and BEYER 1974; ZEITLER 1977; BILD et al. 1989) as demonstrated pathologically and angiographically can be described as follows:

1. Vascular obliterations are localized more peripherally than in non-diabetic patients.
2. In younger patients mostly one artery, but in elderly patients all lower-leg arteries are affected.
3. Multiple arterial stenoses are found in the deep femoral artery, whereas the iliac and superficial femoral arteries are free of arteriosclerotic changes.
4. In patients with additional risk factors (hypercholesterolemia, cigarette smoking, hypertension), additional arteriosclerotic lesions are seen in the superficial femoral artery, but very seldom in the iliac arteries.

Due to the peripheral location of the obliterations, symptoms such as intermittent claudication in the calf muscles are less common. Ischemic lesions (Fig. 26.1) and discomfort in the feet dominate the clinical picture. For example, in patients with impaired glucose tolerance, tissue necrosis is found five times as often as in patients with normal metabolism (HILD 1977). In women, diabetes mellitus is the dominant progression factor in 40% of cases, and in an additional 29% the combination of hypertension and diabetes mellitus (TAUTE et al. 1997).

In many cases, despite severe tissue damage, there is little or no pain, attributable to co-existing diabetic neuropathy. The term 'diabetic foot' (LEVIN and O'NEAL 1973; FLYNN and TOOKE 1992) includes vascular disease, neuropathy and osteopathy. On a metabolic basis, 'autosympathectomy' influences neural and muscle structures and leads also to peripheral vasodilatation. This, with time, results in bone resorption, painless bone necrosis, and foot deformity (GUTMANN et al. 1987; ALEXANDER 1993; WETZ 1998). Radiographs show rapidly progressive, painless osteolyses, predominantly in the region of the metatarsals (Fig. 26.2), but also of the tarsal bones,

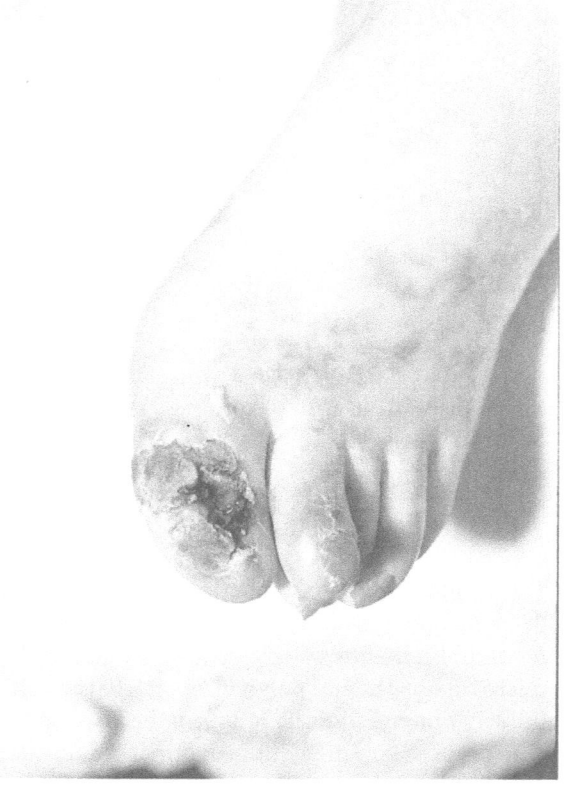

Fig. 26.1. Diabetic foot with gangrene of the first toe: combined macro- and microangiopathy

and can lead to foot deformities. There exist five types of diabetic neuropathic osteo-arthropathies (DNOAP): necrosis of the metatarsophalangeal joints, of the cuneiforms, of the talus and navicular of the talus and superior ankle joint, and of the talus, calcaneum and inferior ankle joint (ZLATHIN et al. 1987; WETZ 1998): The stages of the diabetic foot are, according to SHENAQ (1989):

- No open ulcers, but hyperkeratosis, and deformities of bones.
- Skin ulcers:
  - involving tendons, and joints
  - with bone defects and osteomyelitis
- Localized gangrene
- Extensive gangrene of the whole foot

Diabetic macroangiopathy is exceptional in type I diabetics under 40 years of age, whereas in type II diabetics it occurs independent of the history of diabetes (HAUPT and BEYER 1974). With increasing age, the incidence of obliterative vascular changes in diabetics increases (SCHOOP et al. 1967). Coronary and cerebral arterial occlusions are common findings in type II diabetics in addition to peripheral obliterations (LIEBOW 1955; HILD 1977; APLUND 1980; WIDMER et al. 1981, 1993; ALEXANDER 1983; MANSON et

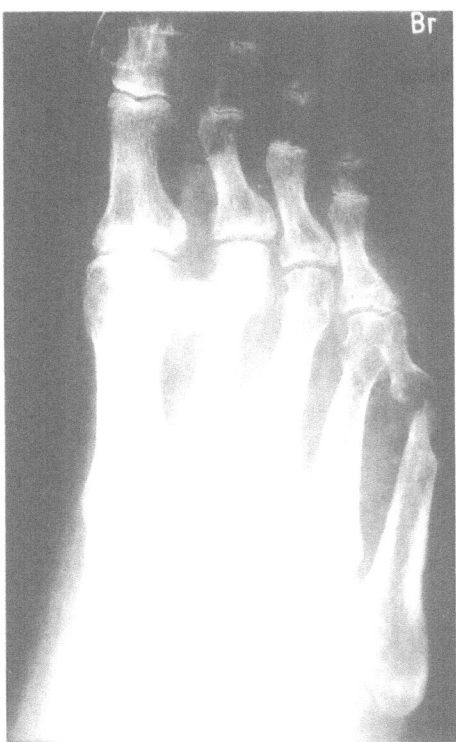

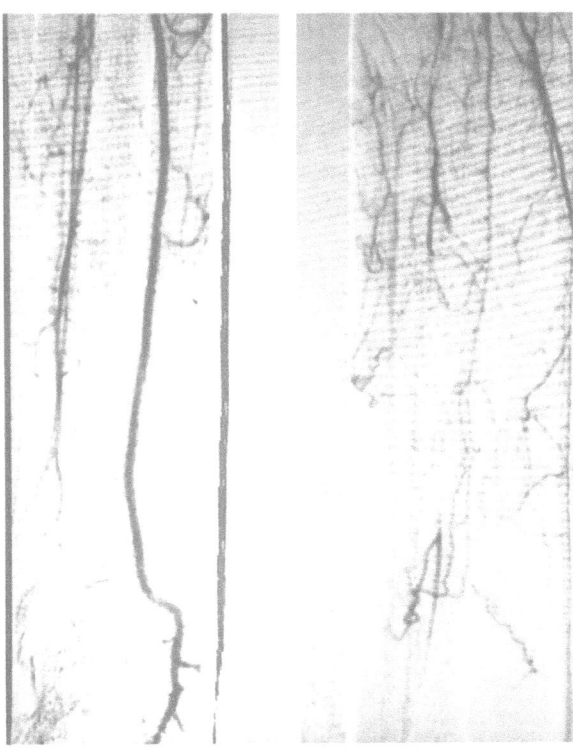

Fig. 26.2. Diabetic osteonecrosis MT V: sugarstick deformity

Fig. 26.3. DSA of calf arteries with occlusion of the anterior tibial and foot arteries: the posterior tibial artery is patent (69-year-old diabetic man with CLI)

al. 1991; TAUTE et al. 1997). Post-mortem studies of 1,214 diabetic patiens out of 50,000 autopsies domonstrated that 40% of them died because of diabetic gangrene (BELL 1950).

Angiography for peripheral obliterations can be limited after clinical examination to needle angiography with puncture of the femoral artery and digital subtraction angiography (DSA), or to prograde angiography with magnification (ZEITLER 1975) to demonstrate the upper thigh, lower leg and feet arteries (Fig. 26.3). Because of the possible combination with an intervention procedure, prograde catheter angiography in patients with diabetic and foot problems (HENNIGES and ZEITLER 1973) is prefered, enabling the use of an optimum contrast agents bolus, to carry out precise morphologic analysis of the foot arteries (Fig. 26.4 and 26.5).

The distribution of the obliterations as found in the different types of occlusion in diabetics and non-diabetics, is shown in Table 26.1. It was based on outpatients in an angiologic department (ALEXANDER 1994). It illustrates the low incidence of upper thigh occlusions in diabetics, compared to non-diabetics, and the higher incidence of occlusions distal of the popliteal artery in diabetic patients.

Figure 26.6 demonstrates the different areas affected as identified by angiography undertaken after clinically established indications.

On magnification arteriography of the foot, we could demonstrate (ZEITLER 1975, 1977; KAMPMANN et al. 1977), in addition to occlusions of the metatarsal and digital arteries, stenotic lesions in very small arteries, microaneurysms and arteriovenous fistulae close to the metatarso-phalangeal joints. Avascularity distal to occlusions is most common in patients with necrosis. Hypervascularity in the area of the metatarsophalangeal joints with more extensive collateral arteries is seen in diabetic patients with gangrene.

Early filling of veins (arteriovenous fistulas) corresponds to a shunt circulation which could be also measured with the integrated capillary pressure (ALEXANDER 1970). Our studies (ZEITLER 1977) based on 161 leg arteriographic studies have been confirmed by DSA techniques for the identification of small AV shunts, as well as hypervascular and avascular forms of diabetic macroangiopathy. An assumption which we could not clearly prove was that hypervascularity mainly occurs in the presence of wet gangrene and co-existing gout, as in the presence

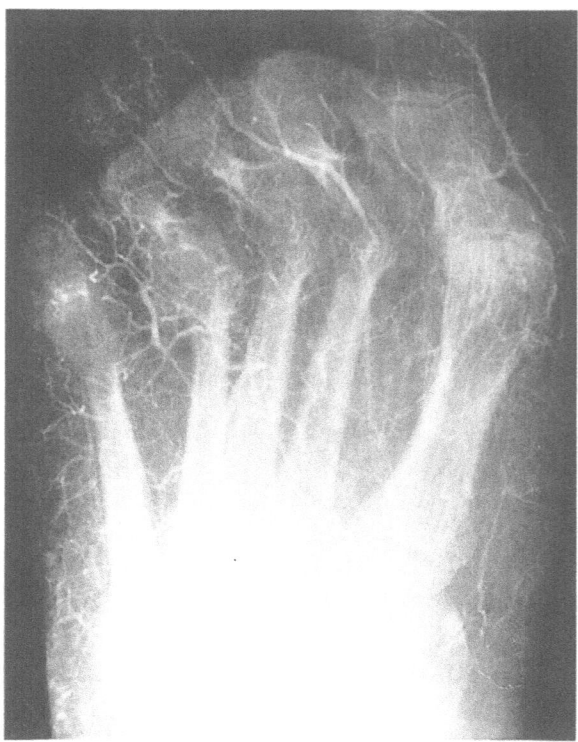

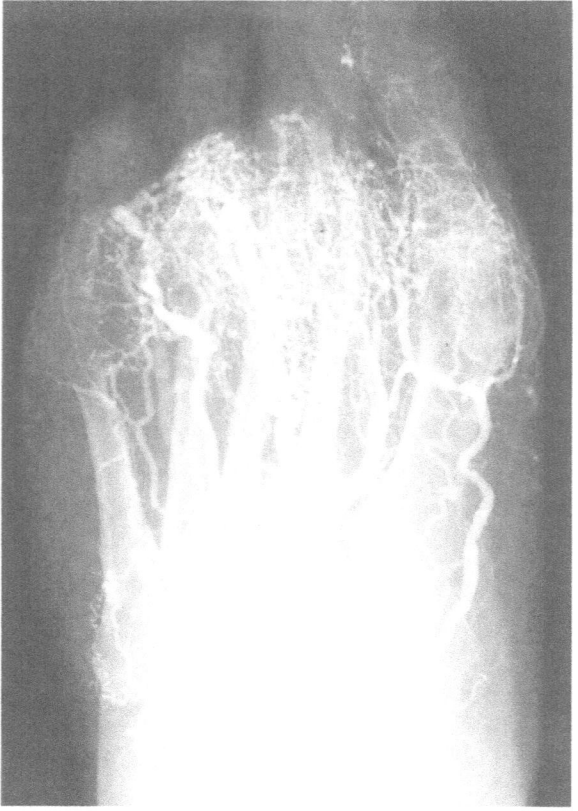

Fig. 26.4. Avascular type of diabetic macroangiopathy. Foot arteriography with magnification, demonstrating multiple occluded foot arteries (76-year-old man with a 25-year history of diabetes mellitus)

Fig. 26.5. Hypervascular type of diabetic macroangiopathy. Foot arteriography with magnification (36-year-old diabetic woman with gangrene of the second and third toes)

of the same factors also avascularity was seen. Whereas occlusions without good collateral arteries in patients with diabetic vascular disease are more common (ALEXANDER 1970; LEVIN and O'NEAL 1973; CLAEYES 1995), well-developed collaterals do not help prevent severe complications.

Diabetes mellitus affects about 2–5% of the general population. The most important complication, apart from diabetic nephropathy and retinopathy, is the formation of ulcers and gangrene of the foot. This occurs in 19–40% of diabetic patients with POVD (BELL 1950; WIDMER et al. 1981; GUTMANN et al. 1987). The age-related rate of lower-limb amputations rate is about 10–15 times higher than that of patients without diabetes (MOST et al. 1983; DORMANDY 1996). The perioperative mortality rate in this population is as high as 25%, with only 50% alive after 3 years.

Clinically, two additional problems exist:
1) The neuropathic foot (NPF)
2) The neuroischemic foot (NIF)

Neuropathy results in a loss of sensory perception of foot trauma, peripheral vascular tissue leads to gangrene, and poor healing of foot lesions. Infection is a frequent complication, which aggravates tissue damage.

The neuroischemic ulcer is defined by:
1) Ulceration or gangrene at the foot
2) Persistently recurring rest pain requiring analgesia
3) Absence of ankle pulses

Peripheral neuropathy has a high prevalence in diabetic patients, and involves sensory, motor and autonomic nerve fibres (Claeys 1995; WETZ 1998). The sensory impairment is characterized by reduced sensation of pain and temperature, resulting in pseudo-syringomyelic patterns. The symptomatic differences are shown in Table 26.2.

In advanced stages of diabetic vascular disease, obliterations of the popliteal and superficial femoral artery manifest themselves as effects of other simultaneously existing risk factors. These segmental occlusions or stenoses are possibly amenable to inter-

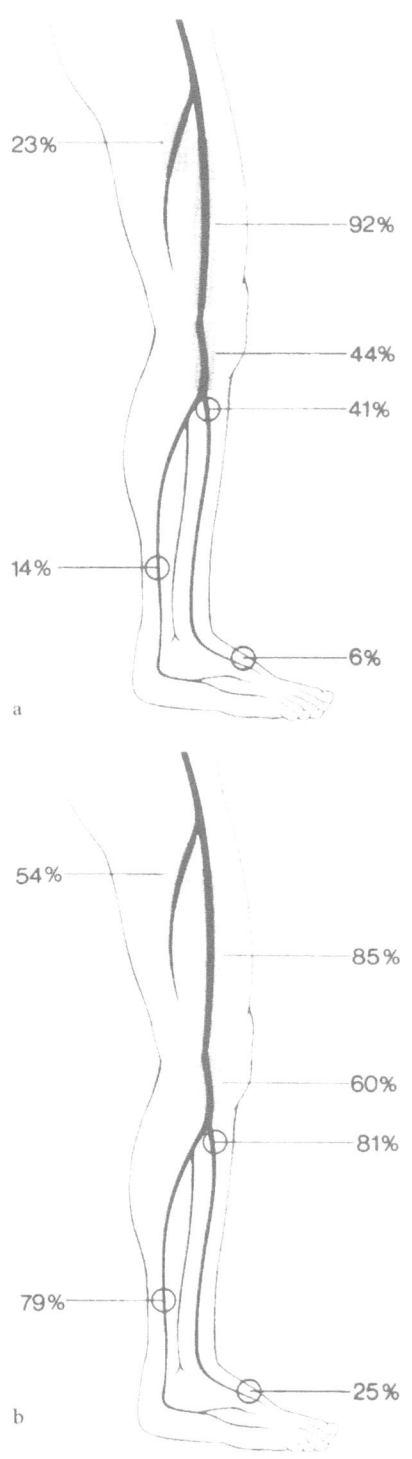

ventional therapy, bringing about a long-lasting palliative effect. In the case of extensive occlusions, femoro-crural and femoro-pedal bypass implantations can help avoid an above-knee amputation, and result in the patient undergoing only amputation of a toe/toes or the forefoot. Amputations should, therefore, not be performed without first performing angiography (ALEXANDER 1993; CLAEYS 1995; VOLLMAR 1996).

Since the introduction of improved catheter techniques using 3- and 4-French catheters, high-torque guidewires with special tip configurations, and balloon diameters of 2–4 mm, percutaneous interventional techniques have gained acceptance, even by vascular surgeons in the treatment of tibioperoneal occlusions causing critical limb ischemia (SAAB et al. 1992; CRIADO et al. 1998). In a group of 26 patients, the follow up limb salvage rate was 80% at 23 months (CRIADO et al. 1998). Interventional radiologists and cardiologists have published increasingly good results for the treatment of below knee occlusions (See Chap. 33). Thus, in specialist vascular centres where skilled personnel employ optimum techniques, percutaneous interventional procedures using selective arteriography and angioplasty should be used as the first-line therapy. However, venous bypass techniques provide a satisfactory alternative in several situations.

Table 26.1. Distribution of obliterations in patients with POVD (%) (According to ALEXANDER 1994)

Type of occlusion	Diabetic patients	Non-diabetic patient
Pelvic	3.1	20.4
Thigh	18.8	45.5
Peripheral	68.7	22.7
Shoulder	9.4	11.4

Table 26.2. Clinical features of neuroischemic foot (NIF*) and neuropathic foot (NPF*) (according to Claeys 1995)

NIF	NPF
Cold foot	Warm, dry foot
No pulse	Pulse present
Painful Ulcer	Painless ulcer
Claudication or	Calluses
Rest pain	Loss of pain

*NIF = Neuroischemic foot
*NPF = Neuropathic foot

Fig. 26.6. Occlusive peripheral artery disease: differences in the location of occlusions in patients **a** without diabetes and **b** with diabetes

References

Alexander K (1970) Die diabetischen Angiopathien. Münch Med Wochenschr 12:690-696

Alexander K, Cachovan M (1977) Diabetische Angiopathien. Witzstrock, Baden-Baden

Alexander K (1983) Mikro- und makroangiopathische Veränderungen bei Diabetes mellitus. Hämostasiologe 4:3-27

Alexander K (1993) Diabetische Angiopathien. In: Alexander K (ed) Gefäßkrankheiten. Urban & Schwarzenberg, Munich, pp 515-531

Aplund K, Hägg E, Helmers C, et al. (1980) The natural history of stroke in diabetic patients. Acta Med Scand 207:417-424

Bell ET (1950) A post-mortem study of 1214 diabetic subjects with special reference to the vascular lesions. Proc Diab Assoc 10:62-72

Bild DE, Selby JV, Sinnock P, et al (1989) Lower-extremity amputation in people with diabetes mellitus. Epidemiology and prevention. Diab Care 12:24-31

Claeys L (1995): Management of the diabetic foot. In: Horsch S, Claeys L (eds) Critical limb ischemia. Steinkopff, Darmstadt

Criado FJ, Twena M, Abdul-Khoud O, et al (1998) Below-knee angioplasty: Misguided aggressiveness or reasonable opportunity. Invasive Cardiol 10:415-424

Dormandy JA (1996) The natural history of peripheral arterial disease. In: A textbook of vascular medicine. Arnold and Oxford University Press, p 162-175

Egner E, Kraus-Huonder B, Markmann HU (1997) Grundlagen der Pathomorphologie der Blutgefäße. In: Zeitler E (ed) Arterien und Venen. Springer, Berlin Heidelberg New York, pp 3-56

Flynn MD, Tooke JE (1992) Aetiology of diabetic foot ulceration: a vote for the microcirculation? Diabet Med 9:320-329

Gutmann M, Kaplan O, Skornicky Y, et al (1987) Gangrene of the lower limbs in diabetic patients: a malignant complication. Am J Surg 154:305-308

Haupt E, Beyer J (1974) Gefäßkrankheiten bei Diabetes mellitus. In: Mehnert H, Schöffling K (eds) Diabetologie in Klinik und Praxis.Thieme, Stuttgart

Henninges D, Zeitler E (1973) Angiopathie der Füße. Fortschr Röntgenstr 118:663-667

Hild R (1977) Klinik der diabetischen Makroangiopathie. In: Alexander K, Cachovan M (eds) Diabetische Angiopathien. Witzstrock, Baden-Baden, pp 150-163

Kampmann B, Berger H, Vogelberg KH, Zeitler E (1977) Arteriographische Befunde bei Vergrößerungsangiographie der Beine bei Diabetikern. In: Alexander K, Cachovan H (eds) Diabetische Angiopathien. Witzstrock, Baden-Baden, pp 248-257

Kerner W (1998) Classification and diagnosis of diabetes mellitus. Dtsch. Ärtzebl 95:3144-3148

Levin ME, O'Neal LW (1973) The diabetic foot. Mosby, St. Louis

Liebow JM, Hellerstein HK, et al (1955) Arteriosclerotic heart disease in diabetes mellitus. Am J Med 18:438-447

Lindner J (1977) Pathomorphologie der diabetischen Makroangiopathie: In: Alexander K, Cachovan M (eds) Diabetische Angiopathien. Witzstrock, Baden-Baden, pp 91-127

Lundbaek K (1954) Diabetische Angiopathie – ein spezifisches Krankheitsbild. Schweiz Med Wochenschr 84:538

Lundbaek K (1973) Diabetic angiopathy. Acta Diabetol Lat 10:183-207

Manson JE, Colditz GA, Stampfer MJ, et al (1991) A prospective study of maturity-onset diabetes mellitus and risk of coronary heart disease and stroke in women. Arch Intern Med 151:1141-1147

Most RS, Sinnock P (1983) The epidemiology of lower extremity amuptations in diabetic individuals. Diabetes Care 6:87-92

Pense G, Panzram G, Pissarek DD (1973) Qualität der Stoffwechselführung und Angiopathie bei 180 Langzeitdiabetikern mit mindestens 20-jähriger Krankheitsdauer. Schweiz med Wochenschr 103:1125-1129

Saab MH, Smith DC, Aka PK, et al (1992) Percutaneous transluminal angioplasty of tibial arteries for limb salvage. Card Vasc Intervent Radiol 15:211-216

Schoop W, Gerhard HJ, Roth U (1967) Häufigkeit klinisch nachweisbarer Lumeneinengungen großer Arterien beim Diabetiker. Med Klin 621:825-829

Schoop W (1988) Praktische Angiologie. Thieme, New York

Shenaq SM (1989) Diabetic foot ulcers. Postgrad Med 85:323-328

Taute BM, Hänsgen K, Fechner L, Große L, Podhaisky H (1997) Untersuchungen zum Progressionsrisiko der peripheralen arteriellen Verschlußkrankheit. Vasomed 9:8-15

The Expert Committee on the Diagnosis and Classification of Diabetes Mellitus (1997) Report of the expert committee on the diagnosis and classification of diabetes mellitus. Diabetes Care 20:1183-1197

Vollmar J (1996) Rekonstruktive Chirurgie der Arterien 4th ed. Thieme, Stuttgart

Wetz HH (1998) Diabetisch-neuropathische Osteoarthropathie. Dtsch Ärtzebl 95:A2701-2705

Widmer LK, Stähelin HB, Nissen C, da Silva A (1981) Venen-Arterien-Krankheiten, koronare Herzkrankheit bei Berufstätigen. Prospektiv-epidemiologische Untersuchung. Basler Studie I-III 1959-1978. Huber, Bern

Widmer LK, da Silva A, Widmer MT (1993) Epidemiologie und sozialmedizinische Bedeutung der peripheren arteriellen Verschlußkrankheit. In: Alexander K (ed) Gefäßkrankheiten. Urban & Schwarzenberg, Munich, pp 16-24

Zeitler E (1975) Die selektive Katheterangiographie der A. femoralis superficialis. Electromedica 5:167-178

Zeitler E (1977) Angiographische Röntgndiagnose bei diabetischer Makroangiographie. In: Alexander K, Cachovan M (eds) Diabetische Angiopathien. Witzstrock, Baden-Baden, pp 128-136

Zlathin MB, Pathrin M, Sartoris DJ, Resmick D (1987) The diabetic foot. Radiol Clin North Am 25:1095-1105

27 Non-Arteriosclerotic Arterial Diseases

E. Zeitler

The arterial vascular diseases not caused by arteriosclerosis have different known and also unknown aetiologies and occur considerably less often (ALLEN 1935; FONTAINE 1967; ALEXANDER 1993). The major underlying pathology is vascular changes in the smaller arteries of the lower leg, distal arms, or fingers. In 1972, KAPPERT described the different forms by noting the features which differentiated them from arteriosclerotic vascular diseases. Most of these vascular diseases are inflammatory in nature (angiitis), are a component of collagenoses, (e.g., scleroderma, lupus erythematosus) or are one of the arterial compression syndromes or vasospastic syndromes. The latter will be described in the chapter "Functional Diseases". RATSCHOW, in 1959, defined some of them as angioneuropathies. In the framework of functional diseases, also the drug-induced, but also iatrogenic arteriopathies (HESS 1972) are dealt with, in as far as they play a role in radiologic differential diagnosis. Under this heading are also summarized: radiotherapy, intraarterial injection of

EBERHARD ZEITLER MD, Professor, University Erlangen-Nürnberg, Germany
address for correspondence:
Virchowstraße 13, D-90409 Nürnberg, Germany

different pharmaca (thiopental, dexamethasone and others). All of these should lead one to consider an imaging diagnosis.

27.1
Buerger's Syndrome - Thrombangiitis Obliterans

The inflammatory vascular diseases present few specific histological findings (LEU 1985). Giant cell panarteritis preferentially affects medium to large arteries and takes a prolonged chronic course. Temporal arteritis has a similar course but mainly occurs in aged patients.

Periarteritis nodosa mainly affects small arteries and veins, with a periodic course of recurrent acute symptoms. The affected vessels develop necrosis or show fibrinoid necrosis of the wall. There may also be microaneurysms of small arteries. Their demonstration in renal, mesenteric, pancreatic, or finger arteries by selective angiogram is considered characteristic and indicated whenever skin biopsies do not provide a clear diagnosis. Muscles biopsies only provide a positive diagnosis in 20–35% of cases (BOLLINGER 1979).

Thrombangiitis obliterans (also called 'Buerger-von Winiwarter's disease') for the most part affects small arteries and veins of the extremities; the inflammatory endothelial reaction causes early thromboses (LEU 1976; SHIONOYA 1978; LYSAK and WELLING 1980; GUILMONT and LASFARGUES 1988; JOYCE 1990). Additionally, larger arteries and superficial veins are affected. Involvement of the media and adventitia results in early thromboses and marked revascularization. Because secondary arteriosclerosis develops rapidly, histological differentiation is only possible with sufficient material, usually from amputated legs (LEU 1988). This fact underlines the importance of differentiating selective angiography (Fig. 27.1) from aortoarteriography, which provides important additional information (McKUSSIK et al.

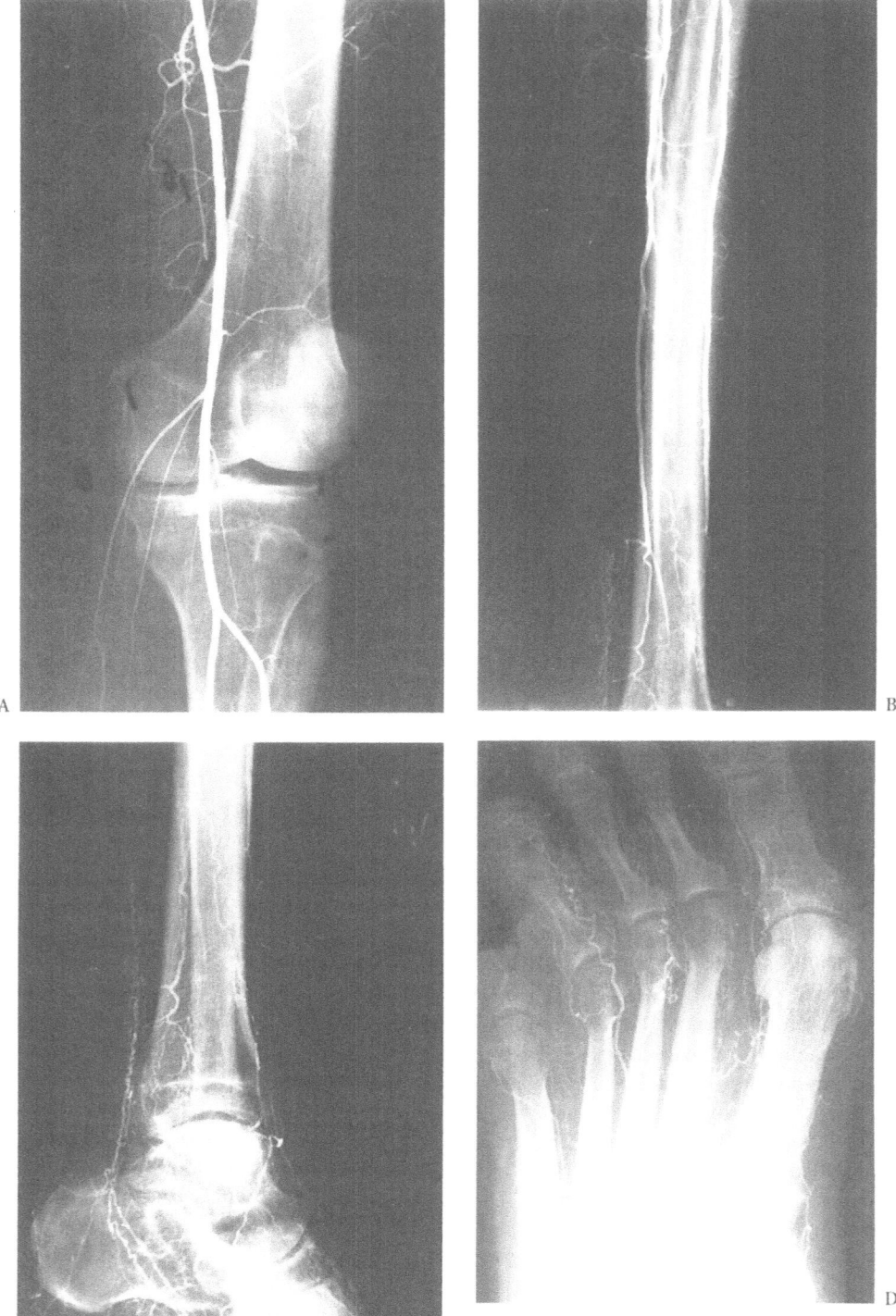

Fig. 27.1 A-D Thrombangiitis obliterans - Buerger (27-year-old man, heavy cigarette smoker, gangrene fourth and fifth toes, history of phlebitis saltans). Angiography demonstrating proximal arteries normal, distal occlusion of all tibioperoneal arteries, and most foot arteries. Typical cork-screw collaterals along the posterior tibial artery: **A** Femoropoplitea arteries **B** calf arteries **C** ankle arteries **D** foot arteries

1962; SELDINGER 1964; SZILAGY et al. 1964; LAMBETH and YONG 1970; CORELLI 1973; RIVERA 1973; HENNINGES and ZEITLER 1979; SUZUKI et al. 1982; HAGEN and LOHSE 1984; LAMBRECHT et al. 1984; KAUSHIK et al. 1986; DIEHM and SCHÄFER 1993).

The history of thrombangiitis obliterans is varied. Even though it was first described pathologically as 'endoarteritis' and 'endophlebitis' with gangrene of the foot by VON WINIWARTER in 1879, BUERGER published the clinical picture in 1908, and expanded the description in subsequent years; he is also regarded as the 'father' of angiology. The monographs by HEIDRICH (1988) and DIEHM and SCHÄFER (1993) give highly detailed information on the different interpretation as regards history and clinical features, and whether the condition is a disease or a syndrome. Nowadays, it is an entity equally recognized by morphologists, clinicians and radiologists, whose etiology has largely remained unclear (KINMONTH 1948; SCHATZ et al. 1966; KAPPERT 1972; MÜLLER-BÜHL et al. 1981; RATSCHOW 1959). The consensus is to define the clinical picture as 'Buerger's syndrome' (MCKUSICK et al. 1962; SCHOOP 1972; DIEHM and SCHÄFER 1993).

In the past two decades, apart from the identified influence of cigarette smoking as a risk factor (STRANDNESS 1969; INADA 1972; CORELLI 1973; SHINOYA et al. 1977; MARTORELL 1958; HEIDRICH 1988), immunologic parameters, such as the anti-elastin-titer have been increasingly suspected as underlying factors in the development of the disease (BOLLINGER et al. 1979; HORSCH et al. 1977; HORSCH 1988; SANDRART et al. 1988). Cigarette smoking is a feature in 92-99% of patients with Buerger's syndrome (HEIDRICH 1988).

Clinically, Buerger's syndrome is defined as follows (SCHOOP 1972; HORST et al. 1980; CACHOVAN 1988; HEIDRICH 1988; ALEXANDER 1993; DIEHM and SCHÄFER 1993):

1. Peripheral arterial occlusions of extremity arteries
2. Developing in individuals before the age of 40 years
3. Previous or co-existing phlebitis, manifesting itself as 'migrating phlebitis' or 'phlebitis saltans'

Apart from pain in the feet, there occurs sensation of coldness in the area of the palmar or plantar site of the hand and foot, which is defined as 'in-step claudication' (STRANDNESS 1987) or 'plantar claudication' (KUMMER et al. 1977). Trophic lesions are observed in about 54% of patients (DIEHM and SCHÄFER 1993). Involvement of the upper extremities occurs in up to 90% of affected Japanese (OHTA et al. 1988), but only in 5–40% of those in Europe and

the USA (MONTOESI and GHIRINGELLI 1961; JANEVSKI 1982; DIEHM and SCHÄFER 1993).

The clinical difference between arteriosclerosis and thrombangiitis obliterans is demonstrated in Table 27.1. While age, sex, pulse and laboratory parameters can be documented, arteriography gives precise information about localization, type of occlusion, and different variations of collateral vessels. The typical patterns that have been described (SZILAGYI et al. 1964; CORELLI 1973; RIVERI 1973; SUZUKI 1982; HAGEN and LOHSE 1984) and which indicate the existence of Buerger's syndrome are listed in Table 27.2.

Figure 27.1 demonstrates the smooth vessel wall in the femoral, popliteal and proximal tibiofibular arteries, cut-off occlusion in the anterior tibial artery and filum terminale appearance of the posterior tibial artery. In the distal calf, 'cork-screw' collaterals go from the occluded posterior tibial artery to the plantar artery. Multiple skip lesions, occlusions and direct collateral vessels go to the fourth toe. Fig. 27.2 (a DSA examination) demonstrates a wide net of collaterals of cork-screw, spider-leg and direct types, but in addition stenotic lesions in the popliteal artery. This patient developed trophic lesions, as a sign of his peripheral vascular disease, 15 years previously. The necrotic lesions subsequently healed, this being the picture of 'burned-out' Buerger's syndrome with residual arteriosclerosis.

The location and incidence of arterial obliterations and collateral formation which we observed in the angiograms of 71 patients is demonstrated in

Table 27.1. Differences between arteriosclerosis and thrombangiitis obliterans (according to LEU 1985)

Criterion	Arteriosclerosis	Thrombanggiitis obliterans
Age at diagnosis	Older	Before age of 40
Sex	Before age of 60: ♂ From age of 60: ♀	
Localization	Major arteries and aorta, coronary and cerebral arteries	Only distal and small arteries
Spread	Generalized, particularly at bifurcations	Skip lesions
Veins	No relation	Phlebitis very common
Formalgenetic	Degenerative, with inhibition of cholesterol and lipids in intima	Inflammation in intima
Immunopathologic results	Without	Can be positive

Table 27.2 Angiographic symptoms of thromboangiitis obliterans

1   Absence of arteriosclerotic lesions
2   Multiple segmental obliterations: "skip lesions" (SZILAGYI et al. 1964)
3   Smooth vessel wall in unaffected arteries
4   Cut-off nature in femoro-popliteal occlusions
5   Tortuous, "cork-screw type" collaterals alongside the occluded artery (SUZUKI et al. 1982)
6   Direct collaterals (Martorell sign) (MONTORSI et al. 1961)
7   "Standing waves" pattern (MAYALL 1964; ISHIKAWA et al. 1973)
8   Tapered occlusion and filum terminale aspect in distal arteries
9   "Tree-root", "spider's leg", "vinetendril" type of collaterals (RIVERA 1973)
10 Corrugated pattern of involved arteries: "rippling sign" (CORELLI 1973)

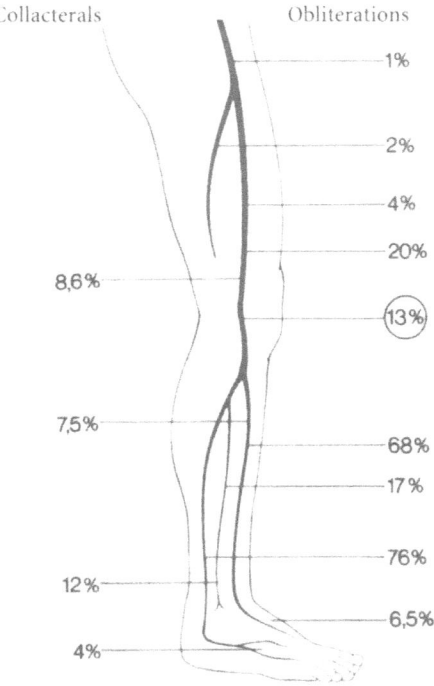

Fig. 27.3 Localization and frequency of arterial obliterations in 71 patients with the clinical diagnosis of Buerger's syndrome, and typical collateral vessels

Fig. 27.3. These patients had been suspected of having Buerger's syndrome using the clinical criteria of SCHOOP(1972). In Fig. 27.4, the distribution of the radiographic signs 'stationary waves' and 'corrugated arteries' is marked. These were observed as either solitary or multiple phenomena, and could always be found 15 and 50 cm proximal to an abrupt arterial occlusion. They mainly occurred during femoral arteriography and did not occur in abdominal aortoarteriography using a catheter.

The incidence of Buerger's syndrome varies between 0.5% and 5% of all patients with peripheral occlusive disease (POVD) (HAGEN and LOHSE 1984; DIEHM and SCHÄFER 1993). Whereas in a clinic for vascular diseases, 5% of 1,400 patients with POVD had Buerger's syndrome (SCHOOP 1972), the incidence in a community hospital in Berlin was only 0.7% (HAGEN and LOHSE 1984). In an analysis of 140

patients with thrombangiitis obliterans out of 20,000 arteriographic studies (Table 27.3) only 7 of 13 angiographic signs had an incidence of more than 70%. The 'rippling sign' and 'standing-wave pattern' (MAYALL 1964; ICHIKAWA et al. 1973; ZEITLER 1976), together with other signs were seen less commonly in their patient population. The incidence should increase with the increased use of catheter angiography compared to needle angiography. The influence to the arterial wall is less important when the contrast medium injection or needle position is in the aorta instead of one of the direct inflow arteries of an extremity.

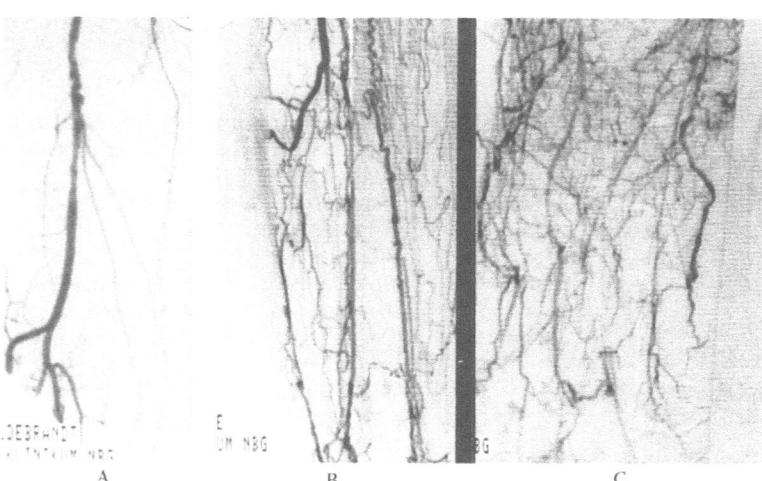

Fig. 27.2 A-C Arterial DSA, Thrombangiitis obliterans, Buerger. POVD of popliteal type (45-year-old man, risk factor cigarette-smoking). Small ulcer on fifth toe. Arterial DSA demonstrating tibioperoneal obliterations, popliteal artery stenoses, foot artery occlusions, good collateral circulation. Buerger's disease with secondary arteriosclerosis. **A** Popliteal artery stenosis **B** occluded tibioperoneal arteries, typical collateral vessels **C** foot arteries with several occlusions

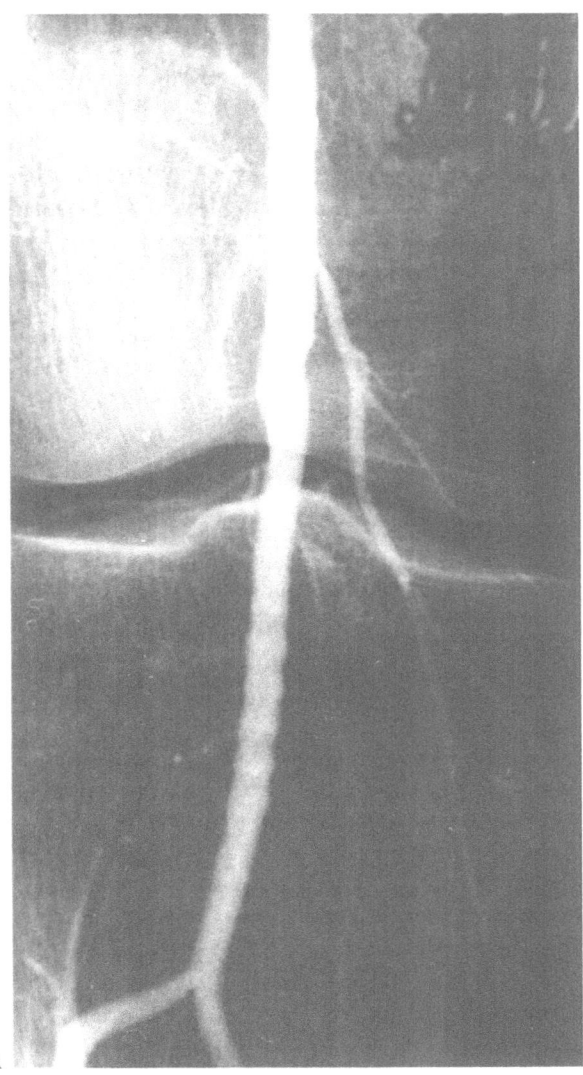

A

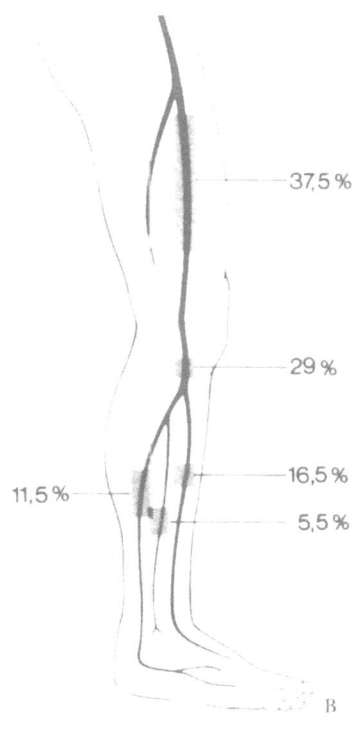

Fig. 27.4 A „Stationary waves" in the popliteal artery (synonyms: corrugated arteries, accordion-like shadows, Pearl-necklace phenomenon) B localization of this sign in 200 angiographic demonstrations in the literature (according to ZEITLER 1976)

Table 27.3. Incidence of angiographic signs of Buerger's disease (According to HAGEN)

Multiple, segmental, discontinuous lesions: "skip lesions"	100 %
Smooth-lined vessels in non-affected arteries	100 %
"Cut-off" type of femoro-popliteal occlusions	100 %
Cork-screw direct (Martorell) and indirect collaterals	100 %
Absence of typical arteriosclerotic lesions	90 %
"Standing waves" pattern: "goose-trachea-like appearance"	75 %
Bilateral incidence with symmetric distribution	70 %
"Filum terminale" feature of distal vessels	40 %
Tortuous, "Spider-leg" or "tree-root" collaterals	40 %
Corrugated pattern of involved arteries; "rippling sign"	20 %

It is therefore of great importance to the interpretation of angiography, to know the underlying cause of the symptoms prior to the selection of the angiographic technique (VAN DER STRICHT et al. 1973; SHINOYAet al. 1978; SUZUKI et a.l 1982; LEU 1988).

Thrombangiitis obliterans needs to be clearly distinguished from other forms of inflammatory vascular disease (MONTORSI et al. 1961; FONTAINE et al. 1959; LAMBRECHT et al. 1984). There are those that affect the major arteries: aorto-arteritis of Takayasu's type and giant-cell arteritis. The medium-size visceral arteries of the kidneys, heart, and pancreas are involved in panarteritis nodosa and Kawasaki's disease. Vasculitis preferentially affecting small vessels in the respiratory tract occurs in Wegner's granulomatosis. Capillary involvement occurs in capillaries in Henoch's purpura, Churg-Strauss's syndrome, and others. These, in general, are characterized by clinical, laboratory, or immunologic parameters (GROSS 1993, 1995). Henoch's purpura requires the documentation of immunologic factors (immunoglobulin, antinuclear antibodies, etc.) in the vascular wall, and in most patients also changes of the complement factors in the circulating blood. Only in large and medium-size vessels is angiography capable of providing some additional information.

27.2
Arterial Diseases in Patients with Collagen Diseases: Progressive Systemic Scleroderma (PSS) and Systemic Lupus Erythematosus (SLE)

Scleroderma is a generalized disease of small arteries and connective tissue (Peller et al. 1985). In the early stages, the fingers are thickened by edema and Raynaud's syndrome is very common. In well-documented series it can be seen in 60–90% of patients (ALARCON-SEGOVIA 1965; DABICH et al. 1973; CAMPBELL and LEROY 1975; ANSARI et al. 1986). The obliterative vasculopathy of arterioles and capillaries can be visualised by capillary microscopy (MAHLER and BOLLINGER 1978; BOLLINGER 1979; RANFT et al. 1986). The vascular condition mainly affects small-diameter arteries of patients with scleroderma of the finger arteries, and this has been demonstrated by arteriography in several publications (SCHOBER and KLÜKEN 1966; POKIESER et al. 1971; DEPALMA et al. 1972; DABICH et al. 1973; ZEITLER 1979; KAUFMANN et al. 1983; JANEVSKI 1986; WAGNER and ALEXANDER 1993). On the basis of several angiographic studies in patients with Raynaud's syndrome and scleroderma, CAMPBELL and LE ROY (1975) postulated the vascular pathogenesis of the disease. Before the development of sclerodactyly, angiography shows small arteries and later irregularities, stenoses and occlusions of digital arteries. The ulnar artery and the superficial palmar arcade of the hand arteries are affected with stenoses and occlusions in a high percentage (up to 45%) of cases (WAGNER and ALEXANDER 1993; SCHMITT and LANZ 1996).

Of 125 hand arteriographies, we diagnosed ulnar artery occlusion in 19 patients. Of these, 15 had scleroderma, 3 had thrombangiitis obliterans with concomitant impairment of the leg arteries, and 1 had Dupuytren's contraction. Obliteration of several digital arteries was the most common result (ZEITLER 1979).

Hand arteriography requires a special technique, with warming and cooling before sequential contrast medium injection and filming, in addition to optimum vasodilatation (RÖSCH et al. 1977; ZEITLER 1976). Cooling in icy water is important to control vasospasm in patients with primary Raynaud's syndrome. This technique of cryodynamic pharmaco-angiography (Table 27.4) helps differentiate between primary and secondary Raynaud's syndrome.

Table 27.4. Technique of angiography of hands and feet

1.	Warming up
2.	CM injection
	a) via catheter in subclavia
	b) via retrograde puncture in brachial artery, elbow
	c) MR: i.v. application
3.	Vasodilation
4.	Angiography with magnification
	a) conventional, with long series
	b) DSA
5.	Angiography after cooling with ice: pharmaco-cryodynamic angiography

In the angiograms of scleroderma patients, in addition to the obliterations of the ulnar arteries, the digital arteries of the second to fourth fingers are of narrow diameter and taper distally, despite optimum vasodilatation. A remarkable fact is lack of the H-shaped communicating arteries at the level of the proximal and middle phalanges between the ulnar and radial digital arteries. If there are collaterals, they, too, have a narrow diameter. In accordance with the reduced soft-tissue mantle of the fingers, the vessels of the finger pulp are markedly attenuated. The cause of this is a thickening of the media and intima, manifesting itself in the digital arteries, particularly in scleroderma, cold injuries and vibration trauma (THULESIUS 1979). Pathologic changes on microscopy are rarefaction, avascular areas, and single giant capillaries (MAHLER and BOLLINGER 1978).

Fluorescein angiography (LUND et al. 1979) allows the demonstration of findings comparable to those of angiography, if organic changes of the digital arteries are present.

In patients with lupus erythematosus, acral gangrene is identifiable in 1% (ALARCON-SEGOVIA 1965; METZ 1971; NORTON and NADO 1970). In about 25%, secondary Raynaud's phenomenon is detected (BOLLINGER 1979). The indication for an arteriography of the hand is easily justified if the diagnosis is confirmed locally by microscopy and by serologic tests (LE-cell phenomenon, and elevated titers of antinuclear antibodies) (DuBois and Arterberry 1962; Tan et al. 1982; Kaufmann et al. 1986; Bakker et al. 1989).

27.3
Compression Syndromes

Arterial compression syndromes are constrictions of vessels caused by the exogenous effects of muscles, tendons and bones. This mainly occurs in special situations, such as congenital variations, marked muscle formation in athletes, and in asthenic individuals under the influence of extreme body positions (Weibel and Fields 1967; Bollinger et al 1979;. Gruss et al. 1982; Schunn 1997).

Of clinical importance, particularly in the context of angiographic technique and interpretation are:
- The Thoracic outlet syndrome (TOS)
- The Popliteal artery entrapment syndrome (PAES)
- The Brachial compression syndrom.(BES)
– Tibialis anterior syndrome (TAS)

27.3.1 Thoracic Outlet Syndrome

At their passage into the arm, the subclavian artery, the neural structures and the subclavian vein cross the scalenus narrowing, the costoclavicular narrowing, the coraco-pectoral narrowing, and the hyperabductional narrowing. The term 'thoracic outlet syndrome' comprises all compression phenomena of the posterior scalenus gap, costoclavicular narrowing, coraco-pectoral narrowing and pectoralis minor tendon (Peet et al. 1956). Dependent on the clinical situation and the dominance of compressed neural structures, it has to be distinguished from the more common neurogenic TOS with compression of the brachial plexus, affecting about 80–95% of patients, and the less common vascular syndromes (Schunn 1997). The arterial TOS with compression of the subclavian artery including its branches results in thrombembolic complications and can be observed in 5% of all examinations for TOS (Adler and Hoschmann1973). The neurologic symptoms are paraesthesia, numbness, prickling, and weakness in the arm and hand. The vascular syndromes are cold hands, ischemic pain, and loss, or reduction of pulse. The venous thrombosis, also described as 'thrombose par effort', could be observed in 5–15% of this patient population (Makhoul, Machleder

1992). The causes of the TOS (Peet et al. 1956; Adler and Hoschmann1973; Roos 1976; Kobinia et al. 1980; Sanders and Haug 1991) are summarized in Table 27.5.

Table 27.5. Causes of thoracic outlet syndrome

Congenital
• Cervical rib
• Hypertrophy of transverse processus from seventh cervical vertebra
• Abnormal first rib
• Dysostosis craniocleidalis
• Atypical fibromuscular ligaments or muscles
• Scalenus minimus muscle

Acquired
• Exostosis of first rib
• Pseudarthrosis and/or callus after clavicular fracture
• Tonus reduction of muscles in shoulder girdle
• Fibrosis and scar formation after radiotherapy or operation in axilla
• Hypertrophy of scalenus muscles

In the angiographic diagnosis it has to be obsrved that in all patients with suspected arterial TOS the angiographic examinations need to be performed not only in the normal position, but also with elevated arms. Three types of stenosis in the subclavian and axillary artery have been defined by Huguet et al. in 1967. Type I is located medially and caused by fibrotic structures, between the first rib and a cervical rib. A ligament from the processus transversus of the seventh cervical vertebra, crossing the subclavian artery above the first rib is type II. Type III is located lateral of the first rib.

In X-ray examinations, the identification or exclusion of a cervical rib, abnormally large processus transversus of the seventh cervical vertebra, or variations of the first rib in the native image is important. As to acquired causes of a TOS, extreme callus or pseudarthrosis after fracture of the clavicle, exostosis, and bone tumors of the first rib and clavicle deserve special attention.

Soft-tissue changes, in contrast, are more likely to be identified by means of US or MRI. Attention should then focus on anomalies of the scalenus muscles regarding their insertion or hypertrophy, on soft-tissue tumors and postoperative changes.

Neurological cervical plexus symptoms in the patient can be clinically induced by the Roos test (Roos

1976). After abduction to an angle of 90° and external rotation, the shoulder reproduces, after 3 min, the neurologic and vascular symptoms well known to the patient. By this technique angiography and US studies can also localize intermittent stenoses.

A common history obtained from these patients is trauma to the shoulder and neck, particularly whiplash injury and injuries to the first rib and clavicle.

The disappearing radial pulse when turning the head to the healthy side, dorsiflexion of the cervical spine, deep inhalation and comfortably resting elbows (ADSON's test) are unreliable indicators for TOS, because they are observed in many healthy individuals (MAKHOUL and MACHLEDER 1992), but can be utilised during functional testing and also with color-coded Duplex sonography (LONGLEY et al. 1992).

Most patients with TOS demonstrate compression in the area of the posterior scalenus gap, which can result in a local thrombotic stenosis of the subclavian artery. The effect in many patients is peripheral emboli to the digital arteries. Microthrombi can also cause vasospastic phenomena resulting in Raynaud's phenomenon. As a result of arterial compression, poststenotic dilatation or aneurysm formation in the subclavian artery may occur. Poststenotic turbulence has been accused of causing these.

The diagnostic examination is best performed with Doppler US (LONGLEY et al. 1992); SANDERS et al. 1991; SCHUNN 1997). The impact of dynamic compression processes during the abduction manoeuvre of the shoulder can be very well analyzed using Duplex sonography.

Angiography should be performed using the transfemoral catheter technique and include documentation of the aortic arch vessels on both sides. Comparison of both sides should take place not only in the normal shoulder position, but also in abduction, external rotation and retroversion. Only under these conditions can compression of the subclavian artery (Fig. 27.5) be precisely documented, provided that no morphologic pathologic situation (stenosis and poststenotic dilatation) yet exists.

Due to the varying causes of compression the therapeutic options need to be carefully considered in every case. The principle aim of surgical treatment is removal of the cause of external vessel compression due to bones, fibrotic structures, or muscles. Furthermore, the pathologic vascular changes, such as stenoses or occlusions, also need to be treated. This can be achieved either simultaneously with surgical therapy (thrombendarterectomy), or in an interventional way, by implantation of a self-expanding stent (COHEN et al. 1976), after elimination of the cause of the external compression.

27.3.2
Popliteal Artery Entrapment Syndrome

Under normal conditions, the popliteal artery lies between the two heads of muscle of the gastrocnemius. In the presence of anatomic variations of either the course of the artery, or the enthesis, the popliteal artery gets under a tendon band and is compressed during muscle contraction, or from severe angulation of the knee joint. Three types of PAES (Fig. 27.6) have been defined (MAHLER et al. 1969; INSUA et al. 1970; LAUBACH and TREDE 1973; KOGEL et al. 1990).

Instead of accompanying the vein and nerve, the artery coils around the insertion of the medial head of the gastrocnemius muscle and finds itself between tendon and bone. This variation is mostly observed in patients with normally inserting muscle, is that most commonly seen, and has been defined as type I. Less commonly (11%) is the abnormal lateral insertion of the tendon (type II). Whenever the artery is compressed by an aberrant muscle part, or the vessel perforates a normally inserting muscle, this is defined as the anatomic variation type III (LAUBACH et al. 1973). In 20% of the affected patient population, the anomaly is bilateral (BIEMANNS and VAN BOKEL 1977).

The entrapment is identifiable by functional tests and on angiography (Fig. 27.7) by the convex vascular course in a medial direction. PAES often occurs bilaterally. The atypical course of the muscle can be documented preoperatively by means of US, CT or MRI, if necessary. Special attention should be paid to identification of an aberrant course of the medial head of the gastrocnemius muscle.

The characteristics of each type of PAES can be documented at surgery (KOGEL et al. 1990):
Type I: The artery courses around the medial normally inserting head of gastrocnemius muscle. The mean age of the patients with the common type I is 22 years of age. Prior to the occurrence of a thrombotic occlusion, in the stage of compression of the popliteal artery, the compression occurs during the muscle contraction, which presses the artery against the medial femoral condyle.
Type II: The artery runs around the abnormal laterally inserting head of gastrocnemius muscle. Type II has been mainly observed in men of average age 33

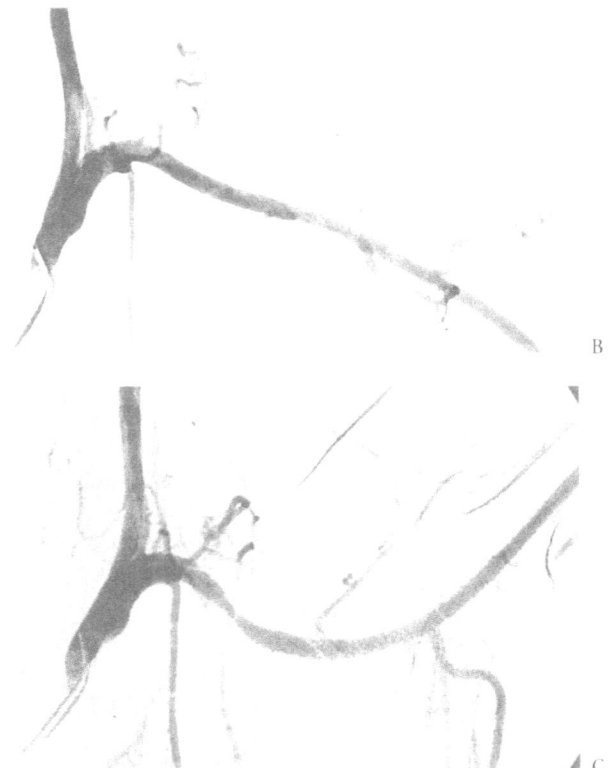

Fig. 27.5 TOS in a 37-year-old woman. **A** With embolus in the brachial artery **B** normal subclavian artery in angiography (standard position) **C** compression of the subclavian artery at elevated arm

years. Marked medial transposition is not typical in these cases (Fig. 27.7).

Type III: The artery runs through the muscle and is compressed by an aberrant muscle part. Men are affected 5–10 times more often than women. This marked variation results from the small patient numbers in attending clinics and reported in different series. PAES has to be suspected:

1) When there is acute ischemia in younger men, particularly if the latter occurs during or after physical strain
2) When there is chronic ischemia, with onset in adolescence, or early adult age (HAMMING and VINK 1965).

The main clinical sign is palpable foot pulses that vanish under maximum plantar flexion (BOLLINGER 1979). In the angiographic examination, medial transposition of the popliteal artery may be lacking.

Early confirmation of the diagnosis is very important in view of the prognosis. Timely surgery can prevent secondary thromboses and the risk of peripheral embolization. Therefore, mainly in young patients, it is of vital importance to clarify questionable intermittent ischemic syndromes by angiography, and to back up the findings by an ex-

amination with other imaging modalities, if necessary. This is in the interests of avoiding an unsuitable therapy.

It is quite possible that a patient with a thrombosed popliteal aneurysm (Fig. 27.8) is referred for imaging of a suspected 'deep phlebothrombosis'. In the phlebogram, the delayed run-off and superficial collateral veins are identifiable, but also an extensive transposition of the popliteal vein, lateral and ventral (Fig. 27.9). Confirmation must then be undertaken either by arteriography, US or MR angiography.

27.3.3
Brachial Entrapment Syndrome

This was first described by SCHULZE-BERGMANN (1977) who had detected it in a young man who had experienced an acute ischemic syndrome in the left arm, during wood cutting. Arteriography revealed an occlusion and at surgery there was an unusually strong medial biceps. This biceps head is demonstrated by US in about 10% of patients. BOLLINGER (1979) added another observation – a 26-year-old woman who developed ischemic symptoms in the

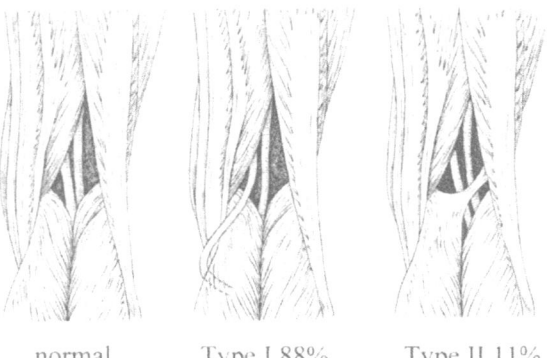

normal   Type I 88%   Type II 11%   Type III < 1%

Fig. 27.6 Variations of the popliteal artery entrapment syndrome – Different types and incidences – (schematic drawing, according to KOGEL et al. 1990)

right hand after a tennis match. On the arteriogram, multiple occlusions at the level of the elbow joint were identifiable. In the lower-arm arteries, parietal thrombi were found, and under isometric contraction of the biceps muscle, the previously palpable radial pulse at stretched elbow vanished. This change in pulse could be objectively assessed by Doppler US. At operation there was a strong bicipital aponeurosis at the elbow joint level. This demonstrates, that in patients with embolic occlusions of the lower-leg, arm and hand arteries, the source of embolism must not only be suspected in the area of the heart and the subclavian artery, but also in more distal arteries with local thrombosis.

27.3.4
Tibialis Anterior Syndrome

The tibial artery is surrounded in its muscle lodge by strong fasciae. During swelling from edema or bleeding, the interstitial pressure in the tissue increases. As soon as the latter exceeds the internal pressure of the capillaries and venules, ischemic necrosis of the muscle develops (BRADLEY 1973; GIERKE and KREBS 1972; MUMENTALER et al. 1960). The pulse of the anterior tibial artery may disappear, or only be palpable on the dorsum of foot. The isolated clinical picture is observed after trauma and unusual physical strain, but can also have iatrogenic causes. On the angiogram, failure to visualize, or diffuse constriction of the anterior tibial artery can be found. Clinical examination is important and there may be a history of overstrain. The surgical therapy is fasciotomy (BRADLEY 1973; BRUNNER and HEINZ 1974). Among the imaging modalities, MRI is capable of documenting oedema of the anterior tibial muscle and extensor digitorum and extensor hallucis longus muscles, and differentiates it from fresh hemorrhage or old hematoma. The muscle swelling and possible flow changes in the anterior tibial artery can also be detected by means of duplex sonography. The differential diagnosis may, however, pose some problems, and an interdisciplinary consultation is recommended.

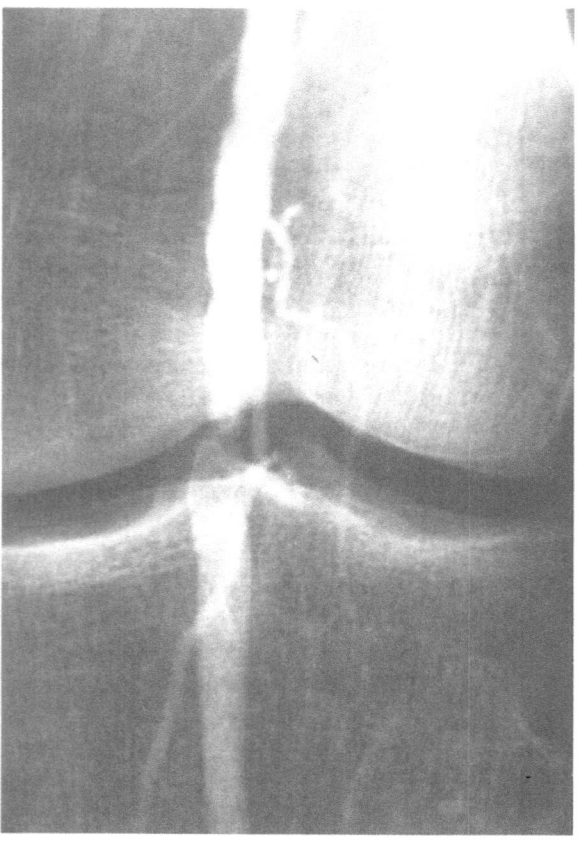

Fig. 27.7 Arteriography with popliteal stenoses and proximal irregulations. Operation demonstrated PES type II, and local thrombus formation. (surgeon: Dr. Gießler)

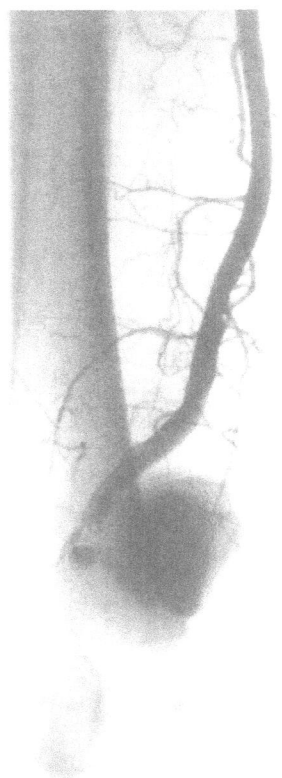

Fig. 27.8 Acute thrombotic occlusion in a 51-year-old patient with popliteal artery aneurysm

27.4
Cystic Adventitial Degeneration

So-called cystic adventitial degeneration (CAE) (ATKINS and KEY 1947; HIERTONN and LINDBERG 1957; SPERLING et al. 1972; LEU et al. 1977; VOLLMAR 1963) is an intramural cyst formation with secondary compression of the arterial lumen. The cysts can be uni- or multilocular (ARLART 1997) and solitary or multiple. The wall consists of mucin-producing cells. The popliteal artery is by far the most affected artery (LEWIS et al. 1967; DUNANT and ENGENIDIS 1973; ALART 1997), but cystic adventitial degeneration has also been observed in the external iliac and common femoral arteries (LEU 1977; ATKINS and KEY 1947). An association with ganglions has been discussed and this theory is supported by the documentation of synovial epithelium inside the cyst (LEU et al. 1977). LEU et al. have also described cases from the literature of cystic adventitial degeneration in the radial and ulnar arteries and in the small saphenous vein.

While VOLLMAR (1996) described a male/female ratio of 8:1, LEU et al. observed nearly equal inci-

dence among 59 patients. The condition has been observed between 11 and 70 years of age, the mean age being 40 years. The typical symptom with localization in the popliteal artery is intermittent claudication. A patient with intermittent symptoms was explained by the increase and decrease in the volume of cystic fluid during systemic thrombolysis (EHRINGER et al. 1969). In this patient the claudication disappeared, but reoccurred after several days or weeks. Improvement during thrombolytic therapy led to the false conclusion that symptoms had been due to local thrombosis. However, surgery performed after recurrence of symptoms confirmed an adventitial cyst.

On angiography, the identification of a smooth-walled unilocular stenosis (Fig. 27.10) is a clear indication for a possible cystic adventitial degeneration. To confirm the diagnosis, US or MRI (GÖRRES et al. 1995) can be helpful. Whenever a cyst is clearly identified, intravascular therapy is contraindicated and surgical removal is appropriate (DUNANT 1973; LEU

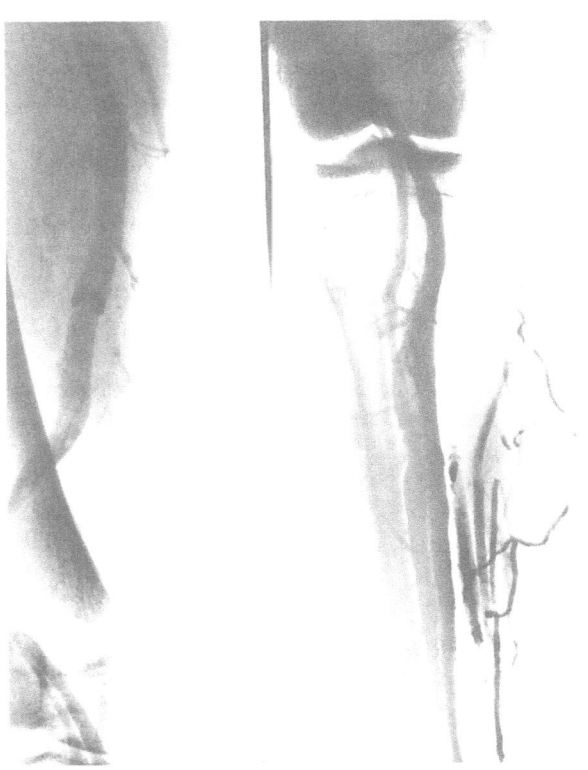

Fig. 27.9 Same patient as Fig. 27.8: Before arteriography, a phlebography was indicated because of severe lower-leg swelling. Phlebography demonstrated the compression to the popliteal vein, reduced flow and partial thrombotic formation. Treatment: aneurysmectomy and femoro-crural bypass, followed by anticoagulation

et al. 1977; SPERLING 1979; VOLLMAR 1996). CT-controlled puncture of the cyst and simple aspiration of cyst contents has been advised as an alternative approach (DEUTSCH et al. 1985; WILBUR and SPIGOS 1986). If the cyst cannot be completely removed, segmental resection with creation of a venous bypass is possible.

For the interventional radiologist, familiarity with cystic adventitial degeneration is important so that it may be distinguished from isolated arteriosclerotic stenoses and the wrong diagnosis and therapy avoided. If an adventitial cyst cannot be excluded by US or MRI, intravascular US (IVUS) or angioscopy are very helpful, before employing atherectomy, balloon dilatation or thrombolysis.

27.5
Fibromuscular Dysplasia

Fibromuscular dysplasia (FMD) is a non-arteriosclerotic non-inflammatory disease of unknown etiology (McCORMACK et al. 1966; MEANEY et al. 1968). It is based on a proliferation of the smooth musculature and the fibrous tissue of the media and intima, with concomitant formation of gaps in the internal elastic lamina. The effect of this is identifiable both morphologically and angiographically as a succession of luminal narrowings and dilatations, which, on angiography, produces the picture of an artery resembling a string of pearls (Fig. 27.11). The disease was first described in renal arteries (LEADBETTER and BURKLAND 1938, McCORMACK et al. 1966). The most common sites are still the renal arteries, followed by the internal carotid, cranial mesenteric, and external iliac arteries (Fig. 27.12) (ARLART 1997). Extrarenal sites, in addition to the internal carotid artery (CONNETT 1965; CORRIN 1981), are the subclavian, iliac (NAJAFI 1966; DRURY 1982), and multiple arteries (NYLIE 1966; CLAIBORNE 1970; LÜSCHER et al. 1980).

FMD mostly affects women in their younger and middle ages. The sex ratio is male: female, 1:3 to 1:8 (HUNT et al. 1965; NYLIE et al. 1966). The right kidney can be located in the pelvis, similar to a floating kidney, with a very long renal artery.

An evaluation of 92 patients with FMD (LÜSCHER et al. 1986) revealed the following distribution of locations: renovascular arteries 89%, cerebrovascular arteries 26%, visceral and subclavian arteries 9%, iliac arteries 5%, and coronary arteries 2%. Twenty-six

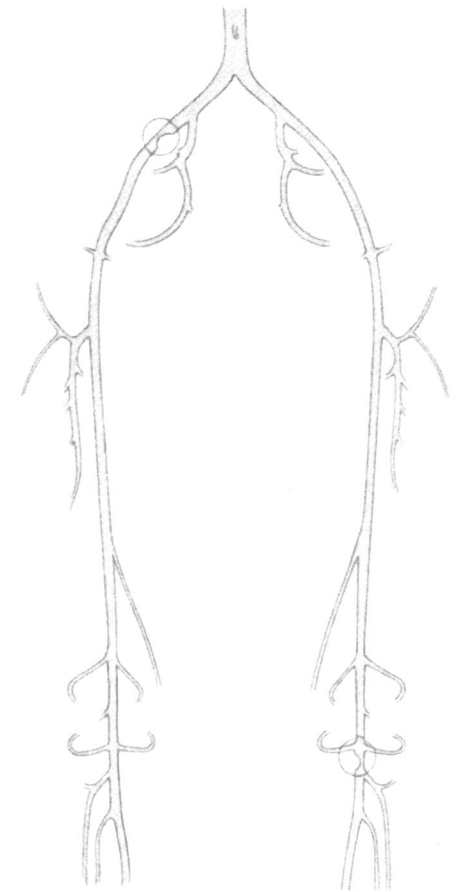

Fig. 27.10 Cystic adventitial degeneration. Localizations and type of stenosis in the popliteal and iliac arteries (schematic drawing)

percent of these patients had a multifocal disease. The right renal artery is affected more frequently than the left, but bilateral renal artery disease is common.

The morphologic classification of FMD (McCORMACK et al. 1966; HARRISON and McCORMACK 1971; STANLEY, et al. 1975) differentiates between changes in all three laminae of the arterial wall (Fig. 27.13). Intimal fibroplasia was identified in 1–2%, FMD of the media in about 96%, and peri-adventitial fibroplasia in 1–2%.

On the angiogram, the media-type FMD, characterized by its string-of-pearls picture, is most readily identifiable (Fig. 27.11). The types affecting the intima and adventitia show segmental, often smoothly limited stenoses, which in the angiogram cannot be clearly differentiated from arteriosclerotic changes. Aneurysms of the renal artery can also be due to FMD in view of the histology. In the differential diagnosis, ostium stenoses are almost exclusively of arteriosclerotic nature, whereas FMD is preferentially located distal to the ostium, both in the renal arteries as well as at other sites.

The most common site of FMD is in the renal artery territory, providing one of the causes of renovascular hypertension (HUNT et al. 1965; HARRISON and MCCORMACK 1971; LÜSCHER et al. 1986; ALART 1997). In the presence of renal artery FMD, FMD of the pelvic arteries should be excluded by catheter angiography at the same time as renal angiography and involvement of the internal carotid arteries should be excluded, at least by means of duplex sonography. MR angiography instead of conventional arteriography is the method of choice for the imaging diagnosis. However, angiography remains an important part of treatment when angioplasty is undertaken by percutaneous transluminal renal dilatation (PTRD).

In patients with renovascular hypertension caused by FMD, balloon dilatation is preferred as the primary treatment (MAHLER et al. 1979, 1992; SOS et al. 1983; ZEITLER et al. 1993; ALART 1997). Stent-assisted angioplasty or surgical therapy (VOLLMAR 1996) should also be considered should PTRD fail or in the treatment of ostium stenoses, which are always arteriosclerotic. FMD in the iliac arteries only needs to be treated when intermittent claudication occurs. A detailed overview on the topic has been provided by ALART (1997).

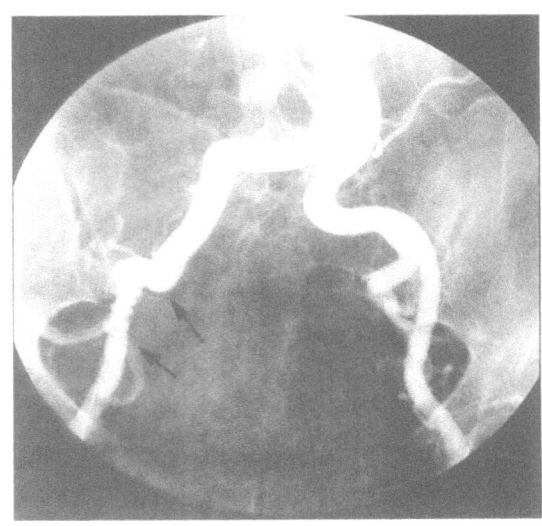

Fig. 27.12 Arteriography of the pelvic arteries with FMD on the right external iliac artery (→)

27.6
Hypothenar-Hammer Syndrome

This condition is due to mechanical trauma to the ulnar part of the superficial palmar arch and to the distal ulnar artery. These may occur whenever the hand is used as a hammer (CONN et al. 1970). The underlying anatomical cause is the close vicinity of the artery to the hamate bone. When the palmar arch, particularly on the hypothenar side, repeatedly hits a solid object, the artery is chronically traumatized. Typically affected professions are manual workers, mechanics and farmers; less often sportsmen. The clinical complaints are confined to the dominant hand. The clinical symptoms are ischemia in the region of fingers 3 to 5, which worsen with cold. Trophic changes have also been observed.

Angiographically, irregular changes of the arteries of the superficial palmar arch, of the distal ulnar arteries, and the finger arteries can be identified (HORVATH et al. 1970; POULIADES et al. 1977). Stenoses, aneurysms, and occlusions of the ulnar artery and the ulnar digital arteries are found. The latter may be the result of arterio-arterial emboli. In motor vehicle mechanics the prevalence is 14% (MILES LITTLE and FERGUSON 1972). In examinations employing Doppler US, no similar changes of the ulnar artery were identified unless the hand had been used as a hammer. The syndrome occurs only after many (>20) years of exposure. Comparison with angiography has shown that the severe changes are identifiable

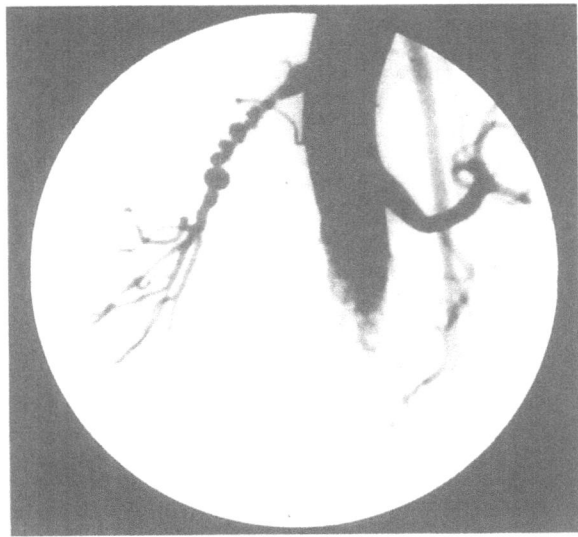

Fig. 27.11 Arteriography of FMD of the right renal artery, „media type"

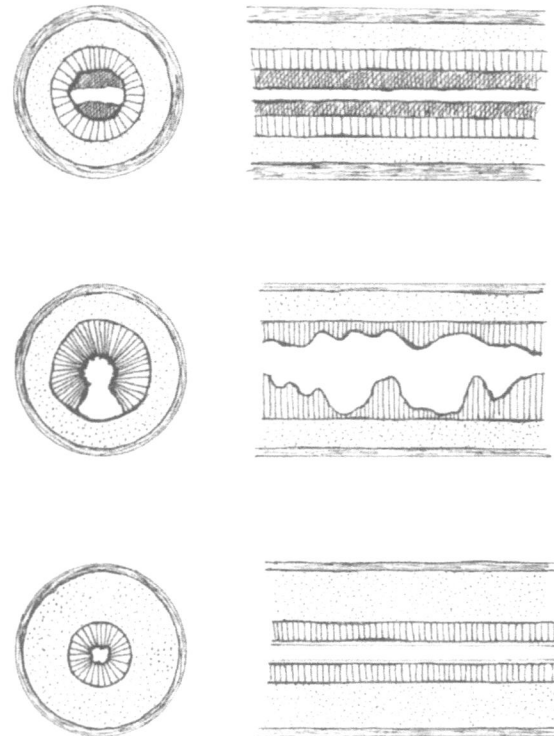

Fig. 27.13 Histomorphologic classification of FMD (modified according to HARRISON and MCCORMACK 1971). TOP: Intimal fibroplasia. MIDDLE: FMD of the media type, with aneurysm and dissection. BOTTOM: Adventitial and periadventitial fibrosis

using Duplex sonography, but mild changes are better documented with angiography, and this technique is sometimes improved when the hand is positioned in extension and with radial abduction (BOLLINGER 1979).

27.7
Chronic Vibration Trauma

Due to chronic vibration trauma caused by working with vibrating machines, the hand and finger arteries may develop primary vasospastic syndromes, which later change into chronic fibrous occlusions (BOLLINGER 1979). Affected professions are chainsaw workers, machine grinders, pneumatic hammer workers, and farmers (TAYLOR 1979; THULESIUS 1979; RADEMACHER et al. 1994). The changes are

often limited to one to three fingers. The onset of such changes is hastened by working in the cold; foresters are exposed to both factors, vibration and cold (HYVÄRINEN et al. 1973). Necrosis of fingertips may also be seen (DENK 1966; TAYLOR 1994). An important aspect in industrial medical care is early diagnosis and the use of so-called 'antivibratory' saws.

The clinical symptoms are similar to Raynaud's syndrome. Initially only one or two fingertips are affected, later two to three fingers, and finally the whole hand with ischemia and cyanosis. The ischemic attacks vary between 5 and 15 min. Several non-invasive methods are not very sensitive or specific (TAYLOR 1979) and angiography with magnification to analyze the hand and finger arteries can be recommended in the same way as in all patients with unclear Raynaud's syndrome.

References

27.1

Alexander K (1993) Thrombangiitis obliterans. In: Alexander K (ed) Gefäßkrankheiten. Urban & Schwarzenberg, Munich, pp 532-540
Allen EV, Camp JD (1935) Arteriopathy. JAMA 104:618
Bollinger A (1979a) Angiitiden, Thrombangiitis obliterans (Morbus von Winiwarter-Buerger). In: Bollinger A (ed) Funktionelle Angiologie, Lehrbuch und Atlas. Thieme, Stuttgart, pp 88-91
Bollinger A (1979b) Oberflächliche Thrombophlebitis, Thrombophlebitis saltans (migrans). In: Bollinger A (ed) Funktionelle Angiologie, Lehrbuch und Atlas. Thieme, Stuttgart, pp 206-208
Bollinger A, Hollmann B, Schneider E, Fontana A (1979) Thrombangiitis obliterans: Diagnose und Therapie im Licht neuer immunologischer Befunde. Schweiz Med Wochenschr 109:537-543
Buerger L (1908) Thrombangiitis obliterans: A study of the vascular lesions leading to presenile spontaneous gangrene, Am J Med Sci 136:567-580
Buerger L (1924) Thrombangiitis obliterans. In: The circulatory disturbances of the extremities. Saunders, Philadelphia, pp 213-385
Cachovan M (1988) Epidemiologie und geographische Verteilungsmuster der Thrombangiitis obliterans. In: Heidrich H (ed) Thrombangiitis obliterans, Morbus Winiwarter-Buerger. Thieme, Stuttgart, pp 31-36
Corelli F (1973) Buerger's disease – cigarette smoker disease may always be cured by medical therapy alone – uselessness of operative treatment. J Cardiovasc Surg 14:28-36

Diehm C, Schäfer M (1993) Das Buerger-Syndrom (Thrombangiitis obliterans). Geschichte, Epidemiologie, Pathologie, Klinik, Diagnostik und Therapie. Springer, Berlin Heidelberg New York

Fontaine R, Kim M, Kieny R (1954) Die chirurgische Behandlung der peripheren Durchblutungsstörungen. Helv Chir Acta 21:499-515

Fontaine R (1967) La Thrombangiose. Presse Medicale Paris, 148

Gross WL (1993) Vaskulitis. Internist 34:599-614

Gross WL (1995) Vasculitiden. Dtsch Arztebl 92:A1372-1381

Guilmot JL, Lasfargues G (1988) Maladie de Buerger ou thrombo-angéite oblitérante. Rev Prat 38:349-356

Hagen B Lohse S (1984) Clinical and radiological aspects of Buerger's disease. Cardiovasc Intervent Radiol 7:283-293

Heidrich H (1988) Thrombangiitis obliterans. Morbus Winiwarter-Buerger. Thieme, Stuttgart

Henniges D, Zeitler E (1979) Die Angiographie bei der Differenzierung der arteriellen Verschlußkrankheit. Verh Dtsch Ges Inn Med 85:1408-1411

Hess H (1972) Iatrogene Arteriopathien. In: Kappert A (ed) Nichtdegenerative Arteriopathien. Huber, Bern, pp 125-131

Horsch AH, Brechmeier D, Robert L, Horsch S (1977) Anti-Elastin-Antikörper bei der Thrombangiitis obliterans. Verh Dtsch Ges Inn Med 83:1758-1761

Horsch AK (1988) Laborchemische und immunologische Befunde bei der Thrombangiitis obliterans. In: Heidrich H, (ed) Thrombangiitis obliterans, Morbus Winnewarter-Buerger. Thieme, Stuttgart, pp 69-71

Horst W an der, Nier H, Florack G (1980) Diagnostische und therapeutische Probleme der Endangitis obliterans. Akt Chir 15:361-368

Inada K, Katsumura T (1972) The entity of Buerger's disease. Angiology 23:668-687

Ishikawa K, Mishima Y, Morioka Y, Hara K (1973) Accordion-like arterial shadows observed on the arteriogram. Angiologie 29:398

Janevski BK (1982) Angiography of the upper extremity. Martinus Nijhoff. The Hague, p 200

Joyce JW (1990) Buerger's disease (Thrombangiitis obliterans). Rheum Dis Clin North Am 16:463-470

Kappert A (1972) Nichtdegenerative Arteriopathien. Huber, Bern

Kaushik NK, Sarin NK, Mahant TS, Bhartwaj BK (1986) Arteriographic observations in cases of Buerger's disease (thrombangiitis obliterans). Ind J Radiol Imag 40:217-222

Kinmonth JB (1948) Thrombangiitis obliterans. Results of sympathectomy and prognosis. Lancet 2:717-719

Kummer A, Widmer KH Da Silva A, Hug B (1977) Thrombangiitis obliterans - zum Morbus Winewarter-Buerger. VASA 6:384-396

Lambeth JT, Yong NK (1970) Arteriographic findings thrombangiitis obliterans with emphasis in femoro-popliteal involvement. Am J Roentgenol. Radium Ther Nucl Med 109:553-562

Lambrecht R, Freitag J, Heinrich P, Freitag G (1984) Zur klinischen und angiologischen Differenzierung der Endangitis obliterans von der Arteriosclerosis obliterans. Dtsch Gesundheitsw 39:1740-1743

Leu HJ (1976) Thrombangiitis obliterans von Winiwarter-Buerger. Dtsch Med Wochenschr 101:113-114

Leu HJ (1985) Thrombangiitis obliterans Buerger. Pathologisch-anatomische Analyse von 53 Fällen. Schweiz med Wochenschr 115:1080-1086

Leu HJ (1988) Organmanifestation der Endangiitis aus pathologisch-anatomischer Sicht. In: Heidrich H (ed) Thrombangiitis obliterans. Morbus Winewarter-Buerger. Thieme, Stuttgart, pp 106, 17-19

Lysak SZ, Welling RE (1980) Buerger's disease: a distinct clinical entity. Vasc Surg 14:346-351

Martorell F (1958) Enfermedades de los vasos perifericos. In: Pons PA (ed) Tratado de patologia y clinica médicas, 2nd edn. Salvat, Barcelona

Mayall GF (1964) Arterial waves. Clin Radiol 15:355

McKusick VA, Harris WS, Ottesen OE et al (1962): Buerger's disease: a distinct clinical and pathological entity. JAMA 181:5-12

Montorsi W, Ghiringhelli C (1961) A case of Buerger's disease in women. Angiology 12:376-381

Müller-Bühl U, Diehm C, Hübsch-Müller C, Eckstein HH, Werner U (1988) Kritische Aspekte in Diagnostik und Therapie der Thrombangiitis obliterans (v. Winiwarter-Buerger). Inn Med 15:18-23

Ohta T, Shionoya S (1988) Fate of the ischemic limb in Buerger's disease. Br J Surg 75:259-262

Ratschow M (1959) Angioneuropathien. In: Ratschow M (ed) Angiologie. Thieme, Stuttgart, pp 553-572

Rivera R (1973) Roentgenographic diagnosis of Buerger's disease. J Cardiovasc, Surg 14:40-46

Schatz IJ, Fine G, Eyler WR (1966) Thrombangiitis obliterans. Br Heart J 28:84-91

Schoop W, Morlinghaus JL (1960) Arterielle Thrombose bei Phlegmasia coerulea dolens. Med Welt 37:1926

Schoop W (1972) Thrombangiitis obliterans. In: Kappert A (ed) Nichtdegenerative Arteriopathien (Aktuelle Probleme in der Angiologie, Vol 17). Huber, Bern, pp 74-79

Seldinger SJ (1964) Arteries of the extremities. In: Diethelm L, Olsson O, Strnad F, Vieten H, Zuppinger A (eds) Handbuch der Medizinischen Radiologie. Springer, Berlin Heidelberg New York

Shionoya S, Matsubara J, Kamiya K (1977) Fortschreiten des Verschlußprozesses bei Thrombangiitis obliterans. VASA 6:249-254

Shionoya S (1978) Pathologie der Thrombangiitis obliterans. Frühläsion und Verlaufsform. VASA 7:253-257

Shinoya S, Ban J, Nakata G, Matsubara J, Hirai M, Kawai S (1978) Involvement of the iliac artery in Buerger's disease. J Cardiovasc Surg 19:69-76

Strandness DE (1969): Peripheral arterial disease – a physiological approach Little, Brown, Boston, pp 241-251

Strandness ED (1987) Vascular diseases of the extremities, thrombangiitis obliterans (Buerger's disease). In: Braunwald E, et al (edes) Harrison's principles of internal medicine. McGraw-Hill, New York, pp 1042-1043

Suzuki S, Mine H, Umehara I, Yoshida T, Okada Y (1982): Buerger's disease (thrombangiitis obliterans). An analysis of the arteriograms of 119 cases. Clin Radiol 33:235-240

Szendro G, Golcman L, Cristal N (1988) Study of the factors affecting viscosity in patients with thrombangiitis obliterans. J Vasc Surg 7:759-762

Szilagyi DE, DeRusso FJ, Elliot JP (1964) Thrombangiitis obliterans. Clinico – angiographic correlations. Arch Surg 88:824-835 van der Stricht J, Goldstein M, Flamand JP, Belenger J (1973) Evolution and prognosis of thrombangiitis obliterans. J Cardiovasc Surg 14:9-16

von Winiwarter F (1879) Über die eigentümliche Form von Endarteriitis und Endophlebitis mit Gangrän des Fußes. Arch Klin Chir 23:202-206

Zeitler E (1976) Das Perlschnurphänomen bei Arteriographie der Extremitätenarterien. In: Zeitler E (ed) Aspekte der Extremitätenangiographie. Huber, Bern, pp 110-115

27.2

Alarcon-Segovia D, Osmundson PHJ (1965) Peripheral vascular syndromes associated with systemic lupus erythermatosus. Ann intern Med 62:907-919

Ansari A, Larson PH, Bates HD (1986) Vascular manifestations of systemic lupus erythematosus. Angiology 37:423-432

Bakker FC, Rauwerda JA, Bernelot-Moens HJ, van den Broek AA (1989) Intermittent claudication and limb threatening ischemia in systemic lupus erythematosus and in SLE-like disease: a report of two cases and review of the literature. Surgery 106:21-25

Bollinger A (1979) Kollagenkrankheiten. In: Bollinger A (ed) Funktionelle Angiologie. Thieme, Stuttgart, pp 95-100

Campbell PM, Le Roy EC (1975) Pathogenesis of systemic sclerosis. Semi Arthr Rheum 4:351-368

Dabich L, Bookstein JJ, Zweifler A, Zarafonetics CI (1973): Digital arteries in patients with scleroderma. Arteriographic and plethysmographic study. Arch intern Med 130:708

De Palma RG, Moskowitz RW, Holden WD (1972): Peripheral ischemia and collagen disease. Arch Surg 105:313-316

Dubois EL, Arterberry JD (1962): Gangrene as a manifestation of systemic lupus erythematosus. J Am med Assoc 181:366-368

Janevski B (1986) Arteries of the hand in patients with scleroderma. Diagn Imaging 55:262-265

Kaufmann GW, Reinhold WD, Hagedorn M (1983) Röntgenmorphologische Befunde bei Sklerodermie. Fortschr Röntgenstr 138:607-610

Kaufmann JL, Bancilla E, Slade J (1986) Lupus vasculitis with tibial artery thrombosis and gangrene. Arthr Rheum 29:1291-1292

Lund F, Cronestrand K, Hardstett C (1979): Fluoreszin-Angiography beim Raynaud-Syndrom. In: Ehringer H, Betz E, Bollinger A, Deutsch E (eds) Gefäßwand, Rezidivprophylaxe, Raynaud-Syndrom. Witzstrock, Baden-Baden, pp 480-487

Mahler F, Bollinger A (1978) Die Kapillarmikroskopie als Untersuchungsmethode in der klinischen Angiologie. Dtsch med Woschenschr 103:523-526

Metz G (1971) Peipheral gangrene in lupus erythematosus. Munch Med Wochenschr 113:729-732

Norton WL, Nardo JM (1970) Vascular disease in progressive systemic sclerosis (scleroderma). Ann Intern Med 73:317-324

Peller JS, Gabor GT, Porter JM, Bennet RM (1985) Angiographic findings in mixed connective tissue disease. Arthr Rheum 28:768-770

Pokieser H, Meixner M, Czembirek H (1971) Röntgenbefunde

im Rahmen der Sklerodermie. Med Welt N F 22:883-886

Ranft J, Lammersen T, Heidrich H (1986) In-vivo capillarymicroscopical findings in patients with thrombangitis obliterans, progressive systemic scleroderma and rheumatoid arthritis, respectively. Klin Wochenschr 64:946-950

Rösch J, Antonovic R, Porter JM (1977) The importance of temperature in angiography of the hand. Radiology 123:323-326

Schmitt R, Lanz U (1996) Bildgebende Diagnostik der Hand. Hippokrates, Stuttgart

Schober R, Klüken N (1966) Angiographische Befunde bei Sclerodermia progressiva. Fortschr Rontgenstr 105:239-244

Tan EM, Cohen AS, Fries JF et al (1982) The 1982 revised criteria for the classification of systemic lupus erythematosus. Arthr Rheum 25:1271-1277

Thulesius O (1979) Physiologie und Pathophysiologie der Fingerdurchblutung. In: Ehringer H, Betz E, Bollinger A, Deutsch E (eds) Gefäßwand, Rezidivprophylaxe, Raynaud-Syndrom, Witzstrock Baden-Baden, pp 475-460

Wagner HH, Alexander K (1993) Durchblutungsstörungen der Hände. Thieme, Stuttgart

Zeitler E (1976) Zur sicheren Darstellung von Digitalarterien an Händen und Füßen in Lokalanästhesie nach oraler Akoholgabe. Fortschr Rontgenstr 123:67-68

Zeitler E (1979) Angiographische Befunde beim Raynaud-Syndrom. In: Ehringer H, Betz E, Bollinger A, Deutsch E (eds) Gefäßwand, Rezidivprophylaxe, Raynaud-Syndrom, Witzstrock, Baden-Baden, pp 471-479

27.3

Adler J, Hosshmand I (1973) The angiographic spectrum of the thoracic outlet syndrome: with emphasis on mural thrombosis and emboli and congenital vascular anomalies. Clin Radiol 24:35-42

Biemans RGM, van Bockel JH (1977) Popliteal artery entrapment syndrome. Surg Gynecol Obstet 144:604-607

Bollinger A (1979) Neurovaskuläres Schultergürtel-Kompressionssyndrom und Kompressionssyndrom der A. poplitea und der A. brachialis. In: Bollinger K (ed) Funktionelle Angiologie. Thieme, Stuttgart, pp 137-142

Bradley EL (1973) The anterior tibial compartment syndrome. Surg Gynecol Obstet 136:289-292

Brunner U, Heinz CH (1974) Akuttherapie und Wiederherstellungschirurgie beim Tibialis-anterior-Syndrom. Helv Chir Acta 41:277-281

Cohen GS, Braunstein L, Ball DS, Domeracki F (1996) Effort thrombisis effective treatment with vascular stent after unrelieved venous stenosis following a surgical release procedure. Cardiovasc Intervent Radiol 19:37-40

Gierke W, Krebs FA (1972) Tibialis-anterior-Syndrom. Dtsch Med Wochenschr 97:469-471

Gruss JP, Bartels D, Vargas H et al (1982) Shoulder girdle compression syndrome. J Cardiovasc Surg 23:221-224

Hamming JJ, Vink JM (1965) Obstruction of the popliteal artery at an early age. J Cardiovasc Surg 6:516-519

Huguet JF, Mercier C, Houel F (1967) L'ischemie transitoire du membre supérieur (thoracic outlet syndrome). Schweiz Rundsch Med 65:142-146

Insua JA, Young JR, Humphries AW (1970) Popliteal artery entrapment syndrome. Arch Surg 101:771-776

Kobinia GS, Olbert F, Russe OJ, Denck H (1980) Chronic vascular disease of the upper extremity: radiologic and clinical features. Cardiovasc Intervent Radiol 3:25-41

Kogel H, Vollmar J, Hutschenreuther S (1990) Neue Variante eines Kompressionssyndromes der A. poplitea. Langenbecks Arch Chir 375:171-174

Laubach K, Trede M, Pererea R, Saggau W (1973) Das Kompressionssyndrom der A. poplitea. Chirurg 44:74-79

Longley DG, Yedlicka JW, Molina EJ, et al (1992) Thoracic outlet syndrome: evaluation of the subclavian vessels by color duplex sonography. AJR 158:623-626

Mahler F, Brunner U, Bollinger A (1969) Das Kompressionssyndrom der Arteria poplitea. Dtsch Med Wochenschr 15:786-788

Makhoul TG, Machleder HI (1992) Developmental anomalies at the thoracic outlet: an analysis of 200 consecutive cases. J Vasc Surg 16:534-538

Mumenthaler M, Baasch E, Ulrich J (1960) das Tibialis-anterior-Syndrom. Schweiz Arch Neurol 86:137-140

Peet RM, Hendriksen MD, Anderson TP (1956) Thoracic outlet syndrome: evaluation of a therapeutic exercise program. Mayo Clin Proc 31:281-288

Roos DB (1976) Congenital anomalies associated with thoracic outlet syndrome: anatomy, symptoms, diagnosis and treatment. Ann Surg 132:774-782

Sanders RJ, Haug C (1991) Review of arterial thoracic outlet syndrome with a report of five new instances. Surg Gynecol Obstet 173:415-420

Schulze-Bergmann G (1977) Das Kompressionssyndrom der A. brachialis. VASA 6:30-33

Schunn C (1997) Neurovaskuläre Kompressionssyndrome des "thoracic outlet" und Schultergürtels. In: Zeitler E (ed) Arterien und Venen. Springer, Berlin Heidelberg New York, pp 655-673

Weibel J, Fields WS (1967) Arteriographic studies of thoracic outlet syndrome. Br J Radiol 40:676-681

27.4

Arlart IP (1997) Zystische Adventitadegeneration. In: Zeitler E (ed) Arterien und Venen. Springer, Berlin Heidelberg New York, pp 360-368

Atkins HJB, Key JA (1947) A case of myxomatous tumor arising in the adventitia of the left external iliac artery. Br J Surg 34:426-427

Deutsch AL, Hyde J, Miller SM, Diamond CG, Schanche AF (1985) Cystic adventitial degeneration of the popliteal artery: CT demonstration and directed percutaneous therapy. AJR 145:117-118

Dunant JH, Engenidis N (1973) Cystic degeneration of the popliteal artery. VASA 2:156-158

Ehringer H, Denck H, Wuketich SE, Brunner E (1969) Intermittierender Verschluß der Arteria poplitea durch zystische Adventitia-Degeneration. Dtsch Med Wochenschr 94:2107-2108

Görres G, Gückel C, Steinbrich W (1995) Diagnostische Möglichkeiten der Magnetresonanztomographie (MRT) und Magnetresonanzangiographie (MRA) beim Popliteal artery Entrapment-Syndrom (PAES). Acta Radiol 5:31-35

Hiertonn TK, Lindberg L (1957) Cystic adventitial degeneration of popliteal artery. Acta Chir Scand. 113:72

Leu H, Bollinger A, Pouliadis G, Brunner U, Soyka P (1977) Pathologie, Klinik, Radiologie und Chirurgie der zystischen Adventitia-Degeneration peripherer Blutgefäße. VASA 6:94

Lewis GJT, Douglas DN, Reid W, Watt JK, (1967) Cystical adventitial disease of the popliteal artery. Br Med J II:441-443

Sperling M, Schott H, Rüppell V (1972) Die zystische Adventitia-Degeneration der Blutgefäße. Chirurg 43:57

Vollmar J (1963) Die zystische Adventitia-Degeneration der Schlagadern. Z Kreisl Forsch 52:1028-1030

Vollmar J (1996) Rekonstruktive Chirurgie der Arterien 4th, edn. Thieme, Stuttgart, p 244

Wilbur AC, Spigis DG (1986) Adventitial cyst of the popliteal artery: CT-guided percutaneous aspiration. J Comput Ass Tomogr 10:161-163

27.5

Arlart IP (1997) Fibromuskuläre Dysplasie – Zystische Adventiadegeneration – Gefäßwandtumoren. In: Zeitler E (ed) Arterien und Venen. Springer, Berlin Heidelberg New York, pp 355-368

Claiborne TS (1970) Fibromuscular hyperplasia: report of a case with involvement of multiple arteries. Am J Med 49:103-105

Drury JK, Pollock JG (1982) Fibromuscular dysplasia of the iliac arteries. Vasc Surg 15:133-136

Harrison EG jr. McCormack LJ (1971) Pathologic classification of renal arterial disease in renovascular hypertension. Mayo Clin Proc 46:161-167

Hunt JC Harrison EG jr, Sheps SG et al (1965) Hypertension caused by fibromuscular hyperplasia of the renal arteries: Postgrad Med 38:53

Lüscher TF, Vetter H, Studer A, et al (1980) Extrarenaler Gefäßbefall bei fibromusculär bedingter renovasculärer Hypertonie. Klin Wochenschr 58:493-500

Lüscher TF, Keller HM, Imhof HG, et al (1986): Fibromuscular hyperplasia: extension of the disease and therapeutic outcome. Nephron 44, [Suppl 1]: 109-114

Mahler F, Krneta A, Haertel M (1979) Treatment of renovascular hypertension by transluminal renal artery dilatation. Ann intern Med 90:56-57

Mahler F (1992) Long-term-results of percutaneous transluminal renal angioplasty. In: Lüscher TF, Kaplan NM (eds) Renovascular and renal parenchymatous hypertension. Springer, Berlin Heidelberg New York

Mc Cormack LJ, Poutasse EF, Meaney TF et al (1966) A pathologic-arteriographic correlation of renal arterial disease: Am Heart J 72:183-198

Meaney TF, Dustan EP, McCormack LJ (1968) Natural history of renal arterial disease. Radiology 91:881-887

Najafi H (1966) Fibromuscular hyperplasia of the external iliac arteries: Arch Surg 92:394

Nylie EG, Binkley FM, Palubinskas AJ (1966) Extrarenal fibromuscular hyperplasia. Am J Surg 112:149

Sos TA, Pickering TG, Sniderman K, et al (1983) Percutaneous transluminal renal angicplasty in renovascular hypertension due to atheroma or fibromuscular dysplasia. N Engl J Med 309:274-279

Stanley JC, Gewertz, Bl., Bove, El., et al. (1975): Arterial fibrodysplasia: historical character and current etiologic concepts. Arch. Surg. 110:561-566

Vollmar J (1996) Rekonstruktive Chirurgie der Arterien 4th edn. Thieme, Stuttgart

Zeitler E, Richter EI, Wachter G (1993): Renovaskuläre Hypertonie: invasive perkutane Diagnose- und Therapie-möglichkeiten. Wien Klin Wochenschr 105:365-370

27.6

Conn J, Bergan JJ, Bell JL (1970) Hypothenarhammersyn-drome: posttraumatic digital ischemia. Surgery 68:1122

Horvath F, Sztankay C, Kavossy T (1970) Angiographische Untersuchungen vibrationsbewirkter Gefäßveränder-ungen. Fortschr Rontgenstr 113:164-167

Miles Little J, Ferguson DA (1972) The incidence of the hy-pothenar hammer syndrome. Arch Surg 105:684-687

Pouliadis G, Bollinger A, Brunner U (1977) Das arterio-graphische Bild des Hypothenar-Hammer-Syndroms. Fortschr Rontgenstr 127:345-347

27.7

Bollinger A (1979) Funktionelle Angiologie. Thieme, Stuttgart

Denk R (1966) Fingerkuppennekrose bei einem Preßluft-werkzeugarbeiter. Med Welt 1595-1597

Hyvärinen J, Pyykkö I, Sundberg S (1973) Vibration frequen-cies and amplitudes in the aetiology of traumatic vaso-spastic disease. Lancet I:791

Rademacher A, Küffer G, Spengel FA (1994) "Vibration-White-Finger"-Syndrom bei 8 Turbinenschleifern. In: Spengel FA, Altmann E (eds). VASA Suppl 43:85

Taylor W (1974) The vibration syndrome. Academic Press, London

Thulesius O (1979) Berufstraumatisches sekundäres Raynaund-Syndrom. In: Ehringer H, Betz E, Bollinger A, Deutsch E (eds) Gefäßwand, Rezidivprophylaxe, Raynaud-Syndrom. Witzstrock, Baden-Baden, pp 503-506

28 Vasospastic Syndromes

E. Zeitler

CONTENTS

Spasms in extremity arteries can appear as long segmental contractions of large vessels (femoral, popliteal, brachial and other arteries), but also as short segments of the arteries of the brain, lower leg, kidneys, and others. There are many underlying causes. The mechanical causes can be: emboli, punctures and mechanical manipulation of guidewires, angiography catheters or other intra-arterial instrumentation (Fig. 28.1). They can also be caused by drugs such as ergotamine, betablockers, digitalis and others; by thermal stimuli, especially cold and congelation; by polyneuropathy; and radicular stimulation syndromes. (VÖLPEL 1957; BOLLINGER 1972; GREMMEL 1976). Puncture of the brachial artery results in spasm more frequently than puncture of the femoral or popliteal arteries. Vasospasm can be differentitated into an early reversible stage and a late stage with secondary thrombotic complications or associated with embolism.

The drugs used for intra-arterial prophylaxis or therapy of vasospasm are nitroglycerin 50–100mg, tolazoline 25 mg (Ciba-Geigy, Wehr, Germany). Verapamil 10 mg (Ratiopharm, Ulm, Germany) can be administered intravenously, while nitrolingual (Pohl, Hohenlockstedt, Germany) and nifedipine can be given orally.

In this chapter, mainly vasospastic clinical syndromes of extremity arteries willbe discussed. The empahsis is not on segmental spasms that may occur

Eberhard Zeitler MD, Professor, University Erlangen-Nürnberg, Germany

address for correspondence:
Virchowstraße 13, D-90409 Nürnberg, Germany

in the framework of punctures, catheterizations and interventions, but on the vasospastic syndromes which were previously called 'angioneuropathies' (RICHTER 1974) and are mainly due to exogenous causes. These are Raynaud's syndrome and ergotism. RATSCHOW (1959) characterized these as clinical syndromes with disturbances of blood flow in the vascular periphery which were beyond normal phys-

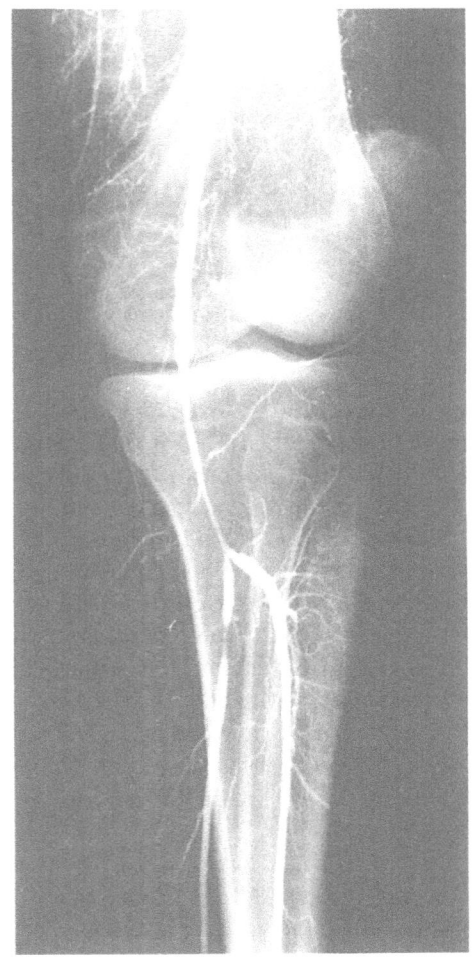

Fig. 28.1: Spasm in the popliteal and posterior tibial arteries after mechanical irritation with a (0.038 in.) guidewire at the time of femoral artery angioplasty

iology and which occur under neural influences. The typical sites of manifestation are the hands and fingertips, more often than the feet, but spasm due to ergotism involves the long arteries (brachial and superficial femoral arteries). The incidence of this disease in patients with vessel pathology has been reported to be less than 6% (RICHTER 1974).

The various, neurally induced, functional perfusion disorders in patients with lumbar or cervical spondylopathy, or after traumatic nerve damage will not be dealt with here. The vasospastic syndromes of importance to the radiologist, caused by exogenous influences such as cold, drugs, and other toxic substances, clearly require a thorough history, in addition to the diagnostic examination with imaging systems (duplex US, angiography and others). In many cases, further history may be necessary in order to interpret correctly the angiographic study. This is essential to avoid incorrect treatment, such as vascular surgical reconstruction using bypass techniques, or angioplasty with balloon catheter or stent for functional clinical situations (SLANINA et al. 1971). Furthermore, unnecessary pharmacological therapy can be avoided because in many cases adequate conservative therapy is successful (HEIDRICH 1979; CREUTZIG 1993).

28.1
Raynaud's Syndrome

Typical of Raynaud's syndrome is intermittent ischemia of fingers 2 to 4, caused by cold or emotional factors (ALLEN 1937; HEIDRICH 1979; JAMIESON et al. 1971; KAPPERT 1985; CREUTZIG 1993). It begins with deadly pallor of the fingers, mostly up to the middle phalanges, accompanied by pain and paraesthesiae and followed by cyanosis and terminal erythrochromia. This 'tricolor syndrome' which is usually bilateral and associated with weakened pulses, is a sign of primary vasospastic Raynaud's syndrome. Women are affected up to 9 times more than men (KAPPERT 1985; CREUTZIG 1993). The prevalence in women is about 5%, in men about 3% (WEINRICH et al. 1990).

Primary vasospastic Raynaud's syndrome differs from secondary Raynaud's syndrome, where organic causes in the hand and finger arteries, or other morphologic changes, e.g. thoracic outlet syndrome (TOS), are identifiable (BOLLINGER and BUTTI 1976). The differentiation is of practical importance for the selection of appropriate therapy.

According to ALLEN and BROWN (1932), the signs of primary vasospastic Raynaud's syndrome are as follows:

* Paroxsysmal vasospasms
* Symmetric affection of the fingers
* Absence of trophic disturbances
* No primary disease
* Symptoms and signs for at least two years.

According to several authors (ERIKSON 1965; GIFFORD 1971; BOLLINGER 1972; HEYDRICH 1979) symptoms can be predominantly unilateral and, in exceptional cases, the thumb can be involved. The latter is also associated with hypotension, Prinzmetal's angina, and migraine (CREUTZIG 1993). An essential aspect in all patients with digital perfusion disorders and "tricolor" hue changes (blue, white and red) is exclusion of organic disorders. Whenever organic causes of Raynaud's symptoms can be identified, this is termed secondary Raynaud's syndrome (BOLLINGER and BUTTI 1976, PRIOLETT et al. 1987). There are many diseases that may cause secondary Raynaud's phenomenon; the most common are:

* Collagenoses (progressive systemic scleroderma and systemic lupus erythematosus)
* Arteriosclerotic arterial obliterations
* Chronic intoxications (polyvinyl chloride, ergotamine, and others)
* Drugs, e.g. hormones, cytotoxics, betablockers.

In patients with scleroderma, Raynaud's symptomatology is one of the cardinal symptoms, occurring in about 90% of patients. It also occurs in about 30% of patients with systemic lupus erythematosus.

For diagnosis, acral electronic oscillography (KAPPERT 1976) can be used. In patients with cold fingers, no swing is registered. After a warm water bath, normal pulse curves with rapid pulse wave increase and sawtooth waves appear. At angiography, peripherally tapering finger arteries are visible. The vessels are not discontinuous and collaterals are not identifiable if optimum vasodilatation prior to angiography is performed. The extreme vasoconstriction in the periphery found in many patients can be removed by careful preparation of the patient with rest and warmth. Intra-arterial administration of the vasodilator tolazoline hydrochloride (Priscol 10 mg, Ciba-Geigy, Wehr, Germany), or oral alcohol (ZEITLER 1976) can help achieve this (WAGNER and ALEXANDER 1993).

The optimum angiographic diagnosis (see Table 27.4) is accomplished by combined cryodynamic angiography (PORTER et al. 1975; RÖSCH et al. 1977; ZEITLER et al. 1979). The principle is to induce extreme vasospasm by hypothermia of the fingers using icy water, whereupon it is eliminated by warmth and vasodilators to visualize morphologic pathologic changes, such as occlusions, stenoses and microaneurysms. If in the future, angiography with contrast medium and X-rays will be less common, cooling and vasodilatation will still be required for functional analysis. This also applies to analysis of the capillary circulation using videodenistometry (MAHLER et al. 1979), or MR angiography. In the evaluation of 125 angiographic studies of the hand (ZEITLER 1979), secondary Raynaud's syndrome could be demonstrated in 78 patients, through identification of morphologic pathologic changes and asymmetric vasospastic changes. The ratio of women:men was 1:2.5. The ratio of women:men with primary Raynaud's syndrome but without any morphologic pathologic changes of the hand arteries, was 9:1 (HEYDRICH 1979; CREUTZIG 1993).

Among the morphologic pathologic changes, occlusions of the digital arteries, as well as an occlusion of the ulnar artery were most common. Occlusions of the superficial palmar arch were observed both in patients with chronic traumata (vibration-induced ischemia) and Dupuytren's contracture.

In the framework of secondary Raynaud's syndrome, particularly in patients with scleroderma, there is a typical, tapered distal narrowing of the digital arteries, which becomes more apparent as the soft-tissue mantle is reduced. In addition, the communicating branches between radial and ulnar digital arteries at the level of the phalanges are not visible on the angiogram.

28.2
Ergotism

Ergotism appears as functional long-segment stenoses, typically in the truncal arteries (Fig. 28.2) of the legs (BOLLINGER and PRAETER 1973), but also of the brachial artery (BOLLINGER and ZEITLER 1976; HEINZ et al. 1994).
Epidemic ergotism caused by contamination with ergot is largely historical. Cases mainly occurred after prolonged intake of submaximal doses of medications containing ergotamine, either for the treatment of gynecological disorders or, more commonly for migraine (JATER et al. 1936; VAGERBERG et al. 1967; JOHNSON 1972; CRANLEY et al. 1963; FELIX

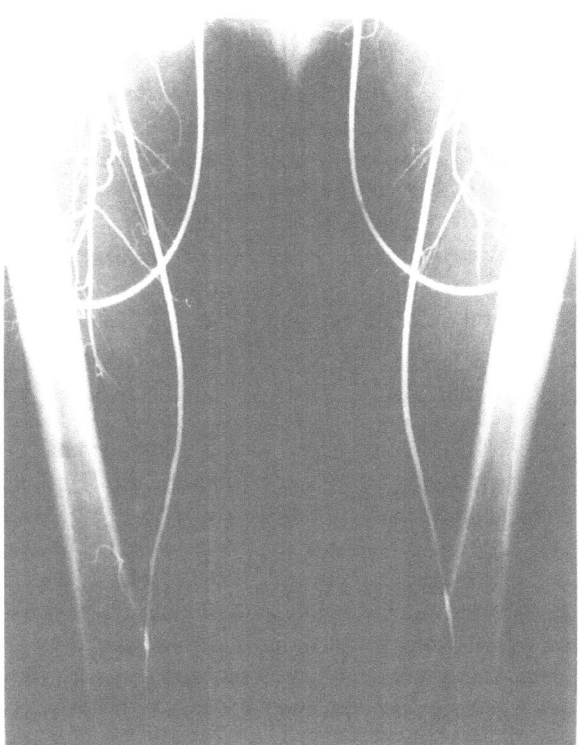
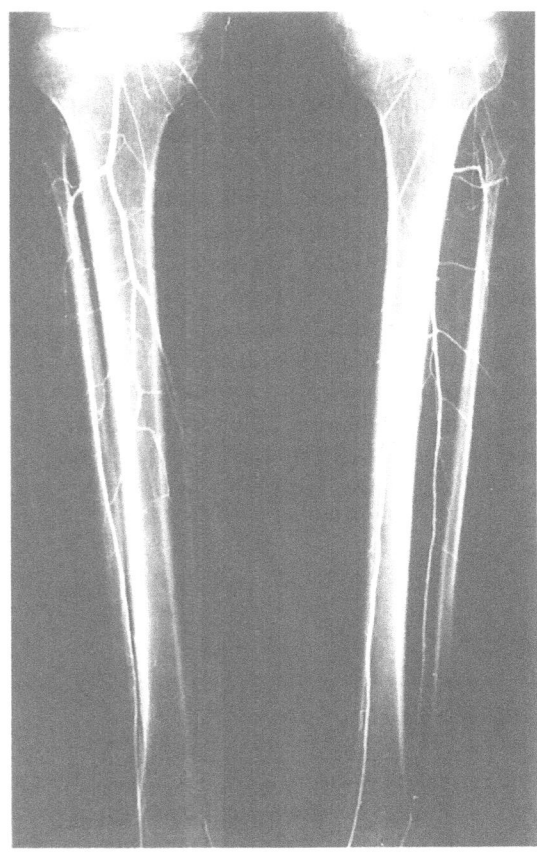

Fig. 28.2: Longsegmental vasospasm after 10 years of abuse of ergotamine tartrate (A 38-year-old woman with migraine for more than 10 years)

1976; BOLLINGER and PRATER 1973; BOLLINGER and ZEITLER 1976). Most were women in our series (BOLLINGER and ZEITLER 1976) in the ration of 18:1 and with a mean age of 37 years (range 23–51 years). They had taken ergotamine tartrate, either in tablet form or, more commonly, as a suppository. In 11 cases the femoral arteries were affected by the vasospastic clinical picture; in 2 cases the brachial arteries were affected. Extreme vasospasm of truncal arteries of several extremities, with gangrene, has been observed after intake of vasodilators, lumbar sympathectomy, and vascular surgery (YATER and CAHILL 1936; CRANLEY et al. 1963).

For the diagnosis of ergotism, the history, analysis of ingested drugs, and the angiographic findings (Fig. 28.3) are decisive (HEIDRICH 1997; BOLLINGER and ZEITLER 1976). An important observation was made by HEINZ et al. in 1994 who showed, by duplex sonography, an occlusion of the brachial artery, but on selective brachial arteriography an extensive typical vasospastic stenosis could be demonstrated. With catheter therapy, the residual stenosis was dilated.

Use of nitroglycerin, tolazoline and hemodilution have not been therapeutic in ergotism. Only strict abstinence from ergotamine leads to an improvement of the clinical picture and elimination of vasospasm. Improvement is not achievable in long-standing cases with secondary thrombosis. A crucial diagnostic sign is the demonstration of smooth, long-segment vasospastic femoral or brachial arteries, with occasional involvement of the radial and tibial arteries, at least in one extremity. The aim in every case of ergotism is to eliminate the vasospasm in a conservative way, through termination of the intake of drugs containing ergotamine. To support the diagnosis, an angiographic diagnosis may be helpful, and the likelihood of therapeutic success can be assessed by the appearances during optimum vasodilatation.

28.3
Hypersensitivity Syndromes and Drug-induced Arteriopathies

Hypersensitivity vasculitis is an immune-complex disease. In most cases, it is an inflammation of small and smallest vessels affecting the skin (SCHELLUNG 1993). In the framework of panarteritis, however, segmental arteries are also affected. Femoral artery

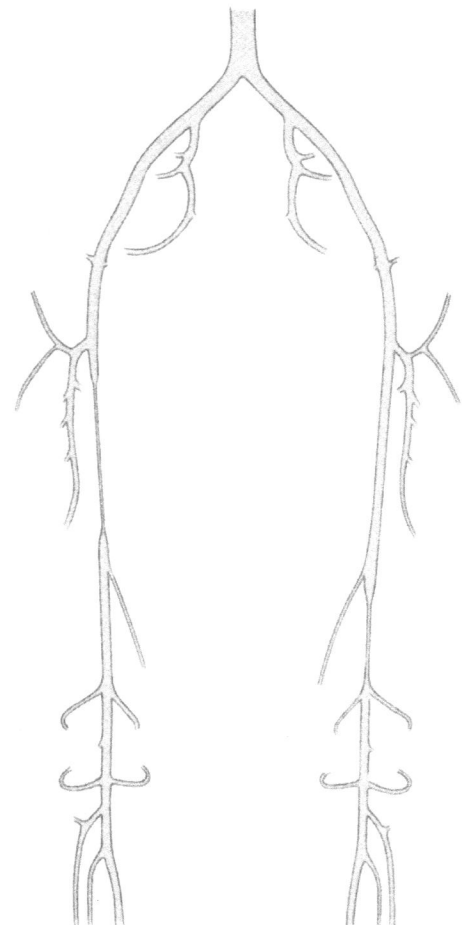

Fig. 28.3. Smooth longsegment stenosis, mainly due by vasospasm or intimal hyperplasia

occlusions have also been documented after antibiotic therapy (MARTIN et al. 1973). The underlying cause is probably a hyperallergic reaction of the intermediate type. Such femoral or brachial artery occlusions can be reversible if the diagnosis is made early and the causative toxic substance can be excluded.

Other drugs which are causes of arteriopathies are steroidal and non-steroidal antirheumatic drugs (cortisone and indomethacin), tranquillizers, ovulation inhibitors, and sympathomimetics. Antibiotics known to cause arteriopathy are erythromycin, tetracycline, and penicillin (HESS 1972, MARTIN 1973). Several exogenous antigens can produce hypersensitivity vasculitis. In addition to laboratory parameters, a chest X-ray and, if there is more than just skin involvement, angiography of the renal or extremity arteries, may be indicated.

References

Allen EV (1937) The peripheral arteries in Raynaud's disease: an arteriographic study of living subjects. Mayo Clin Proc 12:187

Allen EV, Brown GE (1932) Raynaud's disease: a critical review of minimal requisites for diagnosis. Am J Med Sci 183:187

Bollinger A (1972) Klinik und Therapie der vasospastischen Syndrome. In: Kappert A (ed) Nichtdegenerative Arteriopathien. Huber, Bern, pp 154-169

Bollinger A, Butti P (1976) Primäres und sekundäres Raynaud-Syndrom. Schweiz Med Wochenschr 106:415

Bollinger A, Preter B (1973) Spasmen der muskulären Stammarterien der Extremitäten nach Einnahmen von ergotamintartrathaltigen Medikamenten. Dtsch Med Wochenschr 98:825

Bollinger A, Zeitler E (1976) Klinisch-angiographische Probleme bei der Erkennung pharmaka-induzierter Veränderungen der Extremitätenarterien. In: Zeitler E (ed) Aspekte der Extremitätenangiographie – Fehldiagnosen und Fehlinterpretationen. Huber, Bern, pp 121-131

Cranley JJ, Krause RJ, Strasser ES, Hafner CD (1963) Impending gangrene of four extremities secondary to ergotism. N Engl J Med 269:727

Creutzig A (1993) Raynaud-Syndrom. In: Alexander K (ed) Gefäßkrankheiten. Urban & Schwarzenberg, Munich, pp 611-625

Erikson N (1965) Peripheral arteriography during bradykinin induced vasodilatation. Acta Radiol (Stockh) 3:193-201

Fagerberg S, Jorulf H, Sandberg CG (1967) Ergotism, arteriospastic disease and recovery, studied angiographically. Acta Med Scand 182:769

Felix RH, Carroll JD (1970) Upper limb ischemia due to ergotamine tartrate. Practitioner 205:71

Gifford RW (1971) Reserpin and Raynaud's phenomenon. New Engl J Med 285:290

Gremmel H (1976) Arterieller Spasmus, Ursache für Fehldeutungen bei der Arteriographie. In: Zeitler E (ed) Aspekte der Extremitätenangiographie. Huber, Bern, pp 116-120

Hagen B (1986) Gefäßveränderungen bei sporadischem Ergotismus. Epidemiologie, Pathogenese, Klinik und Diagnostik unter besonderer Berücksichtigung der angiographischen Dokumentation. Radiologie 26:388-394

Heidrich H (1979) Konservative Therapie des Raynaud-Syndroms. In: Ehringer H, Betz E, Bollingr A, Deutsch E (eds) Gefäßwand, Rezidivprophylaxe, Raynaud-Syndrom. Witzstrock, Baden-Baden, pp 515-520

Heidrich H (1979) Raynaud-Phänomen. TM-Verlag, Bad Oynhausen

Heidrich H (1997) Funktionelle Gefäßerkrankungen. In: Zeitler E (ed) Arterien und Venen. Springer Verlag, Berlin Heidelberg New York, pp 377-380

Heinz M, Theiss W, Golder W (1994) Unilaterale akute Armischemie als ungewöhnlicher Ausdruck eines Ergotismus. In: Spengel FA, Altmann E (eds) 23. Tagung Deutsche Ges. Angiologie. VASA [Suppl 43]:12

Hess H (1972) Iatrogene Arteriopathien. In: Kappert A (ed) Nichtdegenerative Arteriopathien. Huber, Bern, pp 125-131

Jamieson GG, Ludbrook J, Wilson A (1971) Cold hypersensitivity in Raynaud's phenomenon. Circulation 44:254

Johnsson KA (1962) Angiography in two cases of ergotism. Acta Radiol Stockholm 57:280

Kappert A (1985) Raynaud-Syndrom und akrale Oszillographie. In: Kappert (ed) Lehrbuch und Atlas der Angiologie. Huber, Bern, pp 211-216

Mahler F, Meier B, Bollinger A (1979) Kapillardurchblutung im menschlichen Nagelfalz beim Raynaud-Syndrom. In: Ehringer H, Betz E, Bollinger A, Deutsch E (eds) Gefäßwand, Rezidivprophylaxe. Raynaud-Syndrom. Witzstrock, Baden-Baden, pp 466-470

Martin M, Schulte P, Sobbe A, et al (1973) Multiple Verschlüsse größerer Arterien nach Penicillin-Gabe. Dtsch Med Wochenschr 98:1333

Olbert F, Russe OJ, Ender HG, et al. (1976) Fehlbefunde von Angiographien im Bereich der oberen Extremitäten. In: Zeitler E (ed) Aspekte der Extremitätenangiographie. Akute Probleme in der Angiologie, Vol. 34. Huber, Bern, Bd. 34, pp 150-156

Porter JM, Snider RL, Bardane E, Rösch J, Eidenmiller LR (1975) The diagnosis and treatment of Raynaud's phenomenon. Surgery 77:11-17

Priolett P, Vayssairat M, Housset E (1987) How to classifiy Raynaud's phenomenon: long-term follow-up study of 73 cases. Am J Med 83 494-499

Ratschow M (1959) Angiologie, G. Thieme Verlag, Stuttgart

Raynaud M (1862) De l'asphyxie locale et de la gangréne des extremités. L. Leclerc. Thése de Paris, Paris

Richter H (1974) Angioneuropathien. In: Heberer G, Rau G, Schoop W (eds) Angiologie, 2nd ed. Thieme, Stuttgart, pp 372-384

Rösch J, Porter JM, Gralino BJ (1977) Cryodynamic hand angiography in the diagnosis and management of Raynaud's syndrome. Radiology 55:807-810

Schellong S (1993) Hypersensitivitätsvaskulitis. In: Alexander RH (ed) Gefäßkrankheiten. Urban & Schwarzenberg, Munich, pp 549-551

Schmitt R, Lanz U (1996) Bildgebende Diagnostik der Hand. Hippokrates, Stuttgart

Slanina A, Baumeister L, Blümchen G (1971): Spastischer Verschluß der A. poplitea nach Angiographie. Fortschr Rontgenstr 114:797-799

Völpel W (1957) Der arterielle Spasmus im arteriographischen Bild. Fortschr Rontgenstr 86:79-82

Weinrich MC, Maricq HR, Keil JE, et al (1990) Prevalence of Raynaud phenomenon in the adult population of South Carolina. J Clin Epidemiol 12:1343-1347

Yater WM, Cahill JA (1936) Bilateral gangrene of feet due to ergotamine tartrate used for pruritus of jaundice. J Amer Med Ass. 106:1625

Zeitler E (1976) Zur sicheren Darstellung der Digitalarterien an Händen und Füßen in Lokalanästhesie nach oraler Alkoholgabe. Fortschr Rontgenstr 123:67-68

Zeitler E (1979) Angiographische Befunde beim Raynaud-Syndrom. In: Ehringer H, Betz E, Bollinger A, Deutsch E (eds) Gefäßwand, Rezidivprophylaxe, Raynaud-Syndrom. Witzstrock, Bader.-Baden, pp 471-479

Zschiedrich M, Heidrich H, Dieners HP (1985): Ergotismus: Diagnostik und Therapie. Med Klin 80:721-727

29 Blood-Cell Diseases

E. Zeitler

CONTENTS

Polycythemia and thrombocythemia are rare causes of microemboli and local thromboses. They have also been summarized under the term "hemorheologic diseases" (ALEXANDER 1997). For interventional radiologists and angiologists, familiarity with the risk of spreading of thrombotic wall-adherent material, or cholesterol crystal emboli is very important. This applies to the identification of the respective clinical symptoms and their prevention in the framework of endovascular intervention. Particularly important are the so-called 'blue-toe syndrome', 'cholesterol crystal embolisms', and peripheral perfusive disorders in the presence of severe thrombocythemia and Osler's disease.

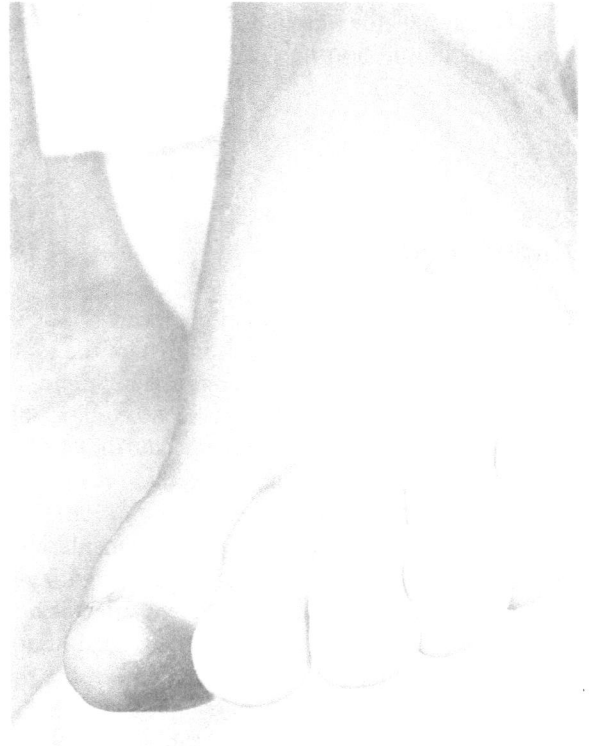

Fig. 29.1   Blue-toe syndrome

29.1
Blue-toe Syndrome (BTS)

The blue-toe syndrome (KARMODI et al. 1976; CRANE 1967; FISCHER et al. 1984) is characterized by the spontaneous onset of acute pain, local sensitivity to touch and blue-reddish discoloration of one toe (Fig. 29.1). Foot pulses are normal. The cause are often microemboli, either from thrombotic material on arteriosclerotic changes in the aorta and pelvic arteries, or from aneurysms of the aorta and more distally located arteries. The differentiation from cholesterol crystal embolism is clinically nearly impossible. Correlation with previous catheter manipulations for cardiac and peripheral vascular diseases or renal diseases is possible (COLT et al. 1988; HYMAN et al. 1987). On selective angiography, vascular occlusions well into the periphery can be demonstrated. The identification of occlusions of the peripheral digital arteries of the toes is also possible with acral oscillography and Doppler US. Histomorphologic studies on autopsy material have shown that cholesterol crystal emboli occur more often than clinically recognised (FEIN et al. 1987; KENNEDY et al. 1989). Studies using high-resolution Duplex US have not been systematically presented to date.

Eberhard Zeitler MD, Professor, University Erlangen-Nürnberg, Germany
address for correspondence:
Virchowstraße 13, D-90409 Nürnberg, Germany

29.2
Osler's Disease

Ten to 20% of patients with Osler's disease suffer occlusions of the cerebral arteries with neurologic deficiency. The higher blood viscosity can, in the presence of peripheral arterial occlusive disease, additionally lead to intensification of the clinical symptoms. On angiography, occlusions of the peripheral digital arteries are hardly identifiable and only capillary microscopy can provide further differentiation. Therapy of the vascular complications entails the use of blood clotting and erythrocytopheresis (RASTÄTTER 1993).

29.3
Thrombocythemia

Thrombocythemia occurs 10 times more often in women in their fifth decade than in men of the same age. Between 50 and 70 years of age, the incidence in men and women is equal (HEHLMANN et al. 1988). Thromboembolic complications occur in 84% of patients, disorders of the microcirculation in 67%, and gangrene in 26%. (HEHLMANN et al. 1988). The spectrum of clinical findings may vary considerably (ALEXANDER 1997) and physicians dealing with peripheral vascular diseases should consider severe thrombocythemia as an underlying cause. Laboratory parameters should be assessed to determine the underlying cause, and the question as to either a hematologic or hemorheologic pathology should be discussed by an multidisciplinary team. To date, selective arteriography with optimum vasodilatation and with magnification has proven to be the most suitable modality for the identification of peripheral arterial occlusions (ZEITLER 1994).

References

Alexander K (1997) Hämorheologische Erkrankungen: Thrombozytose – Polyzythämie – lokale Thrombose – Mikroembolie. In: Zeitler E (ed) Arterien und Venen. Springer, Berlin Heidelberg New York, pp 369-375

Barbui T, Finazzi G (1997) Risk factors and prevention of vascular complications in polycythemia vera. Semin Thromb Hemost 23:455-461

Buss DH, Cashell AW, O'Connor ML, et al (1994) Occurrence, etiology and clinical significance of extreme thrombocytosis. A study of 280 cases. Am J Med 96:247-253

Colt HG, Begg RJ, Saporito JJ, et al (1988) Cholesterol emboli after cardiac catheterization. Medicine 67:389-400

Crane L (1967) Atherothrombotic embolism to lower extremities in arteriosclerosis. Arch Surg 94:96-100

Fenaux P, Simon M, Caulier MT, et al (1990) Clinical course of essential thrombocythemia in 147 cases. Cancer 66:549-556

Fine MJ, Kapoor W, Falango V (1987) Cholesterol crystal embolization: a review of 221 cases in the Englisch literature. Angiology 38:769-784

Fisher DF, Clagetti GP, Brigham RA, et al (1984) Dilemmas in dealing with the blue toe syndrome: aortic versus peripheral source. Am J Surg 148:836-839

Hehlmann R, Jahn M, Baumann B, Köpcke W (1988) Essential thrombocythemia. Cancer 61:2487-2496

Hyman B, Landas SK, Ashman RF, et al (1987) Warfarin-related purple toes syndrome and cholesterol microembolization. Am J Med 82:1233-1237

Karmody AM, Powers SR, Monaco VJ, Leather RP (1976) "Blue to" syndrome. Arch Surg 111:1263-1268

Kennedy A, Cumberland D, Gaines P (1989) The pathology of cholesterol embolism arising as a complication of intra-aortic catheterization. Histopathology 15:515-521

McIntyre KJ, Hoagland HC, Silverstein TS, et al (1991) Essential thrombocythemia in young adults. Mayo Clin Proc 66:149-154

Rastetter J (1993) Die chronischen myeloproliferativen Erkrankungen (CMPE). In: Bergmann H, Rastetter J (eds) Klinische Hämatologie, 4th edn. Thieme, Stuttgart, pp 548-564

Zeitler E (1994) Angiographische Diagnostik und digitale Subtraktionsangiographie bei peripheren Gefäßprozessen. Internist 35:456-464

Lower Extremity Arterial Diseases

30 Iliac Artery Diseases

E. ZEITLER and W. RITTER

CONTENTS

30.1
Normal Anatomy and Variations

The iliac arteries arise directly from the abdominal aorta (Fig. 30.1), by reduction of the vascular lumen. The aortic bifurcation in women is located somewhat more caudally than in men. The aortoiliac bifurcation in men is, therefore, is at a slightly more acute angle, at about 65°, than in women, at about 75° (RAUBER-KOPSCH 1941). With advancing age – particularly in patients suffering from arterial hypertension – not only a dilatation, but also elongation of the arteries develops, whereby the bifurcation may be shifted more in a caudal direction. The common iliac arteries are 3–6 cm in length and bifurcate on both sides into the external and internal iliac arteries, with a further reduction of the arterial diameter. The infrarenal aortic diameter (IAD) in men varies between 20 and 24 mm, in women between 16 and 21 mm. The lumen of the common iliac arteries is between 6 and 9 mm. Only in older age groups was an increase in IAD seen, by means of ultrasound, in 3066 women and 8270 men (WILMINK et al. 1998).

While the internal iliac artery supplies the pelvic viscera, such as the urinary bladder, as well as the buttock muscles, the external iliac artery is a transport artery for the perfusion of the leg. It runs down to the inguinal ligament, with direct transition into the common femoral artery. At the level of the inguinal ligament, both the epigastric caudal and the deep circumflex iliac arteries arise. Both these vessels

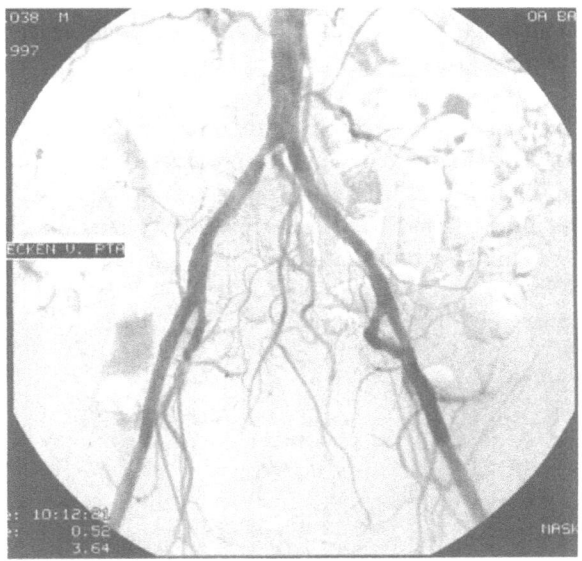

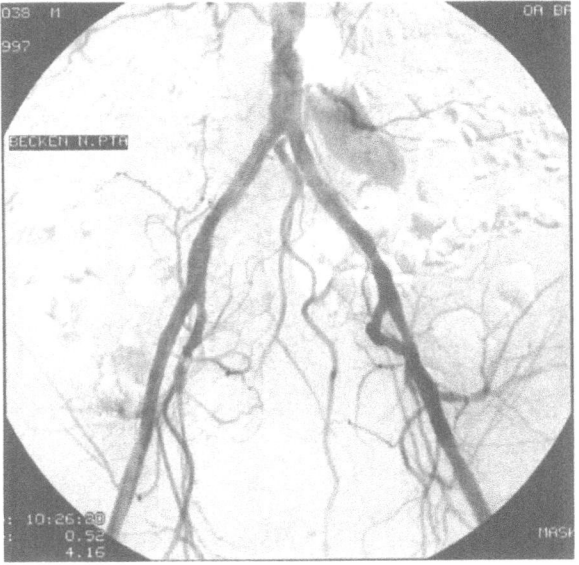

Fig. 30.1 a,b. Acute y-angled aortic bifurcation with caudal aorta and stenoses of the right common iliac artery stenoses (59-year-old male patient). **a** before Balloon-PTA. **b** after successful POBA

E. ZEITLER, Professor, MD, Virchowstraße 13, D-90409 Nürnberg, Germany
W. RITTER, MD, Institut für Diagnostische und Interventionelle Radiologie, Breslauer Straße 201, D-90471 Nürnberg, Germany

can also originate from the deep femoral artery. The common femoral artery is 3–4 cm long and ends at the ramification into the deep femoral and superficial femoral arteries.

The peripheral arteries of the internal iliac artery are important in obliterating vascular diseases for the formation of collateral vessels. Thus, the communications between the caudal mesenteric artery, the lumbar arteries, and the internal iliac artery play an important role as bridges in upper aortoiliac artery occlusions (Fig. 30.2), and in isolated internal iliac artery occlusions. On the other hand, the communications between the internal iliac artery branches from one side to the other are important for bypassing unilateral iliac artery obliterations. The pudendal arteries come from the internal iliac artery and go to the penile arteries on each side. The obturator artery is a common bridging collateral pathway to the deep femoral artery in occlusions of the external iliac and common femoral arteries. The caudal epigastric artery, in contrast, is to the cranial epigastric artery the distal part of the collateral pathway in aortic obliterations (Winslow's pathway) in a cranio-caudal direction, and in aortic arch disease in a caudo-cranial direction (BOYD and JEPSON 1950; GOTTLOB 1952; CHAIT 1976; PRAGER et al. 1977; VOLLMAR 1996).

30.2
Unilateral Iliac Artery Diseases

Isolated iliac artery obliterations are seen in 10%–15% of all peripheral occlusive vascular diseases (POVDs). The majority of iliac artery diseases are the result of arteriosclerotic lesions, followed by local thrombotic occlusion (MÜNSTER et al. 1966; HASSE 1974; LOOSE 1976). A smaller number are embolic diseases at the common iliac bifurcation. Nonarteriosclerotic iliac artery diseases are found very seldom: One is fibromuscular dysplasia (NAJAFI 1966; POLLIT et al. 1972; BOLLINGER 1979) of the external iliac arteries, which is seen mainly bilaterally; another is iliac artery obliteration following radiotherapy for gynecological tumors and cystic degeneration of the adventitia. Typical findings (small

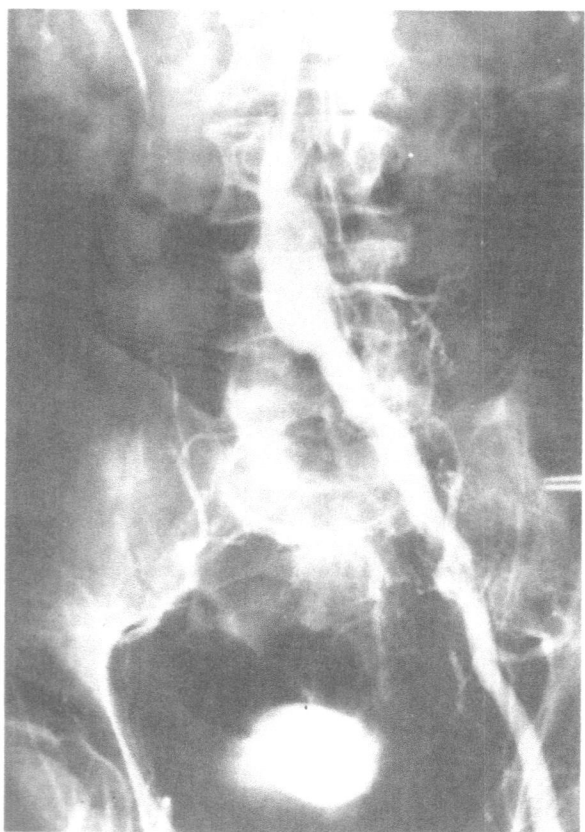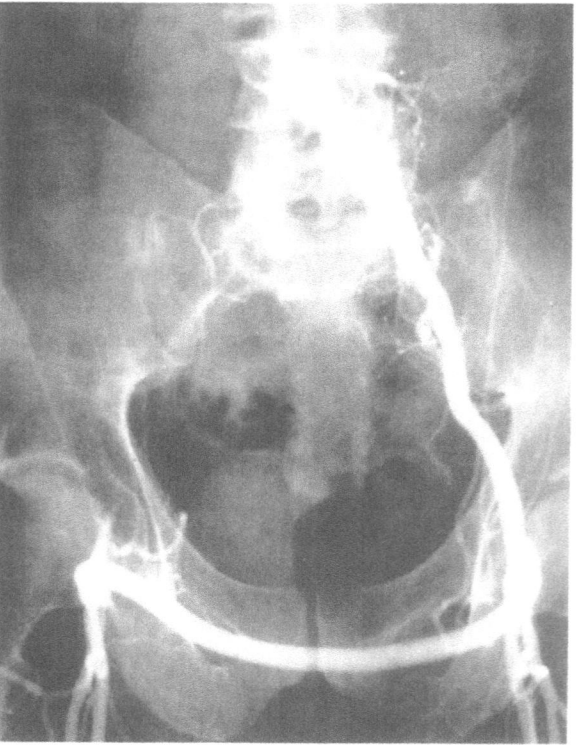

Fig. 30.2 a,b. Common and external iliac artery occlusions [type I according to WELLAUER (1957)] right-side and external iliac artery stenoses with occlusion of the left internal iliac artery (56-year-old man), bilateral claudication, and ulcer on the right big toe, male impotence. **a** Transaxillary pelvic arteriography. **b** Transbrachial arteriography after balloon dilatation on the transaxillary route and femoro-femoral bypass (no change in impotence)

pulse in the groin, claudication, pathologic oscillography, and ankle pressure reduction) of pelvic obliterations were found in 33.3% of all patients with POVD (ALEXANDER 1993).

MÜNSTER et al. (1966) detected isolated iliac artery obliterations in 10.2% of patients on angiography, compared to no more than 3.5% of isolated aortic occlusions. More frequently, these authors identified combined obliterations in the iliac and superficial femoral arteries (15%), in the iliac and tibiofibular arteries (2.7%), and obliterations in all parts of the leg, the pelvis, thigh, and calf in 4.9%.

In earlier years, mainly occlusions of one or more iliac arteries were angiographically identified in the framework of aorto-arteriographies using the translumbar or catheter techniques, which was then only an indication prior to surgical interventions (WELLAUER 1957; ZEITLER 1974; VAN DONGEN 1976). Nowadays, the larger spectrum of therapies, including angioplasty and improved clinical diagnosis using the Doppler technique and duplex sonography, enables obliterations in the area of the pelvic arteries to be identified as early as in the stage of stenosis. This was one intention of the modern angiologists (SCHOOP and LEVY 1969; BOLLINGER 1979; ALEXANDER 1993).

WELLAUER (1957) differentiated between six typical aortoiliac types of occlusion (Fig. 30.4), the first two of which are defined in detail as follows:

- *Type I* is the occlusion of the common iliac artery beginning at the aortic bifurcation, extending down into the inguinal area, including an occlusion of the external iliac artery. Unilateral occlusion of the pelvic arteries can be a thrombotic occlusion developing from either arteriosclerotic stenoses with formation of a thrombosis in a caudo-cranial direction (Fig. 30.2), or a thrombosed aortoiliac aortic aneurysm. They can also develop from a dissecting aneurysm which splits the artery into a true and false lumen down to the iliac artery, and leads to occlusion at the end of the dissection, at the level of the iliac bifurcation.
- *Type II* demonstrates isolated occlusions of the common iliac artery, contrasting the external iliac artery via collaterals. In such cases, collaterals are identifiable between the lumbar arteries, the inferior mesenteric artery, and the internal iliac artery (Fig. 30.3), which underlines the fact that the occlusion had developed slowly. Depending on the degree to which the internal iliac artery is involved in the obliteration, varying forms of collaterals are identifiable, running from the nonaffected, or less affected, side to the contralateral side.

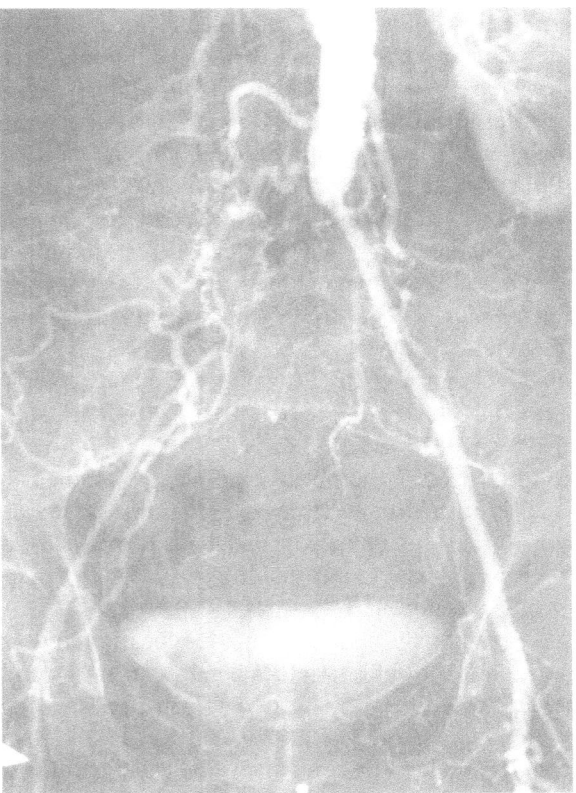

Fig. 30.3. Common iliac artery occlusion [type II according to WELLAUER (1957)]. Right side with collateral vessels, movable right kidney, occlusion of the left internal iliac artery (58-year-old female)

Isolated iliac artery stenoses are localized either in close vicinity to the aortic bifurcation (Fig. 30.1), or at the level of the bifurcation of the common iliac artery into the external and internal arteries. The stenosis may be found either in front of, or distal of, the branching point of the internal iliac artery, or may involve the latter in the arteriosclerotic process (Fig. 30.6). The typical clinical picture of unilateral iliac artery disease is intermittent claudication, with pain in the region of the gluteal, hip, and upper thigh muscles (ROB and VOLLMAR 1959; VAN DONGEN 1976), often in combination with pain in the calf muscles (HASSE 1974).

In patients with unilateral obliterations of the common or internal iliac arteries, impaired potency is an absolute exception. Clinically, the diagnosis of iliac artery disease can be suspected from a lack of pulse and a weakened pulse in the groin, with a simultaneous, auscultable stenotic murmur above the inguinal ligament (SCHOOP 1988). Although by determining the pressure with the Doppler technique and defining the ankle–arm pressure gradient unilateral arterial obliteration can be confirmed, a precise determination of location requires additional stress tests (stress oscillography, or systolic blood pressure measurement using the Doppler technique after knee-bends and/or tiptoe stands) (Schoop 1988; Bollinger 1979). Stenoses of over 50% can be detected with functional stress tests, whereas stenoses of less than 50% – defined as plaques – can only be diagnosed with imaging methods such as angiography, color-coded duplex sonography, or similar techniques (Bollinger 1979). Stress tests can be defined, according to Rutherford and Becker (1991), Durham and Rutherford (1994) (Chap. 5, Table 5.10A), or Bollinger (1979) as follows: (a) 200 m on the treadmill (3.2 km/h) at a gradient of 12.5%; or (b) oscillography after 40 tiptoe stands and 20–30 knee-bends (according to Schoop 1988); or (c) Doppler control at the ankle after 20–30 tiptoe stands (according to Carter 1972).

Angiography then confirms the location and extension of the obliteration. Whenever an occlusion is identified, it is important to define its precise extension and collateral circulation. In the case of stenosis, morphologic analysis regarding existing thrombi which are still amenable to lysis (verrucous iliac artery stenosis), or a smooth, non-lysable stenosis

(smooth iliac artery stenosis) may provide valuable hints for further therapeutic measures. Only angiography, however, is capable of diagnosing a fibromuscular dysplasia (Najafi 1966; Pollit et al. 1972; Sauer et al. 1990) of the external iliac artery.

Isolated external iliac artery occlusions (Boyd and Jeoson 1950) are often the result of embolic disease with a riding embolus on the common femoral bifurcation with ascending thrombosis, or the result of local thrombosis in the inguinal arteries with descending thrombosis (Colapinto et al. 1982; Auster et al. 1984; Ginsburg et al. 1989; McNamara et al. 1991; Vorwerk et al. 1995), if not the result of several types of intervention in the groin. External iliac artery obliterations are very seldom the result of radiotherapy and compression from metastatic lymph node disease. Given such situations, axial scanning methods, such as computed tomography (CT) or magnetic resonance imaging (MRI), and even ultrasound, can provide more information about the course of the obliteration than angiography, which can only demonstrate the arterial occlusion. In unilateral iliac artery disease (Fig. 30.5 and 30.6), several options exist for treatment (Guidelines for Percutaneous Transluminal Angioplasty 1990; Brewster et al. 1989):

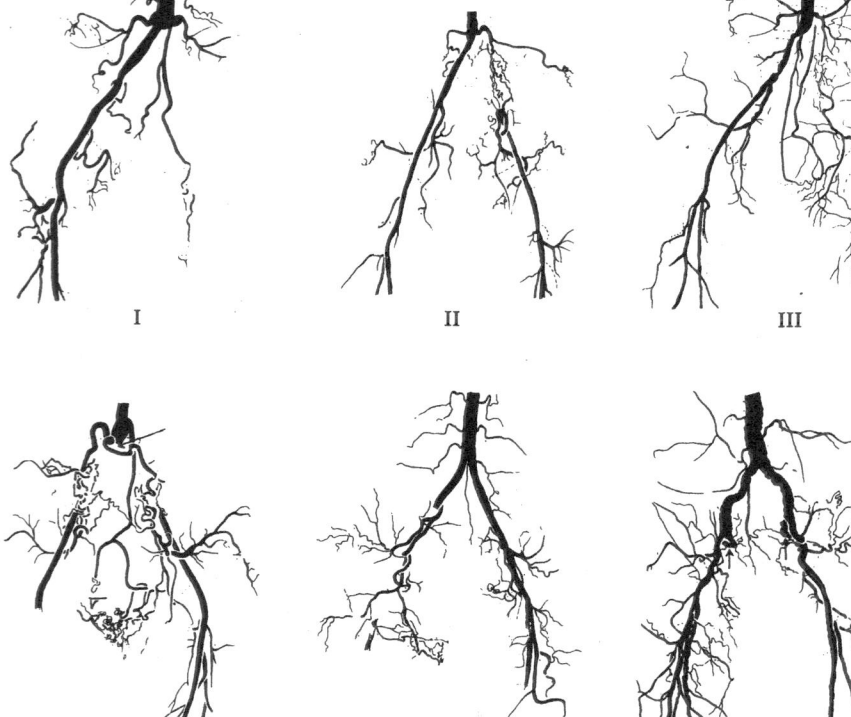

Fig. 30.4. Typical aortoiliac obliterations [according to Wellauer (1957)]. Type I, common iliac and external iliac artery occlusion; type II, common iliac artery occlusion; type III, common iliac artery occlusion and contralateral external iliac artery stenoses; type IV, aortobiiliacal bifurcated occlusion; type V, external iliac artery occlusion; type VI, dilating and obliterating changes in aorta and iliac arteries, plus internal iliac artery obliteration

- Balloon angioplasty
- Balloon angioplasty in combination with femoropoplited bypass surgery
- Thromboendarterectomy
- Femorofemoral bypass from the patent artery to the diseased site and conservative therapy with controlled walking therapy
- Thrombolysis (systemic or intraarterial).
- Stent-assisted PTA

In the early years, we treated iliac artery stenoses (ZEITLER et al. 1971a) first with the Fogarty balloon catheter, then with the Porstmann caged-balloon catheter, and finally with the Grüntzig balloon catheter. Since 1980, and given the modern balloon catheters available, I have preferred non-compliant balloon catheters for iliac artery dilatation.

In the years up to 1976, our team was able to treat iliac artery stenoses with a very low complication rate. There were only 15 complications out of 168 patients, and only one required surgical treatment for a pulsating hematoma in the groin (8.9% complications, 0.6% operations). Clinical success was defined, together with the angiologist and vascular surgeon, as: Angiographically confirmable reduction of the stenotic diameter to below 30%; improved oscillography at rest and after exercise, and improvement by at least one class according to the Fontaine classification. This was achieved in 144 out of 186 cases (77.4%), whereas only in 29 did we achieve a technical, but no clinical success, and in 13, no technical success was achieved. We dilated two or more unilateral iliac artery stenoses in 24 patients, with clinical success in 20, no clinical success in two, and no technical success in a further two cases.

One risk associated with iliac artery dilatation is the occlusion of the internal iliac artery, which is very often stenosed and still an important collateral artery. We observed this in the early years in 2%–5% of patients.

Surgically, local thromboendarterectomy and femorofemoral bypass are very common. The latter operation has a very low complication rate and good hemodynamic results with long-lasting patency rates.

If the patient's history is shorter than 6 months, intraarterial local thrombolysis with a multiple side-hole catheter can be a promising alternative, mainly followed by balloon angioplasty or stent implantation. Only the risk of embolism in the femoropopliteal arteries (AUSTER et al. 1984;

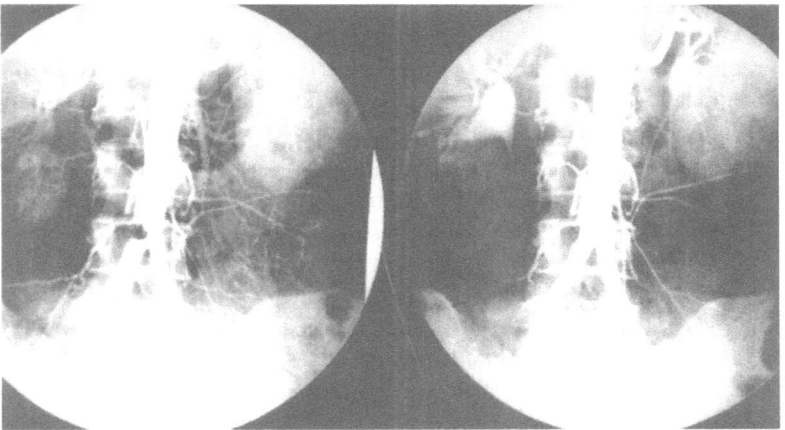

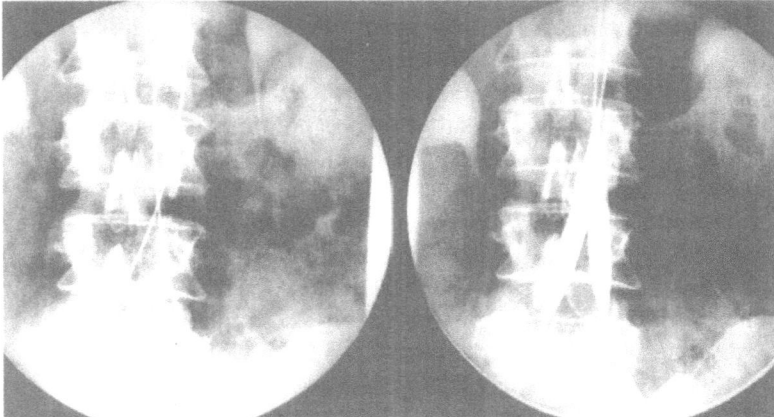

Fig. 30.5. Isolated common iliac artery stenoses on the right. **a** Before treatment. **b** After balloon dilatation. **c,d** Demonstrating the kissing-balloon technique (57-year-old man with claudication)

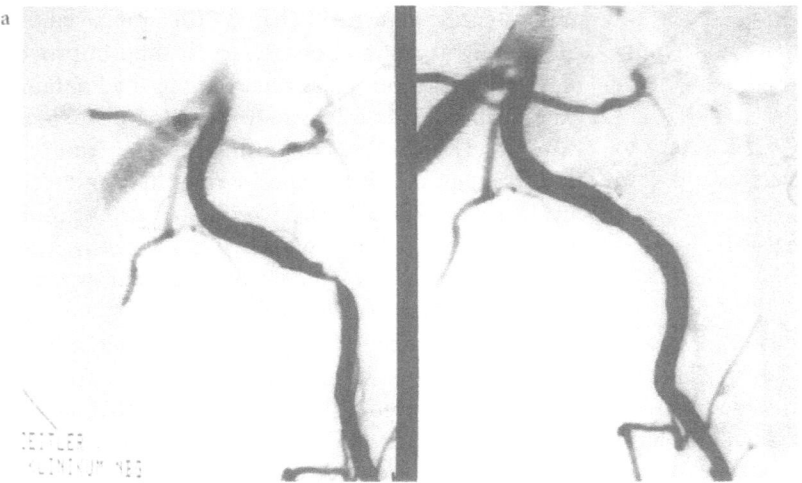

Fig. 30.6. a,b. Unilateral external iliac artery stenoses and internal iliac artery occlusion (69-year-old man), with hypertension and claudication, and additional tibioperoneal obliterations. **a** Before treatment **b** After implantation of a Wallenstent (8-mm diameter, 40-mm length)

McNamara et al. 1991) makes it necessary for this type of therapy to be performed by experienced interventionalists alone.

While in patients with unilateral iliac artery stenoses, single or double stenoses are excellent indications for balloon angioplasty, mainly in combination with the insertion of an uncovered stent, in most patients with combined occlusions in the iliac and femoropopliteal arteries, the treatment of the inflow arteries has priority, irrespective of whether it is a surgical or interventional measure (Dormandy and Stock 1990). In many cases, the removal of the obliteration in the iliac arteries alone produces a sufficient improvement in the clinical situation.

During the years up to 1987, in most cases of iliac artery percutaneous transluminal angioplasty (PTA), we measured the blood pressure in the common femoral artery and in the aorta before and after angioplasty. Our intention was to bring the hemodynamic pressure gradient below 10 mmHg. If this failed, we used a second balloon with a larger diameter in several cases. It was observed that dilatations with balloons of larger diameters resulted in dissections and irregularities more often. Therefore, the balloons we used very seldom exceeded a diameter of 8 or 9 mm. With ever increasing bilateral angioplasties and balloon dilatations from the contralateral side, the pressure measurement was not precise in some cases. Therefore, we stopped measuring the gradient in all cases.

The ankle blood measurement in most patients with iliac artery disease is precise, unless the peripheral arteries are calcified. The ankle/brachial index (ABI) clearly demonstrates the success rate, which can be defined according to the Rutherford classification (Kaufmann et al. 1982; Rutherford and Becker 1991). Today, I would recommend ma-

nometer measurements of the intraarterial pressure only for prospective trials, additionally in view of the economic situation in general (Wilson et al. 1989; Richter et al. 1991). On the other hand, if it is important to inspect the artery more accurately, angioscopy or intravascular ultrasound (IVUS) provide more precise information than intraarterial pressure measurements alone. The latter control methods, however, involve considerably higher costs and, thus, do not favor economical medical practice. A control digital subtraction angiography (DSA) on two or three planes is less expensive, faster, and provides the same result, i.e., in the majority of cases, a second balloon dilatation or the implantation of a stent become necessary (Rees et al. 1989; Ronsseau et al. 1989; Richter et al. 1991).

Detailed information regarding long-term patency after balloon dilatation can be obtained from the German–Austrian Multicenter Study (GAMS) II. This was a double-blind randomized study evaluating long-term results following successful iliac artery PTA, with clear inclusion and exclusion criteria. The primary success rate in iliac artery stenoses, including excluded patients, was 97%.

The study was aimed at comparing adjunctive medicamentous treatment [acetylsalicylic acid (ASA) plus Dipyridamol, versus placebo]. A total of 170 patients (50.9%) received ASA plus Dipyridamol, and 164 patients (49.1%) received a placebo. Of these, 78.8% were males with a mean age of 54.5 years, and 21.2% were females, with a mean age of 57.1 years. In total, 95.2% were in Fontaine class IIb and 4.8% in Fontaine class III/IV. Follow-up controls took place every 3 months, for up to 36 months, and each year one compliance control with urine testing of Dipyridamol was carried out. There was no statistically significant difference between the two groups in 52 parameters.

The cumulative patency rate according to the life-table method can be found below. Success as defined in the study protocol was: ABI above 0.8, or improved by at least 0.15 compared to before treatment, and additional improvement by at least one category.

With thrombocyte function inhibitors (TFI), the patency rate was 60% after 3 years; with placebo, the patency rate was 53% after 3 years. There was no significant difference. In the same patient population, using the Rutherford criteria category +3, and clinical improvement by one category, the 3-year patency rates with TFI were: Rutherford criteria, 48%, improved clinical stage, 66%; with placebo only: Rutheford criteria, 37%, improved clinical stage, 60%.

The comparison of these results from the same collective shows that, even taking into consideration the same criteria in different groups carrying out studies, many factors can influence the result. These include, of course, the run-off situation, the clinical stage, possible additional risk factors of the patient, the instrumentation used, and the skill of the physician or physicians in one team. The application of precise criteria is therefore of great importance for the evaluation of an own collective, and for quality control in the case of a change of staff or change in technical instrumentation. Less favorable results do not always mean that work was poor, just as better results do not necessarily imply that these could also have been achieved by others, if different criteria had been applied. Attempts to achieve an objective and quantitative definition should nevertheless always be made.

In patients with peripheral gangrene, however, a combination of iliac and femoropopliteal reconstruction will become necessary as a rule (ZEITLER et al. 1987; BREWSTER et al. 1989). The latter can be performed either following initial dilatation of the iliac atery stenosis with balloon alone (or stent-assisted), followed after a certain interval by creation of a femoropopliteal bypass. On the other hand, and simultaneously during one setting, intraoperative balloon dilatation via the retrograde route, followed by the creation of the femoropopliteal bypass can be carried out (ROTH et al. 1988; BREWSTER et al. 1989; PICUS 1994; STECKMEIER et al. 1995).

Isolated aneurysms of the iliac artery occur both in the region of the common iliac artery (see Fig. 30.14), or internal iliac artery. These are not very promising indications for a surgical approach. On the other hand, the risk of perforation and peripheral embolization cannot be satisfactorily assessed. Therefore, percutaneous therapy of iliac artery aneurysms by applying covered endovascular grafts should be increasingly favored (HENRY et al. 1997). At the level of the common and external iliac arteries, these endovascular grafts can be applied using a retrograde technique, from the ipsilateral groin. For use in the internal iliac artery, transaxillary access may become necessary.

In the region of the iliac arteries, congenital arteriovenous (av)-malformations, or av-fistulas (see Chap. 16), can be present as a result of complications from other diseases (Fig. 30.7).

Case history. An 81-year-old woman with post-thrombotic syndrome on the left leg. The patient received a veno-venous crossover bypass (8-mm gore graft). After thrombotic occlusion of the common and external iliac veins, bleeding from the large pudendal lips requiring blood transfusion, occurred. The mesenteric and internal iliac arteries had developed into an av-fistula system causing recurrent intestinal and gynecological bleeding. We performed a super-selective embolization and occlusion using Gelfoam, whereby the bleeding could be successfully stopped.

Isolated stenoses of the common and external iliac arteries represent optimum indications for balloon angioplasty well accepted by angiologists and vascular surgeons.

DOTTER et al. 1974; ZEITLER et al. 1976; KADIR et al. 1982; SCHNEIDER et al. 1982; ROTH et al. 1988; GÜNTHER et al. 1989; ANDREANI et al. 1991; KASHDAN et al. 1992; LIERMANN et al. 1992; PALMAZ and ENCARNACION 1992; PICUS 1994; HENRY et al. 1995; ROUSSEAU et al. 1996; STRECKER et al. 1996; VORWERK and GÜNTHER 1997

30.3
Bilateral Iliac Artery Disease

Bilateral iliac artery disease exists in both symmetric and asymmetric forms. The most common forms are iliac artery stenoses on both sides. These stenoses can be located in the common iliac artery close to the aortoiliac bifurcation (Fig. 30.8), but also asymmetrically (Fig. 30.13), sometimes with a very smooth surface and poststenotic ectasia simulating a local aneurysm. If such stenoses are not treated early enough, the result may be an aortobiiliac bifurcated occlusion (Fig. 30.10). Because of the condition's long history, several collateral vessels can meanwhile reduce the symptoms of peripheral leg ischemia, but in men the result is very often impotence. The clinical situation can be diagnosed due to reduced arterial penile circulation using the Doppler technique. This situation presents a clear Leriche's syndrome

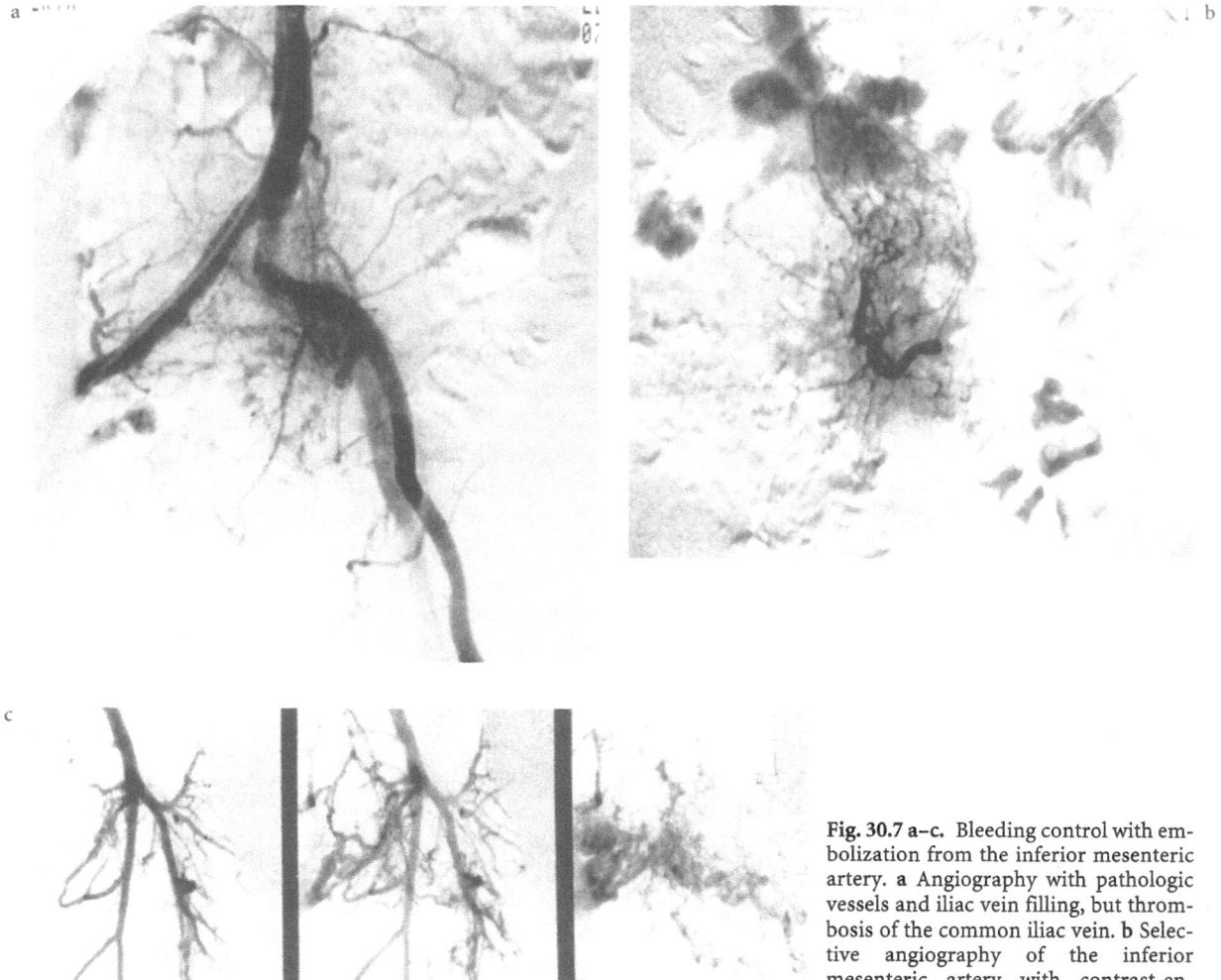

Fig. 30.7 a–c. Bleeding control with embolization from the inferior mesenteric artery. **a** Angiography with pathologic vessels and iliac vein filling, but thrombosis of the common iliac vein. **b** Selective angiography of the inferior mesenteric artery with contrast-enhancement of pathologic vessels. **c** Angiography after occlusion of the atypical vessels and the internal iliac artery with Ethibloc

(Fig. 30.10) with bilateral claudication and male impotence.

Whereas iliac artery stenoses sometimes have a verrucous surface demonstrating still existent clotting on the atherosclerotic plaque which can be lysed, the occlusions with strong collateral circulation mainly suggest that no nonorganized thrombus is present. However, in isolated cases, parts of the occlusion can contain nonorganized thrombus.

After systemic thrombolysis, control angiography mainly shows very smooth borderlines of the inner lumen, demonstrating that all parts are organized or atherosclerotic plaque. More commonly, angiographies demonstrate bilateral iliac artery diseases (Fig. 30.11) with total occlusion of one iliac artery axis, and stenotic lesions on the contralateral side (type III according to WELLAUER). In this situation,

the clinical symptoms depend on the collateral circulation.

If there is a well-developed collateral circulation on the side with total occlusion of the iliac axis, it may be the case that the clinical symptoms are dominant on the contralateral side with an iliac artery stenosis at the iliac bifurcation (Fig. 30.13). This, however, is more evident if there are also occlusions and stenotic lesions distal of the inguinal ligament in the femoropopliteal axis.

This extensive arteriosclerotic disease with thrombotic occlusions exists mainly in patients with generalized arteriosclerosis, including coronary heart disease or stenoses of the renal arteries. Therefore, even if the clinical situation seems to be clear, angiologic documentation of POVD with occlusions in the pelvis and thigh requires an angiographic ex-

Fig. 30.8. Bilateral common iliac artery stenoses. Pretreatment angiography with irregular surface of the stenoses. Control after simultaneous treatment with Strecker stents and balloon dilatation

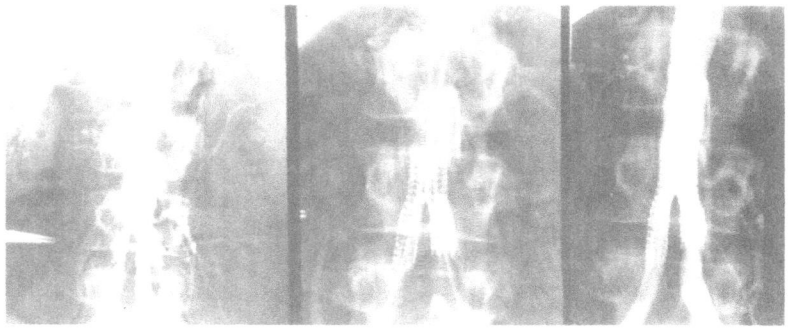

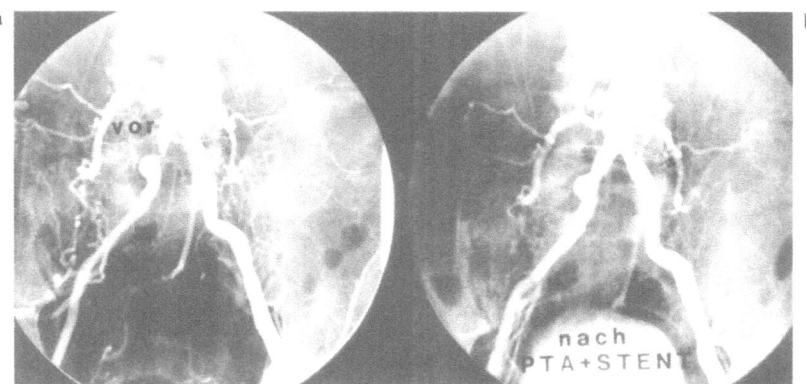

Fig. 30.9 a,b. Bilateral iliac artery stenoses. **a** Pretreatment. **b** After balloon dilatation

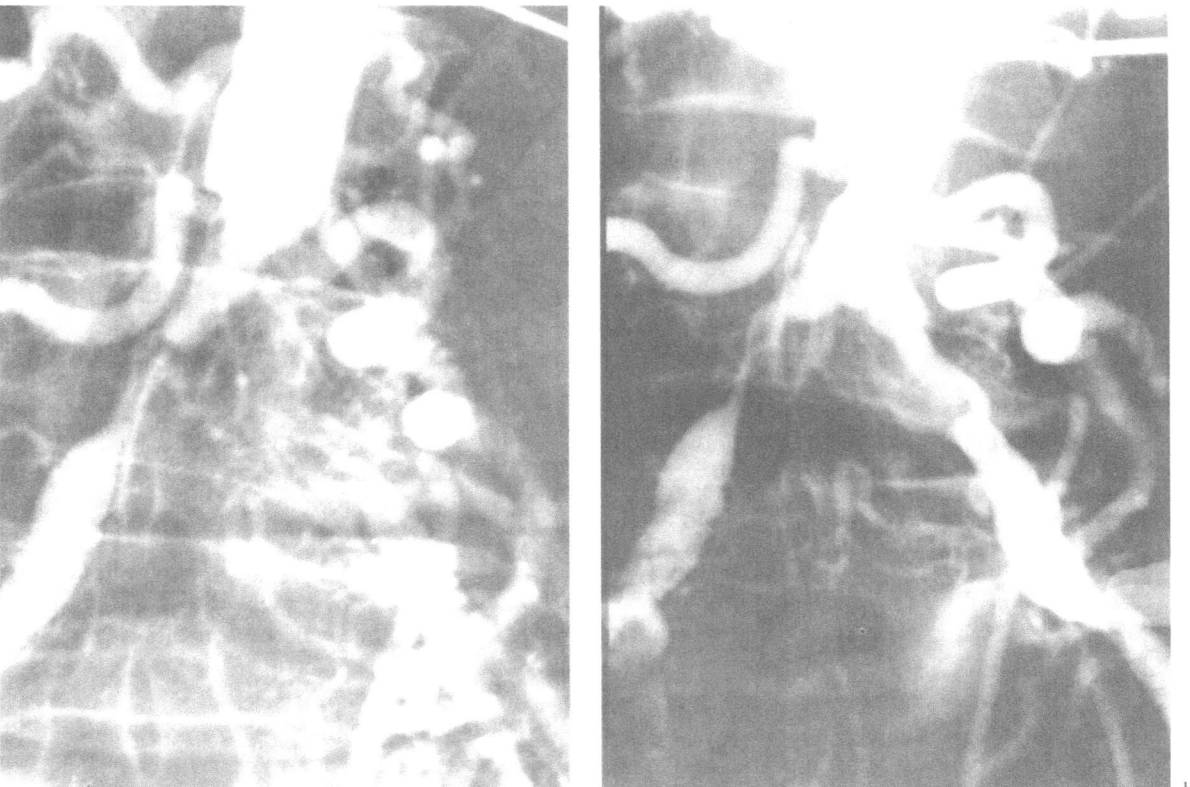

Fig. 30.10 a,b. Aortoiliac bilateral occlusion [type IV according to WELLAUER (1957)]. **a** Pretreatment with good collateral artery. **b** After systemic thrombolysis with streptokinase (operator, Prof. Martin) no further occlusion, but long-distance stenoses with smooth surfaces. No good indication for balloon percutaneous transluminal angioplasty alone, but stent-assisted

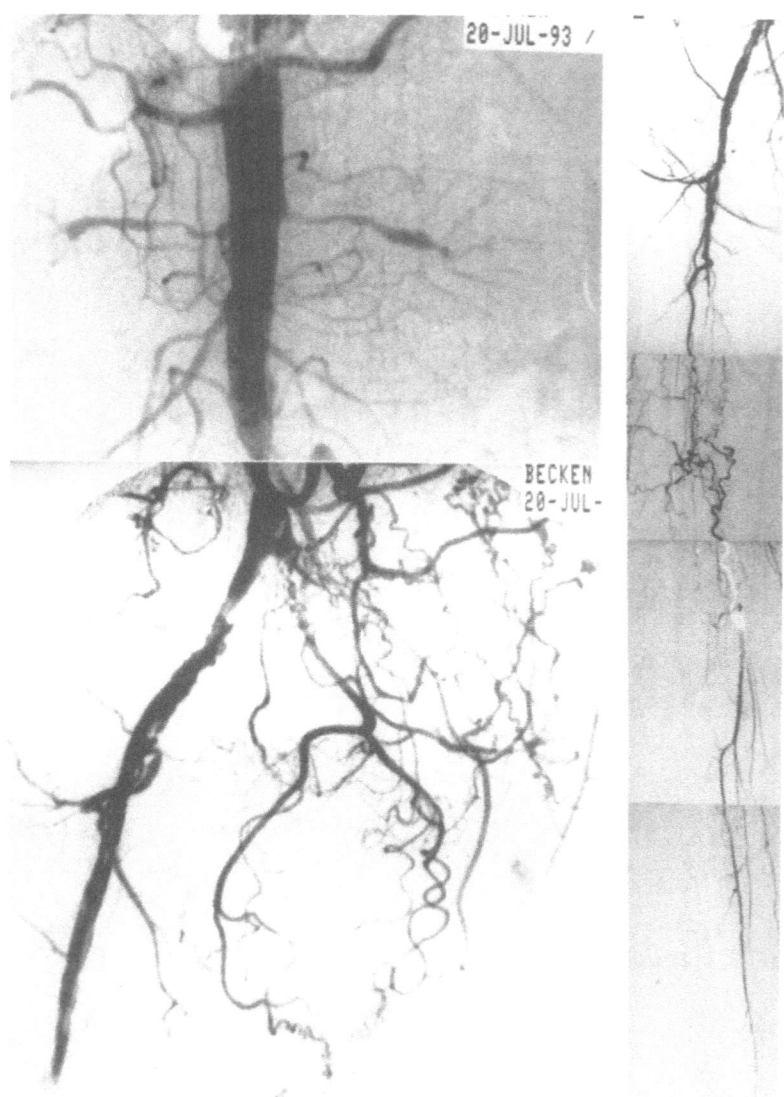

Fig. 30.11 a,b. Aortobiiliac obliterations after amputation of left leg (65-year-old man). Risk factors: heavy smoking, arterial hypertension, diabetes mellitus. a Common external iliac artery occlusion on the left, irregular iliac artery stenoses on the right; aortic stenoses, bilateral renal artery stenoses. b Digital subtraction angiography of the right leg with superficial femoral artery occlusion, good run-off

amination from the renal artery level to the lower leg arteries prior to planning surgical or interventional treatment (Loose and Loose 1976; Raithel 1987; Vollmar 1996).

This was already a state-of-the-art standard both at the time of translumbar aortography with table-top shifting (Wenz 1972; Zeitler 1974; Wenz and Beduhn 1975; Van Dongen 1976; Loose and Loose 1976) and arterial digital subtraction angiography (DSA) with step-by-step documentation. In view of the amount of contrast agent required and the relatively high radiation exposure in the abdominal and pelvic vascular territory, one or other part of the arterial system can be spared whenever the clinical situation is clear with duplex sonography or magnetic resonance angiography (MRA). With fully automatic shifting of the imaging system, however, arterial DSA nowadays also enables visualization of the entire vascular system. Another significant advance is the possibility of producing contrast-enhanced MR angiograms by table-top shifting. If the obliterations have not developed uniformly on the two sides, the velocity of the blood flow is different on either side. For this reason, a serial examination is necessary, sometimes also including a second contrast medium injection. With MRA, this problem has been reduced, but other technical problems still exist (see Chap. 12).

Isolated external iliac artery occlusions, or extensive stenoses (Fig. 30.12), are less common than occlusions of the common iliac artery. In the differential diagnosis, it should be borne in mind that congenital hypoplasia of the external iliac artery may also exist, a situation whereby the internal iliac, obturator, and inferior gluteal arteries bridge collaterals to the thigh (VAN DONGEN 1976). Such conditions, however, are mainly taken into consideration in children, not in the adult patient examined for suspected arteriosclerotic degenerative vascular disease. In the case of asymmetric obliterations of the iliac and femoropopliteal arteries, reliable of the occlusion in a distal or proximal direction should also be taken into consideration, and which may typically occur following operations including vascular reconstruction, as well as after amputation (VOLLMAR 1996).

In external iliac artery occlusions, the angiographically identifiable collateral circulation can only be demonstrated via the internal iliac arteries.

Independent of this, however, it can be assumed that there is also a supply over collaterals from a cranial direction via the caudal epigastric and circumflex iliolumbar arteries, counterbalancing perfusion in the leg.

A smooth, or concave, end of the occlusion indicates that there is a fresh, nonorganized thrombus (see Fig. 30.12), as demonstrated by the result of systemic lysis which achieved a complete restitution of the external iliac artery, whereas on the side with convex ends of the occlusion, lysis is only partially successful. Stenoses distal of the end of the occlusion, however, can also be fresh parietal thrombus.

All these fine morphological distinctions need to be taken into account both in the angiographic interpretation and in interdisciplinary discussions, to

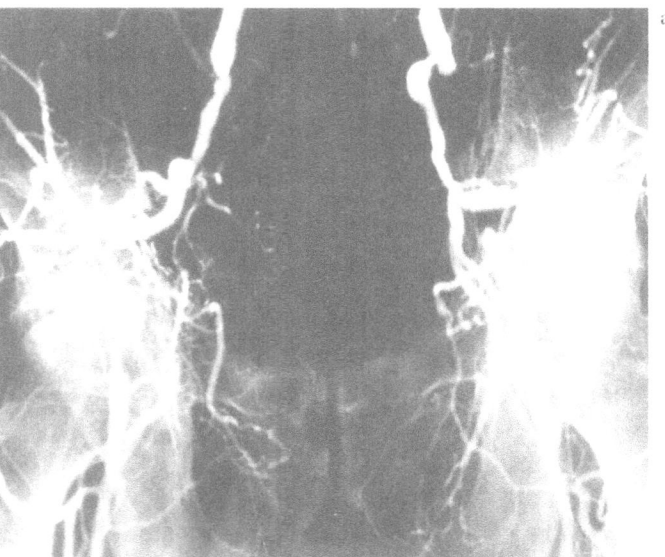

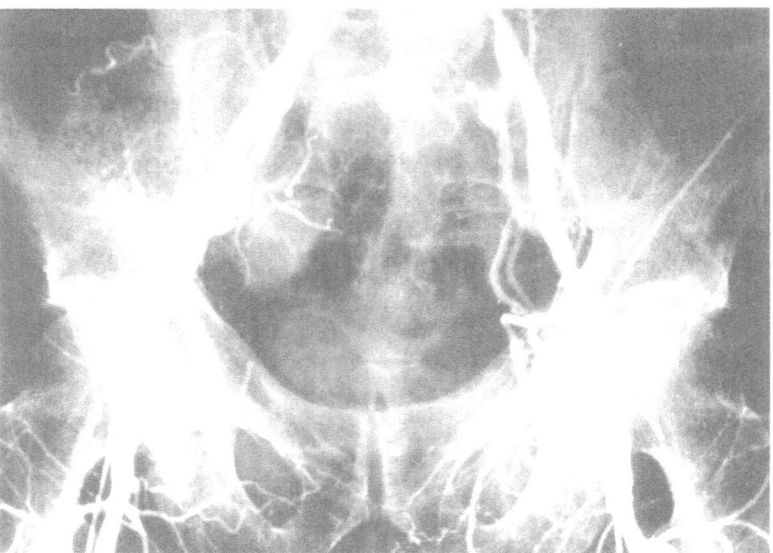

Fig. 30.12 a,b. Bilateral iliac artery occlusion (type V according to WELLAUER (1957)]. **a** Pretreatment. **b** After systemic thrombolysis (operator, Prof. Martin)

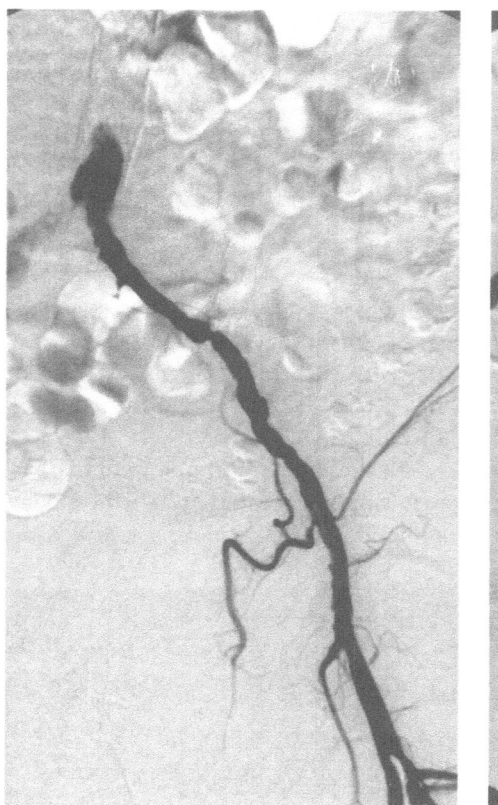 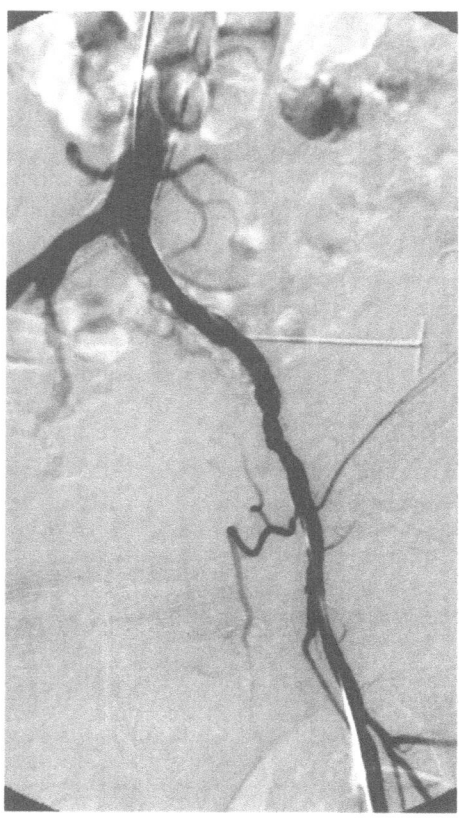

Fig. 30.13 a,b. Balloon angioplasty of an iliac artery stenosis. Additionally existing occlusion of internal iliac artery and superficial artery with collateral circulation from the deep femoral artery. **a** Digital subtraction angiography (DSA). Retrograde contrast medium injection through a vascular 5-F sheath. **b** DSA. Successful balloon angioplasty, small internal dissection. This is the controversial situation: Stenting or not? We did not stent! We treated with heparin for 3 days and later with ASA 100. Follow-up controls indicate stenting in restenoses of over 50% and if the documented ankle/brachial index has worsened by 0.2. In all other situations, further conservative treatment is recommended

jointly establish an optimum therapeutic concept suited to the individual situation (HEYDEN et al. 1980; ZEITLER et al. 1987). Regardless of all recommendations, establishing a diagnosis and treatment protocol is an individual problem, particular to each patient.

The variety of iliac artery stenoses, short or long-segmental (Fig. 30.15), can be the result of formation of arteriosclerosis, poststenotic turbulent flow, as well as petering-out flow distal of an aneurysmatic or dilated artery in a proximal direction (see Fig. 30.14). Table 30.1 shows the distribution of arterial stenoses and occlusions of the aortoiliac arteries, as detected in 50 patients with 98 obliterations of the pelvic arteries who were continuously followed up. Of these, 22 were occlusions and 76 stenoses in the region of the iliac arteries. This is attributable to the changed situation, i.e., angiography being associated with an essentially lower risk than 30 years ago, and the opportunities offered by interventional radiology in the form of active, recanalizing treatment. One third each of the occlusions were located close to the aortic

bifurcation in the common iliac artery, in the external iliac artery, and occlusions of the complete axis, including the common plus external iliac arteries. Distribution among the stenoses varies considerably. The most common type of angiographically identified stenoses in the region of the iliac arteries were found in the common iliac artery and the aortic bifurcation (41%), followed by stenoses of the external iliac artery, for the most part located closely distal of the branching point of the internal iliac artery, or at the level of the branching point. Complete occlusions of the axis of the common and external iliac arteries were a relatively rare finding (17%), and occlusions of the common femoral artery were rather the exception in this population.

This distribution explains the increase in patients receiving interventional treatment for pelvic artery obliterations. The latter are mainly single or double stenoses, uni- or bilateral. Occlusions, in contrast, were treated primarily with catheters in significantly lower numbers. In such cases, either the pull-through approach (GINSBURG et al. 1989) or local,

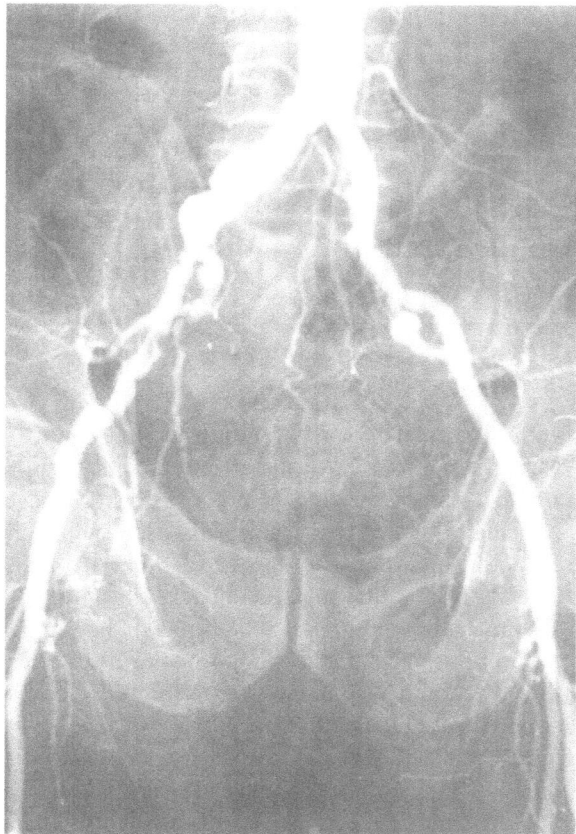

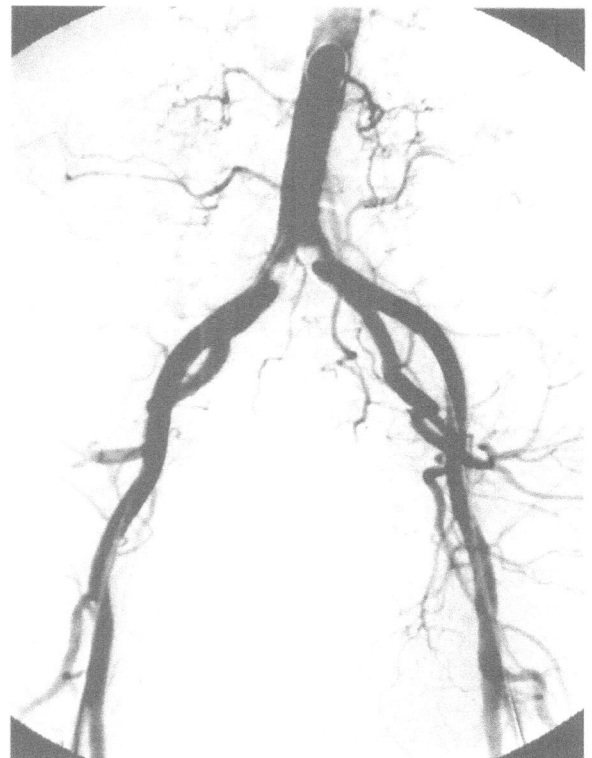

Fig. 30.14. Long-distance stenoses of the right external iliac artery and aneurysmatic formation of the right common iliac artery [type VI according to Wellauer (1957)]

catheter-guided thrombolysis, followed by balloon angioplasty and stent implantation, is appropriate. An alternative, although performed, in only a few centers, can be systemic thrombolysis, completed by balloon angioplasty.

In recent years, the use of interventional percutaneous therapies also for isolated iliac occlusions has been justified to an increasing extent, since even after only partial success, stent implantation can improve the hemodynamic outcome, confirmed by angiography (Richter et al. 1991; Palmaz and Encarnacion 1994; Rousseau et al. 1996; Strecker et al. 1996; Tetteroo et al. 1996; Vorwerk and Günther 1997; Raza et al. 1998). Also, with less important long-term results following stent placement in iliac arteries (Strunk et al. 1994), an improvement could be observed following a second intervention (Henry et al. 1995). Similarly, the combined techniques of PTA and vascular surgery (Walker et al. 1991) can improve primary patency over years, which is recommended in all patients with critical limb ischemia.

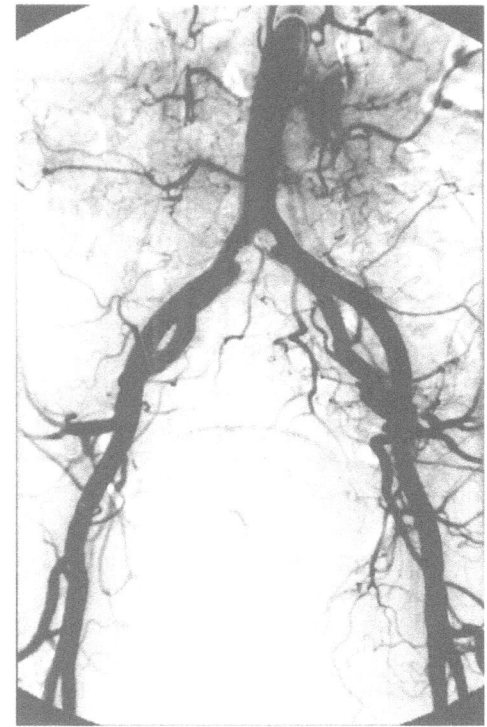

Fig. 30.15 a,b. Aortobiiliac bifurcational stenoses. **a** Digital subtraction angiography (DSA) after bilateral retrograde guiding with the glidewire Naviguide. **b** DSA after bilateral application of two Memotherm nitinol stents, still small residual stenoses. Follow-up treatment with heparin for 3 days followed by ASA 100 three times daily

Table 30.1. Incidence of aortoiliac obliterations; 50 patients (angiographic studies) within 3 months

Number of stenoses (%)		Localization	Number of occlusions (%)	
3	(4)	Aorta	2	
5	⟩ (41)	Bifurcation	–	⟩ (27)
26		Common iliac artery	4	
23	(30)	External iliac artery	7	(32)
6	(8)	Common femoral artery	1	(5)
13	(17)	Combined common + external iliac artery	8	(36)
76	(100)	in summary	22	(100)

Bilateral obliteration in 19 patients

30.4
Classification of Aortoiliac Occlusive Disease

The clinical situation of patients with POVD was first classified by Fontaine et al. in 1954 into four stages, which can only be defined by the clinical situation. The progress of vascular surgery has meant that, both in view of the indication for or contraindication to surgery, and in the interests of a clear delimitation of a conservative therapy, stage II was divided into stages IIa and IIb (moderate or significant claudication). Likewise, it seemed useful to divide stage IV into a stage with mild and severe necrosis, as well as good perfusion, or lacking perfusion detectable on Doppler examination (Cachovan 1991; Vollmar 1996).

Criticism on the Fontaine classification (Andreani et al. 1991; Cachovan 1991) resulted in its modification (see Table 2.2). This revised classification, which largely corresponded to the European Consensus Document (Dormandy and Stock 1990), then served as a guideline to making the indication for either operative reconstructive vascular surgery, conservative, or interventional treatment. Durham and Rutherford (1994) recommended modern definitions of the different categories of acute and chronic limb ischemia, determined by means of a clinical examination, ankle pressure measurement, and treadmill criteria. In several points, such as the differentiation between claudication (moderate and severe) and peripheral necrosis, similar ideas are part of the modified Fontaine classification.

The categories according to treadmill criteria are more complex, as not only the additional use of ankle blood pressure, but also the result of treadmill testing are included. These categories are demonstrated in Table 30.2 (see also Table 5.10). The increasing elderly population suffering from POVD,

with additional diseases of the hip and knee joint and vertebral column, however, is one patient group in whom treadmill testing is not possible. However, patients with cerebrovascular disease, hemiplegia, and other neurological diseases also have to be excluded from this method of classification. For scientific study programs, this means that an important number of patients cannot be enrolled. Therefore, the modified Fontaine classification which can be applied without treadmill testing is useful in all patients. Without question, the problem of comparing different types of treatment, or results obtained in different departments, requires a highly precise definition of the criteria for enrolment and evaluation.

Important are the outcome-endpoints, which were also defined by Durham and Rutherford in 1994 (Table 30.3). Improvement by at least one category of ischemia defines a successful treatment result, regardless of the therapy used. The definition is as follows: +1 denotes minimal improvement, +3 marked improvement. Given this, the definition of primary success and later deterioration (over a defined period of time) is very important. We determined a triple definition for several prospective studies:

1. The angiographic result should demonstrate a residual stenosis smaller than 20%. Biplane documentation in iliac artery stenoses provides a more precise definition than an anteroposterior projection alone.
2. The hemodynamic definition by checking the ABI: The treatment is successful if the ABI is above 0.8, or has at least improved by 0.15 compared to before treatment, or by 0.1 if obliterations in the femoropopliteal arteries are present in addition to the iliac artery obliterations (Zeitler and Oldendorf 1996) (GAMS Study Protocol and Report).
3. Improvement by at least one Fontaine class or Rutherford category.

Table 30.2. Rutherford's clinical categories

O	Asymptomatic
I and II	Mild or moderate claudication
III	Severe claudication
IV	Rest pain
V	Minor tissue loss
VI	Major tissue loss

Table 30.3. Rutherford's scale for gauging degree of improvement, recommended for scientifically controlled studies

Grading	Definition	Results
+1	Increase of ABI by more than 0.1 No categoric improvement	Minimally improved
+2	ABI increased by more than 0.1, and improvement by at least one category Still symptomatic	Moderately improved
+3	ABI increased above 0.9 Symptoms gone or markedly improved	Markedly improved

ABI, ankle/brachial index.

In patients with claudication, improvement in the painless walking distance, under metronome control or by treadmill exercise, can be controlled from the third day after PTA, or after removal of the compression bandage at the earliest. Definite improvements in walking distance can be determined after 1 month. Subsidence of pain at rest can be determined during the first 2–3 days, but is often observed immediately after angioplasty. The improvement in the clinical stage of patients with necrosis, however, cannot be defined earlier than from the third month following the intervention.

When comparing these improvement criteria with those of the Rutherford scale, a clear convergence of the two standpoints becomes obvious. Independent of this, it should be stressed that the results of vascular surgical therapy of *occlusions* of the aortoiliac arteries are at least equal to, or even better than, those of percutaneous interventions as regards patency, as well as the clinical situation. The long-term results of vascular surgery are better, as has been demonstrated in many studies, with a lethality of 1%–2% over the last decade (EDWARDS and LYONS 1959; Voss et al. 1980; RAITHEL 1987; VOLLMAR 1996).

In patients with isolated aortoiliac obliterations, the published results of bypass surgery or thromboendarterectomy have demonstrated 5-year patency rates of 90%–93%. However, following combined treatment of iliac and femoropopliteal obliterations with the "Triaden operation", the 5-year result was 73%, and after a combined operation with aortoiliac and femoropopliteal bypass, only 39% (Voss et al. 1980; VOLLMAR 1996). The principles of surgery for combined arterial obliterations as defined by surgeons (HEYDEN et al. 1980) has meanwhile restricted surgery to the treatment of single obliterations, and are more limited to exclusive obliterations untreatable with interventional techniques.

In patients with focal stenoses, in contrast, the primary results are equally good, and despite shorter long-term patency, the patient suffers no loss in quality of life. Possible restenosis can be treated again with angioplasty using balloon angioplasty, or

additional stent implantation, and even if critical limb ischemia should develop after a further period of time, the latter can be managed without problems by vascular surgery. The advantages of angioplasty in carefully established indications include lower invasiveness, shorter hospitalization times, the possibility of performing out-patient procedures, the lack of general anesthesia or intensive-care, and no scaring, thus precluding the problems of scar healing and wound infection. Large scars can interfere with a patient's professional life, and influence his attitute towards his disease. In view of these aspects, and the complex problem of a precise definition of comparable collectives, it is of little use to discuss extensively the advantages of vascular surgery versus those of angioplasty in all its modifications. The majority of focal lesions, and 85% of patients with intermittent claudication, have good chances of successful percutaneous treatment, whereas other, more severe types of long-distance multiple stenoses and occlusions are still clear indications for vascular surgery. Only if there is a general contraindication to vascular surgery, or the latter should be contraindicated because of a special situation at that time, and if the prospects of vascular surgery to prevent leg amputation do not seem promising, the various types of interventional radiology (GAINES 1989; GINSBURG et al. 1989; PICUS 1994; RAZA et al. 1998; STECKMEIER et al. 1995), including clot lysis, aspiration thrombectomy, Rotablator recanalization, balloon angioplasty, and stent implantation, can be helpful tools. The risk of complications is generally less with these techniques compared to surgery in risk patients (GALLINO et al. 1984; LONG et al. 1991; RICHTER et al. 1991; JOHNSTON 1993; PICUS 1994; ROUSSEAU et al. 1996).

ROTH et al. (1988) reported a mortality rate of 0.05% out of 2054 angioplasties of the pelvic and leg arteries in patients younger than 65 years of age, and a mortality rate of 0.3% out of 614 patients older than 65 years of age who received the same treatment (not including catheter lysis). Complications requiring surgery were also observed more frequently in older patients (0.5% versus 0.05%). According to the German registry of interventional radiology data, major complications necessitating surgery, and the mortality rate, were higher in patients undergoing intraarterial thrombolysis than those who underwent a simple balloon technique or stent-assisted angioplasty.

30.5
Iliac Artery Interventions

30.5.1
Balloon Angioplasty

In the European Consensus Document (DORMANDY and STOCK 1990), PTA of iliac artery stenoses is described as a successful method (in up to 90%), with a 3-year patency rate of 85%. PTA is therefore recommended in patients with iliac artery stenosis and short occlusions, and in patients with critical limb ischemia, following interdisciplinary discussion with the vascular surgeon and angiologist.

Table 30.1 shows that the majority of iliac artery diseaes in developed countries are iliac artery stenoses. Whereas isolated unilateral stenoses of the common and external iliac arteries can be treated after ipsilateral retrograde catheterization, problems arise in patients with aortobifurcational stenoses, or stenoses close to the inguinal ligament (JOHNSTON et al. 1987; BECKER et al. 1990; KASHDAN et al. 1992; PALMAZ et al. 1992; DYET et al. 1993; PICUS 1994; ROUSSEAU et al. 1996).

While the kissing-balloon technique is indicated in patients with bifurcational stenoses (see Fig. 30.5)

following retrograde catheterization from both groins, and the bifurcation can be stabilized by stent application from both sides (Fig. 30.8), there are alternatives in bilateral or unilateral iliac artery stenoses and occlusions, as well as contralateral stenoses. In contralateral stenoses, retrograde catheterization of the stenosed iliac artery is the easy wire-loop (GAINES 1989), or pull-through (GINSBURG et al. 1989) technical way. Bilateral stenoses or multilateral occlusions can be recanalized using the cross-over, techniques. Local thrombolysis, in combination with stent-assisted balloon angioplasty, is the alternative treatment for iliac artery occlusions. If the guidewire, with the help of a Cobra or sidewinder catheter, succeeds in passing the total obstruction, a small-diameter catheter with a tapered tip can easily follow. After successful passage of the occluded area, exchange for a stronger guidewire (Teflon-coated safety-J guidewire, or Amplatz guidewire) ensures that the balloon catheter can follow. Primary dilatation only up to a reduced diameter (6–7 mm) prepares the passage for safe stent application. While the Wallstent and other self-expanding stents can be implanted easily from the contralateral side, the application of balloon-expandable stents is predominantly performed from the ipsilateral side.

Therefore, in addition to contralateral puncture following successful recanalization of segmental occlusions, additional retrograde catheterization on the formerly occluded iliac artery side can follow. This pull-through approach (GINSBURG et al. 1989), or a catheter guidewire loop, can help reduce complications of local thrombolysis.

The cross-over technique (BACHMANN et al. 1979; ROTH 1978; ROTH and CAPPIUS 1983) is the preferred method to treat contralateral iliac artery stenoses, and stenoses in the distal external iliac

Table 30.4. Long-term patency rate (%) results after balloon percutaneous transluminal angioplasty of iliac artery stenoses

Patients (n)	Patency rate (%)	Follow-up (years)	Reference
200	85	5	SCHNEIDER et al. 1982
131	87	5	GALLINO et al. 1984
226 Fontaine Class II	89	5	ZEITLER 1985
96 Fontaine Class III/IV	65	5	ZEITLER 1985
176	87	5	TEGTMEYER et al. 1985
148 TFI 72[a]	49[b]	3	ZEITLER and OLDENDORF 1996
150 Placebo 67[b]	38[b]	3	ZEITLER and OLDENDORF 1996
667	57	5	JOHNSTON 1993
124	74[b]	4	RICHTER et al. 1995, personal communication

[a] 36-Month patency. Definition according to protocol (Rutherford +2 and +3 included).
[b] 36-Month patency. Definition according to Rutherford (+3).
TFI, thrombocyte function inhibitors.

and common femoral arteries. The primary results following dilatation of iliac artery stenoses using the ipsilateral and cross-over technique are equally good (87% versus 84%) (ROTH and CAPPIUS 1983; ROTH et al. 1988).

In 85 obliterations of the common femoral, and 77 stenoses of the deep femoral artery. ROTH et al. (1988) were able to achieve a primarily successful dilatation with clinical improvement in 75% and 88% of patients, respectively, using the cross-over technique. Only 1% of patients suffered a major complication requiring surgical repair. In early publications on angioplasty of the pelvic arteries (ZEITLER et al. 1971a; PORSTMANN 1973; DOTTER et al. 1974; VAN ANDEL and KREPEL 1979; COLAPINTO et al. 1982; RING et al. 1982), attempts to recanalize iliac artery occlusions were initially successful in no more than 30%–40% of cases.

According to publications by TEGTMEYER et al. (1979) and COLAPINTO et al. (1981), attempts at percutaneous recanalization of occlusions, as well as at angioplasties of extensive, long-segmental stenoses, increased in number, which resulted first in a deterioration in both the primary and long-term results. Only the use of combined therapies, such as intrathrombotic thrombolysis (MCNAMARA and BOMBERGER 1986), followed by balloon angioplasty, achieved some improvement in contrast to systemic thrombolysis, which had until then been a primary therapy (see Figs. 30.10, 30.12). The combination of thrombolysis, balloon angioplasty, and stent implantation was capable of achieving better technical primary success rates (VORWERK and GÜNTHER 1992; ROUSSEAU et al. 1996), which, together with the implantation of stents, can also yield satisfactory long-term results (ZEITLER et al. 1995; VORWERK and GUENTHER 1997). An undoubted fact, however, is that mainly short occlusions of the common or external iliac arteries are acceptable indications for interventional therapy, whereas unilateral long-segmental obliterations can be successfully managed by the various vascular surgical techniques (VOSS et al. 1980; VOLLMAR 1996). But also the combination of angioplasty of stenoses on one arterial axis, and femorofemoral bypassing to the totally occluded contralateral axis, can be an efficient therapy with good long-term results, without the need for a major transperitoneal intervention.

Without the use of stent grafts, catheter therapy of extensive iliac artery obliterations, such as those demonstrated in Fig. 30.10, is in my opinion not indicated. Even though – as in this case – a limited improvement was achieved by thrombolysis, since

vascular surgical treatment was contraindicated, this was disputable on initial development of systemic thrombolysis. In general, however, such conditions, particularly in patients with critical limb ischemia, are a clear indication for vascular surgical therapy, including the minimally invasive transfemoral application of endografts.

Angioplasty of focal unilateral iliac artery stenoses is the ideal opportunity for physicians trained in angiography to begin with angioplasty as a therapeutic method, under the guidance, of course, of an expert. Puncture is performed in the same way, retrogradely, which the operator is familiar with, but the critical point is to safely cross the stenosis and to avoid any dissection by the guidewire or catheter. This first step often causes dissections and the formation of two lumina. DSA has facilitated a safe passage of stenoses using the roadmapping technique and a contrast agent, and of guiding catheters through the placed vascular sheath, followed by a Terumo guidewire or a flexible-tip guidewire.

If this procedure is successfully mastered with the help of a contrast agent injected into the aorta, the aim is to place the balloon catheter precisely and to use the balloon catheter of the appropriate diameter and length, selected on the basis of previous angiographic findings. It is recommendable to use a short balloon catheter, as this best transmits the pressure on the stenosis, resulting in dilatation, and in focal lesions only a small segment of the neighboring arterial wall is mechanically traumatized. We prefer the 2-cm balloon with a diameter of 8–9 mm to treat stenoses. We use the 6-mm balloon of 4–6 cm in length after recanalization and before stent application.

In the region of the aortoiliac arteries, it is useful to determine the arterial pessure gradient before

Table 30.5. Results of balloon- and stent-assisted percutaneous transluminal angioplasty (PTA) in a prospective multicenter trial (RICHTER et al. 1999, personal communication)

Number	Months	Cumulative success rate		Number
		Balloon	Stent	
145	0–1	88.9%	98.6%	141
33	48–60	60.5[a]	79.3[a]	52
36	48–60	62.6[b]	75.7[b]	44

[a] Primary morphologic success, angiographically determined lumen >50%.
[b] Clinical success, improvement by at least one clinical Fontaine class (Rutherford +2).

and after balloon dilatation (ZEITLER et al. 1971a,b; KAUFMANN et al. 1982). Also, new results have demonstrated that angiography alone is inadequate to diagnose residual stenoses. Stent application is indicated in all patients with pressure gradients above 10 mmHg (TETTEROO et al. 1996; STRECKER et al. 1996; RICHTER et al. 1991; ZEITLER et al. 1995).

Angioplasty is successful whenever the pressure gradient drops to less than 8 mmHg. The procedure always causes injury to the intima in the form of a dissection or small intimal rupture. It is important, then, that the intima adheres again to the wall with the blood flow, not forming an intimal flap. If the latter should happen, larger dissections, bleeding into the arterial wall, or a collapsing artery may be the result, requiring correction. We have observed this more frequently after use of a long, rather than a short balloon catheter. This explains why, after dilatation of long iliac artery lesions, extensive intimal dissections, which absolutely require subsequent stent implantation, occur more often.

30.5.1.1
Results of Treatment

The technical primary success rate in focal iliac unilateral stenoses is nearly 100%, decreasing to 88% in bilateral stenoses using the cross-over technique. Adjunctive medication corresponds to that described in Chap. 6. Before and after angioplasty, ASA 100 once a day, 5000 IU of heparin administered during the procedure, and low-molecular heparin (e.g., Fraxiparin Sanofi 0.4, Winthrop, Munich) for the subsequent 3 days is our general recommendation. Following treatment of iliac artery occlusions and/or stent placement, similar to post-stent-assisted PTCA, treatment with the ADP-antagonist Clopidogrel (Iscover, Bristol-Myers Squibb, Munich; Plavix, Sanofi, Munich), 75 mg daily as secondary prevention is recommended.

Despite the varying definitions of success in the publications, PICUS (1994) reported a 5-year patency rate of 72%, ranging from 30% to 90%, based on over 6000 iliac artery angioplasties. The marked variations are certainly not only attributable to varying technical skill, the use of the appropriate balloon catheter (we, for example, prefer the non-compliant balloon catheters for iliac artery stenoses), and the additional peri- and postprocedural care. The highly varying results in the literature can more likely be explained on the one hand by the inclusion of short and long-segmental stenoses – without differentiat-ing between stenoses and occlusions – as well as by the inclusion of patients with different clinical conditions in the collective to be studied.

Table 30.4 shows a selection of published results. The 5-year patency rate of 57% published by JOHNSTON (1993) is one of the least favorable results, representing a long period of time with varying stages of development of the angioplasty instrumentation.

When comparing the results achieved in iliac artery stenoses and in patients in the stages of claudication to those in patients with rest pain and gangrene, it transpires that under these conditions, a 5-year patency rate of no more than 65% in the one collective, while a 5-year-patency rate of 89% in the primarily more promising collective with focal lesions were achievable. An aspect of great importance is the follow-up treatment after successful angioplasty. It should not only consist in medication with thrombocyte aggregation inhibitors, anticoagulants, or other medication, but rather specifically include the treatment of risk factors. The patient should be motivated to give up smoking, existing arterial hypertension should be strictly treated, and walking exercise with the achievable pain-free walking distances should be documented in writing. Thus, patient guidance forms a valuable part of the whole treatment. Within this framework, regular follow-up-controls including talks between the patient and physician, supervision of the angiologic parameters, and determination of the ABI, should motivate the patient to cooperate. If necessary, a duplex sonography to inspect the site where angioplasty has been performed is not only important for the early detection of possible restenoses, but also to win the patient's confidence. The foremost aim of angioplasty for aortoiliac obliterations, as after operative therapy (thromboendarterectomy, bypass surgery with alloplastic endoprostheses) is, in addition to a hemodynamic improvement in peripheral flow, not only prolonged life expectancy, but also an improvement in the quality of life and the avoidance of amputation. For this reason, regular controls are important for the early detection of possible restenoses, or new stenoses at another location, which are then amenable to easily performed percutaneous therapy.

30.5.2
Stent Implantation

Among the great variety of metallic stents available (ADAM et al. 1997) (Tables 5.4 and 5.5, Chap. 5), the following have been widely employed in the extremity arteries:

- The balloon-expandable Palmaz stent in its primary form, and improved modifications
- The balloon-expandable Strecker stent made out of tantalum, and the improved version
- The self-expanding Wallstent, followed by the improved "Easy Wallstent"
- The self-expanding Nitinol stents produced by different manufacturers (Cragg Stent, Memotherm, Instent), and other companies.

Figure 30.16 demonstrates very clearly the different implications for results using the Strecker stent. Indications for stent implantation include: (a) Post-PTA dissections, (b) elastic recoil after PTA, (c) recanalization of iliac artery occlusions, and (d) subintimal guidance as a result of balloon PTA.

The role of stents in the prevention of restenosis after primarily successful PTA has been discussed controversially (REES 1994). The positive results obtained in several trials (RICHTER et al. 1991; PALMAZ et al. 1992; VORWERK and GUENTHER 1992; VORWERK et al. 1995; DYET et al. 1993; HENRY et al. 1995; SHAW 1996; STRECKER et al. 1996; RAZA et al. 1998) point to stent application to treat all restenoses.

Between 1990 and 1994, 46 patients received stents at the Nuremberg General Hospital for common iliac artery lesions, and 36 for external iliac artery lesions. Both the Strecker stent and the Wallstent were used (ZEITLER et al. 1995). In the area of stenoses in the aortic bifurcation (Fig. 30.8), and common iliac and external iliac arteries, technical and primary clinical success rates were 95% and 92%, respectively (Fig. 30.17). Similarly, in multiple and long lesions in the common and external iliac arteries, only in 80% could a primary successful result be achieved. According to the German registration of interventional radiologic interventions performed between 1990 and 1994, 886 patients received stents in the iliac arteries. The primary success rate was 89.5%, the complication rate 6.9%. The prospective results published by RICHTER et al. (1991) (Table 30.5) demonstrate the improved results of stent implantation.

In the literature (Table 30.6), stents in iliac arteries were implanted in more than 1800 patients, with a complication rate of 7%, and an 8% rate of restenoses. The average technical success after use in the common iliac artery was reported to be 95%, and 90% for the external iliac artery. Successful primary patency after common iliac artery stenting was reported to be 94%, and 88% after stenting in the external iliac artery (literature search "Medline").

The treatment of aortoiliac obliterations with stents is possible in the form of secondary stenting (Fig. 30.19): Stent application after balloon angioplasty, or with primary stenting, i.e., implantation of the stent after successful guiding of the obstruction. In most situations, the homolateral retrograde application of stents through vascular sheaths is used in the treatment of iliac artery obliterations after dissection (Fig. 30.20) or unsuccessful balloon angioplasty, in addition to single-segmental iliac artery occlusion. The contralateral approach is technically feasible, but necessitates crossing the aortic bifurcation. Whereas each type of stent can be used with the homolateral technique, the contralateral approach is less common with balloon-expandable than with self-expanding stents, such as the Easy Wallstent and the Nitinol stents.

The contralateral approach is preferred for the treatment of external iliac and common femoral artery obliterations. In several situations after a contralateral approach, it is necessary to catch the guidewire by a retrograde homolateral approach (GAINES 1989). This technique is useful in the same way as catching foreign bodies before extraction.

There are various types of intravascular retrieval instruments that can help achieve a perfect and successful contralateral angioplasty. Typical retriever sets can consist of a snare which forms a loop (Curry Intravascular Retriever Set, CRS 100), helical-loop baskets (Dotter Intravascular Retriever Set, DRS 100), and angled-wire loop retrievers (COOK: AWLR-6.3-100-25). In patients with no pulse in the groin, with scar formation, or with inflammation, the transbrachial or transaxillary approaches can be used not only for balloon dilatation, but also for stent implantation. Under these circumstances, a longer catheter and very long guidewires are necessary, and self-expanding stents with a very smooth surface on the long-distance passages best prevent complications such as embolization of atherosclerotic plaque or thrombus.

Whereas in balloon angioplasty the intention is to dilate with a catheter, the diameter of which is equal to or 1 mm greater than that of the free arterial lumen, in situations with primary stenting, the bal-

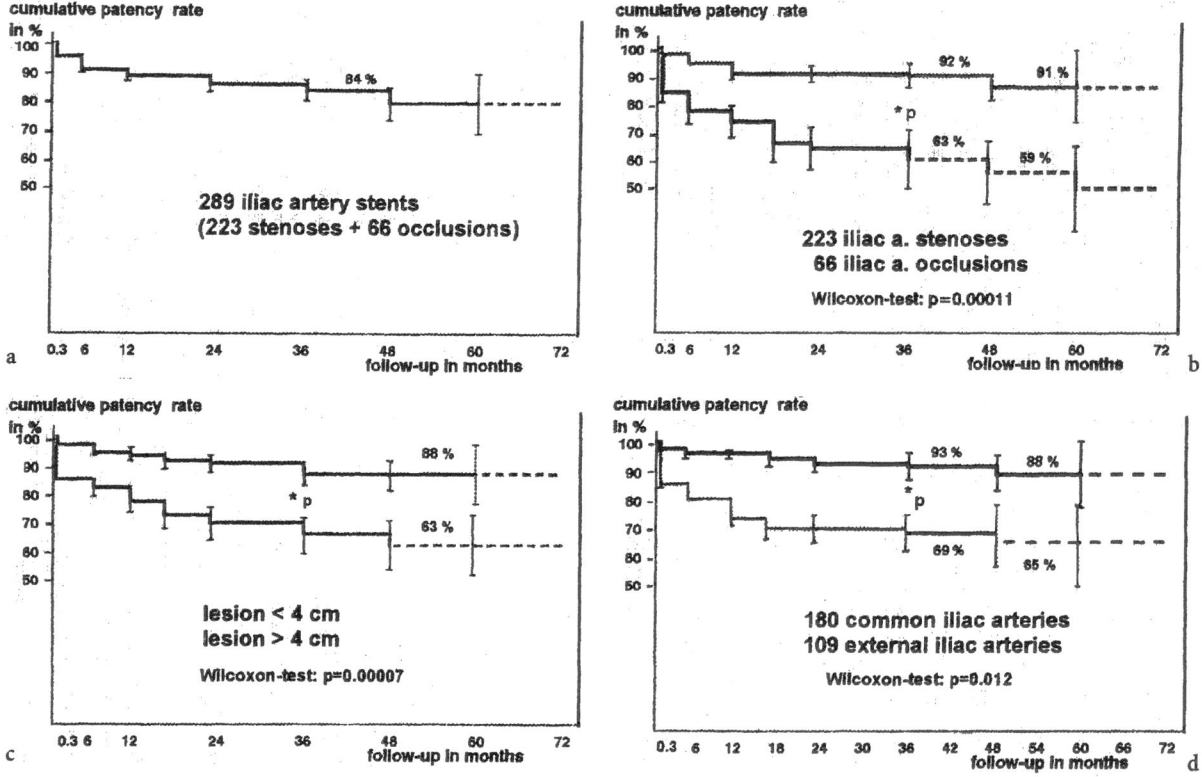

Fig. 30.16 a–d. Iliac artery stenting with tantalum Strecker stent. Primary cumulative patency rates assessed with the Kaplan-Meier life-table analyses with percentage standard error (*solid lines,* standard error less than 10%; *dotted lines,* standard error more than 10%). **a** Patency rates for 289 iliac artery stents. **b** Patency rates for 223 iliac artery stenoses and 66 iliac artery occlusions. **c** Patency rates for 189 short (<4 cm) and 100 long (>4 cm) lesions. **d** Patency rates for 180 common iliac arteries and 100 external iliac arteries after stent implantation. [From STRECKER et al. (1996)

loon dilatation only achieves a free passage for the folded stent, and secondary balloon dilatation is done after stent placement.

Angioplasty of iliac arteries, with balloons in stenotic obstructions, can be accomplished more precisely under manometric control, with a pressure of 5–8 atm. With greater pressure, the risk of dissection followed by collapsing arteries, is higher. Such cases are clear indications for stent application (Fig. 30.20).

In the treatment of iliac occlusions, a strong differentiation regarding history needs to be made. Acute occlusions – thrombotic or embolic – in standard situations, are indications for vascular surgery. Only if contraindications exist, or several technical, individual, or organizational problems in view of the vascular surgical treatment arise, is a combined angioplasty with local thrombolysis or systematic thrombolysis, together with stent application and balloon dilatation, possible. Whereas peripheral embolisms with normal groin pulse are excellent indications for percutaneous aspiration thromboembolectomy (PAT), or clot lysis, the primary

technique in patients suspected of having aortoiliac embolic occlusion is surgical embolectomy. If this should be contraindicated, percutaneous combined treatment, including immediate placement of endoprostheses, followed by balloon dilatation, is recommended (ROUSSEAU et al. 1996; LONG et al. 1991; VORWERK and GUENTHER 1997).

Among the different types of vascular stents, primary and long-term results have been published for the Palmaz stent, Wallstent, Strecker stent, and, with a smaller number of long-term results, the Memotherm stent (Table 30.6).

While an overview of the literature shows a remarkably wide range of long-term success rates varying between 30% and 90% (PICUS 1991; ROUSSEAU et al. 1996; VORWERK and GUENTHER 1997), it is important to bear in mind that different patient selection criteria exist. There is no question that primary technical and clinical success, in addition to the long-term patency rate, is different in the situation involving iliac artery focal stenoses, long-distance stenoses, or iliac artery occlusions (see Fig. 30.16). It has been demonstrated (STRECKER et al.

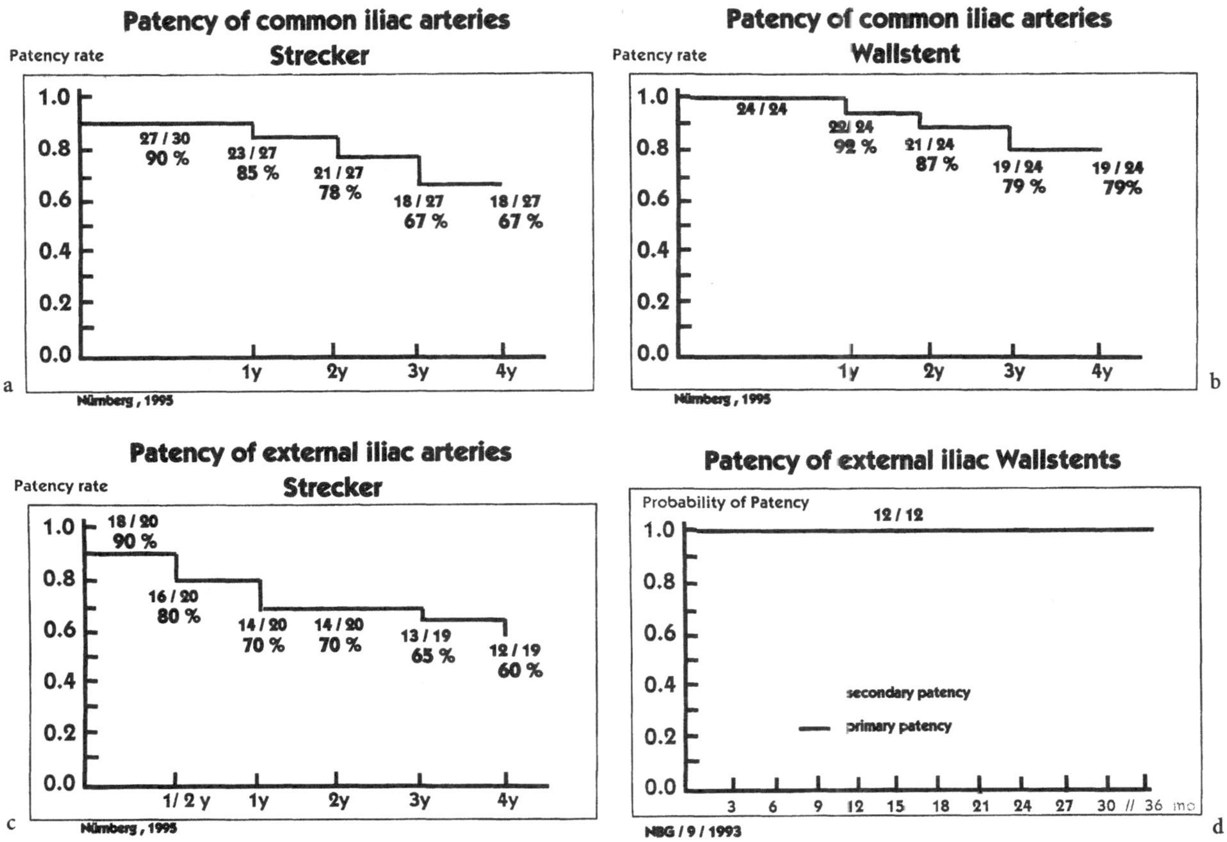

Patency of common iliac arteries
Strecker

Patency rate

```
1.0
     27/30
0.8  90%    23/27
             85%    21/27
0.6                 78%    18/27   18/27
                           67%     67%
0.4

0.2

0.0
            1y     2y     3y     4y
```
Nürnberg, 1995

a

Patency of common iliac arteries
Wallstent

Patency rate

```
1.0  24/24
             22/24   21/24
0.8          92%     87%    19/24   19/24
                           79%     79%
0.6

0.4

0.2

0.0
            1y     2y     3y     4y
```
Nürnberg, 1995

b

Patency of external iliac arteries
Strecker

Patency rate

```
1.0  18/20
     90%
0.8        16/20
           80%    14/20  14/20
0.6               70%    70%    13/19   12/19
                               65%     60%
0.4

0.2

0.0
         1/2 y  1y    2y     3y     4y
```
Nürnberg, 1995

c

Patency of external iliac Wallstents

Probability of Patency

```
          12/12
1.0

0.8

0.6

0.4       ----- secondary patency
          ___ primary patency
0.2

0.0
   3  6  9  12 15 18 21 24 27 30 // 36 mo
```
NBG / 9 / 1993

d

Fig. 30.17. Results of stent – assisted angioplasties in the iliac arteries, with STRECKER – and Wall stents differentiated into common and external iliac artery (According to ZEITLER and BEYER-ENKE 1997)

1996; HENRY et al. 1995; VORWERK and GUENTHER 1992) that the long-term result is better in obliterations with short focal lesions (<4 cm), and statistically less important in longer stenotic lesions. Also, in external iliac arteries, STRECKER et al. (1996) published better long-term results after 5 years, with a patency rate of 88% in common iliac artery stenoses, in contrast to 65% in external iliac arteries. In addition, the situation in the run-off vessels – which is the superficial femoral artery for iliac artery obliterations – also has an influence on the long-term outcome. Therefore, in most cases, the question of whether, in combined obliterations after treatment of iliac artery stenoses, a secondary treatment of the obliteration in the femoropopliteal arteries should follow, needs to be discussed. This can also be an angioplasty technique, or, in longer lesions, bypass surgery.

The problem of restenosis in iliac arteries is less significant than in the femoropopliteal and coronary arteries. One reason is the wider diameter of the artery and the high flow. Nevertheless, in about 20% of cases, follow-up controls are also very impor-

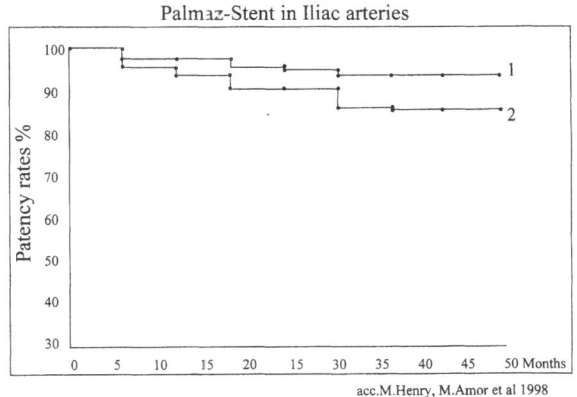

Palmaz-Stent in Iliac arteries

acc.M.Henry, M.Amor et al 1998

Fig. 30.18. Primary (*1*) and secondary (*2*) patency rates for 310 patients determined according to the KAPLAN-MEIER method. The *solid lines* indicate estimated patency rates with a standard deviation of less than 100%. Primary patency rate after 1 year, 94% ± 1.8, after 4 years, 86% ± 4.1; secondary patency rate after 1 year, 98% ± 1%, after 4 years 94% ± 2.8

tant after stent-assisted iliac artery angioplasty to prevent a total iliac artery thrombotic occlusion. Therefore, good cooperation between the patient and his family doctor is essential. In the case of recurrent claudication, with earlier pain onset or other symp-

Table 30.6. Long-term results after stent percutaneous transluminal angioplasty in iliac arteries

Stents	Patients (n)		Primary patency rate (%)	Follow-up (months)	Reference
Palmaz	486		Stenoses 78	48	PALMAZ et al. 1992
Strecker	239		Stenoses 83 Occlusions 76	48	STRECKER et al. 1996
Wallstent	221	118	Stenoses 82 103	48 Occlusions 78	VORWERK and GUENTHER 1997
Palmaz	123		Stenoses 92[a]	48	RICHTER et al. 1995, personal communication

[a]Patient population from one randomized trial. Patency definition, exclusion of >50% restenoses; clinical improvement, minimum 1 category (Rutherford +2).

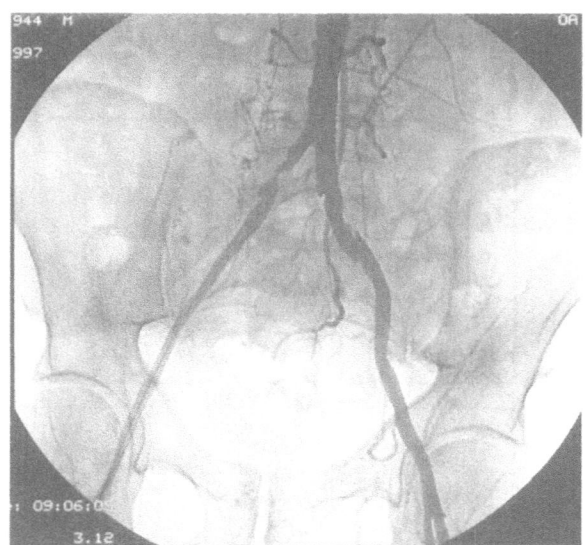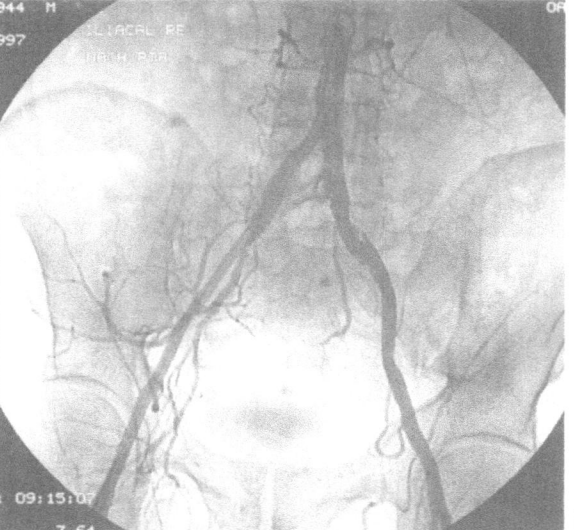

Fig. 30.19 a,b. Bilateral iliac artery stenoses, right common iliac artery stenoses, left iliac bifurcational stenoses. **a** Before balloon percutaneous transluminal angioplasty (PTA) on the right. **b** After PTA on the right: left iliac artery with small dissection, excellent indication for primary stenting

toms, an imaging control by means of duplex sonography or DSA is mandatory. Only in this way is timely stent-assisted balloon angioplasty, or secondary stent implantation, possible with a reduced complication risk. Furthermore, these conditions are the basis for early secondary treatment, if required, resulting in an improved secondary patency rate (see Fig. 30.18).

30.5.2.1
Complications

Complications may arise at the puncture site, or at the site where angioplasty was performed. At the puncture site, the complications are similar to those after most catheter techniques for diagnosis and treatment; these include hematomas, false aneurysms, and acute thrombotic occlusion. In non-coronary angioplasty procedures started in the groin, false aneurysms are the result in 0.3%–0.5%, while acute thrombosis in 1%–3% of patients was observed (PICUS 1994; PALMAZ et al. 1992; JOHNSTON 1993; ROUSSEAU et al. 1996; KADIR et al. 1982; JOHNSTON et al. 1987; HENRY et al. 1995). Major complications requiring subsequent vascular surgery have been published at rates of between 0.5% and 2.7% of cases. In recent years, the complication rate has decreased as a result of the use of small-diameter vascular sheaths and catheter instrumentation, in addition to improved control at the puncture site, made possible by puncture-hole closure systems (see Chap. 17).

The treatment of common femoral artery stenoses or occlusions (Fig. 30.21) with modern, small-diameter catheter systems can best be guided from

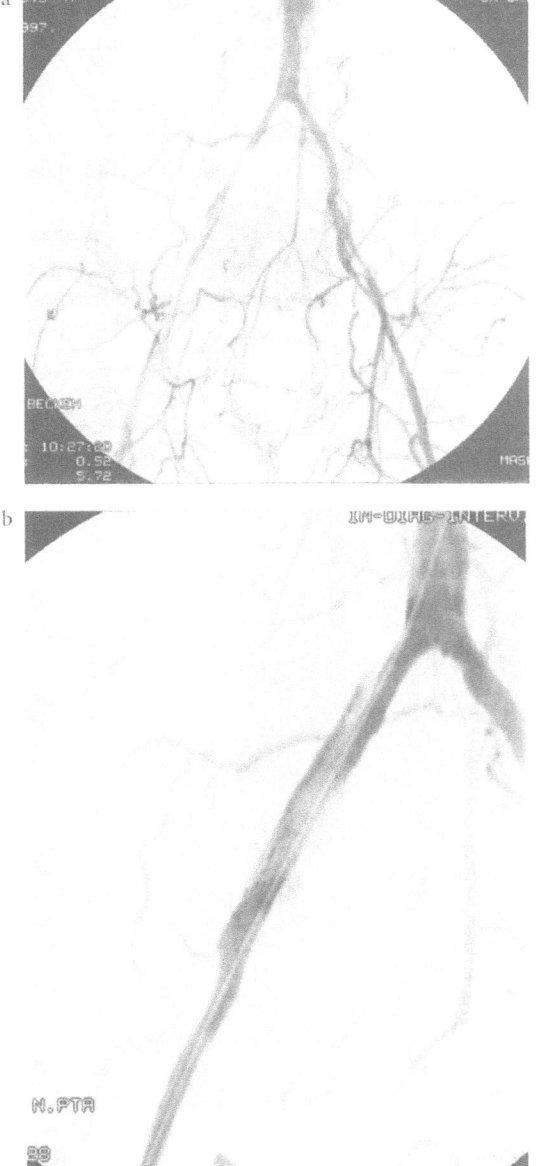

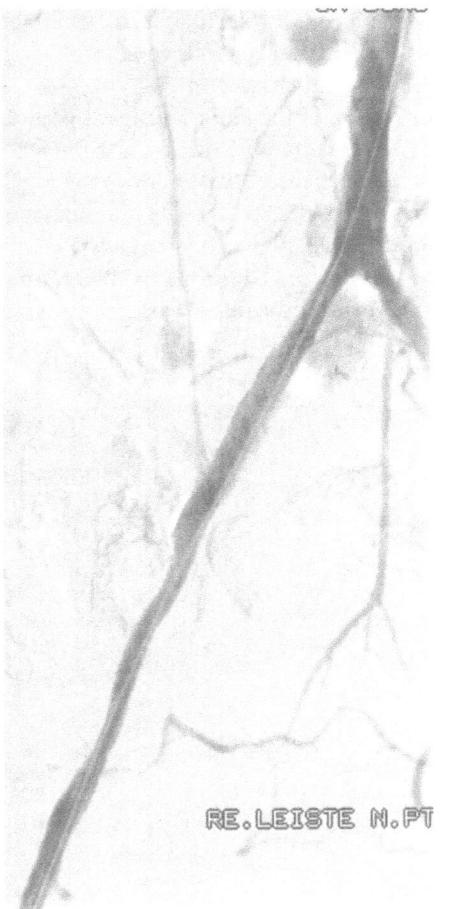

Fig. 30.20. a Long-distance common and external iliac artery stenoses on the right (52-year-old patient). **b** After balloon percutaneous transluminal angioplasty, long distance dissection. **c** Successful recanalization after application of two Wallstents

the contralateral side, but also retrogradely following transpopliteal access. If, however, and very seldom in this area, the indication for stent application arises because of dissection or collapsing arteries, contralateral application with Wallstents or self-expanding Nitinol stents should be preferred. But in most patients with stenoses or segmental occlusion, only balloon angioplasty, in experienced hands, is indicated. Otherwise, common femoral artery obliterations, in the same way as deep femoral artery obliterations, are preferred indications for vascular surgical treatment with patch plasty. Vascu-

lar surgeons emphasize that the deep femoral artery is the important collateral circulation to the whole leg.

30.5.2.2
Indications

The treatment of arterial vascular diseases in aortoiliac arteries has to be established within a framework interdisciplinary cooperation and taking the multiple forms of localization of generalized arteriosclerosis into consideration. Thus, it is not

solely a mechanical principle of treatment, but is composed of all of the following:
- Treatment of risk factors
- Motivation of the patient towards greater physical activity and suitable diet
- Active mechanical treatment of the local obliteration – focal ones preferably percutaneously, long-distance ones preferably surgically
- Meanwhile, or additionally, techniques of systemic or local thrombolysis are available

- Finally, long-term treatment to prevent restenosis, and stop the progression of arteriosclerosis.

This last measure is still under development with systemic or local application of different agents which provide the potential to reduce the natural progression.

In addition to the diagnostic modalities involving different imaging modalities, the interventional methods are a very important part of the treatment

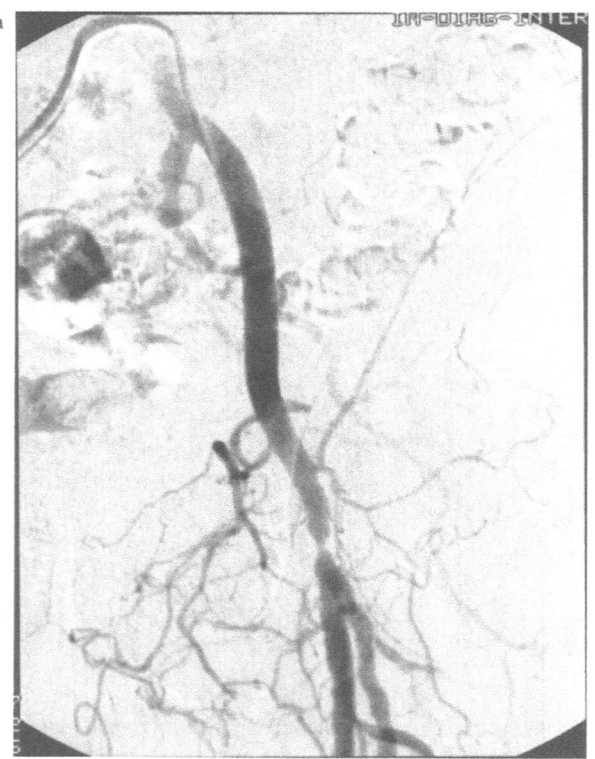
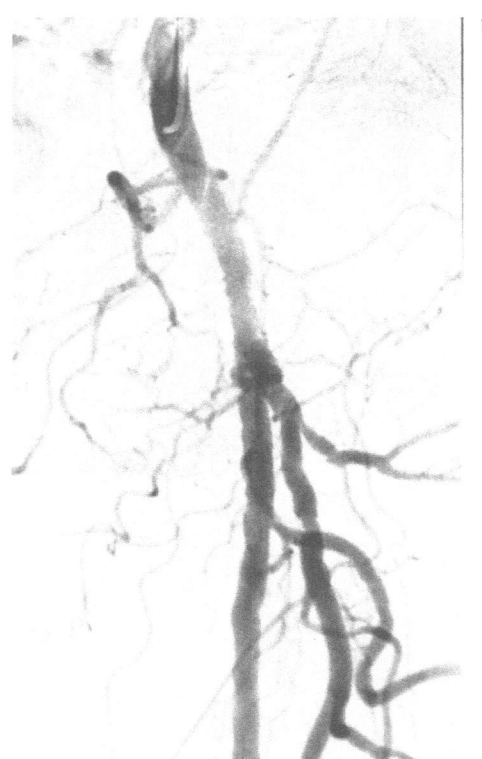

Fig. 30.21 a,b. Common femoral artery stenoses, left side. **a** Angiography before percutaneous transluminal angioplasty (PTA). **b** Digital subtraction angiography after contralateral PTA (85-year-old patient)

of iliac artery obliterations, whereas extensive diseases require the optimum surgical therapy. Some patients, following previous vascular surgery using iliofemoral or femoropopliteal bypass techniques, followed by local thrombosis or stenotic lesions at or behind the anastomosis, can be treated with reduced risk by balloon dilatation or local thrombolysis. This type of therapy, in qualified hands, carries low risk (SCHNEIDER et al. 1982; MCNAMARA et al. 1991; MAHLER 1990; PICUS 1994). The indications for the different types of interventional or surgical treatment are summarized in Chap. 5, Fig. 5.23.

The importance of balloon angioplasty, as well as stent implantation in pelvic arteries with focal and

short-segmental obliterations, is that these can be managed without general anesthesia. Only reduced prediagnostic measurements of the clotting parameters [partial thrombin time (PTT)] and Quick's test are required, and only in situations of thrombolysis is it important to measure thrombocyte counts and fibrinogen levels. Even critically ill patients can be treated under local anesthesia and follow-up in patient care is only necessary for 1–3 days in most cases. Patients with category-I and -II indications can very often even be treated with balloon angioplasty on an outpatient basis.

References

Adam A, Dondelinger RF, Mueller PR (1997) Textbook of metallic stents. Isis Medical Media, Oxford

Alexander K (1993) Typische Symptome bei arteriellen und venösen Durchblu-tungsstörungen. In: Alexander K (ed) Gefäkrankheiten. Urban and Schwarzenberg, Munich, pp 111–124

Andreani D, Bell P, Bollinger A, Breddin K, Cumberland D, Dormandy J, Fagrell B (1991) Second european consensus document on chronic critical leg ischemia. Circulation 84 (Suppl 4):··

Auster M, Kadir S, Mitchell SE, et al. (1984) Iliac artey occlusion: management with intrathrombus streptokinase infusion and angioplasty. Radiology 153:385–388

Bachman DM, Cassarella WJ, Sos TA (1979) Percutaneous iliofemoral angioplasty via the contralateral femoralBrewer MC, Kinnison ML, Perler BA, White RI (1988) Blue toe syndrom: treatment with anticoagulants and delayed percutaneous transluminal angioplasty. Radiology 166:31–36

Brewster DC, Cambria RP, Darling RC (1989) Long-term results of combined iliac balloon angioplasty and distal surgical revascularization. Ann Surg 210:324

Cachovan M (1991) A critique of the Fontaine classification. Crit Limb Ischemia 1:7–9

Carter SA (1972) Response of ankle systolic pressure to leg exercise in mild questionable arterial disease. N Engl J Med 287:578–579

Chait A (1976) The internal mammary artery: an overlooked collateral pathway to the leg. Radiology 121:621–624

Colapinto RF, Harries-Jones EP, Johnston KW (1981) Percutaneous transluminal recanalization of complete iliac artery occlusions. Arch Surg 116:277–281

Colapinto RF, Stronell RD, Johnston WK (1982) Transluminal angioplasty of complete iliac obstructions. Am J Roentgenol 146:859

Dormandy JA, Stock G (1990) Critical leg ischemia. European consensus document, Springer, Berlin Heidelberg New York

Dotter CT, et al. (1974) Transluminal iliac artery dilatation – non-surgical catheter treatment of atheromatas norrowing. JAMA 230:117–124

Durham JD, Rutherford RB (1994) Standards for reporting lower extremity ischemia. In: SCVIR – Syllabus Peripheral Vascular Interventions US Nr. 94-0696675, pp 206–218

Dyet JF, Shaw JW, Cook AM, Nicholson AA (1993) The use of the Wallstent in aortoiliac desease. Clin Radiol 48:227–231

Edwards WSt, Lyons C (1959) Problems in surgery of occlusive disease of the aorta and iliac arteries. Ann Surg 149:675

Fontaine R, Kim M, Kieny R (1954) Die chirurgische Behandlung der peripheren Durchblutungsstörungen. Helv Chir Acta 5/6:499–533

Gaines PA (1989) The WIRE LOOP technique. Radiology 168:275–276

Gallino A, Mahler F, Probst E, Nachbur B (1984) Percutaneous transluminal angioplasty of the arteries of the lower limbs: a 5 year follow-up. Circulation 70:619–623

Ginsburg R, Thorpe P, Bowles CR (1989) Pull-through approach to percutaneous angioplasty of totally occluded common iliac arteries. Radiology 172:111

Gottlob R (1952) Thrombosen der Aorta und Iliakalarterien. Langenbecks Arch Z Chir 272:408

Guenther RW, Vorwerk D, Bohndorf K (1989) Iliac and femoral artery stenoses and occlusions: treatment with intravascular stents. Radiology 172:725

Guidelines for Percutaneous Transluminal Angioplasty (1990) Standards of practice committee of the CVIR. Radiology 177:619–626

Hasse HM (1974): Chronische arterielle Verschlußkrankheiten der Extremitäten-arterien. In: Heberer G, Rau G, Schoop (eds) Angiologie. Thieme, Stuttgart, pp 397–431

Henry M, Amor M, Ethevenot G, et al. (1995) Palmaz stent placement in iliac and femoropopliteal arteries: primary and secondary patency in 310 patients with 2–4 year follow-up. Radiology 197:167–174

Henry M, Amor M, Henry I, et al. (1997) Application d'une novelle endoprothese couverte au treatment des artéropathies peripheriques occlusives et anevrismales. Arch Mal Coer 90:953–960

Heyden B, Vollmar J, Voss U (1980) Principals of operation for combined aorto-iliac and femoro-popliteal occlusive lesions. Surg Gynecol Obstet 151:519–524

Johnston KW (1993) Iliac arteries, reanalysis of results of balloon angioplasty. Radiology 186:207–212

Johnston KW, Rae M, Hogg-Johnston SA (1987) 5 year results of a prospective study of percutaneous transluminal angioplasty. Ann Surg 206:403

Joseph N, Levy E, Lipman S (1987) Angioplasty-related iliac artery rupture: treatment by temporary balloon occlusion. Cardiacvasc Intervent Radiol 10:276–278

Kadir S, White RI, Kaufmann SL (1982) Long-term results of aortoiliac angioplasty. Surgery 94:10

Kashdan BJ, Trost DW, Jagust MB (1992) Retrograde approach for contralateral iliac and infrainguinal percutaneous transluminal angioplasty. Experience in 100 patients. J Vasc Intervent Radiol 3:515–519

Kaufmann SL, Barth KH, Kadir S, et al. (1982) Hemodynamic measurements in the evaluation and follow-up of transluminal angioplasty of the iliac and femoral arteries. Radiology 142:329–336

Liermann D, Strecker EP, Peters J (1992) The Strecker Stent: indications and results in iliac and femoro-popliteal arteries. Cardiovasc Intervent Radiol 15:298–305

Long AL, Page PE, Raynaud AC (1991) Percutaneous iliac artery stent: angiographic long-term follow-up. Radiology 180:771–774

Loose KE (1976) Development of angiography, puncture and injection. In: Loose KE, van Dongen RAJM (eds) Atlas of angiography. Thieme, Stuttgart, pp 1–6

Loose KE, Loose DA (1976) Upper and lower extremities. In: Loose KE, van Dongen RJAM (eds) Atlas of Angiography. Thieme, Stuttgart, pp 74–122

Mahler F (1990) Katheterinterventionen in der Angiologie. Thieme, Stuttgart

McNamara TO, Bomberger RA (1986) Factors affecting initial and 6 month patency rates after intraarterial thrombolysis with high dose urokinase. Am J Surg 152:709–711

McNamara TO, Bomberger RA, Merchant RF (1991) Intraarterial urokinase as the initial therapy for acute ischemic lower limbs. Circulation 83 (Suppl 1):106–119

Mehigan JT, Stoney RJ (1987) Arterial microemboli and fibromuscular dysplasia of the external iliac arteries. Surgery 81:484–486

Münster W, Wierny L, Porstmann W (1966) Lokalisation und Häufigkeit arterieller Durchblutungsstörungen der unteren Exremitäter. Dtsch Med Wochenschr 91:2073–2079

Najafi H (1966) Fibromuscular hyperplasia of the external iliac arteries. Arch Surg 92:394

Palmaz JC, Encarnacion LE (1994) Intraluminal stents: general principles. In: SCVIR-syllabus: peripheral vascular interventions. US Catalog-Nr 94-0696675

Palmaz JC, Laborde JC, Rivera FJ, et al. (1992) Stenting of the iliac arteries with the Palmaz stent. Experience from a multicenter trial. Cardiovasc Intervent Radiol 15:291–297

Picus D (1994) Aortic and iliac angioplasty: technique and results. In: Berge JM (ed) SCVIR-syllabus: peripheral vascular interventions, US-Catalog-Nr 94-069675, pp 36–49

Pollit J, Bolino A, Kukral JC (1972) Symptomatic fibromuscular hyperplasia of the external iliac artery. Vasc Surg 6: 159–161

Porstmann W (1973) Ein neuer Korsett-Ballonkatheter zur transluminalen Rekanalisation nach Dotter unter besonderer Berücksichtigung von Obliterationen an den Beckenarterien. Radiol Diagn (Berlin) 2:239–244

Prager RJ, Akin JR, Akin G, Binder JR (1977) WINSLOW'S PATHWAY A rare collateral channel in infrarenal aortic occlusion. Am J Roentgenol 128:485–487

Raithel D (1987) Operative Therapie bei Beckenarterien-verschlüssen. In: Trübestein, G (ed) Therapie der arteriellen Verschlußkrankheit. Zuckschwerdt, Munich

Rauber-Kopsch F (1941) Lehrbuch und Atlas der Anatomie des Menschen, Bd II: Eingeweide - Gefäße. Thieme, Leipzig, pp 456–497

Raza Z, Shaw JW, Stonebridge PA, et al. (1998) Management of iliac occlusions with a new self-expanding endovascular stent. Eur J Vasc Endovasc Surg 15:439–443

Rees CR (1994): Iliac Stent Placement. In: SCVIR-syllabus: peripheral vascular intervention. US-Catalog-Nr 94-069675, pp 184–205

Rees CR, Palmaz JC, Garcia O (1989) Angioplasty and stenting of complet occluded iliac arteries. Radiology 172:953–959

Richter GM, Roeren TH, Noeldge G, et al. (1991) Superior clinical results of iliac stent placement versus percutaneous transluminal angioplasty: four-years success rates of a randomized study. Radiology 181:161 (abstract)

Ring EJ, Freimann DB, McLean GK, Schwartz W (1982) Percutaneous recanalization of common iliac artery occlusions. AJR 139:587–589

Rob CG, Vollmar JF (1959) Die Chirurgie der Bauchaorta. Ergeb Chir Orthop 42:569

Roth FJ (1978) Die Dilatation von Stenosen der A. femoralis communis nach der Dotter-Technik von der Gegenseite aus. Dtsch Ges Angiologie, Heidelberg 1978 (report)

Roth FJ, Cappius G (1983) Angioplasty of the iliac and inguinal arteries. In: Dotter CT, Grüntzig AR, Schoop W, Zeitter E (eds) Percutaneous transluminal angioplasty. Springer, Berlin Heidelberg New York, pp 115–126

Roth FJ, Heimig T, Berliner P, et al. (1988) Perkutane Rekanalisation peripherer Gefäße. In: Guenther RW, Thelen M (eds) Interventionelle Radiologie. Thieme, Stuttgart

Rousseau H, Joffre F, Raillat C (1989) Iliac artery endoprosthesis: radiologic and histologic findings after 2 years. Am J Roentgenol 153:1075

Rousseau H, Joffre F, Tregant P, et al. (1996) Endovascular treatment for iliac disease. In: Sigwart U, Bertrand M, Serruys PW (eds) Handbook of cardiovascular interventions. Churchill Livingstone, New York, pp 813–886

Rutherford RB, Becker GJ (1991) Standards for evaluating and reporting, the results of surgical and percutaneous therapy for peripheral arterial disease. Radiology 181:277–281

Sauer L, Reilly LM, Goldstone J, et al. (1990) Clinical spectrum of symptomatic external iliac fibromuscular dysplasia. J Vasc Surg 12:488–496

Schneider E, Grüntzig A, Bollinger A (1982) Langzeiterebnisse nach perkutaner transluminaler Angioplastie (PTA) bei 882 konsekutiven Patienten mit iliakalen und femoro-poplitealen Obstruktionen. VASA 11:322–326

Schoop W (1988) Praktische Angiologie, 4th edn. Thieme, Stuttgart

Schoop W, Levy H (1969) Messung des systolischen Blutdrucks distal eines Extremitätenarterienverschlusses mit Hilfe der Ultraschall-Dopplertechnik. Verh Dtsch Ges Kreislaufforsch 35:456–458

Shaw JM (1996) Management of aortoiliac occlusive vascular disease with the Memotherm self-expanding nitinol stent. J Interven Radiol 11:119–127

Steckmeier B, Parzhuber A, Reininger C, et al. (1995) Combined endoluminal and surgical vascular reconstructions. In: Horsch S, Claeys L (eds) Critical leg ischemia. Steinkopff, Darmstadt, pp 105–114

Strecker EP, Boos Irene BL, Hagen B (1996) Flexible tantalum stents for the treatment of iliac artery lesions: long-term patency, complications and risk factors. Radiology 199: 641–647

Strunk HM, Dueber C, Thelen M (1994) Five-year-results after endovascular stent placement in iliac arteries. RSNA-Abstr 882

Tegtmeyer CJ, Moore TS, Chandler JG, et al. (1979) Percutaneous transluminal dilatation of a complete block in the right iliac artery. AJR 133:532–535

Tegtmeyer CJ, Kellum CD, Kron JL, Mentzer RM (1985) Percutaneous transluminal angioplasty in the region of the aortic bifurcation; the two-balloon technique with results and long-term follow-up study. Radiology 157:661–665

Tetteroo E, van Engelen AD, Spithoven JH, et al. (1996) Stent placement after iliac angioplasty: comparison of hemodynamic and angiographic criteria. Intervent Radiol 20:155–159

Van Andel GJ, Krepel VM (1979) De behandeling van stenosen in de arteriae iliacae met dilatie catheters (DOTTER-Methode). Ned Tiolschr Geneeskol 123:873–878

Van Dongen, RJAM (1976) Aortoiliac occlusive disease and abdominal aneurysm. In: Loose KE, van Dongen RJAM (eds) Atlas of angiography. Thieme, Stuttgart, pp 123–163

Vollmar J (1996) Aorto-iliakale Arterienverschlüsse. In: Vollmar J (ed) Rekonstruktive Chirurgie der Arterien. Thieme, Stuttgart, pp 207–241

Vorwerk D, Guenther RW (1992) Stent placement in iliac arterial lesions: three years of clinical experience with the Wallstent. Cardiovasc Intervent Radiol 15:285–290

Vorwerk D, Guenther RW (1997) Arterial stent placement. In: Adams A, Dondelinger RF, Mueller RP (eds) Textbook of metallic stens. Isis Medical Media, Oxford

Vorwerk KD, Guenther RW, Schuermann K, et al. (1995) Primary stent placement for chronic iliac artery occlusions: follow-up results in 103 patients. Radiology 194:745–749

Voss EU, Vollmar J, Heyden B, et al. (1980) Chirurgische Therapie der chronischen aortoiliakalen Arterienverschlüsse. Aktuel Chir 15:77–94

Walker PJ, Harris JP, May P (1991) Combined percutaneous transluminal angioplasty and extraanatomic bypass for symptomatic unilateral iliac artery occlusion with contralateral iliac artery stenosis. Ann Vasc Surg 5:209–213

Wellauer JC (1957) Die abdominale Aortographie. In: Schinz HR, Glauner R, Uehlinger E (eds) Röntgendiagnostik, Ergebnisse 1952-1956. Thieme, Stuttgart, pp 161–209

Wenz W (1972) Abdominale Angiographie. Springer, Berlin Heidelberg New York

Wenz W, Beduhn D (1975) Extremitätenarteriographie. Springer, Berlin Heidelberg New York

Wilmink ABM, Pleumeekers HJCM, Hubard SC, et al. (1998) The infrarenal aortic diameter in relation to age. Eur J Vasc Endovasc Surg 16:431–437

Wilson SE, Wolf GL, Cross AP (1989) Percutaneous trans-luminal angioplasty versus operation for peripheral arteriosclerosis, report of prospective randomized trial in a selected group of patient. J Vasc Surg 9:1–9

Zeitler E (1974) Aortoarteriographie. In: Heberer G, Rau G, Schoop W (eds) Angiologie. Thieme, Stuttgart, pp 243–302

Zeitler E (1975) Behandlung mit Kathetern bei peripheren arteriellen Durchblutungsstörungen. Med Welt 26:2863–1869

Zeitler E, Oldendorf M (1995) GAMS II Forschungsbericht an BMFT Bonn. The GAMS-Study (1991–1995). 2nd international congress and course, Zermatt-Heidelberg

Zeitler E, Hüring HG, Schoop W, Schmidtke I (1971a) Mechanische Behandlung von Beckenarterienstenosen

31 Femoral Artery Disease

D. Liermann and J. Kirchner

CONTENTS

31.1
Anatomy and Variations

Distal to the passage of the lacuna vasorum at the level of the inguinal ligament, the main artery trunk of the leg is called the common femoral artery. At fluoroscopy, this artery is projected to the medial edge of the head of the femur. The femoral nerve is located lateral to the common femoral artery; proximally, the femoral vein is located medial and changes to a dorsal course more distally.

At about 4 cm distal to the inguinal ligament, the deep femoral artery (DFA) originates dorsolaterally. Two main branches (arteria circumflexa femoris lateralis and medialis) supply the head of the femur. Further distal, many vessels originate to supply the

muscles. In the case of an occlusion of the superficial femoral artery (SFA), the DFA becomes larger and develops into the most important collateral vessel of the leg, sufficient for the main femoral and crural circulation – superficialization of the DFA.

Distal to the origin of the DFA, the common femoral artery is called the SFA. It runs a course at the ventral medial femur. A few branches supply the surrounding muscles. Following the musculus adductor longus, the SFA enters medial of the musculus vastus medialis and dorsal of the membrana vasto adductoria into Hunter's canal. Before its entrance into Hunter's canal, the arteria genus descendens originates. Below Hunter's canal (lacuna, built by both parts of the musculus adductor magnus), which inserts into the linea aspera femoris and at the epicondylus medialis (hiatus adductorius), the main arterial trunk is called the popliteal artery.

Rarely, no common femoral artery is present because both the SFA and the DFA take the same origin of the external iliac artery. In a few cases, there is a very short common femoral artery, "high bifurcation", which may cause difficulties in antegrade puncture management. In about 40% of patients, the DFA is located directly behind the SFA, which can also cause difficulties in antegrade puncture.

Another rare variety (0.14%) is a persistent arteria ischiadica. In this situation, a common femoral artery or a SFA cannot be found. The arteria ischiadica takes its origin from the internal iliac artery, while the DFA originates from the external iliac artery in such cases. This variety can also be seen as an unilateral variant. Another variety is the double SFA, which reunites to one artery in Hunter's canal.

31.2
Incidence and Types of Obliteration

In any classification of arterial vascular disease of the lower extremity, a differentiation should be made between acute arterial occlusion and chronic arterial vascular disease. Acute arterial occlusion shows a

D. Liermann, MD, Professor, Direktor der Klinik für Radiologie und Nuklearmedizin, Universitätsklinikum der Ruhr-Universität Bochum, Marienhospital, Hölkeskampring 40, 44625 Herne, Germany

sudden interruption of the blood supply caused by a coagulum (Fig. 31.1). This is an important angiological emergency. The most common cause is an embolus (75%), originating mostly from the heart, and, more rarely, from a proximally located aneurysm or an ulcerated plaque. An autochtonous thrombosis following chronic arterial vascular disease is the cause in less then 25% of cases. Other causes of acute occlusion include injury (mainly iatrogenic) or spastic occlusions after intraarterial injections.

Chronic arterial vascular disease is mainly caused by arteriosclerosis (80%–90%) or inflammatory diseases (angiitides), such as thromboangitis obliterans Buerger-Winiwarter (also known as Buerger's disease).

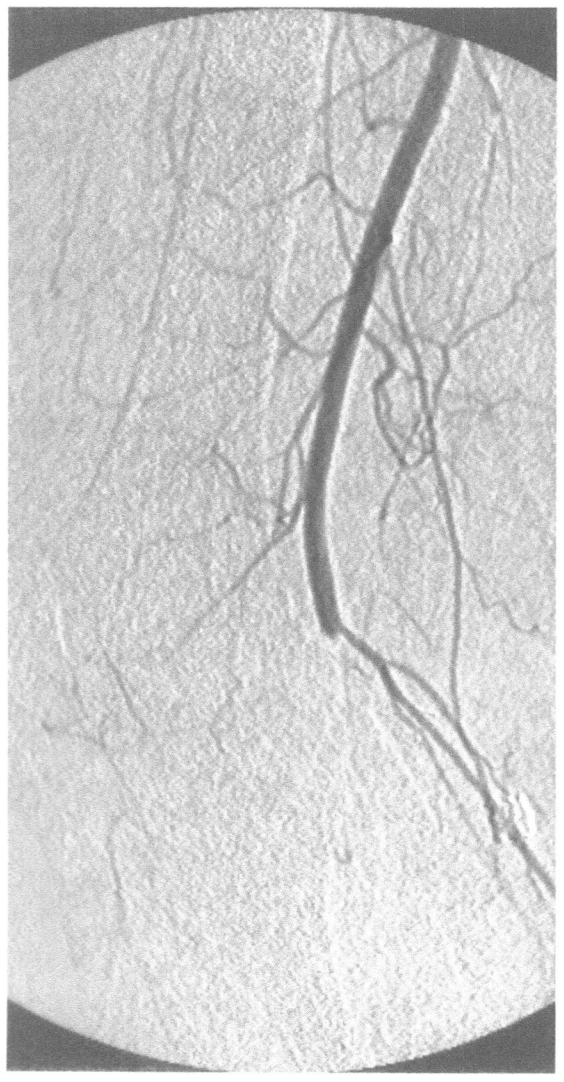

Fig. 31.1. Acute embolic occlusion of the femoropopliteal artery showing a cut-off sign

31.3
The Rutherford Classification

Two systems are used to classify the degree of chronic arterial vascular disease. The Fontaine's classification divides arterial vascular disease into four categories. The differentiation between Fontaine's category IIa and IIb is the tested walking distance below and above 250 m. Because of varying data, it is often difficult to compare studies. Therefore, the additional use of ankle-brachial systolic pressure index (ABI) above and below 50 mm Hg can also prove helpful.

More important are the results of the ad hoc commitee of the Society of Vascular Surgery (RUTHERFORD et al. 1987). They developed a classification differentiating arterial occlusive disease into acute and chronic limb ischemia: While acute limb ischemia is divided into three categories (mild, threatening, and irreversible ischemia), chronic limb ischemia is split into six different categories and three main divisions (claudication, pain at rest, and tissue loss) (see Table 31.1).

31.4
Segmental Superficial
Femoral Obliteration

Angiographic examination shows relatively typical signs of the underlying arteriosclerotic process and its different grades (Fig. 31.2). Thus, narrowing of the contrast column indicates intimal edema, while irregularities show atheromatous lesions, plaques, and ulcerations. Calcifications are better seen in plane views than on angiograms. It may result in the so-called natural road-mapping aspect showing vessels' course already under fluoroscopy. In particular, the mixture of segments with more or less severe pathological changes demonstrates common atherosclerotic disease. Stenoses can be classified (LIERMANN and KIRCHNER 1997) as ring-like, hour-glass-shaped, symmetric or asymmetric. In the SFA, we often find segmental stenosis. A sequence of several stenoses is called a "string of beads". Occlusion caused by arteriosclerosis shows, for the most part, well developed collaterals. Collaterals can be divided according to their course and shape. Direct collaterals have their origin in the occluded SFA, indirect collaterals in proximate feeders. Collaterals due to stronger perfusion of the vasa vasorum result in corkscrew-shaped vessels. The latter are commoly seen in thromboangitis obliterans Buerger-Winiwarter.

Table 31.1. Clinical classification of chronic arterial vascular disease according to Rutherford

Grade	Category	Clinical Symptoms	Objective criteria
I	0	Asymptomatic	Normal walking test
	1	Mild claudication	Completed walking test
			ABI >50 mmHg but >25 mmHg below normal
	2	Moderate claudication	Between 1 and 3
	3	Severe claudication	Interrupted walking test
			ABI <50 mmHg
II	4	Pain at rest	ABI at rest <40 mmHg
	5	Focal gangrene	ABI at rest <60 mmHg
III	6	Extensive tissue loss	ABI at rest >60 mmHg

Analysis of segmental occlusion may help to differentiate chronic occlusion from acute occlusion caused by arterial embolism. The latter shows a clearly depicted cut-off of the contrast column, and less often a gap washed round by contrast medium. There are only rare collaterals in such cases. The cut-off in an otherwise unaltered SFA is a significant sign of embolic occlusion. Most often, emboli in the femoral arteries are found in the region of the bifurcation and Hunter's canal.

It is useful to divide segmental occlusions of the SFA into two groups: those of less and those of more than 10 cm in length. The latter show poor prognosis after recanalization and stenting. Stenosis, as well as occlusion, are most commonly located in bifurcations and those parts which undergo increased mechanical stress – the SFA and Hunter's canal. Stenosis of the SFA near to its origin often leads to total SFA obliteration (see Sect. 31.5).

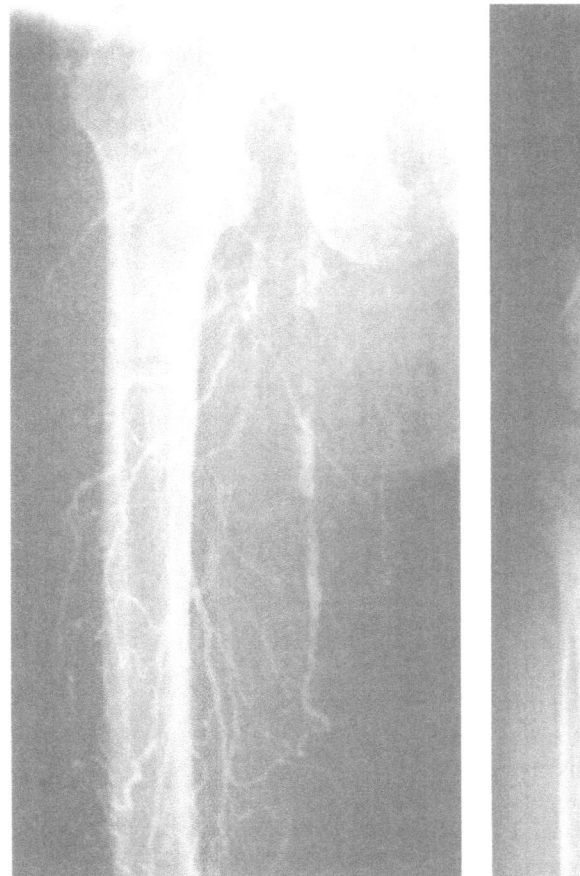
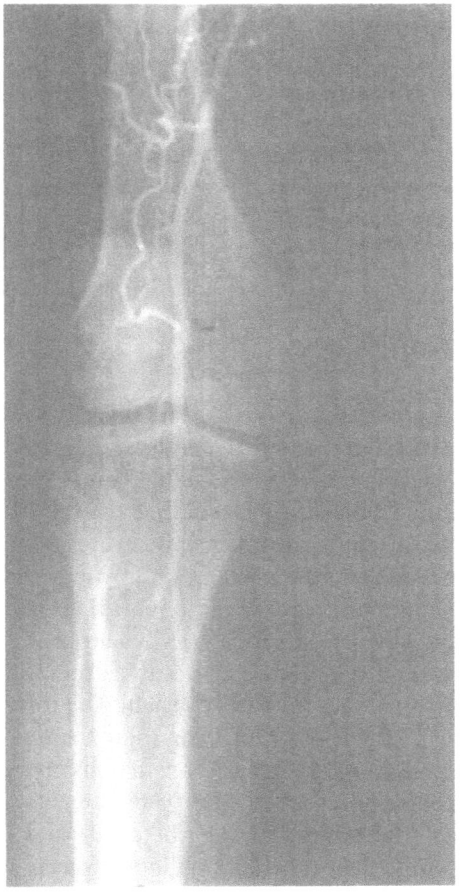

Fig. 31.2. Chronic occlusion of the superficial femoral artery showing multiple collateral vessels and severe changes of the persistent patent vessels segments

The correct information about a segmental obliteration requires a correctly performed angiographic examination in two projections with late spots showing collateral filling, as well as possible retrograde filling of the occluded segment. Incomplete filling of the distal SFA may simulate longer occlusion. On the other hand, side superposition of vessels may obscure the real length of segmental occlusion as filiform stenosis may be imitated by direct collaterals in such cases.

31.5
Total SFA Obliteration

Total SFA obliteration is no proven indication for interventional recanalization. One reason for this is that an intervention can only be successfully carried out in such cases where an origin of the SFA can be probed. Additionally, recanalization of a complete SFA obliteration has such a poor prognosis for primary patency that it should be not recommended.

If there is no short proximal segment and blind probing has failed, retrograde catheterization of the SFA via a popliteal approach may facilitate the advancement of guidewires through the obliterated SFA. Road-mapping after puncture of the common femoral artery and ultrasound guidance (5–10 MHz linear transducer with a sterile cover) are helpful for popliteal artery puncture.

31.7
Femoral Aneurysms

Alongside the occlusion-type diseases, there is a second group of arterial vascular diseases: the ectatic type, also called dilatative arteriopathy. This is found mostly in connection with aortal or iliac ectasy of the vessels or aorto-iliac aneurysms. Real aneurysms of the peripheral arteries are rare, in most cases affecting the common femoral and popliteal arteries. Often, the aneurysms are bilateral. Aneurysms of the lower extremity are seen clinically as pulsating tumors, sometimes accompanied by pain. They often cause sudden occlusion. More common than real aneurysms are findings of false aneurysms in the region of the femoral artery after puncture of the common femoral artery. To describe aneurysms in the region of the femoral artery, oblique projections should be performed. Because the angiographic picture in cases of partial thrombosis of the aneu-

rysm appears to be normal, a computed tomography or ultrasound examination should be performed to show the real size of the aneurysm.

31.8
Interventional Radiology of the Femoral Arteries

31.8.1
Plain Old Balloon Angioplasty (POBA)

Percutaneous transluminal angioplasty (PTA) (Fig. 31.3) was introduced by Dotter and Judkins in 1964. After the development of double-lumen single-end hole balloon catheters by Grüntzig, PTA has gained wide acceptance in the therapy of SFA disease over the last two decades.

Lesions of the common femoral artery are frequently thick, calcified, and do not yield optimal results with PTA. If not, contralateral PTA is possible or successful for common femoral obliterations therefore they are related to previous surgery. In contrast, PTA of the SFA has become the domain of interventional radiology.

While PTA of the common femoral artery usually requires a contralateral approach with passage around the aortic bifurcation, the optimal approach for stenosis or occlusion of the SFA is an ipsilateral

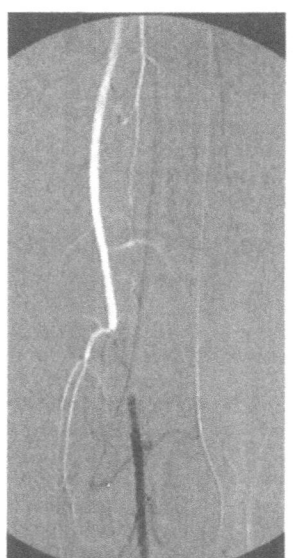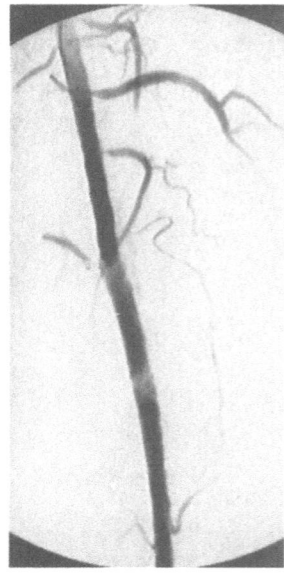

Fig. 31.3. Percutaneous transluminal angioplasty (PTA) of a segmental occlusion of the superficial femoral artery (SFA). **a** Occlusion in the Hunter's canal over a length of 4 cm. **b** After recanalization and PTA, we found excellent flow conditions in the SFA

antegrade puncture of the common femoral artery or SFA. To avoid retroperitoneal bleeding, puncture must be performed distal of the inguinal ligament which extends from the anterosuperior iliac spine to the pubic tubercle. The artery usually bifurcates at the level of the inferior margin of the femoral head. Because the artery below this point is posteriorly uncovered by bony structures (femoral head), effective compression can fail in such punctures. Moreover, a distal puncture may be complicated by arteriovenous fistulas between the SFA and femoral vein.

A vascular approach is performed under local anesthesia. To minimize traumatization of the vessel wall, we prefer an open needle (20-gauge). After catheterization of the SFA by means of a guidewire, a sheath (commonly between 5 and 7 F) is introduced. If the guidewire repeatedly enters the DFA, a 45-degree preshaped catheter should be advanced over the wire. After road-mapping, the catheter can be directed to the origin of the SFA (commonly a point medial and anterior).

In cases of high bifurcation of the common femoral artery, direct puncture of the SFA is recommended, if necessary under ultrasound guidance.

In cases of failure of antegrade methods, retrograde catheterization of the SFA via a popliteal approach (see Sect. 31.5) or the method of conversion of a retrograde puncture by means of a side-winder catheter as proposed by Shenoy (SHENNOY 1983) can be attempted. Pretherapeutic angiography should include the complete arterial system up to the periphery (also for forensic reasons).

The proximal and distal limits of the occluded segment may be identified with opaque markers. In the following, a 5-F catheter is advanced over a straight hydrophilic wire. Crossing the stenosis/occlusion is undertaken under fluoroscopic control, optimally with the road-mapping technique. Following passage of the occluded segment, the wire is left distal to the angioplasty site until the very last control following completion of PTA. Any attempt to recross the dilated site carries a high risk of dissection and occlusion.

Once the stenosis has been passed, a balloon catheter of appropriate diameter and length is advanced over the guidewire and positioned within the lesion. In the case of multiple stenoses, more than one catheter may be necessary due to the increasing diameter of the SFA. The diameter of the balloon used depends on individual factors and should be chosen according to pretherapeutic angiographic findings. Ballon catheters with a diameter of 5–7 mm are usually used in the SFA.

Inflation of the balloon is performed with contrast medium under fluoroscopic control. There is no standardized inflation time: we prefer 120 s. To avoid gaps, it is useful to demonstrate the limits of the inflated balloon on the patients by means of opaque markers.

In cases where an occlusion cannot be passed by means of guidewires, the so-called ROTACS system (VALLBRACHT et al. 1989) is another promising tool in recanalization of the SFA. The device consists of an oval-shaped burr with a diameter a of 7 F and can be advanced to the occlusion over a guidewire. Under rotation at a moderate speed of up to 500 rpm – for example, the TRAC-Kensey catheter (see Sect. 31.8.3) up to 100 000 rpm – the device is advanced under mild axial pressure. The results of our own studies show that recanalization after failed guidewire passage is successful in more than 60% of cases when using the ROTACS system (VALLBRACHT et al. 1993).

31.8.1.1
PTA of Deep Formal Artery (DFA) Disease

PTA of the DFA can be performed using an ipsilateral or contralateral approach. Clinical experience with PTA of the DFA is scant, and is mostly performed only in cases of occlusion of the SFA and severe claudication or rest pain.

Simultaneous dilatation of the SFA and the DFA is possible with an antegrade approach for PTA of the SFA and a contralateral approach for PTA of the DFA. We can place two guidewires simultaneously, which remain in place until a satisfactory result has been obtained. This procedure is promising in cases of severe stenosis at the origin of both the DFA and SFA. Results (HOFFMANN et al. 1992) show clinical success in 66%.

31.8.2
Atherectomy

Atherectomy is defined as the removal of atheroma from vessel walls. We differentiate between cutting and rotating systems (for a description of the latter, see Sect. 31.8.3). In PTA, the stenotic vessels are dilated without removing the occluding atheroma, while the aim of atherectomy is to extract the occluding lesions of the vessel wall without destroying nonpathologic parts of the vessel.

Indications for atherectomy include high-grade excentric calcified lesions, especially excentric re-stenosis, and stent stenoses which have a poor prognosis with POBA.

On the other hand, atherectomy may improve the results of PTA alone, especially in cases with intimal flaps after balloon dilatation.

Atherectomy methods include the following: the well-known *Simpson atherectomy catheter* is a double-lumen catheter with a cylindrical cutting chamber (Fig. 31.4). Below the open end of the cutting chamber, there is an inflatable balloon to fix the cutting device over the lesion. The cutting device is a rotating blade; debris is collected in a reservoir on the end of the catheter, which is available in sizes of 6–11 F. The *TEC system* consists of rotating cutting blades with a pyramidal-shaped tip and a vacuum device to remove atheromatous debris.

The *pull-back atheretomy catheter system*, in contrast, uses a proximal inner rotating blade over which a distal outer cutting cannula is pulled back, removing plaque material, which is collected in the cutting chamber.

The rigidity of atherectomy systems requires large-sized catheter sheaths; furthermore, the angle under which the sheath enters the vessel shoud be flat for easy passage of the catheter system through the SFA. If the atherectomy catheter is unable to pass a stenotic vessel segment primarily, initial passage can be achieved with a smaller angiographic catheter through which a stiff guidewire can be inserted across the stenosis more distally. For exact positioning of the atherectomy system, road-mapping should be used. The available follow-up results show that initial technical success can be achieved in up to 92% of patients (SAWADA et al. 1994; WILDENHAIN et al. 1994). SAWADA et al. reported success in 80.3% of lesions in a group of 48 patients.

31.8.3
Rotablator

Another method of plaque elimination is rotational angioplasty in which a fast rotating catheter tip (up to 190 000 rpm) pulverizes the atheroma, similar to, but faster than, the Rotax which is used for recanalization of occluded segments (s.a.). The most common devices include the TRAC-Kensey catheter (KENSEY et al. 1987) and the Auth rotational atherectomy devise (also called "rotablator"). The TRAC catheter consists of a flexible polyurethane

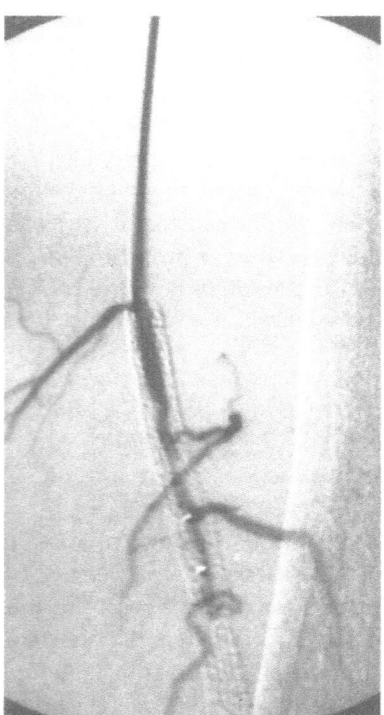 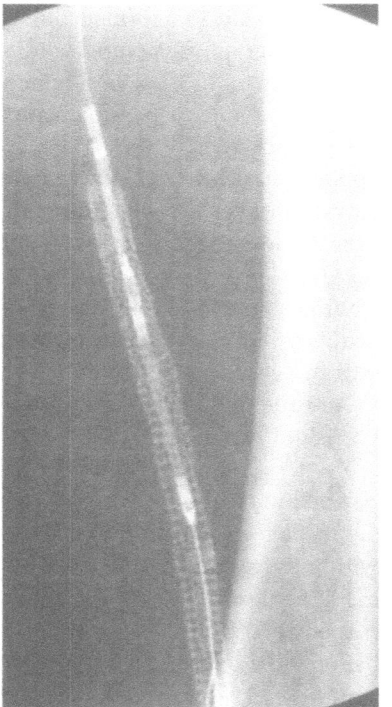 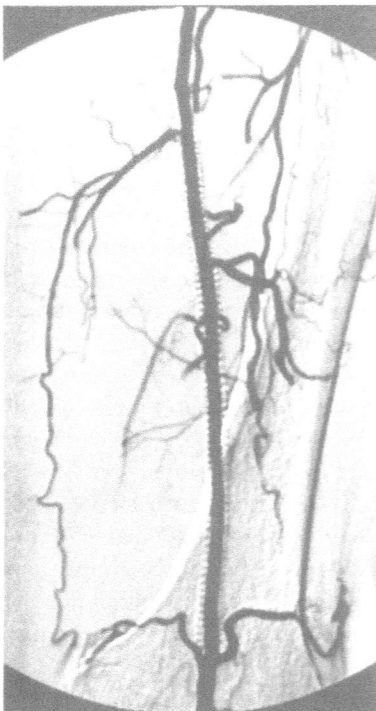

Fig. 31.4 a–c. Atherectomy using the Simpson atherectomy device. **a** Hyperplastic formations in the stented segment of the superficial femoral artery. **b** Simpson atherectomy device during atherectomy in the same segment. **c** Resulting excellent flow conditions

catheter and spinning cam driven by a power unit. It is available in sizes of 5–10 F. To keep the catheter tip centered within the vessel lumen, the device has been designed to direct fluid jets laterally against the arterial wall under rotation. It is common to use a mixture of a contrast medium, heparin, and a thrombolytic agent (urokinase), as well as HAES or dextran. The rotation catheter is moved backwards and forwards in the occluded segment.

In contrast to the TRAC catheter, which uses fluid jets to stabilize the catheter in the center of the vessel, the Auth rotablator needs a guidewire. The exchangeable tip for the Auth rotablator is available in different sizes.

Patency rates for recanalization with rotational angioplasty have been reported at between 53% (SCHILD et al. 1990) and 96% (TRILLER et al. 1992). Both studies combined a TRAC catheter with balloon angioplasty. The high complication rates with both the TRAC catheter (73%) (SCHILD et al. 1990) and the rotablator (70%) (AHN et al. 1992) showed the method's limitations. The most common complications included perforation of the vessel and hemolysis caused by high rotational speed. The significance of the debris produced of unclearly defined size remains unclear. The long-term progno-sis is poorer than the primary patency rate. Early reocclusion caused by intimal hyperproliferation following severe vascular trauma is common. In our opinion, the only indication for these methods is for the treatment of extensive calcified and excentric stenoses which are untreatable by balloon angioplasty (SCHMITZ-ROHDE 1995).

31.8.4
Laser-Assisted PTA

The use of lasers is recommended only in combination with balloon dilatation. In addition to the risk of displacement of debris to the periphery during the procedure, there is not sufficient recanalization of the lumen of the vessel after laser alone. If other recanalization techniques in the SFA have failed, lasers might be a complementary additional tool to recanalize an occlusion to enable a PTA procedure (Fig. 31.5).

The term "laser" is an acronym, standing for "light amplification through stimulated emission of radiation" (GOODKIND J et al. 1993). Energy delivery may be in two forms: continuous-wave or pulsed-laser. The latter is preferred for intravascular appli-

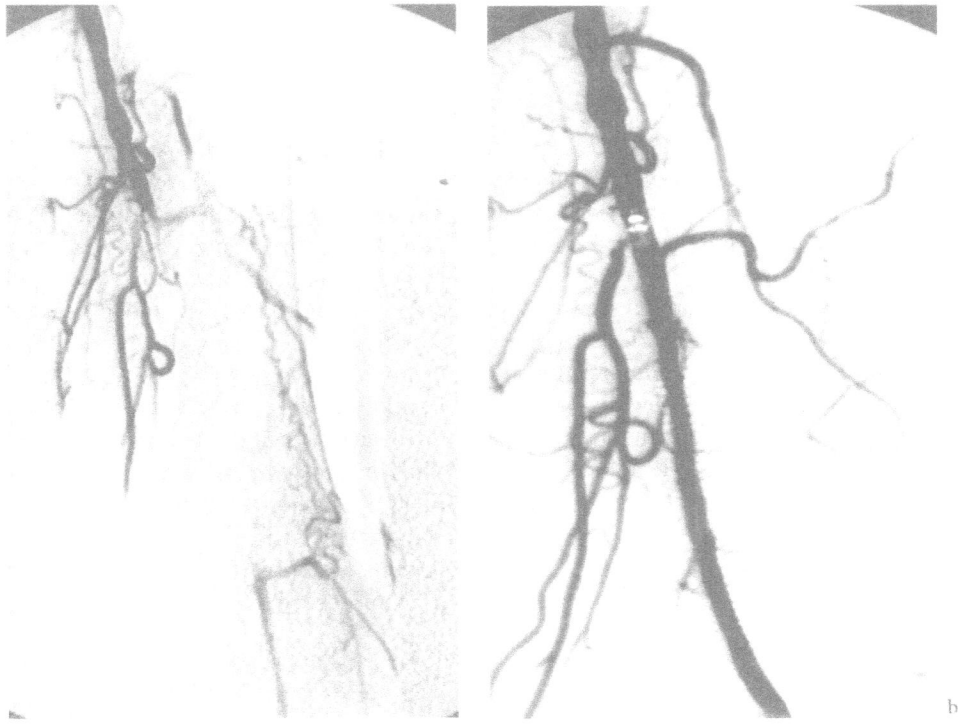

Fig. 31.5. a Segmental occlusion of the superficial femoral artery in the Hunter's canal. **b** In the following treatment with the matted laser, percutaneous transluminal angioplasty, and stenting

cations. The following types of delivery systems are common:

- Argon lasers, which are readily available and economical, but have a relatively low peak energy and continuous-wave output.
- Nd-YAG (neodymium: yttrium aluminium garnet) lasers, which can operate in continuous or pulsed modes and which offer higher energy and relatively easy transmission along optical fibers.
- Excimer lasers, which operate in short pulses and wavelength, generating high peak energy, and which can also be used for calcified lesions; however, these lasers are expensive and difficult to operate.

Thus, all laser systems have specific drawbacks and catheter as wire techniques offer a reduction in the size of the sheath and lower costs. Laser angioplasty cannot be accepted as a routine procedure and must remain an investigational method until better results are demonstrated (FERRAL et al. 1992; HUPPERT et al. 1992, 1994). They offer only the possibility of greater primary patency rates in SFA occlusions of longer than 10 cm (LAMMER and KARNEL 1988). Long-term results, however, are still not promising.

31.8.5
Mechanical Thrombectomy and Clot Lysis

While the mechanical removal of an acutely occluding clot using a balloon catheter can promptly restore arterial perfusion (Fig. 31.6), chemical fibrinolysis is also an effective treatment for vascular thromboses. Both methods have potential drawbacks.

Regarding the first method, we often see wall injuries and dislocation of thrombotic material. The second method – lysis – may cause a systemic lytic-state effect with an increased risk of bleeding in cases of prolonged perfusion. The following sections describe the devices for mechanical thrombectomy, as well as for thrombolysis.

31.8.5.1
Mechanical Thrombectomy

The following devices are commonly used for mechanical thromectomy:

- Starck percutaneous aspiration thromboembolectomy catheter

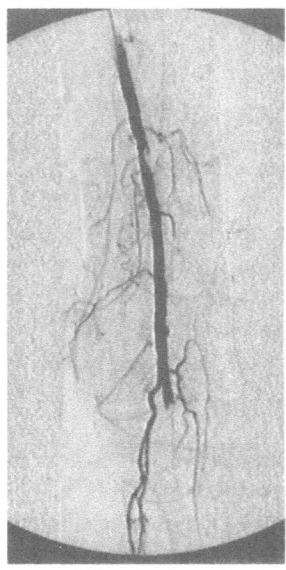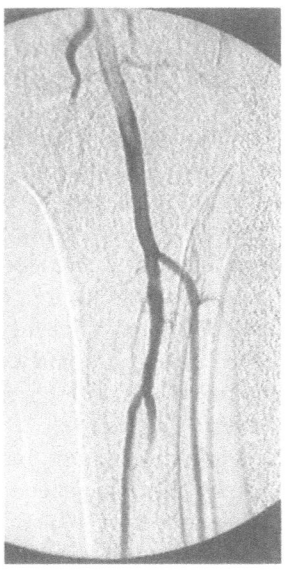

a,b

Fig. 31.6. Acute femoropopliteal occlusion before (**a**) and after percutaneous aspiration thrombectomy (PAT) (**b**). After PAT, good flow conditions are seen in the femoropopliteal segment and the vessels of the lower limb

- Amplatz mechanical thrombectomy catheter
- TEC (transluminal extraction catheter)
- Günther expiration thromboembolectomy catheter
- Rheolytic thrombectomy catheter
- Saline-jet aspiration thrombectomy catheter
- Rotational thrombectomy catheter
- Impeller basket catheter
- Sonic thrombolysis.

These procedures can be divided into those which remove the thrombotic clot completely (percutaneous aspiration thrombectomy, PAT) and those which fragment and partially remove the thrombotic clot (rotational and aspirating thrombectomy, RAT). From a clinical point of view, it is important to determine the size of residual particles generated by the devices which fragment the thrombotic material. The clinical significance of this debris, which potentially does not pass the capillary bed, is unknown. While PAT and RAT (STARCK et al. 1985) have become established procedures, the so-called hydrodynamic procedures are still in a stage of clinical trials.

The device used for PAT (STARCK et al. 1985) includes an 8-F sheath with a detachable hemostasis valve, an aspiration catheter (thin-walled and only minimally tapered) in sizes of 5–9 F, guidewires, and a 50-ml syringe. First, the aspiration catheter is advanced over the guidewire to the site of occlusion until the catheter comes into contact with the thrombus. Aspiration is performed manually using the 50-ml syringe. The catheter is then withdrawn under aspiration through the sheath after disconnection of the hemostasis valve. Clinical practice has shown that a clot can be easily aspirated. Thus, PAT is a valuable tool in cases of soft thrombotic material located proximal to a stenosis causing an acute thrombotic occlusion of the femoral artery. PAT, balloon dilatation, and lysis are often combined.

31.8.5.2
Clot Lysis

As early as in 1974, Dotter inaugurated the idea of intraarterial thrombolysis. Until now, no final conclusion regarding this method has been drawn. A fundamental basis for successful lysis with strepto- or urokinase seems to be the existence of plasminogen in the intravasal thrombus. While new thrombotic stenoses have a relatively high plasminogen content, this is not predictable for embolic occlusions. Before starting lytic therapy, precise knowledge of the hematologic and coagulation parameters is needed. Under therapy with high-dose thrombolytic agents, a control of coagulation parameters every 4h is a condition sine qua non (LIERMANN et al. 1997). In cases of local intraarterial lysis, the puncture of the common femoral artery should be kept as untraumatic as possible. To this end, an open needle should be used and perforation of the contralateral wall should be avoided.

Following diagnostic angiography, a guidewire is inserted over a small sheath (5 F) and is advanced to the occlusion. Using the guidewire, the tip of the lysis catheter is carefully set in the first third of the thrombotic occlusion.

Initially, we administer 100 IU heparin/kg body weight. The thrombosis is then infiltrated with a 100 000 IU urokinase over the lysis catheter. Then, 80 000 IU urokinase/h is administered over a maximum of 48h. During this time, high-dose heparinization is administered to avoid disseminated intravascular coagulopathy, usually 1000 IU heparin/h.

Angiographic controls of lytic results should be performed 2, 6, and 24h after starting lytic therapy. Supervision of the patient in an intensive care unit is essential. During this supervision period, the sheath is covered with an attachable clear plastic foil which enables constant control of the puncture site.

A further development of local thrombolytic therapy by means of mechanically accelerated fibrinolysis was introduced by Bookstein (BOOKSTEIN 1994). Thus, pulse-spray lysis was developed, whereby a solution of urokinase/heparin is sprayed into the center of the thrombus through lateral slit-like openings in a special catheter. The multiple contraindications for local arterial fibrinolysis are shown in Table 31.2.

Table 31.2. Absolute and relative contraindications for intraarterial fibrinolysis

Absolute contraindication for local intraarterial fibrinolysis
- Hemorrhagic bleeding
- Sepsis
- Endocarditis

Relative contraindications
- Diabetic retinopathy
- Gastric/intestinal ulcers
- Intracerebral aneurysm
- Hypertensive crisis
- Extensive surgery within the previous 6 weeks
- Craniocerebral traumatization within the previous 4 weeks
- Cardiac thrombi

31.8.7
Stenting

31.8.7.1
General Considerations

Stenting (Fig. 31.7) in femoral arteries was performed very early on in the history of stenting (ROUSSEAU et al. 1989; STRECKER et al. 1990; SAPOVAL et al. 1992). The reason for this was the poor results following PTA alone. The first femoral artery stent procedure was performed by DOTTER more than 20 years ago. Because of the small diameter of this form of stent (3 mm), reocclusion occurred relatively soon. Nearly 20 years later, self-expanding spring-metal stents (Wallstent) and balloon-expandable stents (Palmaz stent, Strecker stent) were implanted in the SFA, with promising early results. In the early 1990s, memory-alloy stents and stent grafts were introduced to improve the discouraging long-term results in interventional SFA therapy.

Wallstent (Schneider, Bulach, Switzerland). The Wallstent is a self-expanding spring-metal stent which shortens itself significantly on delivery. The Wallstent endoprosthesis has a tight meshwork of stainless steel filaments arranged in a spiral pattern

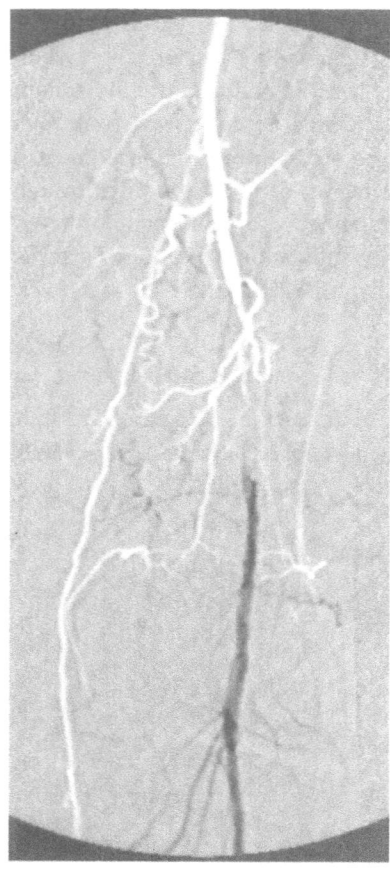
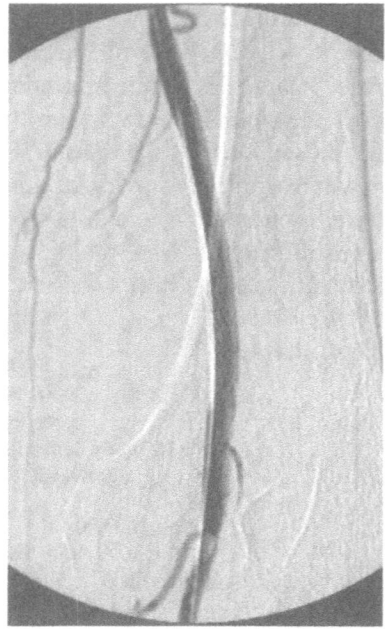
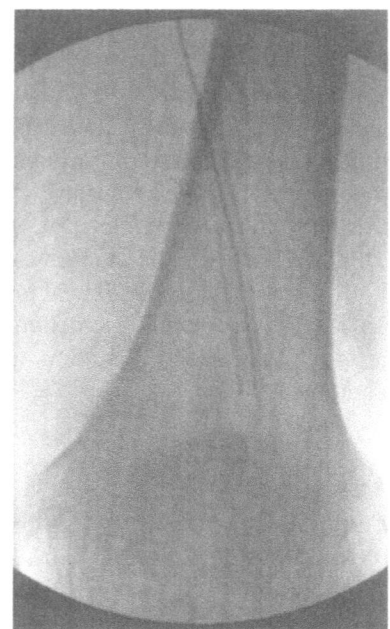

Fig. 31.7 a–c. Percutaneous transluminal angioplasty (PTA) and stenting of a segmental occlusion of the superficial femoral artery (SFA). **a** A 5-cm long occlusion of the SFA in Hunter's canal. **b-c** After PTA with an insufficient result and implantation of a femoral stent excellent flow conditions in the SFA

which transmits its expanding force on to a considerably greater surface area. The hoop strength of the stent filaments is relatively strong. The delivery procedure is difficult and time-consuming. The new model the "Easy Wallstent", is easier to use and can be delivered with greater accuracy.

Palmaz and Strecker Stents. The Palmaz Stent (Johnson and Johnson, Warren, USA) consists of a single segment tubular stainless steel mesh with a wall thickness of 120 μm. The circumference of this stent type consists of four slots, each 4.5 mm long. The diameter in the non-expanded state measures 3.1 mm. The stent is attached to a 7-F balloon catheter. The stent is a non-flexible, rigid stent type which exerts plastic forces on the vessel wall after expansion. The stent shortens on delivery depending on the diameter chosen.

The Strecker Stent (Boston Scientific, Natick, USA) is a meshwork knitted from tantalum wire. The stent is therefore very flexible. It is expanded by inflation of the introducer balloon. The Strecker stent shows only minimal shortening on delivery.

Self-Expanding Nitinol Stents. Nitinol is a binary alloy of nickel and titanium, the physical properties of which were first discovered at the Naval Ordinance Laboratories in Maryland, USA. After mechanical deformation, a wire made of this material regains its original configuration at temperatures above 20°C. We used the Memotherm Stent (Angiomed, Karlsruhe, Germany). The stent is released by withdrawing a plastic sheath constraining the endoprosthesis. The stent then begins to expand and establishes contact with the vessel wall. The memory-metal effect, which has been set at body temperature, compels the stent to assume its designated preprogrammed size and shape (STARCK 1995).

The covered Cragg Endopro Stent (Mintec) is a nitinol stent covered with a woven fabric graft. The stent cover is a prosthetic graft of ultrathin (0.1 mm thickness), low-porosity woven dacron which is coated with a low-molecular-weight heparin.

31.8.7.2
Indications

Because of the high frequency of restenosis in femoral stents within the first 6 months (see also Sect. 31.8.7.3), some authors (VORWERK and GÜNTHER 1997) recommend a conservative policy for the use of stents in the SFA and limit their use to patients with severe flow-impairing dissection or other complications of PTA. Our indications (LIERMANN 1995) for stent implantation in the SFA are shown in Table 31.3.

31.8.7.3
Results

In extended segment occlusions (longer than 5 cm) of the SFA, long-term results of PTA, as well as of stenting, are less than optimal. Our own results, as well as those of most authors (ROUSSEAU et al. 1989; Do et al. 1992; SAPOVAL et al. 1992; VORWERK and GÜNTHER 1997), show that Wallstent placement is not particulary encouraging. SAPOVAL et al. reported early stent thrombosis in 19% of cases and a primary patency rate of 67% after 6 months and 63% after 1 year. VORWERK (VORWERK and GÜNTHER 1997) reported 12% subacute thromboses and primary patency rates of 83% (6 months) and 55% (12 months). Do (1992) found no significant benefits from stenting in a prospective study comparing PTA and stenting of the SFA. Also in this study, the early thrombosis rate was nearly 20% following Wallstent placement. In contrast, the author did not see any rethrombosis in the group which underwent only PTA.

The reported results after placement of Palmaz and Strecker stents in the femoral arteries seem to be better. PINOT et al. (1994) described a low restenosis

Table 31.3. Indications for stenting in the superficial femoral artery

- Acute dissection with subsequent vascular occlusion that cannot be sufficiently controlled by repeated, long-term use of PTA
- Reocclusion of a vascular segment that has been successfully opened by the same intervention through PTA due to vascular wall deficiency
- As an exception in cases of persistent restenosis after PTA with an expected occlusion in the near future due to the considerable slowing down of blood flow

PTA, percutaneous transluminal angiosplasty.

rate of 19%, HENRY et al. (1994) reported a primary patency rate of 72% after a period of 3 years (both studies used Palmaz stents). STRECKER et al. (1990) found a patency rate of 80% after 12 months in a series of 84 femoropopliteal stents.

My own long-term follow-up study (LIERMANN 1995) on a series of 89 patients over a period of 37 months (mean follow-up) showed a patency rate of 82% in proximally placed stents and of 46% in the distal SFA.

There are only few reports as yet on clinical experience with memory-alloy stents in the SFA. STARK reported on his first clinical experience with 243 femoropopliteal Memotherm stents; he found a high degree of damaged stents and no better long-term results in comparison with other stents (STARCK 1995, 1997).

31.8.7.4
Temporary Stenting

The idea behind temporary stenting, which was first performed by the author (LIERMANN et al. 1995), is to avoid the so-called response-to-injury-effect on the vessel wall. In contrast to permanent stent implantation with reactive myointimal hyperplasia as a response to the pressure of the stent on the vessel wall, temporary stenting is performed within a limited time period of 24 h. Moreover, long-term anticoagulation is no longer necessary in these patients. The stent type used in temporary stenting is the Strecker tantalum stent, which was the only one that could be removed with forceps after 24 h without damage to the vessel wall (LIERMANN 1995). In the technique described above, the placed stent is removed after a period of approximately 24 h with commercially available polyp-removal forceps (Boston Scientific, 7 F; Cook Europe, London, UK, 9 F) through the introducer sheath (7- or 9-F Terumo sheath). Thus, the three branches of the forceps are opened after insertion through the sheath and advanced to the implanted stent. The branches are rounded on the outside and at the tip to avoid vascular damage, but have a sharp hook on the inside which snares in the mesh of the stent. After ensnaring the stent, the arms of the forceps are re-closed and the stent is pulled carefully back into the sheath (Fig. 31.8). In a series of 45 patients with dissection of the SFA in Hunter's canal treated by means of prolonged dilatation, 13 cases led to temporary stent implantation. Of these cases, 11 were treated successfully; only in two cases permanent stent implantation was neccessary. When using the relatively stable Terumo sheath, it was always possible to pull the stent – forceps combination completely into the sheath without damaging the sheat.

Minor clinical experience in the use of the Isostent (a memory-alloy stent of extreme elasticity with a spiral configuration) in temporary stenting was reported by HENRY et al. (1994).

31.8.7.5
Prevention of Restenosis: Intravascular Radiation

Treatment of stenoses in the SFA causes injury to the vascular wall, almost always resulting in intimal hyperplasia. Some authors presume that the use of stents alone does not appreciably improve patency rates compared to PTA – POBA.

One possible alternative is to combine the methods available for treating intimal hyperplasia. The good results obtained in treating keloids by means of irradiation therapy (BUENSCH 1937) was the basis for our therapeutic concept for the prophylactic irradiation of hyperproliferative vascular wall reactions (LIERMANN et al. 1994, 1997) (Fig. 31.9). The de-

velopment of small-caliber probes for afterloading therapy in the bile duct enabled us to use such probes for therapy in the vascular system. Indications for endovascular afterloading therapy should be restricted to clinically-relevant stenoses or recurrent occlusions in the stented vascular segment occurring within less than 8 months after previous, repeated PTA treatment.

Technique. The entire treatment is carried out under heparin therapy (100 IU/kg body weight). After recanalization and PTA of the restenosed vascular segment, a 9-F recanalization catheter is inserted through the positioned 9-F sheath via a guidewire, and positioned so that its tip is just below the affected vascular segment. The inner diameter of the catheter permits insertion of a special catheter with a diameter of 5 F. The pointed tip of the catheter means that the measuring rod and special catheter can only be pushed forwards to just before the tip of the recanalization catheter without being able to pass through the catheter opening. This particular feature allows an exact measurement and calculation of the length of the afterloading probe under stable, reproducible conditions.

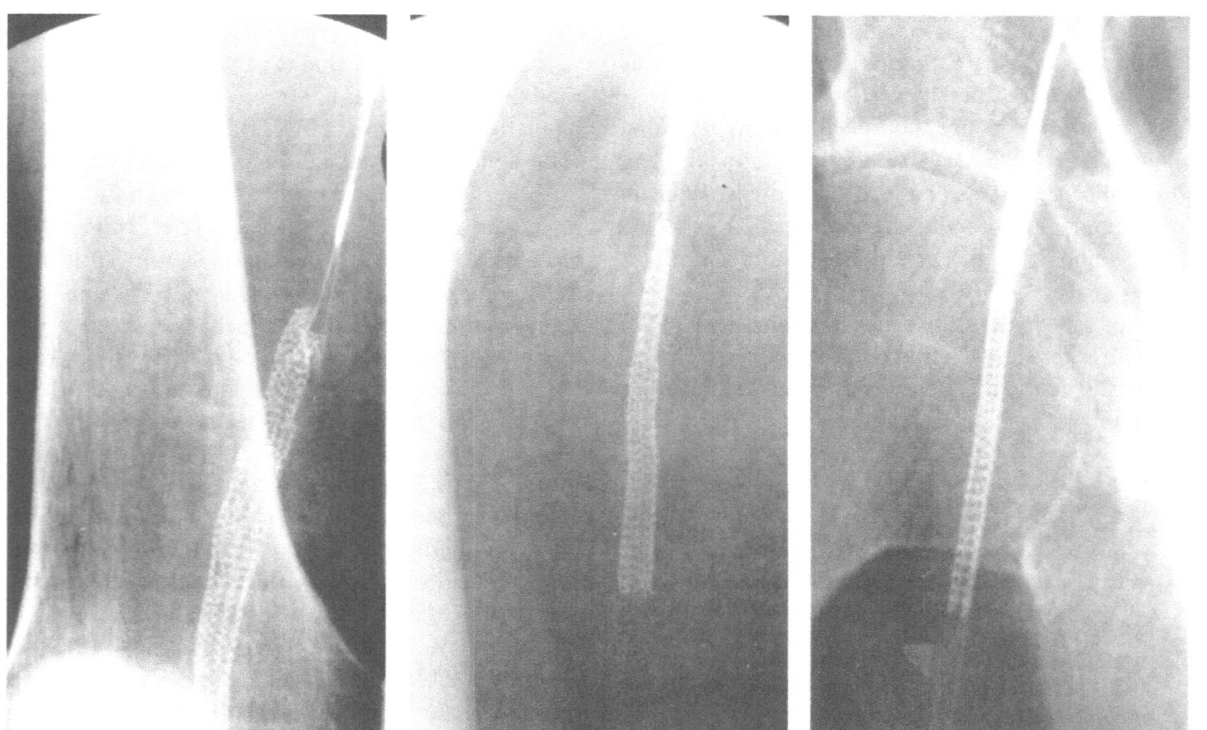

a   b,c

Fig. 31.8 a–c. Temporay stenting. Extraction of a temporarily placed stent in the superficial femoral artery showing the Boston remover with opened branches (**a**), during removal (**b**), and withdrawal back into the introducer sheath (**c**) using a Cook system

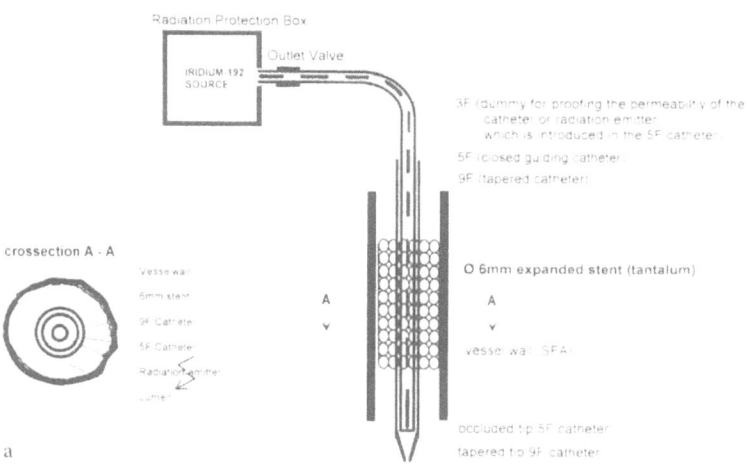

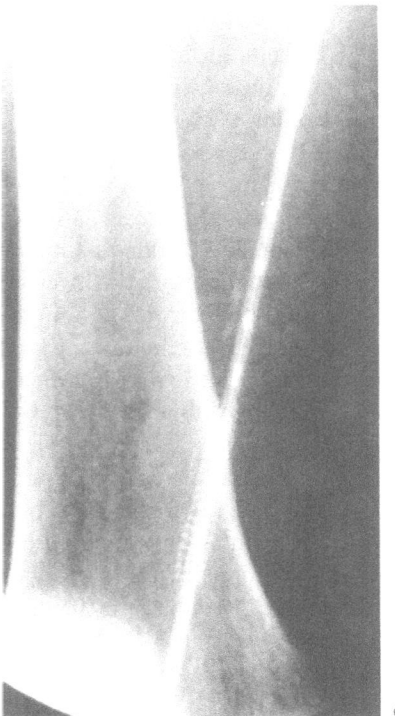

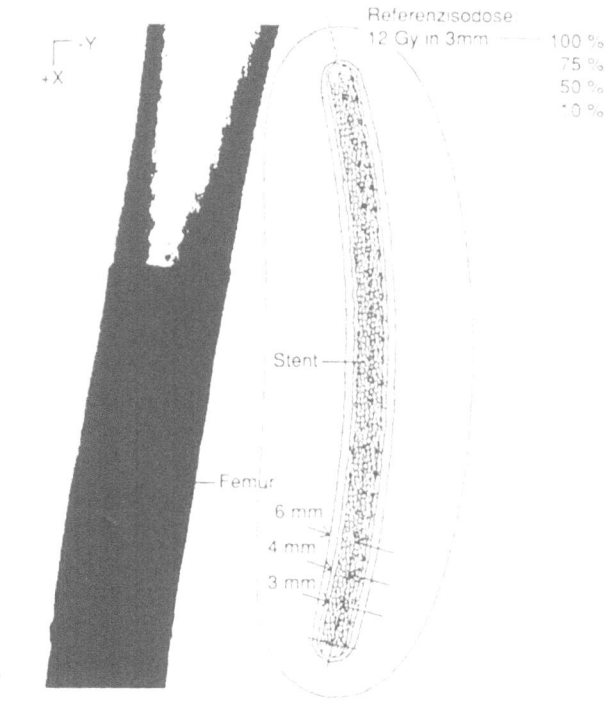

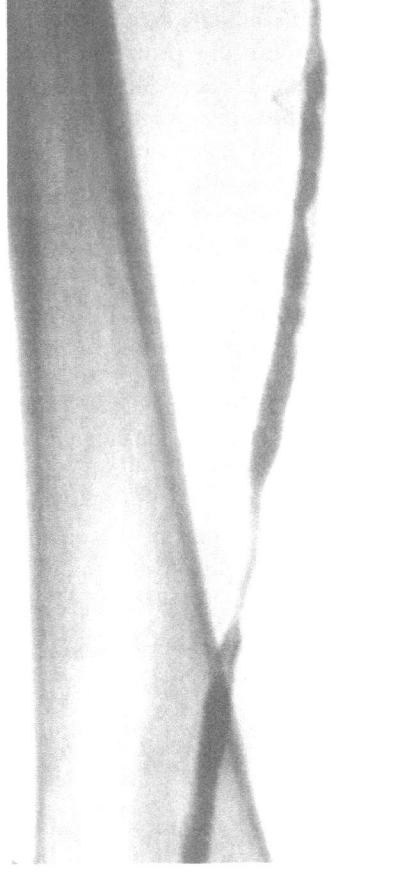

Fig. 31.9 a–d. Iridium-192 afterloading irradiation within a superficial femoral artery (SFA) stent. **a** The catheter and loading system for endovascular irradiation. **b** Distribution of the isodosis in the region of the stented SFA. **c** Calibration probe in the SFA planning the irradiation in the region of two stents. **d** Three-year follow-up shows patency in the stented and irradiated segments and restenosis in the surrounding areas of the SFA

The 5-F special catheter is inserted through the 9-F catheter as far as possible with its independently-sealed tip, which will later accommodate the iridium (iridium 192 with a strength of 10 Ci) probe with its 1.1-mm diameter which is inserted during the afterloading procedure. The reference dose should be 1200 cGy. After calculation of the exact irradiation dose for the afterloading method, the program controls and monitors the insertion and removal of the iridium probe from the source into the special catheter through to the tip, and monitors the irradiation duration. The exposure time depends on the condition of the source and is approximately 200 s.

Material. In a study of 40 patients over a follow up period ranging from 4 to 90 months, we had, in total, clinical findings of reocclusion in 16%. Follow-up examinations revealed no evidence of nerve lesions following irradiation therapy. ZEITLER and colleagues, who also used our procedure, indicated a higher recurrence rate than our group using a single dose of 10 Gy applied to the vascular wall. Our application of 12 Gy also gives rise to doubts as to whether the dose is always homogeneously distributed in the vascular wall, achieving the same antiproliferative effect overall, or whether certain adjacent areas may be differentially exposed as a result of the uncentral position of the probe. In order to minimize this effect, we developed a catheter which can accommodate the probe system with an inner lumen of just 6 F, but which has an outer diameter of approximately 8 F (Optimed).

Afterloading irradiation is a therapeutic concept for treating recurrent intimal hyperplasia in stented vascular segments, which must be applied under extremely strict provisos. In contrast to percutaneous irradiation, which must be applied in a fractionated mode to avoid severe side effects to the surrounding tissue, the endovascular afterloading method achieves the same effect in the vascular wall with only a single application lasting 200 s, with a strong dose decrease for the surrounding tissue. The drawbacks of intravascular irradiation lie in the organization between angiology and radiotherapy. In addition, the method is not available in all clinics.

31.8.7.5
The Future Developement of Interventional Therapy of the SFA

Alternative techniques, such as balloon-mediated drug delivery, drug-coated and-covered stents, taxol stents or gene therapy, are still at the stage of experimental studies or early clinical studies. Results, therefore, are not as yet available.

31.9
Conservative and Additional Pharmacotherapy

In addition to the surgical and non-surgical interventional therapy of arterosclerosis of the limbs, one must consider the possibilities of conventional and pharmaceutical therapy. Above all, the treatment or better avoidance of risk factors which lead to the developement of arteriosclerosis need to be mentioned. One condition sine qua non is to abstain from cigarette smoking. Also, possible arterial hypertension needs to be controlled, whereas hypotension should be avoided in a crictical ischemic situation. A very important aspect of the conservative treatment of patients with intermittent claudication is continuous training up to the pain limit. Once the pain limit has been reached, training should be interrupted. By constant physical training, which should initially be performed under supervision, one can significantly push forward collateralization.

31.91
Pharmacological Therapy

In contrast to the treatment of coronary heart disease, the pharmaceutical therapy of peripheral arteriosclerosis is of only minor importance. Vasodilators have proven ineffective in patients with peripheral arterial sclerosis. Better effects can be shown by using prostaglandin and pentoxifylline. Long-term treatment with aspirin and other inhibitors of platelet aggregation are of importance. Even though these substances are known to reduce the risk of progression of the disease, an improvement in exercise tolerance could not be shown.

In the case of acute arterial occlusion and pre- and post-surgical phase the patient should be treated with heparin to avoid thrombus growth. Dosage is set by doubling the partial thromboplastin time.

31.10
Vascular Surgery

Surgical therapy of femoropopliteal vessels is orientated by the stage and morphology of peripheral occlusive vascular diseases (POVD). These can be divided into three basic types: the segmental type (20%), the intermediate type (20%), and the long-distance type of femoral occlusions (60%). Additionally, the situation and condition of the DFA are of considerable importance. In the case of a patent DFA and patent arteries of the lower limb, the prognosis for the spontaneuos developement of the disease does not justify active surgical treatment in stage II Fontaine classification or stage I.1 and I.2 of the Rutherford classification. Regarding relative stenosis of the DFA, the performance of surgical enlarging of the same using patch-transplant therapy is often combined simultaneously with sympathectomy. Surgical therapy of POVD in the femoropopliteal segment is performed only in stages III–IV of the Fontaine classification or II and III of the Rutherford classification. These stages are mostly accompanied by obliterations in the tibiofibular arteries also. There are various surgical methods of treatment.

31.10.1
Thromboendarterectomy of the SFA

After arteriotomy of the popliteal artery, the occlussion cylinder should be isolated and dissected at the most useful level for dissection, introducing the ring stripper intramurally (VOLLMAR 1975). The occlusion cylinder should be removed under rotational movement of the obliteration device in the direction of its origin. Concomittent intraoperative arteriography and endoscopy are helpful. The complications and limitations of these methods are clearly caused by the method itself: destruction of the origins of side branches and collaterals, injuries to vessel walls causing thrombotic aggregation, hyperplastic repair mechanism, and weakness of the vessel wall resulting in aneurysm and reocclusion. The distal surgical arteriotomy entrance must be closed by stitches, which often also causes dissection.

The embolectomy of acute thrombotic or embolic occlusion using a Fogarty catheter remains a proven surgical treatment (FOGARTY et al. 1963). The high rate of complications requires strict supervision after surgical treatment by radiological means.

31.10.2
Bypass Surgery

The cephalic or great saphenous veins are the most suitable for performing bypass surgery. The veins need to be explanted and reimplanted in a reciprocal fashion to avoid problems with the valvular apparatus of the veins. The valves must be positioned in a flow direction. The use of artificial grafts, such as Dacron or gore, should not be implanted in joint-crossing areas. Therefore, combinations between artificial and autologous vein materials – so-called composite grafts or hitch-hike bypass and jump-bypass (MÜLLER et al. 1995) – have been inaugurated.

Anatomical bypass procedures (HORSCH and CLAEYS 1995) are orientated towards the original position and location of the vessels (aortofemoral, iliacofemoral, femoropopliteal, femorocrural, popliteopedal). Extra-anatomical bypass procedures are less time-consuming, but are performed less often because of the long-term results.

31.10.3
Results of Surgery with Critical Limb Ischemia

Autologous saphenous vein was shown to be the best material for bypass grafting in several randomized studies. VEITH et al. (1990) showed a 4-year patency rate of 49% against a rate of 12% with polytetrafluoroethylene grafts. With reconstruction of the bypass to the isolated popliteal segment, RAITHEL (1995) saw a 5-year patency rate of 58% and an operative mortality rate of 1.9% (5-year survival rate, 46%). ALLENBERG and ECKSTEIN (1995) published their results with limb salvage in 62% and cumulative patency in 40% of patients with critical limb ischemia after 4 years. With these results, together with an analysis of the literature, he concludes that pedal bypass grafting still provides limb salvage in about two thirds of patients with crural occlusive disease and limb-threatening ischemia. Autologous vein bypass as mono-vein bypass or as a jump-graft is the method of choice. Aggressive surgical management, including selective angiography, is necessary even in the presence of a popliteal pulse. Therefore, particularly in patients with critical limb ischemia, close cooperation between the vascular surgeon and the interventionalist is necessary (VEITH et al. 1990).

References

Ahn SS, Eton D, Yeatman LR, Deutsch LS, Moore WS (1992) Intraoperative peripheral rotary atherectomy: early and late clinical results. Ann Vasc Surg 6:272–280

Allenberg JR, Eckstein HH (1995) Critical limb ischemia – does the limb salvage rate justify the time-consuming reconstruction of pedal arteries? In: Horsch S, Claeys L (eds) Critical limb ischemia, diagnosis and treatment. An interdisciplinary approach. Steinkopff, Darmstadt, pp 135–238

Baensch W (1937) Über die Strahlenbehandlung der Keloide. Strahlentherapie 60:204–209

Cox JL, Gottlieb AL (1986) Restenosis following percutaneous transluminal angioplasty: clinical, physiological and pathological features. Can Med Assoc J 136:1129–1132

Do DD, Triller J, Walpoth B, Stirnemann P, Mahler F (1992) A comparison study of self-expandable stents vs balloon angioplasty alone in femoropopliteal artery occlusions. Cardiovasc Intervent Radiol 15:306–312

Ferral H, Fernando CC, Castaneda-Zuniga WR (1992) Lasers in peripheral vascular disease. In: Castaneda-Zuniga WR (ed) Interventional radiology, 2nd edn. Williams and Wilkens, Baltimore, pp 609–620

Fogarty TJ, Cranley JJ, Krause RJ, Strasser E, Hafner C (1963) A method for extraction of arterial emboli and thrombi. Surg Gynecol Obstet 116:241–244

Goodkind J, Coombs V, Golobic RA (1993) Excimer laser angioplasty. Heart Lung 22:26–35

Günther RW, Vorwerk D (1990) Aspiration catheter for percutaneous thrombectomy: clinical results. Radiology 175:271–273

Henry M, Amor M, Ethevenot G, et al. (1994) Primary and secondary patency of stented peripheral arteries. Three years follow-up. A single center experience. Cardiovasc Intervent Radiol 17:57 (abstr)

Hoffman U, Schneider E, Bollinger A (1992) Percutaneous transluminal angioplasty (PTA) of the deep femoral artery. VASA 21:69–74

Horsch S, Claeys L (eds) (1995) Critical limb ischemia, diagnosis and treatment. An interdisciplinary approach. Steinkopff, Darmstadt

Huppert PE, Duda SH, Helber U, Karsch KR, Claussen CD (1992) Comparison of pulsed laser assisted angioplasty and balloon angioplasty in femoropopliteal artery occlusions. Radiology 184:363–367

Huppert PE, Duda SH, Kalighi K, Baumbach A, Seeboldt H, Claussen CD (1994) Periphere gepulste Laserangioplastie – Erfahrungen nach 4jährigem Einsatz. Rofo 160:125–131

Kensey KR, Nash YE, Abrahams C, Zarin CK (1987) Recanalization of obstructed arteries with a flexible, rotating tip catheter. Radiology 165:387–389

Laerum BF, Vlodaver Z, Castaneda-Zuniga WR, Edwards E, Amplatz K (1982) The mechanism of angioplasty. Fortschr Röntgenstr 136:573–576

Lammer J, Karnel F (1988) Percutaneus transluminal laser angioplasty with contact probes. Radiology 168:733–737

Liermann D (1995) Stents in lower extremity arterial vessels. In: Liermann D (ed) Stents – state of the art and future developments. Polyscience, Morin Heights, pp 50–58

Liermann D, Kirchner J (1997) Angiographische Diagnostik und Therapie. Thieme, Stuttgart

Liermann D, Zegelmann M (1995) Extraction of misplaced or occluded endovascular stents. In: Liermann D (ed) Stents – state of the art and future developments. Polyscience, Morin Heights, pp 371–378

Liermann D, Schopohl B, Herrmann G, Kollath J, Böttcher HD (1992a) Endovaskuläres Afterloading als Therapiekonzept zur Prophylaxe der intimalen Hyperplasie in peripheren Gefäßen nach Stentimplantation. In: Kollath J, Liermann D (eds) (1992) Stents II. Schnetztor, Konstanz, pp 80–92

Liermann D, Strecker EP, Peters J (1992b) The Strecker stent: indication and use in iliac and peripheral arteries. J Cardiovasc Intervent Radiol 15:298–305

Liermann D, Böttcher HD, Kollath J, et al. (1994) Intimal hyperplasia after stent implantation in peripheral arteries: treatment by endovascular afterloading. J Cardiovasc Intervent Radiol 17:12–16

Liermann D, Bauernsachs R, Schopohl B, Böttcher HD (1997) Five year follow-up after brachytherapy for restenosis in peripheral arteries. Semin Intervent Cardiol 2:133–137

Liermann D, Kirchner J, Bauernsachs R, Schopohl B, Böttcher HD (1998) Brachytherapy with iridium-192 HDR to prevent from restenosis in peripheral arteries. An update. Herz 23:394–400

Müller P, Rückert R, Bürger K, et al. (1995) Principles of infragenicular vascular reconstruction in patients with critical limb ischemia. In: Horsch S, Claeys L (eds) (1995) Critical limb ischemia, diagnosis and treatment. An interdisciplinary approach. Steinkopff, Darmstadt, pp 141–149

Pinot J, Langlois J, Touze J, Bergeron J (1994) SFA Palmaz stent: long term results. Cardiovasc Intervent Radiol 17:67 (abstr)

Raithel D (1995) Bypass to the isolated popliteal artery. In: Horsch S, Claeys L (eds) Critical limb ischemia, diagnosis and treatment. An interdisciplinary approach. Steinkopff, Darmstadt, pp 135–140

Roeren T, Palmaz JC, Garcia O, Rees CR, Tio FO (1990) Percutaneous vascular grafting with a coated stent. Radiology 177:202

Rousseau H, Raillat C, Joffre F, Knight C, Ginestet M (1989) Treatment of femoropopliteal stenoses by means of self-expandable endoprotheses: mid-term results. Radiology 172:961–964

Rutherford RB, Backer JD, Ernst C, Johnston KW, Porter JM, Ahn S, Jones DN (1987) Recommended standards for reports dealing with lower extremity ischemia: revised version. J Vasc Surg 26:517–538

Sapoval M, Long A, Raynaud A, Beyssen B, Fiessinger J, Gaux J (1992) Femoro popliteal stent placement: long-term results. Radiology 184:833–839

Sawada SJ, van Crups AC, Michel SE, et al. (1994) Percutaneous transluminal atherectomy of the superficial femoral and popliteal arteries: long-term results in 48 patients. Cardiavasc Intervent Radiol 17:312–318

Schild H, Zocholl G, Kopp H, Schmiedt W, Schunk K, Hake U, Jakob H, Thelen M (1990) Klinische Erfahrungen mit dem Kensey-Katheter-System. Komplikation und Ergebnisse. Rofo 152:168–172

Schmitz-Rhode G (1995) Rotationsangioplastie. In: Günther RW, Thelen M (eds) Interventionelle Radiologie, 2nd edn. Thieme, Stuttgart, pp 148–153

Shenoy SS (1983) Sidewinder catheter for conversion of retrograde into antegrade catheterization. Cardiovasc Intervent Radiol 6:112–113

Simpson JB, Selmon MR, Robertson GC, et al. (1988) Transluminal atherectomy for occlusive peripheral vascular disease. Am J Cardiol 61:96–101

Starck E (1995) First clinical experience with the Memotherm vascular stent. In: Liermann D (ed) Stents – state of the art and future developements. Polyscience, Morin Heights, pp 59–62

Starck E (1997) Mechanical instability of femoropopliteal

arterial stents because of kinking. Importance of lateral inflection angiography. Radiology 205(S):557 (abstr)

Starck E, McDermott JC, Crummy AB (1985) Percutaneous aspiration thromboembolectomy. Radiology 156:61–66

Strecker EP, Liermann D, Barth KH, et al. (1990) Expandable tubular stents for treatment of arterial occlusive diseases: experimental and clinical results. Radiology 175:97–102

Strecker EP, Hagen B, Liermann D, Kuhn FP (1993) Komplikationen bei der Implantation arterieller Tantalstents und deren Behandlung. Zentralblatt der Radiologie. Radiology 147:799 (abstr)

Triller J, Do DD, Maddern G, Mahler F (1992) Femoropopliteal artery occlusion: clinical experience with the Kensey catheter. Radiology 182:257–261

Vallbracht C, Liermann D, Prignitz I, Süss B, Awiszus H, Paasch C, Landgraf H, Beinborn W, Stickelmann G, Kollath J, Roth FJ, Schoop W, Breddin HK, Kaltenbach M (1989) Rotationsangioplastik – Wiedereröffnung chronischer Arterienverschlüsse mit einem langsam rotierenden Katheter. Rofo 151:574–587

Vallbracht C, Liermann D, Landgraf H, Kollath J, Roth FJ,

Breddin KH, Hartmann A, Schoop W, Kaltenbach M (1993) Recanalization of chronic arterial occlusions: low-speed rotational angioplasty. 5 years experience in peripheral and coronary vessels. Eur J Med 2:232–238

Veith JF, Gupta SK, Wengerter KR, et al. (1990) Changing arteriosclerotic disease patterns and management strategies in lower limb threatening ischemia. Ann Surg 212:402–413

Vollmar J (1975) Rekonstruktive Chirurgie der Arterien, 2nd edn. Thieme, Stuttgart

Vorwerk D, Günther RW (1997) Arterial stent placement. In: Adam A, Dondelinger RF, Mueller PR (eds) Textbook of metallic stents. Isis Medical Media, Oxford, pp 3–19

Wildenhain PM, Wholey MJ, Jamulowski CR, Hill KL (1994) Infrainguinal directional atherectomy: long term follow up and comparison with percutaneous transluminal angioplasty. Cardiovasc Intervent Radiol 17:305–311

Zollikofer CL, Cragg AH, Hunter DW, Yedlicka JW, Castaneda-Zuniga WR, Amplatz K (1992) Mechanism of transluminal angioplasty. In: Castaneda-Zuniga WR, Tadavarthy SM (eds) Interventional radiology. Williams and Wilkins, Baltimore, pp 249–298

32 Popliteal Artery Diseases

J. Lammer

CONTENTS

32.1
Anatomy and Variations

The anatomic proximal origin of the popliteal artery is at the distal end of the adductor canal (Hunter's canal). The artery runs together with the vein in a connective tissue sheath. The artery and vein are in an anterior-posterior position. Thus, dorsal access to the popliteal artery usually involves a transvenous puncture of the popliteal artery, which increases the risk of an arteriovenous fistula after a transpopliteal intervention. Side branches of the popliteal artery supply the arterial network of the knee (rete articulare genus). Major side branches are the medial

and lateral superior genual arteries and the medial and lateral inferior genual arteries. The popliteal artery terminates at the trifurcation, where it divides into the anterior tibial artery and the tibiofibular trunk, which further ramify into the posterior tibial artery and the peroneal artery.

Functionally, the popliteal artery is divided into three segments:

1. Segment P1 extends from the adductor canal to the superior genual branches, taking the major collateral arteries from the deep femoral artery if the superficial femoral artery is obstructed
2. Segment P2 extends from the superior to the inferior genual artery; this segment is bent during flexion of the knee
3. Segment P3 lies between the inferior genual arteries and the trifurcation. This segment is functionally important because an obstruction may cause occlusion of the trifurcation and proximal calf arteries.

Variations of the distal popliteal artery can be observed in 8% of cases. The most common variation is a high origin of the anterior tibial artery.

32.2
Acute Embolic Occlusion

Embolic occlusion of the popliteal artery may be caused by an embolism from the left atrium due to atrial fibrillation, from the left ventricle after myocardial infarction, or from any aortic aneurysm. Recanalization procedures performed in the iliac or femoropopliteal arteries may also cause embolic occlusion of the popliteal artery. Usually, the embolus stops at the trifurcation. Obstruction of popliteal flow by the embolus will result in a retrograde thrombosis of the P3 segment up to the inferior genual arteries.

Clinically, the patient reports an acute onset of pain and a cold, numb sensation in the calf and foot. The skin might be cold and pale, with reduced

J. Lammer, MD, Professor, Universitätsklinik für Radiodiagnostik, Klinische Abteilung für Angiographie und Interventionelle Radiologie, Währinger Gürtel 18-120, 1190 Vienna, Austria

capillary and venous filling. Emergency catheter angiography with puncture of the contralateral femoral artery should be performed. Angiographic signs of embolic occlusion of the popliteal artery are as follows: In the case of an incomplete occlusion, angiography demonstrates the embolus at the trifurcation, surrounded by contrast medium. Total occlusion will cause acute arrest of contrast column (meniscus sign). Additional signs of an embolic event include a proximally normal arterial system without severe stenoses, lack of collateral arteries, or additional emboli in other arteries, such as the hypogastric or deep femoral arteries. The patient's clinical history may also provide information on a potential embolic event. A bilateral angiography should be performed to identify emboli in the contralateral limb.

32.3
Arteriosclerotic Stenoses and Occlusions

Arteriosclerotic obstructions may occur in all three segments of the popliteal artery. Stenoses in the P2 segment (e.g., stenoses of the common femoral artery) may be more fibrotic or calcified and, therefore, more resistant to balloon angioplasty. Since diabetes causes obstructions and mediasclerosis of the tibial arteries, diabetics are at higher risk of stenoses or occlusions in the popliteal artery.

Intermittent claudication may be caused by an isolated obstruction of the popliteal artery. Additional obstruction of the tibial arteries, which is a common occurrence in diabetic patients, may cause rest pain or gangrene. Assessment of the walking distance and ankle-brachial Doppler index is necessary before any imaging modality is used. Color Doppler ultrasound may demonstrate the obstruction of the popliteal artery. However, intraarterial angiography is necessary to demonstrate inflow obstructions and, furthermore, the exact status of the tibial arteries down to the pedal arch. In some cases, oblique or lateral views of the popliteal artery are necessary for the correct assessment of a stenosis.

32.4
Popliteal Artery Aneurysm

An arterial aneurysm is defined as a localized fusiform or saccular enlargement of the artery, the diameter of which is more than twice that of the normal lumen of the artery. Aneurysms of the popliteal artery are usually seen in patients with arteriosclerotic dilatative arterial disease or in patients with aneurysms at other sites, such as abdominal aortic or iliac artery aneurysms. Bilateral popliteal artery aneurysms are observed in 50% of cases, while aneurysms in different localizations are observed in 25% (GRAHAM et al. 1980). Of course, connective tissue disorders, such as Marfan's disease or the Ehlers-Danlos syndrome, may also cause popliteal artery aneurysms. Posttraumatic pseudoaneurysms are much less frequent.

The aneurysm may be symptomatic – a local mass in the popliteal fossa may cause pain or compression of the popliteal vein. Chronic embolization from the aneurysm to the foot or tibial arteries may cause ischemic symptoms. Thrombosis of the aneurysm can cause acute thrombotic obstruction of the popliteal artery. Therefore, ultrasound should be performed in all cases of popliteal artery occlusion to rule out a thrombosed aneurysm. It has been suggested that fibrinolysis of thrombosed popliteal artery aneurysms should be performed before bypass surgery to unmask normal segments of the popliteal artery. This may avoid the need for a femorocrural bypass instead of a femoropopliteal bypass in selected patients (DAWSON et al. 1991; CARPENTER et al. 1994). Fibrinolysis may be even more useful once a thrombosed popliteal artery aneurysm is associated with embolic tibial artery occlusions.

Rupture of a popliteal artery aneurysm is rare. A popliteal artery aneurysm can be diagnosed by ultrasound. Angiography may only show the perfused lumen of the aneurysm. Thus, angiographically, the true diameter can be assessed only if there are additional calcifications in the wall. Computed tomography (CT) and magnetic resonance imaging (MRI) may be helpful in selected cases (Fig. 1).

32.5
Adventitial Cystic Disease

Adventitial cystic disease of the popliteal artery was first described by Ejrup and Hiertonn in 1954 in Sweden. It mainly affects men. Adventitial cystic disease is a degenerative disorder of unknown etiology. Proposed etiologies include repeated trauma causing degeneration of the arterial wall or a generalized degenerative process with mucinous arterial wall degeneration. A third theory postulates

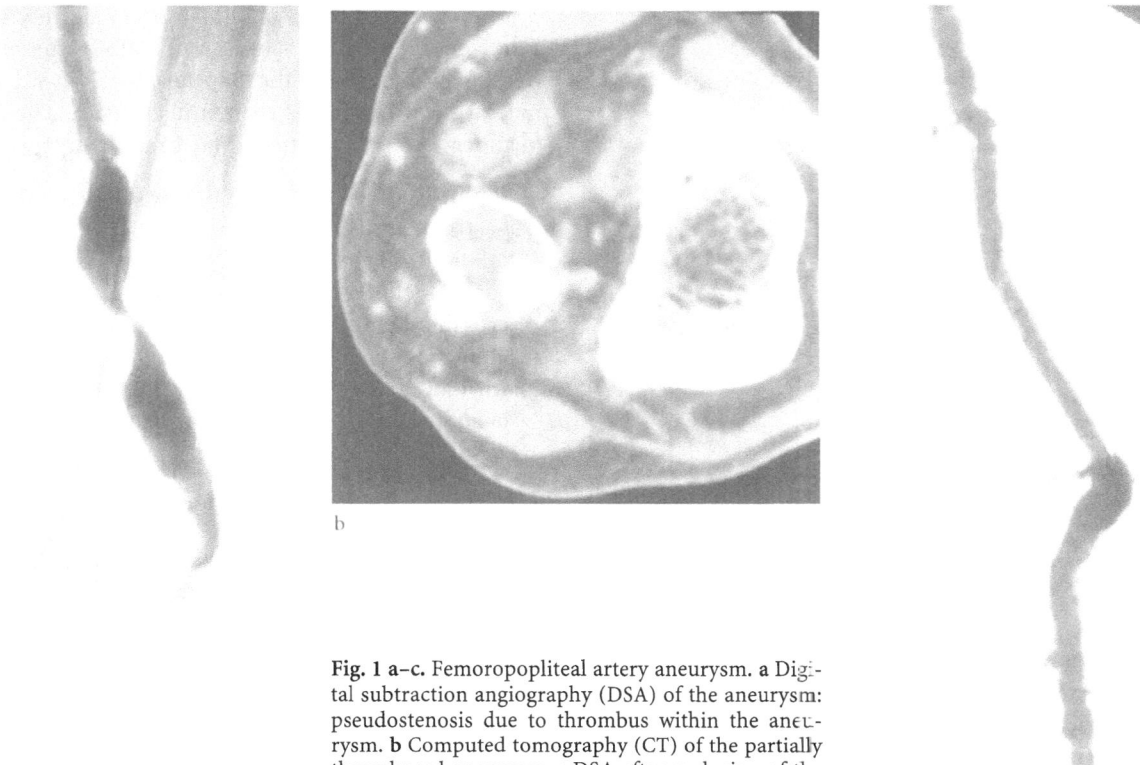

Fig. 1 a–c. Femoropopliteal artery aneurysm. a Digital subtraction angiography (DSA) of the aneurysm: pseudostenosis due to thrombus within the aneurysm. b Computed tomography (CT) of the partially thrombosed aneurysm. c DSA after exclusion of the aneurysm by a stent graft

the inclusion of mucin-secreting cells within the adventitia of the popliteal artery. These cells possibly originate from the synovia of the knee joint (RICH 1982).

The typical clinical presentation is sudden onset of claudication in the mid-forties of a man's life. Angiographically, a smooth wall stenosis or occlusion in the midportion of the popliteal artery with an otherwise normal arterial system is a strong indication of adventitial cystic disease (Fig. 2). Duplex sonography and CT may be helpful in some cases.

Percutaneous aspiration of cystic fluid has been described as one treatment modality. However, surgical intervention by way of enucleation of the cyst or venous interposition is commonly used (WILBUR et al. 1995; JUNG et al. 1997).

32.6
Popliteal Compression Syndromes

Popliteal compression syndromes are uncommon causes of lower extremity claudication in young adults.

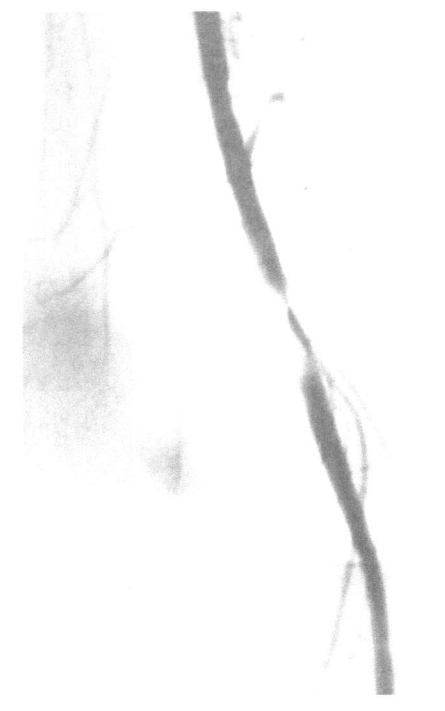

Fig. 2. DSA of a patient with intermittend claudication. Popliteal artery stenosis due to adventitial cystic disease

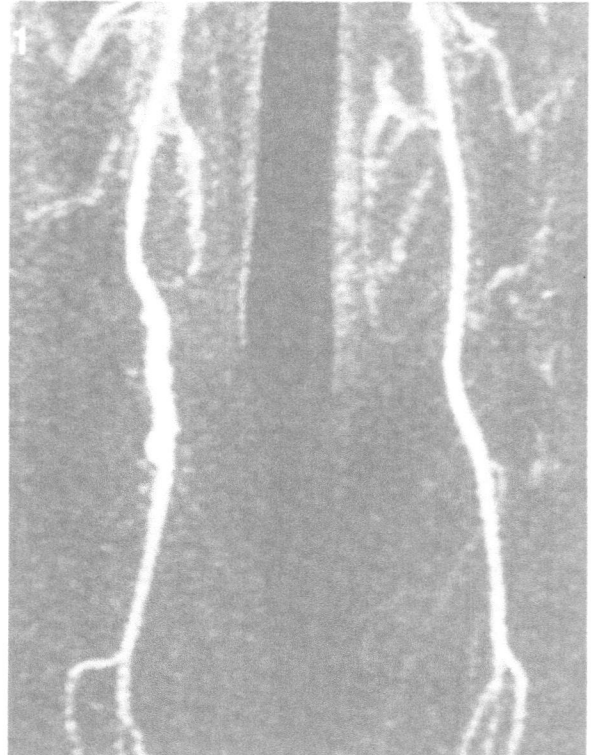

a

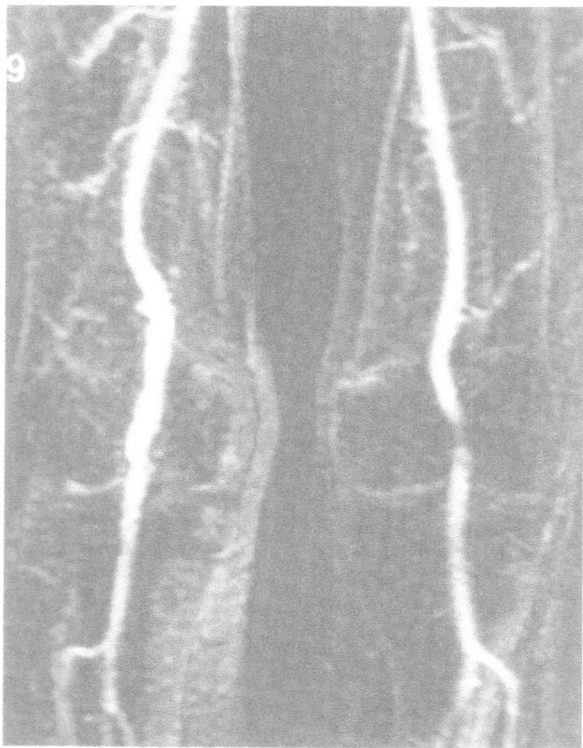

b

Fig. 3 a,b. Contrast-enhanced magnetic resonance angiography (MRA) of a marathon runner with claudication during exercise. **a** Status post venous interposition because of functional entrapment of the right popliteal artery; normal left popliteal artery at rest. **b** Compression of the left popliteal artery during plantar flexion

The classic form of popliteal artery entrapment syndrome is attributed to an anomalous anatomic relationship between the popliteal artery and the medial head of the gastrocnemius muscle. The following anatomic variations may cause compression:

- Popliteal artery medial to the medial head of the gastrocnemius muscle
- Small fibrous band linking the medial head of the gastrocnemius muscle to the lateral condyle and crossing behind the artery
- Same anomaly as that described in association with an abnormally high insertion of the medial head of the gastrocnemius muscle (ROSSET et al. 1995).

A functional form of entrapment has also been observed in athletes. This form of popliteal artery compression is believed to be related to hypertrophy of the calf muscles. It can occur at two sites: (1) Above the knee between the plantar muscle and the medial head of the gastrocnemius muscle; or (2) below the knee between the plantar and popliteal muscles.

The classic form of entrapment is seen on angiography at rest as a medial deviation of the popliteal artery from its normally straight course, and occlusion of the artery during plantar flexion of the foot. Aneurysmal changes may be present. In the functional form, the artery follows a normal course at rest but is compressed and deviated laterally during plantar flexion. CT or MRI of the popliteal fossa at rest and during plantar flexion will permit exact delineation of the muscular origin of the entrapment (CHERNOFF et al. 1995) (Fig. 3). The popliteal vein may also be involved.

Surgical correction with musculo-tendinous release is recommended for the treatment of popliteal compression syndromes.

32.7
Interventional Radiology of Popliteal Artery Disease

32.7.1
Percutaneous Transluminal Angioplasty of Peripheral Arterial Occlusive Disease

Percutaneous transluminal angioplasty (PTA) is applied in cases of lifestyle-limiting claudication due to peripheral arterial occlusive disease (PAOD). A trial of monitored exercise therapy, cessation of smoking, and a reduction of risk factors are warranted before PTA is performed. However, patients with rest pain or gangrene require immediate intervention.

The American Heart Association (AHA) (PENTE-COST et al. 1994) has related clinical outcome to the morphology of lesions as follows:

Category 1 PTA is the procedure of choice; it produces a high rate of technical success with complete relief from symptoms

Category 2 Generally well suited for PTA, complete relief or improvement can be expected

Category 3 Amenable to PTA; however, because of location, extent, or severity, surgery offers a better chance of technical success and lasting patency

Category 4 Surgical options are superior to PTA.

For femoropopliteal artery disease the following lesion morphologies were allocated to the four categories:

Category 1 Lesions are single stenoses up to 3 cm in length, not located at the origin of the superficial femoral artery or the distal popliteal artery

Category 2 Lesions are:
  (a) Single stenoses 3–10 cm in length, not involving the distal popliteal artery
  (b) Heavily calcified stenoses up to 3 cm
  (c) Multiple lesions, each less than 3 cm

Category 3 Lesions are:
  (a) Single, 3–10 cm in length, involving the distal popliteal artery
  (b) Multiple, each 3–5 cm, with or without heavy calcification
  (c) Single stenoses or occlusions over 10 cm

Category 4 Lesions are complete common femoral and/or superficial femoral artery occlusions, or complete popliteal and proximal trifurcation occlusions.

Thus, with regard to the popliteal artery, PTA is well suited for segmental stenoses in segments P1 and P2. Lesions of the distal P3 segment are amenable to PTA; however, patency may be of short duration. Occlusions of the popliteal artery, especially those of the distal segment, including the trifurcation, should be treated by surgery.

This categorization is based on morphology, not on clinical indications. Of course, a more aggressive approach is recommended if the patient has critical limb ischemia.

32.7.2
Popliteal Artery Balloon Angioplasty

In the majority of patients an antegrade approach from the ipsilateral common femoral artery is used. A 5-F sheath is placed antegradely; 5000 units of heparin and 100 µg of nitroglycerin are injected intraarterially. Using "road mapping", the lesion is crossed with a hydrophilic guidewire and balloon dilatation is performed. Balloons of between 4 and 5 mm are commonly used for the popliteal artery. Some patients with ectatic arteries require a 6-mm balloon in the proximal popliteal artery. After PTA, the balloon is withdrawn, but the guidewire remains in place. A control angiogram is performed through the sideport of the introducer sheath. Documentation of the tibioperoneal arteries down to the foot is mandatory before termination of the procedure. If high-grade stenoses or occlusions of the P2 segment are to be recanalized, it is important to place the knee in a strictly extended position to avoid anterior wall dissection of the popliteal artery (Fig. 4).

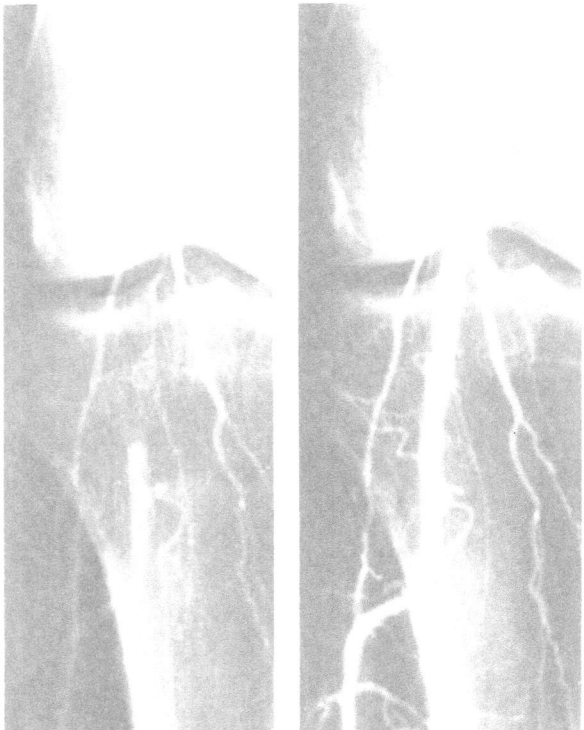

Fig. 4 a,b. PTA of an occlusion of the popliteal artery. **a** Four-centimeter-long occlusion of the middle popliteal segment (P2): AHA category 2 lesion. **b** Control angiogram after PTA

32.7.3
Atherectomy and Lasers

Atherectomy may be necessary in eccentric plaques or large lumen-obstructing flaps following PTA. Lasers play a limited role in the recanalization of total occlusions.

32.7.4
Stents

Experience with stents in popliteal artery disease is limited. In general, immediate and early results following stent placement have been excellent, and many cases of angioplasty failure have been converted to an early success due to the use of stents. However, restenosis as a result of intimal hyperplasia in the stented segment is quite common in the first 3–9 months after treatment. At present, stents would appear indicated only for the salvage of failed PTA due to dissection or marked recoil (Fig. 5).

Self-expandable, as well as balloon-expandable, stents have been used in the popliteal artery. However, it has been reported that balloon-expandable stents have been crushed at the adductor canal due to muscular compression (ROSENFIELD et al. 1997). Care should also be taken if stents are used in the P2 segment. A lateral angiogram with 90° flexion of the knee clearly demonstrates the bending zone of the popliteal artery, which is usually above the joint space. This zone should not be stented as far as possible. A segment of the distal popliteal artery should be kept stent-free so that femoropopliteal bypass surgery can be performed in case the stent reoccludes.

In order to keep the stented segment as short as possible, the stent should be placed under "road mapping". Balloon-expandable stents, such as the Palmaz stent (Johnson and Johnon Interventional Systems, Warren, N.J.) should be mounted on an Olbert balloon catheter (Boston Scientific, Natick, Mass.) since dislocation during antegrade insertion of the stent-balloon assembly does not occur. Balloon dilatation is also necessary after placement

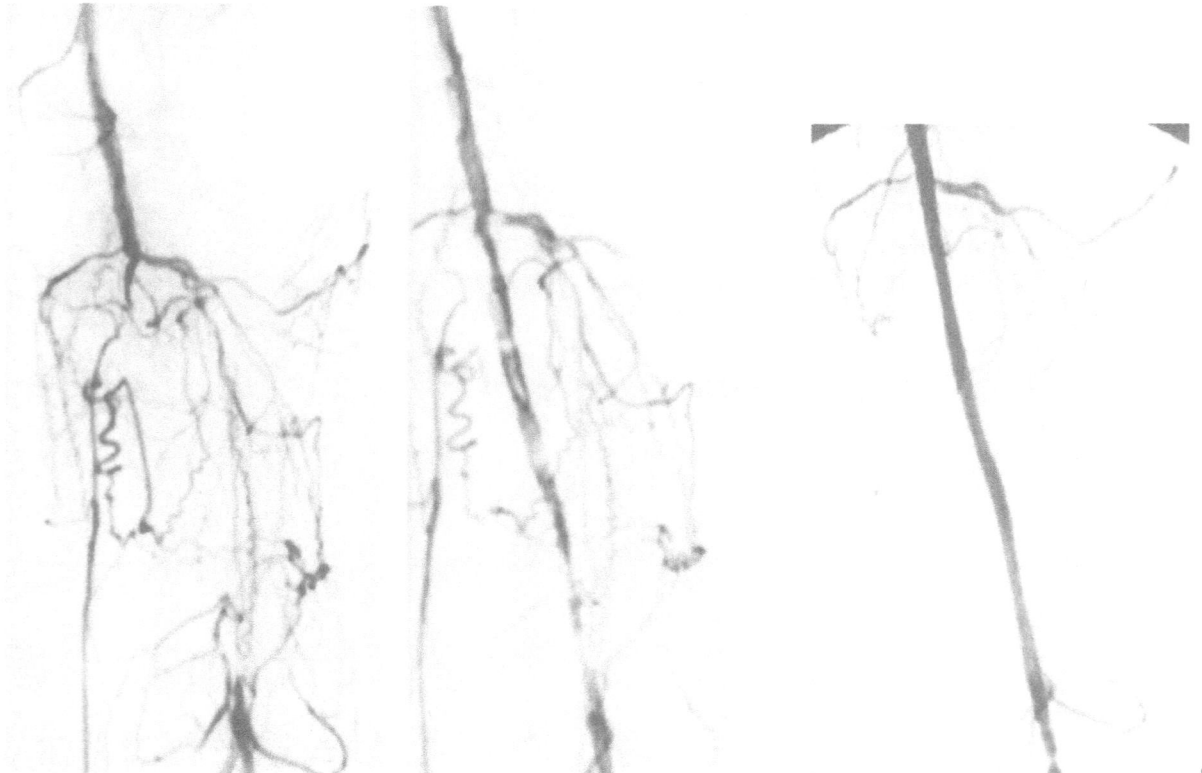

a,b

c

Fig. 5 a–c. PTA and stent placement for an occlusion of the popliteal artery. **a** Ten-centimeter-long occlusion of the P1 and P2 segment of the popliteal artery. **b** Dissection and vascular recoil after PTA. **c** Homogeneous patency of the popliteal artery after placement of a Wallstent

of self-expandable stents to correctly press the stent against the arterial wall. An aggressive anticoagulation and platelet inhibition regimen should be administered in order to prevent early rethrombosis of the stented segment; 5000 Iu of heparin intraarterially and heparin anticoagulation for 2 days (a partial thromboplastin time of 60–80 s) is recommended. In addition, oral ticlopidine hydrochloride in a dose of 500 mg per day for 4 weeks and acetylsalicylic acid 100 mg/day for life should be administered.

32.7.5
Stent Grafts

More recently, endoluminal stent grafts were introduced for the treatment of peripheral arterial occlusive disease and aneurysms (CRAGG and DAKE 1993, 1997; HENRY et al. 1996). Conventional graft materials such as polyester (Dacron) and polytetrafluoroethylene (PTFE) have been used to manufacture the stent grafts. However, alternative materials such as polycarbonate urethane have also been used. The graft fabric is reinforced by a self-expanding metal stent made of a steel alloy or nitinol wire. The main objective of stent grafts in PAOD is to reduce intimal hyperplasia within the grafted segment. However, thrombosis within the grafts and intimal hyperplasia at the proximal and distal ends of the stent graft due to chronic injury by the stent graft and due to compliance mismatch may cause early reocclusion. The use of stent grafts in the P2 segment is not recommended since disintegration of the endograft has been observed. If popliteal artery aneurysms are treated by stent grafts the proximal and distal ends of the aneurysm should be surpassed by 1.5–2 cm to avoid leakage into the aneurysm.

32.7.6
Primary and Long-Term Results

With the use of steerable guidewires, road-mapping technology, and low profile balloons the technical success rate of PTA of popliteal artery stenoses approaches 100%. However, recanalization of popliteal artery occlusions can be difficult, especially if the occlusions are located in segment P2 or P3. Therefore, the advantages and disadvantages of PTA versus infragenual bypass surgery should be

carefully weighed against each other in patients with distal popliteal artery occlusion.

Important variables for the assessment of long-term outcome after PTA include lesion length, distal run-off, grade of residual stenosis, improvement of the Doppler index, and medical conditions such as diabetes or nicotine abuse (CAPEK et al. 1991). Patients with claudication generally do better than those with critical leg ischemia. Primary patency rates after PTA in claudicants after 3 and 5 years are reported to range between 50% and 60%. ADAR et al. (1989) reported a 3-year femoropopliteal PTA patency rate of 62% in claudicants and 43% in critical ischemia. HUNINK et al. (1993) showed that claudicants after PTA of a femoropopliteal stenosis had a 5-year patency rate of 55% versus 29% in patients with critical ischemia. Thus, for symptomatic patients with popliteal artery stenosis, PTA is the preferred initial strategy. PTA provides quality-of-life and lifetime expenditure advantages over a strategy of initial bypass surgery. Studies comparing PTA and bypass surgery are rare since PTA is usually applied in patients with stenotic or short occlusive lesions, while bypass surgery is preferred if long obstructions are present. However, the only long-term prospective randomized studies comparing surgery and femoropopliteal PTA in patients with PAOD showed no significant difference. After a median follow-up of 4 years the patency rate in claudicants was 58% versus 60%, and in critical ischemia 56% versus 53% after bypass surgery versus PTA, respectively (BLAIR et al. 1989). HUNINK et al. (1995) developed a model to evaluate patency results, quality-adjusted life expectancy, lifetime costs, and cost effectiveness ratios for patients undergoing bypass surgery versus PTA. They performed a metanalysis of reports on more than 9000 procedures. It was demonstrated that initial treatment with PTA was more effective than surgery in patients with claudication due to femoropopliteal artery stenosis and occlusion, and in patients with chronic critical ischemia due to femoropopliteal stenosis. Only in patients with critical ischemia due to an occlusion was primary bypass surgery the more effective treatment modality.

Furthermore, the Second European Consensus Document on chronic critical leg ischemia (ANON 1991) also recommended PTA as the first option for this group of patients where possible. It was estimated that PTA may be used in as many as 25% of these patients. Popliteal artery stenting as a primary approach is not indicated. However, stents may have a role in the salvage of acute PTA failures. Reports on the stenting of popliteal arteries are limited; however, long-term patency rates do not exceed 50%–76% after 12 months. The U.S. multicenter trial on the Wallstent (MARTIN et al. 1995) showed, in the femoropopliteal segment, a primary patency of 61% and 49% at 1 and 2 years, respectively. HENRY et al. (1995) reported a primary patency of 50% at 1 year after placement of Palmaz stents in the popliteal artery. STRECKER et al. (1997) reported a patency of 76% and 51% at 1 and 2 years, respectively.

Interestingly, the long-term patency rates of stent grafts in femoropopliteal artery aneurysms are much better. DORFFNER et al. (1998) reported a 1-year primary patency rate of 80%.

32.7.7
Complications

Complications may be classified into generalized and localized complications, procedure-related complications within 24h, or delayed and non-procedure-related complications. Major complications are those which prolong hospital stay, increase the level of care, necessitate surgery, or lead to death. Deaths occurring within 30 days after PTA are considered surgical mortality.

The most common complication is a puncture-site hematoma. Particularly the antegrade puncture, which is required for the majority of popliteal interventions, carries a higher risk of groin hematomas. The incidence is reported to range between 0.8% and 8.6% (HUNINK et al. 1993; JOHNSTON 1992). Major hematomas requiring surgery, such as retroperitoneal hematomas or those causing pseudoaneurysms, are much less frequent. Distal embolization is the second most frequent complication. The rate of embolization depends on the number of total occlusions which are recanalized. In PTA of stenoses, embolization of the thrombus or plaque material occurs in less than 3%. However, when total occlusions are recanalized, the rate may approach 10% (MORGENSTERN et al. 1989). Usually, the emboli get stuck at the popliteal artery trifurcation or at the proximal tibial arteries. In case of an antegrade procedure, aspiration embolectomy is the simplest and fastest way to clear the obstructed artery. A thin-wall large-lumen straight catheter, 6–8 F in size, a sheath with a removable valve, and a 50-cc Luer-Lok syringe are the instruments required for performing a successful embolectomy. If catheter thrombectomy fails to completely remove the emboli and the patient has no acute critical ischemia, an overnight fibrinolysis with urokinase (usual dose 60000–100000 units/h) may reopen the distal arteries. If the patient has acute limb ischemia with a cold, pulseless foot, pain, or loss of sensory and/or motor functions, or loss of capillary and venous filling, an acute surgical revascularization is indicated.

Other localized complications such as thrombosis at the dilatation site, vessel rupture, and arteriovenous fistula are less frequent. Systemic complications may be adverse reactions to contrast media, renal failure, congestive heart failure, or myocardial infarction. The total percentage of complications after PTA was reported to range between 3% and 14%. The 30-day mortality rate is less than 1% (JOHNSTON et al. 1992; MORGENSTERN et al. 1989; MATSI et al. 1994).

Stent placement may be associated with an increased complication rate. The U.S. Wallstent study reported a major complication rate of 16.7% following femoropopliteal stent placement (MARTIN et al. 1995). However, in contrast to this unusually high complication rate, HENRY et al. (1995) reported a major complication rate of only 1% in their stent study. Following distal femoropopliteal stent placement, early thrombosis within the first 3 months was observed in 17%.

32.8
Vascular Surgery

32.8.1
Indications and Techniques

Vascular reconstructive surgery is indicated in patients with PAOD causing lifestyle-limiting claudication, rest pain, gangrene, or tissue loss, following acute thromboembolic occlusion, trauma, and in cases of popliteal artery aneurysm, adventitial cystic disease, or entrapment.

Surgical techniques are well established for the various indications. Embolic occlusions may be treated by transfemoral Fogarty catheter embolectomy and/or by transpopliteal thromboembolectomy. Traumatic lesions and aneurysms are treated either by a short vein/graft end-to-end interposition or by a short bypass with end-to-side anastomoses, usually vein. Adventitial cystic disease is usually managed by enucleation of the cyst or venous interposition. Popliteal compression syndromes are treated by musculo-tendinous release.

In popliteal artery obstructions due to arteriosclerosis, bypass surgery is the state-of-the-art treatment. If the obstruction is in a supragenual region and the distal popliteal segment is intact, a femoropopliteal bypass with supragenual anastomosis is preferred. However, the most important determinant of success is the conduit used; an autogenous vein usually provides a more durable conduit than does a prosthetic graft. The great saphenous vein in the in situ technique or reversed configuration is superior to other autogenous veins, including those of the arm, the small saphenous vein, and composite vein grafts.

For infrainguinal arterial reconstruction with prosthetic grafts, PTFE is the preferred material. However, other materials such as polyester (Dacron) and the umbilical vein have also been used.

For above-knee reconstructions in claudicants, the long-term patency rates of PTFE rafts are claimed to be similar to those with the saphenous vein (VEITH et al. 1986). However, in infragenual and crural reconstructions, any prosthetic graft is worse than an autogenous vein. Various kinds of vein interpositions between the graft and the host artery are used when an autogenous vein is not available.

32.8.2
Results and Nortality

As suggested by the standards committee of the International Society of Cardiovascular Surgery/Society of Vascular Surgery, graft patency rates are reported as "primary" if the graft remains continuously patent without any revision. "Primary assisted patency" is used to describe a continuously patent graft that, however, was treated by service operations or PTA to maintain patency in case of stenoses. "Secondary patency" denotes a graft that has been subjected to some revision or intervention after thrombosis.

Primary patency is highly dependent on variables such as graft material, infra- or supragenual distal anastomosis, and outflow through calf arteries. The 5-year primary patency rates of autogenous vein bypass reconstructions range from 63% to 75%, with a weighted average of 70%. The average patency rate is 75% in above-knee reconstructions and 67% in infrapopliteal reconstructions. The operative mortality rate is 2% (range 1%–3%) (TAYLOR et al. 1990; BERGAMINI et al. 1991). A primary patency rate of 50% after 5 years has been reported for arm vein reconstructions.

In claudicants who underwent infrainguinal reconstructions with PTFE above the knee, 5-year primary patency rates of 42%–76%, with an average of 63%, have been reported. In a clinically mixed population, the 5-year primary patency rate above the knee is 38%–63%, with an average of 50% (VEITH et al. 1986; STERPETTI et al. 1985; AALDERS and VAN VROONHOVEN 1992; DAVIES et al. 1991). However, if PTFE is used for infrapopliteal reconstruction, the 5-year primary patency rate is only 12% (VEITH et al. 1986).

32.8.3
Bypass Thromboses and Stenoses

If a bypass reoccludes early in the postoperative period or within the first 1–2 months after surgery, it may be assumed that surgery has failed. This may occur at the proximal or distal anastomosis due to graft kinking, torsion, and remaining valves when the in situ vein graft technique is used. Surgical revision is mandatory in such cases.

The long-term patency of infrainguinal bypass grafts not only depends on the surgical technique, but also on the postoperative surveillance program. Graft stenosis followed by graft occlusion occurs in 20% of cases (range, 8%–35%) (BERKOWITZ et al. 1989; MILLS et al. 1993). The majority of stenotic lesions are diagnosed in the first year. About 75% of stenotic vein graft lesions are located within the graft. In reversed vein grafts, stenoses are most common at or close to the proximal anastomosis where the vein is smallest. In in situ vein grafts the distal anastomosis is more prone to graft stenoses. However, most in situ grafts develop stenoses in the middle third of the conduit. These mostly web-like stenoses are incompletely excised or hypertrophic valve remnants. PTFE grafts develop stenoses mostly at the distal anastomosis. Stenoses at the proximal inflow artery and distal outflow artery may be clamp lesions or de novo arteriosclerotic plaques.

32.8.4
Interventional Radiology After Vascular Surgery

PTA and fibrinolysis are alternative treatment modalities to surgical patch plasty and thrombectomy. PTA is most successful in short segmental stenoses less than 5 cm in length. In cases of proximal lesions in the inflow artery, proximal anastomoses and lesions in the proximal third of the graft, a crossover technique from the contralateral groin is most suitable. However, in distal lesions at a below-knee popliteal or crural anastomosis, a crossover technique may be cumbersome. In such cases an antegrade puncture of the common femoral artery or a direct puncture of the graft is recommended (Fig. 6). The primary patency rate after bypass PTA may be less than 50% after 5 years. However, primary assisted patency rates of 68%–80% are reported after 5 years as long as only short lesions are dilated (BERKOWITZ et al. 1992; BERKOWITZ 1998). In long, diffuse stenoses and valve remnants, surgical revision by patch plasty or a jump graft may be more successful.

Intraarterial fibrinolysis of occluded veins and prosthetic grafts has been reported using urokinase and recombinant tissue plasmin activator (rt-PA). Depending on the location of the proximal anastomosis, a crossover technique or an ipsilateral antegrade technique is used. If the thrombosed bypass can be passed by a guidewire, a catheter should be advanced through the thrombus. During pullback, the thrombus can be infiltrated with a starting bolus of 5–10 mg rt-PA or 60 000–120 000 IU of urokinase. Finally, the catheter is placed within the proximal bypass graft and 3–5 mg rt-PA or 60 000–100 000 IU urokinase/h are infused until antegrade flow through the conduit is established. It has been claimed that rt-PA causes faster fibrinolysis than urokinase. Continuous infusion of 500–1000 IU of heparin (activated partial thromboplastin time of 60 s) is necessary to avoid thrombus formation along the intraarterial catheter.

Complete clot lysis can be expected in 70%–90% of thrombosed grafts. Long-term results are better for vein grafts (70%) than for prosthetic grafts(< 50%), and better if an unmasked stenosis can be identified and corrected by PTA or surgery (70%–80% at 2 years) than if this is not the case (DURHAM et al. 1989; MEYEROVITZ et al. 1990; SULLIVAN et al. 1991).

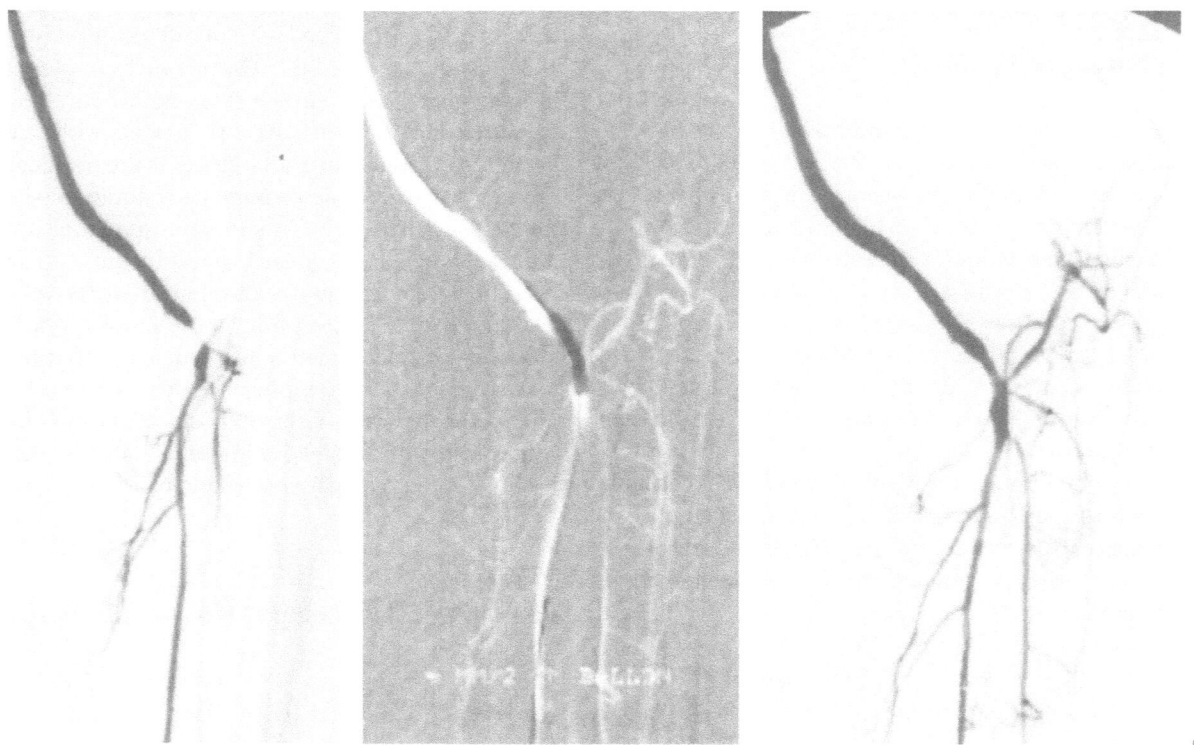

Fig. 6 a–c. PTA of anastomotic stenosis 18 months after bypass surgery. **a** Femoropopliteal infragenual vein bypass, stenosis at the distal anastomosis. **b** Balloon angioplasty with road mapping. **c** Control DSA demonstrates patent anastomosis

References

Aalders GJ, Vroonhoven TJM van (1992) PTFE versus HUV in above-knee femoropopliteal bypass. Six year results of a randomized clinical trial. J Vasc Surg 16:816–823

Adar R, Critchfield GC, Eddy DM (1989) A confidence profile analysis of the results of femoropopliteal percutaneous transluminal angioplasty in the treatment of lower extremity ischemia. J Vasc Surg 10:57–67

Anon (1991) Second European Consensus Document on chronic critical leg ischemia. Circulation 84 [Suppl IV]: IV1–IV26

Bergamini TM, Towne JB, Bandyk DF, et al. (1991) Experience with in situ saphenous vein bypass during 1981 to 1989: determinant factors of longterm patency. J Vasc Surg 13:137–149

Berkowitz HD (1998) PTA of infrainguinal bypass graft stenoses: patient selection and results. In: Perler BA, Becker GJ (eds) Vascular intervention. A clinical approach. Thieme, New York, p 197

Berkowitz HD, Greenstein S, Barker CF, et al. (1989) Late failure of reversed vein bypass grafts. Ann Surg 210:782–786

Berkowitz HD, Fox AD, Deaton HD (1992) Reversed vein graft stenosis: early diagnosis and management. J Vasc Surg 15:130–142

Blair JM, Gewertz BL, Moosa H, et al. (1989) Percutaneous transluminal angioplasty versus surgery for limb-threatening ischemia. J Vasc Surg 9:698–703

Capek P, Mc Lean GK, Berkowitz HD (1991) Femoropopliteal angioplasty. Factors influencing long-term success. Circulation 83 [Suppl I]:I70–I80

Carpenter JP, Barker CF, Roberts B, et al. (1994) Popliteal artery aneurysm: current management and outcome. J Vasc Surg 19:65–72

Chernoff DM, Walker AT, Khorasani R, et al. (1995) Asymptomatic functional popliteal artery entrapment: demonstrations at MR imaging. Radiology 195:176–180

Cragg AH, Dake MD (1993) Percutaneous femoropopliteal graft placement. J Vasc Interv Radiol 4:455–463

Cragg AH, Dake MD (1997) Treatment of peripheral vascular disease with stentgrafts. Radiology 205:307–314

Davies MG, Feeley TM, O'Malley MK, et al. (1991) Infrainguinal PTFE grafts: saved limbs or wasted effort? A report on ten years experience. Ann Vasc Surg 5:519–524

Dawson I, van Bockel JH, Brand R, et al. (1991) Popliteal artery aneurysms. J Vasc Surg 13:398–407

Dorffner R, Thurnher R, Puig S, et al. (1998) Behandlung arterioller Aneurysmen der Becken-Bein-Gefäße mittels Dacron-ummantelter Nitinal-Stents. Fortschr Roentgenstr 168:275–280

Durham JD, Geller SC, Abbott WM, et al. (1989) Regional infusion of urokinase into occluded lower-extremity bypass grafts: long-term clinical result. Radiology 172:83–87

Graham LM, Zelenock GB, Whitehouse WM, et al. (1980) Clinical significance of arteriosclerotic femoral artery aneurysms. Arch Surg 115:502–507

Henry M, Amor M, Etherenot G, et al. (1995) Palmaz stent placement in iliac and femoropopliteal arteries: primary and secondary patency in 310 patients with 2-4 year follow-up. Radiology 197:167–174

Henry M, Amor M, Cragg A, et al. (1996) Occlusive and aneurysmal peripheral arterial disease: assessment of a stent graft system. Radiology 201:717–724

Hunink MGM, Donaldson MC, Meyerovitz MF, et al. (1993) Risks and benefits of femoropopliteal percutaneous balloon angioplasty. J Vasc Surg 17:183–194

Hunink MGM, Wong JB, Donaldson MC, et al. (1995) Revascularization of femoropopliteal disease: a decision and cost-effectiveness analysis. JAMA 274:165–171

Johnston KW (1992) Femoral and popliteal arteries: reanalysis of results of balloon angioplasty. Radiology 183:767–771

Jung EM, Hallermeier J, Schwalbe B, et al. (1997) Zystische Adventitiadegeneration der A. poplitea – Punktion mit Hilfe der Ultraschallangiographie. Rofo 167:423–426

Martin EC, Katzen BT, Benerati JF, et al. (1995) Multicenter trial of the Wallstent in the iliac and femoral arteries. J Vasc Interv Radiol 6:843–849

Matsi PJ, Manninen HI, Vanninen RL, et al. (1994) Femoropopliteal angioplasty in patients with claudication: primary and secondary patency in 140 limbs with 1-3 year follow-up. Radiology 191:727–733

Meyerovitz MF, Goldhaber SZ, Reagan K, et al. (1990) Recombinant tissue-type plasminogen activator versus urokinase in peripheral arterial and graft occlusions: a randomized trial. Radiology 175:75–78

Mills JL, Fujitani RM, Taylor SM (1993) The characteristics and anatomic distribution of lesions that cause reversed vein graft failure: a five year prospective study. J Vasc Surg 17:195–206

Morgenstern BR, Getrajdman GI, Laffey KJ, et al. (1989) Total occlusions of the femoropopliteal artery: high technical success rate of conventional balloon angioplasty. Radiology 172:937–940

Pentecost MJ, Criqui MH, Dorros G, et al. (1994) Guidelines for peripheral percutaneous transluminal angioplasty of the abdominal aorta and lower extremity vessels. Circulation 89:511–531

Rich NM (1982) Popliteal entrapment and adventitial cystic disease. Surg Clin North Am 62:449–465

Rosenfield K, Schainfeld R, Pieczek A, et al. (1997) Restenosis of endovascular stents from stent compression. JACC 29:328–336

Rosset E, Hartung O, Brunet C, et al. (1995) Popliteal artery entrapment syndrome: anatomic and embryologic bases, diagnostic and therapeutic considerations following a series of 15 cases with a review of the literature. Surg Radiol Anat 17:161–169

Sterpetti AV, Schulz RD, Feldhaus RJ, et al. (1985) Seven year experience with PTFE as above-knee femoropopliteal bypass graft. Is it worthwhile to preserve the autologous saphenous vein? J Vasc Surg 2:907–912

Strecker EPK, Boos IBL, Göttmann D (1997) Femoropopliteal artery stent placement: evaluation of long-term success. Radiology 205:375–383

Sullivan KL, Gardiner GA, Kandarpa K, et al. (1991) Efficacy of thrombolysis in infrainguinal bypass grafts. Circulation 83 [Suppl I]:I99–I105

Taylor LM, Edwards JM, Porter JM (1990) Present status of reversed vein bypass grafting: 5-year results of a modern series. J Vasc Surg 11:193–206

Veith FJ, Gupta SK, Ascer E, et al. (1986) Six-year prospective multicenter randomized comparison of autologous saphenous vein and expanded PTFE graft in infrainguinal arterial reconstructions. J Vasc Surg 3:104–114

Wilbur AC, Woefel GF, Flanigan DP, Spigos DG (1995) Adventitial cystic disease of the popliteal artery. Radiology 155:63–64

33 Tibiofibular and Foot Artery Disease

H.-J. Wagner

33.1 Normal Anatomy and Variations

By definition the popliteal artery ends at the origin of the first tibial artery, which typically is the anterior tibial artery. The origin is normally located 4–5 cm below the knee joint (Fig. 33.1). However, in about 4% of cases (BARDSLEY and STAPLE 1970) we find a so-called high origin of the anterior tibial artery at the level of the knee joint or even some centimeters more proximal (Fig. 33.2). Similarly, in a small proportion of the population (about 1%–2%) a high origin of the posterior tibial artery has been described. Normally, the direct continuation of the popliteal artery after the branch of the anterior tibial artery is the tibioperoneal (or tibiofibular) trunk. This vascular segment is about 5 cm long and splits into the posterior tibial artery and the peroneal (or fibular) artery (see Fig. 33.1). As a variation, a

trifurcation of the popliteal artery into all three lower leg arteries at the same point has been observed in 0.4% of patients (BARDSLEY and STAPLE 1970) (Fig. 33.3). The posterior tibial artery may be missing completely in 1%–5% of a normal adult population (BARDSLEY and STAPLE 1970).

Normally, the anterior and posterior tibial arteries are somewhat larger than the peroneal artery. However, if one or two of the vessels becomes diseased and develops a hemodynamically relevant obstruction the unaffected arteries will become hypertrophic and enlarged. The anterior tibial artery continues into the dorsal pedal artery. The posterior tibial artery continues into the plantar artery. Collaterals allow reperfusion of proximally occluded tibial arteries. At the level of the ankle large collaterals are preformed. The peroneal artery, which more often than not is the only patent artery

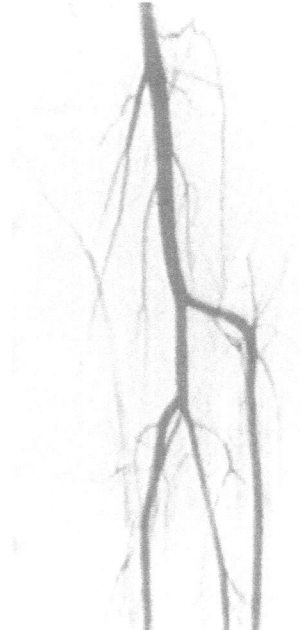

Fig. 33.1. Normal branching of the popliteal artery into the anterior tibial artery, tibio peroneal trunk, peroneal artery, and posterior tibial artery

HANS-JOACHIM WAGNER, MD, Priv.-Doz., Abteilung Strahlendiagnostik, Klinikum der Philipps-Universität, Baldingerstrasse, 35033 Marburg, Germany

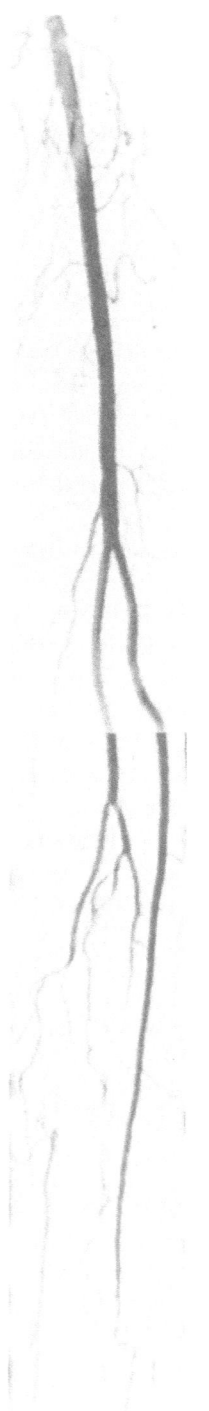

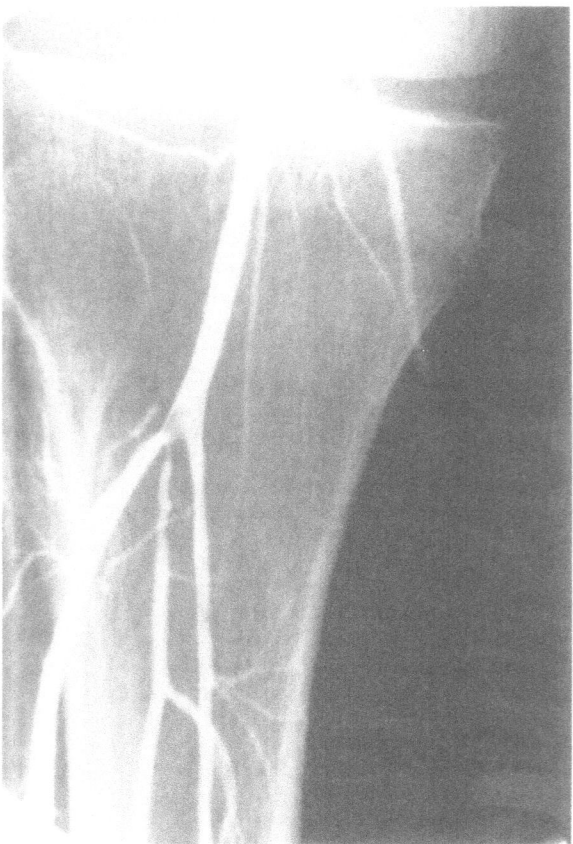

Fig. 33.3. Trifurcation of the popliteal artery into the three calf arteries

anastomoses with the dorsal pedal artery and the ramus communicans with the plantar artery (Fig. 33.4). The dorsal pedal artery and the plantar artery communicate via the plantar arch which is fed medially from the plantar artery and laterally from the dorsal pedal artery (Fig. 33.4).

33.2
Incidence of Lower Leg and Foot Artery Obliterations

Patients presenting with lower-limb-threatening ischemia due to infrarenal atherosclerotic disease generally have diffuse, multilevel disease. However, the stenotic or occlusive disease process involves infrapopliteal arteries in at least one third of these patients (VEITH et al. 1990). In a review of 321 lower extremity angiograms obstructions in below-the-knee vessels alone were observed in 26.5% (HAIMOVICI 1967). In another 50% the tibial arteries

Fig. 33.2. High origin of the anterior tibial artery at the level of the knee joint

in cases of severe peripheral arterial occlusive disease (HAIMOVICI 1967), splits 3–4 cm above the ankle joint into an anterior and a posterior branch, the ramus communicans and the ramus perforans (SCHWARZENBACH et al. 1996). The ramus perforans

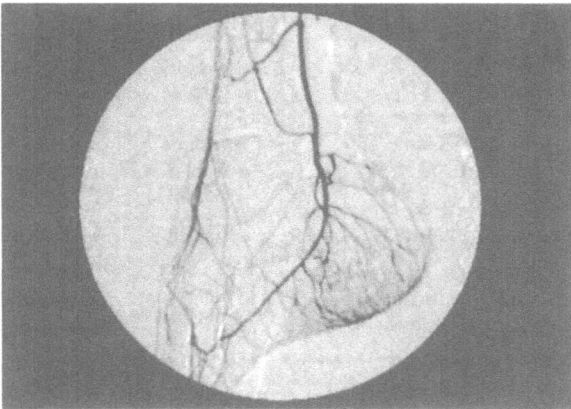

Fig. 33.4. Lateral angiogram of the distal lower leg and foot. Anastomotic communication between the peroneal artery and the anterior tibial artery via the ramus perforans. The ramus communicans posterior anastomoses the fibular artery with the posterior tibial artery. The pedal arch is composed of the dorsal pedal artery and the plantar artery

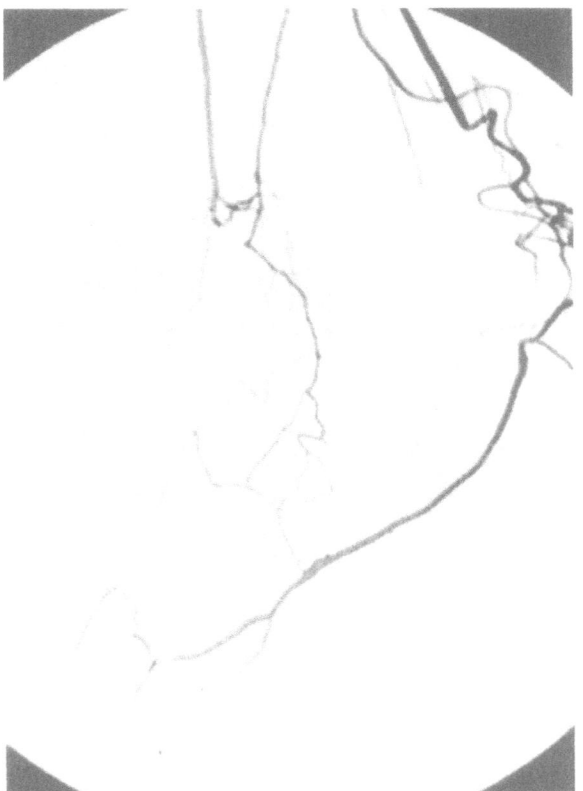

Fig. 33.5. Intraarterial digital subtraction angiography of the foot in lateral projection. Occlusions of the dorsal pedal artery and plantar artery. The plantar arch is perfused through collaterals

were involved in the disease process of more proximal vessels (aorto-iliac and femoro popliteal) (HAIMOVICI 1967). Improvements in imaging modalities over the last two decades have made it possible to routinely visualize arterial disease of distal tibial and pedal arteries, even in cases of proximal multisegmental occlusions. Intraarterial selective digital subtraction angiography (DSA) (Fig. 33.5) and magnetic resonance angiography (MRA) allow the routine visualization of the distal vasculature. An arteriogram of the lower-limb arteries today should demonstrate the entire arteries from the level of the renal vessels to the plantar arch (Figs. 33.4, 33.5).

33.3
Rutherford Gradings

Classification of peripheral arterial occlusive disease in the infrapopliteal arteries follows the guide lines for the grading of lower-limb ischemia (SACKS et al. 1997). Major medical societies (American Heart Association, Society of Vascular Surgery, Society of Cardiovascular and Interventional Radiology) have accepted the guide lines developed by an Ad Hoc Committee of the Society of Vascular Surgery (RU-THERFORD et al. 1986). First, the classification differentiates between acute and chronic limb ischemia. Acute limb ischemia is divided into three categories:

viable ischemia, threatening ischemia, and irreversible ischemia (Table 33.1). Chronic limb ischemia is split into six different categories and three main divisions: claudication, pain at rest, and tissue loss (Table 33.2). By using the criteria described in Tables 33.1 and 33.2 all patients can be easily categorized. A clear definition of the severity of the arterial disease is of major importance since invasive revascularization procedures in vessels below the popliteal artery should be restricted to patients suffering from limb-threatening ischemia (Table 33.2, categories 4–6). However, in diabetic patients with medial wall calcification, who comprise a large proportion of the population requiring infrapopliteal revascularization, grading might be difficult because ankle-brachial artery pressure measurements are useless. For this particular population a different approach for the assessment of severity of peripheral arterial occlusive disease by measuring toe systolic blood pressure (TSBP) and transcutaneous oxygen pressure (tcPO$_2$) is recommended (ORCHARD and STRANDNESS 1992).

Table 33.1. Clinical categories of acute limb ischemia. (From SACKS et al. 1997)

Category	Description	Capillary return	Muscle weakness	Sensory loss	Doppler signals Arterial	Venous
Viable	Not immediately threatened	Intact	None	None	Audible AP more than 30 mmHg	Audible
Threatened	Salvageable if promptly treated	Intact, slow	Mild, partial	Mild, incomplete	Inaudible	Audible
Irreversible	Major tissue loss, amputation required regardless of treatment	Absent (marbling)	Profound, paralysis (rigor)	Profound, anesthetic	Inaudible	Inaudible

AP, ankle pressure.

Table 33.2. Clinical categories of chronic limb ischemia. (From SACKS et al. 1997)

Grade	Category	Clinical description	Objective criteria
0	0	Asymptomatic, no hemodynamically significant occlusive disease	Normal results of treadmill/stress test
I	1	Mild claudication	Treadmill exercise completed, postexercise AP > 50 mmHg but >25 mmHg less than normal
	2	Moderate claudication	Symptoms between those of categories 1 and 3
	3	Severe claudication	Treadmill exercise cannot be completed, postexercise AP <50 mmHg
II	4	Ischemic rest pain	Resting AP ≤ 40 mmHg, flat or barely pulsatile ankle or metatarsal plethysmographic tracing, toe pressure <30 mmHg
III	5	Minor tissue loss, nonhealing ulcer, focal gangrene with diffuse pedal ischemia	Resting AP ≤60 mmHg, ankle or metatarsal plethysmographic tracing flat or barely pulsatile, toe pressure <40 mmHg
	6	Major tissue loss, extending above transmetatarsal level, functional foot no longer salvageable	Same as for category 5

AP, ankle pressure.

33.4
Single and Multivessel Disease

Due to the extensive collateralization of the three different tibial arteries a clinically relevant reduction of blood flow can be anticipated only if all three arteries are diseased. As long as a single tibial artery is patent without a hemodynamic significant stenosis (e.g., >50% diameter reduction) to the level of the plantar arch, symptoms of limb-threatening ischemia will not occur and the indication for a revascularization procedure is not given. Consequently, patients presenting with lower-limb-threatening ischemia due to infrapopliteal disease suffer multivessel obstructions. Very often the only remaining patent artery is the peroneal artery (HAIMOVICI 1967; SCHWARZENBACH et al. 1996). Often two infrapopliteal arteries are completely occluded and the remaining vessel is significantly stenosed. Such short (1 cm or less), single stenoses are ideally amenable to percutaneous transluminal angioplasty (PTA) (Fig. 33.6). According to a guide line issued by the STANDARDS OF PRACTICE COMMITTEE of the SOCIETY OF CARDIOVASCULAR and INTERVENTIONAL RADIOLOGY (1990) such lesions are categorized as a treatment of choice (category 1). However, the majority of patients demonstrate suboptimal or inappropriate lesions

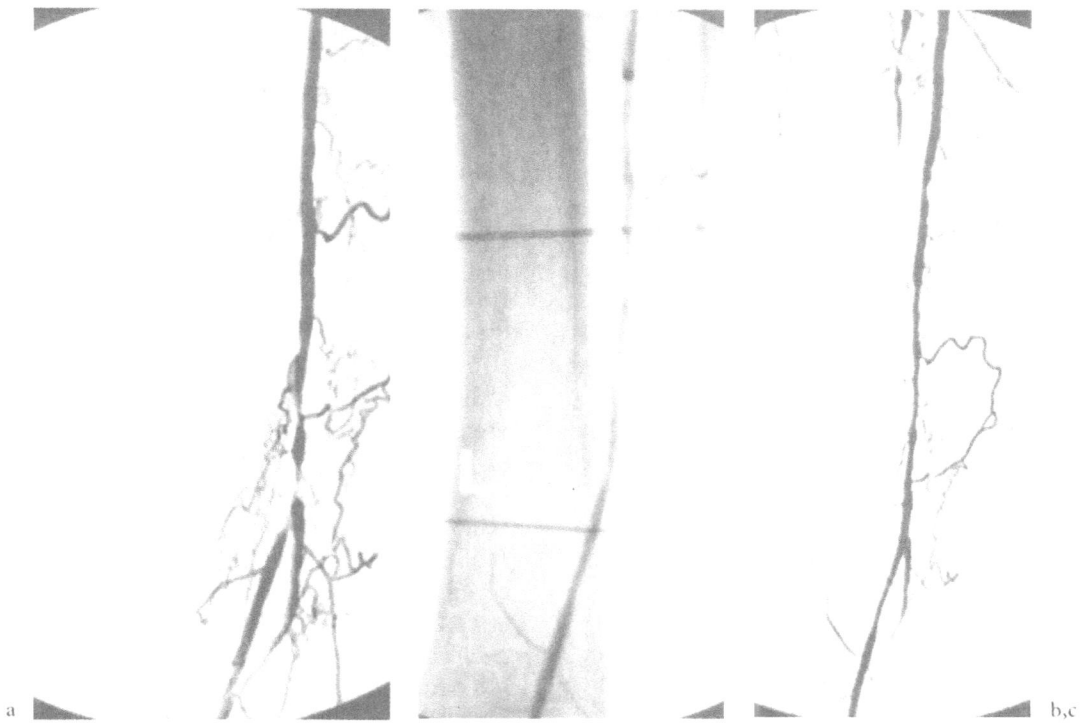

Fig. 33.6 a–c. Balloon angioplasty of the distal anterior tibial artery. **a** Two short high-grade stenoses of the distal third of the anterior tibial artery, which is the only patent calf vessel. **b** Following dilation with a 3-mm diameter balloon (markers denote proximal and distal margin of balloon dilation) sufficient lumen is achieved. **c** Intraarterial digital subtraction angiography after balloon dilatation demonstrating good morphologic results

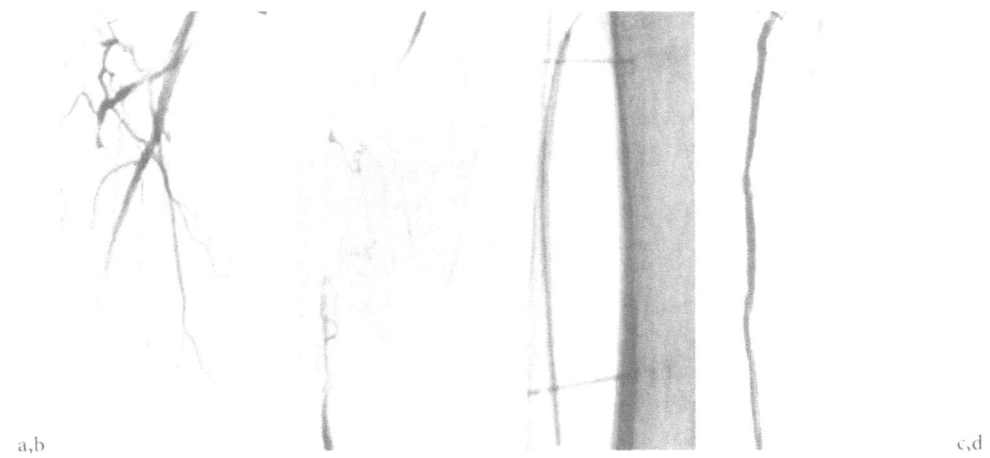

Fig. 33.7 a–d. Percutaneous transluminal angioplasty of a long segment obstruction of the anterior tibial artery. **a, b** A 7-cm long occlusion of the proximal portion of the anterior tibial artery. **c** Balloon dilatation (2-mm diameter, 8-cm length) after recanalization with a hydrophilic guide-wire. **d** Result after angioplasty

for PTA (categories 2–4 of the guide lines) (Fig. 33.7). Nevertheless, a percutaneous transluminal revascularization should be undertaken if a surgical procedure for revascularization is not appropriate because of a failing distal conduit or lack of a suitable saphenous vein. The alternative for these patients would be a primary amputation, which should be avoided under all circumstances according to recommendation No. 29 of the CONSENSUS CONFERENCE ON CHRONIC CRITICAL LEG ISCHEMIA

(1991). There is evidence that a major amputation is not only associated with a 5-year mortality rate of 50%–75% (DORMANDY and THOMAS 1988), but also that amputation significantly decreases quality of life since ambulant rehabilitation is successful only in 9% of major amputees after 5 years (McWHINNIE et al. 1994). Moreover, the total costs of aggressive distal revascularization are outweighed by the total costs of amputation (CHESHIRE et al. 1992).

33.5
Interventional Radiology of Tibiofibular Obliterations

33.5.1
Guide-Wires and Catheters

The development of special material dedicated for use in small vessels had a major impact on interventional radiology below the knee (CASARELLA 1988). This is not only true for low profile balloons, but also for guide-wires and catheters. The introduction of hydrophil-coated wires with a memory-shape metal core of nitinol marked a major progress in PTA in terms of improved recanalization rates. Prospective studies showed a superior recanalization rate with the use of these devices, even in long arterial obstructions (WAGNER et al. 1992). In calf vessels with often extensive disease and long occlusions in relatively small diameter vessels the correct intraluminal recanalization is crucial. Conventional guide-wires, especially if they do not have a straight-tip configuration, tend to create a subintimal channel and may thereby lead to perforation of the vessel wall, which is a complication that occurs more often in this area than at any other peripheral angioplasty site. However, negative clinical sequelae of tibial vessel perforation are rare. Most authors now recommend the use of straight hydrophil-coated guide-wires which will recanalize even long occlusions (more than 10 cm) in >90% (see Fig. 33.7). The use of an angled tip 5-F catheter facilitates the negotiation of the guide-wire into the anterior tibial artery or selectively from the tibiofibular trunk into the peroneal or posterior tibial artery. The angled tip should be short (1 cm) due to the small vessel diameters. Furthermore, the catheter shaft must be braided to achieve enough stiffness to pass the catheter even through long, heavily calcified obstructions. In the distal third of the calf the 5-F catheter might be too large to advance further; therefore, the use of a 5-F catheter

with a tip tapered to 3-F, capable of using a 0.020 in. guide-wire, has been recommended (WAGNER 1994).

33.5.2
Balloon Catheters

Even in the first report on PTA three out of 13 patients were treated in the infrapopliteal region. However, until the development of balloon catheters, these lesions were dilated by tapered catheters (DOTTER and JUDKINS 1964). The first balloon catheters were relatively large and intended for use in the iliac arteries. Since the introduction of small-diameter balloons in the mid 1980s infrapopliteal angioplasty has become a part of the standard PTA procedures (CASARELLA 1988; BAKAL et al. 1996). For a long while some authors also used coronary balloons to dilate the calf vessels (STARCK et al. 1984; HORVATH et al. 1990). To date, we have dedicated small vessel catheters which comprise of low profile balloon catheters with a small, typically sub 4-F shaft and non-compliant balloons with a diameter ranging from 2–5 mm in diameter. The length of the balloon varies from 2–10 cm. The shaft of the catheter is stiff yet flexible to allow advancement in firm, long occlusions. Most of the balloons and shafts are hydrophil-coated to enhance pushability and trackability. Most balloon catheters accept an 0.018-in. guide-wire. Again, for purposes of best advancement guide-wires with a stiff core and a hydrophil coating are preferable (see Fig. 33.7).

33.5.3
Mechanical Devices

Initially, there was great enthusiasm about the use of various types of lasers for angioplasty of tibial arteries. However, there have been only limited reports on the use of laser angioplasty (HORVATH et al. 1990). Lasers have been mainly used for recanalization purposes only, requiring additional balloon dilatation to achieve a sufficient lumen. Also, prospective trials in the femoropopliteal region showed no advantage versus conventional balloon angioplasty.

The rotablator atherectomy system was thought to achieve superior results to balloon angioplasty, particularly in highly calcified lesions and complete occlusions of the infrapopliteal vessels. However, no benefit has been shown as yet. Most published data are discouraging (COMBINED ROTABLATOR

ATHERECTOMY GROUP 1994). Similarly, trans-luminal endarterectomy catheter (TEC) never achieved a significant role in the treatment of occlusive disease below the knee.

Thrombolysis and thrombectomy devices do not play a role in the treatment of chronic athero-sclerotic occlusive disease. Even in cases of throm-botic occlusions the occlusive material will be organized to fibrous tissue within a short period of time due to the small vessel diameter. In contrast, acute arterial occlusion due to a fresh thrombotic or embolic occlusion may be treated with local intraar-terial thrombolysis or thrombectomy (Fig. 33.8) or mechanical thrombolytic systems.

33.5.4
Stents

Although infrapopliteal arteries are of similar size to coronary arteries, stents play a minor or no role in the treatment of obstructions of the tibial vessels. Most authors see contraindications for the use of stents below the knee other than in "bail out" situations. Consequently, there have only been case reports on the use of stents in infrapopliteal arteries (DORROS et al. 1993). However, there have been no prospective or randomized trials to define the status of stent implantation in arteries of the calf. One reason for the caution to implant stents in this

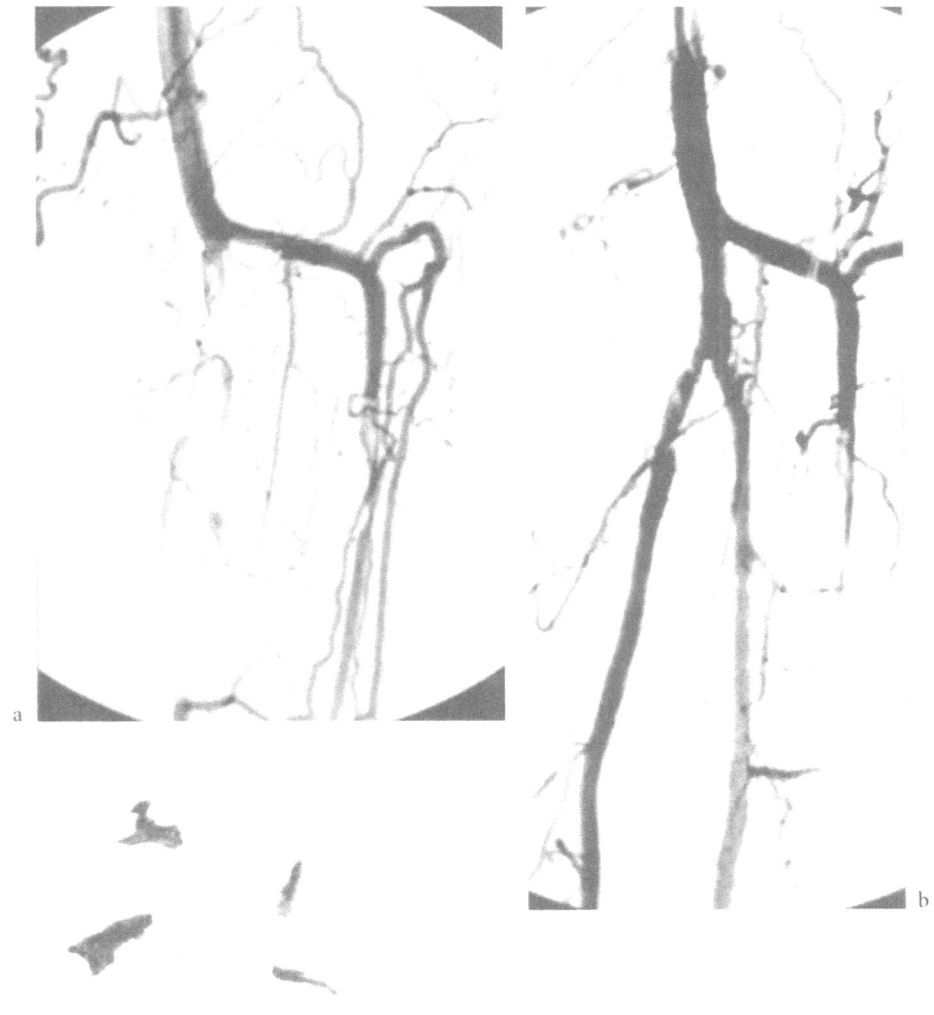

Fig. 33.8 a–c. Percutaneous aspiration thrombectomy. **a** Fresh embolic occlusion of the tibio peroneal trunk after surgery of a popliteal artery aneurysm. **b** Completion angiogram after percutaneous removal of the emboli by suction throm-bectomy with an 8-F catheter. **c** Aspirated emboli

area might be the requirement of an aggressive anti-coagulation regimen to prevent early thrombosis. However, new concepts in stent delivery might lead to a change of this policy such as in coronaries (Co-LOMBO et al. 1995).

33.5.5
Intraarterial Pharmacotherapy

The development of a standard drug regimen before, during, and after the intervention was one of the keys to establishing infrapopliteal angioplasty. In former years, major concerns had been arterial vasospasm and thrombosis. Both complications had been observed frequently in the first attempts at infrapopliteal angioplasty. To overcome these draw-backs an aggressive peri-interventional medication is mandatory. All patients should receive aspirin (ASA), starting at least 1 day prior to the procedure. After placement of the sheath, a bolus of 5000 IU heparin should be administered. If the procedure lasts more than 1 h, a maintainance dose of 1000 IU should be applied every hour. To prevent vasospasm every patient should be given 10 mg nifidepine sublingually immediately prior to the procedure. If spasms occur despite medication with the calcium channel blocker, a dose of 0.1–0.2 mg of nitroglycerin should be administered directly into the affected tibial artery. When the procedure is completed patients should be kept on intravenous heparinization for at least 48–72 h. The dose of heparinization should be adjusted by the prolongation of the partial thrombin time (PTT) to twice the normal value.

Some authors have recommended the use of urokinase at the end of the procedure to dissolve microthrombi. A dose of 100 000 IU was applied as a single shot immediately before withdrawl of the sheath (WAGNER et al. 1993). The role of prostanoids as an adjunctive medication still has to be defined.

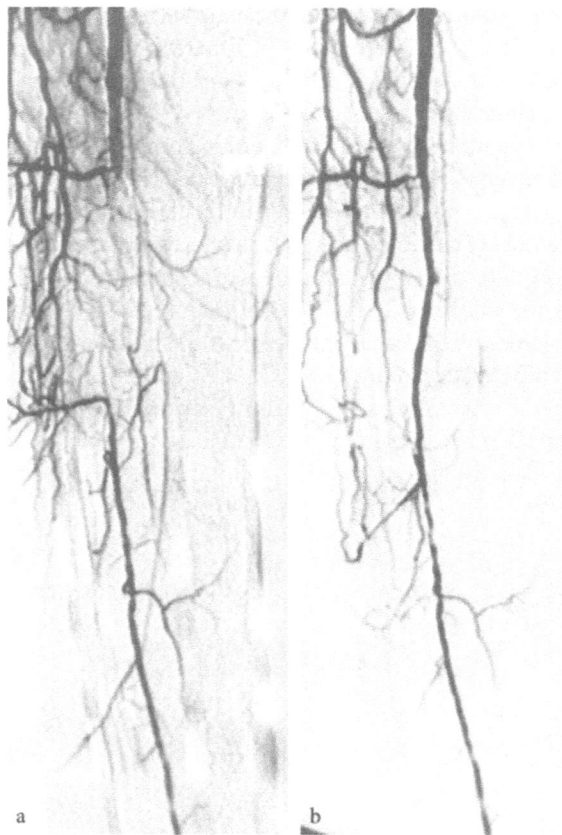

Fig. 33.9 a,b. Infrapopliteal percutaneous transluminal angioplasty after femoropopliteal bypass grafting. **a** The single tibial run-off artery (peroneal artery) shows a segmental occlusion. **b** Result after recanalization and balloon dilation. The procedure was carried out immediately after femoro-popliteal bypass grafting due to a long superficial femoral artery occlusion. The sheath had been placed intraoperatively in the bypass graft

requires excellent angiograms of the tibial and foot arteries (see Figs. 33.4, 33.5).

Postoperative control angiograms after femoro-crural bypass grafting is advocated to reveal residual stenosis and to demonstrate patency of the run-off vessels.

33.6
Perioperative Radiology

Assessing correct vascular status is of major importance before the implantation of distal bypass grafts. To determine the best distal anastomosis site sufficient opacification of distally perfused vascular segments is mandatory. In particular, the creation of distal origin grafts to distal tibial or pedal arteries

33.7
Combined Interventional Radiology and Vascular Surgery

The combination of vascular surgery and percutaneous transluminal revascularization techniques is advantageous in the treatment of multilevel disease. The combination of a long occlusion in the femoro-popliteal region with obstruction in the outflow tract of the tibio-peroneal arteries might be best treated with a combination of a femoro popliteal bypass graft and a subsequent dilatation of the infrapopliteal obstructions (Fig. 33.9). This strategy allows a shorter bypass graft, which might be fruitful if a long homologous vein is not available, and serves for a better bypass graft patency since improved run-off increases the long-term patency rate (MATSI et al. 1993). Such a procedure might be carried out during the same sitting. First, the bypass graft is implanted and then, through a sheath, introduced into the proximal portion of the graft material, the run-off obstruction can be treated by use of the above-described transluminal endovascular technique. The sheath can be safely removed in the operating room and the patient need not undergo a second procedure, nor is the bypass graft endangered by early thrombosis due to diminished run-off flow.

33.8
Results/Prevention of Leg and Foot Amputation

DOTTER and JUDKINS (1964) reported in their historical article in 1964 three cases of infrapopliteal angioplasty out of 13 patients. Even using the old technique of dilating the arterial lumen by tapered catheters amputation could be avoided in one of the three patients. Several reports on the use of tapered 5–7-F catheters to dilate tibial arteries were published in the late seventies and early eighties (MATHIAS et al. 1979; SPRAYREGEN et al. 1980; GREENFIELD 1980; TAMURA et al. 1982; STARCK et al. 1984). The results of these series are mixed. The initial anatomic success was more than 75% in most reports. However, long-term clinical outcome of limb-salvage was either not available or demonstrated limited success of the tibial PTA. The introduction of small-diameter balloons, steerable guide-wires, potent anti-spasmodic drugs, liberal use of heparin, and non-ionic contrast media did not only enable routine PTA of infrapopliteal vessels, but also improved anatomical and clinical results tremendously (CASARELLA 1988; SCHWARTEN and CUTCLIFF 1988; BROWN et al. 1988). The initial report by SCHWARTEN (1991) and the follow-up report described infrapopliteal PTA in 98 and 96 patients with 114 and 112 threatened limbs, respectively. The anatomical success was 100% for treatment of stenosis and 88% of complete occlusions (not longer than 5 cm). The limb-salvage rate of successfully treated patients available for follow-up at 2 years was

83% and 86%, respectively. No major complications were reported.

In the series of BROWN et al. (1988) 11 patients were treated for limb-salvage reasons. The technical success was 75%, the clinical success 67%. During follow-up (1–22 months) 50% remained clinically successful. These results represent the beginning of a learning curve, which was demonstrated as the group published their follow-up results in 1993 (BROWN et al. 1993). In this report 55 infrapopliteal PTAs were carried out on 40 patients; 84% were done for limb-salvage indications. Technical success was now 95%. Limb-salvage rate was 53% at 2-year follow-up (life table analysis). The clinical success rate was quoted 44% at an average follow-up of 26 months.

BAKAL et al. (1990) undertook 57 procedures in 53 patients (98% for limb-salvage reasons). The technical and clinical success rates were significantly higher by use of the balloon technique compared to the tapered catheter method; 29% vs. 86% technical success, 29% vs. 67% clinical success. In a follow-up report the authors quoted a 97% early clinical improvement with 80% limb salvage at 2 years after successful PTA and restoration of straight-line flow to the foot in at least one tibial vessel. In contrast, no patients with obstructed distal outflow achieved any clinical benefit; all such patients required amputation or distal bypass (BAKAL et al. 1996).

In 1990 HORVATH et al. reported on 71 patients with 103 stenosed tibial arteries, 42% treated for limb-salvage reasons. The technical success rate was 96%. Life table analysis of the follow-up showed a 79% patency rate after 1 year, and a 75% rate after 2 years. Limb-salvage rates were not reported.

A small series of 14 limbs of 13 patients treated with tibial balloon PTA were reported by SAAB et al. (1992). All patients suffered limb-threatening ischemia; the technical success was 100% and the limb-salvage rate was 77% at 2-years follow-up. BULL et al. (1992) presented a mixed series of 168 patients with claudication (24%), acute ischemia (11%), and chronic limb-threatening ischemia (65%). Clinical success at 3 years was 83% for a focal stenosis, 76% for multiple stenoses, 44% after local lysis, 36% for occlusions, and 14% for anastomotic stenosis.

MATSI et al. (1993) were the first to publish data from a prospective study on 103 patients with 117 treated limbs. A total of 84 infrapopliteal arteries were dilated and followed for 1–36 months (mean, 12 months). The technical success rate for the entire population was 92% for stenosis and 80% for occlusion. The overall limb-salvage rate was 49% after 2 years. At least one patent calf vessel proved to be statistically significant in predicting limb salvage.

Our own group (WAGNER et al. 1993) conducted a prospective trial on 148 patients with 158 lower limbs, where tibial angioplasty was attempted. A total of 32% of the patients were claudicators, while 68% suffered limb-threatening ischemia. The technical success rate was 94% and the clinical sucess rate 90% at discharge. The mean follow-up period was 17 months. At the end of follow-up all patients primarily presenting with claudication had salvaged limbs, and 80% of the patients with initially limb-threatening ischemia did not undergo a amputation proximal to the tarsometatarsal joint. Diabetic patients had statistically worse results than non-diabetics. Life table analysis revealed a 2-year primary patency rate of 64% for the entire patient group.

WACK et al. (1994) reported in 1993 on 42 infrapopliteal PTAs in 30 patients with single focal lesions of tibial arteries. Later, the same group published their experience of a total of 47 tibial angioplasties in 44 patients with single stenosis (HAUSER et al. 1996); technical success was 80%, follow-up ranged from 1–50 months (mean, 13 months), and the limb-salvage rate was 77% at 2-year follow-up by life table analysis.

DURHAM et al. (1994) treated 14 consecutive diabetic patients with limb-threatening ischemia who were not candidates for surgery. Technical success was 100%. After a mean follow-up of 17 months long-term limb salvage was 77%.

BOLIA et al. (1994) presented results on 21 patients in whom PTA was attempted in a total of 29 occluded tibial arteries with a median occlusion length of 6 cm. Technical success by use of the subintimal revascularization technique was 86%. Long-term results and limb salvage rates were not provided.

SIVANANTHAN et al. (1994) retrospectively analysed 50 tibial PTAs in 38 patients, 20 of whom suffered limb-threatening ischemia. Technical success was 96% and 59% of the patients had clinical improvement by at least one Fontaine stage. Primary patency rates by life table analysis were 60% at 2 years.

VARTY et al. (1995) studied 38 patients with 40 consecutive tibial PTAs. Of these patients 50% had clauducation, the remainder critical ischemia. Technical success was 98%, all technically successfully treated patients demonstrated clinical improvement. Primary and secondary symptomatic patencies were 59% and 79%, respectively. The actuarial limb-salvage rate at 1 year for the limbs presenting with critical ischemia was 77%.

Sos (1996) attempted to treat 81 limbs in 70 patients, 83% of whom suffered from critical ischemia. By using specially designed 3.7-F balloon catheters and steerable 0.018 in. guide-wires infrapopliteal PTA was technically successful in 91.4%. The clinical success rate was 76% after 2 years and 67.5% after 30 months. The amputation rate during the follow-up period (1–48 months, mean 12 months) was 14%.

Table 33.3. Results of tibial PTA

Study	Year	Lower limbs (n)	Critical ischemia (%)	Diabetes (%)	Technical success (%)	Limb salvage (%)	Follow-up (months)
STARCK et al.	1984	46	67	NA	76	NA	NA
SCHWARTEN and CUTCUFF	1988	114	100	60	97	86	24
BROWN et al.	1988	11	100	91	82	73	8
BAKAL et al.	1990	57	98	85	78	NA	NA
HORVATH et al.	1990	71	42	35	96	NA	NA
SAAB et al.	1992	14	100	69	100	79	19
BULL et al.	1992	168	76	52	NA	85	26
BROWN et al.	1993	55	84	64	95	53	26
MATSI et al.	1993	NA	100	77	83	49	24
WAGNER et al.	1993	158	68	46	95	88	17
WACK et al.	1994	30	100	90	83	82	10
BOLIA et al.	1994	24	71	43	86	NA	NA
DURHAM et al.	1994	14	100	100	100	77	17
SIVANANTHAN et al.	1994	41	53	13	96	NA	21
VARTY et al.	1996	40	50	45	98	77	12
HAUSER et al.	1996	47	100	93	80	77	13
Sos	1996	71	83	59	91	86	12

NA, not available from the publication.

The results of the mentioned studies on infrapopliteal PTA are summarized in Table 33.3. In conclusion, the review of the literature clearly demonstrates that since the introduction of small vessel balloon catheters and hydrophilic guide-wires, together with an aggressive pre- and postprocedural medication, the technical results of tibial PTA could be improved enormously. From a technical point of view even complete occlusions longer than 10 cm are today amenable for PTA. However, the clinical improvement in the short-term shows good results, but the long-term results are still characterized by reobstructions.

Nevertheless, since most patients suitable for tibial PTA are poor surgical candidates and often present with several concomitant diseases (e.g., diabetes and end-stage renal disease), PTA should be attempted for limb-salvage reasons according to the Consensus document on chronic critical limb ischemia. However, patients need to undergo careful surveillance to assess the early reobstruction and correctly schedule the reintervention to improve primary assisted and secondary patency rates to achieve better long-term limb-salvage rates.

Finally, there is a definite need for prospective randomized trials comparing the endoluminal percutaneous technique with open surgery to define the future role of both treatment modalities. These trials should include cost-effectiveness analysis and quality-of-life assessment.

33.9
Additional Pharmacotherapy

As already stated above, all patients should be kept on aspirin for life due to the proved secondary prophylactic effect in patients with arterial occlusive disease. In patients with critical limb ischemia the revascularization procedure can be combined with medical treatment by intravenous or intraarterial application of prostanoids for 2–3 weeks. This regimen is recommended particularly in cases with poor run-off and limited success in the revascularization procedure.

Some patients with limb-threatening ischemia might benefit from an adjunctive lumbar sympathicolysis, which should preferably be carried out percutaneously under computed tomography guidance.

The use of oral anticoagulants (vitamin K antagonists) should be restricted to patients with poor run-off or early reobstructions because of the known side-effects in the elderly and multidiseased patient population.

References

Bakal CW, Sprayregen S, Scheinbaum K, Cynamon J, Veith FJ (1990) Percutaneous transluminal angioplasty of the infrapopliteal arteries: results in 53 patients. Am J Roentgenol 154:171–174

Bakal CW, Cynamon J, Sprayregen S (1996) Infrapopliteal percutaneous transluminal angioplasty: what we know. Radiology 200:36–43

Bardsley JL, Staple TW (1970) Variations in branching of the popliteal artery. Radiology 94:581–587

Bolia A, Sayers RD, Thompson MM, Bell PR (1994) Subintimal and intraluminal recanalisation of occluded crural arteries by percutaneous balloon angioplasty. Eur J Vasc Surg 8:214–219

Brown KT, Schoenberg NY, Moore ED, Saddekni S (1988) Percutaneous transluminal angioplasty of infrapopliteal vessels: preliminary results and technical considerations. Radiology 169:75–78

Brown KT, Moore ED, Getrajdman GI, Saddekni S (1993) Infrapopliteal angioplasty: long-term follow up. J Vasc Intervent Radiol 4:139–144

Bull PG, Mendel H, Hold M, Schlegl A, Denck H (1992) Distal popliteal and tibioperoneal transluminal angioplasty: long-term follow-up. J Vasc Intervent Radiol 3:45–53

Casarella WJ (1988) Percutaneous transluminal angioplasty below the knee: new techniques, excellent results. Radiology 169:271–272

Cheshire NJW, Wolfe JHN, Noone MA, Davies L, Drummond M (1992) The economics of femorocrural reconstruction for critical limb ischaemia with and without autologous vein. J Vasc Surg 15 167–175

Colombo A, Hall P, Nakamura S, Almagor Y, Maiello L, Martini G, Gaglione A, Goldberg SL, Tobis JM (1995) Intracoronary stenting without anticoagulation accomplished with intravascular ultrasound. Circulation 91: 1676–1688

Combined Rotablator Atherectomy Group (CRAG) (1994) Peripheral atherectomy with the rotablator: a multicenter report. J Vasc Surg 19:509–515

Consensus Conference on Chronic Critical Leg Ischemia (1991) Consensus document on chronic critical leg ischemia. Circulation 88 Suppl 4:IV1–IV26

Dormandy JA, Thomas PRS (1988) What is the natural history of a critically ischaemic patient with and without his leg? In: Greenhalgh RM, Jamieson CW, Nicolaides AN (eds) Limb salvage and amputation for vascular disease. Saunders, Philadelphia, pp 11–26

Dorros G, Hall P, Prince C (1993) Successful limb salvage after recanalization of an occluded infrapopliteal artery utilizing a balloon expandable (Palmaz-Schatz) stent. Catheterization Cardiovasc Diagn 28:83–88

Dotter CT, Judkins MP (1964) Transluminal treatment of arterial obstruction: description of a new technique and a preliminary report of its application. Circulation 30:654–670

Durham JR, Horowitz JD, Wright JG, Smead WL (1994) Percutaneous transluminal angioplasty of tibial arteries for limb salvage in the high-risk diabetic patient. Ann Vasc Surg 8:48–53

Greenfield AJ (1980) Femoral, popliteal, and tibial arteries: percutaneous transluminal angioplasty. Am J Roentgenol 135:927–935

Haimovici H (1967) Patterns of arteriosclerotic lesions of the lower extremity. Arch Surg 95:918–933

Hauser H, Bohndorf K, Wack C, Tietze W, Wölfle KD, Loeprecht H (1996) Percutaneous transluminal angioplasty (PTA) of isolated crural arterial stenoses in critical arterial occlusive disease. ROFO 164:238–243

Horvath W, Oertl M, Haidinger D (1990) Percutaneous transluminal angioplasty of crural arteries. Radiology 177:565–569

Mathias K, Spillner G, Staiger J, Ahmadi A, Werner JP (1979) Percutane transluminale Revascularisation von Unterschenkelarterien. Chirurg 50:158–163

Matsi PJ, Manninen HI, Suhonen MT, Pirinen AE, Soimakallio S (1993) Chronic critical lower-limb ischemia: prospective trial of angioplasty with 1–36 months follow-up. Radiology 188:381–387

McWhinnie DL, Gordon AC, Collin J, Gray DWR, Morrison JD (1994) Rehabilitation outcome 5 years after 100 lower limb amputations. Br J Surg 81:1596–1599

Orchard TJ, Strandness DE (1992) Assessment of peripheral vascular disease in diabetes: report and recommendations of an international workshop. Circulation 88:819–828

Rutherford RB, Flanigan DP, Gupta SK, et al. (1986) Suggested standards for reports dealing with lower extremity ischemia. J Vasc Surg 4:80–94

Saab MH, Smith DC, Aka PK, Brownlee RW, Killeen JD (1992) Percutaneous transluminal angioplasty of tibial arteries for limb salvage. Cardiovasc Intervent Radiol 15:211–216

Sacks D, Marinelli DL, Martin LG, Spies JB, et al. (1997) Reporting standards for clinical evaluation of new peripheral arterial revascularization devices. J Vasc Intervent Radiol 8:137–149

Schwarten DE (1991) Clinical and anatomical considerations for nonoperative therapy in tibial disease and the results of angioplasty. Circulation 83 Suppl 1:I-86–I-90

Schwarten DE, Cutcliff WB (1988) Arterial occlusive disease below the knee: treatment with percutaneous transluminal angioplastyperformed with low-profile catheters and steerableguide wires. Radiology 169:71–74

Schwarzenbach BP, Groscurth P, Lang A, Schöpke W, Hoffmann U, Bollinger A (1996) Bedeutung von arteriellen Anastomosen am distalen Unterschenkel und proximalen

Fuß zur Kompensation der peripheren arteriellen Verschlußkrankheit. Vasa 25:331–336

Sivananthan UM, Browne TF, Thorley PJ, Rees MR (1994) Percutaneous transluminal angioplasty of the tibial arteries. Br J Surg 81:1282–1285

Sos TA (1996) Infrapopliteal intervention: the Cornell experience. Cardiovasc Intervent Radiol 19 Suppl 2:S104

Sprayregen S, Sniderman KW, Sos TA, Vieux U, Singer A, Veith FJ (1980) Popliteal artery branches: percutaneous transluminal angioplasty. Am J Roentgenol 135:945–950

Standards of Practice Committee of the Society of Cardiovascular and Interventional Radiology (1990) Guidelines for percutaneous transluminal angioplasty. Radiology 177:619–626

Starck EE, McDermott JC, Crummy AB, Heydwolf AV (1984) Angioplasty of the popliteal and tibial arteries. Semin Intervent Radiol 1:269–277

Tamura S, Snidermann KW, Beinart C, Sos TA (1982) Percutaneous transluminal angioplasty of the popliteal artery and ist branches. Radiology 143:645–648

Varty K, Bolia A, Naylor AR, Bell PR, London NJ (1995) Infrapopliteal percutaneous transluminal angioplasty: a safe and successful procedure. Eur J Vasc Endovasc Surg 9:341–345

Veith FJ, Gupta SK, Wengerter KR, et al. (1990) Changing atherosclerotic disease patterns and management strategies in lower-limb-threatening ischemia. Ann Surg 212:402–414

Wack C, Wölfle KD, Loeprecht H, Tietze W, Bohndorf K (1994) Percutaneous balloon dilatation of isolated lesions of the calf arteries in critical ischemia of the leg. Vasa 23:30–34

Wagner HJ (1994) Angioplastie von Unterschenkelarterien. In: Steudel A, Görich J, Götz HJ (eds) Interventionelle Radiologie. Zuckschwerdt, Münich, pp 18–23

Wagner HJ, Reuter P, Alfke H, Starck E (1992) Prospektive Studie zur Rekanalisationszeitbestimmung mit einem Führungsdraht/Rekanalisationskathetersystem bei arteriellen Occlusionen. ROFO 157:477–483

Wagner HJ, Starck EE, McDermott JC (1993) Infrapopliteal percutaneous transluminal revascularization: results of a prospective study on 148 patients. J Intervent Radiol 8:81–90

34 Periamputational Imaging

U. Voss and J. Fernholz

34.1
Indications for and Incidence of Leg Amputation

The goal of treatment in limb salvage is to limit the ischemic tissue loss to the distal foot area. Therefore, a major amputation, as a radical therapeutic principal, should not be undertaken without angiographic evaluation. An interdisciplinary cooperation of radiologists (GAILER et al. 1983), vascular surgeons, and angiologists is mandatory, and may reduce the high rate of major amputation (e.g., 25 000 per year in Germany) by more than 50% (VOLLMAR 1982). Vascular and tissue imaging should contribute to the following therapeutic principals:

- Amputation should be done as distally as possible. In suitable cases, removal of only the necrotic tissue is sufficient.
- Detection of the optimum area of possible healing per primam.
- Selection of patients for revascularization procedures prior to amputation.
- Conditioning of the limb for distal minor or borderline amputation.
- Improvement of circulation by endovascular, reconstructive, or medical treatment to achieve

ULRICH VOSS, Professor, Head of Department of Vascular Surgery, Städtisches Klinikum, Moltkestraße 90, 76133 Karlsruhe, Germany
JOCHEN FERNHOLZ, Professor, Head of Department of Radiology, Städtisches Klinikum, Moltkestraße 90, 76133 Karlsruhe, Germany

transposition of amputation level from above knee to below knee.
- In major amputation myoplastic stump construction takes preference.
- Immediate or early prosthetic management.

34.2
Pathophysiology

Most amputations are necessitated by vascular disease. Other amputations are caused by injury or tumor (Table 34.1).

Table 34.1. Indications for amputation. (KAY and NEWMAN 1975)

Vascular Disease	70%
Trauma	23%
Tumor	4%
Congenital Malformations	3%

More than 90% of vascular cases are due to end-stage arteriosclerosis, or arteritis, and/or sequelae of diabetes mellitus (Fig. 34.1). Rare cases of

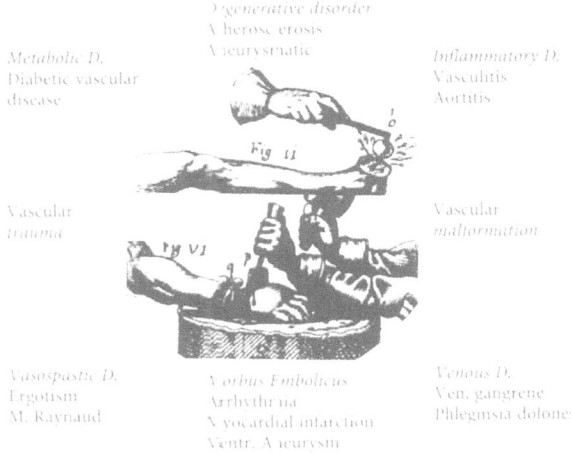

Fig. 34.1. Indications for limb amputation necessitated by vascular lesions

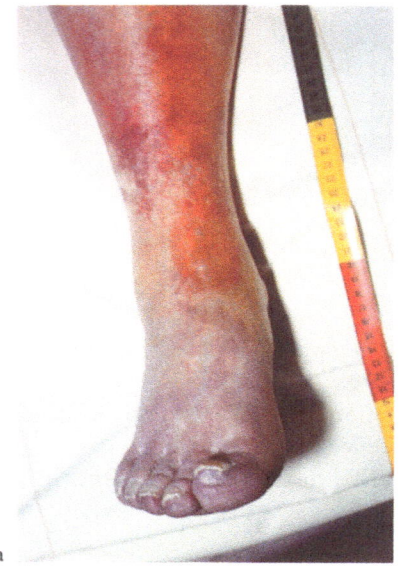 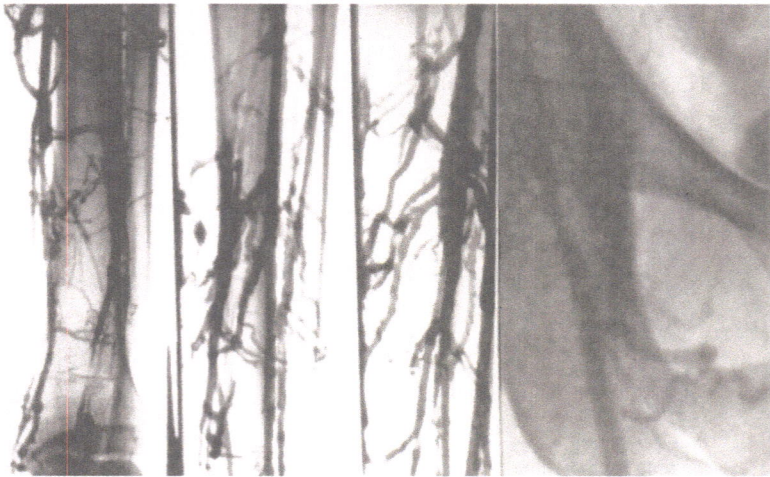

Fig. 34.2. a Phlegmasia coerulea dolens. **b** Ascending phlebography demonstrating poor collateral flow

amputation are caused by vascular malformations such as congenital arteriovenous (AV)-fistulas, or giant hemangiomas with bone destruction (EBSKOV 1983; KAY and NENMAN 1975). Sometimes even venous thrombosis leads to secondary ischemia due to complete obstruction of venous drainage (phlegmasia coerulea dolens; Fig. 34.2).

End-stage disease of progressive vascular occlusive disease results in malperfusions when capillary pressure falls below tissue pressure (40 mmHg). Irreversible tissue damage occurs first of all in the ischemic nervous system. Incomplete ischemia is characterized by loss of sensory function. The main symptoms of complete ischemia is loss of sensory and motory function, as well as pain and paralysis (PRATT 1954; MAHLER 1990).

Most amputation procedures are elective operations (BOHNE 1987). Time should be taken for proper selection of amputation level and for compensation of impaired metabolic and circulatory parameters. A major amputation should never be undertaken when the patient is in a poor or precarious general condition, which includes renal or heart failure and disturbance of water–electrolyte balance. This is important for the reduction of risk of lethal outcome of major amputation in elderly patients (VOLLMAR et al. 1971; VOLLMAR 1982). Emergency amputation is indicated in progressive infection such as anthrax (Fig. 34.3) or Fournier-type gangrene. In cases of rhabdomyolysis and myoglobinuria major amputation can be life-saving or help avoid renal failure (HAIMOVICI 1970; ZÜHLKE and HARNOSS 1988).

Sometimes distal open amputation (Fig. 34.4) is necessary for rapid progressive cellulitis in diabetic patients. Rational therapeutic steps of conservative and surgical treatment to achieve distal amputation is best characterized by infection control, revascularization, and amputation (IRA) principles (VOLLMAR et al. 1966, 1996) (Table 34.2).

Table 34.2. IRA principle

I	Control of infection by abundant incisions. Conversion of gangrene to dry necrosis, mumification
R	Revascularization of perinecrotic tissue (penumbra)
A	Amputation as last step, as distal as possible

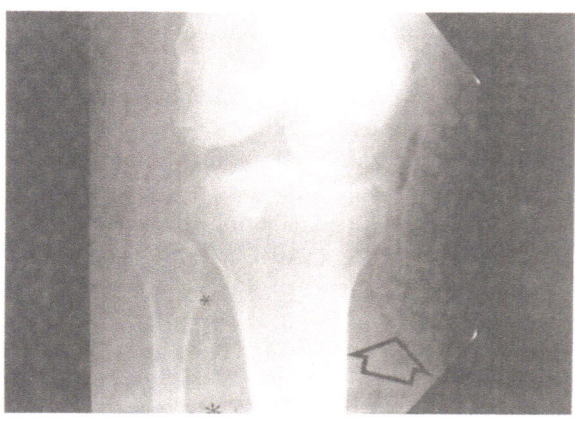

Fig. 34.3. Typical accumulation of gas in a muscular formation (clostridial infection)

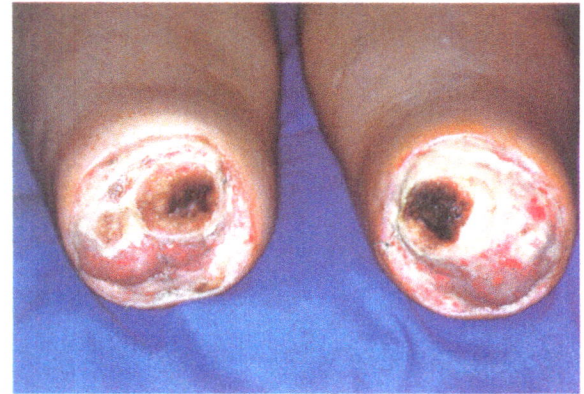

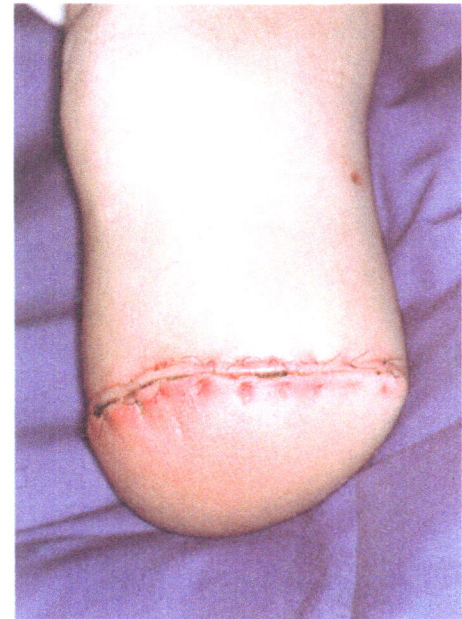

Fig. 34.4. a Distal open amputation for infection control. b Secondary below knee amputation (Burgess-type)

34.3
Angiographic Evaluation

Determining the amputation level and urgency of amputational procedures depends on the degree of arterial insufficiency and the general condition of the patient. Selection of amputation level depends on local and systemic factors, the type of onset of ischemia, the extent of gangrene or ulceration, and severity of pain.

Most of the desired information is obtained by clinical criteria, together with findings such as palpation of arterial pulses, skin color and temperature, and manifestation of myoneural deficit. The definition of critical ischemia needs to be determined using Doppler ultrasound ankle pressure and transcutaneous PO_2 measurement (Table 34.3) as a parameter of microcirculation in the adjacent areas. Despite the fact that clinical findings, and even angiograms, alone are not valid in the prediction of successful amputation (BURGESS et al. 1971; BURGESS and MARSDEN 1974), angiograms fulfill the most important criterion for the best choice of treatment. The complete documentation of morphology of the arterial tree is the best way to ascertain whether recanalization or reconstruction procedures may still be possible for limb salvage

Table 34.3. Definition of chronic critical ischemia

Ankle pressure	<50 mmHg[a]
Transcutaneous PO_2	<30 mmHg

[a] False negative results in media-sclerosis; correction by Thon test.

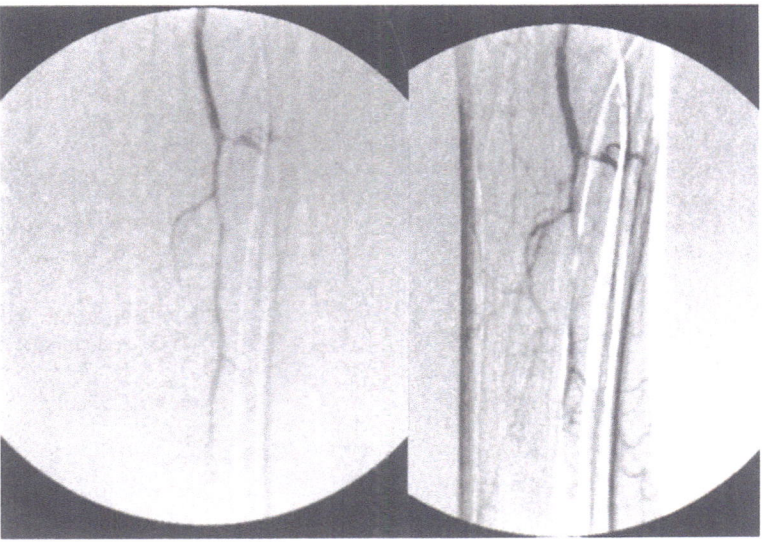

Fig. 34.5. Femoral arteriogram showing non reconstructable vascular morphology; primary amputation indicated

(Fig. 34.5). The transit time of dye gives more functional information on the capacity of collateral flow. The criteria to achieve primary healing of below knee amputations are mainly derived by a complete anatomy of the blood supply (Fig. 34.6).

34.4
Amputation for Trash-Foot Syndrome

Arterio-arterial microembolism to the skeletal muscle does not have the same clinical relevance as is seen in microembolism to the brain resulting in transient ischemic attack (TIA) or even stroke. Nevertheless, the rate of peripheral microemboly is fairly underestimated (BENVEGNA et al. 1990). Sometimes the differential diagnosis of melalgia should refer to muscle infarction as a possible source of pain. The clinical signs are macular spotted necrosis or suggillations in the foot area (Fig. 34.7). Further typical signs of microembolism are blue-toe syndrome and/or deep necrosis or ulcerations. The sources of microembolism are mostly located in a "shaggy aorta" or in an abdominal aortic aneurysm. The capillary circulation is blocked by cholesterol crystals or platelet aggregations originating from an endoaneurysmatic thrombus or "shaggy aorta" (Fig. 34.8).

In cases of acral necrosis in the presence of otherwise good capillary filling of the adjacent tissue an immediate abdominal examination should be carried out clinically and using ultrasound imaging. This is to detect an abdominal aneurysm as a source of arterio-arterial embolism which may necessitate amputation (Fig. 34.9).

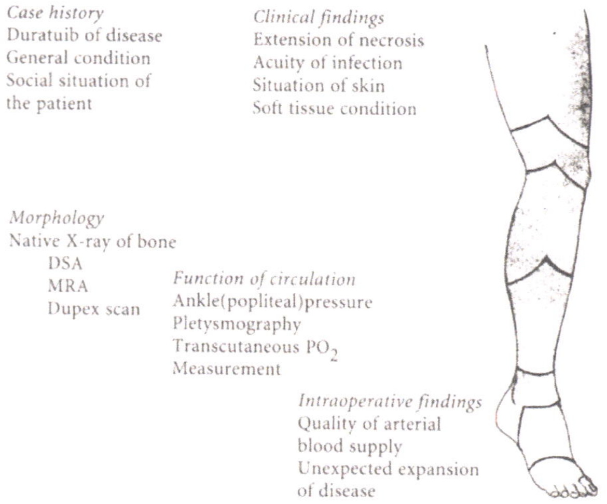

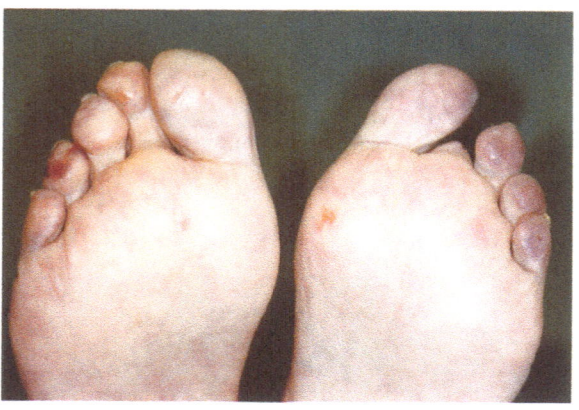

Fig. 34.7. Trash-foot syndrome: arterio-arterial embolization with occlusion of distal vessels (palpable pulses)

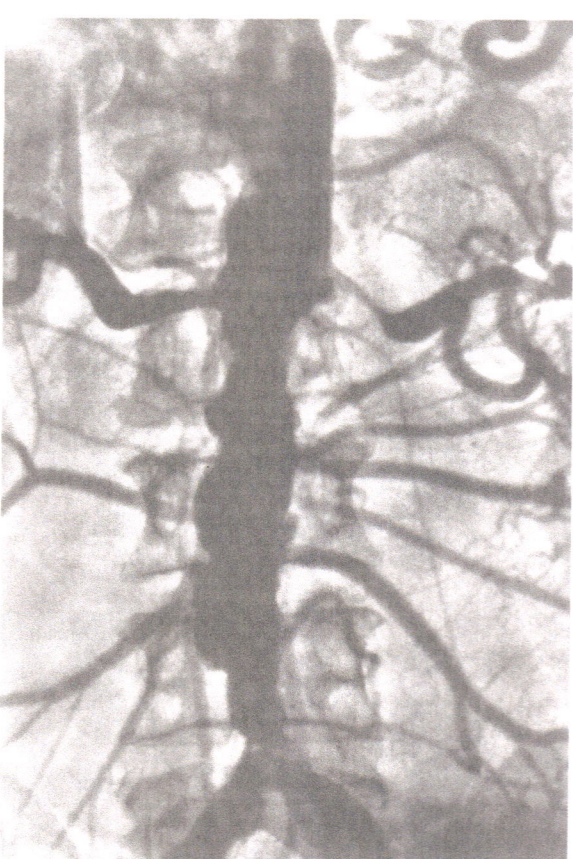

Fig. 34.8. Atheromatous vascular wall as a source of peripheral embolic occlusion ("shaggy aorta")

Case history
Duratuib of disease
General condition
Social situation of
the patient

Clinical findings
Extension of necrosis
Acuity of infection
Situation of skin
Soft tissue condition

Morphology
Native X-ray of bone
    DSA
    MRA
    Dupex scan

Function of circulation
Ankle(popliteal)pressure
Pletysmography
Transcutaneous PO_2
Measurement

Intraoperative findings
Quality of arterial
blood supply
Unexpected expansion
of disease

Fig. 34.6. Choice of amputation levels

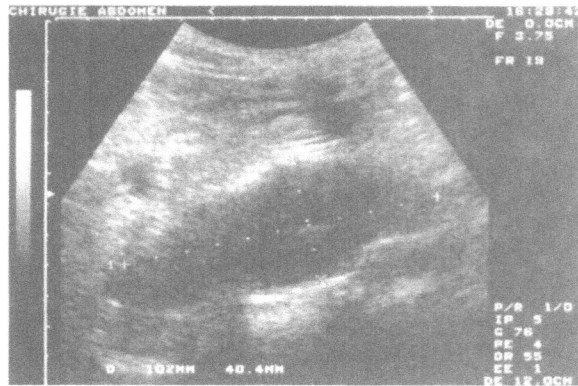

Fig. 34.9. Abdominal B-scan showing infrarenal fusiform aneurysm with mural thrombi as a potential source of distal necrosis

The clinical picture of severe "trash-foot syndrome" is a rare complication (<1%) of interventional procedures (ZEITLER 1985), including open surgery. Intraoperative microemboly from the aorto-iliac segment are due to operative mismanagement such as insufficient flush maneuver or incomplete anticoagulation. Intensive, conservative treatment with heparin and prostaglandin is able to avoid amputation in most of these cases. Nevertheless, amputation following catheter and balloon maneuver, and/or operation are major medical catastrophes. This is especially true in cases indicated for Fontaine stage one or two (non-critical ischemia).

34.5
Magnetic Resonance Imaging for Amputation

Magnetic resonance angiography (MRA) is not yet a substitute for contrast arteriography in most patients. With the current state-of-the-art equipment, femoral MRA could replace contrast angiography adequately in only 57% of cases (QUINN et al. 1993). Future generations of equipment will most probably improve performance. Researchers have stated that, with MRA, important distal surgical target arteries can be detected which are otherwise not visible using contrast arteriography (CAMBRIA et al. 1993).

MRA is a definitive aid to and mandatory for amputation procedures in patients with angiodysplasia. The initial amputation rate of up to 20%

in angiodysplasia type F.P.-WEBER (F.P.-WEBER Syndrome, multiple peripheral AV fistulas) has been reduced by therapeutic measures to 8% over the last decade (Voss 1994). The extent of destruction by abnormal vessels is best visible by MRA (see Fig. 34.8). Thus the decision can be made as to whether a minor distal amputation is feasible. The same is true in cases of giant hemangiomas.

Further indications for MR Imaging prior to exploration of crural vessels are to be recommended in end-stage disease. MR images reflect the water content of tissue. This method might be useful for diagnosing various types of edema. The differentiation between lymphatic edema, venous edema, or ischemic necrosis may be useful for deciding whether amputation is indicated above or below knee (Fig. 34.10). It is generally agreed to maximize the ratio of below knee to above knee amputation in patients with end-stage peripheral vascular disease. Only 26% of patients are able to walk out of the door 2 years after amputation. With an above knee amputation the rate is much lower.

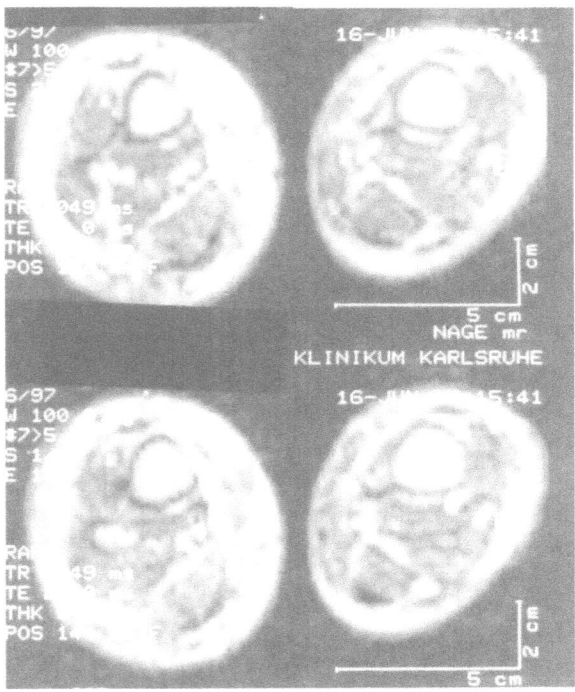

Fig. 34.10. a Magnetic resonance tomography (MRT) showing subcutaneous cellulitis in a diabetic patient (fulminant ascending infection) (b see next page)

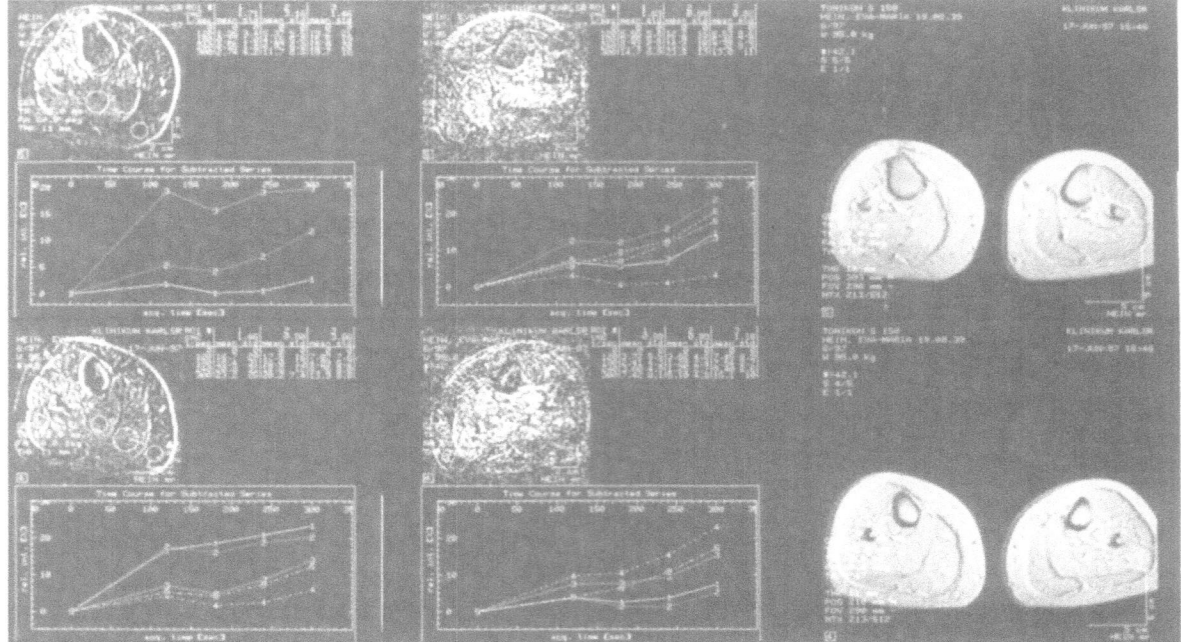

b

Fig. 34.10. **b** MRT perfusion study. Muscular infarctions, left lower leg

References

Benvegna S, Cassina I, Giantini G, Rusigmeols F, Talarico F, Florena M (1990) Atherothrombotic microembolism of the lower extremities (the blue toe syndrom) from atherothrombotic non-aneurysmal aortic plaques. J Cardiovasc Surg (Torino) 31:87–91

Bohne WHO (1987) Atlas of amputation surgery. Thieme, Stuttgart

Burgess EM, Marsden FW (1974) Major lower extremity amputations following arterial reconstruction. Arch Surg 108:655–660

Burgess EM, Romano RL, Zettl JH (1971) Amputation of the leg for peripheral vascular insufficiency. J Bone Joint Surg [Am] 53:874–890

Cambria RP, Yucel EK, Brewster DC, L'italien G, Gertler JP, La Muraglia GM, Kaufman JA, Walfman AC, Abbott WM (1993) The potential for lower extremity revascularisation without contrast arteriography: experience with magnetic resonance angiography. J Vasc Surg 17:1050–1057

Ebskov B (1983) Choice of level in lower extremity amputation nationwide survey. Danish Amputation Register, Copenhagen. Prosthet Orthot Int 7:58–60

Gailer H Grüntzig A, Zeitler E (1983) Late results after percutaneous transluminal angioplasty of iliaca and femoropopliteal obstructing lesions. In: Dotter CT, Grüntzig A, Schoop W, Zeitler E (eds) Percutaneous transluminal angioplasty. Springer, Berlin Heidelberg New York, pp 215–218

Haimovici H (1970) Arterial embolism, myoglobinuria and renal tubular necrosis. Arch Surg 100:639–647

Kay HW, Newman JD (1975) Relative incidences of new amputations. Orthot Prothet 29:3–16

Mahler F (1990) Europäischer Konsensus betreffend chronisch kritische Ischämie der unteren Extremitäten. VASA 19:97–99

Pratt GH (1954) Cardiovascular surgery. Kimpton, London

Quinn SF, Demlow TA, Hallin RW, Eidemiller LR, Szumowski J (1993) Femoral MR angiography versus conventional angiography: preliminary results. Radiology 189:181–184

Vollmar J (1982) Reconstructive surgery of the arteries. Thieme, Stuttgart, p 285

Vollmar J (1996) Rekonstruktive Chirurgie der Arteries. Thieme, Stuttgart, pp 273–277

Vollmar J, Laubach R, Hild R (1966) Schwere chronische Gliedmaßenischämie bei arteriellen Verschlußkrankheiten. MMW 108:894

Vollmar J, Marquardt E, Schaffelder G (1971) Amputation bei arteriellen Durchblutungsstörungen

Voss EU (1994) Chirurgische Behandlung kongenitaler Gefäßläsionen der Extremitäten. In: Balzer K, Brachmann K (eds) Sicherheitsaspekte und Qualitätskontrolle in der Gefäßchirurgie. Steinkopf, Darmstadt, pp 133–142

Weber FP (1907) Angioma formation in connection with hypertroplasty. Brit J Derm 19:231–237

Zeitler E (1985) Die perkutane transluminale Rekanalisation chronischer Stenosen und Verschlüsse peripherer Arterien. Wien Med Wochenschr 135:384–392

Zühlke HV, Harnoss BM (1988) Septische Gefäßchirurgie. Ueberreuter, Vienna, pp 12–13

Upper Extremity Arterial Diseases

35 Subclavian and Brachial Arterial Diseases

E. Zeitler, K. Hüttl and K. Mathias

CONTENTS

The most common locations of arterial occlusive disease in the upper extremities include:

1. In the aortic arch arteries, directly at the ostium (Fig. 35.1)
2. Distal of the latter, before the branching of the vertebral artery (Figs. 35.2 and 35.3)
3. Distal of the vertebral artery, close to the costo-clavicular narrowing (Fig. 35.4).

According to Ratschow (1938), these forms of arteriosclerotic stenoses or occlusions, in the same way as those close to the carotid bifurcation, are typical locations, influenced by the flow pattern. In addition to various risk factors, their formation is essentially influenced by the presence of and change in turbulent flow.

In the case of occlusions of the subclavian artery, there is collateral supply via the vertebral artery and, under physical stress, a subclavian steal syndrome (SSS) (Vollmar 1996) may develop. Formation of this vertebro-vertebral steal effect, however, does not occur if the vertebral artery arises directly from the aortic arch, between the branching point of the left common carotid and left subclavian arteries. These conditions, however, may favor the formation of a perfusive disorder of the arms without cerebral symptoms. A common complication of subclavian stenoses is peripheral embolism into the digital arteries. An additional cause of subclavian stenoses exists in the form of a thoracic outlet syndrome, by chronic constriction of the subclavian artery between the clavicula and the first rib and scalenus muscles (Etter 1944; Sanders et al. 1990; Dawson 1993).

E. Zeitler, Professor, MD, Virchowstraße 13, D-90409 Nürnberg, Germany
K. Hüttl, MD, Department of Vascular Surgery, Semmelweis Medical University, Városmajor u. 68, Budapest, 1122 Hungary
K. Mathias, MD, Stadtische Kliniken, Radiologische Klinik Beurhausstraße 40, D-44137 Dortmund, Germany

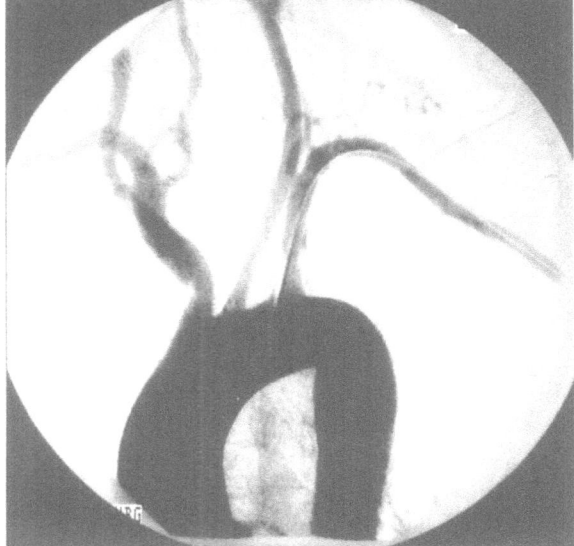

Fig. 35.1. Thoracic aortography (arterial digital subtraction angiography) in left anterior oblique projection. Catheterization from the left brachial artery

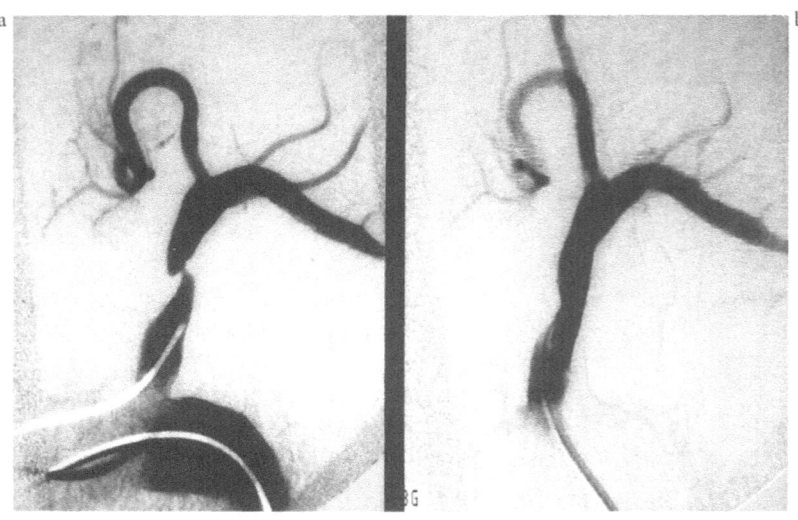

Fig. 35.2 a,b. Selective arterial digital subtraction angiography, left subclavian artery (63-year-old man).
a Stenoses in the second postostial part of the artery proximal to the vertebral artery; no orthograde contrast-filling of the vertebral artery.
b Arteriography after successful balloon dilatation, demonstrating orthograde flow in the vertebral artery

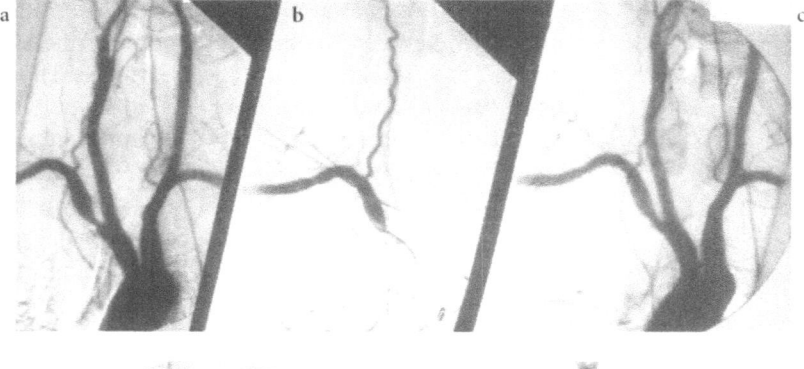

Fig. 35.3 a–c. Stenoses, right subclavian artery (31-year-old woman).
a Thoracic aortography, right anterior oblique projection. b Counterflow arteriography, right subclavian artery, demonstrating high-grade stenosis and collateral neck arteries. c Thoracic aortography after successful balloon percutaneous transluminal angioplasty

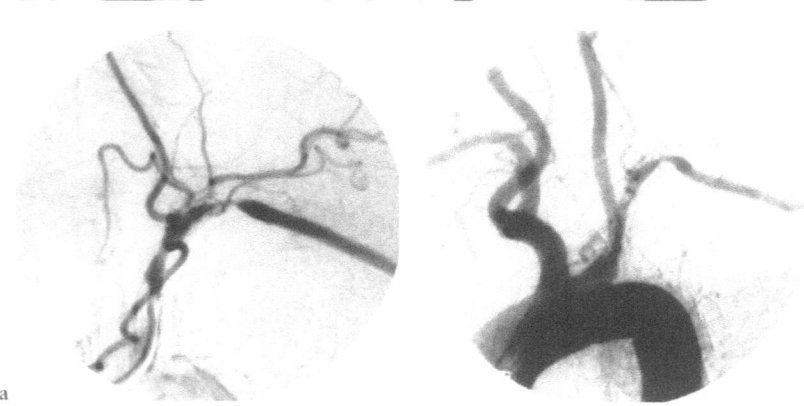

Any angiographic diagnosis, as with diagnoses using other imaging systems, must therefore also consider – apart from the clear diagnostic assessment of arterial obliterations and their location – the possibility of variations in the arteries arising from the aortic arch (ANSON 1963; BEYER-ENKE 1996; LUZSA 1972; HUBER 1979; KADIR 1991; ZEITLER and BÄR 1997) (see also Chap. 17).

In the course of the axillary and brachial arteries, acute thrombotic or embolic occlusions may occur. Arteriosclerotic stenoses, in contrast, are a rare exception in this territory. The most common sites of peripheral arterial disease in the upper extremities are the digital and ulnar arteries (WAGNER and ALEXANDER 1993). Obliterations occur here, especially in the framework of collagenoses, such as sclerodermia, arteriosclerosis, and in the framework of functional vasospastic syndromes, such as Raynaud's disease (ALLEN et al. 1972).

The angiographic diagnosis, therefore, must mainly be oriented by the clinical picture and the objective findings of noninvasive diagnosis with the Allen's test, and additionally with duplex sonography, finger-oscillography, and, if appropriate, also capillary microscopy (BOLLINGER 1979; HEBERER et al. 1966; SCHOOP 1988; STRANDNESS and SUMNER 1975).

Thus, the most important angiographic techniques (EKLÖF and TYLEN 1976; ABRAMS 1983; SCHMITT and LANZ 1996) used for the evaluation of peripheral vascular diseases of the upper extremities include:

- Thoracic aortography with catheter for documentation of the aortic arch and proximal arm arteries
- Selective catheter angiography of the subclavian arteries, with documentation of the shoulder, arm, and hand arteries
- Angiography of the hand and lower arm following retrograde puncture of the brachial artery in the elbow.

Angiographies of the aortic arch are mainly performed in a left anterior oblique projection, if necessary completed with a right anterior oblique or anteroposterior projection, and functional angiographic examinations at elevated arms to identify possible compression in the form of a thoracic outlet syndrome (ROOS 1987; SANDERS et al. 1990; MAKHOUL and MACHLEDER 1992; LINDGREN et al. 1993).

In angiographies of the hand, a cryodynamic angiography may become necessary (RÖSCH et al. 1977) to differentiate between primary and secondary Raynaud's syndrome. The technique consists of a basic angiography after which the hands are cooled in icy water, whereupon another angiography is performed to check the effects of cooling on the arteries. This procedure needs to be complemented by angiography following intraarterial injection of reserpine (0.5 mg) or prostaglandin E1 to check vasodilative effects.

Peripheral perfusive disorders of the upper extremities are found far more seldom than in the lower extremities. The indication for any angiography should therefore be established very cautiously. If, however, angiography should be indicated for planning a therapy, documentation of both sections of the arm arteries close to the aortic arch and of the arteries of the hands and fingers is required.

To perform angiographies of the hand, intraarterial premedication using vasodilators, such as 10 mg tolazoline HCl (Priscol, Ciba), complemented by warming up of the hand(s) and body, or a small alcoholic drink, is always recommended to avoid misinterpretation due to artifacts (ZEITLER 1976a; RÖSCH et al. 1977).

In the case of no documentation of peripheral run-off, angiographies of the aortic arch can be accomplished by retrograde angiography of the brachial artery (see Fig. 35.5), which depicts the run-off distal of an occlusion of the aortic arch.

A common pathologic condition that deserves special attention is aortic arch syndrome (AAS) (TAKAYASU 1908; CACCAMISE and OKUDA 1954; MARTORELL 1961; GREMMEL and SCHULTE-BRINKMANN 1963; RAU 1970; VOLLMAR 1996; ZEITLER and BÄR 1997), also called upper-extremity pulseless disease, or *maladie sans pouls*, where different segments of the arteries arising from the aortic arch show obliterations. The distinction needs to be made in such cases between complete AAS with occlusion of all branches of the aortic arch (brachiocephalic trunk, left common carotid and left subclavian arteries), and incomplete AAS (Fig. 35.5) (RAU 1970). This appearance of a clinical picture of both an inflammatory and an arteriosclerotically degenerative origin has also been called reversed coarctation. RAU (1970) has given a detailed description, including the differentiation of the ten possible combinations of occlusions of incomplete AAS. A scheme by RAU from the same year shows the varying manifestations of incomplete AAS, grouped according to possible combined two or three obliterated aortic arch arteries (Fig. 35.6).

35.1
Normal Anatomy and Variations

The normal anatomy of the thoracic aorta is characterized by the ascending aorta moving up on the

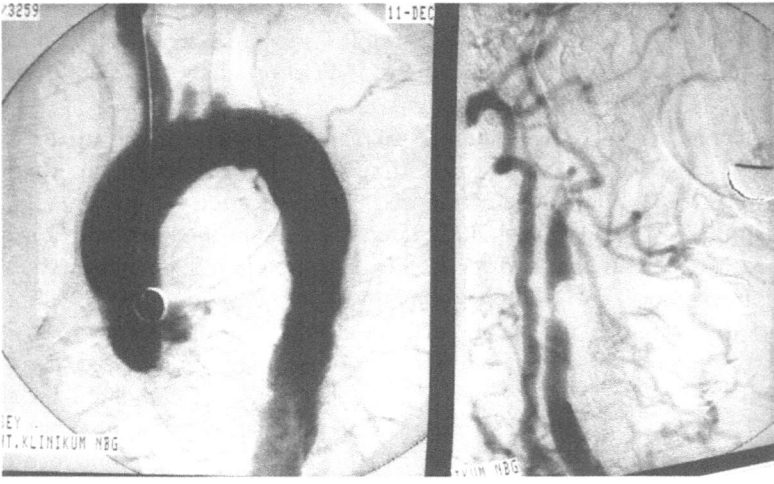

Fig. 35.5 a,b. Incomplete aortic arch syndrome (type 8 with three obliterated arteries). Occlusion of left common carotid, left subclavian, and right common carotid arteries. **a** Thoracic aortography. **b** Retrograde arteriography of the brachial artery. Vertebral artery is patent, common carotid artery stenosed

right – taking a course from ventral to dorso-cranial – the aortic arch, and the descending thoracic aorta in a dorsal direction. The most common vascular ramification of the branching-off aortic arch arteries is found in 70%–84% of the population (RAU 1970), both in anatomic and radiologic studies. In a neuroradiologic collective, HUBER (1979) found this branching-off situation in 64.9%, and the type II, with a joint origin of the brachiocephalic trunk and the left common carotid artery, in 27.1%. In

such situations, the left common carotid artery can branch off either at an acute angle or right-angled (see Fig. 35.4).

The mirror-image symmetrical order with the aortic arch on the right ("high dextroposition of the aorta") and a left-sided brachiocephalic trunk is only found in 0.05%–0.15% of examinations (HEBERER et al. 1966). Figure 35.7 shows the different variations of the aortic arch arteries. Type III deserves special attention with the isolated branching of the left vertebral artery, as well as type V with the atypical branching of the right subclavian artery as the last vessel from the descending thoracic aorta. Other variations include the existence of a right and left brachiocephalic trunk. From the ontogenic point of view, nearly all these variations can also be found as normal variations in mammals.

The right aortic arch is found with and without a complete situs inversus. However, the right aortic arch can also occur with the arteries of the aortic arch in the following order: left carotid artery – right carotid artery, right subclavian artery, and left subclavian artery with retroesophageal course. All branches of the convexity of the aortic arch can be shifted to the right and arise from the ascending aorta. The interspace between the branching points can be equally wide, but also abnormally wide. The origin of the left carotid artery can be located very close to the brachiocephalic trunk, or even form a joint origin, another branching anomaly (RAUBER-KOPSCH 1941; LUZSA 1972; KADIR 1991).

The subclavian artery is a communicating artery contributing (apart from the major supply of the arm) to the cerebral supply via the vertebral artery, and to the arterial supply of the neck and the tho-

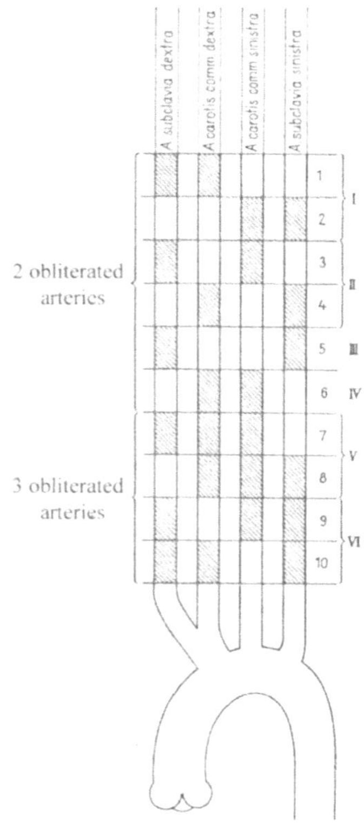

Fig. 35.6. Classification of different types of incomplete aortic arch syndrome (according to RAU 1970)

Fig. 35.7. Incidence of variations in aortic arch arteries. *x*, According to RAU (1970)

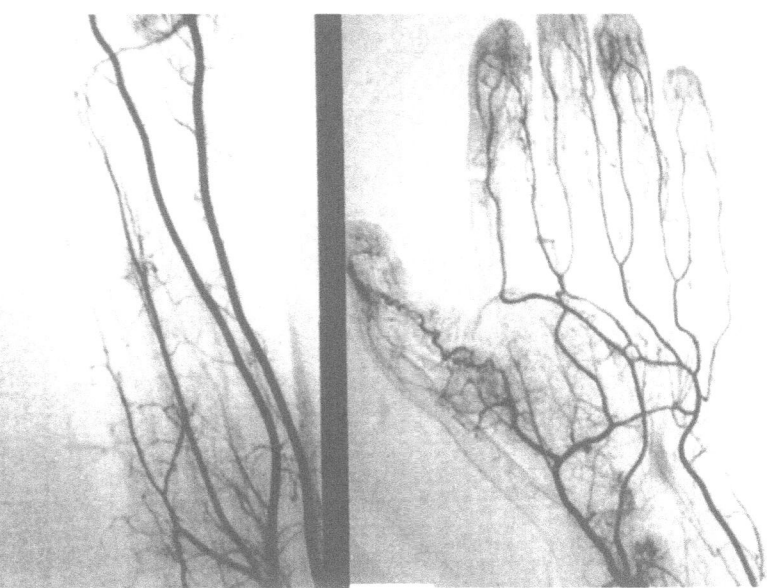

racic wall via the costocervical trunk and the thyreocervical trunk. Thus, it also forms a bridging artery for formation of a variety of collaterals.

Its natural anatomic course above the first rib and between the anterior and medial scalenus muscles may constitute the cause of a compression syndrome (Roos 1987; Sanders et al. 1990). The internal thoracic artery (A. mammaria), as a branch of the subclavian artery, changes into the cranial epigastric artery and joins the caudal epigastric artery at about the umbilical level.

The brachial artery splits distal of the elbow into the radial, ulnar, and common interosseous arteries. The deep brachial artery is by far not as important a collateral vessel as the deep femoral artery in the leg. It only becomes significant as a collateral vessel in the case of the rather rare occlusions of the axial or brachial arteries (see Fig. 35.17). The deep brachial artery gives rise to the proximal ulnar collateral artery according to the literature in 8.6% in Europe (Rauber-Kopsch 1941), and in 16.3% in Japan (Adachi 1928). A high-positioned bifurcation of the brachial artery has been found in up to 10% (Kadir 1991); this is one of the reasons for which an orthograde angiography of the brachial artery with access

from the elbow should be avoided – in order to avoid misinterpretations

In many patients, the radial artery in the lower arm is the vessel with the largest diameter (Table 35.1). Its side branches are the principal artery of the thumb (Fig. 35.8) and the deep anterior arch. Frequently, the ulnar artery has a smaller diameter, which appears differently in the various angiographic techniques. On angiographic interpretation, such differences can be attributed to the type of primarily used vasodilation and reduction of peripheral resistance, the study in plexus anesthesia, or to angiographies performed after cooling of the hands.

Variations in the area of the superficial palmar arch, which is closed in 42% of patients and open in 58%, presenting a differentiated branching situation as described by Lippert and Pabst in 1985, have been documented by Wagner and Alexander (1993). These variations are of importance mainly for surgery of the hand. In the framework of ischemic disorders of the digital arteries, however, the digital artery supply plays an important role. The supply of the digital arteries by the radial or ulnar arteries has been investigated by Hüring (1974) by

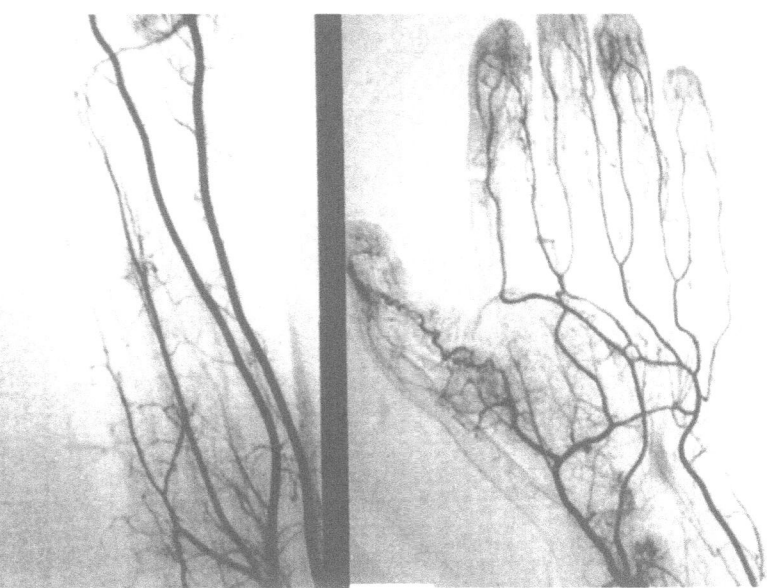

Fig. 35.8. Arterial digital subtraction angiography of left forearm (**a**) and hand (**b**) arteries. Occlusion of first metacarpal artery and thumb arteries. Patient with Dupuytren's contracture. Superficial palmar arch not occluded, excellent digiti indices artery

Table 35.1. Anatomical variations of the hand arteries as demonstrated by various techniques in different countries

Variations	(ADACHI 1928; Japan) Anatomical studies (*n*, 410)	(WEGELIUS 1972; Sweden) Angiography with plexus anesthesia (*n*, 146)	(HÜRING and ZEITLER 1974; Germany) Angiography with local anesthesia (*n*, 118)
Larger radial artery	70%	76%	67%
Larger ulnar artery	14%	2%	21%
Both equal	16%	22%	12%
Superficial palmar arch is complete, documented in angiography	15%	17%	9%

means of angiograms of the hand under optimum vasodilation (ZEITLER 1976).

As far as anomalies of the hand arteries are concerned (Fig. 35.9), all analyses have proven the same result; that the radial artery is the larger hand-supplying vessel (in 67%–76% of patients), whereas the ulnar artery is the artery of larger diameter in only 2%–21%.

The superficial palmar arch could be documented angiographically in only 8%–19% (HÜRING 1974). This is likely to be to some degree the result of angiographic examinations with cut-film documentation under tolazoline (Priscol), without prior special warming up, and cut-films produced at a frequency of between one and two images per second.

Digital subtraction angiography (DSA) has provided the possibility of documenting the whole course of contrast-filling, and the palmar arch is documented with a higher incidence. This is likely to be a result of the intended vasodilation prior to angiography, which results in a higher perfusion of the fingertips, due to which the connections in the region of the wrist are less contrasted. Here, mag-

netic resonance angiography (MRA), in contrast to roentgen angiography, provides the advantage that all perfused arteries are visualized simultaneously, regardless of the functional course of an examination (see Chaps. 12 and 36).

The palmar arch can be fed mainly by the ulnar, but also by the radial arteries, which influences the supply to the digital arteries. Given this, the various types of vascularization of the hand can be differentiated (Fig. 35.9): The ulnar artery as the dominant vessel, e.g. supplying finger arteries 2–5, and only the thumb is supplied by the radial artery.

In type II, digital arteries 1–5 are supplied by the ulnar artery. In type III, these are digits 2–5, and vascularization is effected mostly by the radial artery, and in type IV, these are fingers 3–5. The most common supply pattern is represented by types IV and V, where two and three fingers each are supplied by the radial and ulnar arteries. Type VIII represents the mirror image of type II, where fingers 1–5 are fed exclusively by the radial artery.

In addition to this classification oriented by supply to the digital arteries, there are accessory variations (Fig. 35.10) arising from the metatarsal arteries,

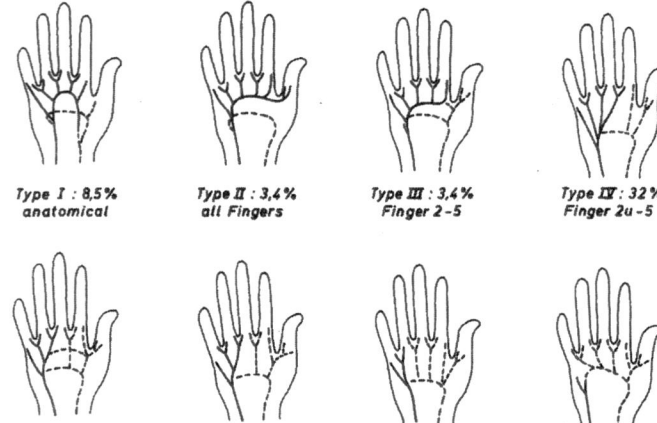

Type *I* : 8,5 %
anatomical

Type *II* : 3,4 %
all Fingers

Type *III* : 3,4 %
Finger 2–5

Type *IV* : 32 %
Finger 2u–5

Type *V* : 40 %
Finger 3u–5
with Anastomoses

Type *VI* : 6,8 %
Finger 3u–5
without Anastomoses

Type *VII* : 1,7 %
Finger 4u–5

Type *VIII* : 4,2 %
no Finger

Fig. 35.9. Variations in hand arteries as defined by finger supply

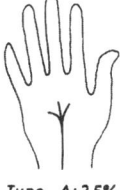 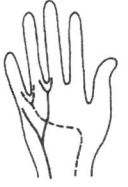 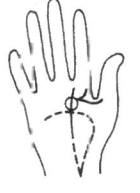 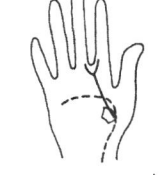

Type A: 2,5%
A. mediana

Type B: 2,5%
crossing over

Type C: 6,8%
origin from Ramus
superficialis radialis

Type D: 6,8%
origin from
A. Metacarpea dorsalis II

Fig. 35.10. Variations of proximal hand arteries

or a crossing-over artery from the radial artery. The incidence of an isolated artery to the index finger (types C and D), either through a side branch from the radial artery or from the dorsal metacarpal artery, is 50%. These modifications illustrate potential pitfalls – false-positive or false-negative diagnoses – in clinical tests performed to evaluate perfusion of the hand with the Allen's test.

Familiarity with the manifold variations in the aortic arch (see Fig. 35.7) at the ramification of the brachial artery into the radial, ulnar and middle interosseous arteries is indispensible, particularly in the planning of surgical or interventional measures and also to avoid misinterpretations following traumata of the hand (Figs. 35.9 and 35.10).

35.2
Unilateral Disease

In the peripheral vascular diseases of the upper extremities, a differentiation between uni- and bilateral obliterating diseases of the upper extremities is easy, based on the patient's complaints and clinical objective findings.

In unilateral diseases, the major discomforts include fatigability, sensation of coldness, and paresthesia of the fingers. Important indications of an obliterating disease within the arm-supplying vessels include varyingly strong pulses and lower systolic blood pressure on one side (CRAWFORD et al. 1962; VOLLMAR et al. 1965; HAAS et al. 1968; MÜLLER-WIEFEL 1975; BUCHWALSKY et al. 1977; MOORE 1987).

Auscultation of the supraclavicular fossa also provides information on a possible subclavian stenosis, which may also manifest itself due to provocation on arm elevation in the form of a thoracic outlet syndrome (STRANDNESS and SUMNER 1975; BOLLINGER 1979; ROOS 1987; SCHOOP 1987; MAKHOUL and MACHLEDER 1992).

The fist-closing test according to RATSCHOW (1938) provides information on possible obliterations of the hand and finger arteries. With elevated arms, about 20 fist-closings by opening and closing

the hands are performed, while the examiner compresses the patient's wrists. If obliterations are present, the diseased hand loses its reddening and turns pale. After opening the fist and releasing compression on the wrists, a new reddening occurs. In the case of segmental arterial occlusions, the renewed reddening of the skin is considerably delayed.

The Allen's test (ALLEN et al. 1972) enables the detection of isolated occlusions of the radial or ulnar arteries (SCHOOP 1937). The fists are also closed, with isolated compression of either the radial or the ulnar artery. If the hand turns pale under compression of the radial artery, an occlusion of the ulnar artery is indicated, whereas the hand turning pale after compression of the ulnar artery indicates an occlusion of the radial artery.

The morphologic identification and localization of morphologic–pathologic changes of aortic arch and arm arteries is successful with angiography, but, given the availability of modern imaging modalities, can also be performed using spiral computed tomography (CT) or MRA (see also Chaps. 9 and 12).

The supraaortic arteries are equally responsible for the cerebral and brachial arterial blood supply. Their intimate vicinity, mainly at the brachiocephalic trunk as their joint run-in to the carotid, vertebral, and brachial circulation, is one of the causes of a combination of symptoms, whereby cerebral vascular diseases often manifest themselves earlier and more predominantly than ischemia in the arms and hands. In such cases, the appropriate noninvasive diagnostic modality is duplex sonography, which preferably serves for the analysis of the extracranial segment of the carotid arteries and of the vertebral circulation.

In the case of an occlusion or severe stenosis in the region of the brachiocephalic trunk (see Fig. 35.15), a vertebro-vertebral steal effect can occur on the right following physical activity of the arm with subsequent antegrade contrast filling of the right carotid artery. This picture of SSS with recovery phenomenon mainly occurs when there are additional intracranial obliterations, or hyperplastic changes in the circulus arteriosus Willisi. Obliterations of the subclavian artery are also often symptom-free in their further course after initial clinical symptoms (BUCHWALSKY et al. 1977). This can be attributed to various adaptative reactions, one of them being the formation of a collateral circulation which does not pass intracerebral arteries, but is fed from the external carotid and other neck vessels.

For preoperative confirmation of a diagnosis – mainly in obliterations close to the aortic arch – angiography is still the easiest and most widely used diagnostic principle (GREMMEL and SCHULTE-BRINKMANN 1963; EKLÖF and TYLEN 1976; HUBER 1979; BAERT et al. 1981; SEYFERTH et al. 1982, 1986), whereas MRA to date has not achieved the same status as regards sensitivity and specificity.

Worldwide, the most common locations of obliterations of the supraaortic branches (Table 35.2; Fig. 35.11) are in the area of the left subclavian artery (10%–17%), followed by the brachiocephalic trunk (3%–10%), and the right subclavian artery (2%–10%). Obliterations in the area of the carotid bifurcation, however, are the most common, with 54% (right) and 67% (left), respectively. Table 35.2 shows the distribution of obliterations of the aortic arch arteries as found in three different collectives (FIELDS et al. 1970; ZEITLER and HOLIK 1977). The joint study carried out by HAAS et al. (1968), BLAISDELL et al. (1969), and FIELDS et al. (1970) represents a collective of patients from mainly neurologic and neurosurgical clinics. The distribution in a clinic specialized in the management of peripheral

vascular diseases (Aggertalklinik) (ZEITLER and HOLIK 1977) demonstrates that patients with acute stroke did not come to this clinic, which can be seen from the smaller group of patients with carotid occlusions. The collective in the vascular surgical department of the University of Erlangen hospital mainly represents patients referred for surgical therapy, with a very low proportion of occlusions, and also the smallest number of obliterations close to the aortic arch (ZEITLER and HOLIK 1977). Independent of one another, these incidences demonstrate that it is important to measure the patient's blood pressure on both arms at the first examination, in order not to overlook unilateral arterial diseases of the upper extremities with basilar insufficiency (ZEITLER and BÄR 1997).

The decisive angiographic examination modality is thoracic aortography, best performed following retrograde catheterization from the groin, with a 4- or 5-F pigtail catheter. Whenever there is some uncertainty as regards the possible existance of an aortic dissection, access from the right brachial artery with a 3- or 4-F pigtail catheter is the preferred route. Only in unclear, special situations, intravenous DSA for an angiography of the heart, with the catheter placed in front of the right atrium, is a less invasive alternative for assessing the thoracic aorta, including the aortic arch arteries (BAERT et al. 1981; SEYFERTH et al. 1986).

For precise imaging of the aortic arch branches, a left anterior oblique projection is preferable. In the case of elongated ectatic arteries, an additional right

Table 35.2. Incidence of aortic arch obliterations (%)

Stenoses	1	2	3	4	Patients (n)
Joint Study (HAAS et al. 1968)	4.2	8.3	4.8	12.4	4748
Aggertalklinik (ZEITLER 1973)	10	10	7	17	443
Erlangen (HOLIK 1976)	2.8	6.7	11.1	10.2	312
	5.6	8.3	7.6	13.2	5503
Occlusions					
Joint Study (HAAS et al. 1968)	0.6	0.8	2.2	2.5	4748
Aggertalklinik (ZEITLER 1973)	2.2	2.7	1.3	6.7	443
Erlangen (HOLIK 1976)	0.3	3.2	0.6	4.1	312
	1.0	2.2	1.3	4.4	5502

1, Brachiocephalic trunk; 2, right subclavian artery; 3, left common carotid artery; 4, left subclavian artery.

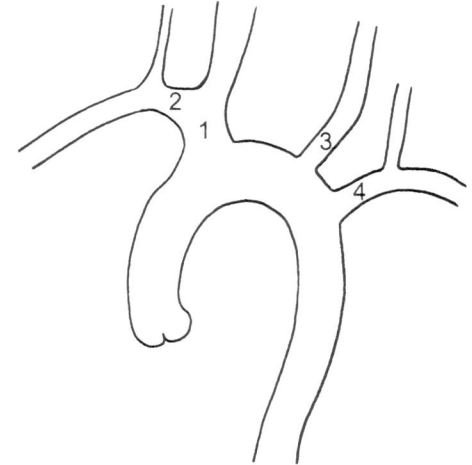

Fig. 35.11. Aortic arch obliterations in patients from 5503 aortic arch angiographies (four-vessel angiography). The numbers indicate the locations of obliteration in Table 35.2

anterior oblique projection may be required, particularly to clearly visualize the branching of the brachiocephalic trunk into the right common carotid and right subclavian arteries.

35.2.1
Obliterations of the Subclavian Artery

The typical symptoms of SSS include vertigo, headaches, impaired sight, syncopes, ataxia, and speech disturbances. The characteristics of peripheral vascular disease of the arm arteries are cold sensation, rapid fatigability, paresthesia and sensation of weakness, livid and or pale skin discoloration, and pain under physical strain (WAGNER and ALEXANDER 1993).

The subclavian artery on the left (see Fig. 35.2) can be divided into three segments: close to the ostium, directly before the branching of the vertebral artery, and distal of the branching of the vertebral artery, on the way into the axillary artery. Analogous to this anatomic distribution, obliterations of the brachiocephalic trunk are localized in direct proximity to the ostium, close to the branching of the right common carotid artery, and after the branching of the common carotid artery in the subclavian artery (see Fig. 35.3), before the branching of the vertebral artery. In addition, there is the segment distal of the branching of the vertebral artery, which is affected if a thoracic outlet syndrome is present (see Fig. 35.22).

35.2.2
Subclavian Steal Syndrome (SSS)

Stenoses on the left subclavian artery are diagnosed between three and five times more often than subclavian occlusions on the left (Fig. 35.12). In the same way, stenoses of the brachiocephalic trunk are diagnosed angiographically between at least five and eight times more often than occlusions (see Fig. 35.18). An aspect that is likely to have some importance here is the wider lumen, with higher flow rates compared to the subclavian artery on the left. SSS (Fig. 35.13) is the most common clinical situation of all aortic arch diseases, with different collateral pathways.

The interaction of the perfusion of the arms and cerebral perfusion becomes obvious in SSS, which occurs in the presence of obliterations to the subclavian artery proximal to the branching points of the vertebral artery and of the brachiocephalic trunk. Reversed flow inside the vertebral artery on the diseased side is caused by a poststenotic pressure decrease provoked, in particular, by physical stress (CONTORINI 1960; VOLLMAR et al. 1965; MÜLLER-WIEFEL 1975). The blood flows from the head to the arm, and is thus withdrawn from the brain. The arterial run-in is then mainly maintained from the vertebral artery of the contralateral side. Thus, there is a vertebro-vertebral collateral circulation (see Fig. 35.12). Only in exceptional cases, the carotido-basilar, or externo-vertebral collateral pathways can be demonstrated with thoracic aortography (see Fig. 35.18). This is possible when selective arteriographies of the right and left carotid arteries are performed.

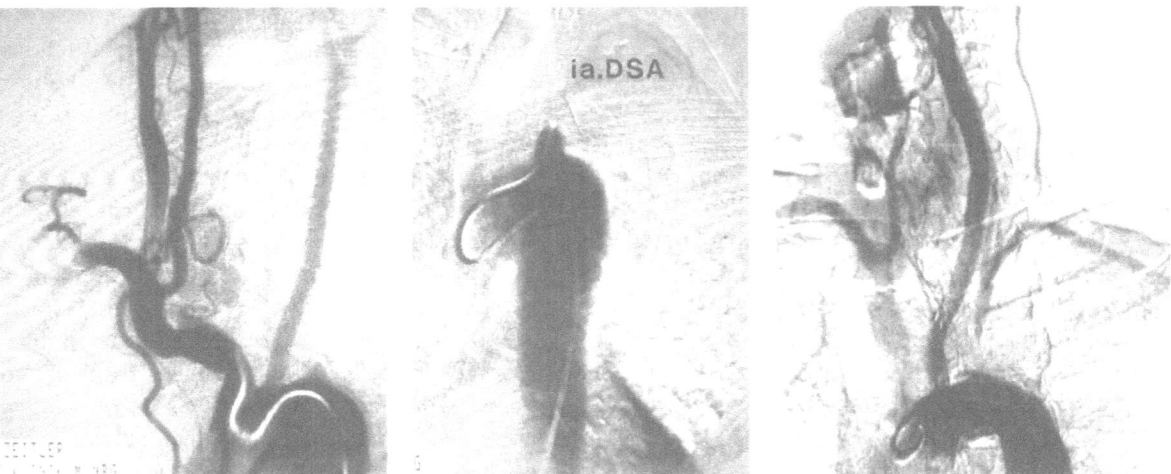

Fig. 35.12 a–c. Left subclavian artery occlusion with subclavian steal. a Semiselective aortic arch angiography. b Occlusion of the subclavian artery; no recanalization possible. c Very late image demonstrating retrograde flow in the left vertebral artery: vertebro-vertebral collateral steal

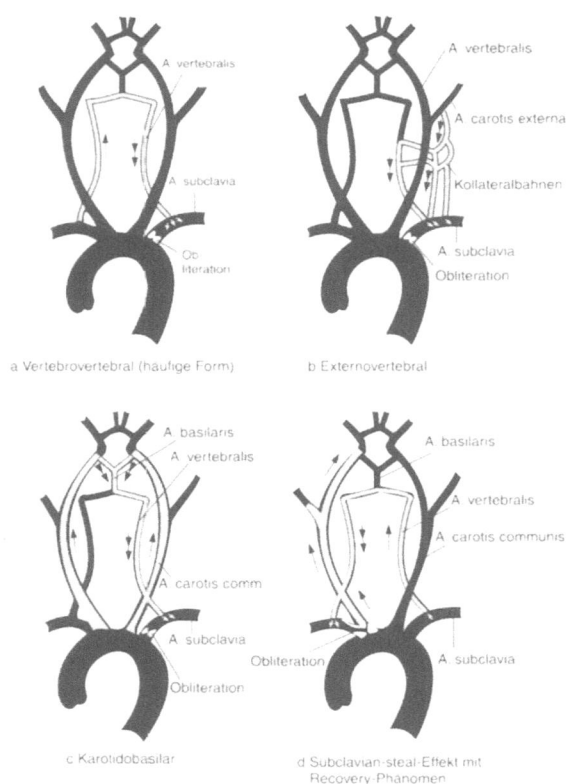

Fig. 35.13 a–d. Collateral circulation in aortic arch obliterations: subclavian steal. **a** Vertebro-vertebral (66%); **b** Externovertebral (6%); **c** Carotido-basilar (26%); **d** Subclavian steal and carotid recovery 2%. *Arrow*, normal flow direction; *double arrow*, reverse flow. (From ZEITLER and HOLIK 1977)

35.2.3
Obliterations of the Brachiocephalic Trunk

As the brachiocephalic trunk is completely occluded far less frequently, the occurrence of a cerebrobrachial collateral circulation – provided there is a normal anatomic vascular supply – on the right is also much less common. If there is an isolated occlusion (see Fig. 35.18), or a high-grade stenosis of the brachiocephalic trunk, the steal effect manifests itself spontaneously or under provoked physical stress. In addition, the subclavian artery may supply the carotid artery. To back up the diagnosis of this subclavian steal effect with carotid recovery phenomenon (Fig. 35.7, "type 4"), long angiographic imaging is required. Provocation prior to angiography is important to confirm a steal syndrome.

As soon as the catheter has been precisely placed in the ascending thoracic aorta, a tourniquet is applied to the upper arm of the affected side and the patient is requested to close his fist several times in succession. After ten such fist-closings, angiographic series can be started under contrast injection, immediately followed by the opening of the arterial clamping. This provokes the steal effect on the left (Fig. 35.12c) and on the right (see Fig. 35.15). It is important, then, to induce the subclavian steal effect during angiography, if necessary through provocation of a steal effect which only manifests itself under physical activity of the arm. For this purpose, the blood-pressure cuff should be applied to the side with the lower blood pressure, with the patient in a left anterior or anteroposterior position. Compression has to be performed exceeding the systolic value. Prior to contrast medium injection, muscle activity of the left arm is stimulated by closing the fist and continued during the injection phase. Immediately after injection has begun, pressure from the cuff is released abruptly.

This situation mimics the collateral circulation as it develops under stress. Figure 35.13 shows the possible collateral pathways. The vertebro-vertebral circulation indicates a subclavian steal effect. Moreover, a cerebral steal syndrome from the carotid artery can occur, causing the same clinical symptoms. This will mainly be the case if the vertebral artery on the right is hypoplastic, or if there are distinct obliterations at its origin or along its course. Mainly asymptomatic forms of subclavian stenoses occur whenever the vertebral artery arises from the aortic arch as isolated vessels between the left common carotid artery and in front of the subclavian artery.

The special angiographic techniques used in the aortic arch are also important for patient follow-up after vascular surgical procedures. In addition to direct reconstruction with neoimplantation of the supraaortic arteries into the aortic arch (see Fig. 35.14), extrathoracic bypass techniques, such as the carotis-subclavia bypass for treatment of SSS in the case of subclavian occlusions (see Fig. 35.4), the cross-over bypass from the left to the right common carotid artery (see Fig. 35.15) or in reverse direction, as well as the subclavia-subclavian bypass in the case of occlusions of the brachiocephalic trunk are common. Reinsertion of the aortic arch arteries is also performed (VOLLMAR 1996), which may cause some difficulty as regards optimum visualization in the angiogram if the angiographer is not familiar with the operational technique performed. This may require

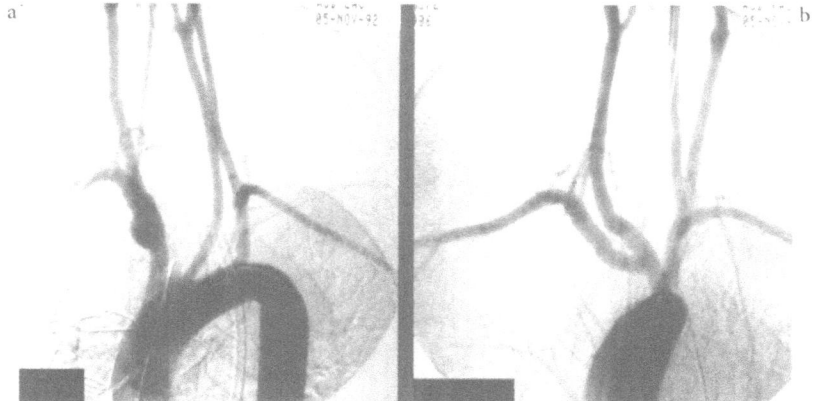

Fig. 35.14 a,b. Thoracic aortography, postoperative (same patient as in Fig. 35.18) after implantation of a new brachiocephalic bifurcation to common carotid and subclavian artery right (operator, Prof. Raithel). **a** Left anterior oblique projection. **b** Right anterior oblique projection

postoperative atypical oblique projections in addition to an anteroposterior projection (see Fig. 35.14).

Transthoracic surgical treatment of stenoses of the aortic arch arteries is becoming increasingly superfluous. Nowadays, balloon angioplasty, either via transfemoral, retrograde transbrachial, or retrograde transaxillary catheterization, completed by stent implantation, particularly for stenoses of the ostium, can be performed with increasing patient safety and very low complication rates (MATHIAS 1988; JIANPIN and ZEITLER 1991) (see Sect. 35.4).

35.2.4
Brachial Artery Disease

The most common occlusions in arm arteries are located in the digital and ulnar arteries. Subjective discomfort is experienced in the rarer forms of occlusion or stenoses (DORMAN et al. 1989) of the brachial artery (Fig. 35.16), and occlusion of the axillary artery (Fig. 35.17). Obliterations of the axillary artery may be the result of extensive lymphadenectomies, radiation therapy, but also of accidents causing dissection, intimal rupture, and secondary thrombosis. In the case of an occlusion of the brachial artery, either no ulnar pulse, or a weakened pulse by collaterals, is palpable. The fist-closing exercise reveals a pathologic result; the oscillogram confirms a marked decrement in the lower arm (SCHOOP 1987). Occlusions of the radial artery present a weakened or lacking radial pulse. The Allen's test reveals a pathologic result, whereas the fist-closing test and the oscillogram do not afford a precise diagnosis.

In the case of ulnar occlusions, only the Allen's test (ALLEN et al. 1972; BOLLINGER 1979) shows a pathologic condition on clinical examination. In pa-

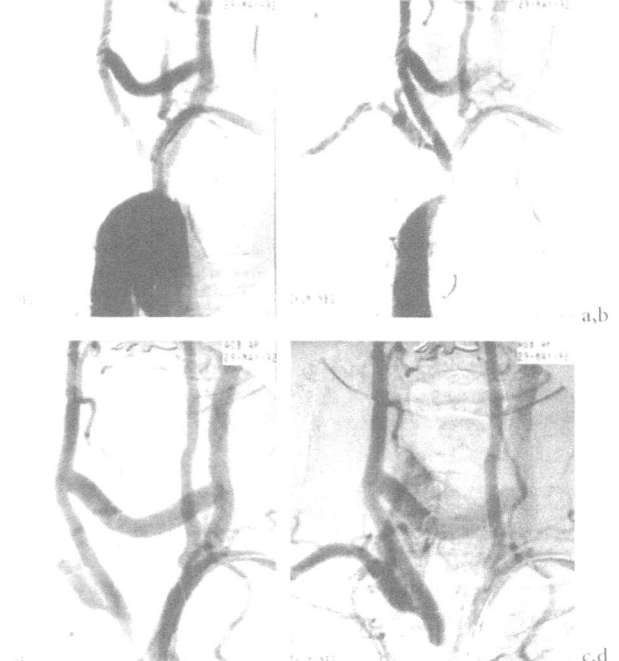

Fig. 35.15 a–d. Thoracic aortography after implantation of an extraanatomic bypass from left to right common carotid artery, with occlusion of the brachiocephalic trunk (52-year-old woman) **a–d** Sequential diagnostic angiographies

tients with sclerodermia, but also thromboangiitis obliterans, an occlusion of the ulnar artery, as well as extensive narrowing of the digital arteries in a distal direction are present in many cases. Angiographic confirmation of the diagnosis is mainly obtained to rule out central obliterations, which would require active therapeutic intervention (see also Chap. 36). Very seldom, fibromuscular dysplasia and ergotism are diagnosed as causes of different types of stenoses (ZEITLER 1976; HAUEISEN et al. 1999).

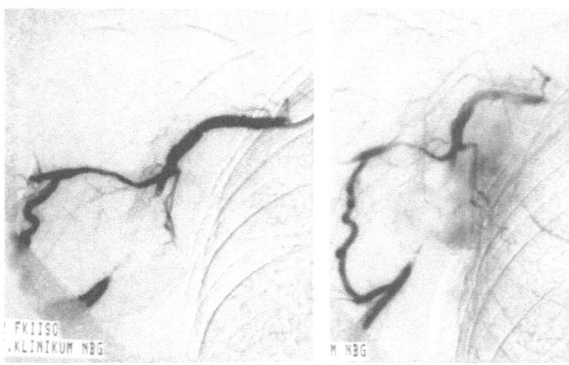

Fig. 35.16. Thrombotic occlusion of the right brachial artery (27-year-old woman, 3 days after complicated birth of twins)

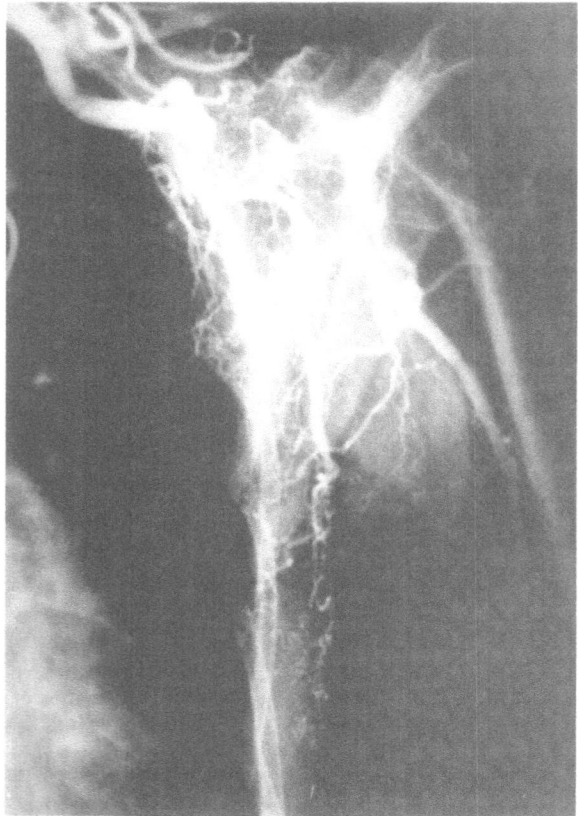

Fig. 35.17. Old occlusion of axillary artery (56-year-old male), left arm

The angiographic diagnostic examination for unilateral arterial perfusive disorders of the arm – including ischemia of one or all fingers – consists of an arteriography to document the aortic arch, down to the finger arteries (ABRAMS 1983; WAGNER and ALEXANDER 1993). This examination makes allowance for the possibility of a digital embolism from

central stenoses in the subclavian or brachial artery, as well as combined vascular diseases of the upper extremities [Raynaud's disease in combination with a thoracic outlet syndrome, fibromuscular dysplasia (DORMAN et al. 1989), or occlusions of the digital arteries in combination with SSS].

This economical examination (EKLÖF and TYLEN 1976) starts with a thoracic aortography in a left anterior oblique projection. Patients with thoracic outlet syndrome are examined with elevated arms to induce the corresponding symptoms. In the case of suspected SSS, angiography is performed after application of a blood-pressure cuff around the arm, with long imaging series. This enables optimum documentation of the peripheral vessels by selective catheterization of the subclavian artery.

In patients with the clinical situation of Raynaud's disease, the thoracic aortography has to be followed by an angiography of the hand, which should initially be performed under maximum vasodilation (ERIKSON 1965; ZEITLER 1976, 1979; RÖSCH et al. 1977; WAGNER and ALEXANDER 1993). This is repeated after cooling of the hand in icy water for 15 min, to differentiate between the vasospastic clinical picture and organic morphologic–pathologic changes. In patients with acute and subacute occlusions of the brachial artery, the application of intraarterial or clot lysis is useful, provided the anamnesis is shorter than 6 weeks. Mechanical recanalization should only be attempted in the case of necrosis of the finger pulps. In the majority of cases, a satisfactory collateral circulation bypassing the brachial occlusion develops (Fig. 35.16).

False diagnoses follwing arteriographies of the arms are mainly the result of insufficient knowledge of the patient's clinical history, inadequate single projection of the aortic arch arteries, and nonobservance of anatomic variations, as well as unsufficient induced vasodilation with in the framework of hand arteriographies (OLBERT et al. 1976).

In patients with peripheral vascular diseases of the upper extremities, the possibility of a differential diagnosis to identify non-thrombotic or arteriosclerotic genesis should be taken into consideration. This mainly comprises the detection of parmaca-induced obliterations. This rather rare cause of arterial perfusive disorders nowadays occurs mainly after the use of barbiturates, penicillin (MARTIN et al. 1973), or drug abuse, either as irreversible occlusions or as vasospastic changes in the form of ergotism, caused mainly by ergotamine tartrate (BOLLINGER and PRETER 1973; BOLLINGER and ZEITLER 1976) (see also Chap. 28). If no obliterations are present, other morphologic changes, such as fibromuscular dyspla-sia, can very rarely be observed, which may also be the cause of a peripheral embolism.

35.3
Bilateral Supraaortic Diseases

Bilateral obliteration syndromes in the supraaortic arteries may be located centrally, directly at the branching from the aortic arch, but also manifest themselves peripherally as a compression syndrome within the framework of thoracic outlet syndrome.

Occlusions of three or four branches of the aortic arch (see Fig. 35.5 and 35.20) always produce a dif-fuse cerebral vascular disease and impaired perfu-sion in both arms. Cerebral symptoms predominate over clinical symptoms in such cases, with vertigo, somnolence, impaired sight, and headaches. In con-trast, a bilateral thoracic outlet syndrome only causes perfusive disorders in both arms, since cerebrovas-cular perfusion is not impaired. The characteristic clinical findings to support the diagnosis include: absent radial pulse, stenotic murmur (supraclavicu-lar and at the neck), and coldness of the hands in certain situations.

35.3.1
Aortic Arch Syndrome (AAS)

AAS (Fig. 35.18) summarizes all acquired diseases with obliterations in the aortic arch and the sup-raaortic artery. According to the patient's com-plaints and the clinical symptoms, as well as the loca-tion and extension of the obliterations, the following types can be differentiated:
– Complete AAS: Occlusions and stenoses in all four supraaortic arteries are present.
– Incomplete AAS comprising: (a) obliterations in the common carotid arteries (carotid syndrome); (b) brachiobasilar syndrome with obliterations in the subclavian and vertebral arteries.

Several combinations of incomplete AAS have been observed, with two or three obliterated supraaortic arteries. Figure 35.6 demonstrates the different modifications of AAS according to Rau (1970). The occlusion of the right subclavian and right common carotid arteries corresponds to the obliteration in the brachiocephalic trunk. In total, there are six combi-nations with two obliterated supraaortic arteries (1–6). Of these, type I – occlusion of the brachiocephalic trunk and subclavian and common carotid arteries (Fig. 35.15) – is very common. Figure 35.5 demon-strates type VII, with obliteration of the left common carotid artery, left subclavian, right common carotid, and intercerebral collaterals from the right vertebral artery.

In contrast to arteriosclerotic AAS, I have seen some patients in whom the definition of Takayasu's disease could be used (Fig. 35.19). This was observed mainly in young women; Ross and McKussick (1953) named it "young females' arteriitis". In these patients, positive inflammatory parameters [el-evated erythro-sedimentation velocity (BKS),

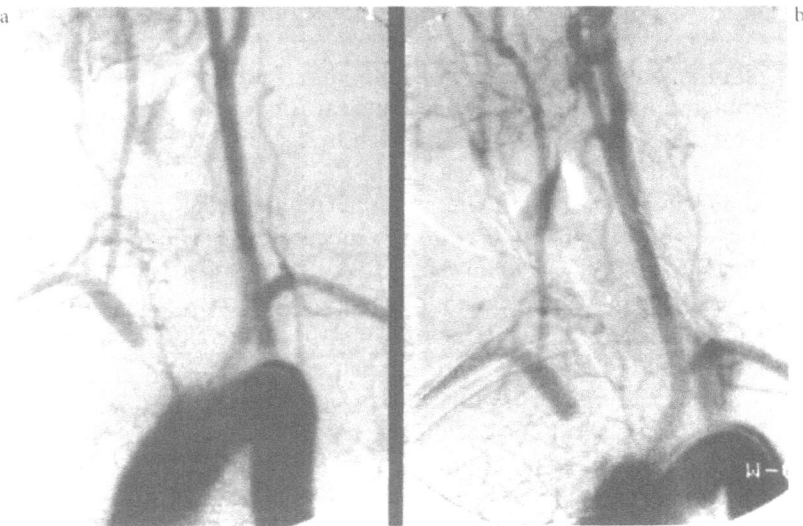

Fig. 35.18 a,b. Aortic arch syndrome, incomplete type I, occlusion of the brachiocephalic trunk and right common carotid artery. Right subclavian steal. **a** Early phase (45-year-old woman). **b** Late phase

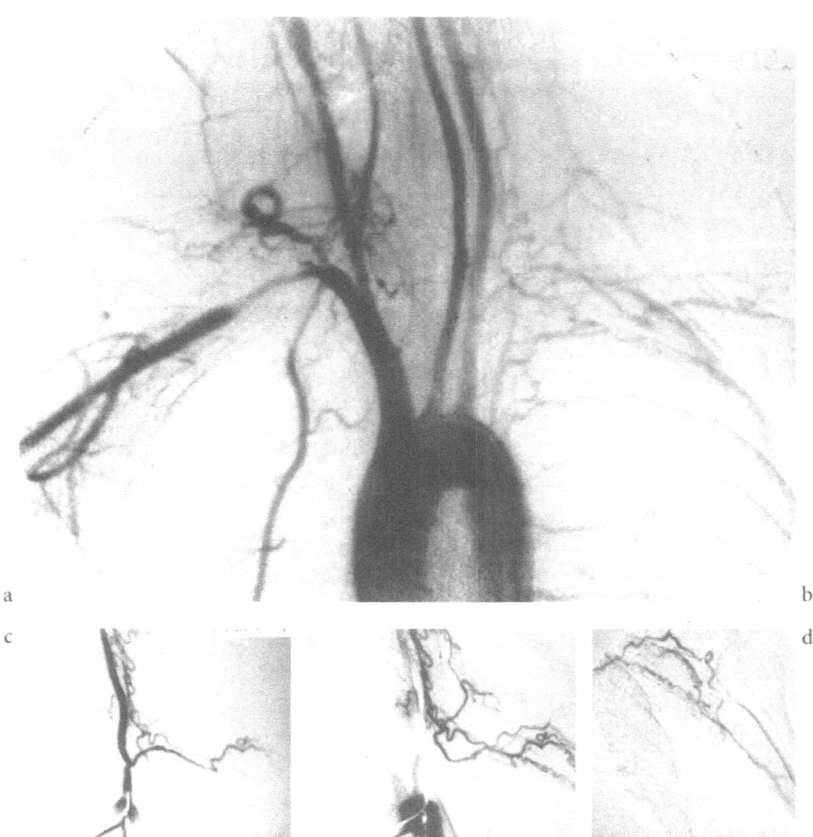

a

c

b

d,e

Fig. 35.19 a–d. Incomplete aortic arch syndrome, type 5 Takayasu's disease (32-year-old Turkish woman). a Aortic arch angiography. b–d Selective subclavian arteriography, peripheral occlusion of left subclavian artery, no SSS

leukocytosis] were identified. In patients with arteriosclerotic AAS, however, the laboratory tests are normal, without taking into consideration, of course, the risk factors associated with arteriosclerosis.

Patients with complete AAS only have a chance of survival if the stenosis develops slowly, and time can be gained to develop a collateral circulation to all brain-supplying arteries. The first description of obliterations of the aortic arch as the cause of circulatory disorders of the eye was given by TAKAYASU (1908). He described embolisms in the eyeground and identified vascular obliterations of an inflammatory nature (in his opinion mostly tuberculosis) as the underlying cause. In most cases, younger women were affected. The aortic arch angiogram typically shows tapering obliterations with direct collateral pathways to the vertebral and external carotid arteries, from the intercostal inferior epigastric arteries to the internal thoracic and subclavian arteries. The collateral circulation pathways are the same as in bypass coarctation, but in reverse direction, not cranio-caudally, but caudo-cranially (Fig. 35.20).

The "syndrome of obliteration of the supra-aortic branches" of any genesis was suggested by MARTORELL (1961). Ross and McKUSSIK (1953) used the term "aortic arch syndrome" only for inflammatory diseases in the sence of "young females' arteriitis". Several authors have published the clinical situations in detail, as well as aortographies with documentation of the collateral circulation (BANGE et al. 1962). Detailed descriptive documentation explaining the spectrum of possible variations of AAS, and AAS as part of a generalized inflammatory disease, was given by RAU (1970). The Japanese literature focuses mainly on inflammatory genesis in the framework of a panaortic syndrome (UEDA et al. 1963), with the subgroups AAS, abdominal aortitis, and extensive aortitis. Of 52 patients with occlusions of the aortic arch branch, arteriosclerosis was identified as the etiologic cause in 48 (92%) (CRAWFORD et al. 1962). RAU (1970) from Cologne determined arteriosclerosis as the underlying cause in 93%, unspecific aortitis in 6%, and syphilis in 1%. Figure 35.19 demonstrates incom-

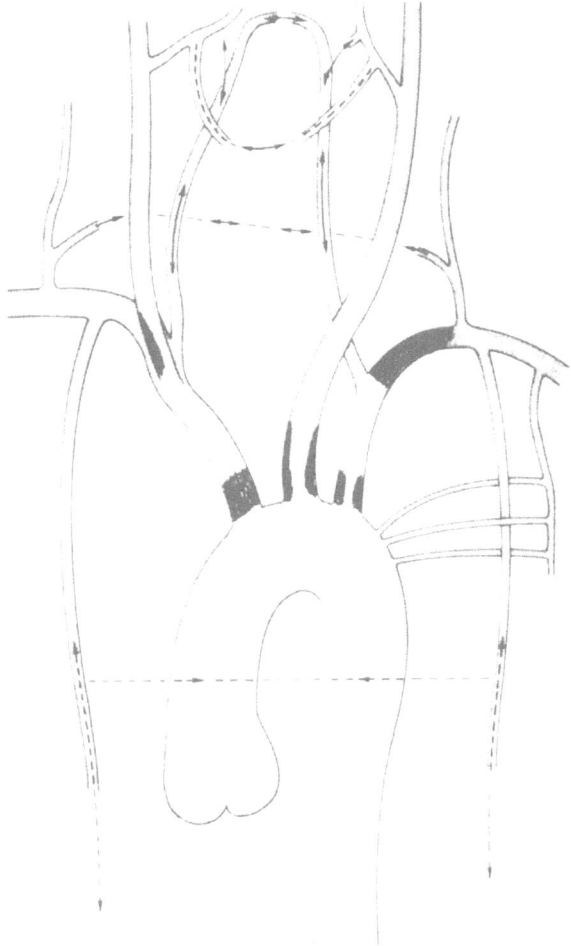

Fig. 35.20. Collateral arteries in aortic arch occlusions: caudo-cranial same as cranio-caudal in coarctation patients. "Winslow's collateral circulation"

plete AAS in a Turkish woman with bilateral subclavian obliterations.

In contrast, of 352 cases in Japan, arteriosclerosis was identified as the cause in 7%, syphilis in 2%, but unspecific aortoarteriitis in 91%. Of the patients with AAS in the western world, only very few present complete AAS. The mean age of the majority of patients is 55 ± 15 years. Most of these are men, in contrast to the inflammatory Takayasu-type aortoarteriitis, which mainly affects women (e.g., 39 out of 44 patients) (SHIMIZU and SANO 1951). Most cases of Takayasu's arteriitis have been published according to a compilation by RAU in Asian countries (Japan, China, India, Vietnam, Thailand, and the Philippines).

Therapy of the arteriosclerotic forms of incomplete AAS is predominantly vascular surgery, whereby extraanatomic bypasses (see Fig. 35.15) are frequently preferred to direct reimplantation (see

Fig. 35.14), to avoid a transthoracic intervention (DE BAKEY et al. 1959; CRAWFORD et al. 1962; BLAISDELL et al. 1969; VOLLMAR 1996).

Stenoses in the area of the brachiocephalic trunk, the subclavian arteries, as well as the common carotid artery, however, are also amenable to a percutaneous approach by means of balloon dilatation, often completed by stent implantation. Combined techniques comprising open surgery and additional interventional techniques are also becoming more common (MATHIAS 1988; JIANPIN and ZEITLER 1991) (see also Sect. 35.4).

The inflammatory forms of aortoarteriitis require, according to predominantly Japanese recommendations, primary corticosteroid and antibiotic therapy until an abatement of the inflammatory parameters is seen. Extraanatomic bypass operations are recommended during this phase. Percutaneous balloon angioplasty for inflammatory stenoses is, in most cases, only of suboptimal value. Should the situation require it, primary stent implantation after abatement of the inflammatory parameters may be justified as a minimally-invasive intervention. In any case, the therapeutic concept has to be established following interdisciplinary discussions between the vascular surgeon and the angiologist.

35.3.2
Thoracic Outlet Syndrome(TOS)

According to a definition by PEET et al. (1956), thoracic outlet sydrome comprises the compression syndromes in the area of the shoulder girdle. Included in these is compression in the area of the posterior scalenus gap and the costoclavicular narrowing, but also the rarer hyperabduction syndrome of the coracoid and pectoralis minor muscles simultaneously. These exert, according to the involved anatomic structures (Fig. 35.21), compression on neurogenic, arterial, or venous structures. While the venous compression syndrome – also known as "effort thrombosis" – is practically a thoracic inlet syndrome, the neurogenic thoracic outlet syndrome mainly results in compression and irritation of the brachial plexus. Neurogenic compression is the most common type (SELKE and KELLY 1988; SCHUNN 1997), observed mainly in young adults, whereby females are more often affected, at a ratio of 4:1 compared to males. Arterial thoracic outlet syndrome with thromboembolic complications caused by compression on the subclavian artery, was only identified in 5% of all thoracic outlet syndromes

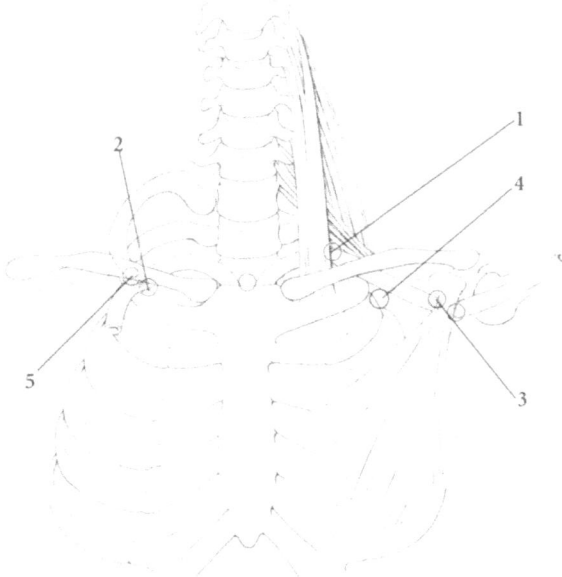

Fig. 35.21. The shoulder with typical compression areas: *1*, scalenus muscles, *2*, costo-clavicular narrowing, *3*, pectoralis muscles, *4*, posttraumatic compression, *5*, cervical rib syndrome

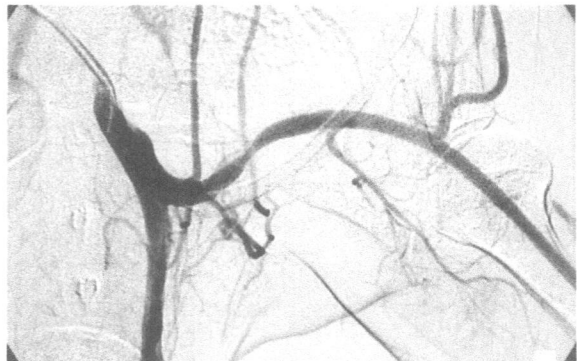

Fig. 35.22. Angiography at elevated right arm with compression of the subclavian artery

according to PEET et al. (1956). Arterial thoracic outlet syndrome affects men almost as often as women. It produces chronic compression of the subclavian artery in the region of the posterior scalenus gap. Also, irritation of the axillary artery between the pectoralis minor muscle and processus coracoideus was observed (SANDERS et al. 1990; FINKELSTEIN and JOHNSTON 1993). A very common cause of arterial thoracic outlet syndrome is a prominent cervical rib, but also the abnormal first thoracic rib compresses the subclavian artery caudally. Also, callus formation after fracture of the clavicula or first rib may induce the compression syndrome. Without the involvement of bones, an arterial compression syndrome cannot be identified in such cases.

During the diagnostic examination, the clamping effect to the artery needs to be investigated by elevating the arms (Fig. 35.22). The radial pulse is no longer palpable then. For angiographies of uni- or bilateral subclavian compression, transfemoral catheterization of the ascending thoracic artery or, in the case of unilateral symptoms, of the subclavian artery, is performed. With the shoulders in a normal position, angiography shows as a rule neither stenoses, nor occlusions. A repeat angiography performed under abduction, external rotation, and retroversion of the shoulder is able to document the compression mechanism as a stenosis in the course of the subclavian artery. In cases of a longer history, an irregu-

larity in the form of a local thrombosis may be present, which may also be the cause of peripheral embolism.

The therapy is very often surgery, mainly in the form of resection of the cervical rib and operative resection of the compressing structures alone. Interventional measures (ROOS 1987; MAKHOUL and MACHLEDER 1992) are not indicated. However, an exercise program may also be successful in some patients (PEET et al. 1956).

35.3.3
Collateral Pathways

The collateral circulation in the presence of supra-aortic obliterations is provided by the same communicating arteries which develop in the case of an aortic coarctation at its classic location. These are the communications between the subclavian, mammary, and caudal epigastric arteries on the one hand, and between the collateral communications between the lumbar and intercostal arteries and the intra- and paravertebral arteries, which bridge connections up to the carotid, vertebral, and external carotid arteries (see Fig. 35.20). In obliterations of the subclavian artery distal of the vertebral artery, the intercostal, as well the as lateral thoracic arteries, become important bridging collaterals, which run in the direction of the axillary artery, and supply blood directly from the descending thoracic aorta from a caudal to a cranial direction. These collaterals, however, can only form if the obliterating changes develop slowly. The essential collateral bridges alongside the aorta include Winslow's collateral pathway in the thorax, Riolan's collateral circulation in the upper abdomen, and the mesenterico-hypogastric collateral circulation in the lower abdomen and in the pelvic area.

Angiographic documentation has been clearly optimized by the new possibilities opened up by MRA and may show the way to new aspects in diagnostics and therapy.

References

Abrams H (1983) Angiography, 3rd edn, vol III. Little Brown, Boston

Adachi V (1928) Cited by Hüring (1974) and Rauber-Kopsch (1941)

Allen EV, Barker NW, Hines NW (1972) Peripheral vascular diseases, 4th edn. Saunders, Philadelphia

Anson BJ (1963) Atlas of human anatomy. Saunders, Philadelphia

Baert AL, Wilms G, Marchall G, et al. (1981) Intravenous digital subtraction angiography. Eur J Radiol 1:97–103

Bange F, Düx A, Lange J, Thurn P (1962) Zum Verschlußsyndrom der supraaortalen Gefäße (sog. Aortenbogensyndrom). Fortschr Rontgenstr 96:597

Beyer-Enke S (1996) Spezielle Diagnostik der großen Gefäße. In: Eichstätt H, et al. (eds) Herz und große Gefäße. Springer, Berlin Heidelberg New York, pp 413–431

Blaisdell WF, Claus RH, Galbraith HG, Imparato AM, Wylie EJ (1969) Joint study of extracranial arterial occlusions. IV. A review of surgical considerations. JAMA 200:1889

Bollinger A, Preter B (1973) Spasmen der muskulären Stammarterien der Extremitäten nach Einnahme von ergotamintartrat-haltigen Medikamenten. Dtsch Med Wochenschr 98:825–827

Bollinger A, Zeitler E (1976) Klinisch-angiologische Probleme bei der Erkennung pharmaka-induzierter Veränderungen an Extremitätenarterien. In: Zeitler E (ed) Aspekte der Extremitätenarteriographie. Huber, Bern, pp 121–131

Bollinger A (1979) Funktionelle Angiologie. Thieme, Stuttgart

Buchwalsky R, Genswein R, Schlosser V, Blümchen G (1977) Subclavian-Steal-Syndrom: postoperativer und spontaner Verlauf bei 27 Patienten über 3 Jahre. Thoraxchir Vask Chir 25:288–290

Caccamise WC, Okuda K (1954) Takayasu's or pulseless disease. An unusual syndrome with ocular manifestations. Am J Ophthalmol 37:784

Contorini L (1960) Il circolo collaterale vertebrovertebrale nella obliteratione dell' arteria subclavia alla sua origine. Minerva Chir 15:268

Crawford ES, De Bakey ME, Morris GC, Cooley DA (1962) Thrombo-obliterative disease of the great vessels arising from the aortic arch. J Thorac Cardiovasc Surg 43:38

Dawson DM (1993) Entrapment neuropathies of the upper extremities. N Engl J Med 329[27]:2013

De Bakey ME, Crawford ES, Fields WS (1959) Surgical treatment of lesions producing arterial insufficiency of the internal carotid, common carotid, vertebral, innominate and subclavian arteries. Ann Intern Med 51:436

Dorman RL, Kaufmann JA, Muraglia LA (1989) Digital emboli from brachial artery fibromuscular dysplasia: a regional cause of peripheral occlusive vascular disease. Angiology 40:108–113

Eklöf B, Tylén U (1976) Rationelle arteriographische Untersuchung bei Finger-ischämie. In: Zeitler E (ed) Aspekte der Extremitätenangiographie – aktuelle Probleme in der Angiologie, vol 34. Huber, Bern, pp 191–198

Erikson N (1965) Peripheral arteriography during bradykinin induced vasodilatation. Acta Radiol (Stockh) 3:193–201

Etter L (1944) Osseous abnormalities of the thoracic cage seen in forty thousand consecutive chest photoroentgenograms. Am J Roentgenol 51:359–368

Fields WS, Maslenikov V, Meyer JS, Hass WK, et al. (1970) Joint study of extracranial arterial occlusion. JAMA 211:1993

Finkelstein JA, Johnston KW (1993) Thrombosis of the axillary artery secondary to compression by the pectoralis minor muscle. Ann Vasc Surg 7:287

Steinkopff, Dresden

35.4
Interventional Radiology

35.4.1
Angioplasty of the Brachial Arteries

K. Hüttl

35.4.1.1
Introduction

Percutaneous transluminal angioplasty (PTA) is performed on the upper limb arteries much more rarely than on the lower limb arteries. The explanation for this is that: atherosclerosis is present on the upper limb much less frequently than in the lower limb. The same degree of stenosis more often presents symptoms on the lower than on the upper limb. This difference can be explained by the rich collateral network on the upper limb and by the fact that the arm is less frequently exposed to physical strain, and the use of the arm can be avoided in more cases than the leg in the every day life. Therefore, usually longer periods of time pass before the patient seeks the help of a physician. Due to the normal interconnections among the brachial and cephalic vessels, a fear of cerebral complications and lack of experience kept, for years, many otherwise aggressive interventionists from doing PTA in the subclavian and innominate arteries.

The most common site for PTA of the arterial system of the upper limb is the subclavian and innominate arteries. Axillary and brachial arteries are less frequent locations for PTA. The forearm arteries are infrequent locations for atherosclerosis and PTA is almost exclusively performed due to the insufficiency of Brescia-Cimino fistulas.

35.4.1.2
Patient Selection

35.4.1.2.1
CLINICAL INDICATIONS

Patient history, physical examination, duplex scan and Doppler examination are usually sufficient to prove the diagnosis of obliterative vascular disease. In case of doubt, a neurologist or angiologist should be involved in the differential diagnosis. The clinical symptoms and examinations necessary are discussed in previous chapters.

We need to answer two basic questions:
- Is the treatment of the occlusive lesion necessary?
- Is PTA the best treatment of choice?

Subclavian and Brachial Artery. The most commonly dilated vessel is the subclavian artery. Patients with asymptomatic subclavian artery lesions require no invasive investigation since there is no evidence that the natural history of such lesions is either harmful or improved by PTA or surgical repair (Herring 1977).

Asymptomatic stenosis is, however, an indication for PTA when a mammary left anterior descending artery (LAD) bypass operation or axillo-femoro bypass operation is planned (Burke et al. 1987; Dorros et al. 1990; Wilms et al. 1987; Vitek et al. 1986). Subclavian artery stenosis resulting in angina pectoris in patients with a previous left internal mammary artery bypass to the LAD can be treated by PTA (Bely et al. 1992; Shapira et al. 1991).

If the stenosis occurs proximal to the origin of the vertebral artery, subclavian steal syndrome may develop, the most frequent indication for subclavian artery PTA. There is no linear correlation between the magnitude of the steal and the degree of vertebrobasilar symptoms (BRANCHEREAU et al. 1990). The symptoms of the subclavian steal become more serious if there are concomitant lesions of the supraaortic branches (HERRING 1977).

Ischemic signs of the upper limb usually occur only if subclavian steal has not, or only insufficiently, developed. Upper limb ischemia is a principal sign in the following cases: (a) The stenosis is distal to the origin of the vertebral artery, (b) the vertebral artery originates from the aortic arch directly (6%–7%), (c) if the vertebral artery on either side is hypoplastic, aplastic, or occluded.

The physical load of the upper limb is smaller and avoidance of usage is less difficult than that of the lower limb. Lifestyle and the degree of symptoms should be considered in order to indicate re-vascularization. If trophic disturbances occur on the hand or rest pain is present, revascularization is necessary.

In cerebrovascular patients, more than one lesion of the supraaortic arterial branches is often diagnosed. In order to increase cerebral perfusion, subclavian artery PTA is indicated in the case of non-operable, severe lesion on the carotid system, e.g., occlusion of the internal carotid artery with concomitant stenosis of the subclavian artery leading to subclavian steal. The angioplasty should be carried out in such patients even if the major symptoms are not due to vertebrobasilar insufficiency.

Innominate Artery. In the case of occlusion of the innominate artery, the symptoms are usually due to the insufficiency in the carotid system, but signs of brain stem ischemia or claudication of the upper

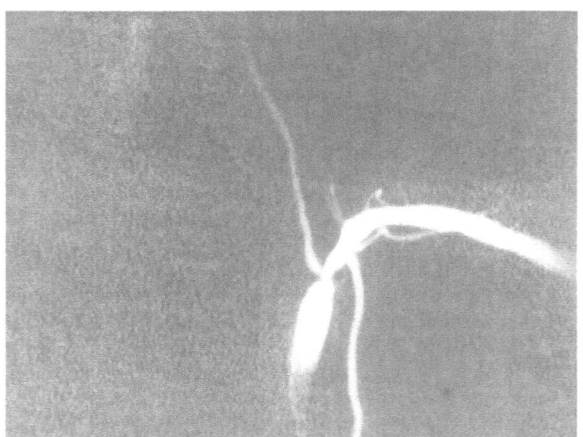

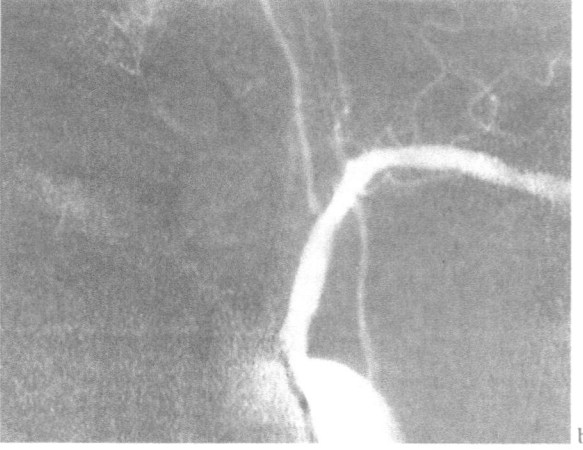

Fig. 35.23 a,b. Subclavian artery percutaneous transluminal angioplasty (PTA) at the vertebral origin. **a** Subclavian artery stenosis is adjacent to the origin of the vertebral artery and antegrade vertebral flow is present. **b** Control angiogram after successful PTA

limb may also occur. The symptoms that develop due to the lesion of the innominate artery are usually not as dramatic as those caused by internal carotid artery lesions. Stroke is a rare consequence. In case of symptoms, PTA is indicated (Table 35.3) (Fig. 35.23).

35.4.1.2.2
ETIOLOGY

In most cases, angioplasty is performed due to an atherosclerotic lesion. Brachiocephalic trunk origin stenosis secondary to Takayasu arteritis is a favorable lesion for PTA (PARK et al. 1989; HODGINS and DUTTON 1984; SADDEKNI et al. 1980). However, PTA is not advised in patients with active inflammation of arteries in case of an elevated erythrocyte sedimentation rate or C-reactive protein levels because arterial stenosis is considered to be progressive and there is a high risk of restenosis.

Angioplasty can be a successful treatment of choice on stenosis of a stenotic anastomosis or myointimal hyperplasia (SADDEKNI et al. 1980) following surgery, or restenosis after angioplasty. Stenosis caused by irradiation is suitable for PTA (SADDEKNI et al. 1980) (PIEDBOIS et al. 1990). These lesions are less likely to release embolic debris. Angioplasty can also be performed on congenital stenosis. Angioplasty of both the coarctic aorta and the stenotic subclavian artery has been performed (HÜTTL et al. 1992). Occlu-

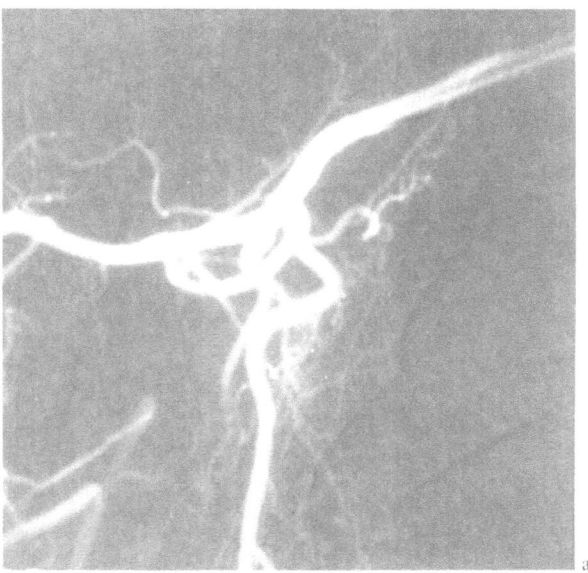
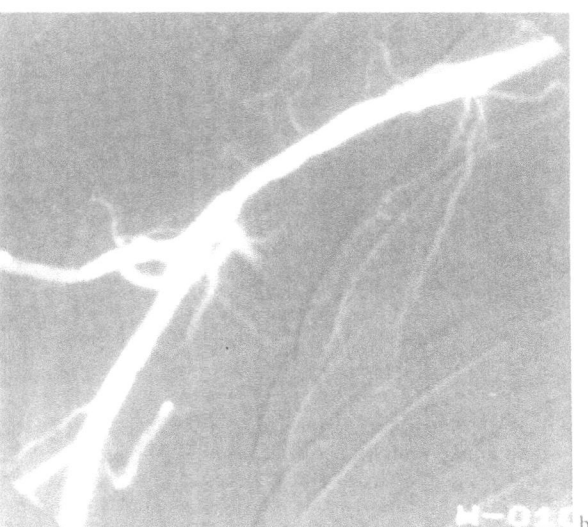

Fig. 35.24 a,b. Axillay artery percutaneous transluminal angioplasty. **a** Selective angiogram shows occlusion of the axillary artery resulting in gangrene of the right hand. **b** After angioplasty a lumen is restored. Patient symptom resolved

Table 35.3. Indications for subclavian and innominate artery percutaneous transluminal angioplasty at the Department of Cardiovascular Surgery of Semmelweis Medical University, Budapest (1979–1996)

Lesion site	Symptoms	n
Subclavian artery	Arm claudication	91
	Rest pain or gangrene	62
	VBI	109
	VBI + arm claudication	141
	TIA maintaining cerebral perfusion through the vertebral artery	13
Innominate artery	TIA	11
	TIA + VBI	33
	VBI + arm claudication	9
	Arm claudication	17
	Asymptomatic (prior to major surgery)	1

VBI, Vertebrobasilar insufficiency; TIA, transient ischemic attack.

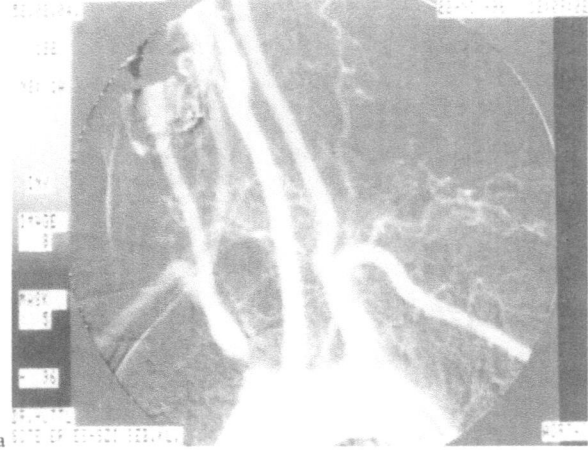

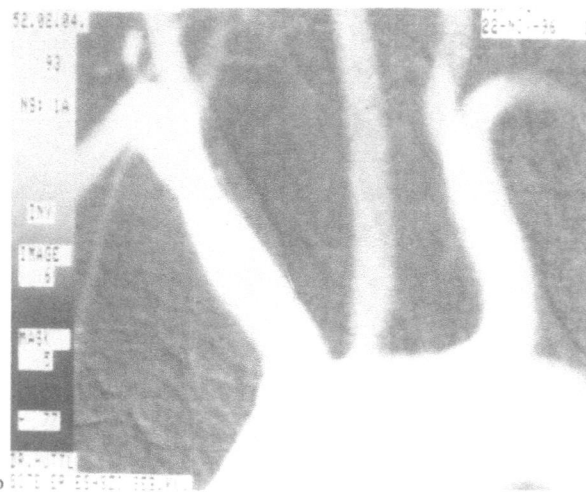

Fig. 35.25 a,b. Percutaneous transluminal angioplasty of innominate artery stenosis. **a** Arch aortogram shows high degree of innominate artery stenosis prior to treatment. **b** Arch aortogram immediately after angioplasty shows increased diameter of the innominate artery

sion due to embolization, external compression (e.g., thoracic outlet syndrome), or lesions of traumatic origin cannot be treated effectively by angioplasty.

35.4.1.2.3
SELECTION BASED ON ANATOMIC FEATURES
The widespread use of PTA on the supraaortic vessels has been delayed due to the fear of embolization of the cerebral vessels. At present, there is no reliable technique available for preventing distal embolization. Therefore, it is important to identify the risk of PTA at different lesion sites. If the vertebral artery is occluded or originates from the aortic arch directly, or if the stenosis of the subclavian artery is located distal from the orifice of the vertebral artery, the risk of cerebral embolization is minimal. In the case of subclavian steal, the risk of embolization is also very

low since the steal phenomenon is reversed only 10–20 s after successful recanalization (RINGELSTEIN and ZEUMER 1984).

Patients with antegrade vertebral flow are at greater risk of cerebral embolization during angioplasty (Fig. 35.24). Some authors consider antegrade flow as a contraindication for PTA (VITEK et al. 1986; BACHMAN and KIM 1980; RINGELSTEIN and ZEUMER 1984; SHARMA et al. 1991). The author agrees with other investigators that subclavian and innominate artery PTA are to the benefit of the patient regardless of the direction of flow in the vertebral artery (DAMUTH et al. 1983; COOK and DYET 1989).

The ideal lesion for angioplasty is a short, round-shaped stenosis. A longer (3–4 cm) or excentric lesion does not constitute a contraindication to PTA (SZLÁVY and TAVERAS 1995; BELY et al. 1992; DORROS et al. 1990; HEBRANG et al. 1990; INSALL et al. 1990). Vertebral artery occlusion can occur if the stenotic plaque is adjacent to the origin of the vertebral artery (THERON et al. 1990; VITEK et al. 1986). Occasionally, even if the vertebral artery is occluded, the symptoms may not be aggravated, but rather ablated.

The indication for PTA on an occlusive lesion of the innominate or subclavian artery is a subject of debate. A possible thrombus on the occluded part may be a source of distal embolization. In the case of occlusion, some authors are against performing PTA because of the high technical failure rate (SHARMA et al. 1991; RINGELSTEIN and ZEUMER 1984; MOTARJAME 1996), while others are in favor of angioplasty in the case of occlusion (DORROS et al. 1990; WHITAKER and GRESON 1991; MATHIAS et al. 1993) (Fig. 35.26). Angioplasty is not suggested if concomitant stenosis and aneurysm are present on the same vessel.

If angiography shows a floating thrombus, or the occlusion has occurred acutely, angioplasty should be carried out following thrombolysis. If the thrombus is situated before the branching of the cerebral vessels, thrombolysis is contraindicated because of the risk of peripheral cerebral embolization during the procedure. When deciding about the indication for angioplasty, the expected risk and benefit to the patient should be weighed against the risk of not performing PTA or surgical treatment. The decision is best made after considering all the above factors by both an interventional radiologist and a vascular surgeon.

35.4.1.3
Technique

The procedure is basically the same as for other vessels, except that this area needs to be approached with caution and only by angiographers with extensive experience in dilatation of other vessels. Prior to angioplasty, aspirin is administered orally. Administration of heparin is advisable as soon as the lesion is crossed. Spasm of the vertebral or axillary arteries can be relieved with the administration of intraarterial nitroglycerin (100–200 μg).

The angioplasty catheter is usually inserted via the femoral artery. The passage of the guidewire through a stenotic lesion is the most critical task where complications and technical problems can occur. Improvements to guidewires (hydrophil, floppy, or steerable guidewires) have helped make crossing the lesion a less traumatic procedure. After exchanging the wire, the balloon catheter is advanced to the stenotic area. Control angiography is preferably performed with the guidewires held in a poststenotic position. In case of ostial occlusion or high grade stenosis, when the guidewire frequently flaps back to the aortic arch, the use of a guiding catheter – providing a firm mechanical support for the guidewire – may be of great help (Fig. 35.26). A brachial or axillary approach is recommended for inserting the catheter if the femoral route is difficult or impossible (e.g., tortuousity of the aorta or Leriche syndrome), or if the lesion is ostial. In the axillary route, the distance between insertion and stenosis is relatively small, therefore it may be easier to maneuver the instruments. On the other hand, the number of local complications is higher and the limb may suffer further from more severe ischemia due to puncture site thrombosis.

Several methodological suggestions have been made to avoid embolization. Concomitant vascular cutdown and arteriotomy with washout of angioplasty debris has been suggested through the arteriotomy site; no debris was seen (HODGINS

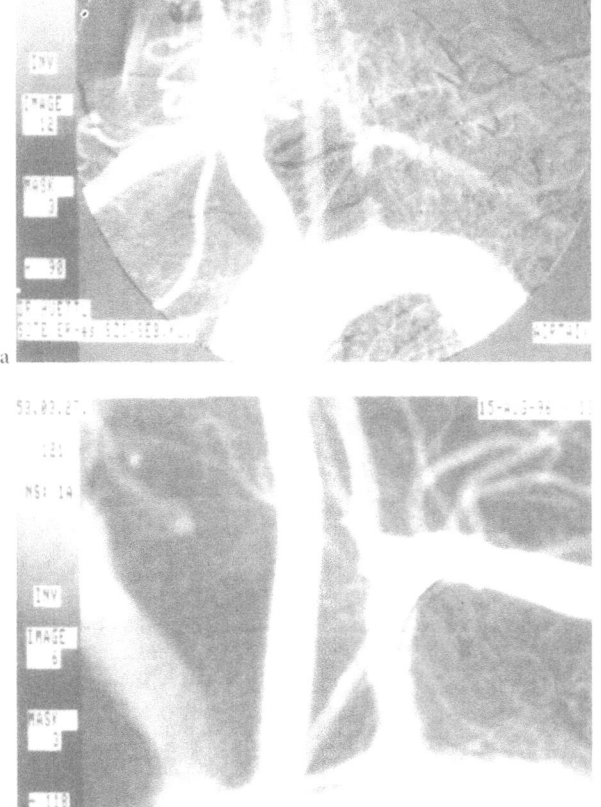

Fig. 35.26 a–c. Percutaneous transluminal angioplasty of subclavian artery occlusion resulting from subclavian steal syndrome. **a** Aortic arch angiogram shows occlusion of the left subclavian artery with retrograde filling of the vertebral artery. **b** Selective angiogram confirms ostial occlusion of the left subclavian artery. **c** Angiogram following angioplasty shows enlargement of origin of the subclavian artery and antegrade filling of the vertebral artery

and Dutton 1984; Derauf et al. 1986). To prevent distal embolization through the vertebral and carotid arteries, blood flow in these vessels was temporarily occluded with balloon catheters (Koike et al. 1992; Theron et al. 1990). However, these techniques are not widely used by interventional radiologists.

35.4.1.4
Complications

Complications related to brachial angioplasty are listed in Tables 35.3–35.5. Cerebral complications are rare occurrences after subclavian PTA with a frequency of less than 1% (Tables 35.4, 35.5). Innominate artery PTA has a very small incidence of neurological complications, though in the literature there is only a small series of patients treated with innominate artery PTA (Dorros et al. 1990; Gobin et al. 1991; Motarjame 1996; Insall et al. 1990; Qi and Zeitler 1991; Vitek et al. 1986). Among our 71 cases, one permanent cerebral complication occurred related to innominate artery PTA (Fig. 35.25). This patient would also have been a high-risk patient for surgery. Acute occlusion of the dilated vessel or the adjacent vertebral artery are also rare complications (Tables 35.4, 35.5).

The frequency of vascular complications at the puncture site does not differ from occurrence with other therapeutic interventions (3%–4%).

35.4.1.5
Results

The technical success rate in the treatment of stenosis is 88%–100% (Tables 35.4, 35.5). PTA on occluded arteries has been tried with varying success, ranging from failure in all cases to 100% success (Table 35.5). Dorros had a 100% success rate with angioplasty on occluded subclavian arteries using brachial insertion. In a recent study (Mathias et al. 1993), an 83% initial success rate of occlusive lesions reflects new developments in balloon-catheter and guidewire technology and expertise in performing angioplasty.

The long-term patency rate in the literature varies between 83%–100%, with a mean follow-up period of 13–37 months (Tables 35.4, 35.5; Fig. 35.28). The patency of the artery and the asymptomatic period do not overlap. In advantageous cases, despite restenosis, the patient can remain clinically asymptomatic due to the collateral network.

Table 35.4. Results of innominate artery percutaneous transluminal angioplasty at the Department of Cardiovascular Surgery of Semmelweis Medical University, Budapest (1979–1996)

Artery	Lesions (n) Stenosis	Occlusion	Technical success rate (%) Stenosis	Occlusion	Long-term patency (%)	Follow-up time (months)	Complications
Innominate	71	4	97	100 (4/4)	94	22 (6–64)	One left occipital lobe infarction Two puncture site thromboses Four transient neurologic symptoms
Subclavian	416	22	96	68	89	33 (9–99)	One subclavian artery occlusion One vertebral artery occlusion (symptomless) Five transient neurological symptoms Three shoulder pain with Six puncture site complications
Axillary and brachial	11	2	90 (10/11)	50 (1/2)	85	23 (9–60)	

Table 35.5. Subclavian artery percutaneous transluminal angioplasty in the literature

Author	Lesions (n)	occl.	Initial success rate stenoses	occl. (%)	Long-term patency (%)	Follow-up time (months)	List of major complications
Burke et al. (1987)	30	2	86		80	37	1 Stroke 1 Hand embolization
Cook and Dyet (1989)	6		100		83	5–20	
Damuth et al. (1983)	9		100		100	13	Occlusion carotid-subclavian artery graft occlusion
Dorros et al. (1990)	30	11	100		95	28	2 Brachial thrombosis
Erbstein et al. (1988)	24	2	88		88	18–26	1 Brachial occlusion
Hebrang et al. (1990)	52	9	45/52	5/6	91	29	
Higashida et al. (1986)	16		100		100	17	–
Insall et al. (1990)	33	3	27/29		96	20	1 Stroke contralateral 2 Puncture site
Kachel and Babche (1991)	44	14	86.5		1/57 2/44	61 58	4 Hematoma, 1 peripheral embolism
Kachel (1993)	57				1/1		1.2%
Koike et al. (1992)	6		100		2/6		
Mathias et al. (1993)	316	46	97	83 38/46	90	36	1 TIA, 1 False aneurysm, 1 bleeding
Mathias (1988)							1.2%
Motarjame (1996)	80	13	92	46	93	60	
Pavone et al. (1987)	83		91				1 Stroke
Qi and Zeitler (1991)	113	7	96.5		98.8	36	1 ITA, 1 peripheral embolism 1.1%
Théron (1992)	55		100				non
Tesdal et al. (1991)	37	1	89		94.4	6–37	8.65% Minor complications
Tournade et al. (1986)	24				87.5	12–18	
Vitek et al. (1986)	13		100				
Wilms et al. (1987)	23		91		80.5	48	1 Embolization to finger artery 1 Axillaris thrombosis
Sharma et al. (1991)	7	3	4/7	0/3	4/4	10	2 Cerebral embolizations
Nicholson (1991)	12	5	11/12				
Ringelstein Zeumer (1984)	12	2	75%	0/2	100	1–7	1 Subclavian artery occlusion
			10/12				1 Hand embolization

35.4.1.6
Comparison of Interventional Radiological and Surgical Treatment

There are numerous advantages and disadvantages of PTA over surgical treatment depending of the location of the lesion.

Advantages of PTA over surgical treatment:
- No need for anesthesia and, therefore, no anesthesiological complications. Employment of local anesthesia enables communication with the patient during intervention. Initial disturbance of the blood supply can be recognized.
- Extremely short interruption (5–10 s) of the arterial blood supply.
- Multifocal occlusive lesions can be treated synchronously by PTA.
- Negligible amount of blood loss.
- There is no wound surface, only a punctured channel, thus the healing process is much quicker. The length of hospitalization is shorter.
- No complications such as inflammation, nerve injury, suture insufficiency, or pseudoaneurysm occur during surgery.
- In the case of an unsuccessful PTA, surgery can be the second option for treatment, but vice versa is not possible.
- In the case of restenosis, PTA can easily be repeated, or reconstructive surgery is indicated. Repeated surgery, however, creates much greater strain on the patient.

Disadvantages:
- PTA can be used only for the treatment of selected arterial lesions.

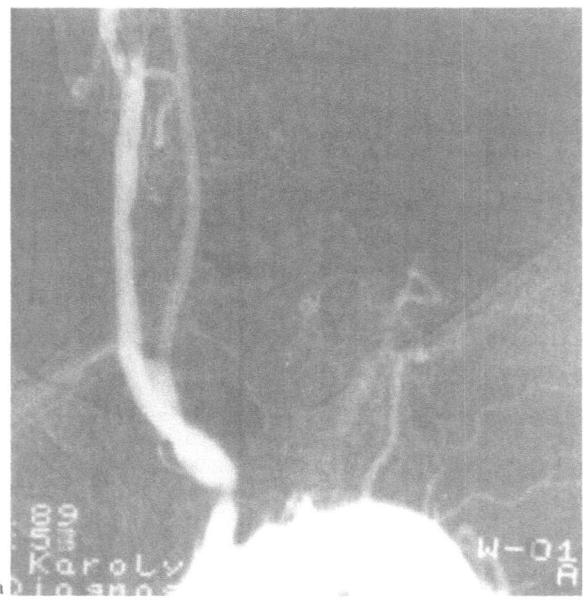
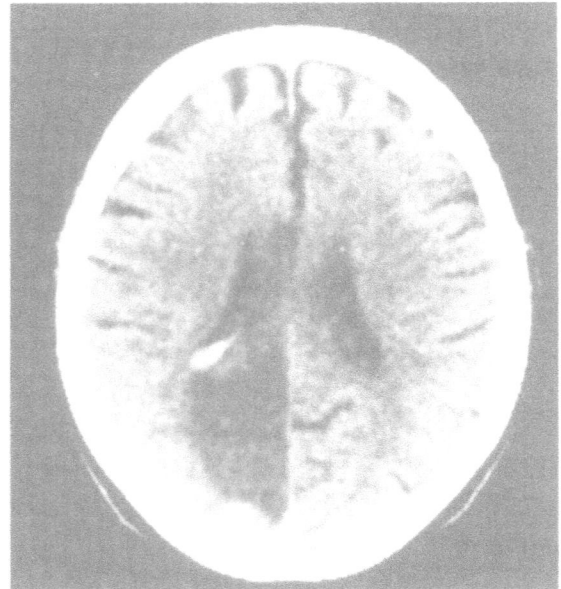

Fig. 35.27 a,b. Cerebral complication following innominate artery percutaneous transluminal angioplasty (PTA). **a** The early phase of the arch aortogram shows atherosclerotic occlusion of the left subclavian and common carotid arteries and high degree of stenosis in the innominate artery. Because of the patient's very severe vertebrobasilar insufficiency syndrome PTA was attempted. The patient lost consciousness immediately after balloon inflation. **b** Computed tomography scan 2 days later shows left occipital lobe infarction

- Prevention of embolization is less effective than with surgery.
- If surgery is chosen, extrathoracic bypass is now the preferred treatment wherever possible. There is lower morbidity and mortality attached to extrathoracic procedures and they are simple, which provides long-term results equal to endarteractomy. The mortality rate for extrathoracal operations is very low, usually less than 1% (BRANCHEREAU et al. 1990) or, as observed in many series, without any lethal complications (KRETSCHMER et al. 1991; RAITHEL 1980). The incidence of neurological complications is less than 1% with good patient selection, but 3% has also been reported (BRANCHEREAU et al. 1990). Other complications (pneumothorax, pleural fluid, chylothorax, lymphatic fistula, wound inflammation, paretic recurrent nerve) may occur in 15%–20% of cases (KRETSCHMER et al. 1991). The 5-year patency rate is 90%–95% (BRANCHEREAU et al. 1990; RAITHEL 1980) and approximately 90% of patients are asymptomatic after 5 years.

35.4.1.7
Summary

PTA of the upper limb arteries is usually a successful treatment of choice because the lesions selected for PTA are usually short segment stenoses. These arteries are of an elastic type, have a relatively large diameter, with a large perfusion, and therefore the risk of restenosis is small. PTA on these arteries is technically feasible, the rate of complications is small, it provides long-term patency, and patients become asymptomatic. It has numerous advantages over surgical treatment. In the case of symptomatic stenosis of the upper extremity arteries – with the restrictions discussed – PTA is the procedure of choice.

References

Bachman DM, Kim RM (1980) Transluminal dilatation for subclavian steal syndrome. AJR Am J Roentgenol 135:995–996

Bely M, Marschall JJ, Cowley MJ, Vetrovec GW (1992) Subclavian balloon angioplasty in the management of the coronary subclavian steal syndrome. Cathet Cardiovasc Diagn 25(2):161–163

Branchereau A, Magnan PE, Espinoza H, Bartoli JM (1990) Subclavian artery stenosis haemodynamic aspects surgical outcome. J Cardiovasc Surg 32:604–612

Burke DR, Gordon RL, Mishkin JD, McLean GK, Meranze SG (1987) Percutaneous transluminal angioplasty of subclavian arteries. Radiology 164:699–704

Cook AM, Dyet JF (1989) Six cases of subclavian stenosis treated by percutaneous angioplasty. Clin Radiol 40:352–354

Damuth H, Diamond AB, Rappoport AS, Renner JW (1983) Angioplasty of subclavian artery stenosis proximal to the vertebral orgin. AJNR Am J Neuroradiol 4:1239–1242

Derauf BJ, Erickson DL, Castaneda-Zuniga WR, Cardella JF, Amplatz K (1986) "Washout" technique for brachiocephalic angioplasty. AJR Am J Roentgenol 146:849–851

Dorros G, Lewin RF, Jamnadas P, Mathiak LM (1990) Peripheral transluminal angioplasty of the subclavian and innominate arteries utilizing the brachial approach: acute outcome and follow-up. Cathet Cardiovasc Diagn 19:71–76

Erbstein RA, Wholey MH, Smoot S (1988) Subclavian artery steal syndrome: treatment by percutaneous transluminal angioplasty. AJR Am J Roentgenol 15:291–294

Gershoni G, Basta L, Hagan AD (1990) Correction of subclavian artey stenosis by percutaneous angioplasty. Cathet Cardiovasc Diagn 21(3):165–169

Gobin Y, Hassani R, Batellier J, Casasso S, Aymard A, Merland J (1991) Transluminal angioplasty of the brachiocephalic artery with cerebral protection. J Mal Vasc 16(2):188–190

Hebrang A, Maskovic J, Tomac B (1990) Percutaneous transluminal angioplasty of the subclavian arteries. AJR Am J Roentgenol 156(5):1091–1094

Herring M (1977) The subclavian steal syndrome: a review. Am Surg 43:220–228

Higashida RT, Hieshima GB, Tsai FY, Bentson JR, Halbavh VV (1986) Percutaneous transluminal angioplasty of the subclavian andvertebral arteries. Acta Radiol Suppl (Stockh) 369:124–126

Hodgins GW, Dutton JW (1984) Transluminal dilatation for Takayasu's arteritis. Can J Surg 4:355–357

Hüttl K, Szlávy L, Szabolcs Z, Repa I, Simonffy Á (1992) PTA of an unusual caorctation of the aorta in adulthood. Orv Hetil 133(23):1437–1440

Insall RL, Lambert D, Chamberlain J, Proud G, Murthy LN (1990) Percutaneous transluminal angioplasty of the innominate, subclavian and axillary arteries. Eur J Vasc Surg 4(6):591–595

Kachel R (1993) Perkutane transluminale Angioplastie (PTA) der A. carotis. Wien Klin Wochenschr 105:187–193

Kachel R, Basche S (1991) Perkutane Transluminale Angioplastik (PTA) im supraaortischen Bereich – eigene Ergebnisse und internationaler Stand. In: Maurer PC, Dörrler J, Sommoggy JS von (eds) Gefäßchirurgie im Fortschritt. Thieme, Stuttgart, pp 242–248

Kachel R, Endert G, Basche S, Grossmann K, Glaser FH (1987) Percutaneous transluminal angioplasty (dilatation) of carotid, vertebral, and innominate artery stenoses. Cardiovasc Intervent Radiol 10:142–146

Kobinia GS, Bergmann H (1983) Angioplasty in stenosis of the innominate artery. Cardiovasc Intervent Radiol 6:82–85

Koike T, Minakawa T, Abe H (1992) PTA of supra-aortic arteries with temporary balloon occlusion to avoid distal embolism. Neurol Med Chir (Tokyo) 32(3):140–147

Kretschmer G, Teleky B, Marosi L, Wagner O, Wunderlich M, Karnel F, Jantsch H, Schemper M, Polterauer P (1991) Obliterations of the proximal subclavian artery: to bypass or to anastomose. J Cardiovasc Surg 32:334–339

Mathias K (1988) Perkutane Rekanalisation der supraaortalen Arterien. In: Günther RW, Thelen M (eds) Interventionelle Radiologie. Thieme, Stuttgart, pp 73–87

Mathias KD, Luth I, Haarmann P (1993) PTA of the proximal subclavian artery occluisons. Cardiovasc Intervent Radiol 16(4):214–218

Motarjame A (1996) Percutaneous transluminal angioplasty of the supra-aortic vessels. J Endovasc Surg 3(2):171–181

Nicholson AA, Kennan NM, Sheridan WG, Ruttley MS (1991) Percutaneous transluminal angioplasty of the subclavian artery. Ann R Coll Surg Engl 73(1):43–52

Pavone P, Castrucci M, Cavallaro A, Rossi P (1987) PTA of subclavian artery: comparative study with surgical procedures. Program of the Cardiovascular and Interventional Radiology Society of Europe, Porto Cervo, Sardinia, Italy, May 27, pp 85–86

Park JH, Han MC, Kim SH, Oh BH, Park YB, Seo JD (1989) Takayasu arteritis: angiographic findings and results of angioplasty. AJR Am J Roentgenol 153:1069–1074

Piedbois P, Becquemin JP, Blanc I, Mazeron JJ, Lange F, Melliere D, LeBourgeois JP (1990) Material occlusive disease after radiotherapy. Radiother Oncol 17(2):133–140

Qi JP, Zeitler E (1991) Katheterdilatation der arteriellen Stenosen supraaortaler Gefäße und Spätergebnisse. RÖFO 155:357–362

Raithel D (1980) Our experience of surgery for innominate and subclavian lesions. J Cardiovasc Surg 21:423–430

Ringelstein EB, Zeumer E (1984) Delayed reversal of verte-bral artery blood flow following percutaneous transluminal angioplasty for subclavian steal syndrome. Neuroradiology 26:189–198

Saddekni S, Sniderman KW, Hilton S, Sos TA (1980) Percutaneous transluminal angioplasty of nonatherosclerotic lesions. AJR Am J Roentgenol 135:975–982

Shapira S, Braun SD, Puram B, Pate G (1991) Percutaneous transluminal angioplasty of proximal subclavian artery stenosis after left internal mammary to left anterior descending artery bypass surgery. J Am Coll Cardiol 18(4):1120–1123

Sharma S, Kaul U, Rajnai M (1991) Identifying high-risk patients for percutaneous transluminal angioplasty of subclavian and innominate arteries. Acta Radiol 32(5):381–385

Szlávy L, Taveras JM (1995) Noncoronary angioplasty and intervetional radiologic treatment of vascular malformations. William and Wilkins, Baltimore, pp 70–145

Théron J (1992) Angioplasty of brachiocephalic vessels. In: Vinuela F et al. (ed) Interventional neuroradiology: endovascular therapy of the central nervous system. Raven, New York, pp 167–180

Theron J, Courtheoux P, Alachkar F, Bouvard G, Maiza D (1990) New triple coaxial cather system for carotid angioplasty with cerebral protection. AJNR Am J Neuroradiol 11:869–874

Tesdal IK, Jaschke W, Haueisen H, Menges HW, Hoffmeister AW, Huck K, Menges V, Georgi M (1991) Percutaneous transluminal angioplasty (PTA) of the arteries of the arm in brachial and cerebral ischemia. ROFO 155:363–369

Tournade A, Zenglein JP, Braun JP, Courtheux P, Tjahmady (1986) Percutaneous transluminal angioplasty of the vertebral and subclavian arteries: an angiographic-velocimetry comparison. J Neuroradiol 13:95–110

Vitek JJ, Keller FS, Duvall ER, Gupta KL, Chandra-Sekar B (1986) Brachiocephalic artery dilation by percutaneous transluminal angioplasty. Intervent Radiol 158:779–785

Whitaker SC, Greson RH (1991) Case report: occlusion of subclavian artery treated by percutaneous angioplasty. Clin Radiol 44(3):199–200

Wilms G, Baert A, Dewaele D, Vermylen J, Nevelsteen A, Suy R (1987) Percutaneous transluminal angioplasty of the subclavian artery: early and late results. Cardiovasc Intervent Radiol 10:123–128

Zeitler E, Bär I (1997) Zerebrovaskuläre Durchblutungsstörungen. In: Zeitler E (ed) Klinische Radiologie – Arterien und Venen. Springer, Berlin Heidelberg New York, pp 431–476

35.4.2
Subclavian Artery Stenting and the Future of IR

K. Mathias

35.4.2.1
Introduction

It is the function of subclavian and innominate arteries to supply the brain and arms with blood. Both vascular territories compete for the distribution of flow in the case of proximal stenosis or occlusion. Therefore, the patient may suffer from symptoms in the arm or the brain (Reivich et al. 1961). The steal of blood from the vertebrobasilar circulation may be without clinical signs – subclavian steal phenomenon – or will be accompanied by symptoms of impaired perfusion of the posterior cerebral circulation and is then defined as subclavian steal syndrome. Clinically manifest vertebrobasilar insufficiency is caused by unilateral obstruction, whereby the dominant vertebral artery is supplied by a stenotic subclavian artery. A stroke as a consequence of subclavian obstruction is a very unusual event when the carotid arteries are patent.

Patients with acute arterial insufficiency of the upper extremity present with the same dramatic signs seen in acute arterial insufficiency of the lower extremities, including pulselessness, pallor, paresthesia, pain, and paralysis. Thromboembolism with acute ischemia of the fingers and hand may have their origins in a subclavian stenosis.

Chronic arterial insufficiency of the upper extremity is more subtle. Disabling discomfort on arm exertion is a common complaint and that reported most frequently by patients.

The subclavian artery may also be used as a donor artery in the surgical treatment of coronary heart disease. Patients with mammary artery anastomosis will develop angina if blood flow in the subclavian artery is impaired (Crowe and Iannone 1993; Edwards 1995; Georges and Ferretti 1993; Kugelmass et al. 1994; Marques et al. 1996; Mufti et al. 1994; Perrault et al. 1993). Also extra-anatomic axillo-femoral bypass grafts are endangered by a proximal subclavian artery obstruction.

The treatment of subclavian and innominate artery obstructions is intended to relieve patients of their complaints and to prevent complications of the disease. We deal mostly with atherosclerotic disease which has its predilection site at the proximal part of

the artery. Atherosclerotic plaque may extend to the aortic arch or involve the origin of the vertebral artery. The stenosis may be short and membrane-like in shape or long and tubular, concentric or eccentric, with or without ulceration of the plaque, and with a varying degree of calcification. The occlusion always extends from the aortic arch to the origin of the vertebral artery. Arm symptoms are more severe when the obstruction is located distal to the origin of the vertebral artery because of poor collateral blood flow via branches of the thyrocervical and costocervical trunk (Mathias et al. 1980).

In addition to atherosclerotic disease, subclavian artery obstruction may also be caused by other disease processes, such as fibromuscular dysplasia, neurofibromatosis, arteritis, radiation damage, posttraumatic scarring, and compression syndromes (thoracic outlet obstruction) (Andros et al. 1996; Hinchcliffe et al. 1995; Mathias et al. 1982; Smith et al. 1995; Tyagi et al. 1996). There are several interventional procedures available to remove stenotic lesions and normalize blood flow, such as balloon dilatation (percutaneous transluminal angioplasty, PTA), stent placement, local fibrinolysis, and thoracic sympathicolysis. Twenty years of experience with subclavian PTA has been the basis for evaluating what has become a widely used method (Bogey et al. 1994; Boer et al. 1994; Gershoney et al. 1990; Gross-Fengels et al. 1990; Harris et al. 1995; Hebrang et al. 1991; Insall et al. 1990; Kumar et al. 1995; Mathias et al. 1993; Millaire et al. 1993; Motarjeme 1996; Qi and Zeitler 1991; Romanowski et al. 1992; Selby et al. 1993; Tesdal et al. 1991; Wilms et al. 1987).

35.4.2.2
Indications

The severity of brachial insufficiency or arm claudication is graded in four stages according to the Fontaine classification of peripheral arterial occlusive disease shown in Table 35.6.

The degree of disability is directly related to the severity of ischemia and to whether the dominant hand is involved. Rest pain and gangrene may be less common manifestations. Tissue loss implies the presence of severe distal obstruction, involving the palmar arch or digital arteries, but it may also occur with multi-segmental disease and recurrent embolism.

Stages II–IV shown in Table 35.6 must be considered as indications for an interventional procedure,

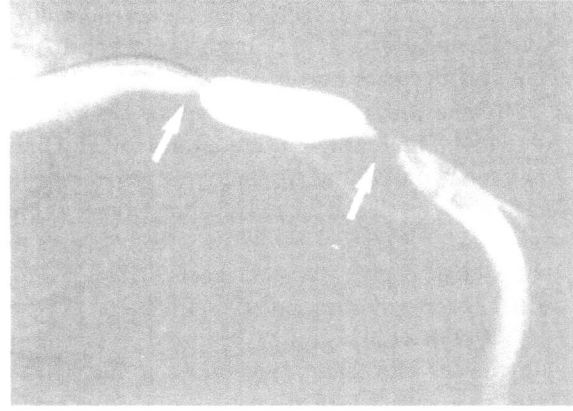

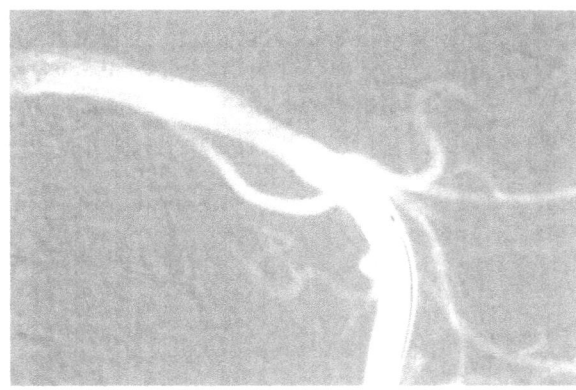

Fig. 35.28. **a** Severe tandem stenosis of the left subclavian artery (*arrows*) without opacification of the vertebral artery and poor filling of the thyrocervical and costocervical trunk. **b** Both lesions were dilated and a Wallstent was placed covering the whole first subclavian artery segment

Table 35.6. Fontaine classification of peripheral arterial occlusive disease

Stage	Symptoms
Stage I	Stenosis of the subclavian or innominate artery without symptoms, even on heavy loading of the arms
Stage II	Work-dependent, intermittent clinical symptoms such as pain, weakness, myasthenia, paresthesia, sensation of cold in combination with verifiable differences in blood pressure between both arms
Stage III	Clinical symptoms as in stage II even at rest
Stage IV	Rest pain, trophic changes in the fingers or even gangrene

but additional examinations should be carried out before any decision regarding the choice of treatment is taken. Relevant history, a thorough clinical examination, pulse status, blood pressure measurement in both arms, and Doppler sonography should be used to document the severity of the disease. In patients with vertebrobasilar insufficiency, cere-bral computerized tomography or magnetic resonance imaging for the assessment of morphological changes of the brain are recommended. To evaluate the morphology of the stenosing process, angiography and intravascular ultrasound are most helpful and should be combined with intraarterial pressure measurements.

35.4.2.3
Techniques

For PTA and stent-PTA of the subclavian and innominate arteries high resolution angiographic equipment and a broad selection of instruments is required to adequately deal with every possible situation. The following list gives an overview of typical materials necessary for the procedure:

- Seldinger puncture needle
- Introducer sheath (6–8 F)
- Guidewires: Teflon-coated, Terumo (Terumo, Frankfurt, Germany), steerable, exchange; diameters 0.018–0.035 in.
- Diagnostic catheter (5 F) with different tip configurations
- Balloon dilatation catheter (5 F) with balloon diameters from 6–10 mm and balloon length of 2–4 cm
- Stents: Easy Wallstent (Schneider, Bülach, Switzerland), Palmaz stent (Johnson & Johnson, Norderstedt, Germany).

The patient is usually under a medication of 100–300 mg aspirin and receives 3000–5000 IU of heparin immediately after cannulation of the artery. Sedative and spasmolytic drugs are not routinely used.

Principally, a femoral, axillary, or brachial approach is possible for the treatment of subclavian and innominate artery obstructions (DORROS et al. 1990; MATHIAS et al. 1993). It is sometimes helpful to use two arterial accesses simultaneously to approach the lesion from both sides. This depends on the type of lesion – stenotic or occlusive – and its location, as well as the patency of the iliac arteries. In the majority of cases, subclavian angioplasty can be accomplished by the transfemoral route. Recanalization of an occluded subclavian artery normally requires an axillary or brachial approach since the femoral route does not provide sufficient support to the catheter to penetrate the occluded artery segment (DORROS et al. 1990; DUBER et al. 1992; MATHIAS et al. 1993). Complications such as axillary hematoma and brachial plexus damage are known sequelae of this approach. Therefore, this route is restricted to patients with subclavian and innominate artery occlusions, severe tortuosity of aorta, iliac, and subclavian arteries, or bilateral occlusion of the iliac arteries.

When the subclavian artery is occluded, a faint pulse can often be palpated. In the case of a pulseless artery, puncture of the brachial or axillary artery is performed with the aid of sonographic or angiographic guidance. Following cannulation of the artery, a diagnostic angiogram is performed to show the disease process, possible additional distal axillary or brachial obstructions, and the collateral pathways. The stenosis is crossed with a steerable guidewire and then with the diagnostic catheter. Pre- and post-stenotic arterial pressures are determined and an exchange-length guidewire is placed. The angioplasty catheter is advanced over the exchange wire. We prefer a 0.020-in. steerable wire with a stiff shaft and J-curved tip. This guidewire is sufficiently stiff to maintain its position while the angioplasty catheter is advanced through the stenosis and permits pressure measurements and control angiograms "on-the-wire" with the use of a Tuohy-Borst adapter (Nycomed, Munich; Bard-Angiomed, Karlsruhe; Cook, Mönchengladbach, Germany).

In subclavian occlusions, recanalization is attempted with a 0.035-in. Terumo J-wire in combination with a multiple-purpose curved diagnostic catheter. Controlled force is often necessary to cross the occluded artery segment, particularly in cases of calcified aortic arches (KUMAR et al. 1995; MARTINEZ et al. 1997; MATHIAS et al. 1980, 1993). After successful passage of the obstruction, the balloon is placed in the lesion and is inflated until fully extended. Where possible we avoid positioning the balloon over the origin of the vertebral artery to prevent vertebral artery occlusion by shifted atherosclerotic material. The risk of permanent vertebral artery occlusion is increased in patients with ostial stenosis of the vertebral artery. In fresh thrombotic subclavian occlusions, primary stent placement can be combined with thrombolysis (AMMORI et al. 1997).

When pressure measurements and control angiograms reveal residual stenosis, stent placement is indicated. The origin of the vertebral artery should not be covered by the stent, but it is not always possible to avoid this in the case of a lesion located close to the vertebral artery orificium. We prefer the Easy Wallstent for this purpose since only a 6-F sheath is needed for the application of this stent and no guiding catheter. With a lesion located at the offspring of the subclavian artery, it is difficult to place the stent

precisely without protrusion in the aortic arch or innominate artery. In our experience, the Palmaz stent can be placed more precisely than the Easy Wallstent in these cases (LYON et al. 1996). As an alternative, the nitinol Memotherm stent (Bard-Angiomed, Karlsruhe, Germany) is also used, but has in our experience the disadvantage that its inner surface is too rough in curved arteries. We were not always able to pass the stent again with a balloon catheter even with the guidewire still in place (WERY et al. 1996). Other groups reported good results with the Strecker stent (Boston Scientific, Hilden, Germany) (KACHEL 1996).

Following angioplasty, the results are documented by an arch angiogram and a pullback pressure measurement. The sheath is removed only when the activated clotting time is not more than 20 s over the baseline value to avoid hematoma formation at the puncture site. The patient is discharged after 24 h on oral aspirin. Usually, no long-term anticoagulation is required.

35.4.2.4
Results

Several reviews have demonstrated the feasibility and efficacy of PTA of subclavian artery stenosis (BOGEY et al. 1994; BOER et al. 1994; GROSS-FENGELS et al. 1990; HEBRANG et al. 1991; INSALL et al. 1990; KACHEL et al. 1991; QI and ZEITLER 1991; ROMANOWSKI et al. 1992; TESDAL et al. 1991; WILMS et al. 1987). A technical and clinical success rate of 90% and more has been well established in small and large series. Presently, PTA of subclavian and innominate artery stenosis is a common procedure in patients with symptomatic subclavian steal syndrome (Figs. 35.29–35.31). The results of angioplasty in cases of subclavian artery occlusion are less favorable. The technical success rate varies from 40% to 90%, but technical developments and growing experience are contributing to improved success rates (DUBER et al. 1992; HARRIS et al. 1995; KUMAR et al. 1995; MARTINEZ et al. 1997; MATHIAS et al. 1993). Bilateral subclavian steal syndrome with subclavian stenosis or occlusion on both sides can be cured by stent-PTA (JÄGER et al. 1994).

Recurrent disease is observed more frequently in subclavian occlusion than in stenosis, with a primary patency rate of between 43% and 90%. Therefore, we prefer to place stents in subclavian artery occlusion routinely with few exceptions (Fig. 35.32). In subclavian artery stenosis, stents are placed after

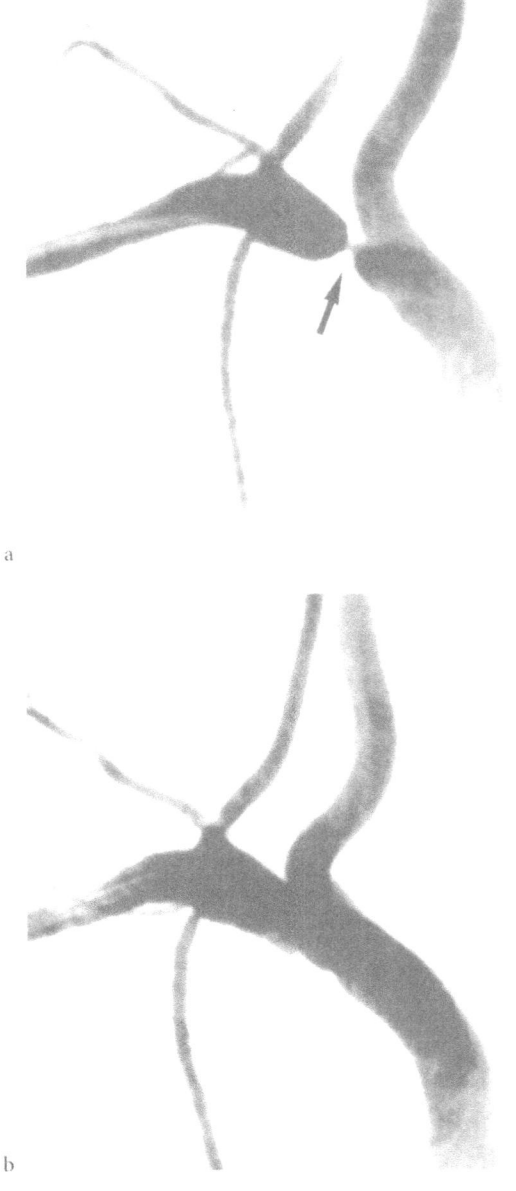

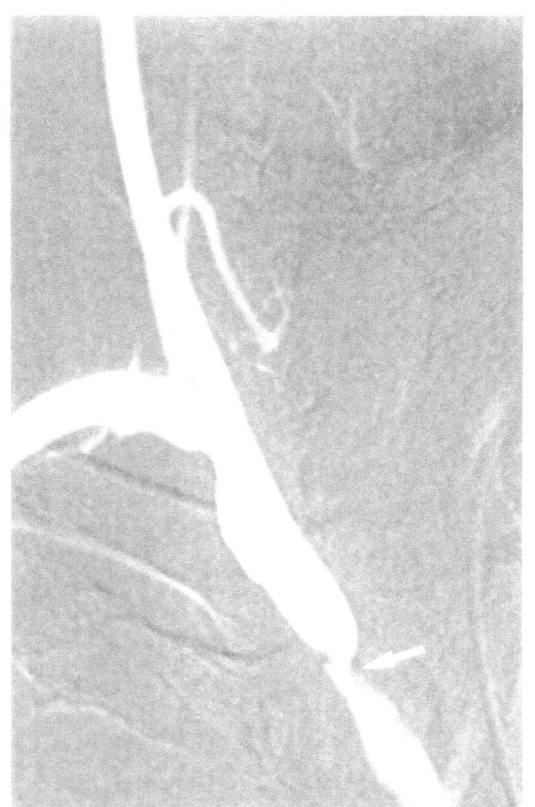

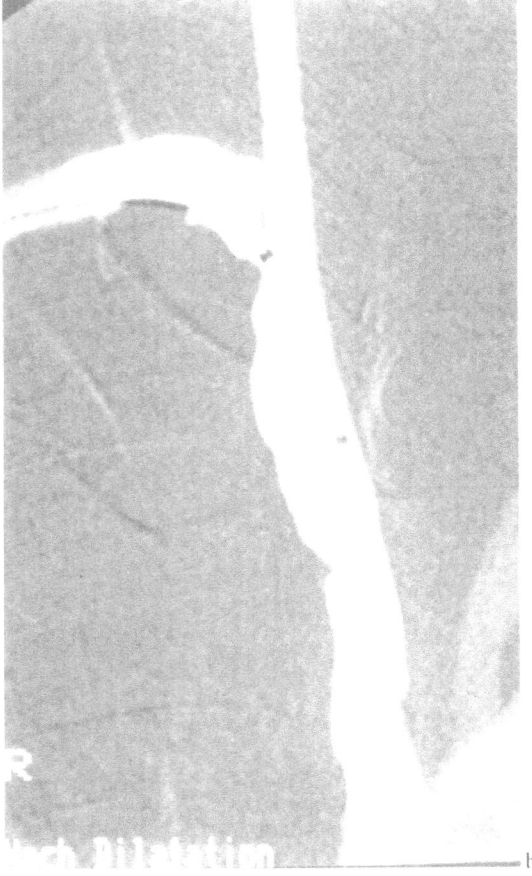

Fig. 35.29. a Stenosis of the right subclavian artery with faint opacification of the vertebral and internal thoracic arteries. An axillary approach was chosen for percutaneous transluminal angioplasty (PTA) of the lesion. **b** Nearly normal diameter of the subclavian artery after PTA with improved filling of the side branches and complete removal of the pressure gradient. For this reason, no stent was placed

Fig. 35.30. a Innominate artery stenosis (*arrow*) with a pressure gradient between both arms of 55 mmHg. **b** The control angiogram reveals some irregularity in the innominate artery, but no pressure gradient was measured after percutaneous transluminal angioplasty

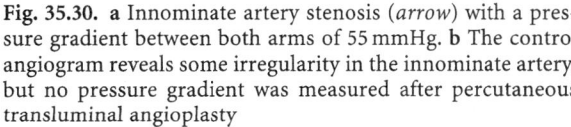

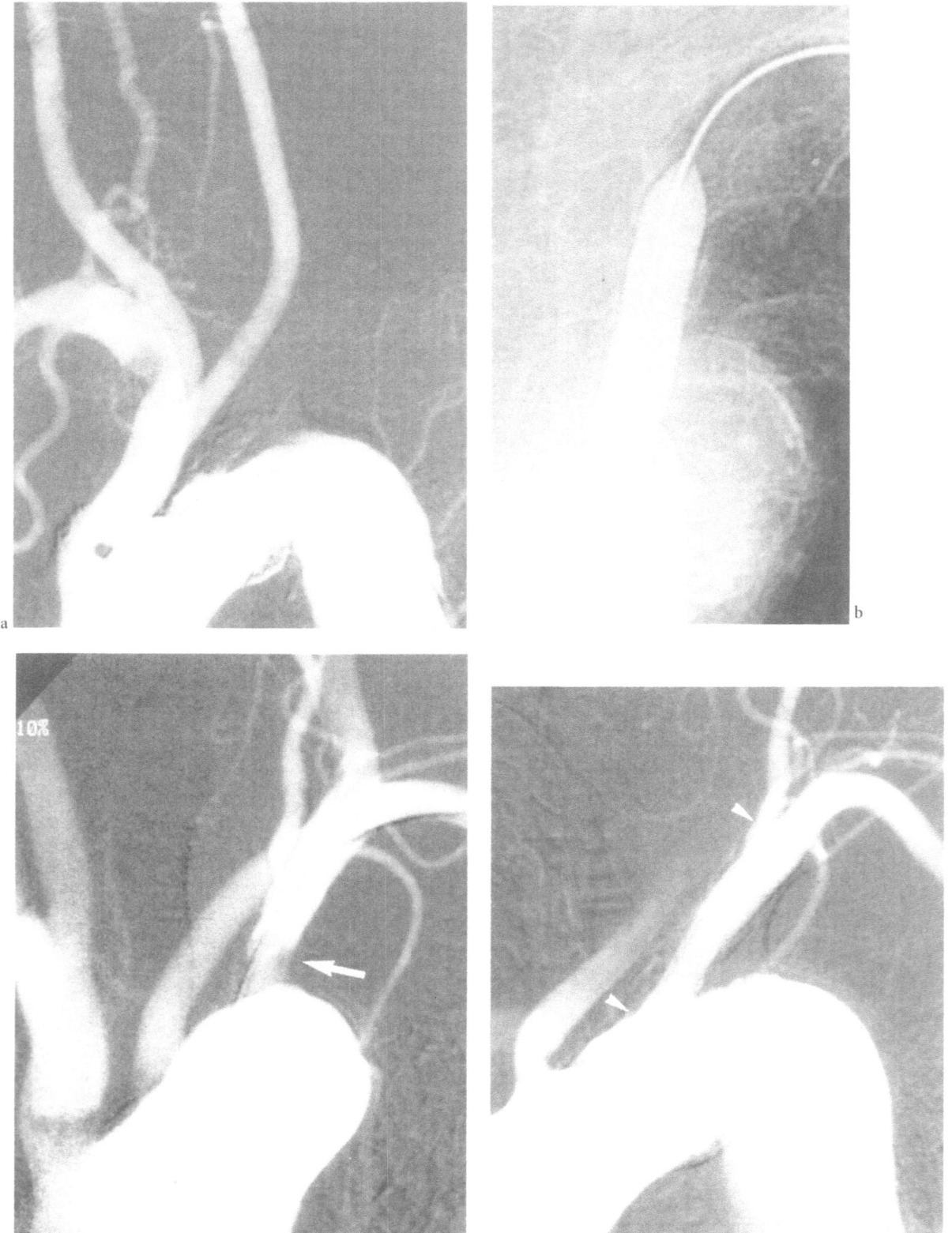

Fig. 35.31. a Left subclavian artery occlusion and calcifying aortic arch atherosclerosis. **b** Transaxillary recanalization with a second catheter in the aortic arch. **c** Significant residual stenosis at the origin of the subclavian artery after percutaneous transluminal angioplasty. **d** Improved result after placement of a Wallstent (*arrowheads*)

PTA when a residual pressure gradient >15 mmHg, intimal flaps, dissection, or intramural hematoma are found. Intravascular ultrasound examinations may be helpful to assess the morphology of the arterial wall.

The risk of vertebral artery embolization during subclavian angioplasty is minimal. This observation is based on the examinations of RINGELSTEIN and ZEUMER (1984). These authors monitored vertebral blood flow during the procedure and were able to demonstrate that the direction of blood flow in the vertebral artery does not reverse immediately. If embolism were to occur, particles would be carried with high probability into brachial arteries. To prevent embolism, various additional techniques were used by other groups with two catheters and the interruption of blood flow to the vertebral artery (CRIADO and TWENA 1996; MEMIS et al. 1997; NASIM et al. 1994). In our experience, these more sophisticated techniques are not routinely necessary.

In 416 patients with subclavian artery stenosis and 68 with subclavian artery occlusion, we attempted to remove the obstruction with PTA and stent-PTA with a primary success rate of 98.8% and 76.5%, respectively. Follow-up examinations with blood pressure measurements, Doppler ultrasound, and intravenous digital subtraction angiography established the efficacy of the procedure with a primary 5-year cumulative patency rate of 74.9% and 58.6% (Figs. 35.32, 35.33). The secondary patency rate is even higher since repeated PTA can be performed with good results and with no increased risk.

In a review of the literature on 1018 subclavian artery angioplasties, KACHEL (1996) reported a complication rate of 2.8% and a stroke incidence of 0.2%. In three of 484 procedures (0.6%), we observed transient ischemic attacks. All of these occurred in the carotid territory and were probably provoked by embolism from the aortic arch. A female patient developed a false subclavian aneurysm after successful dilatation with an 8-mm balloon. The aneurysm was treated surgically at that time. Presently, subclavian aneurysm can be treated by placing prosthetic graft stents (MAY et al. 1993). An 84-year old female suffered irreversible cardiac insufficiency 24 h after the intervention and died of multi-organ failure after 3 days. Other groups encountered complications such as thrombosis of the femoral, iliac, subclavian, and brachial arteries, dissection of the subclavian artery, embolism requiring arm amputation in one case, and temporary median nerve palsy (KACHEL 1996). The complications which we observed are listed in Table 35.7.

35.4.2.5
Perspectives

PTA and stent-PTA of the subclavian artery in patients with brachial or cerebral signs is well established. Further improvements of balloon catheters may increase the success rate of the procedure in subclavian occlusions. Desirable is a self-expanding stent with or without minimal shortening since such a device would make stent placement more precise, particularly when the stent is to be deployed close to the aortic arch or the origin of the vertebral artery. Other endeavors are directed at achieving better long-term results. Many of the attempts to prevent recurrent stenosis, such as intravascular irradiation or local gene therapy of atherosclerosis, are still at experimental stages of development.

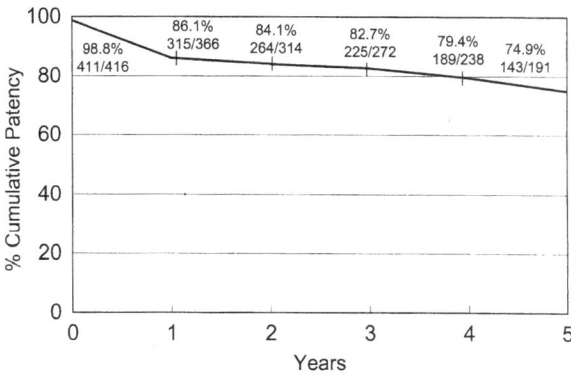

Fig. 35.32. PTA and Stent-PTA of Subclavian Artery Stenosis

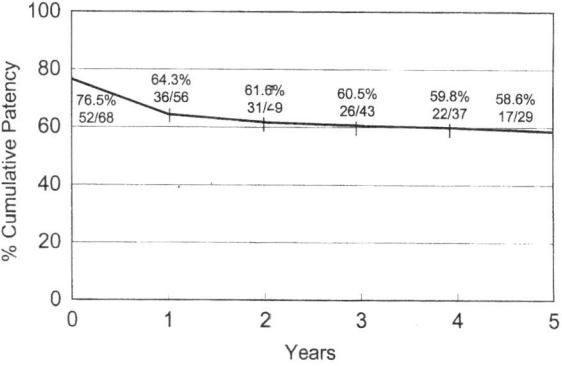

Fig. 35.33. PTA and Stent-PTA of Subclavian Artery Occlusion

Table 35.7. Complications of subclavian artery angioplasty
($n = 484$)

Type of complication	n	(%)
Transient ischemica attack	3	0.6
Digital artery embolism	4	0.8
Axillary hematoma (operative evacuation)	3	0.6
False subclavian aneurysm (operative repair)	1	0.2
Death (multi-organ failure after 24 h)	1	0.2
Total	12	2.4

References

Ammori BJ, Madan M, Chennells PM, Fowler RC, Homer-Vanniasinkam S (1997) Successful stenting of subclavian artery thrombus with intra-arterial thrombolysis. Eur J Vasc Endovasc Surg 13:217–218

Andros G, Schneider PA, Harris RW, Dulawa LB, Oblath RW, Salles-Cunha SX (1996) Management of arterial occlusive disease following radiation therapy. Cardiovasc Surg 4:135–142

Bogey WM, Demasi RJ, Tripp MD, Vithalani R, Johnsrude IS, Powell SC (1994) Percutaneous transluminal angioplasty for subclavian artery stenosis. Am Surg 60:103–106

Boer L, Carrie D, Ribal JP, Glanddier G, Viallet JF (1994) Angioplastie transluminale percutanée des artères sous-clavière, axillaire et du tronc artériel brachiocéphalique. A propos de 18 patients. Arch Mal Coeur Vaiss 87:371–378

Criado FJ, Twena M (1996) Techniques for endovascular recanalization of supra-aortic trunks. J Endovasc Surg 3:405–413

Crowe KE, Iannone LA (1993) Percutaneous transluminal angioplasty for subclavian artery stenosis in patients with subclavian steal syndrome and coronary subclavian steal syndrome. Am Heart J 126:229–233

Dorros G, Lewin RF, Jamnadas P, Mathiak LM (1990) Peripheral transluminal angioplasty of the subclavian and innominate arteries utilizing the brachial approach: acute outcome and follow-up. Cathet Cardiovasc Diagn 19:71–76

Duber C, Klose KJ, Kopp H, Schmiedt W (1992) Percutaneous transluminal angioplasty for occlusion of the subclavian artery: short- and long-term results. Cardiovasc Intervent Radiol 15:205–210

Edwards WH (1995) An unsuspected cause for recurrent angina: subclavian artery stenosis. Am Surg 61:1057–1060

Georges NP, Ferretti JA (1993) Percutaneous transluminal angioplasty of subclavian artery occlusion for treatment of coronary-subclavian steal. AJR 161:399–400

Gershony G, Basta L, Hagan AD (1990) Correction of subclavian artery stenosis by percutaneous angioplasty. Cathet Cardiovasc Diagn 21:165–169

Gross-Fengels W, Steinbrich W, Erasmi H, Neufang KF, Lanfermann H, Zanella FE (1990) Die perkutane transluminale Angioplastie (PTA) der Arteria subclavia: Technik, Ergebnisse, Risiken. Röntgenblätter. 43:203–212

Harris NJ, Cameron I, Beard JD, Gaines P (1995) Percutaneous stenting of proximal subclavian artery occlusion. Eur J Vasc Endovasc Surg 9:479–480

Hebrang A, Maskovic J, Tomac B (1991) Percutaneous transluminal angioplasty of the subclavian arteries: long-term results in 52 patients. AJR 156:1091–1094

Hinchcliffe M, Ruttley MS, Carolan-Rees G (1995) Case report: percutaneous transluminal angioplasty of irradiation induced bilateral subclavian artery occlusions. Clin Radiol 50:804–807

Insall RL, Lambert D, Chamberlain J, Proud G, Murthy LN, Loose HW (1990) Percutaneous transluminal angioplasty of the innominate, subclavian, and axillary arteries. Eur J Vasc Surg 4:591–595

Jäger HJ, Mathias KD, Kempkes (1994) Bilateral subclavian steal syndrome: treatment with percutaneous transluminal angioplasty and stent placement. Cardiovasc Intervent Radiol 17:328–332

Kachel R, Basche S, Heerklotz I, Grossmann K, Endler S (1991) Percutaneous transluminal angioplasty (PTA) of supra-aortic arteries especially the internal carotid artery. Neuroradiology 33:191–194

Kachel R (1996) Subclavian arteries and veins. In: Handbook of cardiovascular interventions. Ed: U Sigwart, M Bertrand, PW Serruys; Churchill Livinstone, New York, p 855–869

Kugelmass AD, Kim D, Kuntz RE, Carrozza JP Jr, Baim DS (1994) Endoluminal stenting of a subclavian artery stenosis to treat ischemia in the distribution of a patent left internal mammary graft. Cathet Cardiovasc Diagn 33:175–177

Kumar K, Dorros G, Bates MC, Palmer L, Mathiak L, Dufek C (1995) Primary stent deployment in occlusive subclavian artery disease. Cathet Cardiovasc Diagn 34:281–285

Lyon RD, Shonnard KM, McCarter DL, Hammond SL, Ferguson D, Rholl KS (1996) Supra-aortic arterial stenoses: management with Palmaz balloon-expandable intraluminal stents. J Vasc Interv Radiol 7:825–835

Marques KM, Ernst SM, Mast EG, Bal ET, Suttorp MJ, Plokker HW (1996) Percutaneous transluminal angioplasty of the left subclavian artery to prevent or treat the coronary-subclavian steal syndrome. J Cardiol 78:687–690

Martinez R, Rodriguez-Lopez J, Torruella L, Ray L, Lopez-Galarza L, Diethrich EB (1997) Stenting for occlusion of the subclavian arteries. Technical aspects and follow-up results. Tex Heart Inst J 24:23–27

Mathias K, Schlosser V, Reinke M (1980) Katheterrekanalisation eines Subklaviaverschlusses. RöFo 132:346–347

Mathias K, Heiss HW, Gospos C (1982) Subclavian-Steal-Syndrom – operieren oder dilatieren? Langenbecks Arch Chir 356:279–283

Mathias KD, Luth I, Haarmann P (1993) Percutaneous transluminal angioplasty of proximal subclavian artery occlusions. Cardiovasc Intervent Radiol 16:214–218

May J, White G, Waugh R, Yu W, Harris J (1993) Transluminal placement of a prosthetic graft-stent device for treatment of subclavian artery aneurysm. J Vasc Surg 18:1056–1059

Memis A, Oran I, Ozbek SS (1997) A simple method to avoid vertebral artery embolism during subclavian percutaneous transluminal angioplasty: provocative maneuver [letter]. AJR 168:569–570

Millaire A, Trinca M, Marache P, de Groote P, Jabinet JL, Ducloux G (1993) Subclavian angioplasty: immediate and late results in 50 patients. Cathet Cardiovasc Diagn 29:8–17

Motarjeme A (1996) Percutaneous transluminal angioplasty of supra-aortic vessels. J Endovasc Surg 3:171–181

Mufti SI, Young KR, Schulthesis T (1994) Restenosis following subclavian artery angioplasty for treatment of coronary-subclavian steal syndrome: definitive treatment with Palmaz-stent placement. Cathet Cardiovasc Diagn 33:172–174

Nasim A, Sayers RD, Bell PR, Bolia A (1994) Protection against vertebral artery embolization during proximal subclavian artery angioplasty. Eur J Vasc Surg 8:362–363

Perrault LP, Carrier M, Hudon G, Lemarbre L, Hebert Y, Pelletier LC (1993) Transluminal angioplasty of the subclavian artery in patients with internal mammary grafts. Ann Thorac Surg 56:927–930

Qi JP, Zeitler E (1991) Katheterdilatation der arteriellen Stenosen supraaortaler Gefässe und Spätergebnisse. Röfo 155:357–362

Reivich M, Holling HE, Roberts B, Toole JT (1961) Reversal of blood flow through the vertebral artery and its effect on cerebral circulation. N Engl J Med 265:878–885

Ringelstein EB, Zeumer H (1984) Delayed reversal of vertebral artery flow following percutaneous transluminal angioplasty for subclavian steal. Neuroradiology 26:189–198

Romanowski CA, Fairlie NC, Procter AE, Cumberland DC (1992) Percutaneous transluminal angioplasty of the subclavian and axillary arteries: initial results and long term follow-up. Clin Radiol 46:104–107

Selby JB Jr, Matsumoto AH, Tegtmeyer CJ, Hartwell GD, Tribble CG, Daniel TM, Kron IL (1993) Balloon angioplasty above the aortic arch: immediate and long-term results. AJR 160:631–635

Smith TP, Halbach VV, Fraser KW, Teitelbaum GP, Dowd CF, Higashida RT (1995) Percutaneous transluminal angioplasty of subclavian stenosis from neurofibromatosis. AJNR 16(4 Suppl): 372–874

Tesdal IK, Jaschke W, Haueisen H, Menges HW, Hoffmeister AW, Huck K, Menges V, Georgi M (1991) Perkutane transluminale Angioplastie (PTA) der armversorgenden Arterien bei brachialer und zerebraler Ischamie. Röfo 155:363–369

Tyagi S, Gambhir DS, Kaul UA, Verma P, Arora R (1996) A decade of subclavian angioplasty: aortoarteritis versus atherosclerosis. Indian Heart J 48:667–671

Wery D, Dussaussois L, Golzarian J, Tack D, Delcour C, Struyven J (1996) Mise en place de la prothèse en Nitinol Memotherm: notre expérience. J Belge Radiol 79:223–226

Wilms G, Baert A, Dewaele D, Vermmylen J, Nevelsteen A, Suy R (1987) Percutaenous transluminal angioplasty of the subclavian artery: Early and late results. Cardiovasc intervent Radiol 10:123–128

36 Radio-ulnar and Hand Artery Diseases

H. Berger and P. Pickel

36.1
Normal Anatomy: Variations

36.1.1
Arteriography: Examination Technique

Since digital subtraction angiography (DSA) with intraarterial injection of contrast media is clinically standard, small amounts of contrast agents are sufficient for entire vascular visualization. Contrast material can be injected by direct vessel puncture with small cannulas (20–22G). A two-component needle with an inner metal cannula and a thin-walled plastic covering, which can be advanced coaxially to achieve a stable endovascular position, is the preferred needle type.

36.1.1.1
Percutaneous Needle Angiography

Both the axillary and brachial arteries are commonly used for percutaneous needle puncture since at this location the vessels are most regularly palpable.

H. Berger, MD, Professor, P. Pickel, MD, Institut für Röntgendiagnostik der Technischen Universität München, Klinikum rechts der Isar, Ismaninger Str. 22, D-81675 München, Germany

Axillary Access. The artery is located by palpation in the axilla with the arm abducted. A retrograde puncture is made and a stable position of the needle secured. The arm is then exposed to the X-ray unit for angiography and the contrast medium injected by hand with a flow rate of 4–6 cc/s.

Brachial Access. The brachial artery is commonly punctured just above the elbow, where it is located superficially and is easily accessible. The brachial artery is more liable to local spasm than the axiallary artery and, therefore, careful puncture technique using small-needle cannulas is advisable. Hand injection of contrast medium is sufficient for optimal visualization.

36.1.1.2
Catheter Techniques for Angiography

Transfemoral Access. The transfemoral route is the most common access for catheter angiography of the upper extremities. If the entire vessel from the origin at the aortic arch to the hand needs to be examined, this type of angiography provides the most reliable information. Pre-shaped catheters (4–5 F), such as the head-hunter configuration, are used for selective catheterization. The catheters are negotiated with the use of appropriate guidewires. The catheter tip can be sited at a level appropriate to the particular examination. For more selective catheter positions, coaxial catheter systems with 2–3 F outer diameter are available.

Transaxillary Access. This approach is less commonly used since the catheter can be passed retrogradely towards the aortic arch only. In some cases, however, for example obstruction of the subclavian artery, this technique can be useful.

Any angiographic technique used for arm or hand arteriography needs to take anatomic variations of the arm/hand arterial supply into consideration. Due to the small caliber of the punctured vessel, vasospasm induced by the catheter tip or the puncture itself should to be kept in mind in the interpretation of pathologic morphology. A liberal use of pharmacoangiography can be recommended to overcome this problems in arm/hand arteriography.

36.1.2
Normal Anatomy

36.1.2.1
Normal Anatomy: Arm

The left subclavian artery arises directly from the aortic arch and passes upward in the thorax, where it leaves the intrathoracic space and continues to the axillary artery. The right subclavian artery arises from the innominate artery and follows a similar course on the right side.

The axillary artery is the direct continuation of the subclavian artery; it begins at the outer border of the first rib and becomes the brachial artery behind the teres major muscle.

The radial and ulnar arteries are the terminal branches of the brachial artery, originating in the cubital fossa opposite the neck of the radius. The radial artery is the smaller vessel with muscular side branches and the radial recurrent artery. It ends in the palm of the hand by anastomosing with the deep branch of the ulnar artery to form the deep palmar arch. Before ending in the palmar arch, it gives off the posterior carpal arch and the princeps pollicis artery.

The ulnar artery as the dominant artery at the origin, gives off the ulnar recurrent arteries, the anterior and posterior interosseous artery, and muscular branches, before terminating with the anastomoses to the radial artery in the superficial and deep palmar arches.

Variations of the brachial artery are rare. The axillary artery can divide into the radial and ulnar arteries in the axillary fossa or, more commonly, the forearm arteries arise from a high bifurcation of the brachial artery in the upper arm. Either the radial or the ulnar artery may be absent and then replaced by branches of the remaining artery or by the interosseous artery. All these variations are of some importance for angiographic techniques using direct puncture of the axillary of brachial artery.

36.1.2.2
Normal Anatomy: Hand

In most cases, the digital arteries follow a standard pattern; however, there is a considerable variation in the distribution of the hand arteries (HÜRING 1974).

The deep palmar arch is formed primarily by the terminal portion of the radial artery after supplying the princeps pollicis artery. A complete deep arch is found in approximately 95% of cases; either the superficial arch or the deep palmar arch may be absent, however. The arch gives rise to palmar metacarpal arteries that frequently anastomose with the common palmar digital arteries from the superficial arch.

The superficial palmar arch is usually the more prominent and distal of the two palmar arches. It is anatomically complete in approximately 80% of cases; in approximately 50% the anastomosis with the very small superficial branch of the radial artery is angiographically visualized only with the compression angiotechnique (Fig. 36.1). The superficial arch is typically the terminal branch of

Table 36.1. Causes of radio-ulnar and hand artery diseases

Arterial disease
Atherosclerosis, thromboangiitis obliterans, angiodysplasia

Collagen disease
Scleroderma, rheumatoid arthritis, periarteritis nodosa, Wegener's granulomatosis, lupus erythematosus, giant cell arteritis, mixed connective tissue disease, dermatomyositis

Hematologic disease
Polycythemia, cold agglutinins

Arterial embolic and thrombotic disease
Cardiac disease, septicemia, heparin-induced thrombocytopenia

Compression syndromes
Thoracic-outlet syndrome, pectoralis minor syndrome, neoplastic disease

Traumatic disease
Vascular trauma, burns, hypothenar hammer syndrome

Toxic disease
Heavy metal, polyvinyl chloride

Medication-induced disease
B-blocker, sympathomimetics, oral contraceptives, cytostatic agents, secale alkaloids, salazosulfapyridine

Miscellaneous
Intravenous drug use, paraneoplastic syndromes, Sudeck's dystrophy, chronic renal failure, chronic hepatic disease, hypothyroidism, diabetes mellitus

Fig. 36.1. Compression angiography demonstrating regular vascular anatomy with closed arch (*left*) and impairment of acral perfusion in case of obstruction or interruption of the arch (*right*)

the ulnar artery. The common palmar digital arteries arise from the convex side of the superficial palmar arch. Each of the palmar digital arteries is joined before it divides by a palmar metacarpal branch of the deep palmar arch. The posterior carpal arch on the back of the carpus is formed by the union of the posterior carpal branches of the radial and ulnar arteries. It gives off the dorsal metacarpal arteries.

36.2
Functional Artery Diseases

36.2.1
Vasospasm

Hand and finger arteries serve as a thermal regulatory organ. Arterial blood flow exhibits cyclical increases and decreases, which are determined by environmental temperature. This thermoregulatory flow is modulated by arteriovenous anastomoses and contributes to body temperature control. Nutritional blood flow, which is provided by capillaries, maintains tissue viability. Modulation of acro-blood flow is determined by sympatic innervation of the blood vessels, regulated by norepinephrine release at the myoneural junction in the vessel wall. Smooth muscles of the arterial wall control this vasomotoric mechanism and reflect the individual sympatic tone (Fig. 36.2) (EBERT et al. 1995).

In its typical form, drug-induced arterial ischemia presents as long segmental vasospasm rather than short segmental vasomotoric changes. Major locations besides the femoropopliteal arteries are brachial and forearm vessels, including hand

arteries. For differentiation of organic lesions, both an anamnestic history of medication with specific drugs and the reversibility of symptoms of the vasospastic changes are diagnostic key points. In its clinically most severe course, vasospastic segments occlude completely, causing arteriosclerotic-like ischemic tissue alterations. Drugs which are known to alter vasomotoric tone are numerous. It is not uncommon to observe vasospasm during angio-graphy induced by angiographic catheters or contrast agents. Antibiotics such as penicillin, coffee ergotamine, and methysergide are reported to induce vasospasm (MILLER and MORGAN 1993).

Early angiographic signs include a diffuse pattern of long segmental stenosis, smooth wall structures without irregularities, and a completely normal aspect of unaffected vessels. Thrombotic segmental occlusions develop in chronically affected vessels.

To differentiate functional disorders from organic vessel obstructions, several tests can be performed. Most effective in the differentiation of both entities is the use of vasoactive drugs applied orally, intravenously, or intraarterially during angiography (HÄNSGEN et al. 1990).

Sympathic nerve interruption decreases the release of norepinephrine at the myoneural junction. Both total flow and nutritional flow increase, resulting in a significant temperature elevation and augmented tissue perfusion (KOMAN et al. 1995). Quantitative Doppler laser flow and temperature measurements pre- and postoperatively assessed in patients with peripheral sympathectomy prove this regulatory mechanism. Color Doppler flow sonography of digital arteries has demonstrated increases in vessel diameter, cross section area, and a significant rise in blood flow velocity after axillary brachial plexus block in patients without organic arterial disease.

36.2.2
Raynaud's Disease

Raynaud's phenomenon is a pathological vasomotor reaction of the digital vasculature, the etiology of which is still unclear. Altered vasomotoric tone, increased blood viscosity, and adrenergic dysfunction have been described in association with Raynaud's phenomenon. Drugs may additionally predispose a patient to this kind of vasospasm. Most patients with Raynaud's phenomenon present clinically with paresthesia, pain, and white discoloration of one or several fingers. Exposure to cold or

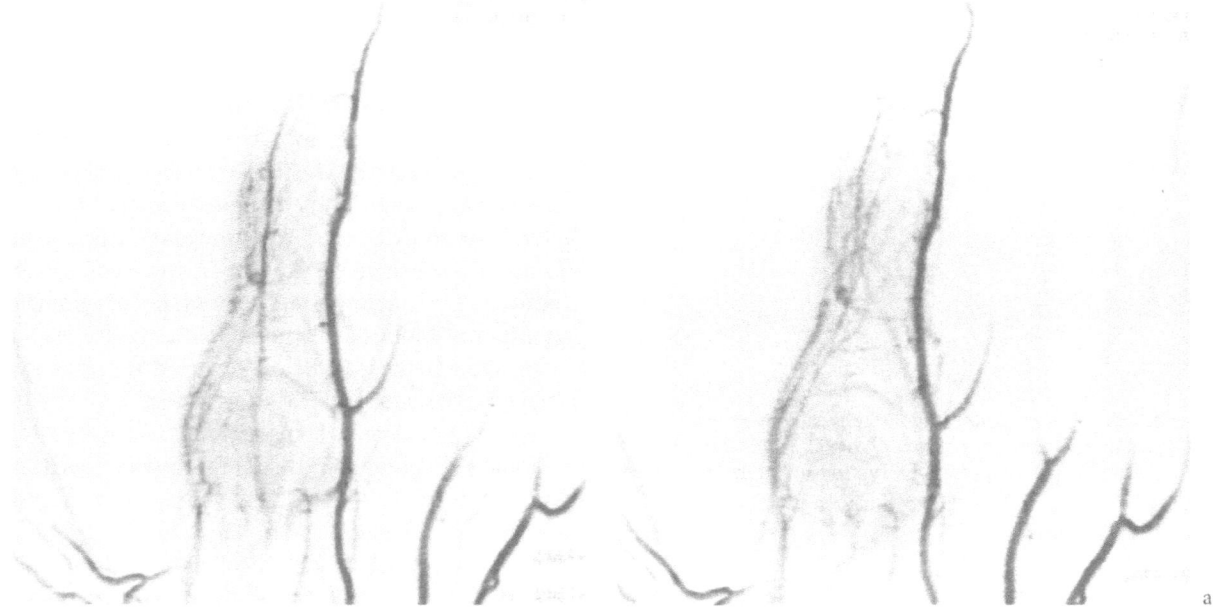

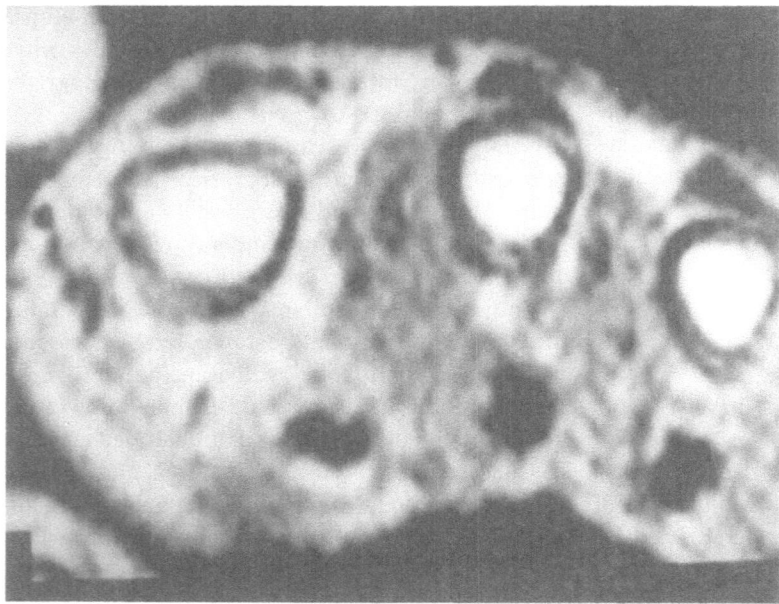

Fig. 36.2. A 32-year-old female patient with histologically proven capillary arteriovenous malformation at the base of D2. **a** Angiography shows severe vasospasm of the digital arteries with the exception of the supplying digital artery of the malformation. **b** Diffuse contrast enhancement of the vascular malformation at D2 in angiography and diffuse paraosseous growth pattern on Magnetic resonance imaging

emotional stress are the typical triggers for this disorder.

Raynaud's disease is a term frequently applied to the condition in which there is no underlying disorder associated with Raynaud's phenomenon, the so-called primary Raynaud's phenomenon. When associated with a systemic disorder, these abnormal vasomotoric changes may be referred to as so-called secondary Raynaud's phenomenon.

Raynaud's phenomenon may cause digital alterations or, in its most severe form, tissue necrosis. Connective tissue disease may progress to oblitera-

tive and thrombotic arteriopathy. The mechanism of this arteriopathy is unclear – thrombosis and inflammation are not suspected of playing a major role initially; these changes are secondary to the underlying vasospastic reaction (MILLER and MORGAN 1993).

It has been demonstrated in clinical investigations that nitroglycerine significantly increases the pressure of finger arteries in patients with Raynaud's phenomenon I and slightly less in patients with Raynaud's phenomenon II, whereas patients with organic arterial obliterations or healthy subjects show no statistically significant changes (vasoactive drugs: nitroglycerine, phentolamine, nifedipine) (HÄNSGEN et al. 1990).

36.2.3
Cold Injuries

Exposure to the cold leads to vasospastic stenosis of digital arteries, which can result in ischemic alterations of the skin, muscles, and nerves. Several acral cold injuries may cause permanent dysregulation of the peripheral circulation due to alteration of neurovegetative autoregulation. Secondary phenomena include dys- and paresthesia, hyperhidrosis and acrocyanosis. Clinical presentation includes four stages: (1) skin erythema and edema, (2) additional blisters, (3) superficial tissue loss accompanied by severe pain, (4) tissue necrosis, ulceration.

Angiographic signs are not specific and reflect the stage of injury. The indication for angiographic examination is restricted to therapeutic requirements and needs specific regional analgesia or intraarterial pharmacoangiography (JONES 1991).

36.3
Obliterative Arterial Disease

Obliterative arterial disease of the hands presents a diagnostic challenge even to the experienced diagnostician. Acral and cutaneous vascular regions may often be the end or indicator organs of systemic disease. Perfusion disorders appearing as functional may be early symptoms of segmental vascular lesions. Vascular morphology, as shown angiographically (Fig. 36.3), may permit further classification and facilitate categorization of disease entities (BAUER et al. 1990).

36.3.1
Peripheral Obliterative Vascular Disease-
Arteriosclerosis

Obliterative atherosclerosis develops in relation to concomitant cardiovascular risk factors. The disease occurs only infrequently distal to the axillary artery and, if it does, it goes along with distinct elongation and tortuosity of vessels increasing from the forearm to the acral region. Arteries of the hands and fingers may show a meandering pattern. Occlusions are irregularly distributed and usually found only in

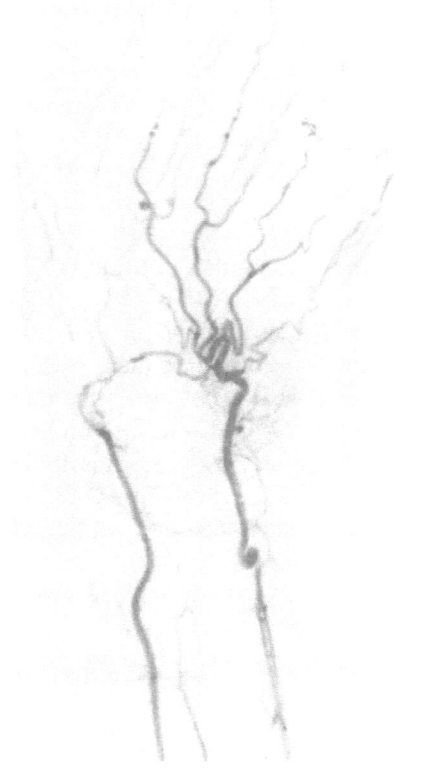

a

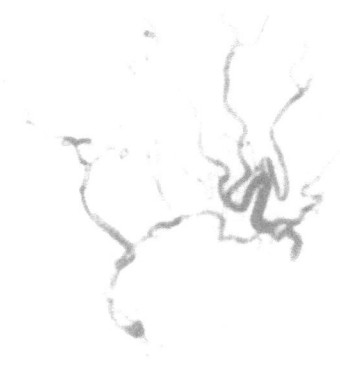

b

Fig. 36.3. A 60-year-old male patient with chronically progressiv ischemia of D1 and D2. No evident risk factors of cardiovascular disease. Angiography reveals diffuse irregularities in the radial segment of the superficial palmar arch and regular vasculature on the ulnar segment of the arch. Rarification of digital perfusion D1 and D2. Early (**a**) and late (**b**) angiographic phase. Histology: intimal hyperplasia, thrombotic occlusions

patients older than 55 years. Involved arteries are the common palmar digital and proper palmar digital arteries. A well developed collateral vascular system is specific for this entity, as are atherosclerotic plaques and intimal changes.

36.3.2
Buerger's Thromboangiitis obliterans

This disease was first discussed in 1908 by Buerger and predominates in young men with nicotine abuse. In recent years, however, the number of female patients suffering from this condition is on the rise. Peripheral arteries are primarily involved. Histopathologic findings vary with the different stages. The early stage presents with a fibrinoid edema of the intima with leukocyte reaction. Consecutively, recurrent thromboses with vessel stenoses or occlusion occur, as well as formation of atherosclerotic plaques. Distal to the plaques, intimal proliferation is found.

Initially, angiography reveals high grade spasm of the main vessels; the hand is perfused via interosseous arteries. The application of vasodilatory agents usually results in the depiction of the radial and ulnar artery with a straight course to the hand. In the early stage, functional impairment with filiform stenoses of the carpal and digital arteries predominates. After vasodilatation, the enhancement of peripheral vessels is slightly delayed, indicating early vessel wall alterations. In the consecutive stages, increasing morphologic changes of the vessels become evident. These are no longer amenable to pharmacologic influence and appear as segmental stenoses and occlusions. In an intermediate stage, the caliber changes and filiform stenoses are localized in the middle and end phalanges. Orthograde vessel run-off is typical. The radial side of the second ray and the ulnar side of the fifth ray are involved in 80% of cases. The more advanced stages present with extensive occlusion in the metacarpus and involvement of the distal regions of the forearm arteries. The ulnar artery is involved predominantly with medium to high grade stenoses. Collateral vessels with a corkscrew appearance, segmental stenoses, and unusual courses are encountered. These classical features of thromboangiitis obliterans may occur in combination with increased tonus of the proximal arteries, smooth contours, corkscrew-like collaterals, and segmental occlusions.

36.3.3
Collagen Diseases

Typical vessel changes associated with collagenoses are intimal proliferations with luminal stenoses, as well as fibroblastic reactions. They may already be detected angiographically in early-stage disease; however, only systemic sclerosis and rheumatoid arthritis present with angiomorphologically unequivocal findings. All other entities show segmental obliteration of the finger arteries with different degrees of vasospasm without pathognomonic patterns.

36.3.3.1
Scleroderma

The incidence of Raynaud's phenomenon in progressive systemic sclerosis is noted at between 35%–100% according to the stage of disease. In late stages, vascular involvement of the hand is present almost invariably.

Histopathologically, vascular stenoses or occlusions are due to acellular intimal hypertrophy and fibrosis with subendothelial edema, edema and focal media fibrosis, as well as sclerosis and hyalinosis of the adventitial tissue.

In the early stage, the vasospastic component is the leading angiographic feature. In more advanced stages, the irregular or anarchic vascular pattern with multiple segmental stenoses and occlusions is pathognomonic. There is only a minor tendency to form collaterals. A vasospastic component is always present and well manageable with pharmacologic agents.

36.3.3.2
Rheumathoid Arthritis

Initially, the vasospastic component predominates, like in all other collagenoses. In advanced stages of the disease, however, in addition to multiple segmental vessel occlusions, areas of hypervascularization may be found adjacent to affected joints. These hypervascularized areas are the hallmark of rheumatoid arthritis. Usually, the lesions are well collateralized; in patients with digital occlusions, perfusion is achieved via acral vessels or the arcuate artery.

36.3.4
Others

The Hypothenar Hammer Syndrome. Occlusions of the ulnar artery due to trauma are well known and were first described by ROSEN in 1934. Usually, these lesions are preceded by chronic vibration trauma due to occupational or athletic exposure. Intimal lesions of the ulnar artery occur in the region of the hamulus ossis hamati or between the volar and transverse carpal ligament. Angiographically, these lesions or occlusions of the distal ulnar artery, the superficial palmar arch, and the third to fifth fingers may be found. Chronic vibration trauma may also lead to the development of ulnar artery aneurysms (VAYSSAIRAT and DEBURE 1987).

Other entities of radio-ulnar and hand artery disease may result from vasospastic as well as morphologic vascular changes without specific angiographic features, which might provide a clue in differential diagnosis.

36.3.5
Heparin-Induced Coagulopathy

Thrombocytopenia may occur during or following heparin therapy. Two different types of heparin-induced coagulopathy (HIT) have been characterized. The literature points to an overall incidence of between 1%-35% among patients treated with heparin. The more infrequent type (1.5%-5%) leads to additional thromboembolic complications in 50%-80% of patients, predominantly in the venous system, but also in major arm arteries (WARKETIN et al. 1995).

References

Bauer T, Rauber K, Rau WS (1990) Differential diagnosis of acral disturbances of blood flow by means of intra-arterial DSA of the hand. RöFo Fortschr Rontgenstr

Ebert B, Braunschweig R, Reik P (1995) Use of colour Doppler sonography for quantitation of the changes in the blood flow following axillary plexus block. Anaesthesist 44:859–862

Hänsgen K, Podhaisky H, Sternitzky R, Preup E-G (1990) Einfluß von Glyceriltrinitrat auf den Fingerarteriendruck. Z Gesamte Inn Med 45:422–424

Jones NF (1991) Acute and chronic ischemia of the hand: pathophysiology, treatment and diagnosis. J Hand Surg 16:1074–1083

Kadir S, Brothers MF (1991) Atlas of normal and variant angiographic anatomy. W.B. Saunders Philadelphia

Koman LA, Smith BP, Pollock FE, Smith TL, Pollock D, Russel GB (1995) The microcirculatory effects of peripheral sympathectomy. J Hand Surg 20:709–717

Loring LA, Hallisey MJ (1995) Arteriography and interventional therapy for diseases of the hand. Radiographics 15:1299

Miller LM, Morgan RF (1993) Vasospastic disorders: etiology, reconstruction and treatment. Hand Clin 9:171–187

Rosen S (1934) Ein Fall von Thrombose in der Arteria ulnaris nach Einwirkung von stumpfer Gewalt. Acta Chir Scand 73:500–506

Vayssairat M, Debure C (1987) Hypothenar hammer syndrome: seventeen cases with long-term follow up. J Vasc Surg 5:838–843

Warketin TE, Levine MN, Hirsch J, Horsewood P (1995) Heparin-induced thrombocytopenia in patients treated with low-molecular heparin or unfractionated heparin. New Engl J Med 332:1330–1335

Venous Diseases

37 Acute Deep Vein Thrombosis

E.-I. RICHTER

CONTENTS

Diagnosis of acute phlebothrombosis without imaging procedures is uncertain. Only in 40% of all cases a clear and accurate diagnosis can be made on the basis of symptoms such as edema, tension pain, and palpable resistance, in addition to other uncharacteristic symptoms which often do not appear at first (MÜLLER 1994; RICHTER and ZEITLER 1980; SPENGEL 1992). This applies in particular to patients confined to bed because of a general medical illness, after an operation, and after childbirth, or to patients lacking general physical exercise. Often only the much-feared complication of pulmonary embolism points to the existence of deep vein thrombosis of the leg. At this stage, 80 of 100 affected patients die within the first 2 h (SCHWING 1994a).

After high-risk operations or during an operation, an acute thrombosis of the lower limbs may develop in 40% of all cases; this means that especially these patients are in danger of incurring pulmonary embolism. The lethality of thromboembolic incidents is indicated to be 7.3/100 000 (SCHUBERT et al. 1992).

The early stage is characterized by a slight cyanotic skin discoloration, as well as hardened, strained muscles. The subfascial edema is palpable in the form of resistance. Additionally, the pulse rate is accelerated (RABE 1993).

If acute thrombosis afflicts a mobile patient while he is still straining, the ensuing disorder of venous flow will lead very quickly to the classical local symptoms with phlebostasis, cyanosis, and the so-called bursting pain in the area of venous drainage.

Most frequently thromboses develop in the lower limbs, the danger of embolism being less with varicothromboses of the superficial veins (MOSER and LE MOINE 1981) (Fig. 37.1).

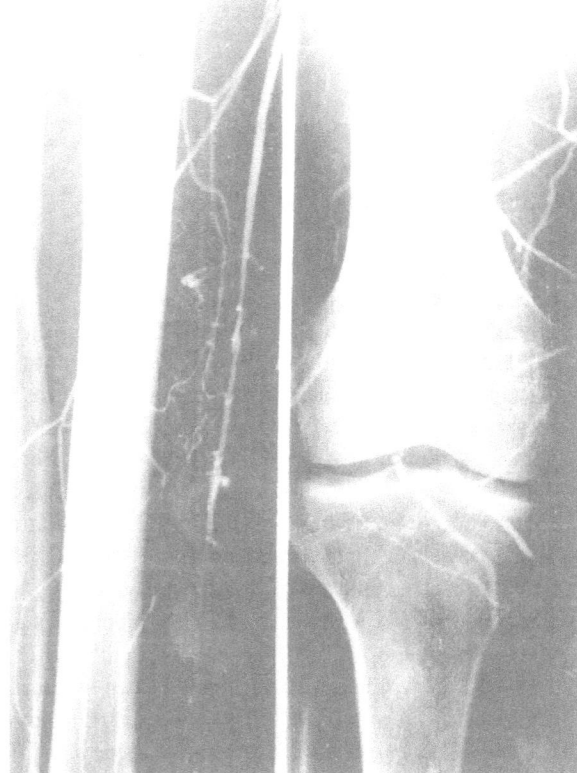

Fig. 37.1. A complete acute deep venous thrombosis of the right leg, with total filling defect of the veins of the lower and upper leg. There is hardly any collateral circulation

E.-I. RICHTER, MD, KH-RD Klinikum Nürnberg Nord, Flurstrasse 17, D-90340 Nuremberg, Germany

37.1
Procedures at Acute Phlebothrombosis

The slightest suspicion of a fresh deep thrombosis demands an immediate examination. In terms of diagnostics, acute phlebothrombosis in the pelvic and lower limb areas stands out because patients are gravely ill and confined to bed. Their weight-bearing capacity is very limited. Often, strict management of ascending phlebography cannot be carried out; for instance, it is impossible to lay a patient in a 60-degree oblique position with hanging lower extremities. Rather he will be laid almost flat on the examination table.

If there is a strong stasis edema, there is no need for a supramalleolar tourniquet, which would otherwise be vital. Puncture should be carried out at a dorsal vein of the foot. A Butterfly needle (21-G) or a Venofix may be used. The perfusory line connected to these instruments as an extension serves for better application and ensures sufficient distance from the X-rays. With a ready-made syringe one can measure out the dose and carefully apply the contrast medium (CM) with manual pressure. With consideration to the general state of the patient, the examination should be carried out as swiftly as possible.

37.1.1
Pelvic Veins and the Inferior Vena Cava

Visualization of the pelvic veins can be achieved by ascending leg phlebography, and possibly also using the digital subtraction angiography (DSA) technique when injecting CM into the dorsal vein of the foot. A good picture can be attained when, in the veins of the lower extremities, not all vascular layers are thrombosed and the thrombus is not located directly at the level of the common femoral vein. Such a situation would demand a percutaneous direct puncture of that vessel on the opposite side under local anesthesia (ZEITLER 1979). In order to visualize the infrarenal inferior vena cava, the CM injection is applied with the help of a 5-F or 6-F short catheter (11-cm dilatator) which is also connected to an extension line (150-cm perfusory tube). If the infrarenal inferior vena cava is free of a thrombus at the level of the caudal inflow, cross-over catheterization of the common iliac vein should be carried out in order to do a retrograde angiography of the contralateral pelvic veins.

Under the condition of undisturbed perfusion in the inguinal veins there is the possibility of bilateral percutaneous puncture of the common femoral vein in local anesthesia. The examination can be carried out as a needle phlebograpy or as a short catheter phlebography. The CM is applied on both sides with the help of a connecting line (maximum 4 bar), joined to a Y-connector. For this procedure the digital technique is ideal; futhermore, it economizes on CM (Fig. 37.2).

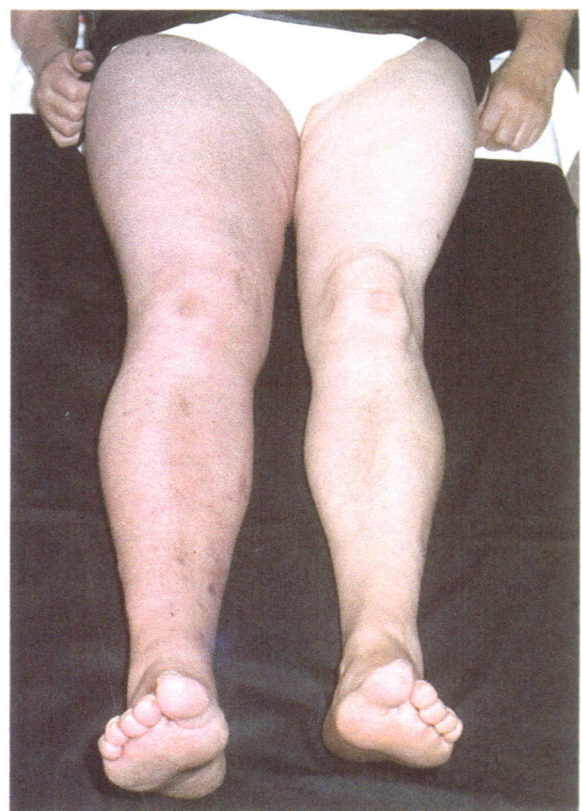

Fig. 37.2. Livid discoloration of the right lower extremity of a 68-year-old woman with concomitant pelvic venous thrombosis

37.2
Phlebographic Diagnostics

The aim of phlebography is to furnish positive proof of thrombi. They can be identified phlebographically by a filling defect after application of CM. The approximate but not exact filling defect does not yield sufficient information to justify the launching of invasive therapy. The whole extremity from foot to the inferior vena cava must be documented in sections. The state of venous drainage from both pelvic sides into the inferior vena cava should be depicted with regard to operative therapy. If the findings are clear and positive, one level is enough. Findings that give rise to doubt or seem to be on the border line should be X-rayed at two levels.

If the tourniquet could be applied at the level of the malleolus, CM should be injected at the end of the phlebography after removal of congestion in order to check up on free perfusion of the anterior tibial veins. Sometimes, only after congestion is removed, can the CM flow into the occluded deep crural veins, so that the extension of the deep vein thrombosis is shown more accuratley.

37.2.1
Radiologic Symptomatology of Acute Deep Leg Vein Thrombosis

The classic direct symptoms of phlebothrombosis include the following:

- Filling defect (Fig. 37.1)
- The cupula sign (see Fig. 37.8)
- The contour sign (Fig. 37.3)
- The "eraser" Phenomenon (Fig. 37.3)
- The monocular or spectacle sign (see Fig. 37.8)
- Collateral circulation, indirect (Fig. 37.3).

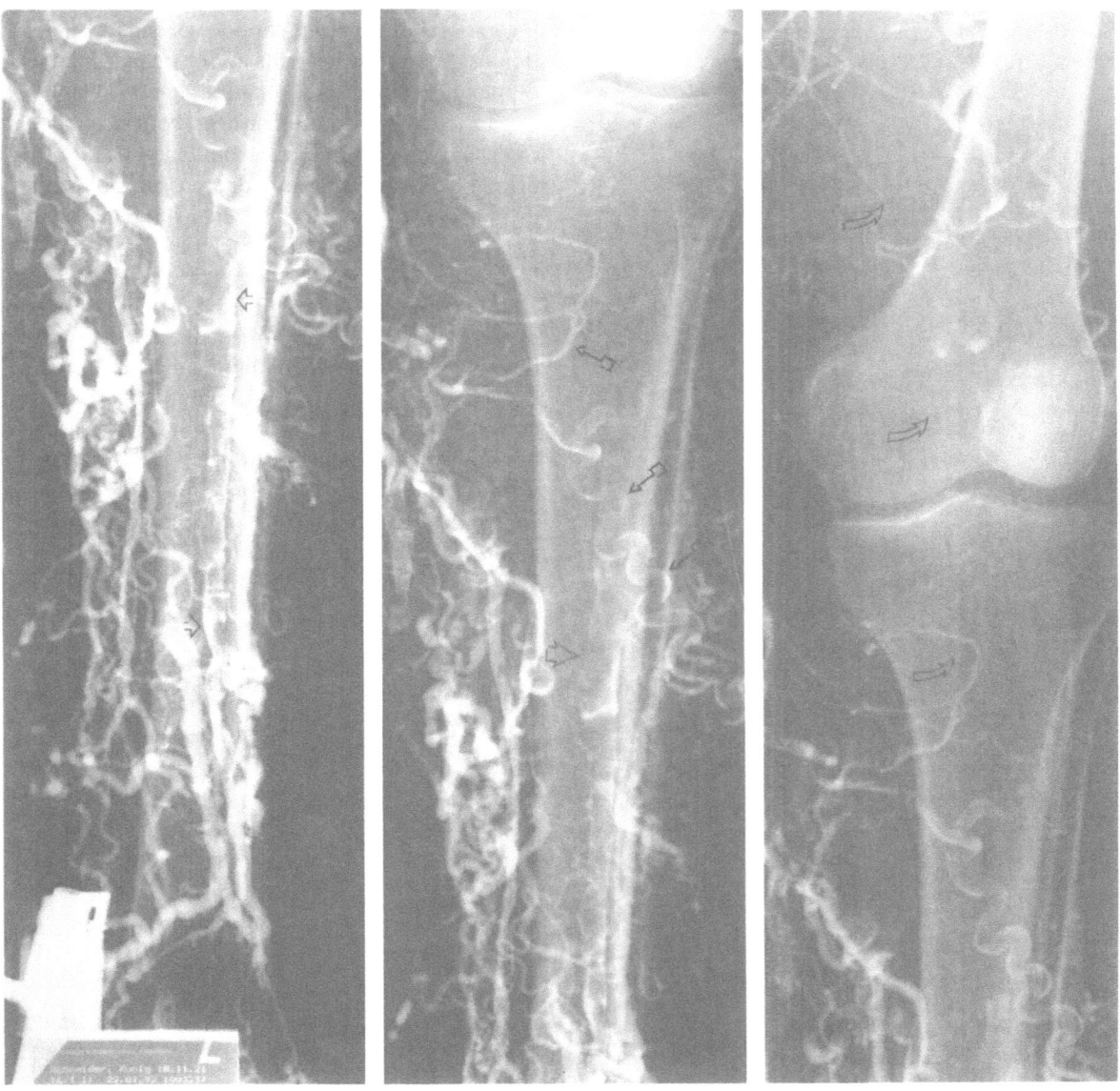

Fig. 37.3. Postthrombotic syndrome with re-thrombosis of both the deep and superficial varicose veins with identified contour signs (↯), rubber phenomenon (↣), and collateral circulation (↳→)

At least two of the above-mentioned defects have to be present, if possible at two levels, in order to ensure an exact diagnosis. The filling defect can be an illusion if, during Valsalva's maneuver, CM dilution occurs caudally of the valves and a concentration of CM in the area of the valve occurs at the same time. This technique is used to check the intactness of the valves (Fig. 37.4).

The outflow of the CM along the great saphenous vein cannot necessarily be interpreted as a sure sign of a filling defect of the deep veins. It can also be a consequence of an insufficient supramalleolar compression, an inadequate oblique positioning of the patient, or an inadequate Valsalva maneuver. Also, a CM injection too near to the drainage area of the great saphenous vein can lead to such a result.

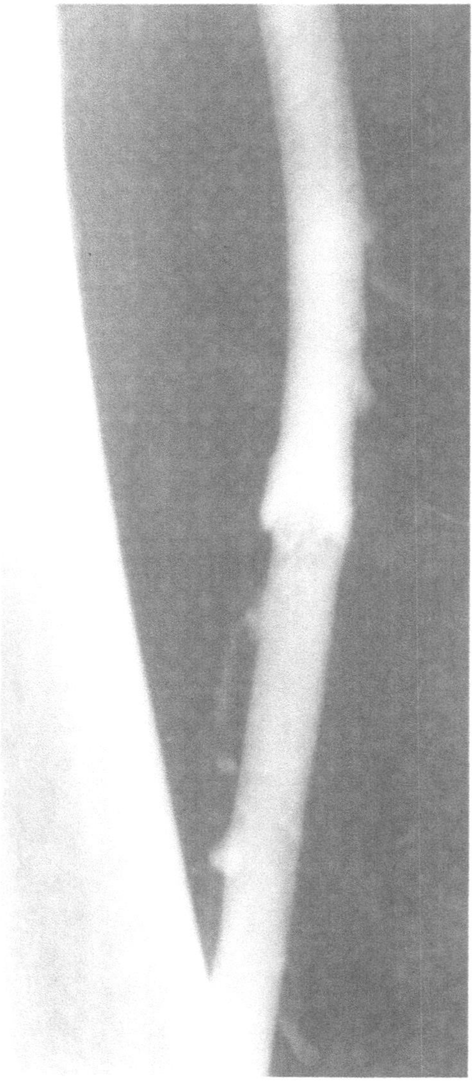

A clear, unequivocal criterion of thrombosis is the local, sharply delineated filling defect. The soft CM outline of a thrombus peripherally surrounded gives the impression of the walls of the vein or the valves having been contoured. This phenomenon is the contour sign.

Differing contrast density within a CM column, in addition to a blurred vessel contour, is called the "eraser" phenomenon. This is believed to be caused by an accelerated CM flow in the veins, by excessively strong compression, or by a firmer adhesion of the thrombus to the vascular walls.

The collateral phenomenon can be shown in acute thrombosis of the deep conducive veins by a depiction of the superficial veins, as for instance the great saphenous vein and the small saphenous vein.

In the case of additional deep collateral connections, one can assume with some justification that a primary varicose condition or a postthrombotic syndrome are already present. In extended collateral vascular connections, it is therefore not unusual to identify a clot thrombosis by filling defects.

When due to a thrombosis, sufficient contrasting of the pelvic veins cannot be achieved. Evidence in the collateral veins in the inguinal region is of primary importance. The suprapubic collateral veins and the "spontaneous palma" with drainage toward the opposite side shown in Fig. 37.5, as well as the infrainguinal depiction of the so-called venous star shown in Fig. 37.6 indicate venous occlusion of the anterior and posterior vascular regions.

Fig. 37.4. Intact venous valves after performance of Valsalva maneuver

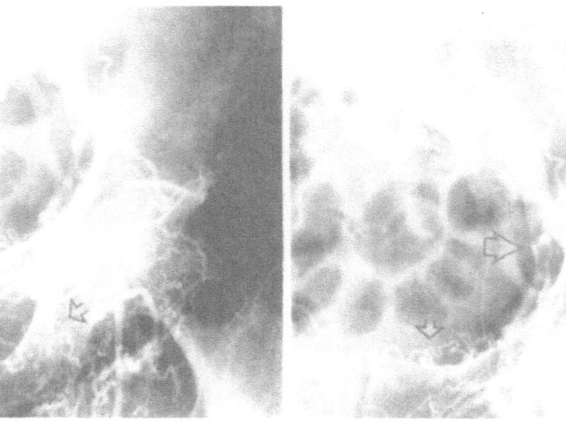

Fig. 37.5. Formation of a "spontaneous Palma" after progressing thrombosis of the lower extremities, involving the external iliac vein on the left (⇨)

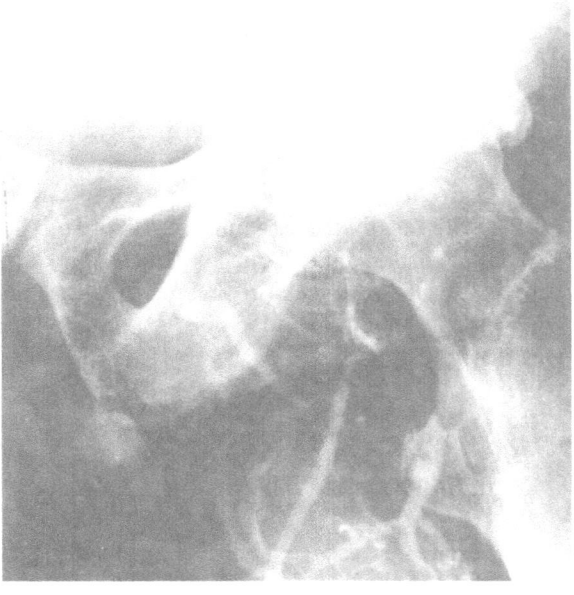

Fig. 37.6. The infrainguinal region of the venous ramification in a patient with deep venous thrombosis on the left

Table 37.1. Most important differential diagnoses of deep venous thrombosis. (From PARTSCH 1996)

- Hematoma (sickle-shaped discoloration behind the inner maleolus)
- Overstretching of musculature/ligament
- Baker's cyst (ultrasound of popliteal fosssa!)
- Postthrombotic syndrome, lipodermatosclerosis
- Superficial thrombophlebitis, vasculitis
- Erysipelas, lymphangitis
- Acrodermatitis chronica atrophicans
- Lymphatic edema, lipedema
- Autocoagulation congestion artefacts
- Cardiac, nephrotic, dysproteinemic edemas
- Compartment syndrome
- Thrombophobia:
  Fear of experiencing a thrombosis, mainly in patients with previous thrombosis

There is frequently a cupular sign at the end of the thrombus. This is a convex-shaped delineation of the thrombus which protrudes into the vascular lumen. The adjacent CM column is of a clear-cut concave shape.

The cupular sign and the contour sign always appear together. Smaller thrombi can be found in the pockets of the venous valves. Through the CM flow pathway an oval gap of the pockets in question emerges. This effect is called a monocular sign when located on one side and a spectacle sign when delineated on both sides in the venous valves. There are sometimes still thrombi at the end of the examination, when the CM has already been washed out with physiological NaCl solution. A late radiograph can provide evidence of this.

The most important differentially diagnostic possiblties of deep vein thrombosis are shown in Table 37.1 according to PARTSCH (1996).

37.2.2
Sources of Error in Phlebography

Possible sources of error or weakness in the phlebography method have been found to be the missing depiction of whole vein groups due to technically inadequate CM fillings. Other possibilities for a false diagnosis can be traced to the inflow of CM-free blood from vein openings. They are called inflow or knot-hole phenomena (Fig. 37.7). The deep femoral vein and the internal iliac vein cannot be sufficiently contrasted. Thromboses of vascular variations can also escape detection (DIEHM et al. 1997).

37.2.2.1
Complications of Phlebography

Generally, the frequency rate of clinically relevant complications with this method of examination is relatively low. General side-effects are caused by the CM which take the form of light, intermediate, or heavy allergic reactions. These should be adequately treated according to their extent. Approximately 2%–3% of all patients examined may suffer a circulatory collapse during phlebography in an oblique position; fresh air ventilation and a horizontal positioning of the examination table are often enough to recover the patient.

The side effects of non-ionic CM with a low osmolality and a low influence on the vascular endothelium are less than 0%–4% (MÜLLER 1994).

The swift process of the examination prevents the CM staying longer in the veins than absolutely necessary. In this way the risk of causing thrombosis of healthy veins is minimized.

Seldom There may occasionally be local complications within the area of puncture in the form of blistering, tissue necrosis, and ulceration (ZEITLER et al. 1983). Initially, the patient may express pain, which arises from CM paravation. In this case the examination should not be continued. Injections

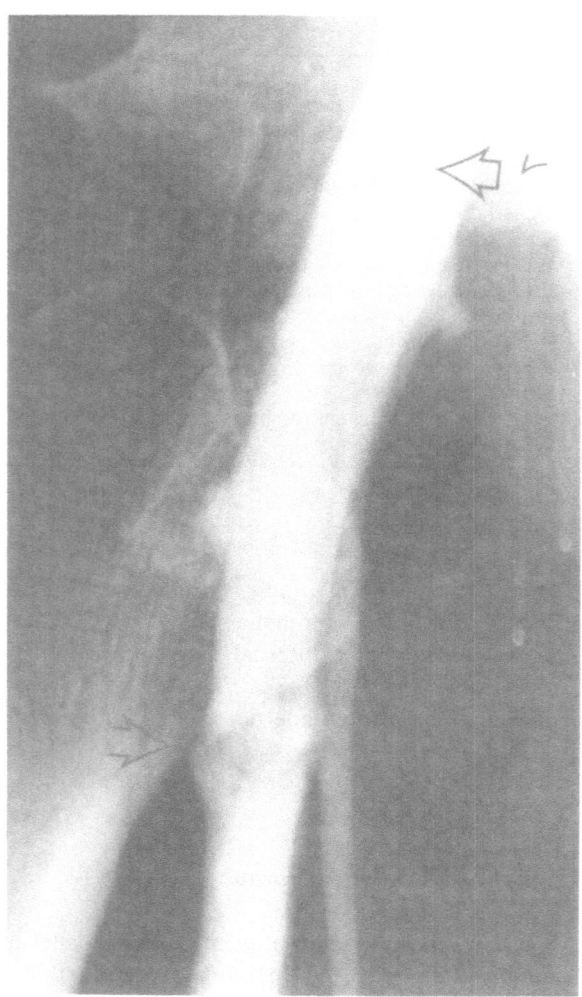

Fig. 37.7. Inflow–knot-hole phenomenon at a typical location

of NaCL solution dilute the paravasate to convey it through the tissue.

Blue discoloration of the toes is a sign of arterial strangulation after application of a very rigid tourniquet. A complete thrombosis of the examined extremity in the presence of peripheral arterial occlusive disease can produce the semblance of the phlegmasia coerulea dolens (Fig. 37.8).

A further possible complication during examination of acute pelvic vein thrombosis may be the transport of thrombotic material through the contrast medium flow. This risk of fulminant pulmonary embolism with lethal outcome increases with the extension of the thrombosis (MARTIN 1993).

37.3
Pathogenesis of Vein Thrombosis

The development of an intravital, intravascular coagulation (thrombosis) is determined by three factors which usually appear in combination. One factor can be predominant, but usually several causes work together. These three factors, also called Virchow's triad, include damage to the intima of the vascular walls, changes in hemodynamics, and changes in blood composition (GEDIGK 1990; GRESKÖTTER 1996).

37.3.1
Changes in Vascular Walls

The behavior of vascular endothelium is of crucial importance in the damage of vascular walls because its defects open up subendothelial structures. This

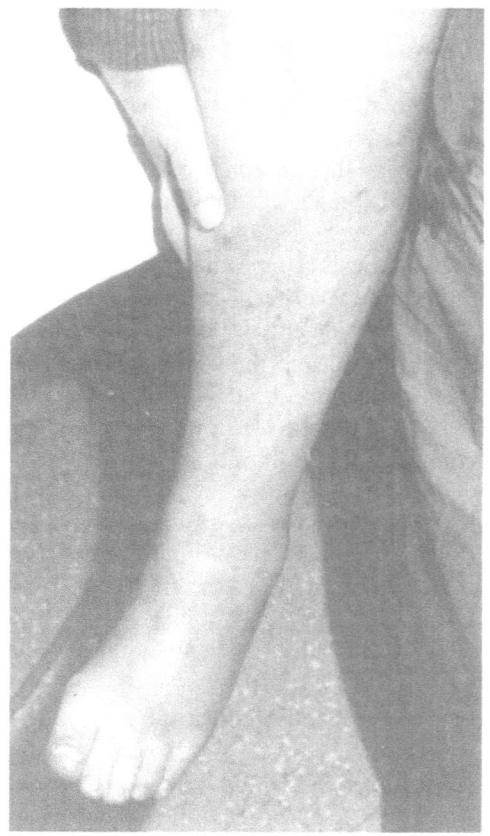

Fig. 37.8. A 65-year-old woman with phlegmasia coerulea dolens

leads to a rough inner surface of the vascular wall to which thrombocytes adhere and agglutinate with the help of the released adenosine diphosphate (ADP). The thrombocytes in turn release thromboplastin. Fibrin coagulation is further enforced by subendothelial connective tissue, adding its tissue thromboplastin through blood contact.

Damaging agents, such as an inflammation in the course of a phlebitis, sclerotic changes as in a phlebosclerosis, or traumata, that is, hypoxic injuries (stasis, general hypoxemia with pulmonary or cardial insufficiency, venous congestion), according to GEDIGK (1990), also contribute their share in damaging vascular walls. Bacteria and bacterial toxins cause direct damage to the vascular endothelium.

37.3.2
Changes in Blood Flow

The development of a thrombosis also depends on local hemodynamic conditions. Changes in the speed of blood flow are followed by an accumulation of thrombocytes in the periphery of the flow. Their contact with the endothelium causes agglutination and the release of thromboplastin. A retardation of the blood flow also leads to agglutination and the development of a laminated thrombus. At a high speed of blood flow on the other hand, thrombocytes, thrombocyte aggregates, and fibrin can be carried away with the blood stream. A general or local congestive hyperemia, a fall in blood pressure, or the failure of muscular transport of venous blood flow, in addition to insufficiency of the venous valves through varicosis, are the most frequent causes of blood flow retardation. Postoperative retardation of venous blood flow in the lower extremities, an especially critical region in terms of hemodynamics, can already be detected after 2–3 h of consequent immobilization (MORGENROTH 1983; GEDIGK 1990; GRESKÖTTER 1996).

37.3.3
Changes in Blood Composition

Changes in blood composition as a prerequisite for the development of a thrombus can involve general as well as local causes. It is, however, difficult to distinguish the individual components. Under normal conditions activated coagulation factors can be relatively quickly deactivated by inhibitors. Coagulation factor and enzyme inhibitor complexes can be assimilated and dissimilated by the macrophages of the vascular system, such as Kupffer's cells, sinusoid cells of the spleen, and medulla macrophages through phagocytosis.

Coagulation defects that have been proven to be risk factors are shown in Table 37.2 (PARTSCH 1996).

A thrombocytosis after a splenectomy leads to an accelerated coagulability of the blood. The greater tendency to thrombosis formation after traumata, child birth, and operations is considered to be due to the combined effects of stasis and a marked inflow of activated coagulation factors, especially of factor Xa. Thrombosis is also more likely to develop when a heightened concentration of free fatty acids in the blood exceeds the capacity of the carrier protein albumin, so that platelet aggregation is increased. Besides these components which influence the coagulability of the blood, there are factors that have a local effect. They especially affect the development of venous congestion and thrombosis by activating the coagulatory system through endothelial damage or through injury to cellular elements of the vascular wall.

Thrombocytes play a special role in this process. Thrombocyte aggregates consolidate through fibrin formation and adhere more strongly to the endothelial defect. By means of additional platelets conveyed by the blood, the thrombus can continue to grow in length and thickness. The initial form of the thrombus is called a laminated thrombus (plain thrombus). Under conditions of complete stasis of the blood column in the veins, but also behind a laminated thrombus, a coagulation thrombus develops. Infiltration with connective tissue, developing 3–4 days after thrombus formation, determines the structure of the thrombus (GEDIGK 1990; GRESKÖTTER 1996).

Table 37.2. Identifiable disturbances of coagulation as a risk factor. (From PARTSCH 1996)

- AT III-, protein C-, protein S-deficiency
- Heparin-Co-factor II- and factor XII-deficiency
- Dysplasminogenia
- Dysfibrinogenemia
- Deficiency of fibrinolysis
- Anticardiolipin antibodies
- Lupus-type anticoagulant
- Resistance to the anticoagulant activity of activated protein C

37.4
Alternative Procedures to Acute Phlebography

The method which has been up to now the most concise and successful in diagnosing thrombophlebitis has to compete today with Doppler ultrasonography and the color-coded blood flow Doppler picture.

The real-time sonographic examination in B-mode undoubtedly has its advantages in screening a proximal vein thrombosis with regard to non-invasiveness and a fast non-stressful procedure (FOBBE et al. 1989; LÖSCH et al. 1993; FÜRST et al. 1990; HABSCHEID 1992). There are different assessments of all ultrasonography methods as regards sensitivity and specificity within thrombosis diagnostics (HACH 1992; HABSCHEID 1992; SPENGEL 1992; THEISS 1992).

In these assessments, the examiner's experience plays a significantr role. With regard to diagnostics of the femoral region, the specificity by means of B-mode as compression sonography is deemed to be 99% and sensitivity 96%. For the deeper pelvic veins, one gets a much poorer result because of inadequate compression and overlay of intestinal gases. For the popliteal vein and the calf veins specificity reaches 99% and sensitiviy 90% (HABSCHEID 1992).

A bidirectional Doppler yields very good results in the pelvic flow region but these results drop to 70% in the popliteal region and to 60% for the crural region (SPENGEL 1992).

Soft, fresh thrombi may lack an echogenic intrinsic pattern in the B-picture, so that only the zero-flow in the Doppler sonogram allows for the diagnosis of a thrombosis (STAPF et al. 1989).

Difficulties may arise with early thrombotic changes because the material is easily compressible and the vascular lumen is only slightly constricted. Only in combination with the color-coded blood-flow Doppler (ccbf), can a better diagnostic result be reached. With this method blood flow and flow direction, including morphological information, can be visualized in an ultrasonic picture. At the same time, it is possible to successfully assess the venous wall including perivascular structures (HACH 1992). The additional effort is considered to be small. Big vessels from the external iliac vein up to the popliteal vein are somewhat easier to diagnose than the deep crural veins, which are of a more complex anatomy and the diameters of the thrombi are too small. Old thrombi present a problem because they shrink. Collaterals can be detected by coloration (Fig. 37.9a,b).

Up to now, fresh thromboses of the big veins have been identified using ccbf with a sensitivity of 96% and a specificity of 97% (Fig. 37.10a–c).

According to pure B-picture diagnostics there is also a lowering of both parameters in the popliteal and crural regions. For surgical partners the documentation of sonographic diagnostics has turned out to be a disadvantage because it is only based on pictures of sections (HACH 1992). For this reason, acute phlebographic diagnostics with their clear, well-organized orientation towards the whole venous system will remain the golden standard in terms of meaningful diagnosis until the newer noninvasive ultrasound methods can come up to par.

Phlebography is a quick, precise, only low-invasive method with a definite diagnostic result. It is possible that, echo contrast medium (Echovist, Schering AG, Berlin, Germany) with ccbf will bring a significant increase in diagnostic information (SCHOTT et al. 1995). For the time being ultrasound methods are considered useful supplementary procedures (HACH 1992; SPENGEL 1992).

Magnetic resonance imaging (MRI) with blood flow analysis is not yet available as a routine method (MARSHALL 1994). MRI requires good cooperation on the part of the patient and is too complicated for acute diagnostics.

37.5
Consequences of Thrombosis

As long as the thrombus is not organized, it can become detached from the vascular wall at any phase of its development. Through localization in different vascular sections, more or less strong obstruction phenomena develop. The heightened internal pressure of the vessel causes the outflow of blood out of the vascular volume into the adjacent tissue. An edema develops, the protein concentration of which will grow with rising venous pressure.

In venous occlusions, serious long-term changes can ensue. Through cicatrization of the venous wall and thickening of the wall that develops from scarring, the muscle pump loses its effectiveness in the discharge of venous blood. Cicatrization mainly affects the venous valves, so that they can no longer counteract the back flow. Also, lateral branches can

Fig. 37.9 a,b. An isolated thrombosis of the lower leg in the tibial anterior vein (▷) on the left and the monocular sign (↙) including the cupula sign of the thrombus (↓). b A color-coded duplex sonography of the same tibial vein

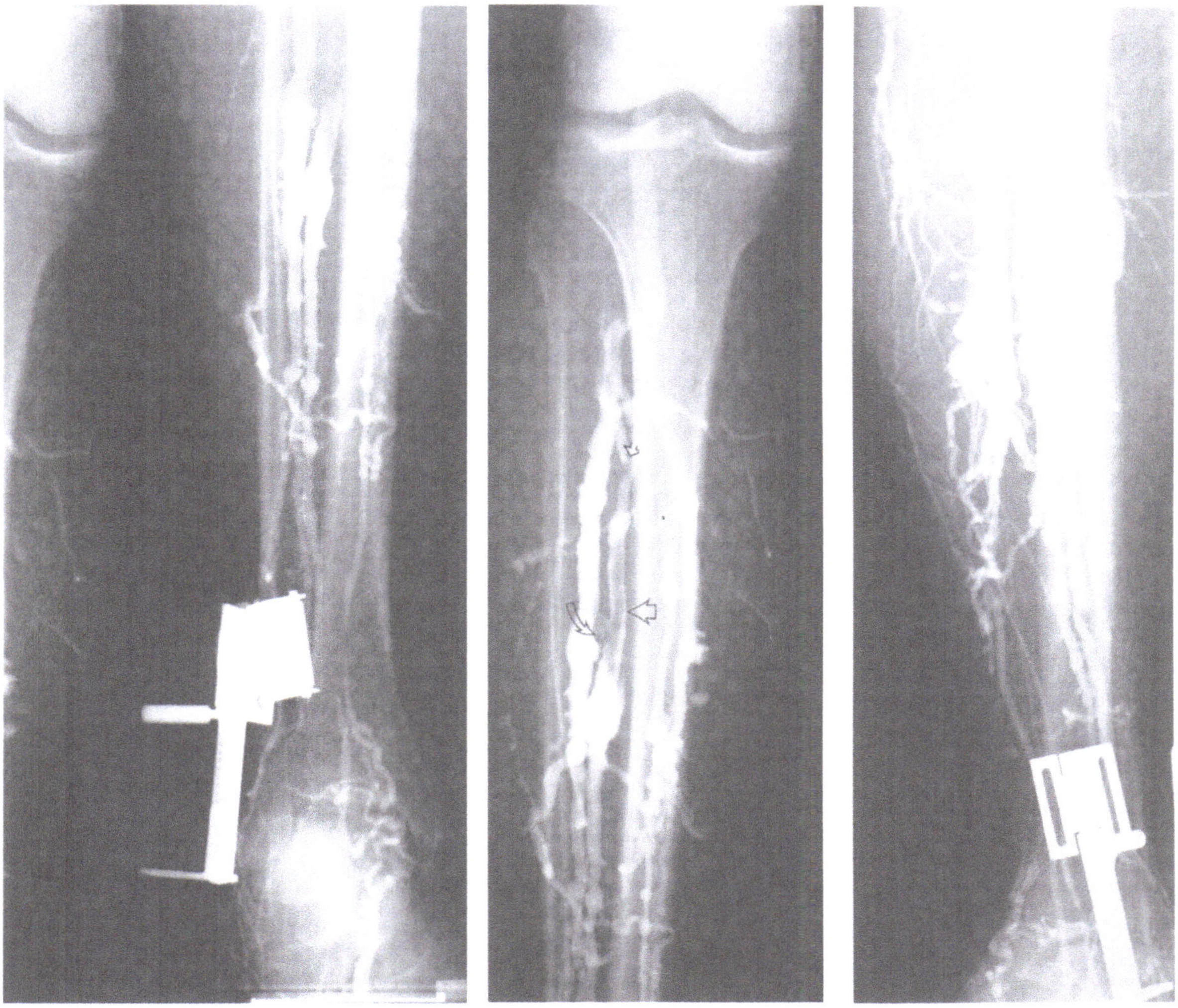

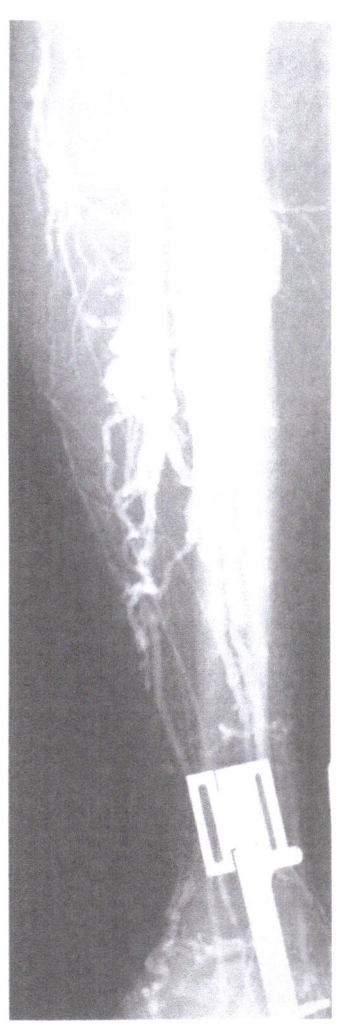

a

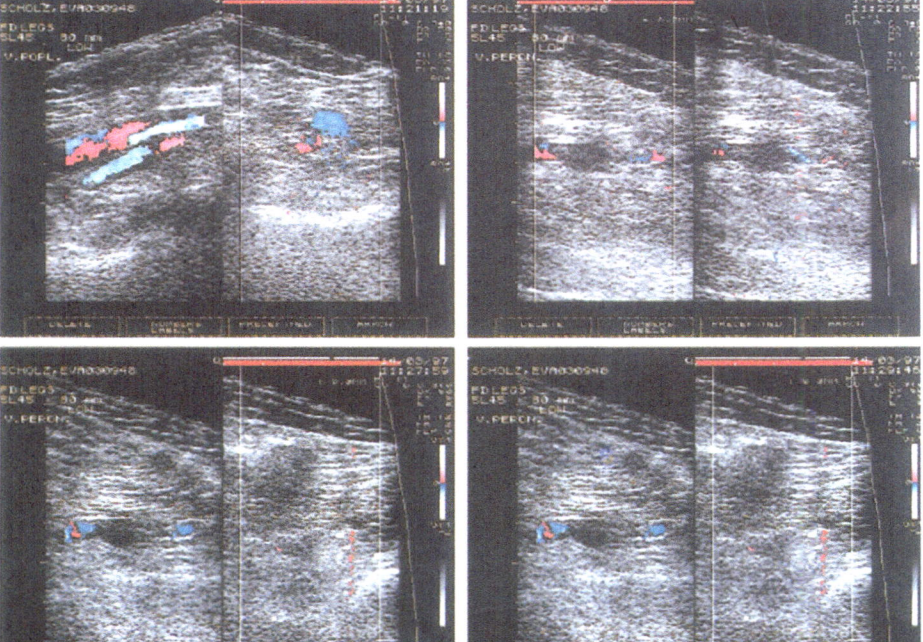

b

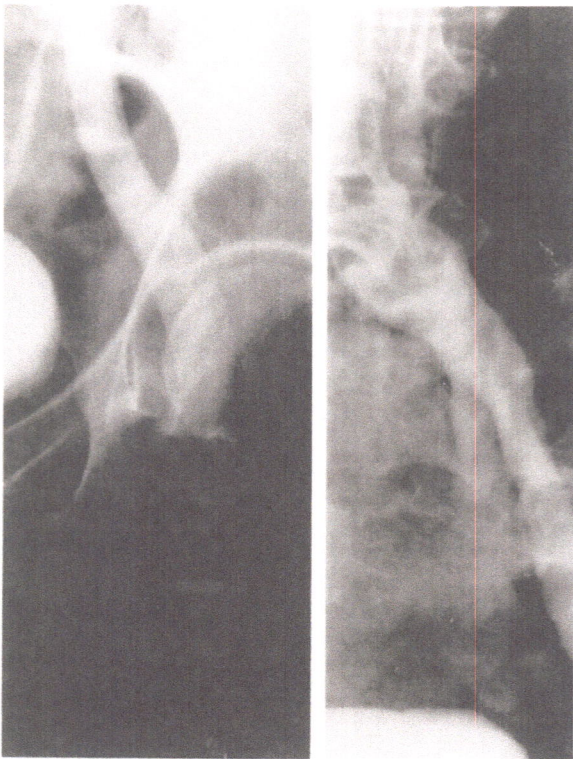

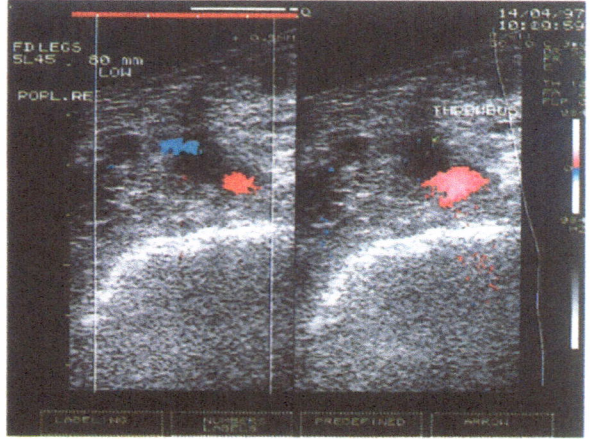

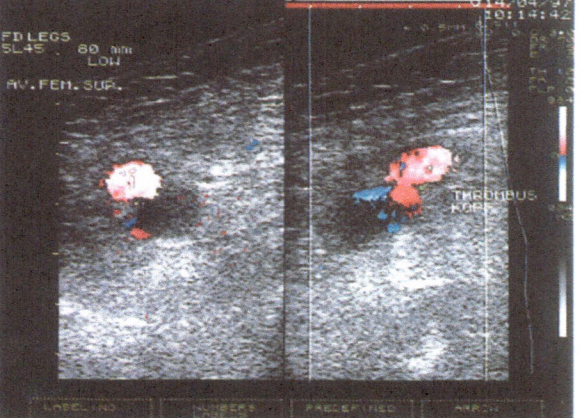

Fig. 37.10. a Recent venous thrombosis of the femoral popliteal vein on the left caused by inguinal lymphadenosis. **b,c** A color-coded duplex sonography identified flow extinction in the course of the superficial femoral vein. The thrombus of the popliteal vein is >180 degrees adherent

be subject to cicatrization, which prevents the opening of the collaterals.

Circulatory disorders in the leg veins become manifest as secondary changes; most frequently in atrophy of the skin. This process leads to the formation of skin ulcerations (ulcus cruris). The venae communicantes of the Cockett group are considered to be responsible for the extension and localization of ulcers. Because they can no longer absorb the heightened venous pressure, circulatory disorders develop, leading to edema. On the basis of the stasis small ulcers form, the blow-out ulcers. A bacterial infection of the ulcer ground is the basis for the development of erysipelas.

A further consequence of venous thrombosis is edema sclerosis with a marked growth in size of the extremity and the appearance of elephantiasis as an expression of the postthrombotic syndrome. For the patient concerned this late consequence of a deep leg vein thrombosis is a severe, permanent ailment, characterized by swelling, pain, trophic skin defects, and secondary varices. Moreover, treatment and therapy implies a considerable social and medical burden.

The biggest danger incurred by a deep vein thrombosis, which is partially life-threatening is pulmonary embolism. According to GRESKÖTTER (1996) it usually occurs 1–2 weeks after the beginning of thrombosis in approximately 30% of all cases. The symptoms of pulmonary embolism include dyspnea, cyanosis, tachycardia, as well as dull retrosternal pain and circulatory collapse.

Fulminant pulmonary embolism leads to a sudden subtotal or total obstruction of the main pulmonary arteries by bigger clusters of emboli. After a fast increase in pressure in the right ventricle reflectory right heart death follows. This applies to 0.4% of all patients in hospital. One fifth of all postoperative cases of death are considered to be caused by pulmonary embolism (BLUM et al. 1996).

Obstruction of the total pulmonary circulatory tract with multiple recrudescent small emboli causes chronic cor pulmonale.

In the periphery of the lung, hemorrhagic pulmonary infarction, partially accompanied by pleurisy, emerges in a wedge-shaped form.

37.6
Risk Factors of Venous Thromboembolism

From the age of 50 onwards, susceptibility to thrombosis increases (incidence, 3/1000). Additionally, degeneration of the valves leads to insufficiency of closure (competence), so that thromboses can develop more easily in the course of unusual mechanical effort. Such venous injuries are the cause of the so-called effort-thrombosis of the popliteal vein (SCHMITT 1996).

Also, immobilization on long car rides and flights (economy-class syndrome), or pareses of the extremities are risk factors. Patients who have already suffered leg vein thrombosis in the past are five times more likely to suffer a re-thrombosis.

Thromboses are more likely to form after traumata; they can accompany tumors and are often even the first evidence of neoplastic disease (paraneoplastic syndrome). Furthermore, a variety of internal diseases or accompanying diseases, as well as the use of certain medication or drugs, can trigger thromboembolism (DIEHM et al. 1997).

37.7
Venous Thrombosis Therapy

In order to prevent serious consecutive damage, immediate adequate therapy should follow an exact diagnosis. If several possibilities of therapy are available for the clinical picture in question, one should choose the method that yields the best results and incurs the fewest complications.

Conservative. If an experienced examiner can exclude with certainty that the popliteal vein is involved by means of sonography, a cautious approach with preventive treatment and sonographic controls is justified (STAPF et al. 1989).

Further conservative measures include rest in bed and high positioning of the affected extremity, if necessary with a compression bandage.

Fibrinolysis. With thrombolysis a therapy is available that shows acceptable long-term results and low lethality. There are, however, quite a few contraindications that limit its use. Table 37.3 shows a list of absolute contraindications to lysotherapy according to WALTER and ERASMI (1997).

Therapeutic alternatives are anticoagulation treatment (SEIFRIED 1993) and venous thrombec-

Table 37.3. The "ABC" of absolute contraindications according to WALTER and ERASMI (1997)

Aneurysm	Intestinal bleeding
Atrial fibrillation	Malignant growth (late stage)
Blood pressure (>180 mm)	Operation (<10 days)
Cerebral sclerosis	Pancreatitis
Cerebrovascular insult (<3 months)	Pregnancy (early weeks)
	Reanimation (<4 weeks)
Diabetes, poor quality of control	Renal insufficiency (severe)
	Sepsis
Epilepsy	Tuberculosis
Gastric ulcer	Vascular puncture (arterial)
General wasting diseases	
Hemorrhagic diathesis	
Hepatic insufficiency	
Injection (intramuscular)	

tomy. A comparison of thrombectomy and anticoagulation shows that the latter produces poorer results.

Thrombectomy. Thrombectomy is surgically indicated in cases of phlegmasia coerulea dolens for fast decompensation in order to save the affected extremity. With attention to risk factors and thrombosis duration – under 5 days – thrombectomy is carried out when thrombolysis is contraindicated. Under these conditions, perioperative lethality can be significantly reduced (POLTERAUER et al. 1989).

Further indications for operating in cases of deep venous leg or pelvic thrombosis include floating thrombus, fresh pelvic vein thrombosis, occlusion in the inguinal region, and massive pulmonary embolism. Postoperative results according to WALTER and ERASMI (1997) are shown in Table 37.4.

37.8
Significance of Thrombosis

Acute thrombosis of the femoral vein and the popliteal vein in the inflow region of several veins is

Table 37.4. Postoperative results of thrombectomy according to WALTER and ERASMI (1997)

Deaths	$n = 397$	9 (2.3%)
Pulmonary embolism		3 (0.8%)
Technique	$n = 278$	Phlebography, on average 22 weeks post operatively
Patency		241 (86.7%)
Postthrombotic syndrome		5 (1.8%)

unfavorable to prognosis. Therefore, in view of developing chronical venous insufficiency and ulcus cruris, evidence in these vascular sections suffices to launch active invasive therapy (HACH 1992).

The frequency of deep leg and pelvic vein thrombosis in the former West Germany was estimated to be about 600 000 a year (WEBER et al. 1989).

Thrombosis does not only significantly affect the life of the patient, but also has social and economic effects because of its long-term consequences, such as postthrombotic syndrome and ulcus cruris. Some 16 million Germans need treatment for varicose veins. Another 9 million suffer from chronic vein deficiency due to advanced venous illness. Two million suffer from leg ulcers, the most serious form of venous illness.

Venous illness is estimated to cost some 1.300 million Deutsche Mark annually in Germany; 835 million DM of this is paid by state-regulated insurances.

Approximately every second a German citizen over the age of 45 must at some point take time off work because of varicose veins. A total of 2% of people aged 35–44 years and 6% of men aged 45–54 years suffer from some illness associated with blocked veins. Approximately 90% of such illnesses affect the legs.

Medicine must in the future move towards early diagnosis of disease to avoid expensive treatment later (SCHWING 1994b).

References

Blum U, Langer M, Spillner G, Beyersdorf F, Buitrago-Telles C, Voshage G, Weinbeck M, Schlosser V, Ehmer M, Cragg A (1996) Die endoluminale Therapie des infrarenalen Bauchaortenaneurysmas. RoFo 164:47–54
Diehm C, Stammler F, Amendt K (1997) Die tiefe Venenthrombose. Dtsch Aerztebl 94(6):29–39
Fobbe F, Koennecke H-C, El Bedewi M, Heidt P, Boese-Landgraf J, Wolf K-J (1989) Diagnostik der tiefen Beinvenenthrombose mit der farbkodierten Duplexsonographie. RoFo 151(5):569–573
Fürst G, Kuhn F-K, Trappe RP, Mödder U (1990) Diagnostik der tiefen Beinvenenthrombose. RoFo 152(2):151–158
Gedigk P (1990) Blutgerinnung und Thrombose. In: Eder M, Gedigk P (eds) Allgemeine Pathologie und Pathologische Anatomie, 33rd edn. Springer, Berlin Heidelberg New York, pp 79–92
Greskötter K-R (1996) Pathologie der Blutgerinnung und der Blutungen. In: Pathologie/Kinische Medizin systematisch, vol 1. Greskötter (ed), UNI-MED, Lorch, pp 234–242
Habscheid W (1992) Diagnostik der tiefen Beinvenenthrombose. Freie Radiol 5/6:26–31

Hach W (1992) Diagnostik der tiefen Beinvenenthrombose. Freie Radiol 5/6:26–31
Heinz M, Theiss W (1996) Lysetherapie venöser Thrombosen. Internist (Berl) 37:567–573
Lösch W, Beyer-Enke S, Rompel O, Zeitler E (1993) Farbkodierte Duplexsonographie (Angiodynographie) im Vergleich zur Phlebographie. Bildgebung/Imaging 60(4):297–300
Marshall M (1994) Die Duplex-Sonographie und die Farb-Duplex-Sonographie in der Phlebologie. Vasomed 78:270–278
Martin M (1993) Phlebothrombose im Alter. Phlebologie 22:225
Morgenroth K (1983) Atlas der Venenthrombose, part I. PVG Pharmazeutische Verlagsgesellschaft, Munich, pp 22–25
Moser KM, LeMoine JR (1981) Is embolic risk conditioned by location of deep venous thrombosis? Ann Intern Med 94:439–444
Müller JHA (1994) Phlebographische Thrombosediagnostik unter Benutzung nicht-ionischer Röntgenkontrastmittel. Vasomed 10:396–402
Partsch H (1996) Diagnose und Therapie der tiefen Venen Thrombose. Vasa Suppl 46:5–41
Polterauer P, Hölzenbein T, Prager M, Kretschmer G, Huk I (1989) Die akute tiefe Beinvenenthrombose. Vasomed 11:39–42
Rabe E (1993) Phlebologischer Bildtalas. Vasomed 8:452–453
Richter E-I, Zeitler E (1980) Die Diagnostik der akuten Phlebothrombose. Radiologe 20:426–433
Schmitt HE (1996) Akute Plebothrombose. In: Zeitler E (ed) Klinische Radiologie. Springer, Belin Heidelberg New York, pp 607–613
Schott U, Laniado M, Duda SH, Seitz D, Claussen CD (1995) Echokontrastmittel für die farbdopplersonographische Diagnostik der tiefen Oberschenkelthrombose. RoFo 162(3):194–198
Schubert U, Blank W, Braun B (1992) Realtime-Sonographie zur Diagnostik der Venenthrombose. Krankenhausarzt 65(4):150–156
Schwing C (1994a) Ultraschalldiagnostik der Beinvenenthrombose. Freie Radiol 8(1):55
Schwing C (1994b) Vascular disease moves up the agenda in Germany. In: Clinica 589 PJP Publications LTD
Seifried E (1993) Tiefe venöse Thrombosen-etablierte Behandlungsvervahren und neue Trends. Z Kardiol 82 suppl 2:49–59
Spengel F (1992) Diagnostik der tiefen Beinvenenthrombose. Freie Radiol 5/6:26–27
Stapf M, Betzl G, Küffer G, Hahn D, Spengel FA (1989) Stellenwert der Duplexsonographie in der Diagnostik der tiefen Bein- und Beckenvenenthrombose. Bildgebung/Imaging 56:52–56
Theiss W (1992) Diagnostik der tiefen Beinvenenthrombose. Freie Radiol 5/6:26–31
Walter M, Erasmi H (1997) Die chirurgische Therapie der tiefen Bein-Beckenvenenthrombose. Herz Kreisl 29(4):116–120
Weber W, Schild H, Kraus W (1989) Diagnostik tiefer Bein- und Beckenvenenthrombose. Med Klin 84(4):196–202
Zeitler E (1979) Roentgenologische und Nuclearmedizinische Diagnostik. In: Venöse Abflußstörungen Ehringer H, Fischer H, Netzer Co., Schmutzler R, Zeitler E (eds) Enke, Stuttgart, pp 302–323
Zeitler E, Milbert L, Richter E-I, Ringelmann W, Strohm CH (1983) RoFo 138(6):670–677

38 Primary Varicosis and Venous Insufficiency

J. WEBER

CONTENTS

38.1
Primary Varicosis

38.1.1
Definition of Primary Varicosis

According to specific conditions of civilized man (upright position and sitting with bent knees, reduction of active muscular training) there is a progressive degenerative process mainly involving the veins of the lower extremities (EHRINGER 1979; GOTTLOB and MAY 1986; NETZER 1979; WEBER and MAY 1990).

Changes in the structure of the venous wall (reduction of muscular and elastic fibers, consecutive enlargement of the calibers of the veins, insufficient closure of the venous valves, and their progressive degeneration and disappearance) lead to reflux and recirculation (BOLLINGER 1979; Fig. 38.1).

J. WEBER, MD, Professor, Institut fur Rontgendiagnostik und Interventionelle Radiologie, DRK-Krankenhaus, Suurheid 20, 22559 Hamburg-Rissen, Germany

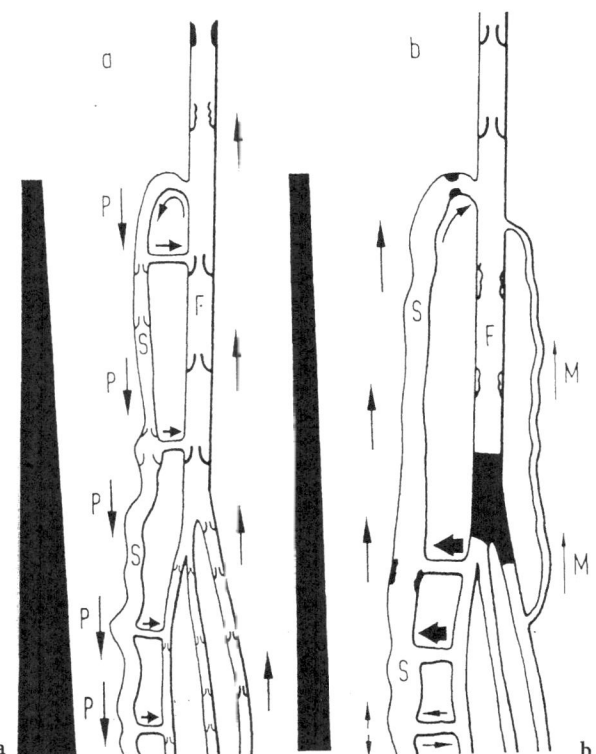

Fig. 38.1 a,b. *Hemodynamics in primary and secondary varicosis* (from WEBER and MAY 1990). a Primary varicosis. Due to the insufficiency of the orifice of the long saphenous vein, there is reflux causing varicose and incompetence of saphenous valves, leading increasingly to peripheral venous hypertension. In the beginning perforators are draining into the deep collecting veins. Recirculation causes later on decompensation of the deep venous system. b Secondary varicosis. Following partial postthrombotic obstruction, the deep veins of the lower leg are draining towards the epifascial saphenous system, causing subsequently incompetence of the perforators and of the saphenous valves (i.e., secondary varicosis). The destruction of valves of the femoral vein does not cause peripheral CVI directly. (The *left wedge* symbolizes increasing peripheral epifascial venous pressure, the right marks the deep venous pressure)

The varicose syndrome consists in 90% of cases of primary varices and in 9.8% of secondary varicose changes caused by thrombotic obstruction and postthrombotic recanalization, including the loss of valves and the persistence of collateralization. Only about 0.2% of varices are related to congenital venous dysplasia (EHRINGER 1979).

38.1.2
Clinical Findings

The typical clinical signs initially deal with enlargement of the subcutaneous epifascial venous calibers showing a tortuous and convoluted pattern. The changes range from small varicose dilatation of the cutaneous veins (capillary ectasis) to reticular enlargement and big truncular varices of the long and short saphenous veins and its side branches, allowing us to identify segments or the whole extent by simple clinical inspection: locally, DOW phenomenon for instance signals the presence of insufficient perforator veins causing epifascial circumscript varices by "blow out" (COCKETT and JONES 1958). Venous aneurysms may be localized close to the orifices or at any other level of the degen-

erated venous trunks, mainly causing dilatation above the level of venous valves (RITTER and LOOSE 1989).

Inspection and palpation of the patient in an erect position and clinical tests (tourniquet tests, Trendelenburg and Perthes; Fig. 38.2) do offer basic information to be confirmed by apparative functional tests (plethysmography, Doppler and duplex ultrasound, phlebodynamometry) and mainly by phlebography.

38.1.3
Topography of the Varicose Syndrome

Following the genesis of a progressive venous degeneration descendent in about 80% of cases (HACH and HACH-WUNDERLE 1997), there are main regions of interest for diagnostic analysis.

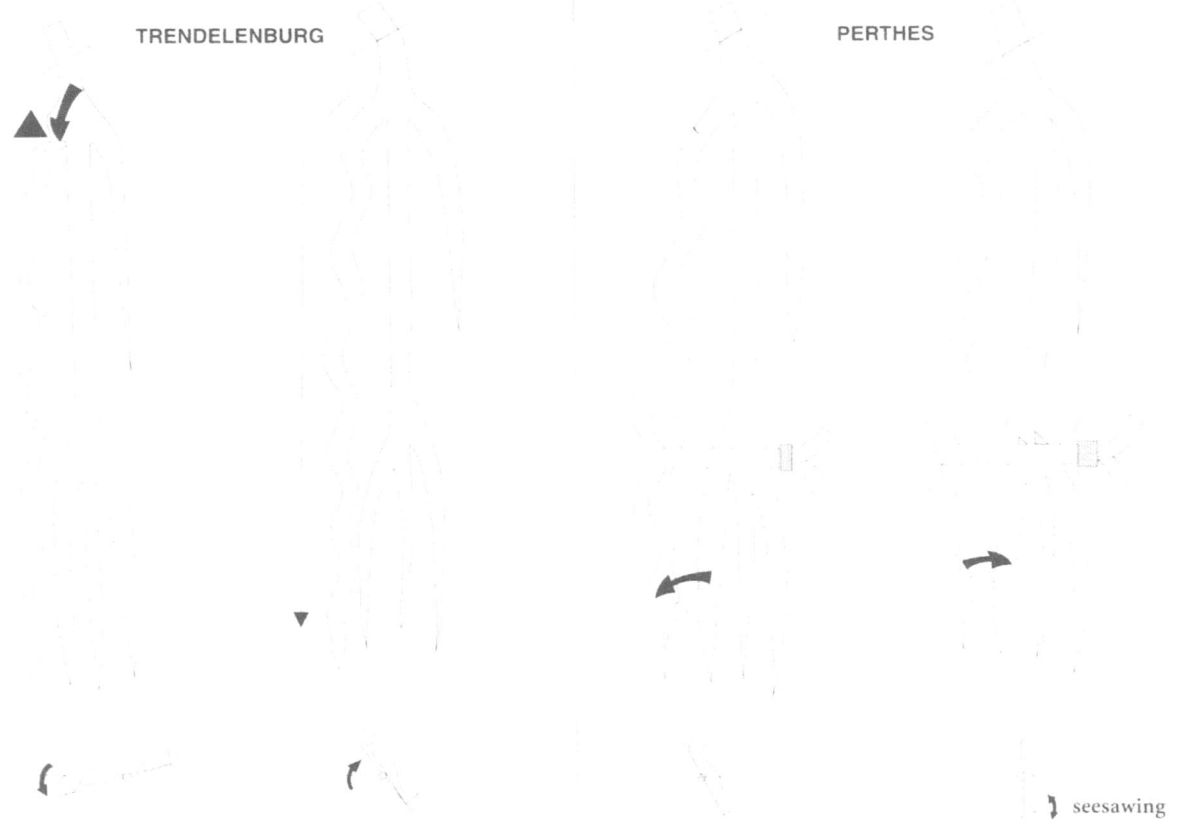

Fig. 38.2 a,b. *Clinical tourniquet tests.* **a** Trendelenburg test: Compression of the previously emptied saphenous trunk. If it fills up rapidly after decompression in an erect position this indicates "Trendelenburg positive" (e.g., the saphenous orifice is insufficient). **b** Pertes test: The tourniquet is closed above an insufficient perforator vein. If the varices remain emptied under exercise, the perforator will be sufficient. If the varices refill while seesawing with the foot, it is insufficient

Orifices of the saphenous veins. Step-by-step venous degeneration leads to an early incompetence of the valves of the orifice to be proven by Doppler and duplex sonography, as well as by phlebography using Valsalva's maneuver (Fig. 38.3).

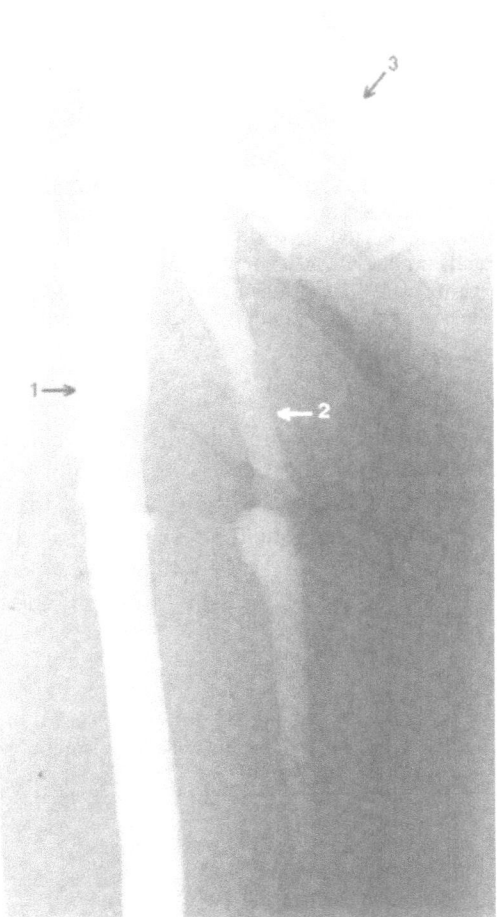

Fig. 38.3. *Phlebography of the orifice of the long saphenous vein.* Reflux of the contrast medium into the insufficient valveless long saphenous trunk, increasing during Valsalva's maneuver. (*1*, Femoral veins; *2*, long saphenous vein; *3*, superficial pudendal vein)

The increased reflux of blood later leads to descendent stages of the saphenous varicosis (long saphenous vein: stages I–IV; short saphenous vein: stages I–III; HACH and HACH-WUNDERLE 1997).

At the level of the orifice of the long saphenous vein there is a large variety of side branches entering the infundibulum of the vein (external pudendal vein, lateral accessorian saphenous vein, superficial epigastric vein, superficial circumflex iliac vein). Most of them cannot be visualized directly by Doppler, duplex, or phlebography as long as there is a direct reflux into the main saphenous trunk. However, following an insufficient crossectomy (e.g., surgical ligation and resection of the venous mouth) local collateralization directly drains over these side branches into persistent segments of the saphenous trunk (or to supplementary steams) causing varicose recurrence (BRUNNER 1979; WEBER and MAY 1990).

Exactly the same problem occurs at the level of the orifice of the short saphenous vein, where patho-anatomy seems to be even more confusing compared to the inguinal area (FISCHER and VOGEL 1987). This is due to the small area of the popliteal space and to the variety of the connectious of the popliteal branches and the terminal short saphenous vein. Further more, the anastomosis with the femoropopliteal vein and the termination of the gastrocnemian veins contribute to a complex local topography in a very limited space. Differentiation of the diseased venous anatomy and of its variations is a difficult task for any imaging modality.

Insufficient Perforator Veins ("Key Perforators"; MAY and NISSL 1973). According to VAN LIMBORGH (1965) there about 150 pairs of transfacial perforator veins connecting the epifascial main trunks and side branches with the deep venous system (Fig. 38.4). However, there is a relatively limited number of perforators tending to insufficiency (e.g., destruction of the valves and the one-way system of venous flow from the epifascial to the subfacial space) (PARTSCH

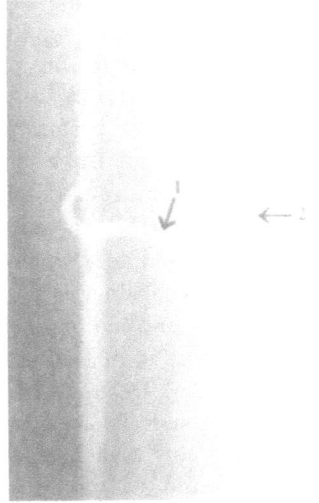

Fig. 38.4. *Perforator veins, varicography.* A perforator vein (DODD group) drains from the enlarged long saphenous vein into a concomitant femoral vein (*2*). Transfascial point (*1*)

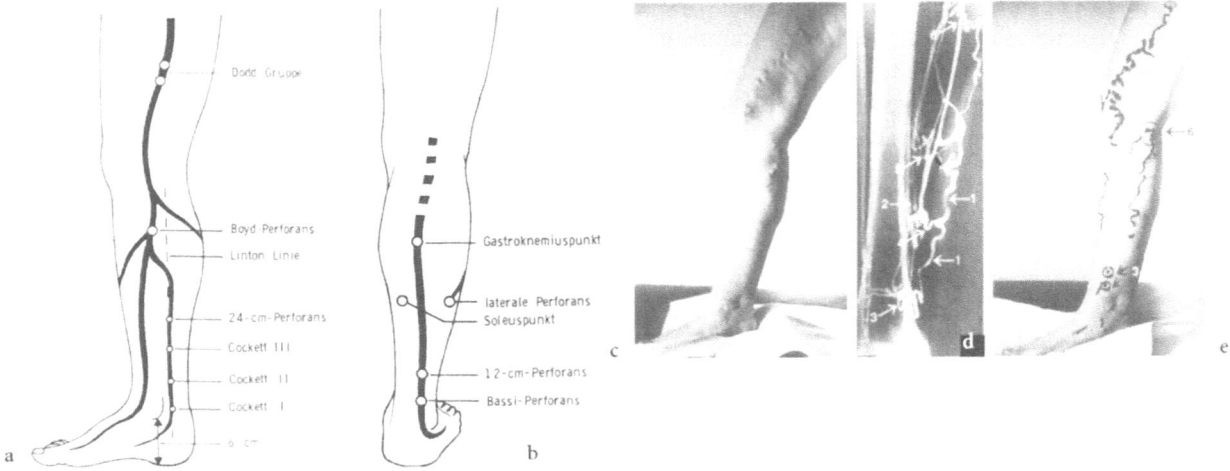

Fig. 38.5 a–e. *Perforator veins of the leg* (From WEBER and MAY 1990). **a** Lateral view. "Key perforators" are more or less positioned along Linton's (imaginative) line, connecting the posterior arcuate vein with the deep venous system. (From WEBER and WAY 1990). **b** Back view. Perforators along the short saphenous vein, soleus and gastrocnemian points. (From WEBER and MAY 1990). **c** Native lower limb, showing the varices at the upper and lower leg. **d** Phlebography showing varices of the posterior arcuate vein (*1*), opacified from the posterior tibial trunk (*2*) via Cockett's perforators: I (*3*), II (*4*), III (*5*) and the Boyd perforator (*6*). **e** Pre-operative marking of the phlebographic findings; only the "blow out" at the level of Cockett I (*3*) and Boyd (*6*) have been seen clinically

and STAUBESAND 1981). In consequence, initially there is a reverse blood flow into the subcutaneous space ("blow out") and a normal "blow in" at rest, whereas a current "blow out" will continuously damage the subcutanous structures later on (BJORDAL 1972; COCKETT and JONES 1983). Together with the "blow down", coming from the varicose saphenous trunk, all this may lead sooner or later to chronic venous insufficiency (CVI).

The incidence of perforator incompetence and the level and site at which it occurs, depend on an average degenerative process. However, there are typical groups of perforator veins, tending to insufficiency, especially at the *inner side* of the lower leg along Linton's line (COCKETT I, II and III; SHERMAN's perforator; BOYD's perforator; Fig. 38.5).

STAUBESAND and HACKLÄUBER have recently demonstrated that there are remarkable variations in the position of the perforator veins along and around this imaginative line (STAUBESAND and HACKLÄUBER 1995). Recording 1000 preoperative phlebograms, we found quite a different distribution of insufficient perforators compared with the literature (Table 38.1; Fig. 38.6). Dealing with the concept of varicose recirculation it is important to know that there is a comparably high rate of insufficient perforators to be found at the *outside* (fibular perforators and mid crural veins) and *backside* (insufficient soleus and gastrocnemian points) of the lower leg. Insufficient perforators, as an origin

or peripheral terminal point of recirculation must be detected by diagnosis (Doppler, duplex and phlebography) and should be treated by surgery as an important component of the varicose syndrome. May has therefore called them "key perforators" (MAY 1973). They also give us the key to understanding peripheral CVI (GOTTLOB and MAY 1986).

Table 38.1. Distribution of insufficient perforator veins in 909 pre-operative phlebograms

1. *Upper leg*		
Dodd's perforators	3.1%	
Hunter's perforators	1.9%	5.05%
Hach's perforators	0.05%	
2. *Knee*		
Giacomini vein	2.1%	
Knee perforator	1.4%	3.5%
3. *Lower leg*		
Boyd's perforator	3.2%	
Sherman perforator	9.7%	
Cockett III	17.5%	46.3%
Cockett II	13.3%	
Cockett I	2.6%	
Mid-crural veins	12.9%	12.9%
Gastrocnemian point	16.9%	
Soleus point	9.3%	29.0%
May's perforator	2.3%	
12-cm Perforator	0.3%	
Bassi perforator	0.6%	0.9%

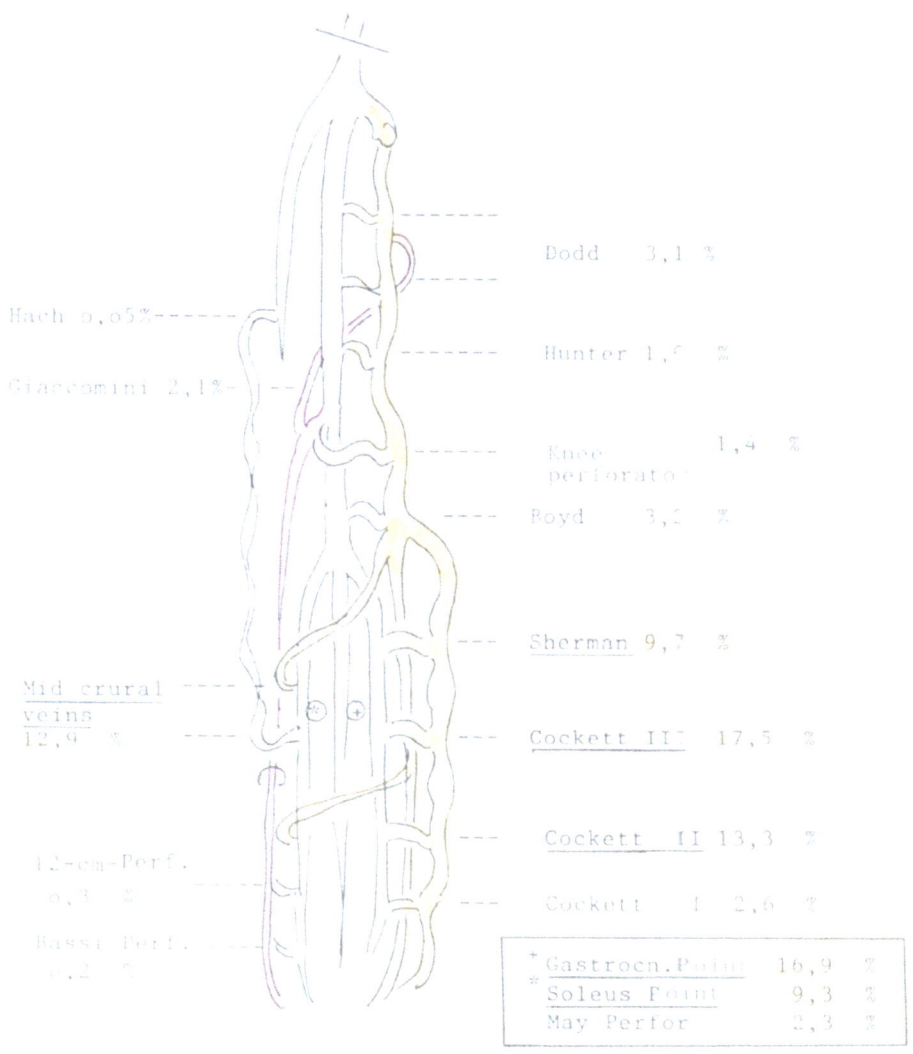

Fig. 38.6. *Perforator veins.* The percentage of insufficient perforators at the back and the lateral border of the lower leg correspond to the number of insufficient Cockett perforators I–III and Sherman's vein at the inner side. (From WEBER and WAGNER 1997, see Table 38.1)

38.2
Definition of CVI

38.2.1
Pathophysiology of CVI

At the level where the venous reflux ends, venous pressure increases more or less permanently, causing venous hypertension (BOLLINGER 1979; NETZER 1979; SCHNEIDER and FISCHER 1979). This may be due to the insufficient orifice of the saphenous veins and to one or multiple incompetent perforators. If the balance of the *blow down* coming from the saphenous trunk, and *blow in* at the level of the basically draining perforators has been lost, the orthostatic pressure and the function of the leg's muscle pumps cause a permanently increased subcutaneous venous pressure sooner or later. There is venous edema inducing infiltration and fibrotic changes of the cutaneous and subcutaneous soft tissues (including the fascia, the ankle joint, and the foot). In consequence, venolymphatic insufficiency leads to cutaneous complications, such as induration, chronic inflammatory and allergic reactions, and chronic venous ulceration (ulcus cruris; EHRINGER 1979; NETZER 1979; SCHNEIDER and FISCHER 1979; WIDMER 1978; WUPPERMANN 1986).

38.2.2
Diagnostic Approach to CVI

Generally, the clinical signs may be evident in a long-lasting varicose syndrome and especially in advanced CVI, showing skin induration, necrosis, and ulceration. However, in earlier stages, showing only slight leg and foot edema, it may be difficult to find a diagnosis (BOLLINGER 1979; WUPPERMANN 1986). Plethysmography can provide information about the disturbances of venous drainage and pump function. Phlebodynamometry, even better allows one to demonstrate the reduced pump function by showing reflux and recovery time, offering quantification of the CVI according to KRIESSMANN (stages I–IV; KRIESSMANN 1975). Doppler and duplex ultrasound can demonstrate the saphenous reflux and blow out coming from insufficient perforators equally as well as phlebography is able to (HACH and HACH-WUNDERLE 1997; PARTSCH 1990; STRAUSS and NEUERBURG-HEUSLER 1997). If one keeps in mind that there are different parameters to be measured by different methods, phlebodynamometry is considered to give the functional "gold standard" by showing the stages of CVI and by applying tourniquet tests which differentiate the various causes responsible for it (PARTSCH 1990; Fig. 38.7).

38.3
Phlebography in Primary Varicosis and CVI

38.3.1
Indications and Contraindications

Phlebography as a so-called invasive method has lost most of its invasiveness since hypo-osmolalic non-ionic contrast media came into use (WEBER and MAY 1990; GOTTLOB and MAY 1986). Nevertheless, anaphylactic (idiosyncratic) reactions may occur in about 1:20000 of patients (WEBER 1991). Also, there are relative contraindications remaining in patients suffering from hyperthyreosis and chronic renal insufficiency (HACH and HACH-WUNDERLE 1997; WEBER 1991).

According to radiation exposure during phleboscopy, pregnant women should not undergo phlebography. Side effects, such as orthostatic reaction following puncture of a foot vein with the patient in an upright position, can be avoided mostly by psychological guidance (Hach and Hach-Wunderle 1997; Weber and May 1990).

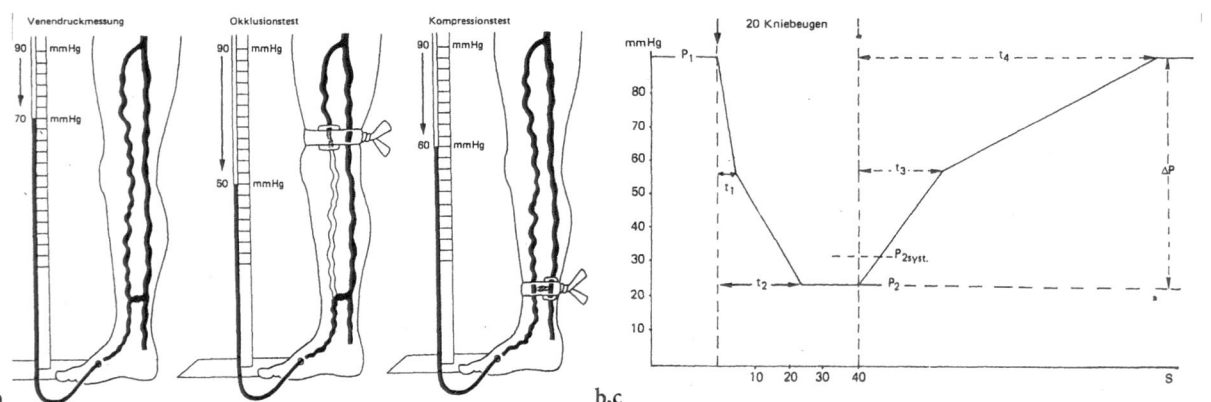

Fig. 38.7 a–d. *Phlebodynamometry* (peripheral direct blood pressure measurements). **a** Testing the peripheral pump function (ankle pump, muscle pump) by bending the knees, the orthostatic pressure decreases to a basic "steady state" (**d**: P_2) and the refilling time at rest (**d**: t_3, t_4) depends on reflux or non-reflux. **b** Occlusion test. By compression (or occlusion) of the insufficient venous trunk reflux is stopped and pressure decreases to the level of the perforator's incompetence. **c** Compression test. Pressure gradient (**d**: ΔP) and refilling time change due to the stop in reflux coming from the compressed perforators (From WEBER and MAY 1990). **d** Phlebodynamometry, standard course. Maximal pump effect during exercise (knee bending, 20 times), P_2; time of refilling of the veins, t_3/t_4; pressure gradient, ΔP. (Phlebodynamometry can be easily associated with ascending leg phlebography, using the needle for both contrast enhancement and pressure measurements; see Fig. 38.8)

38.3.2
Technical Aspects of Phlebography

Basically, the roentgen technique nowadays offers phleboscopy for taking spot films (MAY and NIßL 1973) on a tilted table in a 45-degree upright position of the patient (Fig. 38.8). This is important for making the venous valves visible under fluoroscopy (Fig. 38.9) and for proving the insufficiency of saphenous orifices (see Fig. 38.3) and the incompetence of key-perforators by demonstrating the reflux from the primarily opacified deep venous system to the epifascial space. This may be demonstrated via spontaneous reflux, allthough even better by exercising Valsalva's maneuver (HACH and HACH-WUNDERLE 1997; MAY and NIßL 1973).

Overlapping documentation using plain films at a distance of 1–1.5 m (film:focus) nearly exactly shows pathologic details without magnification.

A standardized documentation technique can be offered; Fig. 38.10 illustrates the strategy of the ascending leg phlebography technique, incorporating Valsalva's maneuver and a "second look" for recording the degree of reflux of contrast medium down to the lowest point of the saphenous veins and its side branches (WEBER and MAY 1990; WEBER 1992).

38.3.3
Ascending Leg Phlebography (ALP) and Varicography (VAR)

Most of the details of primary varicosis needed for an exact planning of surgical therapy can be documented with ALP. However, quality depends on good cooperation between patient and radiologist and from the latter's strategy of contrast injection and current documentation making the varicose findings convincing for the surgeon. Basic information must be offered clearly (Figs. 38.11–38.13). If there are black points in the documentation which do not concur with clinical signs, additional VAR is needed in about 20% of cases (MIGNON 1990). On the whole, details of recirculation via epifascial varicous trunks and side branches (vena saphena accessoria lateralis) and a confusing overlapping of the varicose complex around the soleus and gastrocnemian points can be worked out by direct puncture of the subcutaneous varices (Fig. 38.14). In addition, an unclear anatomy of the central small saphenous vein, as well as recirculation in patients showing post-sclerotherapeutic and post-surgical problems of persistence and recurrence of varices, may indicate VAR (Fig. 38.15).

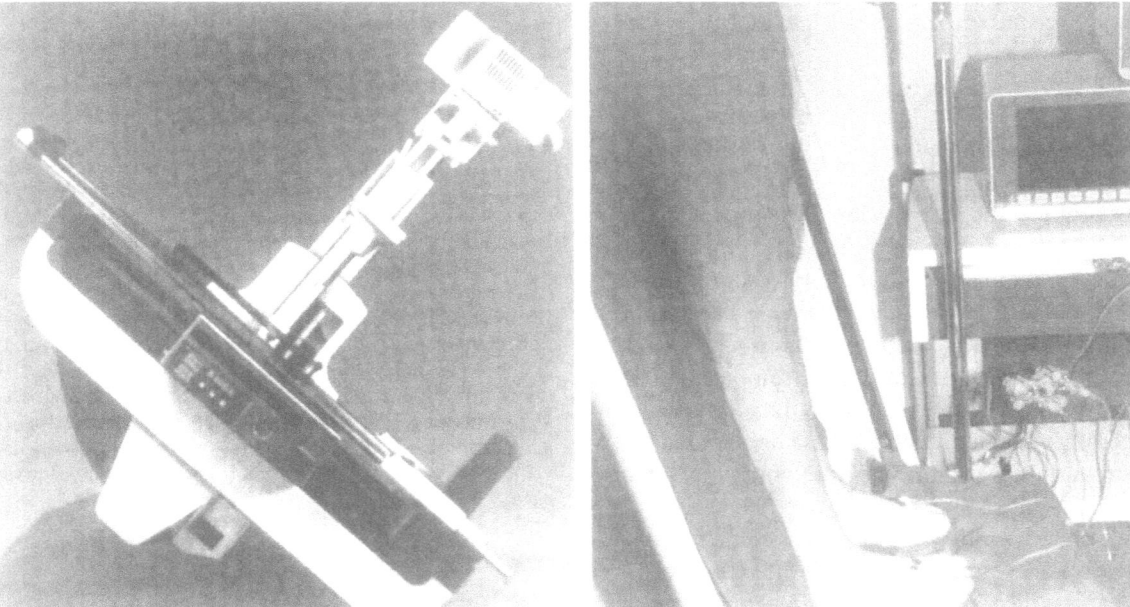

Fig. 38.8 a,b. *Ascending leg phlebography and pressure measurements.* a Overhead postion of the X-ray tube adapted to the tilted table, offering optimal documentation of the venous valves and showing reflux under phleboscopy (MAY and NIßL 1973). b Combination with phlebodynamometry, using the needle on both sides for phlebography (first) and pressure measurements afterwards (see Fig. 38.7d)

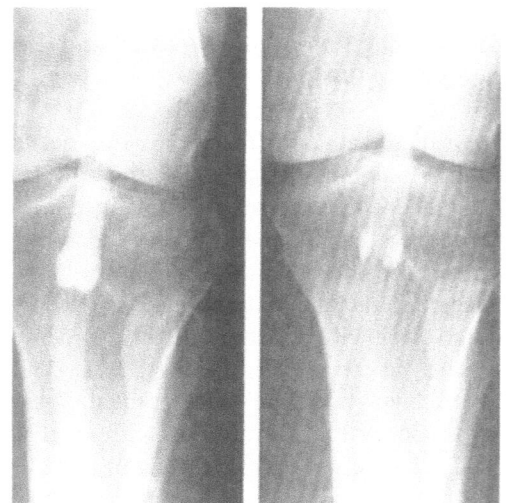

a   b

Fig. 38.9 a,b. *Dynamic phlebography.* Phleboscopy clearly shows the closed functioning valve of the popliteal vein during Valsalva's maneuver (**a**) and the opening wiht venous outflow after (**b**)

However, VAR is considered to be an *additive* method follwing ALP and it should be indicated critically (WEBER and MAY 1990).

Both methods can be performed within one session, and blood pressure measurements may be offered additionally by performing phlebodynamometry subsequently (see Figs. 38.7, 38.8).

38.3.4
Phlebographic Results

It is problematic in our view to compare *accuracy* and *specifity* of phlebography with other methods including Doppler and duplex ultrasound, since all functional tests mentioned above measure different parameters such as volume, venous drainage, and pump function (PARTSCH 1990). Comparing phlebography versus duplex ultrasound, phlebography generally offers more information on pathoanatomy, whereas duplex will primarily demonstrate hemodynamic findings (WEBER and MAY 1990).

Above all, phlebography can demonstrate the whole varicose syndrome, including the deep and superficial diseased veins of the leg, giving an overview of the upper and lower points of insufficiency, showing reflux of blood and signs of the entire recirculation, also allowing direct measurement of the venous calibers, checking the number of

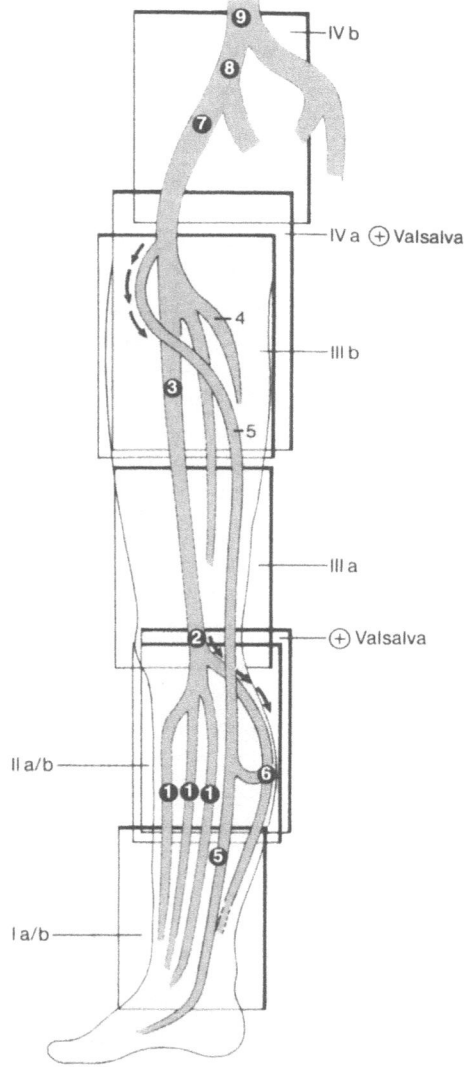

Fig. 38.10. *Ascending leg phlebography, strategy and documentation.* Beginning with the leg *inside*, opacification of the deep veins is achieved using a tourniquet. At the level of the knee a bi-plane documentation serves to detect insufficiency of the short saphenous vein (*arrows*). Valsalva's maneuver is then exercised up to the orifice of the long saphenous vein (*arrows*) in an *outside* position of the leg. Pelvic veins must be documented and reflux to the epifascial varices is followed in a "second look", going backwards down the leg by fluoroscopy (*I–VI*, number of films taken normally). Deep veins, lower leg, *1*; popliteal vein, *2*; superficial femoral vein, *3*; deep femoral vein, *4*; long saphenous vein, *5*; short saphenous vein, *6*; external (*7*) and common (*8*) iliac veins; inferior vena cava, *9*

underestimated (WEBER 1992; WEBER and MAY 1990). In particular, the primary involvement of the deep veins of the leg in venous degeneration and further load, caused by permanent recirculation, can be demonstrated easily with ALP, directly showing the incompetence of venous valves, their reduction, and the level and degree of deep venous reflux under fluoroscopy. Venostasis in the peripheral venous hypertension and all aspects of leakage at the connecting points of the sub- and epifascial veins should be documented and described in primary and secondary varicosis (Fig. 38.17). The degree of peripheral dysfunction, however, should be evaluated by additional functional tests, for instance by combining ALP with phlebodynamometry within one session (WEBER and MAY 1990).

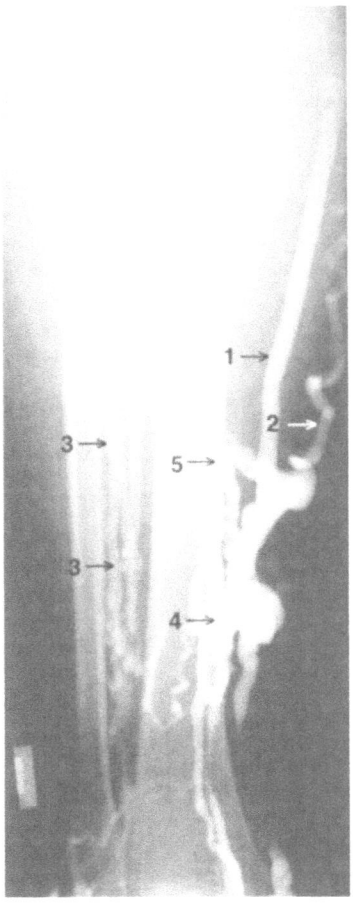

Fig. 38.11. *Cockett perforator's II and III, insufficience.* Primary filling of the deep veins (3) guided by help of a tourniquet. Reflux from perforators Cockett II (4) and Cockett III (5) towards the long saphenous vein (1) and the posterior arcuate vein (2)

functioning and dysfunctioning valves, and showing primary and secondary varicose signs – perhaps in the same patient (Fig. 38.16). Morphometry allows comparison of the de- or re-compensation over time (MELLMANN et al. 1977). According to HACH and HACH-WUNDERLE (1997) the specifity of phlebographic signs ranges from 87% to 96%, and according to NETZER (1979) from 95% to 100%. Varicography helps to complete the preoperative status decisively.

38.3.5
Phlebography and Functional Aspects

In our view, the value of phlebography in its demonstration of hemodynamic changes, has been

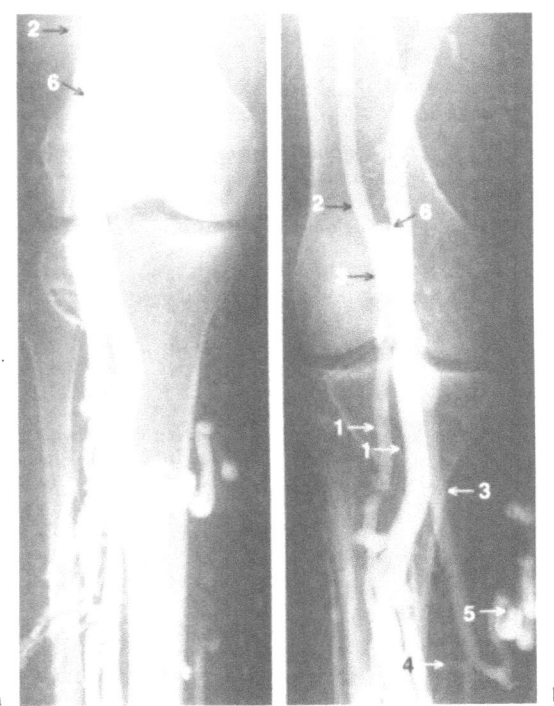

Fig. 38.12 a,b. *Short saphenous vein insufficience.* **a** Sagittal view. Starting with the filling of the popliteal vein, reflux is to be seen under fluoroscopy (6). In an outside lateral view the orifice (6) and the varicose stem of the short saphenous vein (3) are to be seen clearly, separating from the deep veins of the lower leg (1). Varicose side branches at the gastrocnemian point (4, 5). Deep connection of the deep femoral vein with the popliteal vein (2).

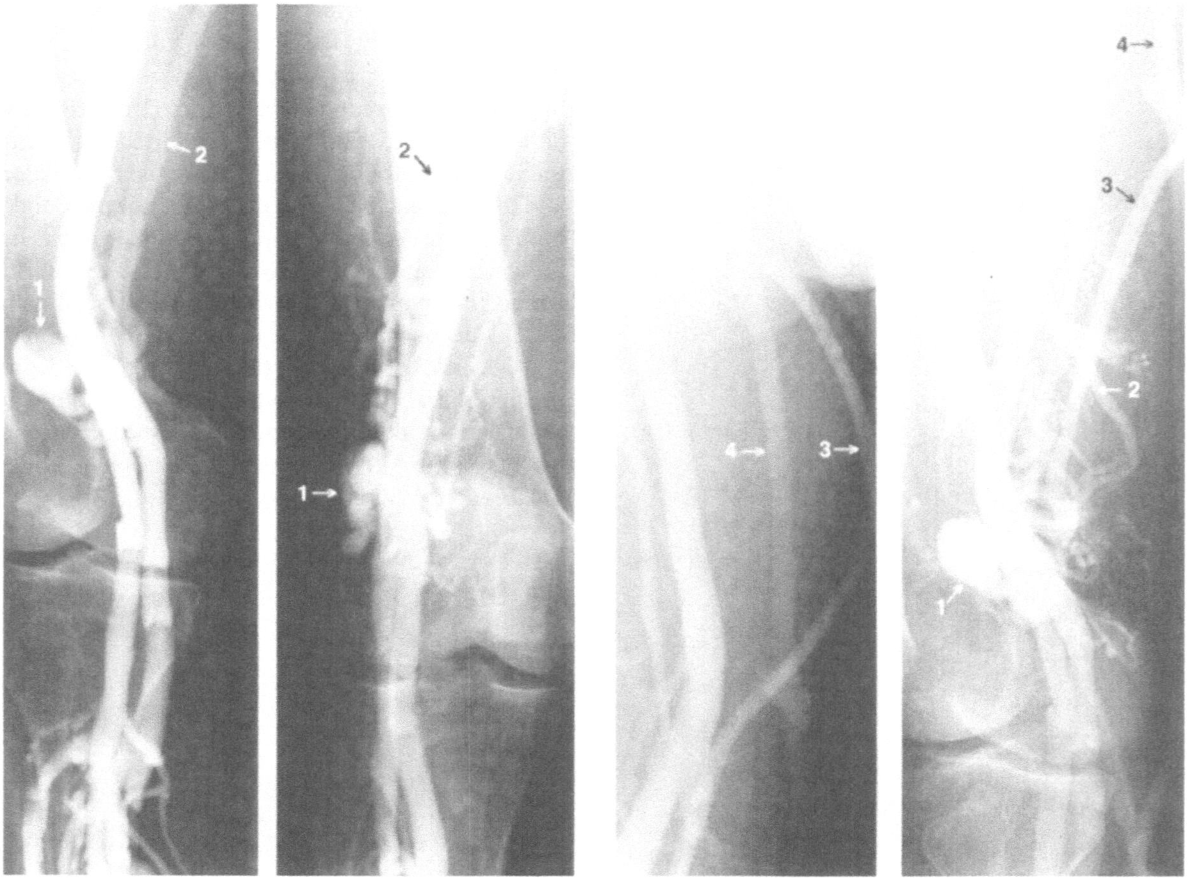

Fig. 38.13 a,b. *Giacomini's varicosis.* **a** In a lateral and sagittal view the popliteal vein shows reflux into an aneurysmatic dilatation of the orifice of the short saphenous vein (*1*) draining into an enlarged ascending venous trunk (*2*). **b** Reflux via the enlarged femoropoplieal vein (*2*) continued via Giacomiani's anastomosis directly to the posterior (medial) accessorian side branch (*3*) of the long saphenous vein (*4*), thus being completely varicosed

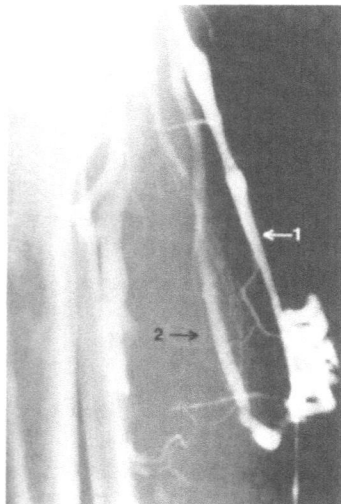

Fig. 38.14. *Gastrocnemian point* (varicography). By direct puncture of the varicose complex at the middle of the calf the dilatated short saphenous vein (*1*) is demonstrated to be insufficient. A perforator may bridge locally to the medial gastrocnemian veins (*2*) subfascially (MAY's perforator)

38.4
Prophylaxis of CVI in Primary Varicosis

38.4.1
Early Diagnosis and Early Adequate Therapy

The clinical discussion of epidemiology – 11% of the average European population show clinical symptoms of varicosis (BORSCHBERG 1967) whereas 57% of adult men and 68% of women show major varices (WIDMER 1978) – tends to differentiate between people with varices and those diseased from varices (MAY 1973). Focusing on many people suffering from CVI over years and even decades and with recurrent complications like phlebitis, thrombophlebitis, phlebothrombosis, and venous ulcer, early diagnosis and active therapy is mandatory (WEBER and MAY 1990). However, the choice of active treatment (sclerotherapy versus surgery, or com-

38.5
Recompensation and Recurrence of Varices

38.5.1
Recompensation of Primary Varices

It is well known in the literature that most of the varices appearing during pregnancy will completely disappear after a while (WUPPERMANN 1986). And in an early stage of varicose syndrome conservative therapy (such as active training, wearing support stockings, etc.) helps to compensate slighter symptoms of reflux and early CVI.

Small varices may be treated successfully by sclerotization. However, in the case of reappearance at the same place, reflux from a distant point of insufficiency (orifice, trunk, main side branches, and insufficient perforators) must be taken into consideration before repeating sclerotherapy. Additional diagnosis is required in this situation to find the leakage and to indicate the appropriate method of therapy.

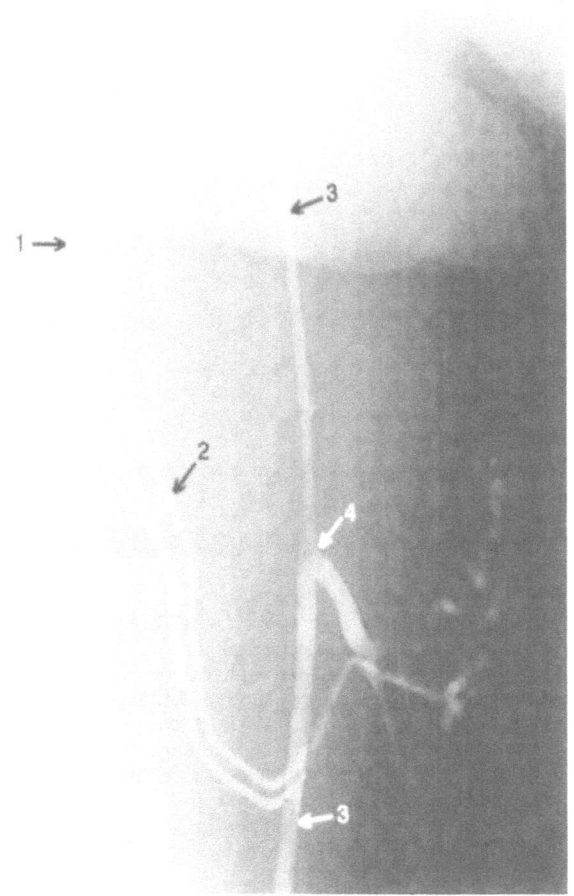

Fig. 38.15. *Incomplete varicosis, long saphenous vein* (varicography). From the superficial femoral vein (*1*) there is a DODD's perforator communication (*2*) connecting with the enlarged middle segment of the long saphenous vein (*3*). The proximal segment is intact. The upper point of recirculation can be clearly identified (*4*)

bined) depends on a precise and systematic diagnostic status of the entire varicose syndrome. Non-invasive techniques may serve to select the diseased patients and to indicate sclerotherapy for the treatment of smaller and limited varices (FISCHER and VOGEL 1987). However, in the advanced varicose syndrome and in patients showing signs of recurrence, phlebography seems to be the method of choice even for the future. It is a "must" if there are hints or clear information about recent deep venous throm-bosis and secondary varicosis as a part of the postthrombotic syndrome (HACH and HACH-WUNDERLE 1997; MAY 1973).

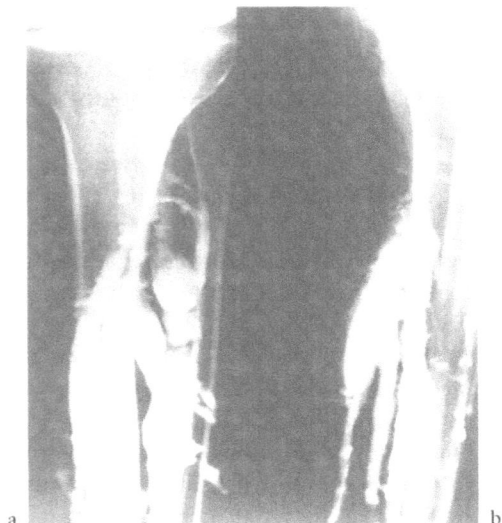

Fig. 38.16 a,b. *Insufficiency of the deep venous system.* Ascending leg phlebography shows a spindle-type enlargement of all deep collecting veins of the lower leg and reduction/dysfunctioning of venous valves. Without manual compression of the ankle area there is direct reflux backwards from the popliteal vein (**a**). Its opacification must be achieved by continuous manual compression (**b**)

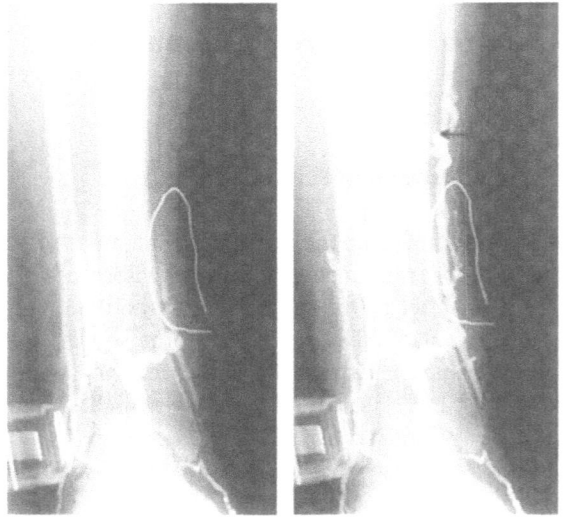

a   b

Fig. 38.17 a,b. *Venous ulcer in varicose syndrome.* A venous ulcer above the medial ankle joint is marked with a preshaped wire. In the early phase of venous contrast filling the deep tibial and fibular veins are opacified above the tourniquet (**a**). As can be seen in a later phase (**b**), an insufficient perforator, type Cockett I, drains back to the epifascial space, filling the varicose long saphenous vein from this point ("blow out"). In addition, Cockett's perforator II (*arrows*) contributes to reflux and chronic venous insufficiency around the skin ulcer

38.5.2
Recurrence of Varices

In the literature the incidence of recurrence of pre-operated varices ranges from 11% to 20% (HACH 1976). There is no literature available, however, quoting the percentage of recurrence following sclerotherapy. Reviewing the different and various surgical techniques which have been applied in the past and which are recommended today, the long-lasting or permanent results of therapy mainly depend on the quality of pre-operative diagnostics and on a corresponding concept and technique of vascular surgery (DODD and COCKETT 1976; HACH 1976; MAY 1973; NETZER 1979).

Special topographical and anatomical problems causing recurrence at the inguinal region and within the popliteal space have been described above (Sect. 38.1.3). Enough time has yet passed to evaluate also the accuracy of Doppler and duplex diagnostic results versus phlebography at these points. But there is no question in our mind that highly qualified ALP (perhaps combined with VAR) can improve the surgical results considerably. It also seems much more evident that there is no real neo-angiogenesis at the level of the ligated and resected vari-

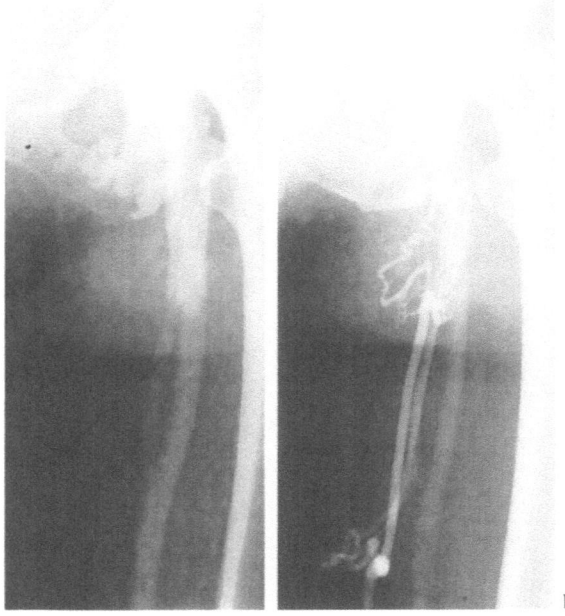

a   b

Fig. 38.18 a,b. *Recurrence of varices.* **a** Three years following crossectomy (e.g., resection of the orifice) and partial stripping of the proximal long saphenous vein, *ascending leg phlebography* shows reflux at the level of the former orifice during Valsalva's maneuver. **b** *Varicography* in addition demonstrates the local inguinal varices guiding reflux towards the persisting proximal part of the lateral ascending side branch, connected with the persisting main trunk of the long saphenous vein at the middle of the upper leg

cose veins against *persistence* of venous structures, leading sooner or later to the recurrence of the primary varicose syndrome (Fig. 38.18).

References

Bjordahl RI (1972) Blood circulation in varicose veins of the lower extremities. In: Schneider KW (ed) Die venöse Insuffizienz. Witzstrock, Baden Baden

Bollinger A (1979) Funktionelle Angiologie. Lehrbuch und Atlas. Thieme, Stuttgart

Borschberg E (1967) The prevalence of varicose veins in the lower extremities. Karger, Basel

Brunner U (1979) Suprainguinaler Zugang zur Krossektomie. In: Brunner U (ed) Die Leiste. Huber, Bern

Cockett FB, Jones DE (1953) The ankle blow out syndrome. A new approach to the varicose ulcer problem. Lancet 1:17

Dodd A, Cockett FB (1976) The pathology and surgery of the veins of the lower limb. Churchill Livingstone, Edinburgh

Ehringer H (1979) Venöse Abflußstörungen. Enke, Stuttgart

Fischer R, Vogel P (1987) Die Resultate der Strippingoperation bei der Vena saphena parva. VASA 16:349–351

Gottlob R, May R (1986) Venous valves. Springer, Vienna New York

Hach W (1976) Ursache und Therapie der Rezidivvarikose. In: Ludwig H, Kurz E (eds) Die Beckenvenen. Schattauer, Stuttgart

Hach W, Hach-Wunderle V (1997) Phlebography and sonography of the veins. Springer, Berlin Heidelberg New York

Kriessmann A (1975) Periphere Phlebodynamometrie. Grundlagen, Technik, Leistungsbreite. VASA Suppl 4:1–35

van Limborgh J (1965) Anatomie der Venae communicantes. Zentralbl Phlebol 4:268

May R (1973) Chirurgie der Bein- und Beckenvenen. Thieme, Stuttgart

May R, Nißl R (1973) Die Phlebographie der unteren Extremität. Thieme, Stuttgart

Mellmann J, Wuppermann Th, Jarosch V, Schweder W (1977) Zur Morphometrie primärer Varizen. Fortschr Rontgenstr 126:205

Mignon G (1990) Technik der Varikographie. In: Weber J, May R (ed) Funktionelle Phlebologie. Thieme, Stuttgart New York

Netzer CO (1979) Die primäre Varikose. In: Ehringer H, Fischer H, Netzer CO, Schmutzer R, Zeitler E (eds) Venöse Abflußstörungen. Enke, Stuttgart

Partsch H (1990) Apparative Funktionstests. In: Weber J, May R (1990) Funktionelle Phlebologie. Thieme, Stuttgart

Partsch H (1991) Compression therapy of the legs. A review. J Dermatol Surg Oncol 17(10):799–805

Partsch H, Staubesand J (1981) Venae perforantes. Urban und Schwarzenberg, Munich

Ritter H, Loose DA (1989) Venous aneurysms and surgical therapy. In: Belov St, Loose DA, Weber J (eds) Vascular malformations. Einhorn Presse, Reinbek

Schneider H, Fischer H (1979) Die chronisch-venöse Insuffizienz. Enke, Stuttgart

Staubesand J, Hackländer A (1995) The topography of the perforating veins on the medial side of the leg. Clin Anat 8(6):399–402

Strauss AL, Neuerburg-Heusler D (1997) Doppler- und Duplex-Sonographie bei venösen Abflußstörungen. In: Zeitler E (ed) Arterien und Venen. Diagnostik mit bildgebenden Verfahren. Springer, Berlin Heidelberg New York

Weber J (1978) Röntgenologische Diagnostik der Varizen der unteren Extremitäten. Langenbecks Arch Chir 347:209–215

Weber J (1991) Kontrastmittel-bedingte Nebenwirkungen und Komplikationen der Phlebographie. Peters PE, Zeitler E (eds) Röntgen-Kontrastmittel, Nebenwirkungen, Prophylaxe, Therapie. Springer, Berlin Heidelberg New York

Weber J (1992) Phlebographie – Qualitätssicherung. In: Peters PE, Zeitler E, Clauß W (eds) Qualitätssicherung bei der Anwendung von Kontrastmitteln. Springer, Berlin Heidelberg New York

Weber J, May R (1990) Funktionelle Phlebologie. Thieme, Stuttgart New York

Widmer LK (1978) Venenkrankheiten. Häufigkeit und sozialmedizinische Bedeutung. Basler Studie III. Huber, Bern

Wuppermann Th (1986) Varizen, Ulkus cruris und Thrombose. Springer, Berlin Heidelberg New York

39 Prevention of Pulmonary Embolism

J. WEBER

CONTENTS

39.1
Incidence of Pulmonary Embolism

According to VOLLMAR (1990) there were approximately 600 000 cases of iliofemoral venous thromboses in Germany in 1982 (23). HEINRICH and KLINK (1981) have calculated that 25%–50% of deep venous thomboses may lead to pulmonary embolism (PE). BENEKE (1973) calculated lethal complications of PE at 24.7%. In the USA the incidence of lethal PE has been estimated at 50 000–200 000 patients every year (ZWAAN et al. 1995). According to SCHWARZ (1965) there is an increasing tendency of severe PE in the First World in spite of mechanical and chemical prophylaxes to be discussed.

PE is generally said to originate from deep venous thrombosis of the lower limb and from the iliofemoral space (BENEKE 1985; BROWSE 1976; GREEN-FIELD et al. 1973; HEINRICH and KLINK 1981; STRAUB 1982; WEBER 1990), two thirds embolizing from the external pelvic veins (BROWSE 1976) and 10%–15% from the inferior vena cava (HEINRICH and KLINK 1981).

One of the most serious problems of PE was pointed out by SCHWARZ: only in 10.6% of patients the diagnosis of PE was made before death (SCHWARZ 1965). According to BENEKE (1985) the diagnosis of deep venous thrombosis was suggested in 17% of patients prior to PE and clearly identified in 24.7% of his patients afterwards. The incidence of recurrent PE was calculated by DE WEESE (1973) at about 5%.

According to SCHLOSSER (1979/1980, in WEBER 1990), the complication of clinically relevant PE must be expected postoperatively in 25%–40% of patients undergoing general surgery, and after surgical intervention in trauma in as much as in 40%–55% of cases.

Nowadays, another patient group must be taken into account: foudroyant PE during fibrinolytic therapy has an incidence of up to 6% (GRIMM et al. 1990; MARTIN and EICKERLING 1990; ZWAAN et al. 1995).

This clinical background indicates prophylaxis for the prevention of PE (Table 39.1) and recurrent embolic complications, originating from acute and subacute deep femoral and iliofemoral venous thromboses. PE originating from other venous spaces is generally considered to be very rare (BENEKE 1985; BROWSE 1976; HEINRICH and KLINK 1981; SCHWARZ 1965; STRAUB 1982).

Table 39.1. Situations of high risk for pulmonary embolism

- Hip surgery
- Prostate surgery
- Heart infarction with complications
- Long hospital stays

39.2
Indications for Active Prevention

39.2.1
Recurrence of PE

The incidence of recurrent PE is generally estimated to be relatively low (DE WEESE 1973; HEINRICH and KLINK 1981; WEBER 1990). This complication, however, must be discussed critically according to the individual situation of the patient (Table 39.2).

JÜRGEN WEBER, MD, Professor, Institut für Röntgendiagnostik und Interventionelle Radiologie, DRK-Krankenhaus, Suurheid 20, 22559 Hamburg-Rissen, Germany

Table 39.2. Indications for active prevention of pulmonary embolism (PE)

- Recurrence of PE
- Floating thrombus in the iliac or superficial femoral veins
- Patients with contraindication against coagulation

According to SCHLOSSER (in WEBER 1990) lethal PE still occurs in 0.1–0.5% of patients who have been operated on. A relatively higher rate of severe PE is estimated in patients undergoing orthopedic hip endoprosthesis (VOLLMAR 1981), abdominal, and thoracic surgical interventions, especially in malignant diseases (GRIMM et al. 1990). Prophylactic filtering of the inferior vena cava is therefore very popular in the USA and in France prior to thoracic, abdominal, and pelvic surgery (WEBER 1990; ZWAAN et al. 1995).

39.2.2
Location and Age of Thrombi

A "floating thrombus" is frequently estimated to be a higher potential risk for causing PE (WEBER 1990). However, Doppler, duplex, and phlebographic findings of a free tip of thrombosis infiltrating the deep veins of the limb or ascending to the iliac veins depend on clinical suspicion leading to diagnosis, and it is well known that the clinical signs of thrombosis are very unclear in the early stages of clotting and venous occlusion (FERRIS 1981; WEBER 1990).

The incidence of PE, however, increases significantly from the level of the popliteal to iliac and iliocaval spaces (BROWSE 1976; HEINRICH and KLINK 1981; ZWAAN et al. 1995).

For this reason the signs of a "fresh" and "floating" thrombus in the ilio-femoral and ilio-caval veins may indicate prophylactic application of vena cava filters, especially in high-risk patients. Focusing the risk of recurrence in patients with acute iliofemoral thrombosis and post-thrombotic syndrome (PTS), pulmonary hypertension is considered an indication for pro-phylactic filtering (GRIMM et al. 1990; MOBIN-UDDIN et al. 1967; VOLLMAR 1981; WEBER 1990).

39.2.3
Arguments Against Filtering

There are many reports of complications of caval filtering, beginning with severe caval thrombosis caused by ligation, clipping, and plication (DE WEESE 1973; WEBER 1990). There are also specific risks of local damage to the veins at the puncture site due to the relatively large calibers of the application catheter devices used (DARCY and CASTANEDA-ZUNIGA 1990; FERRIS 1981; GÜNTHER et al. 1985; WEBER 1990).

Filter damage to the wall of the inferior vena cava, migration and fragmentation of the filters all cause additional risks associated with this method (MIERSCH et al. 1991).

Misplacement of filters also reduces the value of mechanical protection against PE (FERRIS 1981; PRICE et al. 1983). Even under optimal conditions pulmonary transport causing severe and lethal complications have been described (MIERSCH et al. 1991; PERRY and WELLS 1993; ZWAAN et al. 1995). VOLLMAR (1981) therefore recommended restrictive indication of caval filtering, emphasizing his concern about prophylactic handling of permanent filtering devices (VOLLMAR 1981).

39.3
Inferior Vena Caval Filters

39.3.1
Permanent Filters

Starting with MOBIN-UDDIN's umbrella filter in 1967, commercially available filtering devices have been used by surgeons since 1970 with increasing frequency (MOBIN-UDDIN et al. 1967). A high rate of caval thromboses, however, originate from the silastic membrane: a 40% rate of thrombotic complications against 0.3% of recurrent PE was a high price (FERRIS 1981).

The KIMRAY-GREENFIELD filter opened a new area of active prevention of PE (GREENFIELD et al. 1973, 1981). The application of filters was then possible via the transfemoral and transjugular approaches by venae sectio. The risk of caval thrombotic obstruction was reduced to about 3%; however, the rate of PE increased to 8%, caused by widespreading pricks of the filter and its tendency to tilt from its axial position in the middle of the caval space (PRICE et al. 1983). An "autocentring filter" (Fig. 39.1), which modified the Greenfield type, led to a smaller application catheter sheath, offering a percutaneous approach for SELDINGER's technique and for radiologists (WEBER 1990).

The "bird's nest" filter, designed by GIANTURCO, ANDERSON, and WALLACE since 1980 was able to

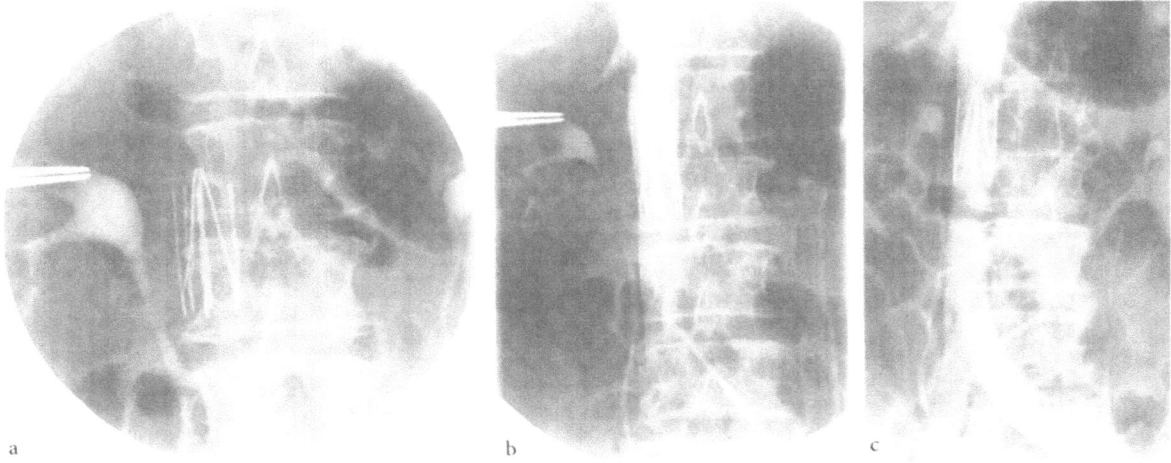

Fig. 39.1 a–c. *Permanent LGM caval filter.* Recurrent pulmonary embolism in post-thrombotic syndrome. **a** *Plain film* showing LGM "autocentring" filter in position. (The connection of the renal veins with the inferior vena cava is marked on the right side). **b** *Cavography* performed via the application catheter clearly shows renal inflow. **c** *Control-cavography* 2 months later: identical position of the functioning filter. No clotting

increase filtering abilities by creating a "nest" of tortuous thin wire, pushed via the application catheter and fixed between two pricks at the level of the subrenal inferior vena cava (ROEHN et al. 1985, Fig. 39.2).

GÜNTHER et al. (1985) designed another type of caval filter in 1985 which offered permanent and temporary placement by means of a small hook to be caught for withdrawal. The convenient design of this filter, however, was complemented by defects in the stainless steel material, causing the disintegration of the filter and the migration of fragments, (MIERSCH et al. 1993) or the whole fiter, into the heart or into pulmonous arteries.

39.3.1.1
Positioning of Filters

When compared with the surgical application of the Kimray-Greenfield filters by means of venae sectio, Seldinger's technique of percutaneous access has several advantages: puncture and insertion of the catheter sheath can be done easily under local anesthesia, using catheter devices of up to maximal 10F.

Under *fluoroscopic* guidance cavography and the positioning of the application catheter can be managed with full control, finding the optimal point at which to unfold the filter. The different types of filters available do require different delivery techniques from the applicator. Today's high resolution x-ray video and digital subtraction angiography (DSA) techniques make it possible to visualize, document, and control the positioning procedure under optimal conditions.

39.3.1.2
Cavography

Contrast enhancement of the inferior vena cava is extremly important prior to filter application. The decision of which way to access depends on the patency of the iliac veins and inferior vena cava or the extent of thrombotic obstruction on this level. If the caval vein is directly affected by thrombus formation, the transjugular or transbrachial approach is obligatory (Fig. 39.3). All filter devices should be applied from the right side if possible in order to avoid kinking and damage to the applicator.

The diameter of the inferior vena cava should be measured in order to apply the appropriate filter size (PRICE et al. 1983). The average diameter of the vein ranges from 13 to 30 mm, and in 3% of cases more than 28 mm must be calculated for. Shifting and migration of filters is mainly due to an inappropriate filter which is too small to become securely attached to the venous wall (PRICE et al. 1983; WEBER 1990).

The optimal position of a permanent filter is just below the orifices of the renal veins (Fig. 39.4) If there are anatomical variations, such as a duplicated inferior vena cava or additional left-sided renal branch as in the so-called "circum-aortic ring", cavography should show this in order to avoid mis-positioning of

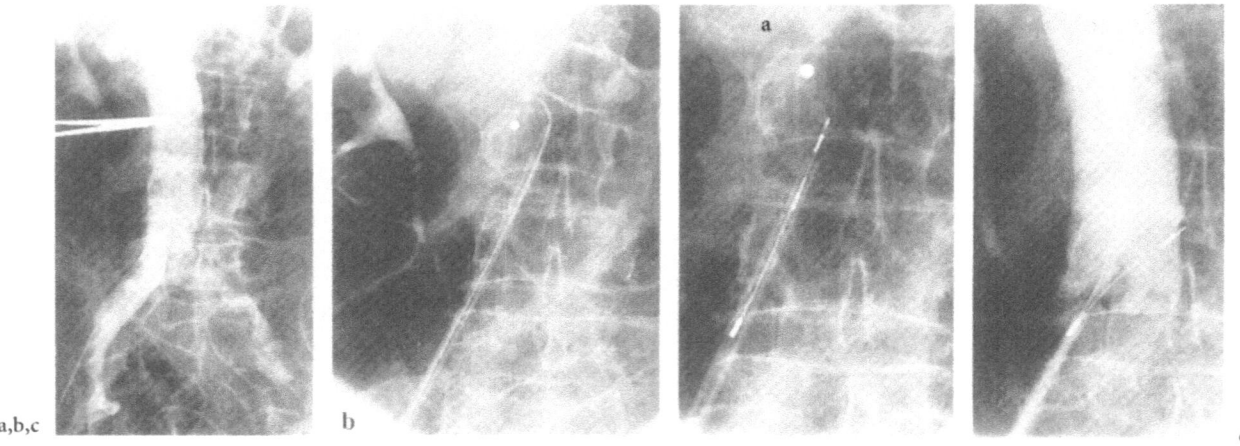

a,b,c   b   d

Fig. 39.2 a–f. *Permanent "bird's nest" filter.* Indication: Recurrent pulmonary embolism following left-sided il- iofemoral venous thrombosis. **a** *Inferior cavography* from the right femoral side: large diameter of the inferior vena cava (∅ 28 mm). Marking of the upper position of the filter to access. **b** Application device and guide wire in position. **c** Compressed filter system inside the applicator in posi- tion. **d** Fixing of the upper prick of the bird's nest filter. **e** Both upper and lower pricks in position, forming the frame of the bird's nest. (The two nearby invisible wires are netting in between the pricks.) **f** Cavography 8 days later shows the functioning of the filter without clotting

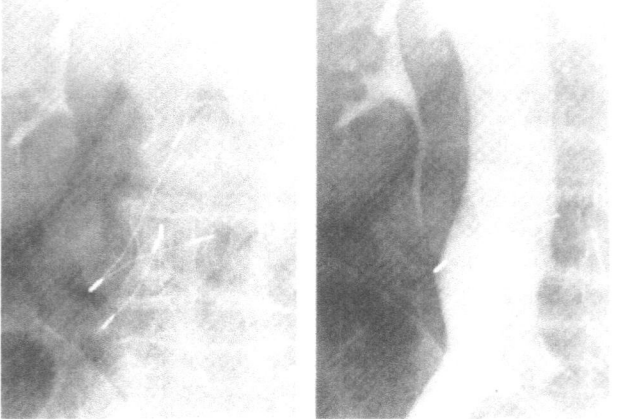

e,f

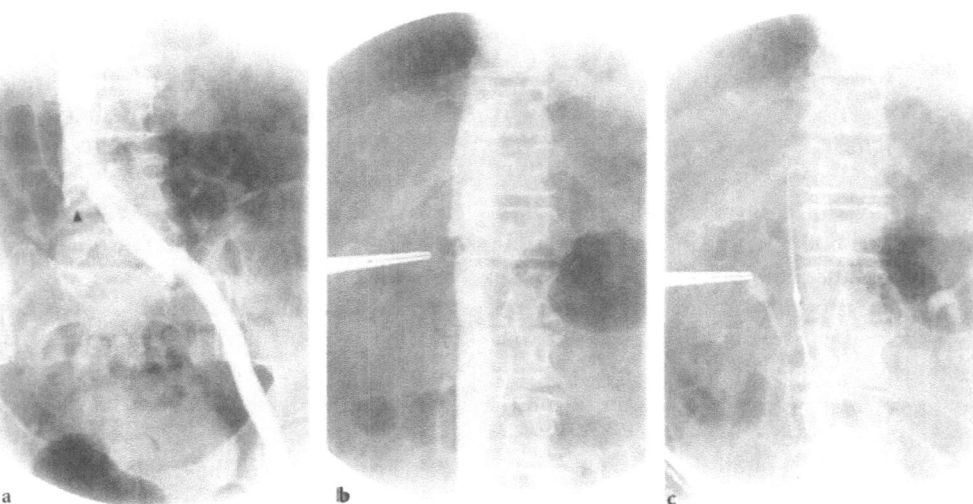

a   b   c

Fig. 39.3 a–c. *Cavography prior to filtering.* **a** *Phlebography* from the left femoral vein, showing the upper point of a right-sided common iliac thrombus. **b** *Cavography* in the following shows a normal caliber (∅ 22 mm) and the inflow from the right renal vein (marking by clamp). **c** *Positioning of the application catheter* on the left-sided transfemoral route

the filter, which in most cases cannot be corrected when using permanent filters without the danger of damaging the intimal wall (WEBER 1990).

Opacification can be managed by ascending leg venography, improving the contrast by DSA. If the situation has been assessed before hand and a superior access on the jugular and transbrachial side has already been decided upon, opacification of the caval vein can be carried out by direct contrast injection via the application catheter.

The long-term results of permanent filter placement have been analyzed comparing different types of filter devices (FERRIS 1981; GREENFIELD et al. 1981; MIERSCH et al. 1991; PERRY and WELLS 1983). For various different types have been presented in the literature (AMPLATZ 1985; DARCY and CASTANEDA-ZUNIGA 1990). In general terms, they all have advantages and disadvantages as regards application, the effect of the filtering and the balance of thrombotic clotting inside the filter (Fig. 39.5) compared with the rate of thrombi passing the filter and causing PE. Temporary filtering, therefore, is gaining increasing attention for the prevention of PE over a certain short period of high risk.

39.3.2
Temporary Filters

Even the very first description of a suitable filter device dealt with this subject. EICHELTER and SCHENK 1968 (in WEBER 1990) experimented with a preliminary, handmade catheter with a pre-shaped, basket-like tip.

The temporary filtering catheters currently available generally originate from the DORMIA basket-catheter principle whereby a metalic basket consisting of six thin branches is opened by pushing them through a co-axial catheter tip (Fig. 39.6).

Having positioned the closed catheter, the basket will be opened under fluoroscopy and fixed to the handle or lock of the catheter outside the patient. Opacification of the caval vein can be repeated by contrast injection into the catheter itself. Fixed to the skin at the level of percutaneous insertion, the catheter even allows the patient to get up. The transjugular approach, therefore, seems to have some advantages over transbrachial access: by elevating the arm the filtering basket will move and shift away from the optimal position. On the other hand, moving prevents thrombotic adaption to the intimal wall.

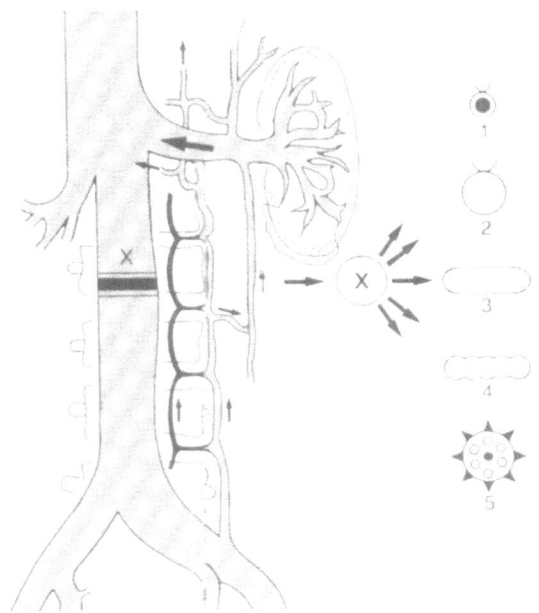

Fig. 39.4. *Caval filtering.* All techniques applied for total caval ligation (*1*), partial ligation (*2*), clipping (*3*), plication (*4*), and filtering (*5*) tend to approach a level of the inferior cava closely below its communication with the renal veins, reducing the incidence of caval thrombotic occlusion

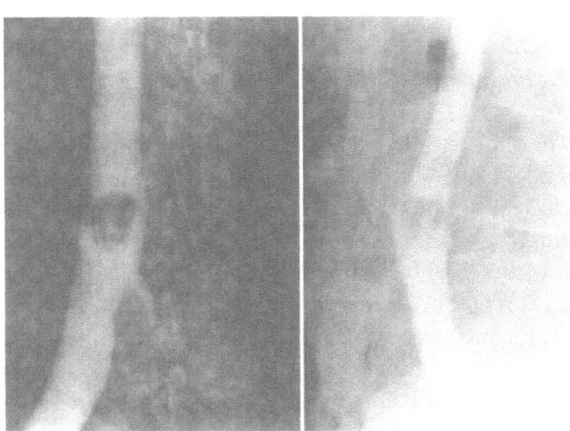

Fig. 39.5. *Filter clotting.* A permanent *Mobbin-Uddin umbrella filter* was positioned 5 days previously. Clotting of a thrombus within the caval filter is shown at the upper level of the silastic membrane in both projections.

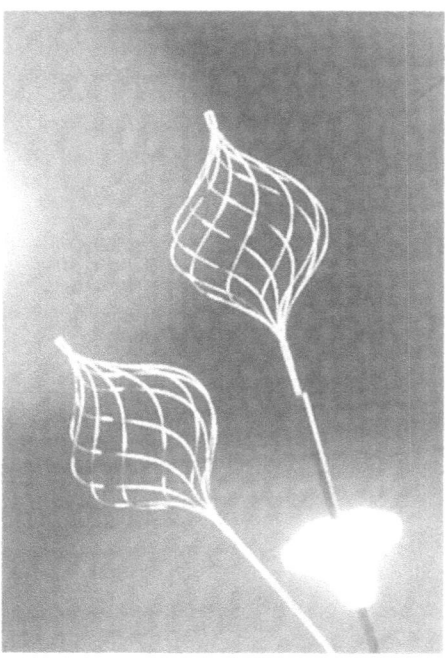

Fig. 39.6. *Temporary caval filtering.* The design of the *Günther-Cook filter* is based on the Dormia basket catheter principle. After withdrawal to the puncture side, the catheter shaft serves as a lock which can be fixed at the skin. Transfemoral, transbrachial, and transjugular approaches are possible

39.3.2.1
Preliminary Results

There have only been a few reports in the literature since 1995; ZWAAN et al. (1995) published their clinical findings among 49 patients using Cook, Angiocor, and Antheor filters in the transjugular, transbrachial, and transfemoral route. ZWAAN and LORCH (1997) completed the report in another multicenter study, including the Cordis filter in a total of 192 patients (43 post-operative patients, 120 patients during fibrinolytic therapy, 31 pre-operative cases).

Vos et al. (1997) reported on 86 patients undergoing temporary filtering with the removable "tulip filter" (GÜNTHER et al. 1985). The technique for inserting and removing the filter is comparable with the former GÜNTHER basket filter (Fig. 39.7a,b); retrieval is carried out by catching the hook at the tip of the filter. The mean follow-up period lasted a total of 136 days. Removal was only carried out in 25 patients over 2–14 days after insertion. The indications for filtering have not been discussed.

39.3.2.2
Prospective Indications

Given VOLLMAR's position (1981) the temporary placement of caval filters may open new perspectives of prophylactic and preventive installations (WEBER 1990). However, there is only a limited time during which temporary filters are safe. In contact with the venous intima the reins of the filter tend to be adapted to the venous wall by local clot formation and sprouting of neo-intima (NEUBURG et al. 1997; WEBER 1990). It has been recommended, therefore, to remove the filtering device at latest 8 days after its incorporation (GÜNTHER et al. 1985; NEUBURG et al. 1997), and heparinization is considered obligatory during application and the time of its functioning (Vos et al. 1997; ZWAAN et al. 1995).

Problems may also occur if there are clot-formations inside the filtering basket at the time of planned removal. This happened in 32 of 192 patients (ZWAAN and LORCH 1997). Besides that, pulmonary transport of major thrombi causing severe PE was reported in 11 patients, and causing death in three of them under fibrinolythic therapy (Fig. 39.8a–e).

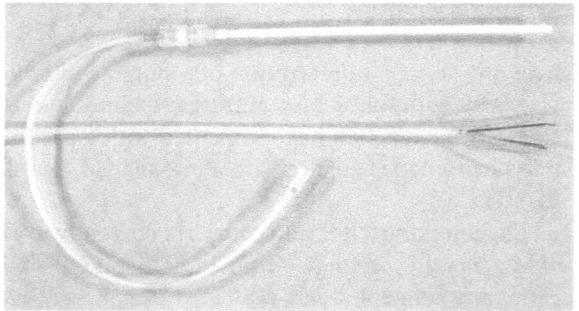

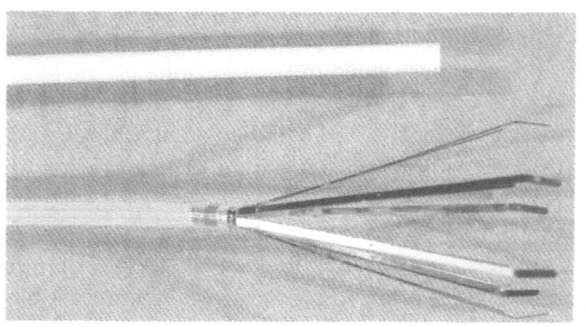

Fig. 39.7 a,b. *Temporary caval filtering.* The configuration and function of the *LGT filter* (Braun, Melsungen) derives from the Kimray-Greenfield filter type. Application is similar to the Günther filter. The internal application catheter can be connected directly to an external catheter, to be used for drug administration and contrast enhancement

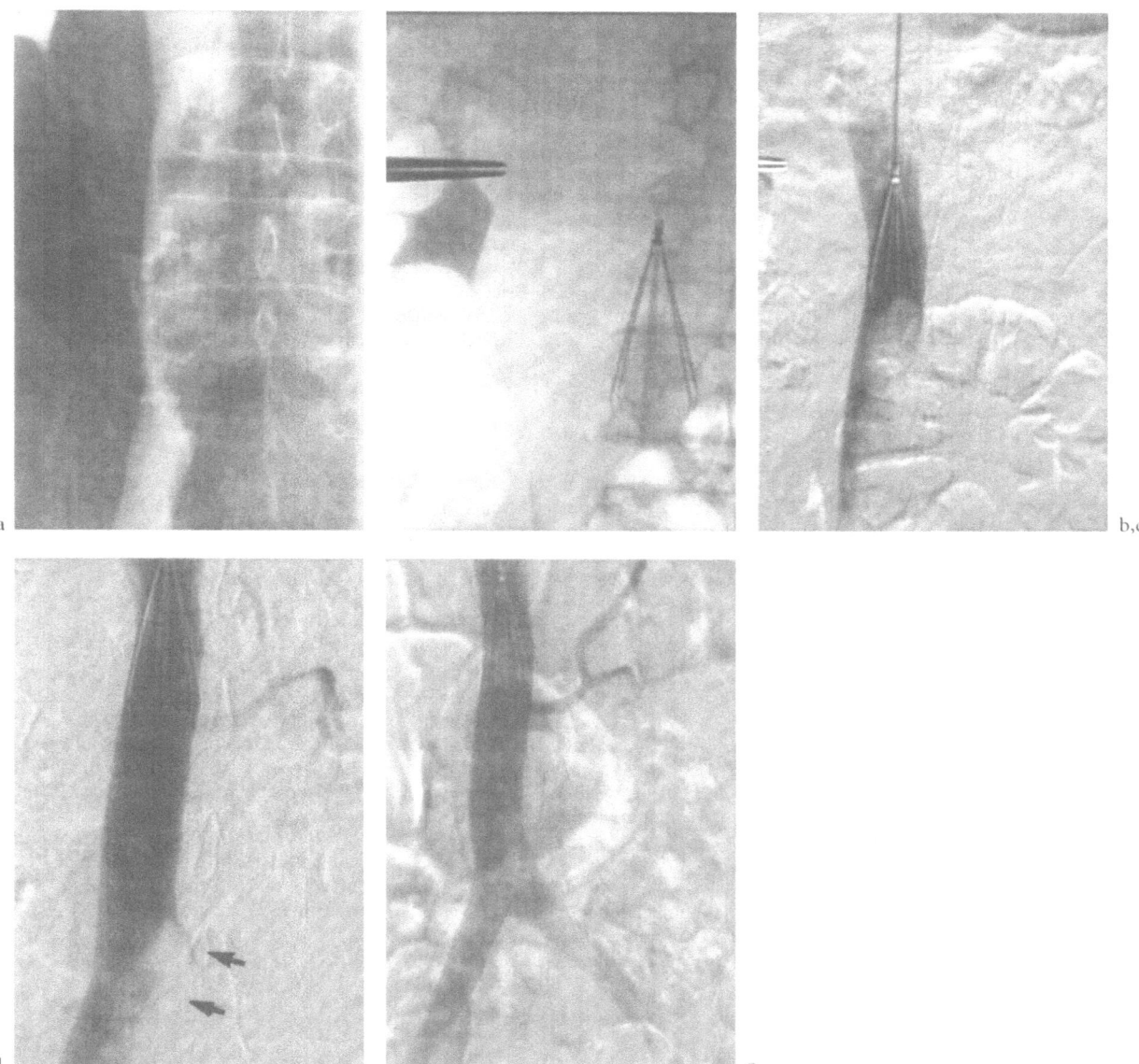

Fig. 39.8 a–e. *Temporary caval filtering.* Recurrent pulmonary embolism in a 46-year-old woman leads to phlebography and streptokinase (SK)-fibrinolytic therapy, protected by a temporary *LGT caval filter.* **a** Large thrombus growing from the left comon iliac vein, as demonstrated from the right side. **b** Transjugular approach and positioning of the filter at the optimal infrarenal level of the inferior vena cava. **c** *Cavography* using the shaft of the filter for contrast enhancement shows the caval thrombus below the filter just after its application. **d** *First control*: during SK-fibrinolysis on the seocnd day the caval thrombus has resolved incompletely. **e** *Second control*: 5 days after filtering and the beginning of the fibrinolytic therapy the caval and comon iliac thrombi have been resolved completely without embolic complications. (Contrast enhancement via the shaft of the filtering catheter using Valsalva's maneuver)

Nevertheless the protective effect of temporary caval filtering seems to reduce the number of cases of severe PE during the most dangerous period of invasive therapy (fibrinolytic and surgical) (GÜNTHER et al. 1985; Vos et al. 1997; ZWAAN et al. 1995; ZWAAN and LORCH 1997) without the various disadvantages of a permanent filter.

In our opinion, however, a restrictive policy for indicating permanent and temporary filtering should be maintained and the handling of filters should be reserved for experienced angiographers and interventional radiologists.

References

Amplatz K (1985) New developements in caval filters. In: Donner MW, Heuck FH (eds) Radiology today 3. Springer, Berlin Heidelberg New York

Beneke G (1985) Pathologie der Venenerkrankungen. In: Haid-Fischer F, Haid H (eds) Venenerkrankungen. Phlebologie für Klinik und Praxis. Thieme, Stuttgart

Browse NL (1976) The general problem of thromboembolism. In: Dodd H, Cockett FB (eds) The pathology and surgery of the veins of the lower limb. Churchill Livingstone, Edinburgh

Darcy M, Castaneda-Zuniga WR (1990) Percutaneous vena cava filtering. In: Dondelinger RF, Rossi P, Kurdziel JC, Wallace S (eds) Interventional radiology. Thieme, Stuttgart, pp 706–716

De Weese JA (1973) Unterbrechung der Vena cava inf. bei Lungenembolien. In: May R (ed) Chirurgie der Bein- und Beckenvenen. Thieme, Stuttgart

Ferris EJ (1981) Mobin-Uddin filter – with emphasis on follow-up results. In: May R, Weber J (eds) Pelvic and abdominal veins. Excerpta Medica, Amsterdam

Greenfield LJ, McCourdy JR, Brown PP, Elkins RC (1973) A new intracaval filter permitting continued flow and resolution of emboli. Surgery 73:599

Greenfield LJ, Peyton R, Crute S (1981) Greenfield technique for catheter pulmonary embolectomy and vena cava filter insertion. In: May R, Weber J (1981) (eds) Pelvic and abdominal veins. Excerpta Medica, Amsterdam

Grimm W, Schwieder G, Wagner T (1990) Tödliche Lungenembolie bei Bein-Beckenvenenthrombose unter Lysetherapie. Dtsch Med Wochenschr 115:1183

Günther R, Schild H, Fries A, Stöckel S (1985) Vena cava filter to prevent pulmonary embolism. Experimental study. Radiology 156:315

Heinrich F, Klink K (1981) Lungenembolie. Springer, Berlin Heidelberg New York

Martin M, Eickerling B (1990) Tödliche Lungenembolien unter ultrahochdosierter Streptokinasebehandlung. Dtsch Med Wochanschr 115:1812

Miersch G, Münster W, Schöpke W, Stobbe G, Kornotzki M, Hasert V (1991) Kavafilter nach Günther. Ergebnisse von Langzeitkontrollen. VASA 32 Suppl:279

Mobin-Uddin K, Martinez LO, Jude JR (1967) A vena cava filter for the prevention of pulmonary embolus. Surg Forum 18:209

Neuburg JM, Günther RW, Vorwerk D, Dondelinger RF, Jäger H et al. (1997) Results of a multicenter study of the retrievable tulip vena cava filter: early clinical erperience. Cardiovasc Intervent Radiol 20:10

Perry JN, Wells IP (1993) A long term follow-up of Günther vena cava filters. Clin Radiol 48:35

Price MR, Novelline RA, Athanasoulis CA, Simon M (1983) The diameter of the inferior vena cava and its implications for the use of vena caval filters. Radiology 149:637

Roehn JOF, Gianturco C, Barth HM (1985) Percutaneous interruption of the inferior vena cava: the bird's nest filter. In: Bergan JJ, Yao JST (eds) Surgery of the veins. Grune and Stratton, Orlando

Schwarz SI (1965) Diagnosis of thrombembolic disease. J Cardiovasc Surg (Torino) 7 [Suppl] p 127

Straub H (1982) Letale Komplikationen der Fibrinolyse. MMW 124:17

Vollmar J (1981) Considerations on the question: V. cava interruption or reconstruction. In: May R, Weber J (eds) Pelvic and abdominal veins. Excerpta Medica Amsterdam

Vos LD, Tielbeek AV, Bom EP, Gooszen HC, Vroegindeweij D (1997) The Günther temporary inferior vena cava filter for short-term protection against pulmonary embolism. Cardiovasc Intervent Radiol 20:91

Weber J (1990) Filterung der unteren Hohlvene bei Thromembolie. In: Weber J, May R (1990) Funktionelle Phlebologie. Phlebographie, Funktionstests, Interventionelle Radiologie. Thieme, Stuttgart

Zwaan M, Lorch H (1997) Multicenterstudie "Temporäre Cavafilter": Vorläufige Ergebnisse. Röfo 166 Suppl 1:17

Zwaan M, Kagel C, Marienhoff N, Weiss H-D, Grimm W et al. (1995) Erste Erfahrungen mit temporären Vena-cava-Filtern. Röfo 163:171

40 Stent Treatment in the Venous Circulation

CH.L. ZOLLIKOFER

CONTENTS

40.1
Introduction

The areas of the venous system most frequently involved in obstructive lesions (Table 40.1) are the superior vena cava (SVC) and brachiocephalic veins, as well as the inferior vena cava (IVC) including the pelvic veins in malignant disease, post-thrombotic obstructions after central venous lines and deep venous thrombosis (DVT), and finally peripheral and central venous outflow obstruction in hemo-dialysis access fistulas. Other, rarer causes of venous obstruction are trauma, infectious diseases, venous anomalies such as "webs" or the pelvic venous spur (May–Thurner syndrome), and finally stenoses of the liver veins in Budd–Chiari syndrome.

Table 40.1. Typical locations of venous stent application

Superior vena cava
Inferior vena cava
Brachiocephalic veins
Common and external iliac veins

CH.L. ZOLLIKOFER, MD, Department of Radiology, Kantons-spital Winterthur, 8401 Winterthur, Swizerland

Because of a high recurrence rate due to continued external compression or elastic recoil and/or complete resistance to balloon dilatation of many of the above-mentioned venous obstructions endovascular stents have been increasingly introduced to overcome these problems. So far the majority of stent procedures have been performed for the treatment of malignant SVC and IVC syndromes (ANTONUCCI et al. 1992; BJARNASON et al. 1997; ELSON et al. 1991; IRVING et al. 1992; NAZARIAN et al. 1996; OUDKERK et al. 1993; RÖSCH et al. 1992, SEMBA and DAKE 1994) and for venous outflow obstruction in hemodialysis access fistulas (BEATHARD 1993; GRAY et al. 1995; QUINN et al. 1992; VORWERK et al. 1995; VORWERK and GÜNTHER 1997; ZOLLIKOFER et al. 1992). But also for benign obstructions such as postthrombotic and post-surgical strictures (BJARNASON et al. 1997; MICKLEY et al. 1993; NAZARIAN et al. 1996; SEMBA and DAKE 1994), the May–Thurner syndrome (BINKERT et al. 1998; JANSSEN et al. 1994) and IVC and hepatic vein stenosis in Budd–Chiari syndrome (WALKER et al. 1990; XU et al. 1996) stents have been successfully used with a low complication rate.

40.2
Indications and Contraindications

Generally speaking all lesions which cannot be satisfactorily dilated by balloon angioplasty alone may be treated by stent implantation. There are practically no absolute contraindications to the method other than those applicable to balloon angioplasty. Relative contraindications (Table 40.2) are coagulation disorders with hypercoagulability

Table 40.2. Relative contraindications to venous stent application

Important coagulation disorders
Decreased in- and outflow
Costoclavicular compression syndrome

and decreased inflow or outflow in a stented venous segment because of an increased risk of thrombotic occlusion. In addition, lesions leaving a significant waist in the balloon even during high-pressure angioplasty should be handled with caution because of the possibility that the stent may not be able to expand enough to relieve the stenosis significantly. Cross-stenting of large venous branches does not represent an absolute contraindication either, since in the majority of cases side branches remain patent. Nevertheless, it is clearly advisable to spare large branching collateral veins and particularly the renal veins if it is technically feasible to do so. Care should be taken of stents in the subclavian vein because of a possible compression of the stent between the clavicle and first rib. A costoclavicular compression syndrome, therefore, is a contraindication for primary stenting.

40.3
Selection of Stents

General recommendations as to which stent is best suited for venous obstructions can be given only to a limited degree. Apart from the anatomical location some important criteria include flexibility and radial force of the stent, maximal stent diameter available, and stent shortening during release. Flexibility and self-expansion have the advantage that they allow the stent to adapt to the natural course of the vessel and compensate to some degree for differences in calibre along the course of the vessel. Moreover, in areas of movement (across joints such as the hip and shoulder) preferably stents of a flexible, self-expanding construction should be used. However, in the vena cava and also the pelvis more rigid stents can be applied successfully.

The most widely used stents in the venous system so far have been the Gianturco or Gianturco–Rösch stents (Cook Europe A/S, Bjaeverskov, Denmark) and the Wallstent (Schneider Europe, Bülach, Switzerland) (Table. 40.3). Occasionally, other self-expandable stents such as the nitinol Memotherm stent (Bard Europe, Trappes, France) and the balloon expandable Palmaz (Johnson and Johnson, Warren, N.J.) and Strecker (Boston Scientific, Watertown, Mass.) stents have also been used, particularly for hemodialysis outflow stenosis (BOSNJAKOVITCH et al. 1992; GRAY et al. 1992; VORWERK and GÜNTHER 1997). However, balloon expandable stents seem to have a higher risk for central embolization and may be permanently deformed by osseous obstacles, particularly at the subclavian junction (GRAY et al. 1992; VORWERK and GÜNTHER 1997).

Table 40.3. Stents recommended for application in the venous system

Wallstent
Gianturco-Rösch (or Z) stent
Strecker stent
Palmaz stent

In our minds, the Wallstent has been most appropriate in most venous lesions because it features the best combination of a small-diameter introducing instrument, large stent lumen, and high flexibility and sufficient expansile force. A potential drawback of the Wallstent is the limited radioopacity during fluoroscopy and the foreshortening of the stent during release and expansion. Stent diameters are selected according to the anatomical site. Apart from these objective criterias, other factors such as personal experience and preference for a certain stent type may influence the selection. So far, no significant differences in clinical results according to the stent design have been published with the exception of a comparatively low secondary patency rate in peripheral hemodialysis outflow stenosis when using Gianturco–Rösch stents as compared to Wallstents (BEATHARD 1993; QUINN et al. 1992; VORWERK and GÜNTHER 1997).

40.4
Adjunctive Medication

As with angioplasty 5000 IU of heparin are also given intravenously with stent implantation. There is no uniform opinion in the literature concerning heparinization and oral anticoagulation following stent placement; however, we favor heparinization with 20 000 IU per 24 h for 2–3 days followed by overlapping anticoagulation with coumarin for 6–12 months if there is no contraindication. Only in high-flow situations such as hemodialysis fistulas no antithrombotic drugs are given.

Analgesic medication may be necessary as the dilatation of both tumor stenosis and dialysis fistula stenosis may be painful. In the latter subcutaneous infiltration of local anesthetics around the stenotic vein can reduce pain significantly.

40.5
Stents in Malignant Venous Obstruction of the Vena Cava, the Brachiocephalic and the Pelvic Veins

Obstruction of the superior vena cava and/or the brachiocephalic veins is responsible for the so-called superior vena cava syndrome (SVCS). In up to 80% of cases it is caused by involvement of mediastinal lymphnodes in bronchogenic carcinoma or by postirradiation fibrosis. Its indicidence in this disease is 3%–15%. The syndrome is hallmarked by severe swelling and edema of the neck, head and upper extremities, headache, orthopnea, and cyanosis (Fig. 40.1). The syndrome may also be seen in mediastinal fibrosis secondary to irradiation. The counterpart of the SVCS for the lower extremities is the IVCS which in the majority of cases is caused by retroperitoneal lymph node involvement in malignant disease with compression of the pelvic veins or the IVC. In some cases the intrahepatic segment of the IVC may be compressed by metastatic enlargement of the liver, particularly the caudate lobe. Symptoms in IVCS are characterized by massive leg swelling, edema of the genitals, and may be accompanied by venous claudication.

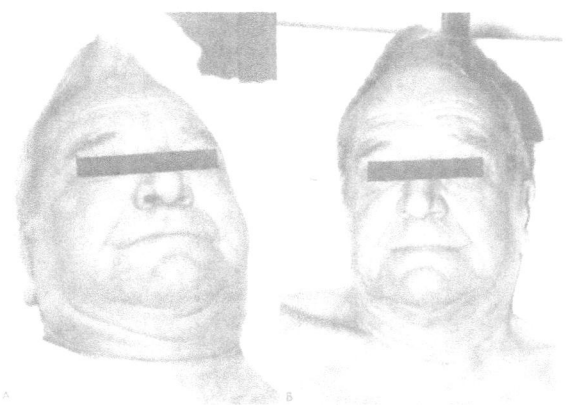

Fig. 40.1 A,B. Patient with severe superior vena cava syndorme due to bronchogenic carcinoma. A Patient shows severe edematous swelling of the face and neck. B Forty-eight hours later the edematous swelling of the head and neck has completely vanished

Traditionally, the treatment of choice for the cava syndrome has been radiation therapy and/or chemotherapy. However, the reponse time to this treatment is usually several days and not all patients will be eligible for this treatment because they have already had maximum tolerance radiotherapy or chemotherapy. On the other hand the severe distress caused by the vena cava syndrome justifies the attempt at intervention with a relatively simple percutaneous technique using endovascular stenting which leads to significant relief of the symptoms within hours. Several hundred cases of palliative stenting in malignant vena cava syndrome have been reported as original articles or in abstract form. In most reports Gianturco–Rösch or Z-stents and Wallstents were used.

40.5.1
Technique and Results

As a first step before stenting a phlebography of the obstructed veins should be obtained. For passing the obstruction of the pelvic veins and the vena cava, as well as for the stent placement itself, a femoral approach is usually used. An additional approach via the anticubital vein may be necessary in occlusion of the innominate and/or subclavian vein. If significant thrombi proximal to the obstruction are found on phlebography, local thrombolysis should be performed before stent placement to prevent pulmonary emboli and/or early reocclusion. In cases of complete occlusion of the SVC and innominate veins it is not necessary to always reopen both innominate veins. In our experience drainage via one of these veins and the superior vena cava is enough to relieve the edema of the head and both extremities as long as collateral pathways such as the internal jugular veins are patent.

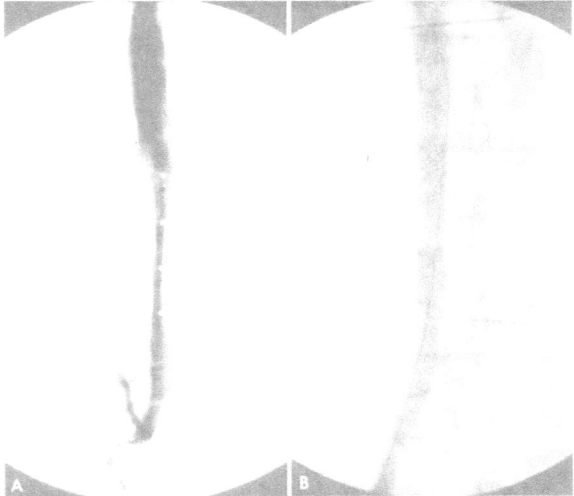

Fig. 40.2 A,B. A 63-year-old patient with metastasizing carcinoma of the prostate. A Cavogram shows high-grade stenosis of the infrarenal vena cava approximately 7 cm in length (note calibrated catheter). B Inferior vena cavogram after placement of a 20-mm Wallstent shows good patency

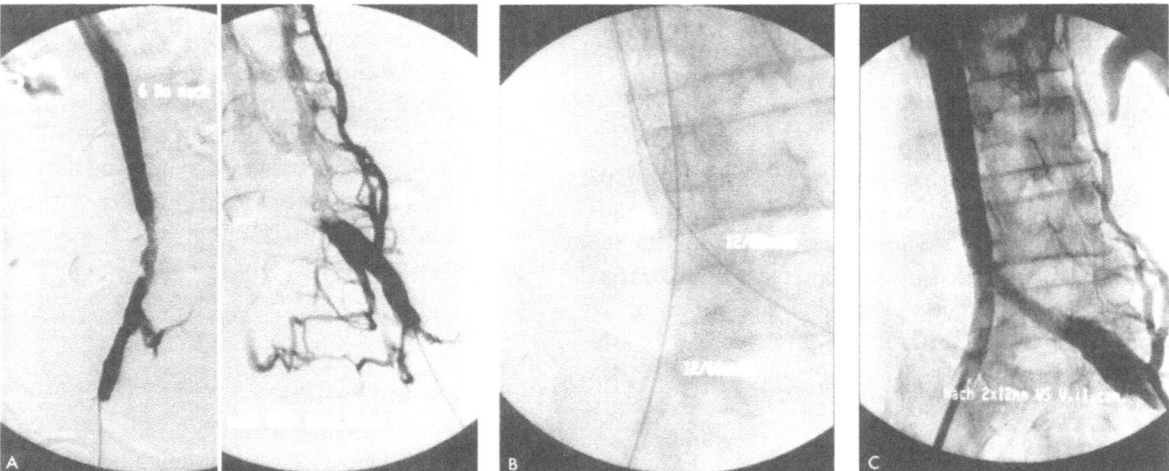

Fig. 40.3. A Same patient as in Fig. 40.2 with recurrent inferior vena cava (IVC) syndrome 6 months after stenting of the IVC. Bilateral phlebography shows tumor progression with stenosis of both common iliac veins. **B,C** After placement of two additional 12-mm stents reaching into the previously placed IVC stent good drainage of the pelvic veins is reestablished

Significant immediate relief of symptoms after stenting can be expected in 70%–100% (Figs. 40.1–40.4). In most cases rapid relief of subjective complaints by the patients are seen within hours followed by disappearance of edematous soft tissue swelling within 1–2 days (see Fig. 40.1). Long-term patency in SCV and IVC stenting ranges from 86%–100%. In the subclavian and pelvic vein patency seems somewhat less and may be related to smaller caliber, decreased inflow and/or tumor overgrowth. However, with secondary interventions patency rates of 60%–100% have been reported (BJARNASON et al. 1997; NAZARIAN et al. 1996; ZOLLIKOFER et al. 1994) (Fig. 40.3). Acute occlusions

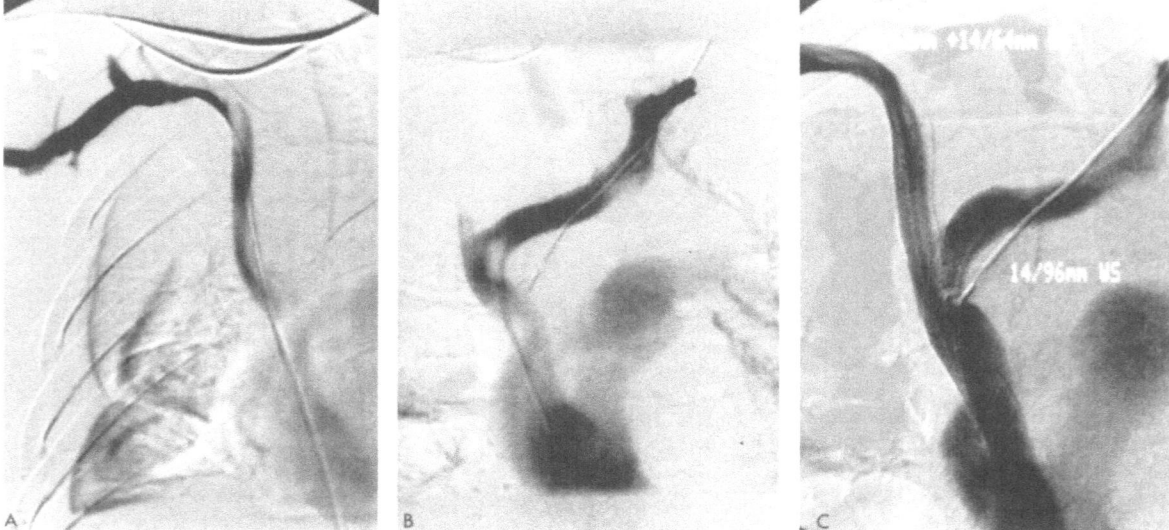

Fig. 40.4 A–C. Same patient as in Figs. 40.2 and 40.3 developed superior vena cava (SVC) syndrome 1 month after the second stent placement for pelvic vein obstruction. **A,B** Bilateral phlebography from an inguinal approach shows high grade stenosis of the right subclavian and innominate vein reaching into the SVC. In addition there is also involvement of the confluence of the distal left innominate vein. **C** After placement of a 12- and 14-mm stent to the right subclavian and innominate vein reaching the confluence of both innominate veins and successive placement of an additional 14-mm stent from the left innominate vein to the SVC, all lesions are satisfactorily stented and rapid drainage of both subclavian and innominate veins, as well as the SVC is reestablished

due to thrombosis occur in 5%–14% and can usually be treated with local thrombolysis and additional stent placement if necessary. Otherwise, significant complications are comparatively rare and include stent migration, stent breakage, and cardiac arrhythmia. Limited migration has mainly occurred with Gianturco stents, but has also been reported with other stent types. To our knowledge the only two deaths related to stent procedures were both due to stent migration to the right heart, one with a Gianturco stent in the IVC and one with a 25-mm Wallstent placed in the intrahepatic segment of the IVC. The problem of tumor ingrowth into the stented segment seems comparatively infrequent, particularly with the Wallstent with its tight wire mesh. We have treated two such cases successfully with additional stents to form a tighter wire mesh which prevented further tumor ingrowth.

We believe that anticoagulation after stent placement is necessary for the following reasons: Increased risk of thrombosis in turmor patients because of paraneoplastic syndromes and definitely delayed or even absent neoendothelialization of the stent surface in patients under radiation or chemotherapy, as demonstrated at autopsy in several of our patients.

40.5.2
Long-Term Results

The mean survival time of all patients is 6 months (the mean survival time of the patients who died is currently 4.8 months). The total patency rate (including enlargement of the stented area for tumor progression, etc., i.e., the secondary patency rate) until death or the last control was 92%. A total of 81% of the patients were symptom-free, 10.5% were partially or temporarily symptom-free, while 8% of the patients did not experience an improvement of the symptoms of obstruction, some of them due to additional lymph edema.

Therefore, the term "long-term patency" actually only applies to a period of 6 months, as only a minority of patients survive for more than 1 year (in the author's institute, five out of 45).

40.6
Stents in Benign Obstruction of the Vena Cava and Large Veins

Most benign obstructive lesions in the SVC and brachiocephalic veins that are not related to hemo-

dialysis fistulas are due to mediastinal fibrosis or postthrombotic states after central venous catheter placement. The most common causes of IVC obstruction are retroperitoneal fibrosis and stenosis in conjunction with Budd–Chiari syndrome. Involvement of pelvic and large femoral veins in stenotic and occlusive disease are most frequently related to postthrombotic complications including iliac venous spur (May–Thurrer syndrome) and surgery or trauma. Furthermore, previous radiation therapy may induce stenotic processes in the vena cava and large central veins after years. Since operative treatment in these conditions usually involves major and difficult surgery and conservative treatment is often of limited success, treatment with endovascular stents is the method of choice today.

40.6.1
Techniques and Results

Provided that dilatation of an obstructing lesion of the vena cava and large veins with a balloon catheter allows enough expansion of the lesion to permit stent implantation practically any benign venous obstruction may be stented. However, adequate in- and outflow of the stented area must be secured before stenting.

A femoral approach is usually employed for stenting but an internal jugular may be indicated for IVC lesions and hepatic veins. For very tight lesions or chronic occlusion of the brachiocephalic or pelvic vessels a double approach from the arm or the internal jugular vein, i.e., a so-called pull-through method, to stabilize the guidewire from both ends may be necessary. For chronic thrombotic occlusions recanalization with a steerable hydrophilic guidewire may be possible even in long-standing occlusion. Additional lysis with urokinase has not been of additional benefit in these cases in our experience. However, aggressive local thrombolysis for acute deep vein thrombosis (DVT) combined with stent placement has been advocated (BJARNASON et al. 1997; NAZARIAN et al. 1996; SEMBA and DAKE 1994). Although data from larger series of stenting in benign disease is still limited at present a very high initial success rate with significant relief of symptoms in up to almost 100% is reported (BINKERT et al. 1998; NAZARIAN et al. 1996; SEMBA and DAKE 1994; ZOLLIKOFER et al. 1994). Also, the long-term patency rates in the vena cava, the liver veins and iliofemoral veins after several years are very promising, with a primary stent patency ranging from 67% to 100% and secondary patency rates of 86%–100% (BINKERT et al. 1998; JANSSEN et al. 1994; NAZARIAN et al. 1996; RILINGER et al. 1997; SEMBA and DAKE 1994; WALKER et al. 1990; ZOLLIKOFER et al. 1994). Iliac vein stenting seems particularly useful in a group of patients suffering from the May–Thurner syndrome where surgery is usually hampered by high recurrence rates (Fig. 40.5). Another group of patients which can benefit from stent placement is iatrogenic stenosis in the region of the common femoral vein after surgical or percutaneous interventional procedures in this region. Using Wallstents crossing the hip joint in the common femoral vein – a critical region for surgical reconstruction – seems to have excellent long-term results (ZOLLIKOFER et al. 1994). In our own exerience bending of the hip has had no adverse effect to the stent and no significant intimal hyperplasia has been noticed (Fig. 40.6). A total of 18 patients with stents in the common femoral and iliac veins showed a primary patency rate of 94% after follow-up of 6 months to 10.5 years (mean 3.3 years) and no late recurrences. The only cases where recurrences from intimal hyperplasia have been reported are cases

were surgical clamping during creation of arteriovenous fistulas after recanalization of pelvic veins has been performed (MICKLEY et al. 1993; RILINGER et al. 1997).

No serious procedure-related complications have been published to our knowledge although strictures resistant to adequate dilatation may end up with thrombotic occlusion even in cases of benign disease.

The only exception where primary stenting is not advocated is the so-called costoclavicular compression syndrome. In these cases stents should only be used after surgical resection of the first rib since otherwise the stents may be severely damaged by the continuous compression between the first rib and the clavicle with elevation of the arms. Stents, however, may be indicated if residual stenosis persists after the operation.

Generally, if there is no contraindication we use anticoagulation with coumadin for 6–12 months after the initial heparinization for the first 3 postoperative days after stent placement. There is no uniform opinion on this topic in the literature.

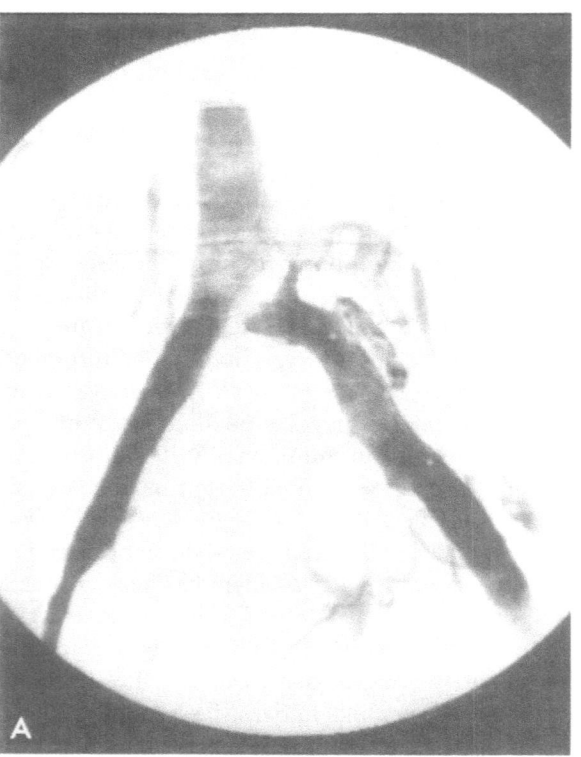 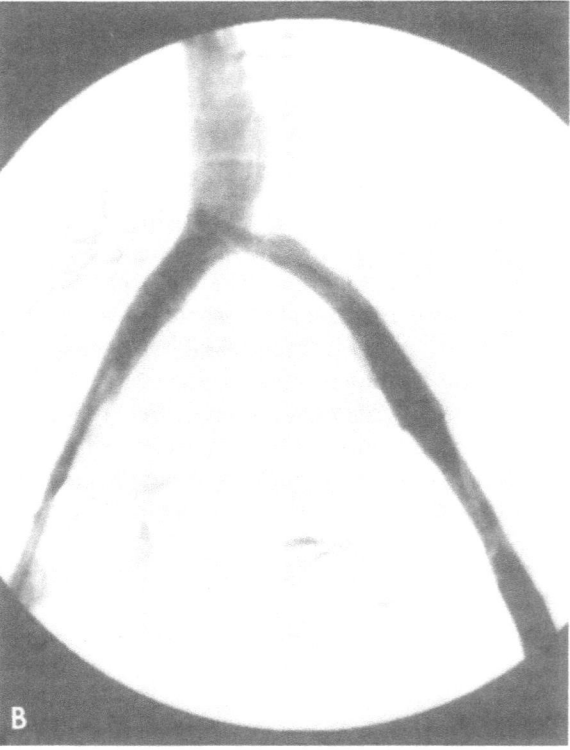

Fig. 40.5 A,B. A 43-year-old patient 4 days after surgical thrombectomy for left deep vein thrombosis. At the time of surgery a resistance in the common iliac vein was felt. The patient was therefore sent for phlebography for diagnosis and treatment of possible May–Thurner syndrome. **A** Antegrade pelvic phlebography shows typical lateral venous spur (May–Thurner syndrome) at the inflow of the left common iliac vein into the inferior vena cava. **B** After placement of a 16-mm Wallstent there is good antegrade flow on the left. The patient is free of symptoms 2 years after the procedure

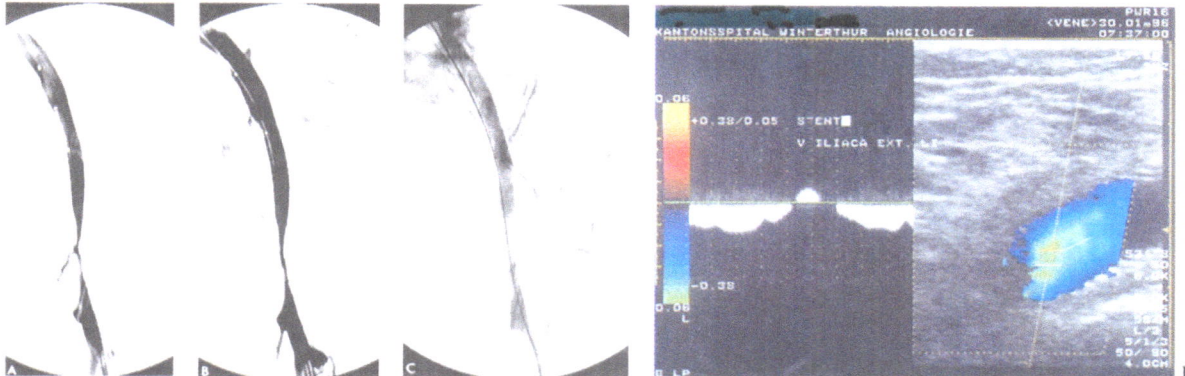

Fig. 40.6 A–D. A 62-year-old patient with leg swelling on the left 3 weeks after percutaneous transluminal angioplasty (PTA) of the superficial femoral artery. **A** Crossover phlebography shows severe stenosis of the distal external iliac and common femoral vein due to hematoma. **B** There is no significant improvement of the stenosis after crossover PTA. Note reflux of contrast into the greater saphenous and femoral vein. **c** After placement of a 12-mm Wallstent and additional PTA within the stent the control phlebography shows rapid flow and no further reflux into the femoral or saphenous vein is seen. **D** Color Doppler ultrasound 4 years after the procedure shows good patency of the stented area and no signs of intimal hyperplasia

40.7
Stents for Hemodialysis Fistula Outflow Obstruction

Percutaneous transluminal angioplasty (PTA) as a non surgical treatment of outflow stenosis in hemodialysis access shunts and graft are hampered by the high rates of restenosis. Therefore, metallic expandable stents have been used in order to improve the results of PTA alone in peripheral, as well as in central, venous obstruction. The typical indications for stent placement are recurrent stenosis or recoiling lesions after PTA along the venous outflow tract and graft vein anastomoses.

Contraindications to stenting include AV shunts which have never matured or functioned poorly, or where the segment for venous or graft puncture would be too short. As a general rule a stented segment should not be punctured in order not to damage the stent wire or filaments (VORWERK and GÜNTHER 1997). Furthermore, treatment of a stenotic AV anastomosis with stents is contraindicated and should be treated with balloon angioplasty only.

40.7.1
Technique and Results

Similarly to PTA the access to the lesion depends on the location of the stenosis. For central and proximal peripheral lesions we prefer a femoral approach. In

peripheral lesions where the stent-introducing instrument would be too short an antegrade approach is selected in such a way that enough space remains for introduction of a hemostatic sheath and manipulation of guidewires and balloon catheters. As a test we always predilate the stenotic segment before stent implantation and repeat dilatation of the stented segment immediately following stent release if adequate stent expansion seems delayed. Generally no antithrombotic regimen is necessary after the procedure.

The initial technical and clinical success rates after stenting of hemodialysis outflow stenosis are very high. Unfortunately, restenosis at some point after stent (usually between 4 and 12 months) is almost the rule, reaching 80%–100% in peripheral lesions and 60%–80% in central lesions (Figs. 40.7, 40.8). Two recent reports (BEATHARD 1993; QUINN 1993) found no differences between two groups of patients treated with either PTA alone or PTA and stenting with Gianturco stents. QUINN et al. (1992) reported primary patency at 2 years of 25%. The secondary and tertiary patency rates were 34% and 42%, respectively. While VORWERK et al. using the Wallstent also had a low primary patency rate of 45% at 2 years their secondary patency rate was considerably higher reaching 77% (VORWERK and GÜNTHER 1997). TURMEL-RODRIGUES et al. (1996) report a secondary patency rate using the Wallstent at 2 years of 82% for grafts and 77% for native veins. Our own experience with the Wallstents shows a secondary and tertiary patency rate at 2 years of 62% and 85%. Generally, the flexible Wallstent seems

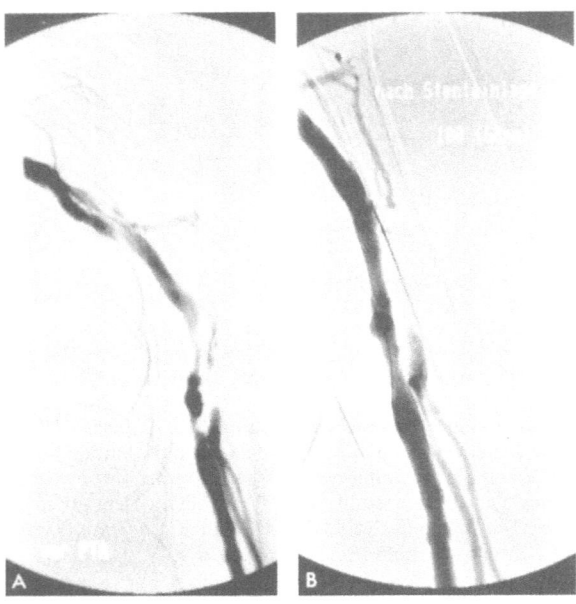

Fig. 40.7 A,B. A 60-year-old patient on hemodialysis. **A** Shuntogram shows high-grade stenosis of the basilic vein in the upper arm after previous percutaeous transluminal angioplasty (PTA). **B** Shuntogram shows good patency after placement of 10-mm stent because of insufficient PTA result. Stent was placed via a femoral, retrograde approach

lesions only after repeated trials of PTA when the intervals between interventions become shorter (2–3 months) or if elastic recoil causes immediate restenosis. In such circumstances stents can significantly improve and prolong shunt function. The patients, however, should be followed closely and the nephrologist must be informed that if venous pressures begin to rise the shunt should be immediately checked for possible restenosis and treated if necessary. Generally, these hyperplastic reactions of the venous wall develop within the stented area or at the transition from the stented to the non-stented vein. These narrowings can generally be redilated by balloon angioplasty quite easily but additional stent placement may be necessary (Fig. 40.8). In addition, however, also the entire venous outflow tract has to be checked since new lesions may develop at a distance from the stent, particularly in the subclavian area. In contrast to peripheral lesions central obstruction and particularly recanalization after chronic occlusion of innominate and subclavian veins should be stented primarily since PTA alone gives unsatisfactory results in the majority of cases.

40.8
Concluding Remarks

Management of venous obstructions with interventional radiological techniques are valuable alternatives to surgical procedures or medical treatment. In many instances PTA and stent implantation are the only means of palliation and also allow long-term curative treatment with minimal risk of complications and highest rates of vessel patency. Stent placement for treatment of malignant as well as

preferable to the rigid Gianturco stent for treating dialysis-related stenosis in the arm and shoulder region where bending of the extremity or the natural curvature of the vein may be disturbed by a more rigid stent like the Gianturco stent (VORWERK and GÜNTHER 1997). Similar to the experience reported by QUINN et al. (1992) and VORWERK and GÜNTHER (1997) we had fewer restenoses in large central veins.

In view of the as yet unsolved problem of intimal hyperplasia we recommend stenting of peripheral

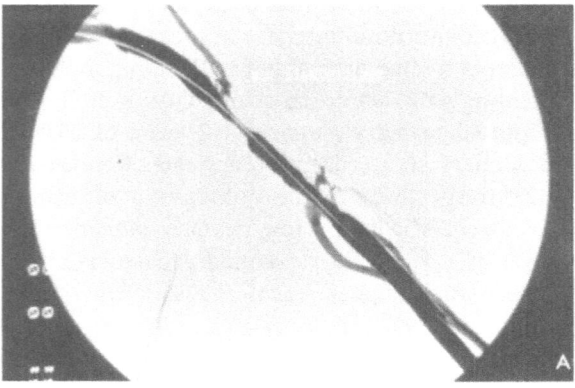
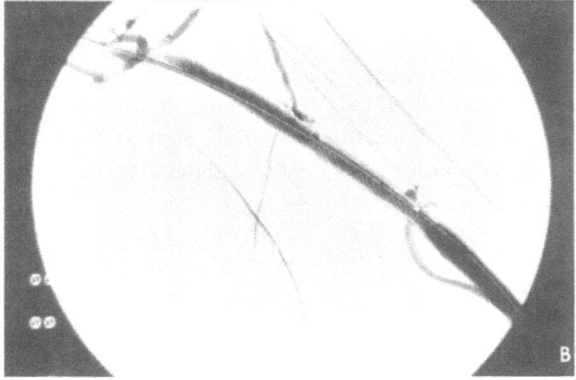

Fig. 40.8 A,B. Same patient as in Fig. 40.7, again showed increased venous pressures on dialysis 14 months later. **A** Retrograde shuntogram via femoral approach shows intimal hyperplasia in the proximal part of the stent and high-grade stenosis at the outflow of the stent. **B** After percutaneous transluminal angioplasty and additional stent placement at the proximal outflow tract good patency is once again reestablished

benign SVC and IVC syndrome is now the general method of choice. A particular group of patients with rewarding results with curative stenting are those suffering from the May–Thurner syndrome or after iatrogenic stenosis and obstruction of the common femoral vein. These patients do badly with surgical treatment and stent placement seems to be the method of choice.

In hemodialysis outflow stenosis of peripheral veins stents should be reserved for repeated recurrences or elastic recoiling lesions because of a high propensity for intimal hyperplasia. In contrast, central lesions can and should be stented primarily. Close follow-up and immediate secondary balloon intervention in the event of intimal hyperplasia or secondary lesions are mandatory and mean that dialysis fistula function can be kept up for years avoiding surgical interventions. Likewise, all other stent placements should be followed regularly in order to be able to intervene if restenosis should occur. No advantage of covered stents (stent grafts) over conventional stents to prevent intimal hyperplasia has been found to date.

References

Antonucci F, Salomonowitz E, Stuckmann G, et al. (1992) Placement of venous stents: clinical experience with a self-expanding prosthesis. Radiology 183:493–497

Beathard GA (1993) Gianturco self-expanding stent in the treatment of stenosis in dialysis access grafts. Kidney Int 4:872–877

Binkert C, et al. (1998) Treatment of pelvic venous spur (May–Thurner syndrome) with self-expanding metallic endoprothesis. Cardiovasc Intervent Radiol 21:22–26

Bjarnason H, Kruse JR, Asinger D, et al. (1997) Iliofemoral deep venous thrombosis: safety and efficacy outcome during 5 years of catheter-directed thrombolytic therapy[1]. J Vasc Intervent Radiol 8:405–418

Bosnjakovitch P, Ivkovic T, Ilic M, et al. (1992) Strecker stent in stenotic hemodialysis Brescia-Cimino arteriovenous fistulas. Cardiovasc Intervent Radiol 15:217–220

Elson JD, Becker GJ, Wholey MH, et al. (1991) Vena caval and central venous stenoses: management with Palmaz balloon-expandable intraluminal stents. J Vasc Intervent Radiol 2:215–223

Gray R, Dolmatch B, Horton K (1992) Metallic stents for hemodialysis access. Radiology 185:134

Gray R, Horton K, Dolmatch B, et al. (1995) Use of Wallstents for hemodialysis access-related venous stenoses and occlusions untreatable with balloon angioplasty. Radiology 195:479–484

Irving JD, Dondelinger RF, Reidy JF, et al. (1992) Gianturco self-expanding stents: clinical experience in the vena cava and large veins. Cardiovasc Intervent Radiol 15:328–333

Janssen HJ, Antonucci F, Stuckmann G, et al. (1994) Behandlung von Venenstenosen und-verschlüssen benigner Aetiologie mit vaskulären Endoprothesen: ein neues, nicht-operatives Therapiekonzept. Vasa. 23:66–73

Mickley V, Friedrich JM, Hutschenreiter S, et al. (1993) Langzeitergebnisse nach perkutan-transluminaler Angioplastie und Stentimplantation bei venösen Stenosen nach transfemoraler Thrombektomie. Vasa 22:44

Nazarian GK, Bjarnason H, Dietz CA, et al. (1996) Iliofemoral venous stenoses: effectiveness of treament with metallic endovascular stents. Radiology 200:193–199

Oudkerk M, Heystraten FMJ, Stoter G, et al. (1993) Stenting in malignant vena caval obstruction. Cancer 71:142–146

Quinn S, Schuman E, Demlow T et al. (1995) Percutaneous transluminal angioplasty versus endovascular sent placement in the treatment of venous stenoses in patients undergoing hemodialysis: intermediate results. J Vasc Intervent Radiol 6:851–855

Quinn S, Schuman E, Hall L (1992) Venous stenoses in patients who undergo hemodialysis: treatment with self-expandable endovascular stents. Radiology 183:499–504

Rilinger N, Görich J, Mickley V, et al. (1997) Long-term results after stenting of stenoses in the iliofemoral veins: 5 years experience. Eur Radiol Suppl S164

Rösch J, Uchida BT, Hall LD, et al. (1992) Gianturco-Rösch expandable Z-stents in the treatment of superior vena cava syndrome. Cardiovasc Intervent Radiol 15:319–327

Semba CP, Dake MD (1994) Iliofemoral deep venous thrombosis: aggressive therapy with catheter-directed thrombolysis. Radiology 191:487–494

Turmel-Rodrigues L, Blanchard D, Pengloan J et al. (1997) Wallstents and Craggstens in hemodialysis grafts and fistulae: results for selective indications. J Vasc Intervent Radiol 8:975–982

Vorwerk D, Günther RW (1997) Stents in hemodialysis fistulas and grafts. Semin Intervent Radiol 14(1):59–69

Vorwerk D, Günther RW, Mann H, et al. (1995) Stenting of venous stenoses and occlusions in hemodialysis shunts: follow-up results in 65 patients. Radiology 195:140–146

Walker HS, Rholl KS, Register TE, et al. (1990) Percutaneous placement of a hepatic vein stent in the treatment of Budd-Chiari syndrome. J Vasc Intervent Radiol 1:23–27

Xu K, He FX, Zhang H, et al. (1996) Budd-Chiari syndrome caused by obstruction of the hepatic inferior vena cava: immediate and 2-year treatment results of transluminal angioplasty and metallic stent placement. Cardiovasc Intervent Radiol 19:32–36

Zollikofer CL, Antonucci F, Stuckmann G, et al. (1992) Use of the Wallstent in the venous system including hemodialysis-related stenoses. Cardiovasc Intervent Radiol 15:334–341

Zollikofer CL, Schoch E, Stuckmann G, et al. (1994) Perkutane transluminale Behandlung von Stenosen und Verschlüssen im venösen System mittels Gefäßendoprothesen (Stents). Schweiz Med Wochenschr 124:995–1009

41 The Surgeon's Requirement for Radiological Information Prior to Venous Surgery

D.A. LOOSE and J. WEBER

CONTENTS

41.1 General Aspects of Surgical Treatment

The curative treatment of varicose veins by surgery mainly deals with the larger subcutaneous main trunks and side branches of the long and small saphenous veins (LOOSE and WEBER 1997; NETZER 1979; MAY 1974). However, the concept of surgical interruption of the venous reflux includes a knowledge of the subfascial muscular and collecting veins of the leg and the pelvic venous outflow. Recirculation by reflux under orthostatic conditions generally means an upper principal point of insufficiency (orifice of the saphenous veins or an insufficient upper perforator vein), a valveless or valve-insufficient segment of the epifascial trunk (including varicose side branches, additional trunks, etc.), and a lower point of insufficiency (varicose perforator veins and the veins of the foot and ankle).

DIRK A. LOOSE, Dr. med. habil., Professor, Zentrum für Gefäßmedizin, Abteilung für Angiologie und Gefäßchirurgie der Chirurgischen Klinik Dr. Guth, Jürgensallee 44, 22609 Hamburg, Germany
JÜRGEN WEBER, Dr.med., Professor, Institut für Röntgendiagnostik und Interventionelle Radiologie, DRK-Krankenhaus, Suurheidstraße 20, 22559 Hamburg-Rissen, Germany

All this must be clearly diagnosed prior to surgery in order to obtain reliable long-lasting or even definitive curative results (LOOSE and FUNCK 1995; WEBER and MAY 1990; ZEITLER 1979). Crossectomy means preparation, ligation, and dissection of the orifice of the saphenous trunk, including all side branches. Stripping of the varicose trunks and side-arms and ligation of the perforator veins involved means a time-consuming and demanding surgical technique which is based on clear and reliable patho-anatomical and patho-physiological diagnostic findings.

41.2 Diagnostic Imaging and Functional Evaluation

41.2.1 Morphologic Aspects

There are many anatomic variations in all venous areas of the leg, including the central pelvic and caval drainage. The main saphenous trunks may be duplicated totally or in segments; other segments of the trunk involved may be intact and collateralized. Varicosis of the long saphenous vein may be associated with a segmental or complete small saphenous vein. In the majority of cases two or more perforator veins are dealing with the venous dysfunction. The main collecting trunks of the deep venous system play an important role in varicose recirculation (degeneration of valves and major reflux of blood) in most instances. The differentiation between "primary" and "secondary" (postthrombotic) changes must be clearly demonstrated in order to indicate or contraindicate surgical intervention (MAY 1974; NETZER 1979; WEBER and MAY 1990; ZEITLER 1979). Phlebectasias and persistent dysplastic embryonal veins (the marginal vein) and diagnostic hints for the presence of arteriovenous-shunting fistulas in congenital vascular malformations must be documented and differentiated from the common varicose syndrome (LOOSE and WEBER 1997).

41.2.2
Functional Aspects

The degree of venous reflux and recirculation and the recovery time during compression tests, etc., may help to find objective criteria to calculate peripheral venous hypertension, e.g., to measure the stages of chronic venous insufficiency (CVI). It is also imperative to find out which degree of re-compensation is to be gained by surgical intervention *prior* to therapy (MAY 1974; WEBER and MAY 1990). Cutaneous damage such as chronic venous leg ulcer due to long-lasting CVI must be correlated to the venous findings locally, as well as in the whole varicose involvement of the leg.

41.2.3
Imaging Modalities and Functional Tests

Among a variety of methods for measuring and documenting individual patho-anatomy and patho-physiology there is a range of screening methods which obtain objective results and which lead to optimal surgical therapy:

Plethysmography. This method provides comparatively precise information about venous drainage and pump function. It may help to indicate surgery and qualify the therapeutic result thereafter.

Doppler Ultrasound. This technique is able to clearly show the points of reflux (orifice of the saphenous veins, insufficient perforator veins) and the functioning/dysfunctioning of venous valves along the subcutaneous varicose trunks and side branches.

Duplex Ultrasound. Duplex ultrasound is an advanced and valuable Doppler technique, demonstrating both morphologic details locally and hemodynamics of the deep and superficial varicose veins, such as reflux and recirculation. This technique also helps to differentiate between primary varicosis and postthrombotic changes (valvelessness, wall thickening, recanalization, perivenous fibrosis).
The drawback of ultrasound techniques, however, is still poor quality of documentation (small sectors

and the absence of overview, and correlating the various aspects of the varicose syndrome simply and clearly enough).

Direct Blood Pressure Measurement (Phlebodynamometry). This clearly shows peripheral venous hypertension and enables classification of CVI. It is also able to show and document the degrees of recompensation following appropriate surgery by adding the compression tests, blocking the superficial reflux of blood from every level of insufficiency (orifice and perforators), and also providing information about the degree of degeneration of the deep venous system of the leg (WEBER and MAY 1990).

Plethysmography can be easily combined with the method of ascending leg phlebography, this improving the morphologic and functional information to be gained.

Phlebography. In the view of vascular surgery this method still represents the "gold standard" in diagnostic imaging of varicose veins as a whole. However, the overall average standard of quality should be improved, documenting and describing all the information which can be presented and documented to prepare an optimal "venous status" prior to surgery.

41.3
Need for Phlebographic Information

41.3.1
Invasiveness

Compared with functional tests (plethysmography, boppler, and duplex ultrasound) phlebography needs a venous puncture. By applying iodinated contrast medium there is a certain risk of side effects (anaphylactic reaction, thyroidal hyperfunction, decompensation in chronic renal failure), meaning relative contraindications.

Modern non-ionic hypo-osmolalic contrast media have almost completely overcome the risk of damaging the venous intima. However, the indication of an invasive method should be limited to those patients who are clear candidates for surgery or for those at risk from postthrombotic syndrome. In addition, the "output" of information gained from phlebography should be adequate or even higher compared with other methods.

41.3.2
Definition of Patho-anatomy and Patho-physiology

Phlebography is able to offer a complete overview of the main veins of the foot, leg, pelvis, and caval outflow. It demonstrates at the same time the sub- and epifascial venous system of the leg, showing functioning and varicose dysfunctioning veins via the reflux of contrast medium applied, defining the varicose syndrome according to its points of leakage.

The parameters of venous calibers, the functioning/non-functioning of venous valves, reflux (seen and documented under fluoroscopy) should enable a precise classification of the entire venous system to be opacified.

41.3.3
Description of Phlebographic Findings

According to its ability to demonstrate morphologic *and* functional findings a systematic description is mandatory. In particular, the regions of interest (orifices of saphenous veins, insufficient perforators) should be documented and described clearly. Opacification of the deep veins of the leg and the direct reflux of the contrast medium back to the sub-cutaneous varices ought to guide the surgeon in his preparation for suitable surgical access and to execute an interruption of reflux (Loose and Funck 1995). Phlebography should also help to avoid over- and under-therapy of the individual complex of varices, reducing side effects and complications in the surgical approach, and also reducing the risk of recurrence of the varices to be operated. A total of 20% of recurrences of varices must be attributed to insufficient diagnosis or to a sub-optimal operative technique resulting from sub-optimal diagnostic information.

41.3.4
Classification of the Varicose Syndrome

Vascular surgery requires the clearest classification in order to repair or protect against CVI. The following information should be available:

Differentiation: primary versus secondary varicosis
Extension of the varices, upper and lower points of insufficience (orifices, perforator veins)

Condition of the deep veins of the leg, the venous inflow at the ankle, the pelvic and caval outflow
Descending and ascending types of truncal varicosis, incomplete involvement, collateralization, side branches to be involved
Definition of "recurrence" of varices, upper and lower points of the pathologic recirculation
All functional aspects of the venous circulation should be documented and described adequate to what the radiologist has seen under fluoroscopy.

41.4
Legal Aspects and Quality Standards

It is extremely important in our eyes to improve the quality of diagnostics and therapy to the level expected nowadays by diseased patients when undergoing surgery. The increasing number of malpractice cases going to court clearly demands *high quality standards*.

Planning operations on varicose patients and improved diagnostic methods must help to win optimal long-lasting therapeutic results and to reduce the charge of "varicose recurrence". Documentation and descriptions must be precise, presenting the complete varicose status and indicating which therapeutic approach is needed to gain optimal surgical results. Phlebography so far mainly enables the surgeon to obtain adequate information on patho-anatomy and the related hemodynamics to improve the surgical results.

References

Loose DA, Weber J (1997) Angeborene Gefäßmißbildungen. Nordlanddruck, Lüneburg
Loose DA, Funck I (1995) Angeborene Venenfehler – Diagnostische und therapeutische Möglichkeiten. Aktuelle Chir 30:329–340
May R (1974) Chirurgie der Bein-und Beckenvenen. Thieme, Stuttgart
Netzer CO (1979) Anatomie und Physiologie der Venen. In: Ehringer H, Fischer H, Netzer CO, Schmutzler R, Zeitler E (eds) Venöse Abflußstörungen. Enke, Stuttgart, pp 1–62
Weber J, May R (1990) Funktionelle Phlebologie. Thieme, Stuttgart
Zeitler E (1979) Röntgenologische und nuklearmedizinische Diagnostik. In: Ehringer H, Fischer H, Netzer CO, Schmutzler R, Zeitler E (eds) Venöse Abflußstörungen. Enke, Stuttgart, pp 297–450

42 Leg Ulcers

K. Gall, R. Möller and E. Paul

CONTENTS

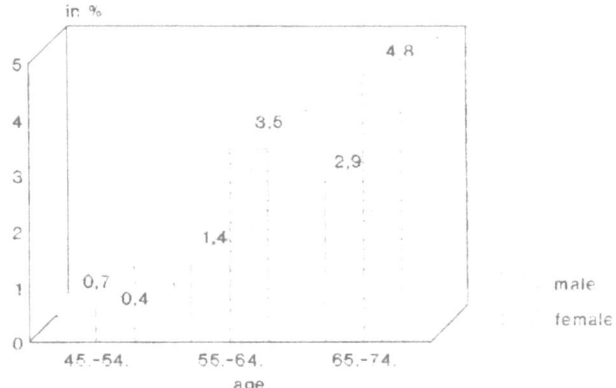

Fig. 42.1. Prevalence of leg ulcers; sex-differentiated graph

42.1
Definition, Epidemiology, and Social Economic Data

Ulcus cruris is defined as a chronic leg ulceration of various disease entities. It can be seen as a polyetiological syndrome associated with numerous diseases with tremendous socio-medical and politico-economic impact. Studies in the former West Germany have estimated that annual leg ulcers have caused economic costs of approximately DM 2–3 billion. Data from 1991 show that more than 2 million days of disability and 1.2 million days of absence from work occurred due to this ailment (Gallenkemper et al. 1996). The prevalence is about 2% of the population, whereas women are afflicted two to three times more often than men (Fig. 42.1). The main factor involved in this frequency is that women have a longer life span (Goldman and

Fronek 1992; Mayerhausen 1988). At 40 years of age the prevalence of chronic leg ulcers among the sexes is approximately equivalent. The graphic presentation of this data is divided into three age classes with respect to sex (Fig. 42.1).

All these factors demonstrate the high priority for a correct therapy, as well as appropriate insurance coverage. In general, the therapy for leg ulcers is considered to be frustrating and demands much effort and attention. Often resignation and therapeutic nihilism are the results for both the patient and the physician. Frequently, the Latin phrase *primum nihil nocere* is heard among specialists treating patients with leg ulcers. So much the more, then, does successful treatment require optimal diagnostics regarding various differential diagnoses.

42.2
Differential Diagnoses of Leg Ulcers

Leg ulcers, as a polyetiological symptom, have numerous causes. Their classification concerning different etiopathogenetic groups is summarized in Table 42.1.

K. Gall, MD, Hautklinik, Klinikum-Nord, Prof.-Ernst-Nathan-Str.1, 90419 Nürnberg, Germany
R. Möller, MD, Hautklinik, Klinikum-Nord, Prof.-Ernst-Nathan-Str.1, 90419 Nürnberg, Germany
E. Paul, Prof., MD, Hautklinik, Klinikum-Nord, Prof.-Ernst-Nathan-Str.1, 90419 Nürnberg, Germany

Table 42.1. Leg ulcers as a polyetiological syndrome (CLAUDE and BURTON 1993; GILLILAND and WOLFE 1991; HAFNER et al. 1996; MARGOLIS 1992)

Vascular ulcers	Non-vascular ulcers
Ulcus cruris venosum	Ulcus cruris infectiosum
Ulcus cruris arteriosum	Ulcus cruris exogenicum/traumaticum
Ulcus cruris mixtum	Ulcus cruris trophicum/neuropathicum
	Ulcus cruris hematopathogenicum
	Ulcus cruris neoplasticum

42.3
Pathophysiology/Etiopathogenesis

42.3.1
Vascular Leg Ulcers

42.3.1.1
Ulcus Cruris Venosum

Due to its high prevalence of about 85% (DOUGLAS and SIMPSON 1995; MAYERHAUSEN 1988) of all leg ulcerations the venous type should be discussed first. In the past it has often been referred to as the absolute *entite morbide*. It is usually painless and develops at sites of previously damaged skin, most typically located on the medial malleolus. Leg ulcers result from chronic venous insufficiency (CVI). One must distinguish between a suprafascial and subfascial insufficiency (GOLDMAN et al. 1994; MOLLARD 1994). This distinction is not only of practical use but also of therapeutic relevance. The suprafascial insufficiency has its cause in the valvular insufficiency at the saphenofemoral junction (SFJ) of the major vein, the long saphenous vein (LSV) flowing into the femoral vein and the short saphenous vein (SSV) flowing into the popliteal vein. In addition, significant insufficiency of hemodynamically important perforating veins can also induce a suprafascial CVI.

An existing varicose vein is not the only relevant pathoetiological factor of ulcer genesis. Disturbed hemodynamics, namely, the degree of venous reflux, determines whether a CVI develops and not the degree of varicosity itself. Depending on clinical findings, an ulceration of the lower limb can be adequately treated by surgery or sclerotherapy. Subfascial CVI is based on occlusion of the hemodynamically important deep venous system, e.g., as a result of thrombophlebitis or deep venous thrombosis. Deep vein blocking (90% of the flow of blood comes from the subfascial venous system) causes an increase in pressure distal to the venous regions and

can give rise to leg ulceration similar to the suprafascial type (CLAUDE and BURTON 1994). The various etiological factors of ulcer genesis can be established (Table 42.2).

Chronic venous hypertension with capillary dilatation and deformation can occur due to venous stasis. This leads to an increase in transendothelial protein and fluid permeability resulting in a high concentration of protein within the fibrous tissue. The consequence is a pericapillary fibrin cuff (disturbed fibrinolysis) that induces disturbances in the microcirculation and local trophism. This gives rise to local hypoxia; accompanied by minimal trauma a leg ulcer can occur.

Table 42.2. Etiological model of the development of ulcera crurum venosa (leg ulcers) (MAYERHAUSEN 1988; MULDER and REIS 1990; VANSCHEIDT et al. 1992)

Valvular incompetence, refluxes
Chronic venous insufficiency
Dilatation of capillaries and deformation
Increase of transendothelial protein permeability
Pericapillary fibrin cuff via disturbed fibrinolysis
Local hypoxia
Necrosis/ulcer

42.3.1.2
Ulcus Cruris Arteriosum

Although arterial ulcers represent only a small proportion of about 4%–30% of all cases (GALLENKEMPER et al. 1996; GOLDMAN and FRONEK 1992), this type of ulcer should receive special notice, since such patients are usually in increased danger. Table 42.3 shows a collection of leg ulcerations due to an underlying arterial disease.

An arterial ulcer, as a consequence of arterial occlusion, is always a late symptom of a vascular process that takes decades to develop. The pathogenesis is usually potentiated by risk factors such as lipometabolic disease, hyperuricemia, diabetes mellitus, hypertension, smoking, etc. The last step

Table 42.3. Types of ulcus cruris arteriosum (FALK and KLÜKEN 1990; MULDER and REIS 1990)

Arterial occlusive disease (including diabetic macroangiopathy)
Pan- (peri-)vasculitis(-arterititis) nodosa
Diabetic microangiopathy
Vasculitides (e.g., vasculitis nodosa, vasculitis racemosa, erythema nodosum, collagenosis)
Necrobiosis lipoidica (diabeticorum)
Essential hypertension (ulcus hypertonicum Martorell)
Arteriovenous anastomosis
Arterial aneurysm

---

in the syndrome – the irreversible necrosis – mirrors a long course of suffering characterized by a decreased duration of walking and pain at rest. If the restrained circulation is reduced more drastically than the compensating collateral mechanism, this will lead to an intracellular lack of oxygen and stimulation of the anaerobic glycolysis within the cell, and subsequently to tissue necrosis despite a compensated increased oxygen uptake. As shown in Table 42.3, several types of special vascular ulcers can be discriminated between based on different diagnostic and therapeutic procedures resulting from various metabolism diseases, vascular abnormalities, and rare angitisies with respect to collagenosis. Their pathogenesis and management are deduced from the underlying disease and cannot be discussed in this context.

The arterial ulcer does not usually occur in regions of physiologically undersupplied tissue such as the toes. Instead, it usually develops on traumatically exposed regions such as the ventral tibial margin and lateral malleolus. In addition to is-chemia, certain trigger factors such as minimal trauma and all types of infections are required for the initiation of arterial ulcers.

42.3.1.3
Ulcus Cruris Mixtum

Approximately 10% of all leg ulcers have a combined pathogenesis (KLÜKEN and ROSENHEIM 1983; SCHULTZ-EHRENBERG and WEINDORF 1984). This manifestation of ulcers is primarily confined to older age groups (age peak 70–79 years) and requires not only an exact diagnosis but also a precise therapeutic regimen adapted to the individual vascular situation. Since the sufficient compressive treatment of venous ulcers is contraindicated for an ulcus cruris mixtum, important and adequate measures, such as compression bandages, cannot be applied.

42.3.2
Non-Vascular Leg Ulcers

Ulcerations of the lower limb unrelated to an underlying vascular disease require a very differentiated diagnostic modality due to their nonhomogeneous origin and rarity (approximately 10% of all leg ulcers). Moreover, a precise therapeutic regimen corresponding to the primary disease is necessary. Due to heterogeneous etiopathogenesis, a satisfactory classification is rarely possible. Since not all ailments with a predispositon to ulcers can be dealt within this chapter, various types of etiopathogenesis for differential diagnosis are listed in Table 42.4.

Table 42.4. Differential diagnosis of the etiopathogenesis of nonvascular ulcer types (BILAND et al. 1984; CLAUDE and BURTON 1993; KLÜKEN and ROSENHEIM 1983)

Ulcus cruris infectiosum:
Ecthymata, necrotized erysipelas, deep mycosis, gummatous ulcer, anthrax, diphtheria, leishmaniasis, lupus vulgaris, fistular and colliquative tuberculosis, atypical mycobacteriosis, sporotrichosis, herpes zoster gangraenosum
Ulcus cruris exogenicum/traumaticum:
Trauma (mechanical, thermic, actinic, chemical), artifacts
Ulcus cruris trophicum/neuropathicum:
Diabetes mellitus, nerve lesions (polymyelitis, leprosy, traumatic), acrodermatitis chronica atrophicans Pick–Herxheimer
Ulcus cruris haematopathogenicum:
Essential thrombocytopenia, sickle cell anemia, polycytemia vera, perniciosa, spherocytosis, familial hemolytic anemia, cryoglobulinemia
Ulcus cruris neoplasticum:
Carcinoma spinocellulare, basalioma, papillomatosis cutis carcinoides, malignant melanoma, aged kaposi sarcoma, hemangioendothelioma, keratoacanthoma, papillomatosis Gottron, venous or osteolytic basis, bone metastasis

---

42.4
Diagnostics

Before treatment, the diagnostic procedure should be initiated according to the following steps. Symptomatic therapy can begin simultaneously, but the final decision on appropriate therapy requires a precise diagnosis.

42.4.1
Individual Case History

1. Family history: Venous diseases, ulcers, lung embolism, heart disease, disturbances of blood-clotting;
2. Past medical history (PMH): Time of occurrence, course, symptoms;
3. Accompanying and preceding illnesses: Varicosis, ulcers, thrombophlebitis, thrombosis, lung embolism, diabetes mellitus, hypertension, arterial occlusive disease, lipometabolism disturbances, heart, liver, and renal diseases;
4. Previous surgery: Venous operations, gynecological surgery, surgery on joints, abdominal surgery, trauma;
5. Pregnancy
6. Occupational history
7. Allergies (e.g., parabenes, lanolin, iodine)
8. Vegetative anamnesis: Nicotine, alcohol, medication (contraceptives, phenprocoumon, etc.);
9. Previous topical therapy.

42.4.2
Clinical Examination

The initial aspect of the examination is a careful observation of the wound. This helps to establish differential diagnostic considerations and gives a clue to therapeutic success. Special attention should be paid to the topographical site of the wound and its attributes such as size, circumference, base, and surroundings. Findings from palpation, temperature, and venous and arterial status should be noted.

In addition to risk factors (adipositas, heart and circulatory disturbances), the general examination should also include neurological and orthopedic findings. Simple functional tests should be performed at the end of the check-up (e.g., Ratschow's test, walking test). Even though an experienced doctor can usually discern the genesis of a leg ulcer

quite accurately, laboratory diagnostic techniques should verify the preliminary diagnosis.

42.4.3
Technical Methods of Examination

Over the past few years the extent of our knowledge of peripheral vascular diseases has grown enormously, mostly due to the increasing use of technical examining methods. On the one hand, angiography displays morphological changes, while on the other, various technical methods mainly assess the functional state of the peripheral vascular system. In the following, according to our own experience, only methods of clinically practical importance for diagnosis will be discussed; scientifically interesting testing methods are not included.

42.4.3.1
Non-Invasive Methods

The Doppler ultrasound transducer represents the basic device for every doctor dealing with vascular problems. This device enables an assessment of the extent and location of vascular occlusions, venous obstructions, and valvular incompetence of the superficial and deep venous systems. The principle of this method is that ultrasound waves are reflected by corpuscles of flowing blood with a change of frequency when they transcutaneously target a vessel. This change of frequency between emitting and reflecting ultrasound waves is detected within an audible range by means of a headset or speakers, and can be graphically registered by an oscilloscope or printer. For daily routine non-directional pocket Doppler devices are sufficient without registration. Directional Doppler devices can detect blood flow velocity as well as blood flow direction.

The venous Doppler signal bears low frequency and is respiratory-dependent, whereas pulse-synchronic arterial signals have a high frequency. Measuring distal malleolar systolic arterial blood pressure makes it possible to recognize consistently hemodynamically relevant stenoses of the main leg arteries. The posterior tibial artery and the dorsal pedis artery are continuously auscultated on a recumbent patient while a blood pressure cuff is inflated above the systolic pressure. After a slow depression the systolic pulse initially heard is registered, which is normally higher than the brachial pressure. Low pressure measurements indicate arterial stenosis. The absolute parameter of systolic pressure correlates well with the degree of perfusion disturbancy. Blood pressure rates under 50 mm Hg endanger the limb. Medial sclerosis of vessels, observed particularly in patients suffering from diabetes and in patients with extensive cuff-formed dermatosclerosis and massive edema, makes an accurate measurement of pressure unreliable due to improper compression of arteries. In these cases an electric oscillometry and photoplethysmographic device have proven useful (FEUERSTEIN 1981; GOLDMAN and FRONEK 1992; JAMIESON 1993).

Oscillography serves as a registration of volume changes of a pulse wave at a certain point on the limb using a blood pressure cuff and manometer by GESENIUS and KELLER (KAPPERT 1987). This method identifies arterial occlusion sites and can be performed not only at rest but also during exertion (SCHOOP 1988). Results of the curves can give information on obliterations and their location, above or below the inguinal ligament (PARTSCH 1982, 1985; SCHOOP 1988).

Photoplethysmography is another non-invasive screening method that assesses the function of limb vessels. Infrared light of a defined wavelength with an absorption maximum in the near infrared region is emitted into the skin. The reflected portion is registered and printed. This reflected portion is dependent on the blood volume of the examined body region. This technique can answer questions concerning the registration of arterial pulse waves, as well as venous volume changes under standardized conditions of exercise (calf muscle pump). With the help of a tourniquet test approximate information on impaired venous function can be provided between the superficial and deep venous systems (Fig. 42.2) (GOLDMAN et al. 1994; JAMIESON 1993; RABE et al. 1996).

The infrared-sensitive diodes of the thermography method measure the superficial temperature of selected body regions. The detection of thermal radiation in the lower limb has become of practical interest with special respect to incompetent perforating veins and deep venous thrombosis. The former indication is easy to perform in practice using thermoplates. For thrombosis diagnostics the extensive telethermography requires a special camera. At a sensitive setting the course of arteries can be followed (PARTSCH 1982).

The venous occlusion plethysmography is another method in which a cuff is placed around the thigh and venous stasis is induced. The volume increase in the calf is measured by means of a strain

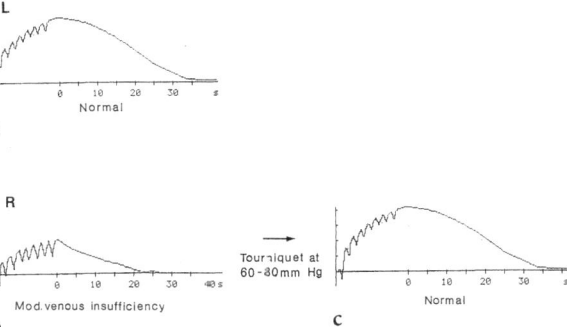

Fig. 42.2 a. Here the left leg is normal with refilling time longer than 25 s after eight dorsiflexions at the ankle [shown as eight slowly rising peaks on photoplethysmography (PPG) tracing]. **b** The right leg indicates venous valvular insufficiency. **c** On the right leg, the test is repeated with an above-knee tourniquet at approximately 60–80 mmHg; repeat tracing shows refill time, which is considered normal. This PPG examination shows the deep valves to be competent with reflux occurring in the superficial veins on the right. A correctable PPG predicts that elimination of varicosities will normalize venous function of the involved leg (comp. SCHULTZ-EHRENBURG 1985)

gauge, and after ending the stasis the decrease is registered. Thus, information is obtained about the venous capacity and the venous reflux. Additional parameters such as the venous elasticity and capillary filtration rate can also be measured. The major disadvantage of this test is its poor reproducibility (JAMIESON 1993; PARTSCH 1982).

An additional method is duplex ultrasound, which is also presented with a color code. This method combines an imaging procedure (B-method, real-time technique) with the capability of a simultaneous Doppler investigation. Flow direction, tachography, and venous filling can be measured non-invasively, while venous valves, wall, and surroundings can also be assessed. Certain questions can be answered without using the invasive phlebography technique. Duplex ultrasound devices have become quite popular despite their high cost.

42.4.3.2
Invasive Procedures

Phlebodynamometry has become the reference method to assess the venous pressure of the calf muscle pump by a direct sanguineous puncture of the dorsal foot, and mainly deals with functional aspects. By outer compression of the vein, mostly by fascial and muscle compression through joint movement, blood is pushed from the distal limb upwards.

The subsequent hydrostatic reflux is hindered by sufficient valve action. The amount of pressure decrease correlates to the function of the calf muscle pump. The pressure measurement is performed by an electromagnetic pressure gauge and graphically registered. No specific diagnosis (varicosis, deep venous thrombosis) can be made, but the severity of the venous pump impairment can be estimated. Phlebodynamometry is still the most precise test method, but due to painfulness and possible complications (hematoma, phlebitis) it is not applied routinely (PARTSCH 1982).

Phlebography permits an assessment of the morphology of the venous system. Its indication is appropriate when prior investigations have not been able to yield reliable data. It remains the standard method for diagnostics and follow-up control of deep venous thrombosis. The contrast medium is injected into a distal vein of the dorsum of the foot which is observed by a fluoroscope under supramalleolar stasis. Continuous radiographs are subsequently taken from the calf, the thigh, and pelvic region tracing the transport of the contrast medium in the veins. Next, the Valsalva maneuver is performed; when the valve is incompetent the retrograde flow of contrast medium will appear at the SFJ or transfascial perforating veins into the superficial venous system. In addition to morphology, venous hemodynamics can be assessed. Contraindications are contrast medium intolerances, serious general ailments, extensive lymphedema, and pregnancy (relative contraindication). Possible complications include the above-mentioned intolerance reactions and allergies, as well as contrast medium-induced thrombophlebitis and deep venous thrombosis (JAMIESON 1993; PARTSCH 1982). Arteriography, with or without digital subtraction, is indicated before surgical or interventional recanalization of occluded arteries and before treatment of arteriovenous (AV)-malformations and special problems of differential diagnosis.

42.5
Therapy

A leg ulcer – a tissue defect as a consequence or end product of a multifactoral cause – is actually merely a symptom of different, pathogenetic, more or less significant, underlying disease. Since the basic heterogenic pathophysiologic findings are quite important for therapeutic procedures, many different treatment strategies exist. The most important therapies will be discussed below, with special regard to the most frequent differential diagnoses (ulcus cruris venosum and ulcus cruris arteriosum). Subsequently, external treatment modalities will be presented and demonstrated on the example of the venous leg ulcer.

42.5.1
Therapy of Venous Leg Ulcers

Conservative, surgical, and combined treatments exist in several modifications.

42.5.1.1
Surgical Treatment

Venous Surgery. The aim is to improve local or general venous function by either eliminating or removing incompetent epifascial veins that overload the deep venous system by reflux. In addition to vein stripping, usually performed on varicosis of the long and short saphenous veins, insufficient interconnecting veins between the epifascial and subfascial venous systems should also be ligated in an additional operation (perforating veins, SFJ) (DOUGLAS and SIMPSON 1995; MOLLARD 1994; NETZER 1979).

Fascial Surgery. A paratibial fasciotomy may be applied to ulcers resistant to therapy, in some cases combined with perforating venous dissection or ligation, or an endoscopic perforating dissection with or without fascial cleavage. Pressure relief in subfascial tissue is obtained by a resulting fascial dehiscence, as well as a broader surface communication between intra- and extrafascial compartments. This enables new capillaries from muscles to grow into the indurate subcutaneous tissue. This improves the microcirculation and increases oxygenization and thus facilitates healing of an ulcer (GLOVICZKI et al. 1996; HACH and HACH-WUNDERLE 1994).

Sclerotherapy. Sclerotherapy can be applied to eliminate epifascial veins. Because of a high recurrence rate sclerotherapy should be confined to lateral and reticular varices. Varices adjacent to the ulcer region (so-called feeding veins) may also be considered to sclerose (GOLDMAN et al. 1994; MOLLARD 1994).

Ulcer Surgery. Besides surgical débridement (ulcer curettage, radial incisions of callous edges) skin surgery is closely associated with free skin grafting. The main goal of plastic covering with

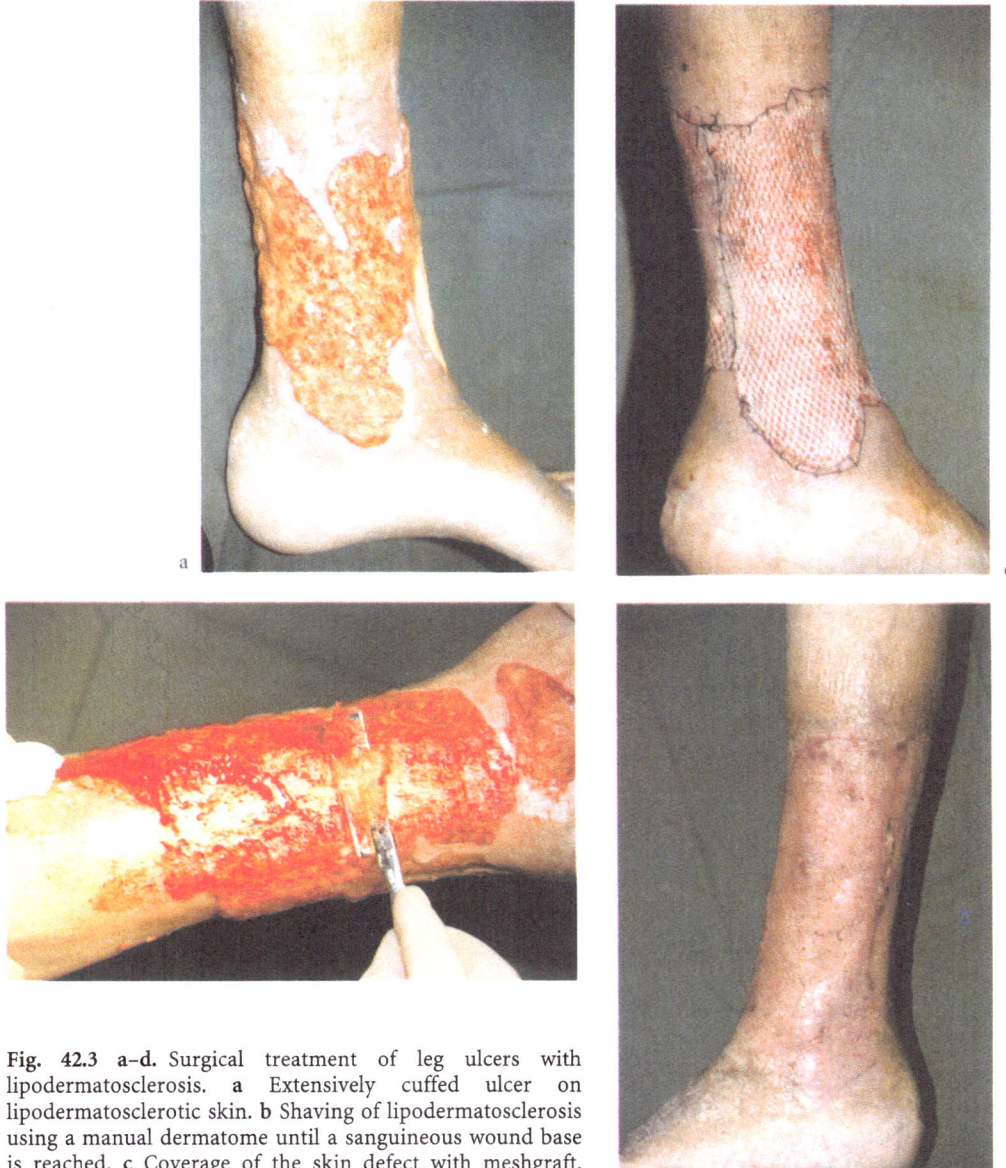

Fig. 42.3 a–d. Surgical treatment of leg ulcers with lipodermatosclerosis. **a** Extensively cuffed ulcer on lipodermatosclerotic skin. **b** Shaving of lipodermatosclerosis using a manual dermatome until a sanguineous wound base is reached. **c** Coverage of the skin defect with meshgraft. **d** Healed skin-graft

meshgraft, split-skin, or (full) skin is to shorten the lengthy phase of epithelization and provide stable wound coverage. The maximal variant of ulcer surgery is lipodermatosclerosis shaving with consecutive split-skin grafting (Fig. 42.3). Superficial scar tissue is removed until the tissue is well supplied with blood. The fresh wound base is covered with meshgraft (split-skin). This enables a stable, durable, and resistant skin coverage with successful long-term results (GALLI et al. 1992). Thus, ulcers which have appeared to be therapy-resistant for years have been healed by this method (DOUGLAS and SIMPSON 1995; KAUFMANN et al. 1986).

42.5.1.2
Conservative Treatment

Physiotherapy. The basic treatment of venous ulcers should not be confined to the mere ulcer, but rather should deal with the complete needs of the patient. This is why not only medical but also physiotherapeutic measures should be considered that take a decreased orthostatic burden into account. Exercises included are controlled walking training and physiotherapeutic mobilization with special regard to adequate mobility of the ankle joint (JAMIESON 1993; PESCHEN et al. 1996). Since the calf muscle pump is not activated at rest, this pump embodies the most important mechanism of venous return besides the supportive compression bandage.

Pharmacotherapy. Some evidence of the efficacy of controversially discussed systemic "preparations for varicosis" has been presented, or at least made plausible, in recent years with the help of more sensitive measuring methods. Besides countlessly combined preparations containing mixtures of diverse and mostly underdosed extracts, three main groups of drugs can be distinguished and are presented in Table 42.5.

The theoretical background for the usage of these drugs is based on their profile of action to counteract abnormalities and risk factors in ulcer patients. It must be stressed that these adjuvant measures are not a substitute for causal treatment. Furthermore, possible side effects and contraindications restrict the use of many drugs.

Compression Bandage Therapy. Medical compression therapy represents the basis of non-invasive treatment. It can be performed as a monotherapy or be used in combination with invasive strategies. The effect of compression therapy on the hemodynamics of ulcer pathogenesis is demonstrated in Table 42.6.

Hereby, we distinguish three main types of compression therapy: (1) Compression bandage; (2) technical compression; (3) compression stockings.

The most important compression therapy is the compression bandage. We distinguish between fixed dressings and changed dressings (Table 42.7).

The various types of compression offer a wide range of individuality and can be suited to therapeutic requirements. Optimal compression is ensured when high work pressure during exertion and reduced pressure during rest are achieved. The resting pressure is exerted on the tissue by the bandage during muscle diastole. Accordingly, the work pressure can be seen as the resistance of the compression bandage against the dilatation of the muscles. Stiff dressings, such as Unna's paste dressing or adhesive dressings, but also "short stretch bandages", demonstrate these attributes most satisfactorily. They exert only slight rest pressure on a recumbent patient, but since walking activates the calf muscle pump, they develop optimal working pressure alleviating the congestion of the limb. Compression therapy can only be successful if the patient contributes actively to the healing process.

Table 42.5. Main groups of systemic pharmacotherapy for leg ulcers (PESCHEN et al. 1996)

Edema-protective drugs
 Plant glycosides, semi-synthetic lavonoids, synthetic monosubstances, combinations
Drugs that lavage the edema
 Diuretics (triamterene, bemetizide, furosemide, combinations)
Venous tone stimulation
 Sympathomimetics, combinations
Antiphlogistic agents

Table 42.6. Effects of compression therapy (MOSCHNER-KUNERT and ZABEL 1992; SCHULTZ-EHRENBURG 1985)

Increase in interstitial pressure
 Reabsorption of edema
Constriction of venous system
 Under some circumstances, valvular insufficiency
 Acceleration of blood low
 Emptying of venous plexus
 Reduction of blood volume
Outer support
 Improvement of calf muscle pump
 Cuff substitute around ulcer

Table 42.7. Types of compressive bandages (MOSCHNER-KUNERT and ZABEL 1992; WULFHORST and KÜLTER 1990)

Fixed dressings
 Self adhesive dressings
 Unna's paste dressing
Changed dressings
 Short-stretch bandages
 Middle-stretch bandages
 High-stretch bandages

HAID (1997) recommends the so-called Fisher bandage to facilitate adequate drainage of venous blood and interstitial edema based on the principle of the ankle-suction-pressure pump. By using this bandage, an increased compression of the distal calf is achieved without impairing ankle joint movement.

An accompanying modality recommended for patients suffering from venous leg ulcers is intermittent pneumatic compression (MOSCHNER-KUNERT and ZABEL 1992). Decongestion of limb edema can be achieved and accelerated by pneumatic pressure devices. This is best suited to immobilized patients. The rhythmic increase and decrease of pressure replaces the active movement of the muscle calf pump. This can be verified by venous functional diagnostics.

Compression stockings maintain the achieved conditions of therapy. They are most suitable for patients with healed ulcers. A suitable compression class is a prerequisite: stockings representing the intermediate superficial effect class II are most commonly used. Wearing compression stockings is usually a life-long condition for patients. General attrition of stockings makes it necessary to prescribe new stockings every half to 1 year.

42.5.2
Treatment of Arterial Ulcers

42.5.2.1
Secondary Prophylaxis

The therapeutic procedures against peripheral occlusion disease initially comprise preventing, discovering, and treating risk factors in addition to providing prophylactic measures that may reverse progress of the disease. This includes leading a healthy life, nicotine abstinence, weight control, optimal nutrition, drug management of diabetes mellitus, hyperlipoproteinemia, hyperuricemia, and hypertension. In order to slow down the progress of a diabetic microangiopathy, it is vital to stabilize blood sugar levels; if necessary to change over to insulin (CREUTZIG 1991).

42.5.2.2
Ergotherapy

An active exercise program is quite important to stimulate own-body compensation mechanisms, especially during the intermittent claudication phase. Interval training induces an increase in muscular metabolic capacity by an increase of myoglobin content. Other effects include an enlargement and increase of mitochondria, an increase in activity of oxidative enzymes, and an increase in the collateralization and blood supply in favor of the tissue's nutritive perfusion.

42.5.2.3
Vasodilatory Measures

Vasodilatory measures should be taken into account in advanced phases of arterial occlusive disease with reduced patient ability to walk (distances generally under 100 m), also showing signs of decompensation of the peripheral circulation under resting conditions (stage III/IV). For this indication percutaneous transluminal angioplasty (PTA) has obtained general acceptance. Stenoses and segmental occlusions in iliac, femoral, popliteal, and proximal tibiofibular arteries are good indications for percutaneous recanalization methods, whereas long occlusions are indications for bypass surgery. The application of stents is recommended for unsatisfactory dilatation because it guarantees more long-term success. Vascular surgery offers a broad spectrum of revasculative modalities. The range of indications begins at stage IIb and is absolute for stages III–IV. Depending on the vessel region, thrombendarterectomy (TEA), vascular prosthesis, or bypass surgery must be considered (HACH 1996; SCHULZ-EHRENBURG 1980).

42.5.2.4
Pharmacotherapy

Drug therapy of arterial occlusive disease is indicative as a prophylaxis for progress of the disease, as a concomitant therapy after catheter angioplasty, or in some cases where revascularization is not possible, undesirable, or unsuccessful. The rheologic measures shown in Table 42.8 can be considered.

Despite all the progress in diagnostics and treatment of arterial occlusive disease, the limb with extensive blood supply disturbances cannot usually be saved. Amputation should not be delayed if extensive necrosis and pain appear, in order to prevent irrepairable damage to the locomotor system by immobilization. Additionally, the patient is endangered by drug dependence and general body decay. The former concept that amputation stops arterial occlusive disease in a negative sense is obsolete. Patients need further intensive medical care since

Table 42.8. Pharmacotherapeutic measures for occlusive arterial disease (HEIDRICH 1997)

Hemodilution

Increase of erythrocyte formability (e.g., pentoxifylline)
Vasoactive pharmacological products (e.g., prostaglandin E1, prostacyclin, naftidrofuryl, bulomedil)
Prophylaxis of thrombosis by anticoagulation and with thrombocyte aggregation inhibitors (e.g., ASA, phenprocoumon, heparin, low-molecular heparin)

ASA, acetylsalicylic acid (aspirin).

arteriosclerosis progresses with a potential danger of circulatory disturbances in other vital organs.

A review of important therapeutic strategies for arterial occlusive disease is summarized in Table 42.9.

Table 42.9. Principles of therapy for arterial occlusive disease (CREUTZIG 1991)

Secondary prophylaxis:
    Prevention/uncovering and treatment of risk factors
    (nicotine abstinence, weight loss, treatment of
    hypertension, diabetes, and hyperlipoproteinemia)
Ergotherapy:
    Increase of reserve circulation of the interval type by
    ambulatory training
Radiological/surgical interventions:
    Arterial recanalization (percutaneous transluminal
    angioplasty)
    Thrombendarterectomy
    Bypass surgery
Pharmacotherapy: (see Table 42.8)
Ablation:
    Borderline amputation
    Lower or proximal leg amputation (as *ultima ratio*)

42.5.3
Dressing of Ulcers

The example given here is that of a venous leg ulcer. A great variety of therapeutics imply that either various types of treatment can heal well or that no specific treatment can ensure success. As regards treatment with an ulcer dressing, it is difficult to decide which interpretation suits best since the etiology of leg ulcers is broadly heterogeneous and the assessment of different therapeutic measures is difficult due to a widely individual healing process of ulcers (LINDEMAYR and SANTLER 1982). In practice, the physician often tends towards polypragmatic treatment with respect to the etiological type of ulcer, wound condition, and pain experienced by the patient suffering from leg ulcers. However, it is advisable that the doctor confine his topical treatment of leg ulcers to a few and, if possible, simple measures. A leg ulcer does not represent merely a common wound on just any part of the body, it is tissue destruction in a problematic region.

The application of systemic antibiotics as treatment for leg ulcers should be restricted to possible complications such as erysipelas and phlegmon (ALINOVI et al. 1986). Moreover, dressings containing antibiotics are usually dispensable. Topically applied antibiotics never really attain sterile condi-

tions of the wound; instead they often induce antibiotic resistance of bacterial colonies and allergy sensibilization. Highly recommended are antiseptic topical agents (chinosol, chloramin, etc.). They have a broad therapeutic range and do not lead to the feared bacterial resistance. Their application – especially by means of wet dressings and baths – is recommended at an initial stage, if discharge and acute inflammation are present.

Wound healing usually takes a three-stage course under physiological condition. First there is the exudative stage, followed by the proliferative and reparative stages, respectively. The differential therapy of ulcers should be accommodated by a phase-adapted treatment (Table 42.10). The different stages of the healing process should be viewed individually; due to overlapping of the different phases they cannot always be readily distinguished from one another. After cleansing and healing of inflammation, granulation of the wound base is immediately stimulated. The danger of dressings, especially over a long period of time, is the external sensibilization and induction of contact-allergic skin damage (PARAMSOTHY et al. 1988). The most common allergies are listed in Table 42.11.

The application of hypoallergic preparations, as well as allergological investigation (epicutaneous test), especially if eczema is present, is the key to success for ulcer dressings. It is often practical to use

Table 42.10. Phase-adapted dressing (SCHULTZ-EHRENBURG 1985)

Ulcer cleaning:
    Mechanical (curettage, scalpel)
    Chemical (trypsine, streptodornase, collagenase)
Stimulation of granulation:
    Chemical/osmotic (Dextromer, Seesand, Actihaemy,
        Granugenol, etc.)
    Mechanical (wound edge incisions, etc.)
Epithelialization:
    Chemical (e.g., gauze)
    Surgical (skin grafting)

Table 42.11. Most common contact allergies of leg ulcer dressings (MAYERHAUSEN 1988)

Perubalsam
Anesthesin
Preservatives (e.g., p-hydroxybensoic acid, sorbic acid)
Neomycin
Bacitracin
Vioform
Formalin
Lanolin

own simple prescription formulas containing simple galenicals, whereas the hypoallergic dressings can be individually prescribed. Only those commercial products which clearly state all ingredients should be prescribed.

In summary, leg ulcers present a clinically complex picture regarding diagnostics, as well as therapeutic regime. In addition to a careful medical history, inspection, and palpation, an angiologic examination of the case is mandatory at the outset and must be supplemented by further steps such as biopsy, laboratory, and allergy tests. Subsequently, a phases-adapted treatment should be applied that suits the clinical findings. In addition to conservative treatments, various surgical modalities are available.

References

Alinovi A, Bassissi P, Pini M (1986) Systemic administration of antibiotics in the management of venous ulcers. J Am Acad Dermatol 2:186–191

Biland L, Widmer LK, Baillod L (1984) Zur Häufigkeit und Bedeutung des Ulcus cruris. Ther Umsch 41:835–845

Claude S, Burton MD III (1993) Management of chronic and problem lower extremity wounds. Dermatol Clin 11:767–773

Claude S, Burton MD (1994) Venous ulcers. Am J Surg 167[1A Suppl]:37–41

Creutzig A (1991) Krankheiten der Gefäße. In: Classen M, Diehl V, Kochsiek K (eds) Innere Medizin. Urban und Schwarzenberg, München, pp 913–949

Douglas WS, Simpson NB (1995) Guidelines for the management of chronic venous leg ulceration. Report of a multidisciplinary workshop. Br J Dermatol 132:446–452

Falk A, Klüken N (1990) Das Ulcus cruris als polyätiologisches Symptom. Phlebol Proktol 19:84–89

Feuerstein W (1981) Bedeutung und Indikation der Dopplerultraschalldiagnostik bei chronischer venöser Insuffizienz. Hautarzt 32:1–7

Gallenkemper G, Bulling BJ, Kahle B, Klüken N, Lehnert W, Rabe E, Schwahn-Schreiber C (1996) Leitlinien zur Diagnostik und Therapie des Ulcus cruris venosum. Phlebologie 25:254–258

Galli KH, Wolf H, Paul E (1992) Therapie des Ulcus cruris venosum unter Berücksichtigung neuerer pathogenetischer Gesichtspunkte. Phlebologie 21:183–187

Gilliland EL, Wolfe HNJ (1991) Leg ulcers. Br Med J 383:776–779

Gloviczki P, Cambria RA, Rhee RY, Canton LG, McKusick MA (1996) Surgical technique and preliminary results of endoscopic subfascial division of perforating veins. J Vasc Surg 23:517–523

Goldman MP, Fronek A (1992) Consensus paper on venous leg ulcer. The Alexander House Group. J Dermatol Surg Oncol 18:592–602

Goldman MP, Weiss RA, Bergan J (1994) Diagnosis and treatment of varicose veins: a review. J Am Acad Dermatol 31 Part 1:393–409

Hach W (1996) Arterien unter Verschluß. Was tun bei AVK? Med Trib 19[Suppl]:11–14

Hach W, Hach-Wunderle V (1994) Die Rezirkulationskreise der primären Varikose. Pathophysiologische Grundlagen zur chirurgischen Therapie. Springer, Berlin Heidelberg New York, pp 62–65

Hafner J, Bounameaux H, Burg G, Brunner U (1996) Management of venous leg ulcers. Vasa 25:161–167

Haid H (1997) Die Kompression als konservative Behandlung venöser Erkrankungen der Extremitäten. In: Zeitler E (ed) Klinische Radiologie Arterien und Venen. Springer, Berlin Heidelberg New York, pp 483–488

Heidrich H (1997) Konservative Therapie peripherer arterieller Durchblutungsstörungen. In: Zeitler E (ed) Klinische Radiologie Arterien und Venen. Springer, Berlin Heidelberg New York, pp 179–183

Jamieson WG (1993) State of the art of venous investigation and treatment. Can J Surg 36:119–128

Kappert H (ed) 1987. Lehrbuch und Atlas der Angiologie. Hans Huber, Bern

Kaufmann R, Vranes M, Landes E (1986) Dermatochirurgische Behandlungsmöglichkeiten des Ulcus cruris. Z Hautk 61:923–939

Klüken N, Rosenheim R (1983) Ulcus cruris venosum und Lebensalter unter Berücksichtigung der arteriellen Beteiligung. Hautarzt. [Suppl VI]:125–127

Lindemayr H, Santler R (1982) Die Lokaltherapie des Ulcus cruris venosum. Z Hautkrankheiten 57:203–211

Margolis DJ (1992) Management of venous ulcerations. Hosp Pract 5:32–44

Mayerhausen W (1988) Therapie des Ulcus cruris venosum. H + G Z Hautk 63[suppl 4]:92–94

Mollard JM (1994) Insuffisance veineuse chronique: prevention et therapeutiques non medicamenteuses. Presse Med 23:251–258

Moschner-Kunert F, Zabel M (1992) Indikation und Kontraindikation der Kompressionstherapie bei Ulcus cruris venosum. Vasomed, pp 614–620

Mulder GD, Reis TM (1990) Venous ulcers: pathophysiology and medical therapy. Am Fam Physician 42:1323–1330

Netzer C (1979) Ulcus cruris. In: Ehringer H, Fischer H, Netzer CO, Schmutzler R, Zeitler E (eds) Venöse Abflußstörungen. Enke, Stuttgart, pp 215–231

Paramsothy Y, Collins M, Smith AG (1988) Contact dermatitis in patients with leg ulcers. Contact Dermatitis 18:30–36

Partsch H (1982) Meßmethoden in der Dermatologischen Angiologie. Z Hautkrankheiten 57:227–246

Partsch H (1985) Apparative Zusatzuntersuchungen bei den häufigsten peripheren Gefäßerkrankungen in der Praxis. Hautarzt 36:203–211

Peschen M, Petter O, Vanscheidt W (1996) Chronisch venöse Insuffizienz – von der Pathophysiologie zur Therapie. Folge 1: Pathophysiologie, Kompressionsbehandlung, systemische Pharmakotherapie. Fortschr Med 26:315–318

Peschen M, Petter O, Vanscheidt W (1996) Chronisch venöse Insuffizienz – von der Pathophysiologie zur Therapie. Folge 4 (Schluß): Behandlung des Ulcus cruris – Therapierichtlinien. Fortschr Med 30:395–397

Rabe E, Berg D, Gerlach E, Seyeck J, Stemmer R, Wienert V (1996) Leitlinien zur venösen Diagnostik mit der Licht-Reflexions-Rheographie/Photoplethysmographie. Phlebologie 25:259–260

Schoop W (1988) Praktische Angiologie. Thieme, Stuttgart, pp 70–88

Schultz-Ehrenburg U (1980) Moderne konservative Therapie der arteriellen Verschlußkrankheit. Hautarzt 31:419–427

Schultz-Ehrenburg U (1985) Aktuelle Behandlungsrichtlinien und Differentialdiagnostik des Ulcus cruris venosum. Hautarzt 36:212–217

Schultz-Ehrenburg U, Weindorf N (1984) Problemsituation Ulcus mixtum. Swiss Med 6:41–44

Vanscheidt W, Laaf H, Lauber A, Schöpf E (1992) Pathogenetische Endstrecke der venösen Ulcera cruris. Phlebol 21:72–76

Vollmar (1996) Rekonstruktive Chirurgie der Arterien (4th ed). Thieme, Stuttgart

Wulfhorst B, Külter H (1990) Untersuchungen der Zugelastizität von elastischen Kompressionsbinden. Phlebologie und Proktologie 19:230–238

Appendix

I
Conversion table

BAR	PSI	ATM	PSI	BAR	ATM
1	14.5	1.02	1	0.1	0.1
2	29.0	2.04	5	0.3	0.4
3	43.5	3.06	10	0.7	0.7
4	58.0	4.08	50	3.5	3.5
5	72.5	5.10	100	6.9	7.0
7	101.5	6.12	200	13.8	14.1
8	116.0	7.14	300	20.7	21.1
9	130.5	9.18	400	27.6	28.1
10	145.0	10.20	500	34.5	35.2
11	159.0	11.22	600	41.4	42.2
12	174.0	12.24	700	48.3	49.2
		800	55.2	56.3	
		900	62.1	63.3	
		1000	69.0	70.3	
	1 bar = 1.02 atm = 14.5 psi	1100	75.9	77.4	
		1200	82.8	84.4	

French	mm	Inches	Gauge	OD (mm)	OD (Inch)
0.5	0.16	0.006	27	0.41	0.016
1	0.33	0.013	26	0.46	0.018
1.5	0.49	0.019	25	0.51	0.020
1.8	0.59	0.023	24	0.56	0.022
2	0.67	0.026	23	0.64	0.025
2.5	0.82	0.032	22	0.71	0.028
3.0	1.00	0.039	21	0.81	0.032
4	1.33	0.052	20	0.97	0.038
5	1.67	0.078	19	1.07	0.042
6	2.00	0.079	18	1.27	0.050
7	2.33	0.092	17	1.50	0.059
8	2.67	0.105	16	1.65	0.065
9	3.00	0.118	15	1.83	0.072
10	3.33	0.131	14	2.11	0.083

1 Fr = 0.0131 inch = 0.33 mm   1 inch = 2.54 cm

II

Bollinger score for evaluating peripheral occlusive vascular disease. *O*, occlusion; *St*, stenosis; *Ir*, irregularities less than 20% diameter reduction; *mult*, more than one stenosis; *n*, normal

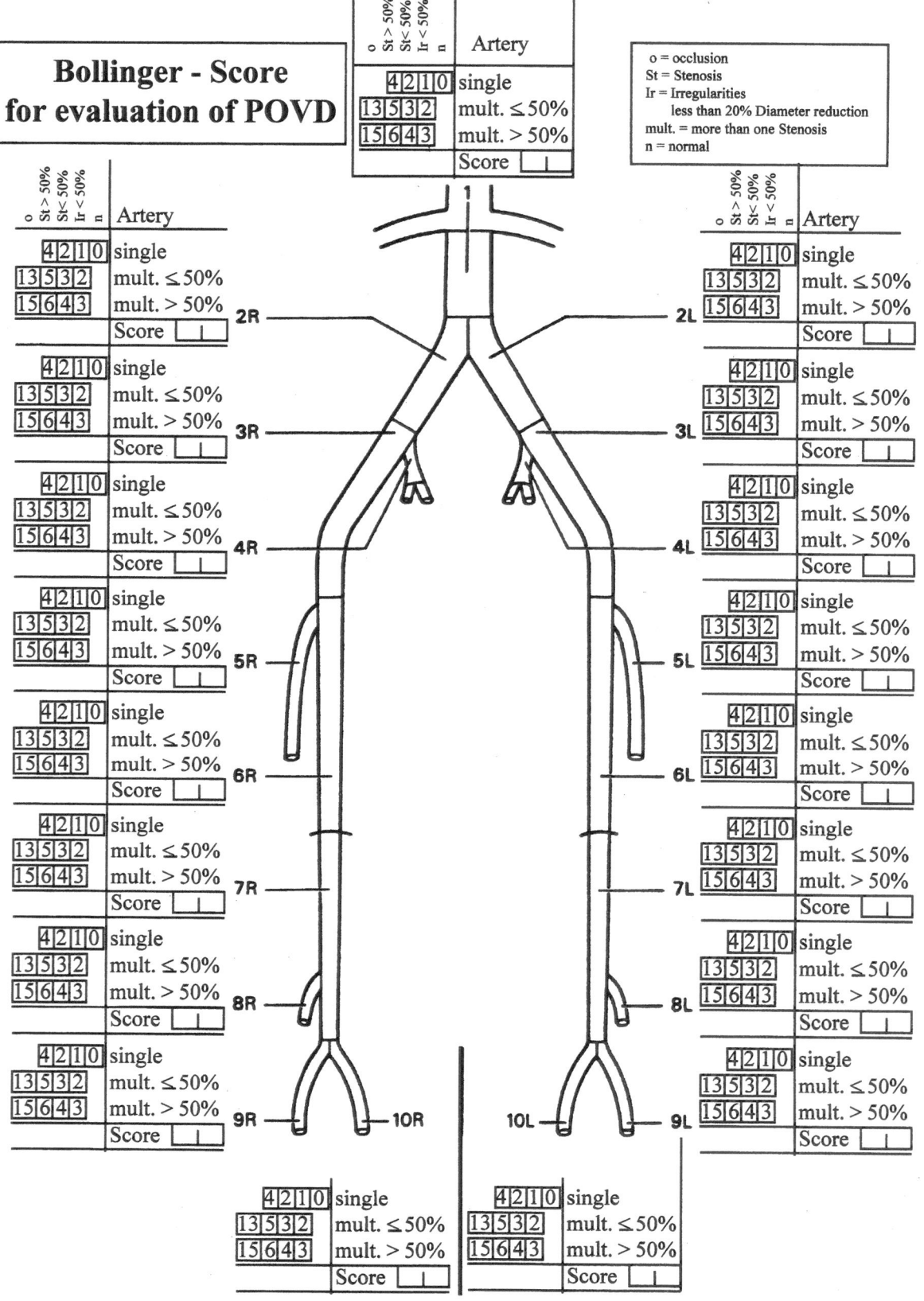

III.
List fo addresses of Companies

A) which develop and/or sale medical instruments for vascular diagnosis and intervention

Angiomed GmbH
Eisenbahnstr. 36
76229 Karlsruhe, Germany

Avalon Medizintechnologie
Leinstr. 33
30159 Hannover, Germany

Bard – Angiomed
C. R. Bard GmbH
Wachhaustr. 6
76227 Karlsruhe, Germany

BARD, C. R. Inc.
Billerica Mass., USA

Becton-Dickinson AG
Tullastr. 8–12
69126 Heidelberg, Germany

Biomedical Technology s.r.l.
Vis Tolstoj, 7/B
20090 Trezzano s/Naviglio (MI), Italy

Boston Scientific International
Schneider / Scimed
Vera 745
1414 Buenos Aires, Argentinia

Boston Sientific Ges.m.b.H.
Schneider / Scimed
Handelskai 388/521A
1020 Wien, Austria

Boston Sientific do Brazil
Schneider / Scimed
Av. Morumbi 6849
Soa Paulo, Brazil

Boston Scientific Nordic AS
Schneider / Scimed
Vestre Strandallé 101
8240 Risskov, Denmark

Boston Scientific International B.V.
Schneider / Scimed
Immeuble Vision Defense
91 boulevard National
92257 La garenne Colombes Cedex,
France

Boston Sientific GmbH
Schneider / Scimed
Christinenstr. 2
40880 Ratingen, Germany

Boston Scientific S.p.A.
Schneider / Scimed
World Trade Center – 10th Floor
Via dei Marini, 1
16149 Genoa, Italy

Boston Scientific, K.K.
Schneider / Scimed
Toho Building 8F
3-3-5, Kita-Shinagawa
Shinagawa-Ku, Tokyo 140, Japan

Boston Sientific International B.V.
Schneider / Scimed
MECC Business Center
Gaetona Martinolaan 85
6229 GS Maastricht, Netherlands

Boston Scientific
Schneider / Scimed
Rua Jose Gomes Ferreira
4, 7A
I-250 Lisbon, Portugal

Boston Scientific Iberia
Schneider / Scimed
Avenida europa 4, Edifico bruselas
Parque Emprasarial "La Moraleja"
28100 Alcobendas (Madrid), Spain

Boston Scientific Nordic A/B
Schneider / Scimed
Floor 4
Bega Alle 1
25452 Helsingborg/Sweden

Boston Scientific AG
Schneider / Scimed
Schneider technology Center
Ackerstr. 6
8180 Bulach, Switzerland

Boston Scientific Limited
Schneider / Scimed
New England House
Sandridge Park, Porters Wood
Sr. Albans Herts
AL3 6PH, UK

B. Braun Melsungen AG
Postfach 110
34212 Melsungen, Germany

BSIC Medizintechnik GmbH
Kölner Str. 67
40723 Hilden, Germany

Cardiovascular Dynamics, Inc.
13700 Alton Parkway
Irvine, California 92618, USA

Cook Incorporated
P.O. Box 489
Bloomington, IN 47402, United States

William, A. Cook Australia Pty. Ltd
Brisbane Technology Park
12 Electronics Street
Eight Mile Plains, Brisbane QLD 4113,
Australia

Cook Belgium NV/SA
Romeinsesteenweg 558 A
1853 Strombeck-Bever, Belgium-Lux-
embourg

Cook (Canada) Inc.
111 Sandiford Drive
Stouffville, Ontario L4A 7X5, Canada

William Cook Europe A/S
Sandet 6
4632 Bjaeverskov, Denmark

Cook France s.a.r.l.
2 rue du Noveau Bercy
94227 Charenton, Cedex, France

W. Cook Europe GmbH
Malmedyer Str. 10
41066 Mönchengladbach, Germany

Cook Italia s.r.l.
Via Raffaelo Sanzio 17/19
20092 Cinisello Malsano (MI), Italy

Cook Netherland B.V.
Eckestrijt 4502
5692 DM SON, The Netherlands

Cook Espana S.A.
Mallorca 27,
08029 Barcelona, Spain

Cook (Switzerland) AG
Schellenrain 5
6210 Sursee, Switzerland

Cook (UK) Limited
Monroe House, Letchworth
Herts SG 6 1 LN, UK

Cordis Corp.
Johnson & Johnson Comp.
PO Box 025700
Miami, Florida 33102-5700, USA

Cordis Division
Johnson & Johnson Comp.
Gunoldstr. 14, Postfach 8
1199 Wien, Austria

Cordis International SA
Johnson & Johnson Company
Waterloo Office Park
Dreve Richelle 161 H
1410 Waterloo, Belgium

Cordis NV / SA
Johnson & Johnson Comp.
Horizon Center
Leuvensesteenweg 510 Bus 42
1930 Zaventem, Belgium

Cordis S.A.
Johnson & Johnson Comp.
Parc de Viry Bátiment A,
Rue de Ris
91178 Viry-Châtillon Cedex, France

Cordis S.A.
Johnson & Johnson Comp.
Rue Camille Des Mouslins 1
TSA 71001
92787 Issy les Moulineaux, France

Cordis Med. Apparate GmbH
Johnson & Johnson Comp.
Rheinische Str. 2
42781 Haan, Germany

Cordis Med. Apparate GmbH
Johnson & Johnson Comp.
Max-Planck-Str. 20–22
40699 Erkrath, Germany

Cordis Hungaria KFT
Johnson & Johnson Comp.
Iranyi utaca 21–23/2
1056 Budapest, Hungaria

Cordis Italia
Johnson & Johnson Comp.
Plazza don Enrico Mapelli 1
20099 Sesto San Giovanni
(M) Italy

Cordis Italia SpA
Johnson & Johnson Comp.
Via Teocrito 36
20128 Milano, Italia

Cordis Europa NV
Johnson & Johnson Comp.
Pb 38 Oosteinde 8
9300 AA Roden, The Netherlands

Cordis Portugal sa
Johnson & Johnson Comp.
Rua Latino Caolho 33 6 Esq
1000 Lisboa, Portugal

Cordis Espana
Johnson & Johnson Comp.
Gronegatan 9
20011 Malmö, Sweden

Cordis Corp.
Johnson & Johnson
Staffansväg 2
19184 Sollentuna, Sweden

Cordis AG
Johnson & Johnson Comp.
Gaswerkstr. 48
4900 Langenthal, Switzerland

Cordis
Johnson & Johnson
Rotzenbühlstr. 55
8957 Spreitenbach, Switzerland

Johnson & Johnson Medical
Cordis Divison
Coronation Road
South Ascot
Berkshire SL5 9EY, United Kingdom

Corotec Medizintechnik GmbH
Am Weinkastell 7
55270 Klein-Winternheim, Germany

Dastascope GmbH
Collagen Products
Zeppelinstr. 2-4
D-64625 Bensheim, Germany

Datascope Collagen Products
14 Philips Parkway
Montvale NJ 07645, USA

Deutsche Abbott GmbH
Max-Planck-Ring 2
65205 Wiesbaden, Germany

Gore-Technologies
W.L. Gore & Associates GmbH
Hermann-Oberth-Str. 22
85640 Putzbrunn, Germany

W.L. Gore & Associates, Inc
Flagstaff, Arizona 86003-3200, USA

W.L. Gore & Associates, Inc.
1327 Oreleans Drive
Sunnyvale, California 94089, USA

Grifols S.A.
Ctra Nacional N 152, km 21
Parets de Vllés, Spain

Johnson & Johnson
Interventional Systems Co.
35 Technology Drive
P.O. Box 4917, Warren
N.J. 07059

Johnson & Johnson
Medical NV/SA Europe
Dréve Richelle
161H–161O Waterloo, Belgium

Jomed Deutschland
Carl-von-Linde Str. 38
85716 Unterschleißheim, Germany

JOMED Netherlands B.V.
Bamfordweg 1
6235 NS Ulestraten, The Netherlands

JOMED Russia
Studencheskaya el. 34, Box 5
121165 Moscow, Russia

JOMED Switzerland AG
Amthauptstrasse
8222 Beringen, Switzerland

JOMED UK Ltd
Tabley Court, Moss Lane
Ober Tabley
Knutfford-Cheshire WA 16 CPL, United
Kingdom

A.D. Krauth
Wandbeker Königstr.
Postfach 701260
22041 Hamburg, Germany

Mallinckrodt Medical GmbH
Josef-Dietzgen-Str. 1–3
Postfach 1462
53761 Hennef/Sieg, Germany

Malinckrodt Medical Co., Ltd
Shuwa Kamiya-Cho Bldg.
3–13 Toranomon 4 – Chome
Minato – Ku, Tokyo 195, Japan

Medcare
Mail du Centre
3, allée Hector Berlioz
95130 Franconville, France

Medico's Hirata, Inc.
3-4-3 Edobori
Nishi-Ku, Osaka 550, Japan

Medtronic AVE, Inc.
3576 Unocal Place
Santa Rosa, CA. 95403, USA

Medtronic Aneu Rx.
1312 Crossmann Avenue
Sunnyvale, CA 94089, USA

Medtronic B.V.
Wenckebachstraat 10
6466 NC Kerkrade, The Netherlands

Microvena Corp. and
RJP International Inc.
P.O. Box 1527, Baldwin
New York 11510 USA

Optimed
Medizinische Instrumente GmbH
Ferdinand-Porsche-Str. 11
76275 Ettlingen, Germany

Perclose, Inc.
199 Jefferson Drive
Menlo Park
CA 94025, USA

Promedics GmbH
Egliweg 10
2560 Nidau, Switzerland

Prague Medical CS s.r.o.
Na Safrance 41
10100 Praha 10, Czech Republic

Sherine Med AG
Kirchstr. 7
3427 Utzendorf, Switzerland

Sherine Med Americas LLC
P.O. Box 51570
Irvine, CA 92619-1570, USA

Sherwood Davis & Geck
Angio-Seal
St. Louis, Missouri, USA

St. Jude Medical GmbH
Daig Division
Marienbergstr. 82
90411 Nürnberg, Germany

Tamro Medical AS
Langebjerg 23
4000 Roskilde, Denmark

Tamro MedLab AB
Danmarkgatan 46
164 40 Kista, Sweden

Targe CMI, Inc.
4-7-1 Aobadai
Meguro-Ku
Tokyo 153, Japan

Target Therapeutics
San Jose, California, USA

Terumo (Deutschland) GmbH
Postfach 710863
60498 Frankfurt
Lyoner Str. 11a
60528 Frankfurt, Germany

Tietze-Medical
Tannerweg 16
91329 Adelsdorf, Germany

Trigon-MTS GmbH
Könneterring 11
41068 Mönchengladbach, Germany

B) Contrast Media

Bracco- Imaging
Bracco. S.p.A.
Via E. Foli 50
20134 Milano, Italy

Byk-Gulden-Lomberg
Byk-Gulden-Str. 2
78467 Konstanz, Germany

Mallinckrodt Medical GmbH
Josef-Dietzgen-Str. 1–3
Postfach 1462
53761 Hennef/Sieg, Germany

Nycomed Arzneimittel GmbH
Postfach 450361
Freisinger Landstr. 74
80939 München, Germany

Schering AG
Müllerstr. 170–178
13353 Berlin, Germany

Subject Index

List of Contributors

ERNST AMANN, Dr. Ing.
Abteilungsdirektor
c/o Siemens AG
Medizinische Technik
Henkestrasse 127
D-91052 Erlangen
Germany

address for correspondence:
Giebelbachstrasse 15
D-88131 Lindau/B
Germany

D. C. BAUMGART, MD
Georgetown University Hospital
Department of Medicine
3800 Resevoir Rd NW
Washington DC 20007-2197
USA

A. BECK, Professor, Dr. med., Dr. theol.
Klinikum Konstanz
Institut für Röntgendiagnostik
und Nuklearmedizin
D-78461 Konstanz
Germany

GARY J. BECKER, MD
Miami Cardiac and Vascular Institute
8900 North Kendall Drive
Miami, FL 33176
USA

H. BERGER, MD
Professor, Institut für Röntgendiagnostik
der Technischen Universität München
Klinikum rechts der Isar
Ismaninger Straße 22
D-81675 München
Germany

S.A. BEYER-ENKE, MD
Institut für Diagnostische
und Interventionelle Radiologie
Klinikum Nord
Flurstrasse 17
D-90340 Nürnberg
Germany

UWE BÖTTCHER, PhD
Siemens AG
Medizinische Technik
Med MRA
Henkestraße 127
D-91052 Erlangen
Germany

DANIEL COLUMBIER, MD
Department of Radiology
CHU Rangueil 1
Avenue Jean Poulhes
F-31054 Toulouse
France

KLAUS DETMAR, MD
Institut für Diagnostische und
Interventionelle Radiologie
Klinikum Nord
Flurstraße 17
D-90340 Nürnberg
Germany

DAI-DO DO, MD
Angiologische Abteilung
Inselspital
CH-3010 Bern
Switzerland

JOCHEN FERNHOLZ; MD
Professor, Head of Department of Radiology
Städtisches Klinikum
Moltkestraße 90
D-76133 Karlsruhe
Germany

T. FRITZSCHE, MD
Universitätsklinikum der Humboldt-
Universität zu Berlin
Campus Charité MiHe
Klinik für Anästhesiologie und
operative Intensivmedizin
Schumannstraße 20/21
D-10117 Berlin
Germany

K. GALL, MD
Hautklinik
Klinikum-Nord
Prof.-Ernst-Nathan-Str.1
D-90419 Nürnberg
Germany

WALTER GROSS-FENGELS, MD
Professor, Abteilung für Diagnostische und
Interventionelle Radiologie
Gefäß-Centrum Hamburg-Harburg (GCH)
Allgemeines Krankenhaus Harburg
Eißendorfer Pferdeweg 52
D-21075 Hamburg
Germany

PETER HEILBERGER, MD
Klinik für Gefäßchirurgie
Städtisches Klinikum Süd
Breslauer Straße 201
D-90471 Nürnberg
Germany

R. HILDEBRANDT, MD
Institut für Diagnostische und
Interventionelle Radiologie
Klinikum Nord
Flurstraße 17
D-90340 Nürnberg
Germany

B. HOLIK, MD
Praxis Drs. Holik-Frank-Meusel-Lösch
Wetterkreuz 21
D-91058 Erlangen-Tennenlohe
Germany

KÁLMÁN HÜTTL, MD
Department of Vascular Surgery
Semmelweis Medical University
Városmajor u. 68.
H-Budapest 1122
Hungary

FRANCIS JOFFRE, MD
Department of Radiology
CHU Rangueil 1
Avenue Jean Poulhes
F-31054 Toulouse
France

BARRY T. KATZEN MD
Miami Cardiac and Vascular Institute
8900 North Kendall Drive
Miami, FL 33176
USA

W. KRAUSE, MD
Professor
Schering AG
Contrast Media Research
Muellerstrasse 170-178
D-13342 Berlin
Germany

J. LAMMER, MD
Professor, Universitätsklinik für Radiodiagnostik
Klinische Abteilung für Angiographie
und Interventionelle Radiologie
Währinger Gürtel 18-120
A-1190 Vienna
Austria

P. LEGER, MD
Department of Cardiovascular Surgery
CHU Rangueil 1
Avenue Jean Poulhes
F-31054 Toulouse
France

DIETER LIERMANN, MD
Professor, Direktor der Klinik für Radiologie und
Nuklearmedizin
Universitätsklinikum der Ruhr-Universität Bochum -
Marienhospital
Hölkeskampring 40
D-44625 Herne
Germany

W. LÖSCH, MD
Praxis Drs. Holik-Frank-Meusel-Lösch
Wetterkreuz 21
D-91058 Erlangen-Tennenlohe
Germany

DIRK A. LOOSE, Dr. med. habil.
Professor, Zentrum für Gefäßmedizin
Abteilung für Angiologie und Gefäßchirurgie der
chirurgischen Klinik Dr. Guth
Jürgensallee 44
D-22609 Hamburg
Germany

R. LOOSE, MD, PhD
Institut für Diagnostische und
Interventionelle Radiologie
Klinikum Nord
Flurstraße 17
D-90340 Nürnberg
Germany

THOMAS F. LÜSCHER, MD
Division of Cardiology
University Hospital Zürich
Rämistrasse 100
CH-8091 Zürich
Switzerland

FELIX MAHLER, MD
Professor, Angiologische Abteilung
Inselspital
CH-3010 Bern
Switzerland

M. MARTIN, MD
Professor
Angiologische Praxis
Klinikum Duisburg
Zu den Rehwiesen 9
D-47055 Duisburg
Germany

K. MATHIAS, MD
Städtische Kliniken
Radiologische Klinik
Beurhausstraße 40
D-44137 Dortmund
Germany

R. MÖLLER, MD
Hautklinik
Klinikum-Nord
Prof.-Ernst-Nathan-Str. 1
D-90419 Nürnberg
Germany

M. MÜCK-WEYMANN, MD
Klinik und Poliklinik für
Psychotherapie und Psychosomatische Medizin
Technische Universität Dresden
Fetscherstraße 74
D-01307 Dresden
Germany

TAKAO OHKI, MD
Division of Vascular Surgery
Montefiore Medical Center
111 East 210th Street
Bronx, NY 10467
USA

F. OLBERT, MD
Professor of Radiology
Department of Radiodiagnostics
Clinical Department of Angiography and Interventional
Radiology
General Hospital
Währinger Gürtel 18-20
A-1090 Vienna
Austria

M. OLDENDORF, MD
Institut für Diagnostische und
Interventionelle Radiologie
Klinikum Nord
Flurstrsse 17
D-90340 Nürnberg
Germany

PHILIPPE OTAL, MD
Department of Radiology
CHU Rangueil 1
Avenue Jean Poulhes
F-31054 Toulouse
France

EBERHARD PAUL, MD
Professor
Leitender Arzt der Hautklinik
Klinikum-Nord
Prof.-Ernst-Nathan-Str. 1
D-90419 Nürnberg
Germany

PIERRE PERREAULT, MD
Department of Radiology
CHU Rangueil 1
Avenue Jean Poulhes
F-31054 Toulouse
France

PETER PICKEL, MD
Institut für Röntgendiagnostik
der Technischen Universität München
Klinikum rechts der Isar
Ismaninger Straße 22
D-81675 München
Germany

T. Pollack, MD
Radiologic Clinic
Städtisches Klinikum Dresden-Friedrichstadt
Friedrichstrasse 41
D-01067 Dresden
Germany

D. RAITHEL, MD
Professor
Klinik für Gefäßchirurgie
Städtisches Klinikum Süd
Breslauer Straße 201
D-90471 Nürnberg
Germany

E.-IRIS RICHTER, MD
Department of Röntgendiagnostic
Klinikum Nürnberg Nord
Flurstrasse 17
D-90340 Nürnberg
Germany

address for correspondence:
Heynestr. 41, Nürnberg

W. RITTER, MD
Institut für Diagnostische
und Interventionelle Radiologie
Breslauer Straße 201
D-90471 Nürnberg
Germany

P. ROMANIUK, MD
Charité - Humboldt Universität
Institut für Röntgendiagnostik
Schumannstraße 20/21
D-10098 Berlin
Germany

HERVÉ ROUSSEAU, MD
Professor, Department of Radiology
CHU Rangueil 1
Avenue Jean Poulhes
F-31054 Toulouse
France

T. SCHMIDT, PhD
Institut für Medizinische Physik
Klinikum Nürnberg
Flurstrasse 17
D-90340 Nürnberg
Germany

C. SCHUNN, MD
Klinik für Gefäßchirurgie
Städtisches Klinikum Süd
Breslauer Straße 201
D-90471 Nürnberg
Germany

PHILIPPE SOULA, MD
Department of Cardiovascular Surgery
CHU Rangueil 1
Avenue Jean Poulhes
F-31054 Toulouse
France

F. Stösslein, MD
Radiologic Clinic
Städtisches Klinikum Dresden-Friedrichstadt
Friedrichstrasse 41
D-01067 Dresden
Germany

Ulrike Szeimies, MD
Institut für Radiologische Diagnostik
Kernspintomographie
Klinikum Innenstadt - Universität München
Ziemssenstrasse1
D-80336 München
Germany

Dr. med. Felix C. Tanner
Cardiovascular Research
University Zürich-Irchel
CH-8057 Zürich
Switzerland

Frank J. Veith, MD
Chief of Vascular Surgical Service
Montefiore Medical Center
111 East 210th Street
Bronx, NY 10467-2490
USA

Ulrich Voss, MD
Professor, Head of Department of Vascular Surgery
Städtisches Klinikum
Moltkestraße 90
D-76133 Karlsruhe
Germany

Kai-Uwe Wagenhofer, MD
Abteilung für Diagnostische und
Interventionelle Radiologie
Gefäß-Centrum Hamburg-Harburg (GCH)
Allgemeines Krankenhaus Harburg
Eißendorfer Pferdeweg 52
D-21075 Hamburg
Germany

Hans-Joachim Wagner, MD
Abteilung Strahlendiagnostik
Klinikum der Philipps-Universität
Baldingerstrasse
D-35033 Marburg
Germany

Jürgen Weber, MD
Professor, Institut für Röntgendiagnostik
und Interventionelle Radiologie
DRK-Krankehaus
Suurheid 20
D-22559 Hamburg-Rissen
Germany

David M. Williams, MD
Associate Professor of Radiology
University Hospitals B1-D530
1500 East Medical Center Drive
Ann Arbor, MI 48109-0030
USA

M. Wucherer, PhD
Institut für Medizinische Physik
Klinikum Nürnberg
Flurstrasse 17
D-90340 Nürnberg
Germany

Eberhard Zeitler, MD
Professor
University Erlangen-Nürnberg,
Germany

address for correspondence:
Virchowstraße 13
D-90409 Nürnberg
Germany

Ch.l. Zollikofer, MD
Department of Radiology
Kantonsspital Winterthur
CH-8401 Winterthur
Switzerland

MEDICAL RADIOLOGY
Diagnostic Imaging and Radiation Oncology

Titles in the series already published

DIAGNOSTIC IMAGING

Innovations in Diagnostic Imaging
Edited by J.H. Anderson

Radiology of the Upper Urinary Tract
Edited by E.K. Lang

The Thymus - Diagnostic Imaging, Functions, and Pathologic Anatomy
Edited by E. Walter, E. Willich, and W.R. Webb

Interventional Neuroradiology
Edited by A. Valavanis

Radiology of the Pancreas
Edited by A.L. Baert,
co-edited by G. Delorme

Radiology of the Lower Urinary Tract
Edited by E.K. Lang

Magnetic Resonance Angiography
Edited by I.P. Arlart, G.M. Bongartz, and G. Marchal

Contrast-Enhanced MRI of the Breast
S. Heywang-Köbrunner and R. Beck

Spiral CT of the Chest
Edited by M. Rémy-Jardin and J. Rémy

Radiological Diagnosis of Breast Diseases
Edited by M. Friedrich and E.A. Sickles

Radiology of the Trauma
Edited by M. Heller and A. Fink

Biliary Tract Radiology
Edited by P. Rossi

Radiological Imaging of Sports Injuries
Edited by C. Masciocchi

Modern Imaging of the Alimentary Tube
Edited by A. R. Margulis

Diagnosis and Therapy of Spinal Tumors
Edited by P. R. Algra, J. Valk, and J. J. Heimans

Interventional Magnetic Resonance Imaging
Edited by J. F. Debatin and G. Adam

Abdominal and Pelvic MRI
Edited by A. Heuck and M. Reiser

Orthopedic Imaging
Techniques and Applications
Edited by A.M. Davies and H. Pettersson

Radiology of the Female Pelvic Organs
Edited by E.K. Lang

Magnetic Resonance of the Heart and Great Vessels
Clinical Applications
Edited by J. Bogaert, A. J. Duerinckx, and F. E. Rademakers

Modern Head and Neck Imaging
Edited by S. K. Mukherji and J. A. Castelijns

Radiological Imaging of Endocrine Diseases
Edited by J. N. Bruneton
in collaboration with B. Padovani and M -Y. Mourou

Trends in Contrast Media
Edited by H. S. Thomsen, R. N. Muller, and R. F. Mattrey

Functional MRI
Edited by C. T. W. Moonen and P. A. Bandettini

Radiology of the Pancreas
2nd Revised Edition
Edited by A. L. Baert
Co-edited by G. Delorme and L. Van Hoe

Radiology of Peripheral Vascular Diseases
Edited by E. Zeitler

Emergency Pediatric Radiology
Edited by H. Carty

Spiral CT of the Abdomen
Edited by F. Terrier, M. Grossholz, and C. Becker

Liver Malignancies
Diagnostic and Interventional Radiology
Edited by C. Bartolozzi and R. Lencioni

Medical Imaging of the Spleen
Edited by A. M. De Schepper and F. Vanhoenacker

Diagnostic Nuclear Medicine
Edited by C. Schiepers

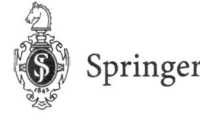

Springer

MEDICAL RADIOLOGY
Diagnostic Imaging and Radiation Oncology

Titles in the series already published

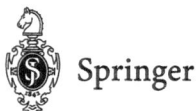
Springer